Medical-Surgical Nursing

Medical-Surgical Nursing:
A Core Text

EDITED BY

Chris Game RN RM DipNEd FCNA

Robyn E. Anderson RN Intensive Care Cert DipNEd FCNA

Jenny R. Kidd RN Intensive Care Cert Dip Hosp Nsng and Unit Management BAppSc(NEd) FCNA

CHURCHILL LIVINGSTONE

MELBOURNE EDINBURGH LONDON AND NEW YORK 1989

CHURCHILL LIVINGSTONE
Medical Division of Longman Group UK Limited

Distributed in Australia by Longman Cheshire Pty
Limited, Longman House, Kings Gardens, 95
Coventry Street, South Melbourne 3205, and by
associated companies, branches and representatives
throughout the world.

First published 1989

ISBN 0-443-02542-8

British Library Cataloguing in Publication Data
Medical-surgical nursing.
   1. Medicine. Nursing – For student nurses
   I. Game, Chris II. Anderson, Robyn E.
   III. Kidd, Jenny R.
   610.73

Library of Congress Cataloging in Publication Data
Medical-surgical nursing: a core text/edited by Chris Game,
Robyn E. Anderson, Jenny R. Kidd.
     p. cm.
   Includes index.
   ISBN 0-443-02542-8
   1. Nursing.   I. Game, Chris. II. Anderson, Robyn E.
III. Kidd, Jenny R.
   [DNLM: 1. Nursing.   WY 100 M4885]
R141.M482 1989
610.73 – dc19
DNLM/DLC
for Library of Congress   88-20233

Produced by Longman Singapore Publishers (Pte) Ltd.
Printed in Singapore

Preface

The planning, writing, and production of this volume – the first comprehensive, integrated, Australian textbook to provide a basis for the nursing management of adults with a medical or surgical condition – has been a lengthy, challenging, and exciting process.

It is an all-Australian work, written largely by nurses. The reader can therefore expect to find information on the medical and surgical conditions found in our hospitals, supported by Australian statistics of morbidity and mortality. Furthermore, the reader will also find that the text reflects the pattern and style of health care delivery in this country.

This is a textbook for student use. We have made a deliberate attempt to present information in an organized, systematic, and concise format. And we believe that the student will welcome a portable and practical text from which information may be easily retrieved. These attributes may also enable the book to be used as a valuable adjunct to refresher courses in general nursing, and as a ready reference in clinical practice settings such as the wards or departments of general hospitals.

This book is not based on a particular nursing theory nor structured around a nursing model. Rather, our intention is to supply the information which underpins this area of nursing practice. Thus we present pathophysiology; disease symptomatology; medical diagnosis and treatment; drug therapy and its indications, contraindications, and toxic effects; and likely outcomes. We also provide general guidelines for the specific nursing interventions and care that must be provided for patients whose conditions have required medical or surgical intervention.

We believe that illness and disease, its causes and effects, and its medical treatment, must be understood and assimilated so that safe and effective nursing care can be practised. A sound knowledge base ensures that the nurse is able to:
• identify all the appropriate information when assessing a patient;
• recognize actual and anticipate potential patient problems;
• select realistic, patient-centred objectives;
• implement appropriate nursing actions to assist the patient to achieve these objectives; and
• revise the plan of care as necessary.

And so this book places the nursing management of the patient in the context of the student's need to be equipped with technical information which may then be applied to any of the various theories of nursing.

The book is presented in 3 unequal parts. Part 1 introduces concepts basic to medical-surgical nursing; Part 2 reviews pathophysiological concepts affecting medical-surgical conditions and nursing practice; and Part 3 discusses common medical-surgical conditions and interventions. Part 3 is organized on a body systems basis, selected in the belief that this is an effective educational approach which allows for the logical and economical presentation of a large amount of information.

It is assumed that the users of this textbook will have completed an introductory year of nursing studies and so be proficient in basic nursing skills and have a sound knowledge of basic human bioscience, microbiology, and physical science. As a consequence, the information provided in Parts 1 and 2, and in the introductory chapters to each

Section in Part 3, is included as a convenient review of basic knowledge, applied specifically to the medical or surgical setting. It should not be regarded as an initial learning resource.

The delivery of health care in Australia is, to a major degree, within hospitals which provide intervention for acute medical or surgical conditions. This textbook reflects that mode by concentrating on medical-surgical nursing in the acute care setting. Consequently there is only superficial discussion of the management of chronic disorders, and scant attention is paid to the vital role of the community-based nurse. Additionally, since this book is intended for the generalist nurse, the editors have resisted the temptation to include detailed discussion of the specialist areas of nursing practice.

It should be noted that whenever drug therapies are mentioned, it is assumed that the medications administered by the nurse are given orally unless otherwise stated and have been prescribed by a physician. It should also be noted that no sexism or gender-specific incidence of occupation or disease is intended or implied by the use of pronouns relating to physicians, surgeons, patients, and nurses in the text.

It was in 1979 that Judy Waters, Publisher at Churchill Livingstone, first approached a number of registered nurses involved with the clinical education of students of nursing to invite views on the desirability and feasibility of producing an Australian medical-surgical nursing textbook. These nurses, from a variety of health agencies, were unanimous in their support for the idea, believing that Australian nurses should not be completely dependent on imported literature for their basic education.

A project committee was established to plan the approach, structure, and contents. Sample chapters were written; a major national survey of nurse education institutions was undertaken inviting comment on the 'bones' of the project; and it was decided to embark on the book.

During the intervening years we estimate that over 1.5 million words have been written (and re-written) as the book developed. It has been a major task involving the energies, goodwill, and generosity of a huge network of Australian nurses who have provided continuing material and/or emotional support.

We hope that their confidence has been justified by the appearance of this volume. And we hope that readers will find it of value.

CG
RA
JK

Melbourne 1989

Acknowledgements

The publishers and editors wish to thank all the nurses, colleagues, and friends who provided help, advice, support, and coffee during the development of this book.

We are grateful to the many nurse educators in schools of nursing around the country who participated in our initial survey and provided ideas, criticism, and encouragement.

Our thanks are also due to staff in many hospitals who willingly provided opportunities for clinical discussions, protocols, and support. In particular, we thank: The Alfred Hospital, Melbourne; The Peter MacCallum Hospital, Melbourne; Prince Henry's Hospital, Melbourne, The Repatriation General Hospital, Melbourne; and The Royal Melbourne Hospital. Staff at the Mayfield Centre also gave generously of their time and expertise, as did the many nurse librarians who assisted with references and bibliographic details.

The following people generously contributed time, information, advice and criticism at various stages throughout the project: Jacqui Baker, Jenny Blundell, Marilyn Coffee, Joy Cruickshank, Marlee Inge, Mary Dadswell, Helen Eastwood, Elaine Fryer, Colleen Goldsmith, Loris Grote, Pauline Lambert, Maria McKenna, Sue McLeod, Daphne Milford, Cheryle Moss, Joan Pawsey, Bobby Pearce, Helen Philp, Bev Scott, Sharolyne Smith, Verna Steele, Helen Tse, Rayner Yudkin.

Special tribute is also due to Graham Joyson, who acted as 'devil's advocate' during the early planning stages, and maintained an advisory role throughout the development of this book. His contribution and positive encouragement are gratefully acknowledged.

The Melbourne office of Churchill Livingstone supported and co-ordinated the development of this book. The editors wish to thank: Judy Waters whose vision became reality by constantly keeping the editors working towards the goal of completion; Jon Murray for his commas, editorial skills, and patience; and Sandra Tolra for her secretarial and word-processing skills – and for the endless supply of tea, coffee, and good humour.

Contributors

Robyn E. Anderson RN Intensive Care Cert DipNEd FCNA
Formerly Hospital Chief Nursing Advisor to South Vietnam; Principal Teacher, Alfred Hospital, Melbourne. Chairman, Victorian Nursing Council Examinations Committee

A. P. Barnett RN BAppSc(Nursing) NEd FCNA MACE
Head, Faculty of Nurse Education, Warrnambool Institute of Advanced Education, Victoria

Peter Allen Braithwaite MB BS FRCS
Formerly Lecturer in Surgery, University of Tasmania. Consultant Surgeon Mid Glamorgan Health Authority, Wales

Jennifer L. Cater RN Onc Cert
Formerly Clinical Nurse Specialist in Oncology, Repatriation General Hospital, Concord, Sydney

Michael Drake FRCPA FRCPath FRACP FIAC
Consultant Pathologist, Melbourne

Helen Farrer RN RM
Midwife, St Vincent's Private Hospital, Melbourne; Sessional Teacher, School of Nursing, St Vincent's Hospital, Melbourne

Chris Game RN RM Dip NEd FCNA
Formerly Lecturer in Medical-Surgical Nursing, Lincoln Institute of Health Sciences, Melbourne. Consultant in Curriculum Design; Sessional Clinical Teacher, Lincoln Institute of Health Sciences, Melbourne

Graham Joyson RN RMN FCNA
Acting Director of Nursing, Royal Southern Memorial Hospital, Caulfield, Melbourne

Jenny R. Kidd RN Intensive Care Cert DipHosp Nsg and Unit Management BAppSc(NEd) FCNA
Formerly Senior Teacher, Alfred Hospital, Melbourne

R. B. Lefroy AM MA(Oxon.) FRACP
Human Ageing Research Unit, University of Western Australia, Perth

Mavis L. Matthews RN BAppSc (Nursing)
Lecturer, School of Nursing, Western Australian College of Advanced Education, Churchlands

Sunita McGowan RN BAppSc (Nursing)
Stomal Therapist
Nurse Researcher, Fremantle Hospital, Perth

Barbara L. Piesse LLB
Barrister and Solictor of the Supreme Court of Victoria; Lecturer in Law, Warrnambool Institute of Advanced Education, Victoria

Helga Sabel RN DipT (Nursing)
Formerly Co-ordinator Post Basic Orthopaedic Nursing Courses, Royal Adelaide Hospital, Adelaide

Dace Shugg RN
Formerly Research Associate, Royal Hobart Hospital Clinical School, University of Tasmania

Mary (Errey) Snell RN Grad Dip Rehab Studies Grad Dip Health Admin
Director of Nursing, Holy Spirit Home for the Aged, Brisbane

John Sullivan MD MRCP(UK) FRACP
Oncologist in Private Practice, Melbourne

Contents

1

The application of a problem-solving method of nursing management

Chris Game

INTRODUCTION

The provision of nursing care needs to be preplanned if all the objectives of both the patient and the attending nurse are to be realized. The haphazard delivery of nursing care almost guarantees unco-ordinated achievement of nursing objectives, if in fact the objectives are reached at all. Lack of planning leads to the stereotyping of care, in that regardless of the needs of the individual or the presentation of their medical and/or surgical condition, the same nursing action is implemented, whether or not it is appropriate. Table 1.1 differentiates the implications for nursing action when care is planned, as against stereotyped in nature.

Over recent years Australian nursing has seen an explosion of ideas relating to the delivery of health care by nurses and other health professionals. Whether the system of nursing care management that is chosen is defined as 'a problem-solving technique', the 'nursing process', an 'individualized or personalized nursing care technique', or 'primary nursing care', all are based on the principles of scientific method and therefore are problem-solving in nature.

The aim of planning nursing care is to produce a written patient assessment and care plan that will: provide a permanent and cumulative record of the physical and psychological health status of patients; produce an accurate communication tool for use between health care professionals; and achieve health care delivery that is consistent, progressive, co-ordinated and scientifically based. A care plan is concerned with the identification of health problems and needs, and the objectives to be reached in attaining optimal health recovery.

The formulation of a successful care plan depends on the nurse working from a sound theoretical and practical knowledge base. The nurse must be equipped with a vast amount of data and skills. This includes information about disease symptomatology; drug therapy and its indications, contraindications, and toxic effects; methods of nursing practice; and perhaps of greatest importance – disease prevention.

Table 1.1 Implications for nursing action

Assessed problem/need	Planned/individualized care	Stereotyped care
Patient has mobility restriction due to painful arthritic joints	Nurse recognizes that patient will require greater assistance in activities of daily living than will a nonaffected person	The patient's degree of dependence may not be identified
Residual aphasia and agnosia following a cerebrovascular accident	Nurse employs special communication aids, as the patient will be severely handicapped regarding his ability to communicate his needs	The patient's handicap may not be recognized, or be even ignored
Anxious about how his family will cope, as he is unemployed	Nursing assessment takes account of the possible effect that his underlying anxiety might have on his ability to contribute effectively to his own care	The 'problem' may be referred to a social worker and the implications for his nursing management/care disregarded

A PROBLEM-SOLVING METHOD

The 4 primary phases, and their interrelationships, (as shown in Figure 1.1) of any scientifically based problem-solving method are:

1. Assessment
2. Planning
3. Implementation
4. Evaluation.

A problem-solving method enables the nurse to set objectives of care; these can be defined as the goals that the individual patient and/or nurse and other health team members aim to achieve whilst the patient is receiving health care. These objectives provide a guide for planning the health care; goals to be achieved when implementing care; and parameters by which to measure whether the care has been effective. The objectives can be stated in either patient terms; that is, what the individual patient must be able to do, (for example: 'Is able to freely expectorate secretions'); or in nursing terms – what the nurse must be able to achieve, for the patient, through his/her nursing care (for example: 'With the use of pharyngeal aspiration maintains a patent airway'). Wherever possible the use of patient-centred objectives should be employed in an effort to promote the independence of the patient. However, where the patient is dependent upon the nurse for the identification and the provision of his daily health care needs (for example, the deeply comatose patient) objectives will need to be stated in nursing terms.

Assessment

In order to implement the appropriate nursing actions for a particular patient, at a specified time of health care need, the nurse must first collect data on those aspects of the patient's environment, condition, and situation that will influence either the success or failure of nursing care delivery.

The collection of such a data base constitutes the assessment phase of a problem-solving method and enables the nurse to consider the variables that he/she will be likely to encounter when implementing nursing care. Information is usually obtained by the nurse on admission of the patient, or when the patient is first visited in the community. This information is then updated as necessary, to reflect the patient's response to treatment and his progress in the course of his condition. The assessment phase continues as an ongoing process throughout the patient's period of health care, being updated continuously and becoming more selective as the patient responds to nursing and health care. Re-evaluation of the total plan, including reassessment of the patient's health status, may take place at the end/beginning of each shift in the acute hospital situation, or on a daily or weekly basis where the patient is nursed in a less acute environment.

Information that needs to be considered includes the patient's past and present medical condition; his current physical and psychological condition; his attitude to health care and health care professionals; his ability to communicate his needs to the nurse; his cultural background; his usual lifestyle, habits, and beliefs; his social and economic status; and perhaps most importantly – his ability to comprehend the nursing and medical interventions either advised or planned for him.

However, each patient has a right to privacy and this right must be respected. So, when embarking on patient assessment the student should beware the seeming ease with which this delicate task is portrayed in some nursing literature. It is not safe to assume that the patient will willingly 'reveal all' during a nursing interview; in fact, it is much more likely that a patient will not reveal all aspects pertinent to the planning of his care. A patient may withhold information for a variety of reasons: he may be totally unaware of the significance to his management of certain information that he holds; he may believe that certain information is of an extremely personal nature and may not wish to reveal it to the inquiring nurse; his cultural beliefs may prevent

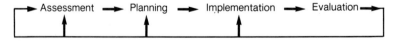

Fig. 1.1 The phases involved in problem-solving.

him from revealing certain information to either a nurse or a doctor; and he may even consider that the nurse should be able to perform his/her function without some, or even any, information from him.

Therefore communication between the patient and the nurse, and between members of the health team, is a vital element in the ability to amass information on which realistic nursing care plans may be based. Thus the data base will be subject to revision as the needs of the patient change, or more information becomes available during the course of nursing management.

During this assessment it is important to attempt to identify the patient's strengths and vulnerabilities, as these will contribute markedly to his ability to cope with his altered health status. Early identification of strengths (for example, a fully supportive family and extended family network, or excellent preoperative physical condition) and vulnerabilities (for example, pre-existing respiratory disease, or a social situation that leaves the patient economically disadvantaged) allows the nurse to preplan care more effectively. Strengths can be maximized in planning nursing actions, and areas of vulnerability can be anticipated and overcome before they adversely affect the patient's progress.

When assessing a patient's abilities and needs, the nurse must utilize all his/her skills of communication and look for both verbal and nonverbal cues from the patient. Time must be set aside so that an adequate assessment can be made and the patient given the time necessary to communicate all his information, requests, and fears. The nurse should be skilled enough to know when not to intrude upon the patient's privacy; be capable of assessing whether or not the patient actually does understand what is happening, and that he is not concealing his inability to comprehend the course of treatment planned for him; and be able to determine if the patient's family are also comprehending the planned course of treatment. A hurried assessment will undoubtedly be inaccurate and incomplete, and will leave the patient apprehensive and unsure of the concern that the nursing staff have for him and his needs. The assessment phase is a valuable opportunity for the nurse to institute health teaching and patient education of the health care course that lies ahead; it then follows that the nurse's skill in communicating nursing actions is paramount. (See also Chapter 2.)

The nurse must draw on his/her knowledge base to ensure that the patient assessment contains relevant and accurate data. The data should be obtained as a written record and retained for future reference, along with all other patient documentation, as it is a valuable adjunct to the patient's medical history. The collection format is as a Nursing Assessment: 'the initial planned systematic collection and recording of the subjective and objective nursing data base (comparable to the physician's history and physical examination) . . . the data gleaned becomes the foundation for plans of nursing care' (Little & Carnevali, 1976). In some health agencies the term 'Nursing History' is used to describe the nursing assessment. There are many examples of these forms and Appendix 1 provides a sample document. A Nursing Assessment or Nursing History form is usually developed, by individual health agencies, with a particular need or nursing model in mind. They vary widely throughout Australia from agency to agency, and especially depending upon the type or format of Quality Assurance Programme that is used by the Nursing Department.

Planning

Following assessment, the information gained enables the nurse to enter the planning phase wherein he/she is able to: identify specific health and/or nursing problems that need to be solved; assign an order of priority to the identified list of problems; set realistic objectives that can be achieved by both the patient and the nursing team; and formulate the appropriate nursing actions to achieve the set objectives.

The patient, and his family where appropriate, is actively encouraged to participate in this process; eventual success of the total nursing care plan hinges on the degree of patient acceptance of, and therefore his involvement in, the decisions made regarding his nursing care. Where possible other health team members should also be involved so that realistic objectives are set for the patient and/or nursing team to achieve; for example, the therapists' input regarding physical therapy and return to independent living is essential when planning the rehabilitation programme for a patient severely handicapped following a cerebrovascular accident. There is very little to be gained by the nurse in isolation formulating objectives of care for either the patient to achieve or other health team members to work towards. Both the patient and health team members must contribute to the planning phase so that the ultimate objectives selected are acceptable to all persons working towards the eventual recovery of the patient.

However, the nurse must again respect the rights of the patient who may not seek this degree of involvement. Some patients hold the belief that the nurse, and other health team members, should know their function well enough to plan care without the input or approval of the patient, and in fact to be involved decreases their confidence in the ability of that health team member.

When documenting the nursing care plan it is necessary to differentiate between problems that are actually present and those which have the potential to develop; for example, an elderly, immigrant, obese patient admitted for major abdominal surgery will have an 'actual' problem of pain postoperatively, and the 'potential' to develop either a deep vein thrombosis or respiratory atelectasis. This differentiation between problems is also known as making a nursing diagnosis. 'A nursing diagnosis describes a combination of signs and symptoms that indicate an actual or potential health problem nurses are licensed to treat and capable of treating' (Dossey & Guzzetta, 1981). Justifying the selection of a problem assists the nurse in determining whether it is actual or potential, and the written care plan should stipulate this where appropriate.

When developing the plan of care the nurse must first list the identified problems in their order of priority; actual problems precede potential problems, and the problem seen as the most crucial would be stated first. Table 1.2 lists the actual and potential problems that may apply to the patient mentioned above.

The second step involves the construction of objectives related to each problem and its solution.

Table 1.2 Planning the Basic Care Plan (i)

Identified problem/need: 'Nursing diagnosis'

1. Pain from abdominal wound and position of drainage tubes (actual)
2. Unable to state his needs as he does not speak English (actual)
3. Restricted mobility due to painful arthritic joints (actual)
4. Anxiousness brought on by his fear of the unknown and how he will cope with the surgery (potential)
5. Deep vein thrombosis due to obesity and postoperative immobility (potential)

Objectives should be seen as guides to action for the patient and/or nursing staff and are stated either in patient terms or in nursing terms, for example:

1. The patient is to be pain-free at all times postoperatively.

or

Ensure analgesia is administered regularly and before the patient experiences pain.

2. The patient is to be able to communicate all his needs whenever necessary.

or

Ensure interpreter service availability when implementing any aspects of the plan.

3. The patient is to achieve independence, within his limitations, before his date of discharge.

or

Assist the patient with activities of daily living only after he has reached his limitations or he requests help.

4. The patient is to understand hospital and preoperative routine and the implications of the surgery.

or

Ensure adequate explanations of all routines and procedures.

5. The patient is to avoid the development of venous stasis or thrombosis.

or

Institute nursing measures to prevent the development of the complication of deep vein thrombosis.

Objectives are of two types: short-term and long-term, and should stipulate a period of time over which it is anticipated the objective will be achieved. (See Table 1.3.)

Table 1.3 Planning the Basic Care Plan (ii)

Identified problem/need: 'Nursing diagnosis'	Objective
1. Pain from abdominal wound and position of drainage tubes (actual)	To be pain-free at all times
2. Unable to state his needs as he does not speak English (actual)	To be able to communicate all his needs whenever necessary
3. Restricted mobility due to painful arthritic joints (actual)	To achieve independence within his limitations, before his date of discharge
4. Anxiousness brought on by his fear of the unknown and how he will cope with the surgery (potential)	To understand hospital and preoperative routine and the implications of the surgery
5. Deep vein thrombosis due to obesity and postoperative immobility (potential)	To avoid the development of venous stasis or thrombosis

The third step is to identify the implications that each objective has for the selection of nursing actions that will assist the patient in achieving the stated objectives. In this way, stereotyping of nursing care management is avoided. Table 1.4 provides an example of a method of this documentation. Appendix 2 provides an example of a fully developed nursing care plan. It should be appreciated that many health agencies using nursing care plans employ a check-list method rather than fully documenting the plan as outlined in Appendix 2.

Implementation

The nurse now enters the implementation phase – the organized and co-ordinated delivery of nursing care aimed at achieving objectives which have been identified with the patient, his family and other members of the health team. The planned nursing actions are implemented as designed, the identified objectives are achieved,

Table 1.4 Planning the Basic Care Plan (iii)

Identified Problem/Need: 'Nursing diagnosis'	Objective	Implications for nursing action
1. Pain from abdominal wound and position of drainage tubes (actual)	To be pain-free at all times	Position of comfort Assistance when exercising Splint wound Administer ordered analgesia strictly 3 hrly
2. Unable to state his needs as he does not speak English (actual)	To be able to communicate all his needs whenever necessary	Use nonverbal cues Use translation lists Use hospital interpreter service when plan is designed, implemented and evaluated
3. Restricted mobility due to painful arthritic joints (actual)	To achieve independence within his limitations, before his date of discharge	Allow all time necessary to enable him to perform those activities of daily living of which he is capable Intervene only when he has reached his limitations or he requests help
4. Anxiousness brought on by his fear of the unknown and how he will cope with the surgery (potential)	To understand hospital and preoperative routine and the implications of the surgery	Involve family members Utilize interpreter services Involve other immigrants Inform OR supervisor regarding need for a preoperative visit Needs to talk out his fears Simplify explanations of routines
5. Deep vein thrombosis due to obesity and postoperative immobility (potential)	To avoid development of venous stasis or thrombosis	Institute active exercises immediately on return from the operating room Encourage fluid intake Prevent obstruction to leg veins Ambulate ASAP Commence reduction diet

and the problems are met and overcome. As examples:

A potential problem of anxiousness is resolved by the patient being informed of the hospital and preoperative routines with the involvement of the OR staff and interpreter services.

An actual problem of postoperative pain is resolved by positioning of the patient, nursing measures to support the wound, and the administration of the ordered analgesia.

Conversely, the plan, regardless of its implementation, may fail to achieve the stated objective(s) and the patient may remain with unresolved problem(s). As examples:

A potential problem of anxiousness is not resolved by explanation, and becomes an actual problem interfering with his postoperative recovery.

An actual problem of pain is not resolved by repositioning for comfort, explanation of treatments, or the administration of analgesia.

Evaluation

Whether the plan succeeds or fails, because of its design it enables the nurse to retrace his/her steps and determine which part or parts were appropriately or inappropriately identified for the patient. If necessary the plan can then be revised or modified.

This evaluation phase allows the nurse to revise the plan at any stage of his/her delivery of patient care, thus ensuring consistent nursing actions designed to assist the patient achieve his stated objectives. As examples:

• An identified problem, or its reason for selection, may be incorrect.
• An objective may require reassessment as it may be stated in such a way as to be unachievable by either the patient or the health team; or a short-term objective may have been inappropriately or ambitiously selected for a long-term health or nursing problem.
• Unrelieved pain may be resolved by a change of analgesia, identification and relief of psychological anxieties, health team acceptance of the cultural determinants of pain expression, or rearrangement of the analgesia administration schedule.
• The onset of a wound infection may be resolved by alteration of the dressing technique, utilization of topically applied antibiotics, or an alteration of the antibiotic used systemically.

The importance of evaluation to all aspects of the nursing care plan is best seen in Figure 1.2.

SUMMARY

The delivery of nursing actions aimed at assisting the patient to achieve the objective of optimal health must be planned and based on a problem-solving method if co-ordination and integration of

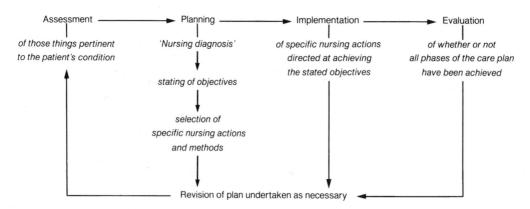

Fig. 1.2 Nursing interrelationships of the phases of problem-solving.

nursing care is to be achieved. Regardless of the method of nursing care delivery chosen, if the technique used incorporates: assessment of each patient as an individual; selection of short- or long-term objectives appropriate to that assessment; planning and implementation of specific nursing actions to achieve those objectives; and evaluation of both the process and the outcome;

then it can be seen that a problem-solving method has been instituted.

The problem-solving method ensures the individualization of nursing care, increases the likelihood that the patient and his family and/or significant others will be involved in that care, and ensures that specific nursing actions are instituted to meet specific problems or needs.

REFERENCES AND FURTHER READING

Texts

Little D E, Carnevali D L 1976 Nursing care planning, 2nd edn. Lippincott, Philadelphia, ch 6, 95–123
Robinson J (ed) 1981 Documenting patient care responsibly: nursing skillbook, 2nd edn. Intermed Communications, Pennsylvania
Roper N, Logan W W, Tierney A J 1985 The elements of nursing, 2nd edn. Churchill Livingstone, Edinburgh
Urosevich P R (ed) 1984 Assessing your patients: nursing photobook, 2nd edn. Springhouse, Pennsylvania

Journals

Baggaley S 1979 Deficiencies in traditional reporting and recording techniques. The Australian Nurses Journal 8 : 9 : 30–31
Baron J A 1985 Computerized record keeping: the good, the bad, and the legalities. Nursing 85 15 : 5 : 19–20
Baskin P 1980 Primary nursing: Australia's emerging patterns. The Australian Nurses Journal 9 : 9 : 28–31
Brill C, Hill L 1985 Giving the help that goes on giving. Nursing 85 15 : 5 : 44–47
Britton C, Lambe M, Madonna M, Sharkey P, Waszczak C 1980 Innovative discharge planning – try it: the results may surprise you. Nursing 80 10 : 10 : 44–49
Bryant R B 1980 Problem-oriented nursing care plans. The Australian Nurses Journal 10 : 1 : 35–36
Cameron J E 1982 'Giant leap forward' begins with the nursing interview. The Australian Nurses Journal 12 : 2 : 47–48
Campbell C 1983 Nursing process: one long round of bother. Nursing Mirror 156 : 7:: 26–28
Campbell S L 1984 Some sound advice for managing a hearing-impaired patient. Nursing 84 14 : 12 : 46
Cuthbert M I 1984 Evaluating patient care: the questionnaire. The Australian Nurses Journal 13 : 8 : 36–38
deJulia N 1980 The nursing interview. The Australian Nurses Journal 19 : 5 : 39
Dettmore D 1984 Spiritual care: remembering your patients' forgotten needs. Nursing 84 14 : 10 : 46
Dixon J, Walker B 1986 Nursing diagnosis: defining the goal of care. The Australian Nurses Journal 16 : 5 : 43–44
Dolan M B 1986 Why nurses should make "medical" diagnoses. Nursing 86 16 : 2 : 50–51

Dossey B 1979 Perfecting your skills for systematic patient assessment. Nursing 79 9 : 2 : 42–45
Dossey B, Guzzetta C E 1981 Nursing Diagnosis. Nursing 81 11 : 6 : 34–38
Eggland E T 1980 Charting: how and why to document your care daily – and fully. Nursing 80 10 : 2 : 38–43
Farrell J 1980 The human side of assessment. Nursing 80 10 : 4 : 74–75
Forsyth D M 1983 Looking good to communicate better with patients. Nursing 83 13 : 7 : 34–37
Galton M 1981 The evaluation stage of the nursing process. The Australian Nurses Journal 10 : 10 : 50–52
Gutierrez K 1985 Home is where the care is. Nursing 85 15 : 11 : 48–49
Hase S 1983 The nursing process – is it idol worship? The Australian Nurses Journal 13 : 1 : 39–40
Hudson M F 1983 Safeguard your elderly patient's health through accurate physical assessment. Nursing 83 13 : 11 : 58–64
Humphris M R 1979 The nursing process: an application of scientific method. The Australian Nurses Journal 9 : 4 : 30–31
Jamison J R 1984 Personal health assessment – a trend of the 80s. The Australian Journal of Advanced Nursing 2 : 1 : 9–13
Martins A C 1985 The dilemma of assessment. The Australian Nurses Journal 14 : 11 : 46–47
McHugh M K 1987 Has nursing outgrown the nursing process? Nursing 87 17 : 8 : 50–51
Mengel A 1982 Getting the most from patient interviews. Nursing 82 12 : 11 : 46–49
Mercer L 1980 Pseudocommunication with patients. Nursing 80 10 : 2 : 19–22
Millers N, Koop A J 1984 A person-oriented view of patient-centred care. The Australian Nurses Journal 13 : 6 : 38–39
Neel C J 1986 Make nursing diagnoses work for you . . . everyday. Nursing 86 16 : 5 : 56–57
Rankin S H, Duffy K L 1984 15 Problems in patient education and their solutions. Nursing 84 14 : 4 : 17–22
Rich P L 1983 Make the most of your charting time. Nursing 83 13 : 3 : 34–39
Rich P L 1985 With this flow sheet, less is more . . . Nursing 85 15 : 7 : 23–29
Roper N, Logan W W, Tierney A J 1983 Nursing process: endless paperwork? Nursing Mirror 156 : 25 : 34–35
Rutkowski B 1985 The perennial problem of problem solving. Nursing 85 15 : 2 : 29–31

Schneggenberger C 1979 History-taking skills: how do you rate? Nursing 79 9 : 3 : 97–101

Shoemaker C A, Schaefer K 1985 In planning Mr Bowen's care, one picture was worth a thousand words. Nursing 85 15 : 12 : 44–46

Smith B 1981 A systems model of the nursing process. The Australian Nurses Journal 11 : 4 : 33

Tartaglia M J 1985 Nursing diagnosis: keystone of your care plan. Nursing 85 15 : 3 : 34–37

Townsend J K 1982 Solving problems means asking questions. The Australian Nurses Journal 12 : 3 : 49–50

Vasey E K 1979 Writing your patient's care plan . . . efficiently. Nursing 79 9 : 4 : 67–71

Wells M I 1983 Discharge planning: closing the gaps in continuity of care. Nursing 83 13 : 11 : 45

Wilson G 1980 Nursing diagnosis (assessment) and changing accountability. The Australian Nurses Journal 9 : 10 : 36–38

2

Psychosocial aspects of illness and hospitalization

Sunita McGowan

INTRODUCTION

Patients are individuals from all walks of life who have been conditioned from an early age to accept certain attitudes, values, and beliefs, and these factors affect their behaviour. Human behaviour itself is a reflection of psychological, social, cultural, spiritual, physical, and biological aspects that encompass each individual and, therefore, influence his response to illness and hospitalization.

THE EFFECTS OF HOSPITALIZATION

If we consider that prior to hospitalization many of our patients have had a period of illness or suspected disease, it is not surprising to realize that the added stress of hospitalization increases anxiety. Worries about 'what to expect' and 'what to do' in hospital, along with possibly increased financial problems, worries about job security, and many other factors, can often precipitate maladaptive responses. Events perceived as harmful or threatening evoke a variety of coping mechanisms. Reality may be discounted by denial, which may manifest as rationalization and self-deception, and is a common way people deal with distressing events. Another coping mechanism often used is withdrawal from the perceived stressful situation. Arnold (1976) states that psychological stress is accompanied by emotions, the most obvious being anger, fear, and grief, and therefore emotion would appear to be a reliable indicator of psychological stress. Robinson (1972) discusses patients' reactions to hospitalization, and he suggests that they react and use defence mechanisms that they normally use in other stressful situations. For example, patients who usually trust people will generally trust the hospital staff, whilst anger, hostility, and criticism may be exhibited by those who normally react to stress in this manner.

Once the initial admission procedure is completed, anxiety may then be compounded by depression. This may be due to a number of reasons which include:

• A feeling of loss of independence and personal identity
• A feeling of helplessness and inability to control personal destiny
• Isolation from family and friends
• Disruption to family, social and business life
• Encounters with unfamiliar medical jargon, and the presence of imposing, unfamiliar scientific machinery.

Be sure to observe and record your patient's appearance on admission, since clothing can reflect socioeconomic differences as well as cultural and ethnic ones. Observe if outdoor clothing is neat, dirty, or shabby. Appearances can also give us a clue to whether a patient is feeling depressed or unwell; for example, the man who is normally clean shaven but has not shaved.

The hospital system, because it is a system, also promotes institutional depersonalization. Hospital clothing, despite the virtues of easy care and cleanliness, contributes towards depersonalization. With an identification band fastened around his wrist, and sitting in a numbered bed, the patient soon begins to feel 'just like everyone else'. This is borne out when discharged patients return to visit, and we do not recognize them in their own clothing. It can also lead to such amusing situations, such as being confronted by a former patient in a cinema queue, and responding with 'I didn't recognize you with your clothes on'! Since clothing makes such a difference, patients should be encouraged to wear their own.

CULTURAL BELIEFS AND HOSPITALIZATION

Patients when admitted to hospital bring with them their cultural beliefs regarding pain, illness, and hospitalization. Whether that cultural baggage is a stumbling block or a support in their care can depend largely upon the nurse. Although a patient's cultural beliefs regarding illness may seem strange to us, we need to be aware that what he believes is not as important as the fact that he does believe it.

Pain

Patients' attitudes towards pain and its acceptance vary considerably depending upon their culture. Patients from Mediterranean countries usually have no difficulty in expressing pain, requesting analgesia, or reporting lack of pain relief. Unfortunately instead of nurses realizing this is a cultural determinant, these patients are often described as having 'a low pain threshold'. Patients who come from a culture which does not admit to pain will find difficulty in reporting pain. The patient who refuses an injection for pain may not necessarily have 'a high pain threshold'; instead he may find it difficult to admit to pain. It is important that we are aware of these different attitudes, and are able to suggest methods of pain relief that are acceptable to our patients. Expression of feelings may or may not be acceptable in certain cultures. Societal attitudes regarding accepted behaviour in males in Western culture prevents many men from expressing their feelings in the form of crying. They are, therefore, more likely to retreat into their room, remain uncommunicative, or play the role of the 'good patient'. Comments such as 'You seem unhappy' may encourage them to communicate their feelings.

Traditional remedies

Many people accept the therapeutic value of the advice offered in 'lay' or traditional remedies for medical problems, and although some may have some benefits, others, such as keeping a pyrexial patient warm, can do more harm than good. Most non-medical people are shocked that nurses will cool a pyrexial patient by tepid sponge, fanning, and removal of bed clothes.

Religious beliefs

Religious beliefs and certain taboos in various cultures often present many problems and these can actually interfere with nursing care, particularly if these beliefs are not understood, or are misunderstood by nursing staff. Some religious sects believe that illness is directly related to a person's spiritual state and so may refuse conventional medical treatment, believing that prayer will cure the illness. Other religious sects may refuse certain aspects of conventional medical treatment, the most publicized being the refusal of blood transfusions by Jehovah's Witnesses. Although it may be difficult not to lose patience with them for refusing blood transfusions in a life-threatening situation, it is important to realize that they are not trying to be difficult, but are expressing a sincere belief that the Bible instructs them to abstain from blood in any form.

Food

Devout members of certain Asian religious groups follow food restrictions. Many Hindus and Sikhs are vegetarians, and those who are not do not eat beef. They also may fast or eat very little on certain days each month. Jews and Muslims do not eat pork or pork products, and may eat other meat only if it is killed in a specified manner. Often patients from these religious groups will refuse all food in case it contains forbidden ingredients, or because it is unfamiliar to them and therefore unappetizing. It is important that the nurse indicates to patients that he/she understands their decisions and is able to help them choose suitable foods which provide the required nutrition. Family and friends can be encouraged to supplement the hospital menu, particularly if the hospital is unable to provide acceptable food.

Death

All of us have to face death at some time and cultural attitudes are very important. As nurses it is our responsibility to be aware of the wishes of patients and their families regarding religious or cultural customs. These wishes should be complied with whenever possible, and should always be respected.

Although cultural and religious beliefs and attitudes may be difficult for us to understand, to the people concerned they are a reality. By developing insight into these areas we will be able to discover what is not acceptable to our patients, so enabling us to accommodate their views when planning nursing care.

PATIENTS' RIGHTS

The patient has an ethical and legal right to be told what is being done. For example, with the insertion of a nasogastric tube, he should be told why the tube is necessary, where it is going, and if possible how long it is likely to remain in situ. Similarly, when a patient is prepared for surgery, he should understand the reasons for the preparations, exactly what the operation consists of, and what to expect postoperatively. Sometimes discretion may be needed in the amount of information given, for if all possible complications of a procedure were mentioned, the patient might not consent. However, when there is a high risk of a complication occurring, the patient must be fully informed. In some cases a person's physical and emotional condition, or his capacity for understanding, will limit what he can be told. For non-English speaking patients an interpreter should always be available. Contrary to the belief of some medical practitioners, most patients wish to be told frankly about their illness and prognosis, and empirical evidence supports this claim. (See also Chapter 3.)

Personal research undertaken with patients in surgical wards revealed that patients who were not given information relating to pre- and postoperative procedures expressed more apprehension and discomfort than those who were given information prior to the events. Patients who were unaware that they would return to the ward with an intravenous infusion, a nasogastric tube, or a wound drainage system in situ, often commented that they thought 'something had gone wrong'. Discussion with staff revealed that these patients were more reluctant to ambulate, to perform deep breathing, coughing and leg exercises, and required more frequent analgesia. Janis (1971) conducted a survey with surgical patients and demonstrated the positive value of advance information in reducing postoperative stress.

BODY IMAGE AND CONCEPT OF LOSS

Body image is the mental picture each of us has of our own body; culture, race, feelings, and attitudes influence our perception of this image. The development of body image commences soon after birth and is repeatedly revised to accommodate the ongoing changes that occur during the life cycle, through puberty, middle-age, and senescence. At birth, infants have no concept of a physical body image, experiencing sensations only at a feeling level; for example, hunger, comfort, warmth, and pain. During the first year of life the infant learns to differentiate between his body and the external world. This awareness that his body is separate from all others is the basis of, and becomes the foundation for, development of body image. Physical growth and development of motor skills allows active exploration and involvement with the environment and so increases differentiation between self and the environment. Other important developmental components of body image include sex role identification and differentiation, and peer and parental attitudes. These create an impression of the child's own concept of himself, his body, and its function. These and other physical, psychological, and social changes that occur during the life cycle are responsible for individuals continually modifying their body image.

Our society is based upon 'physical wholeness' which is continually reinforced by the media, particularly in advertising, where only the attractive and physically complete person is portrayed. It is important that nurses understand the concept of body image, and realize that patients, regardless of their physical or mental state of health, value their wholeness. In cases of sudden illness, trauma, or radical surgery which results in disfigurement, there is often a delay between the change in body image and the person's awareness of this change. The subsequent alteration in body image is capable of creating a crisis.

Many patients go through a period of mourning for their lost body image. The significance to the individual of that lost or altered body part will determine the effect of the alteration of their body image. Women who equate much of their femininity and attractiveness with their hairstyle will view the prospect of alopecia resulting from chemotherapy with far greater significance than will other women. Following a mastectomy, or a diagnosis of infertility, a woman may feel that her usefulness in life has ended and that no one understands how she feels. Patients with cardiac or renal disease, diabetes, or infertility, where there are less obvious changes in body structure, still experience an altered body image or self concept. Adaption and acceptance of this change is influenced by significant people in the patient's life. Female mastectomy patients often express concern that perhaps their partner will be unable to cope with their appearance, and patients following amputation, formation of a stoma, or disfiguring surgery express similar concerns. Changes in personal concepts of sexuality following an alteration in body image, will depend upon a person's view of their own sexual attractiveness and expertise prior to the illness, as well as perception of its importance to their partner.

COMMUNICATION

Learning to communicate effectively with a patient is as important as, if not more important than, learning the intricate details of applying Hamilton Russell traction, or performing a complicated dressing. Unfortunately, it is an area that is frequently neglected, and although nurses often think they are communicating with patients,

they rarely evaluate the process to see if it is being effective. Too often nurses say 'The patient doesn't understand', but very rarely do they consider 'How well have I made myself understood?'

Communication is a complex process involving at least two people: the sender, who is the person imparting the news, or giving the information; and the receiver, the person who receives the news or information. Effective communication occurs only when the receiver provides some sort of response, 'feedback', to the sender. It is an ongoing process, and the quality of the interaction depends largely on the skills developed in interpersonal communication. For effective communication, adaption and modification of messages is required so that they best fit the needs of each individual patient. A message that is carefully adapted to situational factors such as age, intellectual ability, emotional status, or ability to understand and speak English, tends to be more effective because it has been created for each individual patient. Its effectiveness can be measured in terms of whether or not the sender's message has had the desired impact on the receiver.

Although communication is commonly thought of as a verbal process, speech represents only a small portion of human communication. Nonverbal communication is equally as important and we express much more by this method than we care to think. Perhaps the most important aspect of effective communication involves not just what is said, nor just how it is said, but rather the degree of consistency between verbal and nonverbal messages. If there is any conflict between what is actually said and what is transmitted nonverbally the nonverbal message is more likely to be received. For this reason the nurse needs to be aware of all channels of communication and ensure that they are not used to transmit confusing, contradictory, or negative messages.

Nonverbal methods of communication

Facial expressions, eye contact, gestures, tone of voice, and touch are all nonverbal methods of communication; if they conflict with the verbal message they will provide a barrier to communication.

Facial expression. A grimace, smile, or expression of fear are all communicative acts. The patient who is grimacing and clasping his abdomen does not need to tell you that he is in pain, since he is communicating his distress by nonverbal means. The nurse who is frowning whilst interviewing a patient might just be concentrating. However, the patient is more likely to interpret this as the nurse disapproving of what he is saying. He will then be reluctant to communicate any further with him/her.

Eye contact. During conversation, eye contact is maintained for about one third of the time, with the listener maintaining more of the eye contact. Observe if your patient is maintaining eye contact; total lack of eye contact may mean a lack of self-concept or distrust.

Gestures. These also convey important signals. For example, an aphasic patient unable to verbalize his feelings of frustration, will often bang his fist on the bed or table.

Touch. Blondis & Jackson (1977) state that 'in nursing, touch may be the most important of all nonverbal behaviours'. A distressed patient will often receive more comfort and reassurance by a warm touch than by a multitude of words.

Distance. Each of us sets our own 'personal space', an invisible area with a boundary which we do not like others to intrude upon unless invited. In our culture most people have a personal space of about an arm's length. Hall (1959) points out that in France, Mexico, Brazil, and Arabian countries this distance is shorter. A patient's sense of his own 'personal space' will determine how closely you can approach whilst allowing him to remain comfortable and at ease. Communicating from too great a distance can also create a barrier, and the nurse who observes a patient attempting to get out of bed will give the impression he/she has more important things to do if he/she remains at a distance when asking 'Would you like me to help you?'

Useful hints in communicating with patients

1. Try to sit at the bedside, and ensure privacy – this lets the patient know he has your undivided attention.
2. Address him by his name – this helps to avoid institutional depersonalization.

3. Be aware that much of the communication will be nonverbal.
4. Make frequent, brief eye contact – failure to look a patient in the eye is all part of the process of dehumanization.
5. Be prepared to express your own personal thoughts, if necessary, but be careful not to dictate your views.

Techniques to overcome barriers to interpersonal communication

1. Use feedback. Two-way communication allows us to search for verbal and nonverbal cues from our patients. The more complex the information we are trying to communicate, the more essential it is that we encourage our patients to ask questions, and to indicate areas of confusion.
2. Be sensitive to the patient's world. Be aware that patients differ in their values, needs, attitudes, and expectations. Empathy with those differences will improve our understanding and make it easier to communicate.
3. Use direct, simple language. Most patients, however educated they may be, do not understand medical jargon, and it needs to be translated into simple terms that they can understand. Try not to lecture; patients rightfully want to protect their egos, and nurses who lecture their patients instead of talking to them will receive cold, formal replies. Nurses who act as equals and who indicate that they trust and respect their patient's feelings will usually receive honest, less defensive replies.
4. Use the correct amount of redundancy. If the message is important, or complicated, then it is probably necessary to repeat it in several different ways to ensure that your patient understands. It may even be necessary to write instructions down, or get your patient to repeat them.

Nursing approaches to communication

1. Always allow your patients to express their feelings, these may range from despair and hopelessness through optimism and even euphoria, prior to achieving adjustment.
2. Be aware of the importance of predicting and recognizing the occurrence of altered and distorted body image in certain patients.

3. Observe verbal and nonverbal behaviour which may indicate adaption or nonadaption, for example, the patient who refuses to look at a scar.

4. Intervene when necessary and assist patients to cope by rebuilding and intensifying feelings of self worth, rather than allowing them to focus on physical appearance.

5. Discuss their illness with patients, and how it will affect their lifestyle. This can help patients dispense with unrealistic fears and allows them to concentrate on coming to terms with their change in body image. This can begin preoperatively if surgery is anticipated, and a visit from someone who has had similar surgery can help to allay fears of social unacceptability, curtailment of social activities and work, or the inability to wear normal clothes.

COMPLIANCE AND NONCOMPLIANCE

Compliance

The majority of patients when admitted to hospital comply with both medical and nursing instructions, and are seen to behave in an acceptable manner. The 'good patient' is often considered the easiest type of patient to nurse for he rarely asks questions or queries treatment ordered. It is, however, important to realize that compliance does not necessarily equate with acceptance and/or understanding of diagnosis and treatment. When nursing the compliant patient it is important to ensure that he fully comprehends what is happening to him. Patients are silent for many reasons, and among the most common causes are fear that what they might say will lead to disapproval or rejection, and anxiety which can influence the thinking processes. Manifestations of anxiety vary from patient to patient, and several factors may obscure our recognition of their anxiety. For instance, older people have defenses which they have used well for many years, and so are often more able to conceal their anxiety than a younger person. The following behaviours and physiological changes may help you identify an anxious patient:

1. Increased pulse rate and/or blood pressure and ventilations

2. Urinary frequency
3. Insomnia
4. Restlessness – continual wandering
5. Fatigue
6. A change in tempo or tone of voice
7. Hostile or dependent behaviour
8. Chain smoking.

The person who feels he must play the role of the 'good patient' is often hesitant to question the busy nurse, for fear of wasting his/her time. It is therefore important to encourage the seemingly compliant patient to verbalize hidden fears. It is essential that the nurse appears approachable, allowing the patient to recognize that he is an individual and, as such, is important and respected. Often, a question such as 'Tell me how much you understand about your illness' will allow him to express his feelings and clarify areas he does not understand. By being alert to the cues our patients give, both verbal and nonverbal, we are more likely to recognize those compliant patients who may not have accepted their situation.

Noncompliance

Perhaps one of the most frustrating experiences in nursing is an encounter with the patient who refuses to accept treatment and routines. Noncompliance or seemingly inappropriate behaviour may be seen in the form of aggressive or passive behaviour.

Aggressive or violent behaviour

Violent behaviour is more often associated with psychiatric hospitals; however, the violence offered by patients, and sometimes by the public, in general hospitals is as severe and potentially dangerous as that seen in psychiatric hospitals. The most vulnerable staff are those working in an Accident and Emergency department and they should be aware that in certain patients there is a potential for unpremeditated violence. Staff should be particularly careful when nursing:

- Patients regaining consciousness following an overdose

- Diabetics in a precomatose state of hypoglycaemia
- Drug addicts
- Epileptics recovering from a seizure
- Patients with alcohol intoxication.

People who are intoxicated often exhibit aggressive behaviour because of prior involvement in a fight, or because they have been brought in against their will. They often demand attention for minor injuries and refuse to consider patients with more acute emergencies. Anxious relatives and friends may demand immediate treatment for a patient, and these demands may be frequently accompanied by verbal abuse and threats of violence. It is evident that some people will intimidate and use threats of violence, which may be carried out, in order to bend staff and systems to their own advantage.

The confused elderly patient is a recurring problem for ward staff. They frequently insist on getting out of bed at night, dressing, and going home. Attempts to dissuade them from such action can be met with physical and verbal aggression.

Passive or nonviolent behaviour

The behaviour of noncompliant patients, however inappropriate, is not just a mere whim on the part of the patient. There are reasons why patients respond as they do, and often an explanation can be found. Consider the following two examples:

A 30-year-old male, hospitalized with rheumatic heart disease, who despite numerous explanations refused to stay in bed. Often he was found out of bed, staring through the window. Did he fail to understand the seriousness of his condition; was he self destructive, or did he lack common sense? He was considered by the ward staff 'a problem patient'. (See later for discussion.)

A 56-year-old female who was admitted for an elective cholecystectomy. On admission she displayed aggressive behaviour to all staff and, when asked to undergo a routine preoperative electrocardiogram, refused and announced she was going home. This patient was labelled

'difficult' by the staff. (See page 18 for discussion.)

Intellectually handicapped patients often present a problem when admitted to a ward by displaying disruptive behaviour.

Patients with a psychiatric history, or worse still, those who have been labelled with some psychiatric history, (often because of noncompliant behaviour during previous hospital admissions) are often classified as 'difficult', since their presence on the ward seems to create anxiety amongst the staff!

Some reasons for noncompliance

Cultural, ethnic, social, and religious backgrounds are all sources of different responses to illness and treatment. Apparent refusal to follow medical treatment often stems from one of these differentials.

Let us reconsider the 30-year-old male who refused to remain in bed. When someone finally thought to ask him why he persisted in disobeying orders, the explanation was quite simple. As a Muslim he was required to face Mecca five times a day to pray, and for him religious practices were more important than medical orders. The solution was simple; his bed was moved to a position which allowed him to face Mecca and so carry out his religious practices whilst in bed.

Another situation involved a middle-aged Arabian male who presented with carcinoma of the rectum. When it was explained that he would require surgery that necessitated the formation of a stoma, he refused the operation. Despite a visit from a well adjusted ostomate, and being shown a multitude of available appliances, he continued to refuse surgery saying he would never be able to manage the bags. Discussions with his family revealed that in some Arab communities any material classed as dirty, such as faeces or urine, can only be touched by the left hand, the right being kept clean for handling food. No wonder he rightly considered the changing of an appliance with only his left hand as impossible. Once the problem had been identified, colostomy irrigation was suggested as an alternative. This was acceptable because he was able to use both hands to set up the equipment and regulate the fluid, whilst only his left hand was used to introduce the catheter and clean the stoma on completion of the procedure.

Poor or inadequate communication can often be the cause of noncompliant behaviour. If the patient misunderstands or misinterprets the instructions he will not be able to comply. For example, an elderly patient who was prescribed glycerin suppositories for constipation, remarked that he didn't like taking them with his cup of tea because they melted!

Fear and anxiety affect behaviour differently depending upon individual personalities. Some people are able to discuss fear and anxiety related to their hospitalization, whilst other patients may become withdrawn or aggresive. With the female admitted for cholecystectomy, discussion with her husband revealed that her mother had undergone similar surgery which had revealed cancer; the patient was terrified she also had cancer. As her father had died from a heart attack, she had interpreted the taking of a routine electrocardiograph to mean she had something wrong with her heart. After reassurance and dispelling her fears, the patient had the operation and made a safe postoperative recovery with no further displays of aggression.

Insecurity also affects patients' behaviour. This can occur when information regarding diagnosis and prognosis is denied.

Patients who have spent some time in an intensive care unit often exhibit demanding behaviour upon transfer to a ward, as do patients who have received constant attention when critically ill. The demanding behaviour usually presents when the patient's condition is improving, and such patients are often labelled 'hospitalized' by the staff. Insecurity can often be the basis for this behaviour, and discussion with such a patient transferred from an intensive care unit revealed that he was worried that his condition might deteriorate and that without constant observation no one would know. He was also worried that if he went to sleep without a nurse to watch him, perhaps he would not wake up.

Frustration can play a part in patients displaying aggressive behaviour, particularly if they perceive their medical treatment as inadequate. Frustra-

tions for the patient may include: lack of night sedation, inadequate pain relief, and the feeling that they are being unnecessarily disturbed by nurses who are more sensitive to the demands of hospital routine than to the patient's condition.

Loss of personal identity and inability to govern their own destiny will affect patients' behaviour. People, patients included, dislike having to obey orders and respond more congenially if asked to do something. Many nurses tend to treat patients like small children or use familiar terms which may be interpreted by the patient as a sign of disrespect; these thoughtless behaviours lead to resentment. A nurse, overheard referring to an elderly patient as 'Gran', evoked the angry response that she was not this girl's grandmother.

Labelling. Patients once labelled as 'difficult' tend to act out that role. However rigorously we discipline ourselves not to show irritation or anger at patient behaviour, there are a number of ways in which we unconsciously transmit such messages; chief amongst these are tone of voice, or expressive behaviour of the body. Such messages, more meaningful to the patient than is usually recognized, do not ameliorate the situation; rather, they evoke counter responses and our patients continue to be 'difficult'.

Nursing approaches to noncompliant behaviour

1. Listen to your patient and always be alert to verbal and nonverbal cues the patient may express. The patient who denies that he is worried about impending surgery, but is plucking at the bed clothes and gazing nervously around the room is displaying nonverbal signs of anxiety. He needs reassurance as much as, if not more than, the patient who openly expresses anxiety and fear.
2. Identify and attempt to solve immediate worries expressed by your patient.
3. Ensure effective communication. The importance of effective communication between staff and patients cannot be overemphasized. Rather than ignore a patient because he is difficult, try to draw him into conversation.
4. Explain all investigations and procedures. Patients who are fully informed tend to be less anxious and more co-operative.
5. Establish a relationship of trust and under-

standing. This allows patients to express tensions and anxieties, and may well prevent the nurse from becoming the target for pent up feelings.

6. Always be straightforward and truthful. Dishonesty results in lack of trust. Never make a promise you cannot keep, for example 'You can go home tomorrow'. This will only result in someone else having to deal with the problem.

7. Anticipate and plan in advance to prevent potential problems materializing, for example, obtain guidelines for the daily routine of intellectually handicapped patients, and try to arrange for a familiar person to be with them during the day.

8. Make use of all available resource personnel, for example, use an interpreter to relay information and reassurance to non English-speaking patients.

9. Give patients some control over their own care. Encourage them to set their own goals (for example, a decreasing regime of number of cigarettes smoked per day) and to work at their own pace to achieve them.

10. Finally, be aware of the importance and effect of cultural, ethnic, social, and religious backgrounds.

If we use these approaches with all our patients we may prevent problems for, as in many other areas in nursing, prevention is better than cure.

SUMMARY

This chapter provides few answers for the nurse who wants a set of rules with which to nurse patients, as each patient is an individual concerned with his own feelings and beliefs. Awareness of the psychological, social, cultural, and spiritual, as well as physical and biological, determinants of behaviour should motivate nurses to help their patients to identify areas of concern, and to help them find ways of coming to terms with these problems.

REFERENCES AND FURTHER READING

Texts

Arnold M B 1976 Psychological stress. In: Appleby M H, Trumbull R (eds) Stress and Emotion. Appleton Century Croft, New York

Blondis M N, Jackson B E 1977 Nonverbal communication with patients. Wiley, New York

Brown M S 1977 In: Bower F L (ed) Distortions in body image in illness and disability. Wiley, New York

Hall E 1959 The silent language. Fawcett, Connecticut

Janis I 1971 Stress and frustration. Harcourt Brace Jovanovich, New York

Porritt L 1984 Communication: choices for nurses. Churchill Livingstone, Melbourne

Roberts S L 1978 Behavioural concepts and nursing throughout the lifespan. Prentice Hall, New Jersey

Robinson J (ed) 1982 Using crisis intervention wisely. Intermed Communications, Pennsylvania

Robinson L 1972 Psychological aspects of the care of hospitalized patients, 3rd edn. Davis, Philadelphia

Wilson-Barnett J 1979 Stress in hospital. Churchill Livingstone, Edinburgh

Journals

Adams F E 1984 6 very good reasons why we react differently to various dying patients. Nursing 84 14 : 6 : 41–43

Bailey I, Lissenden K, Sagenkahn L E, Paxton L A, Bores J 1985 View from the horizontal side of caring. Nursing 85 15 : 10 : 52–54

Brill C, Hill L 1985 Giving the help that goes on giving. Nursing 85 15 : 5 : 44–47

Burlew C 1981 Communication and nursing. The Australian Nurses Journal 11 : 2 : 41–42

Cave L, Johnson J M, Komar R, Korth C, Meaker C, Patton R M 1985 When families get together. Nursing 85 15 : 2 : 58–61

Cooper J 1979 Actions really do speak louder than words. Nursing 79 9 : 4 : 113–118

Crovella A C 1985 The person behind the disease. Nursing 85 15 : 9 : 42–43

English M (ed) 1983 Ordeal. Nursing 83 13 : 10 : 34–43

Ferszt G G, Taylor P B 1984 The patient's right to cry. Nursing 84 14 : 3 : 10–11

Forbes B J 1984 Let your actions do the talking. Nursing 84 14 : 3 : 32

Friedman H S 1979 Nonverbal communication between patients and medical practitioners. Journal of Social Issues 35 : 1 : 82–99

Giarratana C M 1984 Reach out, reach out and touch . . . Henry. Nursing 84 14 : 2 : 47–49

Gutierrez K 1985 Home is where the care is. Nursing 85 15 : 11 : 48–49

Hagerty B K 1980 Denial isn't all bad. Sometimes not facing facts is helpful. Nursing 80 10 : 10 : 58–60

Jackson S 1985 The touching process in rehabilitation. The Australian Nurses Journal 14 : 11 : 43–45

Johnson S H 1986 10 ways to help the family of a critically ill patient. Nursing 86 16 : 1 : 50–53

Jones M K 1986 Caring for the patient who makes caring difficult. Nursing 86 16 : 5 : 44–46

Kanitsaki O 1983 Acculturation – a new dimension in nursing. The Australian Nurses Journal 13 : 5 : 42–45, 53

Laken D D 1983 Protecting patients against themselves. Nursing 83 13 : 1 : 26–27

Luna M L 1984 The patient who complains. Nursing 84 14 : 11 : 47–49

Margetts D 1984a Crisis intervention – the myth of expertise. The Australian Nurses Journal 14 : 2 : 45–47

Margetts D 1984b Crisis intervention – the myth of expertise. The Australian Nurses Journal 14 : 3 : 46–48, 60

McAuliffe K, McAuliffe D 1984 I care. Nursing 84 14 : 4 : 58–59

Meissner J E 1980 Semantic differential scales for assessing patients' feelings. Nursing 80 10 : 2 : 70–71

Meissner J E 1980 Measuring patient stress with the Hospital Stress Rating Scale. Nursing 80 10 : 8 : 70–71

Mercer L 1980 Pseudocommunication with patients. Nursing 80 10 : 2 : 19–22

Milne J 1984 The pastoral care experience in acute situations. The Australian Nurses Journal 13 : 8 : 39–41

Presley S R 1980 When it came to communicating without words . . . Cyrus was an expert. Nursing 80 10 : 10 : 28–31

Richardson J I, Berline-Nauman D 1984 In the face of anger. Nursing 84 14 : 2 : 8–11

Rowlands D 1984 Therapeutic touch: its effects on the depressed elderly. The Australian Nurses Journal 13 : 11 : 45–46, 52

Rubin R 1968 Body image and self esteem. Nursing Outlook 16 : 6 : 20–23

Searle L (ed) 1985 Honoring the personal side of chronic illness. Nursing 85 15 : 11 : 52–57

Shubin S 1979 Communicating (or, make that noncommunicating) with doctors. Nursing 79 9 : 2 : 12–16

Shubin S 1980 Nursing patients from different cultures. Nursing 80 10 : 6 : 26–29

Steffee D R, Suty K A, Delcalzo P V 1985 More than a touch: communicating with a blind and deaf patient. Nursing 85 15 : 8 : 37–39

Strauch B, Crespo M, McMahon M, Kornblatt J 1980 Caring enough to give your patient control. Nursing 80 10 : 8 : 54–59

Thompson B 1986 Interpersonal skills – learning the importance of listening. The Australian Nurses Journal 16 : 3 : 45–47, 61

Tierney M J, Watson M, Betzold J, Taniguchi D A, Mazique S I 1986 Mr Gomez had a bad case of 'hospital smarts'. Nursing 86 16 : 2 : 44–46

Vago M D 1984 Remember the roommate. Nursing 84 14 : 5 : 51

Valente S 1984 Stalking patient depression. Nursing 84 14 : 8 : 62–64

Wiley L (ed) 1979 Finding – and using – your patient's strengths. Nursing 79 9 : 3 : 40–45

3

Legal principles in the practice of medical-surgical nursing

Barbara Piesse

INTRODUCTION

This chapter does not profess to be an exhaustive and definitive treatment of all the legal principles relevant to nursing. Rather, it is a response to commonly held anxieties and questions raised by nurses in the context of their medical and surgical nursing practice.

Accountability and advocacy

Initially it is important to establish the relevance of law to the practice of nursing. The professionalism of nursing practice is based on two major concepts: accountability and patient advocacy.

In a practical sense accountability requires the nurse to report, explain, and justify both the care provided and the action taken to ensure that the patient obtains appropriate care. Ultimately it means that the nurse is responsible, in both a professional and legal sense, to and for the patient.

The concept of patient advocacy denotes the nurse acting for and on behalf of the patient. The patient will often seek from the nurse information and clarification, as well as reassurance. It is the nurse in many instances who implements care on the patient's behalf.

It is important therefore that the nurse has an understanding of those principles of law relevant to nursing practice which govern the nurse/patient relationship. This is necessary not only from the aspect of patient rights, but also in relation to the potential liability of the nurse.

The need for such understanding increases as the nature of the relationship between patient and nurse changes. Factors which have influenced this change in recent years include the increased educational status of both the patient and nurse and a growing awareness of individual rights evoked by media publicity, consumerism, and legislative encouragement of accountability through access to information under various Freedom of Information Acts.

Sources and functions of law

Prior to discussing specific aspects of law affecting nursing practice, it is useful to consider the sources and functions of such law. Principles of law relevant to the health care area can be found in Acts of Parliament (statutory law) and in the decisions of cases determined by court process (common law).

Law functions not only to prohibit and punish, but to compensate, regulate, facilitate, to create and uphold values, and to provide the means of enforcing rights and remedying wrongs.

In the context of medical and surgical nursing, the law functions to regulate the practice of nursing by registration of professionals, and by delineation of qualifications and areas of practice. Further, it operates to regulate the relationship between the nurse and the patient on an individual basis. It functions to protect both patient and nurse.

Nurses often ask about the functions of law, ethics, and morality, and how these concepts differ. Law is concerned primarily with the well-being of society as a whole and the individual within society. Its principles are applied to all and enforced by the courts as a means of protecting society against conflict. Ethics and morality on the other hand are more limited in function and concern rules of behaviour. Ethics concern the behaviour of an individual, for example in relation to the values of a particular profession. They seek to voluntarily promote professional conduct that is inherently good. Morality concerns value judgements between right and wrong, and thus may determine acceptable behaviour in a community at any particular time.

Law does not and cannot impose and enforce ideals in morality and ethics. The law cannot make 'good' professionals as opposed to bad ones. It can only concern itself with attempting to ensure social well-being by enforcement of minimum acceptable standards of conduct. The law must have certainty as an objective; and were it to establish binding principles that corresponded to all demands of morality, it might be vague and uncertain in operation.

The example of the Good Samaritan provides clear illustration of the three concepts. If an off-duty nurse came across a roadside emergency with injured people in need of help, professional ethics would suggest that, voluntarily, whatever assistance could be rendered should be rendered to those in need. Further, professional qualification would render the nurse appropriate to assist. Morally it is desirable to assist people in need. Legally the nurse is under no obligation to assist. The law cannot and will not dictate that the nurse must help: there is no relationship between nurse and accident victim, and no duty in law to act in these circumstances. If, however, the nurse did proceed to assist, the law would then demand that actions taken accord with standards of reasonable care. (See page 28, Negligence.)

The treatment or continued treatment of terminally ill patients is another example involving legal, ethical, and moral considerations in balancing the notion of sanctity of life against individual rights to self-determination. The nurse as a professional should be able to consider all three aspects.

THE LAW AFFECTING MEDICAL-SURGICAL NURSING

The balance of this chapter concentrates on the relationship between nurse and patient as individ-

uals, and is thus concerned primarily with common law principles in the area of civil law. The categories of civil and criminal law differ in both philosophy and objectives. A crime, for example murder or larceny, is an offence against the values of society as a whole. It is prosecuted by the State on behalf of society, and is sanctioned by punishment of some form to protect society and maintain its well-being.

Civil law, on the other hand, concerns the relationship between individuals, and regulates their behaviour by providing the means of enforcing rights and remedying wrongs. Areas of civil law of concern to nurses include the law of torts (a broad area of civil wrongs including vicarious liability, trespass, negligence), and the law of contract. Liability in tort (in negligence for example) is primarily aimed at compensating the individual who has suffered.

In determining liability the courts attempt to balance differing interests. The patient's interest essentially demands that no harm be suffered as a result of unreasonable risk during hospitalization; and that if harm is suffered, then a right to compensation exists. On the other hand, the nurse's interest would demand that liability be imposed only in clear cases of individual fault. The ultimate outcome in any court situation depends on the legal principles involved, the evidence presented by both sides, and the examination and credibility of witnesses. It is in this area that the quality of nursing documentation is critical in relation to the particular case. (See page 30.)

What the law does is to establish general principles to be applied to varying situations, enabling adaption to differing circumstances coming before the courts. If principles were too narrowly defined, options for further development would be limited.

Vicarious liability

The principle of vicarious liability is relevant to a nurse no matter whether he/she is practising within a hospital environment, in a domiciliary setting, or in a community health facility. In effect this principle renders an employer liable for the torts of an employee committed in the course of employment. It is technically possible for an employer to recover part or all of the damages awarded to the injured plaintiff from a culpable employee. However, as employers almost invariably insure against the risk of vicarious liability, the probability of an employer taking action against an employee is small.

Why is it that the law renders the employer primarily liable, when in fact the employee causes the harm to the plaintiff? The answer seems to lie in economic grounds: the employer, through insurance, is better able to cover the cost of the risk of liability, and thus the plaintiff can sue a defendant who has the assets with which to meet judgement. Through insurance, the cost of liability is distributed widely.

The protection afforded by the concept of vicarious liability only applies where an employment relationship exists. Accordingly, locum and agency nurses would be well advised to check their position and to take out appropriate indemnity insurance where necessary.

Similarly, in emergency situations outside the hospital where a nurse renders assistance voluntarily, and unconnected with employment, the principle of vicarious liability would not apply. Therefore the nurse rendering assistance would be directly liable for his/her actions should the plaintiff have cause for complaint.

Trespass

Trespass is an area of tort law concerned with protecting both personal and proprietary interests from unauthorized and unjustifiable interference. Battery, assault, and false imprisonment are the three significant and distinct areas of trespass to the person which are relevant to nursing practice.

Battery, as the word denotes, involves a direct, intentional, and unauthorized application of physical force or contact to someone else's body. All nursing procedures involving touch potentially fall within this category. These procedures range from the provision of basic bedside care, to the administration of medication, the dressing and care of wounds, and the insertion and removal of catheters.

Assault, on the other hand, involves the apprehension of imminent harmful or offensive contact;

the actual contact being a battery. To succeed, a plaintiff would need to prove that the apprehension was reasonable and that the defendant had an apparent ability to carry out the threat.

Assault is both a crime and a civil wrong. It is thus possible for a person who commits an assault to be sued for damages by the 'victim' and also charged by the police, prosecuted, and dealt with according to the criminal law. The term 'assault' commonly refers to both assault and battery, although it is possible to have one without the other.

False imprisonment involves the complete and total deprivation of someone's freedom of movement without any lawful justification. It thus protects both freedom and personal dignity.

A patient need not be conscious to suffer a trespass. Trespass in the form of battery and false imprisonment can be committed against an unconscious or anaesthetized patient. Consider the use of cot sides and restraints. In what situation is a nurse justified in using them? This issue is considered below under Defences.

If patient rights protected by the law of trespass are infringed, then, in the absence of authorization or justification, the nurse and/or the employer concerned may be liable. It should be noted that it is not only patients who can be victims of assault: nurses too may be assaulted by patients or visitors, and they too have rights to legal redress for the wrongs suffered.

A nurse threatened with assault is entitled to use reasonable, but not excessive, force in self-defence. This is one of the defences or excuses recognized by law as justification for the conduct in question. The defences of consent, necessity, and statutory justification are relevant to medical-surgical nursing.

Defences to trespass

Consent

The defence of consent is based on the premise that no injury or harm can be suffered by someone who is willing and who agrees to participate in, for example, an operative procedure.

How can a patient consent to nursing or operative procedures? Consent may be given impliedly, by conduct or behaviour, or expressly by written or spoken agreement.

A patient who, in a spirit of co-operation, gives no indication of unwillingness to allow administration of an injection, or to allow readings of temperature, blood pressure and pulse to be taken, and who by behaviour positively assists the nurse, would be giving implied consent to such procedures. In such situations the nurse may reasonably infer from the circumstances that the patient consents.

Any indication of withdrawal of consent, be it express or implied, must be treated seriously and documented objectively, informatively, and accurately in the patient record. If the withdrawal of consent relates to medical, as distinct from nursing matters, the physician concerned must be notified accordingly. Failure to notify and to act responsibly in relation to such withdrawal could result in actionable trespass. A patient may expressly agree to a procedure by a statement to such effect. This too should be noted in the record, together with a record of time and circumstances.

In relation to surgical procedures, the usual way of documenting consent is by completion of the appropriate form and signature by the patient. In some hospitals nurses act as witnesses to the patients' signature on the consent form. This is an undesirable situation which may result in ethical dilemmas for the nurse, given that the patient will often direct questions and anxieties to the nurse. It is the responsibility of the physician concerned to obtain patient consent and it is the physician who knows in detail the patient's medical condition, the nature of the procedure, and prognosis.

A completed and signed consent form can be used to support verbal testimony should a case arise and thus documentation is desirable from an evidentiary point of view. Written consent is no different from verbal consent in that it must still be valid to provide a defence to an action.

When a case does arise in which a patient takes legal action in respect of harm that has been suffered, the consent may well be examined for validity. In determining whether the consent in question is valid the courts consider the capacity of the person consenting, whether the consent has been freely and voluntarily given, and also whether it is specific in that it covers the procedure to be performed or something substantially similar in nature.

Obviously a patient must be competent to consent. Capacity in this sense is the recognized legal ability to consent, to decide whether to agree to participate or not. Capacity is determined by the patient's age, mental, and intellectual condition.

Who, then, can consent? Generally a competent adult patient is the only one capable of consenting. Thus the practice of obtaining consent from family members, while it has valid communication aspects, is of doubtful legal value.

Legislation in Victoria deems persons of 18 years to be adults and thus legally competent. However, it is generally accepted that persons aged between 14–18 years can consent if they appear mature enough to understand the nature, risks, and consequences of the procedure involved. In practice this maturity factor is often determined by ascertaining whether the patient is independent, self supporting, and managing alone. The consent of parent or guardian is required for those not in this category.

Sometimes, as a matter of public policy, legislation removes the right of certain individuals to consent, on the basis that they need protection from themselves and from others. Thus, social interest dictates that not all persons are able legally to consent and further that the interest of such persons be safeguarded. Patients under the care and protection of the Mental Health Authority or the Department of Community Welfare Services lack the ability to consent in their own right, and legislation regulates the consent by nominated persons on behalf of such patients. Patients who are intellectually handicapped to the extent that they are not able to decide for themselves and yet are outside the jurisdiction of these departments can have a parent/guardian/spouse consent on their behalf.

Consent must also be voluntary or freely given. Thus, consent will not be valid if it is obtained in circumstances of duress or untoward pressure due to which the patient is not able to respond voluntarily, for example after administration of preoperative medication. Coercion thus might invalidate consent.

In *Beausoleil* v *Sisters of Charity* [1966] 53 DLR 2d 65, the patient agreed to a general anaesthetic. On the day of the operation the anaesthetist decided that a spinal anaesthetic would be preferable. The patient did not agree to this. After premedication had been administered the anaesthetist ultimately persuaded the patient to change her mind and have a spinal anaesthetic. The patient was paralysed and successfully sued for assault on the basis that the consent to the spinal had not been given voluntarily. Each case must be considered on its merits and there may well be premedicated patients who are lucid enough to make such decisions.

Consent must be specific in that it must precisely cover the procedure or operation to be performed, or at least acts of substantially similar nature. It is thus important that the details entered on the documentation and consent form correspond with the procedure or operation to be performed and that identification of the patient, the limb, or the site, be cross-checked for correspondence. In the event of a discrepancy the appropriate person should be notified.

What information should be provided to the patient before requesting consent to a procedure or an operation? Ideally, from a nursing view point, that the patient should receive a clear and unequivocal explanation of the nature of his condition and of the proposed treatment, procedure or operation, the chances of success and failure, the risks and discomforts involved, and an indication of any possible alternative. (These factors constitute in some overseas countries the 'doctrine of informed consent'.)

At a minimum, then, patients should be informed of the inherent nature of the procedure or operation and the real risks involved. Expert medical evidence will assist courts in determining whether the disclosure has been adequate and appropriate.

While the Royal Australian Nursing Federation (Victorian Branch) policy requires that information should be given to the patient regarding the nature of nursing procedures to be performed, nurses often face a dilemma in relation to consent to surgical procedures. The obtaining of consent is the province and responsibility of the physician concerned. It is the nurse, however, who must at

first instance handle the patient's anxieties, doubts, and need for knowledge and information. This dilemma is heightened by the fact that the doctrine of informed consent which is accepted as a legal right of patients in some overseas jurisdictions, does not yet apply in Australia.

The doctrine of informed consent, conveys two notions; not only that the patient has the capacity to agree and has agreed freely and voluntarily; but, more importantly, that sufficient information has been given to the patient to enable a reasoned choice to be made between the risks and benefits involved in the particular procedure proposed.

As yet this doctrine has no parallel in Australia and thus adequacy of the information provided to the patient will be judged by the objective standard of what a reasonable professional would provide in the same or similar circumstances. This view is supported by the case *Hills* v *Potter and Others* ([1983] 3 All ER 716) wherein it was held:

> The standard of care required of a doctor when giving information to a patient who had to decide whether to undergo an operation was the same as that normally required of a doctor in the course of his diagnosis and treatment, namely the exercise of the ordinary skill which a doctor in the defendant's position would be expected to possess. Accordingly, in giving advice prior to an operation a doctor or surgeon did not have to inform the patient of all the details of the proposed treatment or the likely outcome and the risks inherent in it but was merely required to act in accordance with a practice accepted as proper by a responsible body of skilled medical practitioners, and that required the doctor or surgeon to supply the patient with sufficient information to enable the patient to decide whether to undergo the operation.

This reaffirms the rule in *Bolam* v *Friern Hospital Management Committee* [1957] 2 All ER 118, namely that a physician is not negligent if he acts in accordance with a practice accepted as proper by a responsible body of medical opinion. It is further supported by the case of *Sidaway* v *Bethlehem Royal Hospital Governors and Others* ([1985] 1 All ER 643), wherein it was held:

> The test of liability, in respect of a doctor's duty to warn his patient of risks inherent in treatment recommended by him was the same as the test applicable to diagnosis and treatment, namely that the doctor was required to act in accordance with a practice accepted at the time as proper by a responsible body of medical opinion. Accordingly English law did not recognize the doctrine of informed consent.

Mrs Sidaway was severely disabled after a spinal operation. She suffered from persistent pain in her neck and shoulders and on the advice of a neurosurgeon proceeded with a laminectomy and face-tectomy. She was warned of the possibility of damage to the spinal cord. The risk of damage to the spinal cord was estimated at less than 1% and the possible resultant injury could range from mild to very severe.

Mrs Sidaway claimed damages for negligence on the basis that the surgeon breached his duty of care to her by not disclosing the special risks inherent in the operation, and as a result that she had not been in a position to give 'informed consent' to the operation.

The court held that because the physician had acted in accordance with a practice accepted as proper by a body of responsible medical practitioners he had not breached his duty of care to her. The issue of whether she should have consented had full disclosure occurred was not addressed because the 'doctrine of informed consent' has no role in English law.

The New Zealand case *Smith* v *Auckland Hospital Board* ([1965] NZLR 191) concerned an aortogram. The patient specifically asked about the risks involved after receiving a general explanation of the procedure. He was reassured by one of the surgical team members and told that he would have a light anaesthetic and would be home within a couple of days. The outcome of the aortogram was that a small piece of atheroma was dislodged from the wall of the artery causing obstruction to the blood supply and resulting in ultimate amputation of the leg affected. It was accepted that this was a rare but recognized risk of aortography. The plaintiff succeeded in his action for negligence in that the physician breached his duty of care by not answering the patient's questions accurately and reasonably, knowing that the plaintiff was relying on his skill and judgement.

Several points arise from the cases considered. While the duty to take reasonable care is a duty imposed by law, it is the judgement of the medical profession rather than the law that will determine whether the physician concerned provided adequate information to the patient to satisfy the medical profession's requirements.

The defence of consent protects the professionals and the hospital involved from liability in trespass.

It does not exonerate the professionals involved from negligence (see page 27) in the care provided, the procedure carried out, or the obtaining of consent. It is thus open for a patient to take action against the professional involved where there has been negligence in the obtaining of consent.

It is necessary to appreciate that in relation to operative procedures it is the physician's responsibility to obtain consent and that patients who ask questions are entitled to have them answered properly.

What then is the nurse's role in relation to consent to operative procedures? Usually nurses are involved in confirming the identity of the patient, and checking the procedure, limbs and site for compliance with the detail on the appropriate documentation. It is invariably the nurse to whom the patient will direct queries, doubts, and calls for reassurance. Obviously the nurse is a significant reference for information.

Nurses then should encourage patients to ask questions of their physicians, for in asking they are entitled to a reasonable reply. It is obviously difficult to ask questions about unknown risks and often there may be difficulty with an inequality of knowledge between professional and patient. Nurses should be aware of the avenues of appeal within their hospital hierarchy to help a patient in this regard.

As the patient's advocate, a nurse should always respond to indications that the patient is unsure about the procedure to be performed. If the nurse becomes aware that consent has been obtained in such circumstances that it may not be genuine or that consent is refused or withdrawn then appropriate persons should be notified immediately and details documented accurately.

The right of self-determination and control over unauthorized interference is upheld by the law of trespass. It is the patient's right to choose whether to proceed and that choice, regardless of its wisdom, should be respected.

As the patient's advocate the nurse must be conscious of the need to safeguard the patient's right to consent, or withhold or withdraw consent, to an operation or procedures.

The Law Reform Commission of Victoria made the subject 'Informed Consent' its first specific enquiry within its general reference on Medicine, Science and the Law. It is hoped that some legislative initiatives may follow from its work. (Law Reform Commission of Victoria, 1987.)

Necessity

What happens when the patient is unable to consent, unconscious, or admitted in an emergency situation, and the professionals involved are not expressly or impliedly authorized to act? In this situation the professionals involved act as agents of necessity for the patient, as they undertake procedures often in life-threatening situations and to avoid greater harm occurring to the patient. They must however conform to a reasonable standard of care and the defence of necessity does not apply to protect against liability for negligence.

Does the defence of necessity protect nursing staff against liability for trespass where irrational, senile, demented, feverish or postoperative patients are restrained? It appears that the defence will apply only if restraint is necessary for the protection of the patient or others from the risk of injury or harm. What is necessary in any situation is a matter of judgement to be assessed in the light of medical and nursing evidence. In the absence of hospital policy (providing for instance guidance on the use of bed sides for postoperative, elderly or feverish patients) restraints should only be applied on medical orders, and the facts well documented.

Statutory justification

In some circumstances legislation dispenses with the need for consent and provides legal justification for conduct which would otherwise be actionable trespass. For example, legislation authorizing the taking of blood samples from persons admitted to hospital as a result of road accidents, vaccinations and isolation in specialist units for contagious or infectious diseases, and blood transfusions for children regardless of parental consent. In these instances overriding public interest outweighs the individual's rights and the interests of children, in relation to transfusion, are safeguarded.

Negligence

The word 'negligence' is used in two senses: generally, to describe carelessness; and legally, to describe conduct falling below the standard required by law in certain circumstances. Negligence is an area of concern to nurses and from a practical point of view negligent acts by nurses can have the following consequences: harm to the patient, and/or potential harm to both the hospital's reputation and the future career of the nurse. However, adherence to the principles of sound nursing practice, following established policies and acting in the patient's best interest reduce the likelihood of injury to the patient and the concurrent risk of liability for negligence. Negligence as we will consider it is an area of civil law, developed to protect both person and property against unreasonable risk of harm and to compensate persons who have suffered as a result of the negligence of another in the circumstances to be detailed. It should be noted that there is an area of negligence involving the criminal law where the reckless disregard for others is such that society, through the process of the criminal law, imposes sanctions. The instances of criminal negligence are fortunately rare and we thus concentrate on the civil law and the circumstances in which a nurse and the employer involved may be liable in negligence.

It would be useful if the law were to prescribe a definitive statement of principles in relation to all the situations to be confronted at some time in nursing practice. What the law does however, is to establish general principles which are then applied to varying situations thus enabling its adaption and development as new situations come before the courts. What then are the principles of negligence or the elements comprising a course of action in negligence? There are three elements a plaintiff must prove to succeed in an action for negligence, namely:

1. That the defendant owed the plaintiff a duty of care
2. That this duty of care was breached, by failure to conform to the appropriate standard of care
3. That the plaintiff suffered injury as a result of the breach of duty. In this regard there must be a reasonably close causal connection between the

defendant's conduct and the injury or damage to the plaintiff.

A plaintiff must prove these three elements on the 'balance of probabilities'. That is, it must be more probable than not, for example, that the defendant's conduct caused the plaintiff injury. (This burden of proof can be contrasted with the criminal law which requires proof 'beyond reasonable doubt'.)

Duty, breach, and damage are distinct matters for a plaintiff to establish. It is thus possible for someone to be 'negligent' in conduct and yet not liable because no duty of care was owed; and further, for someone to breach a duty owed and yet not be liable because the breach in question did not cause the injury complained of; or that the damage suffered was not a reasonable consequence of the breach.

Duty

The existence of a duty of care is a question of law to be determined according to the principles established by the courts. When, then, will a duty to take care arise? The statement of Lord Atkin (1932 A.C. 562 at p 580) in the famous case of *Donoghue* v *Stevenson* provides some assistance. He stated inter alia:

> There must be, and is, some general conception of relations giving rise to a duty of care, of which the particular cases found in the books are but instances . . . The rule that you are to love your neighbour becomes in law, You must not injure your neighbour, and the lawyer's question, who is my neighbour? receives a restricted reply. You must take reasonable care to avoid acts or omissions which you can reasonably foresee would be likely to injure your neighbour. Who then, in law, is my neighbour? The answer seems to be persons who are so closely and directly affected by my act that I ought reasonably to have them in contemplation as being so affected when I am directing my mind to the acts or omissions which are called in question.

From Lord Atkin's statement it is clear that proximity and foresight are important criteria for determining the circumstances in which a duty of care will be owed. Undeniably, the relationship between nurse and patient is so close that it would be forseeable that harm might be caused to the patient if reasonable care is not taken with nursing practice.

You will recall the Good Samaritan example discussed earlier. Legally the nurse is under no duty to assist in such a situation but once assistance is rendered the close relationship is established, and the duty of care will be owed. Consider an example of a swimmer in distress at an unpatrolled, crowded beach. On whom could the duty of care be specifically placed, of all the people on the beach? If shouts of help are ignored no liability for negligence could exist in the absence of a duty of care. If however, someone proceeded to render assistance, then the duty to take care would apply.

Breach

The plaintiff must prove that the defendant breached this duty of care: that the appropriate standard of care was not applied. The standard of care required is determined by applying the concept of the reasonable person. The standard thus is an objective one and a defendant nurse's conduct will be measured against what the reasonable nurse would have done in the same or similar circumstances. For instance, a nurse acting as a Good Samaritan at a roadside emergency will be judged according to the standard of a reasonable nurse in the same or similar circumstances, not as one acting with the staff and equipment support of an acute hospital.

Knowledge and skill are significant factors to be considered in the application of the standard of reasonable care. The standard of care required will vary according to the special training and experience of the individual involved and this in itself provides a warning. The actual knowledge and skill possessed by the particular defendant is not relevant. The important criterion is the knowledge and skill that the defendant is presumed to have, that is, that of the reasonable nurse in the same or similar circumstances.

If a nurse professes to have special skills that are in fact not possessed, then such a nurse will be judged according to the standard of the reasonable nurse possessing such skills and thus owe a higher duty of care than that for which the nurse is in fact qualified. Student nurses (*Henson & Another* v *Board of Management of the Perth*

Hospital, (1939), 41 WALR 15), and generalist practitioners (*Norton* v *Argonaut Insurance Co.*, 1962, 144 SO 2d 249) must therefore be careful not to carry out procedures beyond their level of qualification and expertise.

Norton's case provides a significant illustration of this point. An Assistant Director of Nursing who had not practised as a clinical nurse for some time was helping out in the children's ward of an American hospital. The ward was busy and the staffing limited. She noticed that a 3-month-old child admitted for observation and treatment of a congenital heart disease had not been given the medication ordered and noted the following change of order on the patient's card: 'Give 3.0 cc Lanoxin today for one dose only'. (The original medication order on admission had specified 'Elixir Pediatric Lanoxin', the dose, and frequency of administration). The change of order did not specify the elixir nor the route of administration. The Assistant Director of Nursing thought the dosage rather excessive for an intramuscular injection and so she consulted the charge nurse and two physicians present in the ward. They advised her to follow the notation. At no stage did she consult the child's physician. She proceeded with the injection and the child died. The injectable form was 5 times as strong as the oral form.

The physician was found to be negligent in relation to the unclear medication order and the Assistant Director of Nursing was also found to be negligent in that she had breached the standard of care required. The court stated:

> A nurse who is unfamiliar with the fact that the drug in question is prepared in oral form for administration to infants by mouth is not properly and adequately trained for duty in a paediatric ward. As laudable as her intentions are conceded to have been on the occasion in question, her unfamiliarity with the drug was a contributing factor in the child's death. In this regard we are of the opinion that she was negligent in attempting to administer a drug with which she was not familiar. While we concede that a nurse does not have the same degree of knowledge regarding drugs as is possessed by members of the medical profession, nevertheless, common sense dictates that no nurse should attempt to administer a drug under the circumstances shown in the case at bar. Not only was Mrs Evans unfamiliar with the medicine in question but she also violated what has been shown to be the rule generally practised by the members of the nursing profession in the community and which rule, we might add, strikes us as being most reasonable and prudent, namely, the practice of calling the prescribing physician when in doubt about an order for medication.

In applying the standard of the reasonable person, the courts try to identify risks that the reasonable person would deem unacceptable and to balance the risks and the likely consequences against the factors and costs involved in averting the risks. As an example the likelihood of injury occurring is considered. If the possibility of harm occurring is small then the reasonable person may be justified in ignoring it. It thus seems that the mere possibility of harm occurring is insufficient: there must be a reasonable probability of harm.

The extent and seriousness of the likely consequences of the conduct in question are also considered. The more serious the consequences, the greater the degree of care required. Thus, 'at risk' patients (for example, those in the recovery phase of the postoperative period) require special attention.

Conformity with common or usual practice and/or with hospital policy is usually sufficient to rebut allegations of negligence. Although not conclusive in itself, failure to adopt the common or accepted practice is often a strong indication of want of care. Similarly, ignorance of hospital policy is no defence. It is thus important that professionals, nurses included, keep abreast of developments in their practice.

In all cases the courts assess the defendant's conduct against that of the standard of reasonableness. Breach of duty is a question of fact and the ultimate outcome in any court action depends on the interpretation of evidence presented, the examination and credibility of witnesses, and, in negligence situations, evaluating the defendant's conduct against the objective standard of what the reasonable man would do in similar circumstances.

Damage

The final element for a plaintiff to prove in an action for negligence is that damage was suffered as a result of the defendant's breach of duty. Damage in this sense is injury or harm including death. The law has gradually developed to recognize as compensable not only physical injury suffered as a result of negligent actions but also pecuniary loss suffered as a result of negligent advice. There must be a reasonably proximate connection between the defendant's conduct and the damage to the plaintiff. This requirement raises two issues for consideration: causation, and remoteness of damage.

Causation. A plaintiff must prove that the type of damage is foreseeable and also that the defendant's conduct caused the damage. *Barnett's case* [1969] 1 QB 428 provides good illustration of the causation elements. Briefly, the facts were as follows. Three men presented at a hospital casualty department on New Year's Day complaining of vomiting after drinking tea. Their appearance was of men who had been drinking alcohol. However, the nurse rang the physician on duty whose advice was to send them home for sleep and then to have them contact their own physicians. Subsequently one of the men died from arsenic poisoning. Without doubt a duty of care was owed and had been breached by the physician but the court held that there was no liability. The physician's failure to examine did not cause the death since this would have happened anyway before completion of diagnostic tests. There was not a sufficiently close connection between the physician's negligence and the patient's death.

In determining causation the courts consider whether the damage would not have been suffered 'but for' the defendant's conduct (*Cork* v *Kirby Maclean* [1953] 2 All ER 402 per Denning L J at 407). Where there are several possible causes of the damage this test can be useful in eliminating factors which did not effect the damage and in identifying breaks in a chain of causation. If sufficient factors are not eliminated then the courts will apply the 'balance of probabilities' test. This is simply that if it is more probable than not that a particular factor caused the damage then such factor is deemed the cause of the damage.

Remoteness of damage. The second issue for consideration is that of remoteness of damage. A defendant will not necessarily be liable for all the consequences of neglect. The courts have thus to delineate compensable and noncompensable consequences on the basis of distinguishing those consequences which the defendant could reasonably have been expected to foresee. The legal principle is that a person will only be liable for damage of a kind that is reasonably foreseeable (*Overseas Tankship, UK, Ltd* v *Morts Docks & Engineering Co* [1961] All ER 404).

Defences to negligence

Consent

The defence of consent has been considered in relation to trespass. It is unlikely to provide a defence to negligence in a nursing or hospital situation as the defendant would need to show that the plaintiff perceived and fully appreciated the existence of the risk of negligence, and voluntarily agreed to accept the risk.

Contributory negligence

In essence this defence involves the plaintiff's failure to meet the standard of care to which he is required to conform for his own protection, thus contributing to his injury. Contributory negligence is not a complete defence to an action in negligence and, as a result, any negligence on the plaintiff's part will result in an apportionment of damages based on the extent of the plaintiff's negligence: his contribution to the injury suffered.

Award of damages

The main objective of an award of damages is, as far as is possible with a monetary award, to restore the plaintiff to the pre-loss position. Legally a plaintiff has a duty to minimize or mitigate the extent of the injury suffered and failure to do so, or aggravation of the extent, can result in a plaintiff being awarded reduced compensation.

A claim for damages in a hospital situation for personal injury or death involves compensation for financial and nonfinancial loss. Medical and rehabilitation expenses and loss of income can be calculated with reasonable precision and are thus claimed as special damages. General damages on the other hand are not capable of such precise calculation, and include such things as pain and suffering, loss of expectation of life, loss of enjoyment of life and amenities, and loss of future earnings. General damages are presumed to arise as consequences of the negligence.

Documentation

In documenting a patient's period of hospitalization many hospitals now use a system of total patient reporting. The system incorporates the traditional nursing notes or records, IV and fluid balance charts, incident reports, pathology reports and all other information relevant to the patient's hospitalization. The advantages of such a system are obvious in relation to holistic care of the patient. Without doubt such reports play a significant role in patient care. As a means of communication they facilitate continuous care by keeping all staff involved with the care of the particular patient accurately informed of condition, observations, medical orders, and monitoring. They form the basis for discharge planning and for research, quality assurance, and patient dependency studies.

In the context of the liability of nurses, reports may provide legal protection or defence. If something goes wrong and a patient takes legal action, such records can provide evidence that the nurses acted according to a reasonable standard of care, and so rebut a claim of negligence or trespass. Thus accurate detailing of all relevant events is essential for valid documentation and to provide adequate explanation to a court of law.

There are many incentives for quality documentation. Legally, patient records are discoverable as evidence in courts of law. This means that hospitals can be compelled to produce their records and that the author of the record can be required to give oral testimony to the court. Further, they are now accessible by patients under the Freedom of Information Act. Accountability becomes a reality. Effective communication in the form of documentation can not only relieve much of the anxiety of facing the risk of accountability, but can also satisfy the concept of professional responsibility of the nurse.

It can be many years before a case is heard and memories do fade; therefore, it is essential that nurses document well since recall will be assisted by the clarity of the record. Documentation provides the evidence that the patient has received the appropriate quality of care; it also provides the means of defence in any potentially litigious situation. In this regard the interests of the patient and the nurse go hand in hand.

Just as nurses are advocates for their patients in relation to the care they provide, lawyers, be they barristers or solicitors, are advocates for their particular client. This means that they must present the best possible case to the court on behalf of their client. Courts are run on an adversary system which gives each party to an action the opportunity to present their case. It provides for the examination and cross examination of witnesses in an attempt to convince the court that, on the facts and according to the legal principles involved, the particular allegation is sustained (or rebutted).

The quality of documentation influences not only recall, but also the ability with which the lawyer can defend a hospital and its staff against an action. Gaps in the records, uncertainties, subjective comments, and equivocal statements can all be utilized to cast the competence and credibility of the staff in unfavourable light. Liability can often arise purely because a hospital cannot show in its documentation that it has not been negligent.

Reports will be read and interpreted by lawyers who are interested in establishing a case against a hospital and its staff and thus they will be used to present the strongest possible case on behalf of the patient, and against the hospital. For example, if litigation arose through problems caused by an intravenous infusion running through in one third of the scheduled time, problems of defence may arise if the separate checklist of observations is not retained. If it does not form part of the record, the gap in explanation may create reasonable doubt that the nurses were in fact checking as required. No proof for defence would exist.

The American case *Darling* v *Charleston Community Memorial Hospital* (1965 211 NE 2d 253) provides a glaring example of deficient documentation, and of deficient care.

In this case a teenage boy was hospitalized with a fractured leg set in a plaster cast. Over a period of days the nursing notes dutifully and accurately describes the symptoms of deterioration in condition in such terms as 'swelling, oedema, pain, warmth in toes, blisters, insensitivity to touch, smell'. The doctor had been notified but no proper action was taken. The records failed to indicate that the nurses had acted in the patient's best interests in that they did not disclose that appropriate steps had been taken to ensure that the patient received the care and attention to which he was entitled.

Thus merely documenting the fact that the doctor has been notified may provide insufficient defence to nursing staff. The records must show proper management of patient care.

The interests of both patients and nurse are thus best served by clear, concise and accurate reporting which is objectively written in unequivocal terms and as far as possible contemporaneous with the facts being recorded.

REFERENCES AND FURTHER READING

Texts

Bullough B (ed) 1980 Law and the expanding nursing role, 2nd edn. Appleton Century Croft, New York

Derham D P, Maher F K H, Waller P L 1986 An introduction to law, 5th edn. Law Book Co, Sydney

Fleming J C 1983 The law of torts,6th edn. Law Book Co, Sydney

Hemelt M D, Mackert M E 1982 Dynamics of law in nursing and health care 2nd edn. Reston, Virginia

Law Reform Commission of Victoria 1987 Symposia 1986: Informed Consent

O'Sullivan J 1983 Law for nurses and allied health professionals in Australia, 3rd edn. Law Book Co, Sydney

Staunton P 1985 Nursing and the law. Saunders, Sydney

Journals

Barnett v Chelsea and Kensington. Hospital Management Committee 1969 1 QB 428

Bennett J A, Korolishin M J 1984 "Nurse, I want to read my chart." Nursing 84 14 : 10 : 20–21

Bolton G 1981 The right to a 'good death'. The Australian Nurses Journal 10 : 10 : 41–43

Cohen M R 1982 Play it safe: don't use these abbreviations. Nursing 82 12 : 10 : 66–67

Cote A A 1981 The patient's representative: whose side is she on? Nursing 81 11 : 1 : 26–30

Cox L 1979 To whom are we accountable? The Australian Nurses Journal 8 : 10 : 35–36, 44

Davidhizar R M, Monhaut N 1985 Guidelines for giving bad news by phone. Nursing 85 15 : 4 : 58–59

Dolan M B 1984 Where do you stand on the coding question? Nursing 84 14 : 3 : 42–48

Doll A 1980 What to do after an incident. Nursing 80 10 : 1 : 15–19

Dunn J M 1985 Warning: giving telephone advice is hazardous to your professional health. Nursing 85 15 : 8 : 40–41

Eggland E T 1980 Charting: how and why to document your care daily – and fully. Nursing 80 10 : 2 : 38–43

Finch J 1983 Breach of duty. Nursing Mirror 156 : 7 : 34

Finch J 1983 Breach of the nurse's legal duty. Nursing Mirror 156 : 8 : 36

Finch J 1983 Negligent but not liable. Nursing Mirror 156 : 9 : 41

Galton M 1980 Emergency resuscitation ethics and legalisms. The Australian Nurses Journal 19 : 3 : 44–45

Helm A 1985 Final arrangements: what you should know about living wills. Nursing 85 15 : 11 : 39–43

Hemelt M D, Mackert M E 1984 Steering clear of legal hazards. Nursing 84 14 : 5 : 12–15

Laken D D 1983 Protecting patients against themselves. Nursing 83 13 : 1 : 26–27

Langslow A 1981–1985 The nurse and the law. The Australian Nurses Journal 19 : 8 through 15 : 6

Meissner J E 1981 Become a patient advocate . . . by asserting your autonomy as a nurse. Nursing 81 11 : 10 : 24–25

Merryman P 1985 The incident report: if in doubt, fill it out. Nursing 85 15 : 5 : 57–59

Misik I 1981 About using restraints – with restraint. Nursing 81 11 : 8 : 50–55

Nurses Reference Library 1984 Keeping clear of charting pitfalls. Nursing 84 14 : 6 : 8–9

On life . . . and death . . . and dots. 1984 Report of the Queens County Grand Jury. Nursing 84 14 : 6 : 52–58

Saunders J M, Valente S M 1986 Code – no code? The question that won't go away. Nursing 86 16 : 3 : 60–64

Smith C E 1986 Upgrade your shift reports with the three R's. Nursing 86 16 : 2 : 62–64

Sparks M R, Robinson J 1984 How the Good Samaritan Act protects you. Nursing 84 14 : 9 : 12–14

Symm N K, Travis J 1985 Discharging the critically injured patient against medical advice. Nursing 85 15 : 4 : 43–45

Vasey E K 1979 Writing your patient's care plan . . . efficiently. Nursing 79 9 : 4 : 67–71

4

Preoperative nursing management

Robyn Anderson

INTRODUCTION

Surgery is controlled trauma. If patients are to undergo such trauma it is obvious that their chances of surviving will be greater and their postoperative problems less if they present to the operating room (OR) in the best possible condition.

The major part of preoperative care is the responsibility of the nurse. The more expertly the nurse performs his/her preoperative care, the smoother will be the patient's preparation for surgery. Part of the patient's preparation for surgery is preparation for the anaesthetic; nowadays the risks associated with anaesthesia can be reduced by thorough preoperative preparation.

Obviously there are minor differences in the preparation of patients for different types of surgery, however, the principles of preoperative care are basically the same. Fundamentally they are to present the patient to theatre in the best possible condition and prevent postoperative complications.

There are two major groups of patients to undergo surgery: elective patients – those who know days or even months in advance that they require an operation; and emergency (or non-elective) patients – those who require emergency surgery.

The type of preparation discussed in this chapter is mainly for the elective patient, and of course as much of this care as possible must be telescoped for the emergency patient.

EARLY PREOPERATIVE CARE

Preparation of the patient is commenced weeks or months before surgery where possible.

Nutrition

Undernourished or poorly nourished persons should have their nutritional status corrected whilst awaiting admission to hospital for surgery. The person should be encouraged to:

- Obtain and maintain ideal body weight
- Identify and supplement nutrients which may be lacking in the diet in order to correct obvious deficiencies
- Lose weight if obese prior to surgery, by adopting a well balanced reduction diet.

Protein malnutrition is often seen in elderly patients, and those with carcinoma. Protein is essential for tissue repair and protein deficiencies take some time to correct, therefore it is obvious that the sooner correction is started the better will be the condition of the patient on the day of surgery.

Eradication of infection

In order to minimize anaesthetic risk, all infections should be treated prior to surgery. Persons with an infection have a raised metabolic rate, and the extra demands placed upon the body systems by anaesthesia and invasive surgery will further compromise physiological adaptive responses (core temperature, pulse and blood pressure), thus increasing the anaesthetic risk. In debilitated persons, chest and urinary tract infections are not uncommon and require attention well in advance of the proposed surgery. Chest physiotherapy is essential preoperatively to assist the patient in removal of retained lung secretions; this will also reduce the likelihood of postoperative chest complications.

Cigarette smoking

Ideally, this should be ceased as long before surgery as possible. Cigarette smoking is responsible for paralysis of the ciliated mucous membrane of the trachea, predisposing to the retention of lung secretions. If the patient is unable to give up smoking, then the number of cigarettes smoked per day should be reduced.

Anaemia

Anaemia should be corrected as soon as possible. This may entail the control of chronic blood loss, blood transfusion, or simply dietary supplementation of the missing or deficient nutrient; the most common being folic acid, vitamin B_{12}, and/or iron.

Dental care

Prior to surgery the person should, if possible, be in optimal dental health. This is particularly important where cardiac surgery is to be undertaken, as damaged teeth or gums can be the portal of entry for bacteria such as *Streptococcus viridans* or *Staphylococcus albus*, which can be the cause of complications postoperatively, the most common being sub-acute bacterial endocarditis.

THE DAYS BEFORE SURGERY

For major surgery the patient is usually admitted to hospital several days prior to operation; however, with modern techniques, greater patient awareness of preoperative requirements, and greater medical and nursing awareness of the patient's need and right to participate in his own treatment, much of this preparation can be done on an outpatient basis.

Psychological factors

Much of the fear associated with surgery is fear of the unknown. If the patient is given an honest, simple explanation of the surgery and its consequences, is told what is expected of him, and is given an explanation of the equipment which will be attached to him in the postoperative phase, he will be far more co-operative and much less frightened.

In some situations, where the patient will be returned postoperatively to an area other than the one he has been in whilst awaiting surgery, it is of great importance to take him to see the postoperative area, and to see a postoperative patient. This is particularly important in cardiac surgery and other specialized surgery for which special postoperative units exist. It can also be of great value to put a frightened preoperative patient in the same room as a successful postoperative patient.

The patient's relatives also require special advice, explanation, and attention as they are often going through the same, and sometimes even greater, stress than the patient.

Patient history

A complete nursing and medical history must be taken from the patient. Relatives can often contribute vital information to the history and should be consulted where possible.

All relevant subsequent information regarding patient progress must be documented.

Diet

In almost all situations the patient should receive a well balanced diet supplemented where necessary with vitamins until the day of surgery, except where this would be specifically contraindicated, for example, in the case of the patient who is to undergo gastrointestinal surgery.

Bowel preparation

If the patient is to undergo gastrointestinal surgery he should present for operation with his bowel as empty and as clean as possible. This will help prevent spillage of bowel content into the peritoneal cavity during surgery.

Bowel preparation may entail a low residue diet for 3 to 5 days preoperatively. This type of diet leaves little or no residue in the patient's bowel.

Chemical cleansing of the bowel may include an antibiotic which will not be absorbed systemically, for example: neomycin, phthalylsulphathiazole, or streptomycin. Any of these will remain in the patient's bowel and help to kill the bowel flora whilst having little or no effect on metabolism. A non-metabolized disaccharide or polysaccharide may be given orally, for example, lactulose or mannitol. Either of these substances will remain in the bowel to irritate the lining and thereby increase peristalsis, and by osmosis increase faecal volume and thus cause faster evacuation of faeces from the bowel. Charcoal adsorbs blood, pus, mucus, toxins, and the remains of dead bacteria, and passes out of the bowel in faeces taking these substances with it.

Suppositories and enemata are prescribed by some surgeons to clean the distal bowel. These are usually given for three or more consecutive days. Bowel washouts are occasionally prescribed. These are used in conjunction with other bowel preparations.

Patients who are to undergo surgery other than bowel surgery usually require only a light aperient, a suppository, or a small disposable enema the night before or early on the day of surgery.

Tests and investigations

The results of all investigations must be filed in the medical history and accompany the patient to the operating room. The following general investigations are performed routinely on almost all patients.

Chest X-ray. Performed to check heart size, and clarity of lung fields, and to establish a baseline for postoperative comparison.

Blood tests. Full blood examination to allow preoperative correction of abnormalities.

Urea and electrolytes to allow preoperative correction where obvious problems exist.

Blood grouping and cross matching. At least two units of cross-matched blood should be held in reserve for any patient undergoing surgery.

Urine tests. Routine urinalysis to detect abnormalities and to establish a baseline for postoperative comparison.

Tape and solution skin tests. These simple skin tests are performed by applying a variety of commonly used tapes and solutions to the patient's inside forearm, removing them 24 hours later, and noting any redness or irritation caused to the skin. If an allergy is detected, this should be recorded in the history and use of the tape or solution should be avoided, hence preventing unnecessary distress and discomfort to the patient.

Physiotherapy

The physiotherapist visits the patient preoperatively to develop rapport with him. The physiotherapist should teach the patient the range of leg and chest exercises and any specific exercises that will be necessary postoperatively. Where a physiotherapist is not available the nurse assumes this responsibility.

Medication

In general, all medication should be continued until the day of surgery and beyond. However, anticoagulant drugs and oral contraceptives should be stopped some days before surgery.

THE DAY PRIOR TO SURGERY

General physical preparation

Shaving

In general, hair should be removed from the proposed surgical area and for a reasonable margin around that area. This is to ensure that bacteria which normally inhabit the area on and around the body hair do not enter the surgical site. It also prevents invagination of hair into the wound, which can cause superficial infection. All surgeons have their own routines but general basic shave areas are:

Head surgery. Head, face and neck shave for males; head only for females.

Chest surgery. Face (males only), neck and body down to umbilicus.

Cardiac surgery. Is usually more extreme, requiring shaving of the whole body anterior and posterior, down to and including the pubic hair. If coronary bypass grafts are to be taken from the leg veins the patient is shaved from neck to ankle.

Abdominal surgery. Body shave from nipple line to pubis, bed line to bed line.

Vaginal surgery. Pubic shave including the labia and perineum.

Limb surgery. The involved limb is shaved as far as is practicable.

Skin preparation

The patient is showered where possible, using an antiseptic soap, and the area is then swabbed with an antiseptic solution. Special attention is paid to skin folds, groin, under breasts, and the umbilicus which must be thoroughly cleaned using cotton buds.

Make-up and nail polish

This must be thoroughly removed so that the true colour of the fingernail beds can be seen by the anaesthetist, enabling him to make a quick and accurate assessment of peripheral blood supply, venous return, and the onset of cyanosis.

Intravenous hydration

Intravenous (IV) fluid therapy may be commenced to ensure adequate hydration until the time of surgery. This is particularly important in elderly, debilitated, and dehydrated patients in order to reduce postoperative hypovolaemic shock.

Urinary catheterization

This is relatively unusual, but an indwelling catheter may be inserted for some types of surgery according to the surgeon's preference. Ideally this should be performed in the OR after induction of anaesthesia.

Observations

Baseline observations of pulse, ventilation, and blood pressure are established prior to surgery. It is important that the patient is resting calmly when these observations are made so that they are an accurate record to which postoperative observations can be intelligently related.

Consent for anaesthesia and surgery

It is a legal requirement that consent for surgery be given by the patient or, in special circumstances, by his legal guardian (see Chapter 3). This should be in the form of a specific consent: the signatory must know and understand the full extent of the surgery to be undertaken, and the consent form should carry a brief description of the procedure for which the patient is giving his consent. An explanation such as: 'Mr X, we are going to do something about that foot' is certainly not adequate when the real explanation should be 'Mr X, we are going to amputate your left leg just below the knee joint'.

The former leaves the surgeon and the nursing staff open to legal proceedings, and the patient totally unprepared for the postoperative phase. *Consent forms must be signed before the premedication is given.*

THE HOURS IMMEDIATELY BEFORE SURGERY

The preoperative check list

Most hospitals have some form of preoperative check list. In the last hours before the patient goes to the OR, the various items are checked off on the list and signed by the appropriate registered nurse. These check lists greatly reduce the possibility of error or omission in preoperative care.

Fasting

It is not necessary for the stomach to be totally dry prior to surgery. The resting stomach contains approximately 160 ml of fluid, and this will be increased if the patient is anxious. For this reason many anaesthetists no longer consider long fasting periods to be intelligent. A reasonable regime is to cease solid foods four to six hours prior to surgery, allowing the patient a small early breakfast if he is scheduled for the OR at 10:00 a.m. or later. Clear fluids in small amounts can be continued up until two hours before surgery. In gastrointestinal surgery a nasogastric tube may be inserted to keep the stomach empty, but this is usually performed in the OR after induction of anaesthesia.

Medication

Important medication, such as digoxin, should be given at the normal times prior to surgery. One small tablet and a mouthful of water will make little or no appreciable difference to the fasting regime. Insulin should always be given as usual to diabetic patients except where there is a specific contradictory order. Diabetic patients are often given intravenous dextrose to supply carbohydrate during the fasting period.

Dress for operation

The patient is dressed in the OR clothes of the hospital, and although these may vary, they should be made of cotton and are designed to preserve the patient's dignity as far as possible, as well as preventing bacteria being taken into the OR. Cotton clothing is important to prevent the accumulation of static electricity in the OR which would occur if synthetic material were used. At the time the patient is dressed for the OR, the bed is made up with clean linen. Patient warmth must be maintained.

Other physical preparation

A special identity card is tied to the patient's wrist and/or ankle. It carries confirmation of the patient's identity and a brief description or title of the operation to be performed to prevent error in the OR.

All jewellery and hairpins are removed to prevent the rare chance of electrical burns from diathermy. If a wedding ring is left on the patient, tape should be wrapped around the ring on the finger to insulate it from the operating table. The shave and skin preparation (including cleanliness of the ears and umbilicus) are checked.

Dentures are removed, but may accompany the patient to the OR if the anaesthetist wishes, as it may make ventilation easier to have the patient's mouth supported by dentures. If they remain in the ward, they are appropriately labelled and stored. Contact lenses and any other prostheses may be removed.

The patient's bladder is emptied and the volume of urine and the time of voiding is recorded on the patient's chart.

Premedication

The final preparation of the patient prior to surgery is the administration of premedicant drugs. The premedication is ordered by the anaesthetist to be given at a specific time, and it usually contains a narcotic, a sedative, and possibly an anticholinergic drug (to supress vagal stimulation); antibiotics may also be given at this time.

The patient should not be disturbed after the premedication is given, however a relative may sit with him, or he may listen to his radio or watch a television set. These distractions will not prevent him from dozing when the medication takes effect, but may help to allay anxiety.

Most patients lie supported on one or two pillows after receiving the premedication, but where the surgery is to be long and involved, or the chest is to be opened, some surgeons prefer the patient to remain sitting and some even have the patient transported to the OR in this position.

Transport to the operating room

This is done with as little disturbance to the patient as possible. He is gently transferred to a trolley and escorted to the OR by a nurse who takes with him/her the patient's medical history, X-rays and, if required, the patient's dentures.

At the door of the OR suite the patient is handed over to an OR nurse.

PATIENTS FOR EMERGENCY SURGERY

These patients can be divided into two groups:

- Nontraumatic
- Traumatic.

The nontraumatic emergency patient

As much as possible of the care described in this chapter is telescoped for this patient. It is vital that the consent form is signed, the skin preparation and shave are performed, and a nasogastric tube is inserted to empty the stomach where necessary. All other immediate physical prep-aration is performed as for an elective patient, prior to the administration of the premedication and the transportation of the patient to the OR.

The traumatic emergency patient

A consent form must be signed or verbal consent obtained, if necessary by telephone from relatives. The patient's condition should be stabilized, bleeding arrested, and as much dirt and blood removed from the patient as possible. The patient is dressed in OR clothing and transported to the operating room as quickly and as efficiently as possible.

REFERENCES AND FURTHER READING

Texts

Bickerton J 1985 Surgical nursing. Heinemann Nursing, London

Brunner L S, Suddarth D S 1984 Textbook of medical-surgical nursing 5th edn. Lippincott Company, Philadelphia

Carey K W (ed) 1984 Caring for surgical patients. Springhouse, Pennsylvania

Duke University Hospital Nursing Services 1983 Guidelines for nursing care: process and outcome. Lippincott Company, Philadelphia

Henderson M A 1980 Essential surgery for nurses. Churchill Livingstone, Edinburgh

Kneedler J A, Dodge G H 1983 Perioperative patient care: the nursing perspective. Blackwell Scientific Publications, Boston

LeMaitre G D, Finnegan J A 1980 The patient in surgery: a guide for nurses. Saunders Company, Philadelphia

Lewis L W 1976 Fundamental skills in patient care, 3rd edn. Lippincott, Philadelphia

Luckman J, Sorensen K C 1980 Medical-surgical nursing: a psychophysiologic approach, 2nd edn. Saunders Company, Philadelphia

Middleton D 1983 Nursing 1. Blackwell Scientific Publications, Oxford

Nash D F E 1980 The principles and practice of surgery for nurses and allied professions, 7th edn. Edward Arnold, London

Saxton D F, Pelikan P K, Nugent P M, Hyland P A 1983 The Addison-Wesley manual of nursing practice. Addison-Wesley, California

Witter Du Gas B 1983 Introduction to patient care: a comprehensive approach to nursing, 4th edn. Saunders Company, Philadelphia

Journals

Aker J G 1985 Communicating effectively: the preoperative interview. A A N A Journal Feb 53 : 1 : 54–9

Anon 1985 Preop education can cut LOS and cost aid PPS delivery. Hospitals Feb 16 : 59 : 4 : 78, 80, 82

Bland B V, Miracle V A 1983 The no-write way to document preop patient teaching. Nursing 83 13 : 12 : 48–49

Burden N 1986 Preoperative assessment of the ambulatory surgery patient. Feb: 1 : 1 : 48–51

Castilo, P 1986 Improving surgical patients' knowledge. Point View Jan 1: 23 : 1 : 4–7

Craig C P 1986 Preparation of the skin for surgery. Todays OR Nurse. May: 8 : 5 : 17–20

Craig C P 1986 Preparation of the skin for surgery. Infection Control. May 7 : 5 : 257–8

Crawford F J 1985 The elderly patient. AORN J Feb: 41 : 2 : 356–9

Dale J 1984 Sterile pursuit. Nursing Mirror 159 : 23 : 14 : 19–26

Dierking L et al 1984 Assessing preoperative information – was it enough? Plastic Surgery Nursing 4 : 4 : 120–5

Fraulini K E, Gorski D W 1983 Don't let perioperative medications put you in a spin. Nursing 83 13 : 10 : 54–57

Fuchs P 1983 Before & after surgery stay right on respiratory care. Nursing 83 13 : 5 : 46–50

Greenwood B S 1982 Check out your patient's presurgery fears. Nursing 82 12 : 7 : 34–35

Gelfant B B 1986a Minimizing the stress of surgery through patient and family orientation and education. Point View Jan 1 : 23 : 1 : 9

Gelfant B B 1986b Preparing acutely ill patients for surgery . . . in the emergency department. Point View 23 : 2 : 12

Justice L A 1986 Skill-sharpening methods in conducting patient interviews. Todays OR Nurse Aug: 8 : 8 : 32–3

Kemp A R et al 1985 Patient anxiety levels. An ambulatory surgery study. American OR Nurses Journal Feb: 41 : 2 : 390–1, 394, 396

Manolio T A 1986 Getting the patient to surgery – and back: choices in pre-op testing Part 2. Emerg Med May 30: 18 : 10 : 77–80

Meckes P F 1984 Preoperative care of the elderly patient. Todays OR Nurse Sep: 6 : 9 : 8–11, 14–5

Mogan J et al 1985 Effects of preoperative teaching on postoperative pain: a replication and expansion . . . brief relaxation training. Int J. Nurs Stud 22 : 3 : 267–80

Quinn J C 1986 Another dimension in postanesthesia nursing . . . preoperative teaching and counselling. J. Post Anesth Nurs Feb: 1 : 1 : 26–30

Rathburn A M et al 1986 Preoperative skin decontamination a study on efficiency and effect. AORN Jul: 44 : 1 : 62–5

Short E A 1983 Peri-operative starvation – an often unrecognized condition. The Australian Nurses Journal 13 : 4 : 47–49 52

Sigmon H D 1983 Trauma: this patient needs your expert help. Nursing 83 13 : 1 : 32–41

Stone M A 1983 Preoperative visiting – part of the OR nurse's role? The Australian Nurses Journal 12 : 7 : 46–48

Sumner S M, Lewandowski V 1983 Guidelines for using artificial breathing devices. Nursing 83 13 : 10 : 54–57

Williams D 1986 Preoperative patient education: in the home or in the hospital? Orthopaedic Nursing Journal Jan–Feb: 5 : 1 : 37–41

Wong J et al 1984 Pre-operative patient education. CONA Journal Sep: 6 : 3 : 7–8. 10–1

5

The nursing implications of anaesthesia

Chris Game

We have now reached the stage where anaesthetic care is considered to include the preoperative preparation and postoperative supervision of the patient. The actual administration of the anaesthetic in [the operating] theatre is only one part of the sequence. While the nurse plays an important part at all stages, the anaesthetist has come to rely on her [/him] to an ever increasing degree in the preparation of the patient and especially in the supervision of the potentially hazardous postoperative phase.

Norris & Campbell, 1975

INTRODUCTION

Until the 1840s surgical anaesthesia, that is, the absence of sensation/insensibility to pain during surgical procedures, was achieved by the overuse of alcohol, with mouth gags and/or body restraints to compensate for the deficiencies of the technique. With the advent of the use of ether and nitrous oxide, surgeons were able at last to operate under conditions wherein patients were not subjected to physiological jeopardy in order to achieve surgical anaesthesia.

As improvements are made in anaesthetic technique and the drugs available for use become more selective and refined in their action, so has the state of anaesthesia become safer for the patients who are its subjects. Today, with highly selective and sophisticated surgical and anaesthetic techniques, it is possible to anaesthetize the chronically ill, elderly or critically ill individual both safely and with minimal side- and after-effects of the anaesthetic intervention. Modern anaesthesiology combines the effects of anaesthesia (loss of sensation) and analgesia (loss of painful impressions without loss of tactile sense), and may also include narcosis (unconsciousness produced by a drug). The major aims of anaesthesiology are to render

a patient insensitive to pain and oblivious to the procedure being performed, and to maintain him in a painfree and safe environment for as long as is possible both during and following the surgical event.

TYPES OF ANAESTHESIA

The major classification of anaesthesia is twofold: general and regional. A large number of factors and conditions determine the type of anaesthetic used for any individual surgical event, for example, the condition of the patient; the patient's size, age, and personality; the type, site, and duration of the operation; anaesthetist preference and where possible patient preference; and the degree of surgical difficulty.

General anaesthesia, that is, the loss of sensation with an accompanying loss of consciousness, is achieved with the use of drugs administered either intravenously or by inhalation. Regional anaesthesia, that is, the loss of sensation in which nerve conduction is blocked and painful impulses fail to reach the brain, is achieved by the application of drugs to nerves or nerve roots by a variety of methods.

General anaesthesia

The aim of any anaesthetic and the purpose of anaesthesia in general is to provide not only a safe environment for the patient but also one of comfort. A pain-free environment provides such a situation and an important aim is that good or optimal operating conditions ensue for the surgeon. If in addition the patient is rendered unconscious, then it can be deduced that a 'general' anaesthetic has been administered. The anaesthetic agent acts upon the central nervous system (CNS) in order to produce functional loss/disruption, that is, consciousness is lost, unconscious cerebral activity ceases, reflex responses are blocked and a degree of muscle relaxation is achieved. Until the early 1950s it was only possible to achieve all these functions by the use of a heavy anaesthetic as only single agents were available, for example, ether, nitrous oxide, and chloroform. Nowadays with the development of adjuvent gases and drugs (for example, halothane, enflurane, thiopentone sodium, and short- and long-acting intravenous muscle relaxants) it is possible to achieve excellent operating conditions whilst administering a 'light' anaesthetic made up of a mixture of anaesthetic agents providing a balanced anaesthesia, without exposing the patient to the physiological risks of deep anaesthesia.

It should be noted however, that general anaesthesia is not risk-free, and in some cases it may have distinct disadvantages. Primarily, general anaesthesia has the capacity to so depress the CNS that circulatory and/or respiratory depression may ensue. Also, gases and volatile liquids are used to administer inhalational anaesthesia, and certain of these are flammable and explosive when in contact with either air or oxygen. Therefore the risks to the patient are potentially large and it is necessary to ensure that informed consent to the operation has indeed been gained by the surgeon and anaesthetist before further preparing the patient for the surgical procedure.

Modern anaesthesia usually commences with the administration of a premedicant drug prior to the patient leaving the ward for the operating room (OR). The purpose of premedication is to assist in alleviating preoperative apprehension or anxiety, to promote relaxation and co-operation, to initiate sleep, and to inhibit secretions from the respiratory tract. Hence the types of drugs that are usually administered as a premedication are a mixture of a narcotic analgesic (for example, morphine, pethidine, or papaveretum) with or without an accompanying sedative (for example, diazepam or promethazine) and/or an anticholinergic (for example, atropine or hyoscine). Prior to the administration of the premedication the patient

should be informed as to the changes to be expected in mood and physical feeling caused by the particular drug administered, as normal defence mechanisms are altered by the action of the narcotics. Suffice to say that the administration of the premedicant drug(s), with subsequent 'euphoric' and anxiety-relieving effects, is not a substitute for the nursing responsibility of providing an adequate and detailed explanation to the patient of the preoperative events. It should also be noted that 'informed' consent does not comply with legal requirements if the patient has been premedicated prior to the obtaining of consent (see Chapter 3).

The four stages of anaesthesia

Stage I – Analgesia. Extends from the beginning of the anaesthetic administration until consciousness is lost. The patient may appear inebriated and drowsy and complain of dizziness; before consciousness is lost the patient can usually indicate the degree of pain loss (depth of analgesia). The sense of touch is retained and hearing is heightened, therefore it is essential that the nurse maintain a quiet induction environment and be prepared to assist the patient, but without any sudden movements.

Stage II – Delerium. Extends from the loss of consciousness until the onset of surgical anaesthesia. The patient is unconscious but may appear agitated or excited, may exhibit automatic movements of the arms and legs, and if excessively stimulated by external noise or touch may even become verbal or aggressive. The nurse should maintain a quiet environment, be alert to prevent injury to the patient, and be well prepared and available to assist the anaesthetist as required.

Stage III – Surgical anaesthesia. This is the maintenance phase of anaesthesia. It commences with the onset of relaxation; this is characterized by regular ventilations, jaw relaxation, pupil constriction, and the loss of eyelid reflexes. Auditory sensation ceases at this stage and the depth of relaxation is controlled by the anaesthetist. Depending upon the type of anaesthetic administered, this stage can extend until vital functions are depressed and normal reflexes cease. The OR nurse should ensure that no part of the surgical procedure commences until the anaesthetist is satisfied that the patient has reached Stage III and is under good anaesthetic control. The nurse may also be responsible for assisting in both observing and monitoring the patient's vital functions; he/she should also be prepared to assist in the event of the patient's condition becoming too depressed.

Stage IV – Medullary paralysis. This stage is reached when ventilation ceases due to depression of the respiratory centre at the end of Stage III, resulting in respiratory and cardiac arrest. Nowadays this complication, due to such CNS depression, would constitute an anaesthetic accident. The nursing responsibilities involved during cardiac arrest would apply.

The induction phase of general anaesthesia is usually accomplished by the administration of an intravenous agent, and the most commonly used drug is thiopentone. Other induction agents are methohexitone, and ketamine. Intravenous induction is pleasant and rapid for the patient and provides a hang-over recovery effect with minimal postoperative nausea and vomiting. The rapid absorption that intravenous induction allows can produce laryngospasm and bronchospasm and in high doses, for example the induction of morbidly obese patients, can lead to hypotension, respiratory arrest and ultimately cardiac arrest. Induction is therefore never attempted without all anaesthetic equipment being present in correct working order.

Following induction and airway maintenance with or without intubation, Stage III anaesthesia is maintained by the inhalational route utilizing gases. The most common gas in use is nitrous oxide (the original anaesthetic), and it is mixed with oxygen in the usual concentrations of nitrous oxide 60–70% with oxygen 40–30%. Under normal circumstances a vaporized liquid is added to these gases in order to provide a stable and safe anaesthetic. The most common vaporized liquid in clinical practice is halothane, a sweet smelling, non-irritant vapor that also has the property of reducing arterial pressure with minimal peripheral vasodilation. For this reason it is commonly used to induce controlled hypotension during the surgical procedure and therefore provide a relatively blood-free operative site. As a degree of hypothermia also occurs with the use of halothane, postoperative shivering can occur and the nurse needs to be prepared for this situation in the immediate and subsequent recovery periods. Another commonly used volatile liquid is enflurane, its actions and properties being similar to those of halothane.

To provide optimal operating conditions it is often necessary to utilize muscle relaxants in order to produce muscle paralysis and decrease interference within the operative field. It is to be noted however that all striated muscle is affected when these drugs are used and it is therefore necessary to artificially ventilate a patient who has received muscle relaxants. These drugs fall into two groups: the depolarizing and the non-depolarizing muscle relaxants.

Depolarizing muscle relaxants are most commonly used during either the induction phase of anaesthesia or for very short-term operative procedures, for example, endoscopic, instrumental, or digital examinations. This is because they are extremely quick-acting but the paralysis effect lasts for only 2 to 3 minutes. The commonest drug from this group in clinical practice is suxamethonium, and it is important to note that there is no known antidote or reversal drug for its effects.

Non-depolarizing muscle relaxants have as their chief constituent the naturally occurring drug, curare. It is available as tubocurarine and synthetic forms in common use are pancuronium, alcuronium and gallamine. They are most commonly used during the Stage III maintenance phase of anaesthesia, taking up to 7 or 8 minutes to have an effect but lasting for up to 45 minutes depending upon the dose given and the condition of the patient. The effect of this group can be terminated or reversed when required by the injection of an anticholinesterase agent, usually in the form of neostigmine.

At the end of the operation and following reversal of the effects of the muscle relaxant, the inhalational agent is ceased and the patient is then ventilated with 100% oxygen. As recovery is fairly rapid the patient should regain control of his own ventilation and gag reflex within a few minutes.

Extubation can then be effected by the anaesthetist when he/she is satisfied with the patient's capacity to maintain his own ventilatory effort, and airway. The patient can then be transported to the recovery room.

Regional anaesthesia

Many students may more readily recognize the term 'local' anaesthesia, however 'regional' is more anatomically correct. The aims of regional anaesthesia are the same as for general anaesthesia with the exception of the fact that the patient is not rendered unconscious and therefore a state of local analgesia is produced, that is, the loss of painful impressions without the loss of tactile sense. This, however, does not mean to imply that this anaesthetic form is risk-free. It is certainly more beneficial under certain circumstances and may in fact be the anaesthesia of choice in certain patients who fall into risk groups for general anaesthesia. Regional anaesthetic agents, like any drug, may adversely react with the patient's body systems and therefore their use carries a degree of risk.

Regional anaesthesia can be applied in a variety of ways using locally-acting anaesthetic agents synthetically derived from the alkaloid cocaine, the most commonly used in clinical practice being lignocaine, procaine, bupivacaine and cinchocaine. Unfortunately, these locally acting agents tend to produce fairly toxic reactions with body systems should they be rapidly absorbed or injected erroneously into the blood stream, for example: pallor, restlessness, anxiety, tremor, convulsions, hypotension, bradycardia, sweating, and respiratory depression.

The aim is to achieve anaesthesia to a limited region of the body without producing systemic side-effects. Thus, any drug which may enhance the anaesthestic locally whilst at the same time reducing the likelihood of high doses of the agent entering the bloodstream and therefore diminishing its side-effects, is extremely welcome. For this reason adrenaline is frequently administered with the anaesthetic agent. Adrenaline produces a reflex vasoconstriction which in turn reduces the blood flow to the anaesthetized area, and therefore delays the absorption of the anaesthetic agent into the bloodstream. It also reduces the degree of bleeding from the operative site. However it needs to be remembered that adrenaline is itself toxic to the human body with symptoms and signs similar to cocaine overdosage, for example, pallor, sweating, hypotension, syncope, and tachycardia; and the side-effects observed in patients undergoing regional anaesthesia may in fact be a reaction to the adrenaline rather than to the anaesthetic agent itself. Due to the vasoconstrictive nature of regional anaesthetic agents that have adrenaline added, they should be used with extreme caution (if at all), in peripheral areas of the body, for example, digits and surface prominences.

Regional anaesthesia can be administered in a variety of ways and the method of choice is dependent upon factors which include the operative site, the patient's condition, the nature of the injury/condition, the presence of local infection; and surgeon, anaesthetist, or patient preference. Techniques include:

Surface/topical. A short-acting form of anaesthesia that is capable of blocking peripheral nerve endings underlying mucous membranes. Strong solutions of the agent are either rubbed into or sprayed or dropped onto the surface, and they enable such procedures as rectal and vaginal examinations, cystoscopy, bronchoscopy, gastroscopy, and male catheterization to be undertaken painlessly. Cocaine applied topically to the conjunctiva or to the mucosa of the nose is frequently used in surgery to the eye or nose.

Infiltration – local block. The anaesthetic agent is injected into the skin and subcutaneous tissue of the operative site. Analgesia takes place only in the area to be incised.

Infiltration – field block. The area surrounding the incision is injected, thus providing a larger area of analgesia. Infiltration can be used for minor surgical procedures such as removal of moles and cysts. As injection takes place in a highly vascular area, the physician must take care not to inject the agent directly into the bloodstream as this could produce an adverse systemic reaction.

Regional nerve block. The agent is injected to selectively block a particular nerve, for example, a digital nerve (anaesthetizing a finger); or used to block an entire plexus of nerves, for example, the brachial plexus (rendering the entire arm anaesthetized). An advantage of nerve blocks is that a relatively small amount of anaesthetic agent can be used to provide a more extensive and longer lasting degree of anaesthesia than either the topical or infiltration methods, and this form of anaesthesia is commonly used for the reduction of distal fractures. However extreme caution must be taken if an agent with added adrenaline is used for a regional nerve block. Although adrenaline constricts the local vessels and slows the absorption rate of the agent used, the action of vasoconstriction in digital nerve blocks could lead to the development of ischaemic necrosis.

A regional nerve block may also involve the application of a tourniquet to occlude arterial blood supply. As this technique also includes limb elevation and venous drainage, the application of the tourniquet helps to achieve a blood-free operative site. However this interruption to blood supply can lengthen even further the anaesthetic effect achieved with the regional block, and the nurse must include this factor in his/her management of the patient's limbs during recovery from this form of regional anaesthesia.

Spinal. This form of regional anaesthesia enables the physician to block the impulses of nerves either from the spinal cord itself or the nerve roots that lie adjacent to the cord. The two most common routes of administration are epidural and intrathecal. In the epidural route, the anaesthetic agent is injected into the bony spinal canal and the solution is 'laid upon' the spinal cord and anaesthetizes the dura mater and the nerves which leave the cord. The lumbar and caudal regions are most often anaesthetized in this way; the lumbar for many general operative procedures including prostatic surgery, pelvic surgery and caesarian sections; and the caudal for the obstetric management of labour.

In intrathecal spinal anaesthesia, the anaesthetic agent is injected into the subarachnoid space and is mixed in with the cerebrospinal fluid. This method is also used for general operative procedures of the lower abdomen, pelvis, and lower limbs. Both intrathecal and epidural spinal anaesthetics are especially valuable as alternative anaesthetic methods in patients who are considered at great risk should they undergo general anaesthesia, for example, patients with moderate or severe cardiac or respiratory disease, the elderly, and chronically or critically ill patients.

Although intrathecal anaesthesia is more readily used due to its ease of administration it does have the side-effects of severe postoperative headache and the capacity to cause meningitis if an aseptic technique is not employed in its administration. Epidural anaesthesia is more difficult to administer but it does not produce severe headache postoperatively and does not lead to the development of meningitis. With correct nursing management postoperatively (for example, keep the patient lying flat on one or two pillows for at least 12 hours and do not ambulate the patient for 24 hours), headaches can be prevented and the patient experience an uneventful recovery from spinal anaesthesia.

Neuroleptanalgesia

This is an 'anaesthetic technique in which the major agents are a neuroleptic and an analgesic drug, allowing the patient to retain the ability to co-operate' (Roper, 1978). Neuroleptics are pharmacological agents which produce a general state of peacefulness and indifference to one's environment. They do not induce sleep and when used in conjunction with nitrous oxide the resultant level of analgesia permits the performance of surgical procedures such as endoscopic, radiological, and digital examinations; and burns dressings which are enhanced by patient co-operation. The neuroleptics most frequently used are phenoperidine and fentanyl, both of which are related to the narcotic analgesic pethidine, but have a shorter action time and a greater action potential than does pethidine. A decided advantage in the use of neuroleptics is their property of producing retrograde amnesia, so that on recovery from the surgical phase the patient has very little or no memory of the actual event, even though he was conscious for the entire procedure. However, in some instances a patient may experience the distressing phenomenon of 'flashback': a momentary rememberance of the surgical episode which is distorted in its detail.

Neuroleptic drugs are more potent analgesics than either pethidine or morphine, and are associated with potential high risks that necessitate their use only under the strictest of medical supervision. Respiratory depression is a feature characteristic of neuroleptics and in addition to having all correctly working anaesthetic equipment immediately at hand, the appropriate reversal agent should also be readily available. The narcotic antagonists nalorphine or naloxone are specific reversal agents for pethidine, morphine, methadone, and other drugs with morphine-like actions.

NURSING IMPLICATIONS

To voluntarily submit oneself to surgery and to the necessity of an anaesthetic creates different feelings and fears in each patient. Even in patients who are admitted for emergency surgical intervention, the prospects of anaesthesia and surgery create feelings and anxieties that must be recognized and understood by the attending nurse. As an extension of the patient, the family or significant others must also be considered when preparing the patient for the surgical intervention. Cultural differences in Australian society will also vastly affect the way the nurse prepares his/her patient and their families for the surgical event.

Most patients harbour some fears of anaesthesia itself, especially general anaesthesia. Some people are fearful that they will not wake up after the surgery, or that they may even die whilst anaesthetized. Others are afraid that they may wake up during the operation itself and that no-one will know, because they will be unable to communicate this fact. Many people may be embarrassed by previous occasions when they behaved uncharacteristically when affected by the premedicant drugs or when recovering from the anaesthesia. A common anxiety among some patients is that prostheses which support a positive body image (such as dentures) will not be replaced before they once again are in control. The science of anaesthesia is still at a stage where many potential surgical patients have either experienced early attempts at inhalational anaesthesia with ether or chloroform, or have memories of parents or other relatives who underwent this form of anaesthetic. Thus an understandable fear of many individuals is the likelihood of induction claustrophobia or postoperative nausea and vomiting.

Culturally, surgery is viewed very differently by many ethnic groups and the nurse needs to be aware of the differing perspectives in order to meet the needs of the individuals in his/her care. Some groups see surgery as a last resort, whereas others do not believe that they have been completely 'cured' unless they have undergone some form of surgery – no matter how minor the surgery may have been. Most groups in society hold views somewhere between each of these extremes and it is therefore necessary that the nurse assesses each of his/her patients and their individual beliefs and needs before planning any nursing management.

Each and every patient in the nurse's care will benefit from the informed support that he/she can provide. It is therefore essential that nurses acquaint themselves with their patient's condition and take responsibility for only those patients for whom they have prepared themselves to care. Preparation of the patient for anaesthesia is not just informing him of what the premedication will do to him and what is likely to occur in the OR. The nurse needs to be conversant with the patient's condition, the proposed treatment schedule, the drugs which have been ordered for him and any aspects in his nursing or medical history which may have a bearing upon the safe administration of the anaesthesia, in order to determine whether the patient is giving informed consent to the procedure for which he is being prepared.

Anaesthesia necessitates the patient relinquishing control to those who care for him in the preoperative, operative and postoperative stages. All forms of anaesthesia place the patient at risk to some degree and the following factors need to be carefully considered by the nurse when assessing and caring for his/her patient throughout the surgical situation.

Loss of protective responses to pain

Regardless of whether general or regional anaesthesia or neuroleptanalgesia has been employed, the patient's awareness of pain or changes in the external environment is greatly diminished or totally absent, and the nurse becomes especially responsible to protect the patient from any injury or harm, such as the hyperextension of a joint, leading to disarticulation. It is the responsibility of the attending nurse to anticipate any such occurrence and be adequately prepared to prevent and/or treat any emergency situation that may arise. An anaesthetized patient should never be left unattended as injury or death could negligently result from an unobserved situation such as the aspiration of vomitus.

Loss of normal reflexes

Diminished or absent responses occur after any form of anaesthesia is administered and the patient should be closely observed to prevent trauma to himself, for example, burns due to sensory loss following spinal anaesthesia, joint or limb damage following a nerve block to an extremity. Patients admitted for minor surgery or examination under anaesthesia as 'day patients' should be accompanied home by a relative/friend or encouraged to take a taxi. To allow the patient to transport himself home is to ignore the residual effects of the anaesthetic agent that may interfere with his normal ability to respond to his environment. For this reason also, the patient should be advised against the drinking of alcohol for a 24 hour period.

Cardiovascular and respiratory disturbances

The general effect of anaesthesia is one of depression to the body systems in general and the patient, regardless of preoperative condition, is at risk of physiological dysfunction during and after surgery. Situations which the nurse must observe for and prepare against include: cardiac dysrhythmias, myocardial infarction, cardiac arrest, heart failure, venous pooling, venous thrombosis, haemorrhage, shock, peripheral shutdown, respiratory depression, respiratory acidosis, and airway obstruction.

Drug interactions

A wide range of drugs may be administered to a patient during surgery and the patient may also have been on some form of drug therapy preoperatively. Adverse drug reactions are always a possibility and patient idiosyncracy may increase the likelihood of drug interactions. Any previous history of allergy should be noted in the patient's nursing and medical history, and the nurse should ensure that the anaesthetist is aware of such allergies. An uncommon condition that may arise during general anaesthesia is called malignant hyperpyrexia. This is usually attributed to the interaction of halothane and suxamethonium and the mortality rate is extremely high if the condition is not recognized and treated rapidly by the anaesthetist.

REFERENCES AND FURTHER READING

Texts

Ballinger W F, Treybal J C, Vose A B 1972 Alexander's care of the patient in surgery, 5th edn. Mosby, St Louis
Birch A A, Tolmie J D 1976 Anesthesia for the uninterested. University Park Press, Baltimore
Craig S (ed) 1985 MIMS annual 1985, 9th edn. Intercontinental Medical Statistics, Sydney
Havard M 1986 A nursing guide to drugs, 2nd edn. Churchill Livingstone, Melbourne
Laurence D R, Bennett P N 1980 Clinical Pharmacology, 5th edn. Churchill Livingstone, Edinburgh
Luckmann J, Sorensen K C 1980 Medical-surgical nursing: a psychophysiologic approach, 2nd edn. Saunders, Philadelphia
McFarland J (ed) 1980 Basic clinical surgery for nurses and medical students, 2nd edn. Butterworths, London
Norris W, Campbell D 1975 A nurse's guide to anaesthetics, resuscitation and intensive care, 6th edn. Churchill Livingstone, Edinburgh
Roper N (ed) 1978 Nurses dictionary, 15th edn. Churchill Livingstone, Edinburgh
Society of Hospital Pharmacists of Australia 1985 Pharmacology and drug information for nurses, 2nd edn. Saunders, Sydney

Journals

Chitwood L B 1987 Unveiling the mysteries of anaesthesia. Nursing 87 17 : 2 : 53–55

Fraulini K E, Gorski D W 1983 Don't let perioperative medications put you in a spin. Nursing 83 13 : 12 : 26–30

Fraulini K E, Murphy P 1984 R.E.A.C.T. a new system for measuring postanaesthesia recovery. Nursing 84 14 : 4 : 12–13

Fuchs P L 1983a Before & after surgery stay right on respiratory care. Nursing 83 13 : 5 : 46–50

Fuchs P L 1983b Providing endotracheal tube care. Nursing 83 13 : 9 : 6–7

Hogan P, Bell S 1986 How to handle postanesthetic hypertension. Nursing 86 16 : 5 : 58–63

McConnell E A 1983 After surgery: how you can avoid the obvious . . . and the not so obvious . . . hazards. Nursing 83 13 : 3 : 8–15

Norheim C 1986 Spinal anaesthesia – as bad as it sounds? Nursing 86 16 : 4 : 42–44

Seaman D J 1983 Shortcuts to a more complete postanaesthesia room transfer summary. Nursing 83 13 : 9 : 47–49

Stevens M 1977 Anaesthetic Agents. The Australian Nurses' Journal 6 : 11 : 26–27

Sumner S M, Lewandowski V 1983 Guidelines for using artificial breathing devices. Nursing 83 13 : 10 : 54–57

6

Postoperative nursing management

Robyn Anderson

INTRODUCTION

Postoperative care of the patient begins the moment the operation is completed.

The patient is gently transferred from the operating room (OR) into the recovery room. This area is staffed by nurses who are responsible to the OR supervisor. It is important that the recovery room be in close proximity to the OR as it is likely that any complication directly related to the anaesthetic will occur within a thirty minute period.

The responsibility of the recovery room staff is to care for the patient and monitor his progress until he is in a stable condition and ready to be returned to the ward.

The recovery room is a small intensive care unit. It should contain emergency equipment, and a complete range of oxygen and aspiration equipment should be available and in close proximity to the patient. The lighting should be indirect where possible and the walls and ceiling acoustically tiled to reduce noise levels.

Staff in the recovery room should perform their nursing care with a minimum of noise as postoperative patients are extremely sensitive to sound. They should be spoken to in a soft voice – shouting at postoperative patients will not cause them to wake up faster!

CARE OF THE PATIENT IN THE RECOVERY ROOM

General condition

At the time the recovery room nurse receives the patient from the OR, he/she must be given a brief history of the patient's condition and a complete description of the surgery the patient has just undergone. He/she must ensure that the history contains postoperative orders. These are usually relatively standard and include:

- An order for the half-hourly monitoring and recording of temperature, pulse, ventilation, blood pressure, and conscious state
- Orders for intravenous fluid and/or blood replacement for the next 24 hours and the period during which the patient must continue to fast
- An analgesic prescription.

Airway

On admission to the recovery room the patient may still be unconscious, therefore it is necessary to keep the patient's jaw forward and to keep the airway open. If vomiting occurs (which, due to improved anaesthesia, is nowadays unlikely) the patient's head is turned to the side and vomitus aspirated. A Guedall's airway may be used to help keep the airway open and to allow free access for oropharyngeal aspiration. Oxygen may be given to the patient if the nurse considers it necessary.

Patient position

Generally the patient is placed in a recumbent position whilst in the recovery room, supported on one or possibly two pillows. If the patient is to be nursed in a more upright position, it is important to sit him up gradually so that his blood pressure does not fall, leading to dizziness or even loss of consciousness.

Observations

A set of baseline observations including vital signs are established as soon as possible after the patient arrives in the recovery room. The purpose of these observations is to enable the nurse to assess deterioration or improvement in the patient's condition and to warn of impending shock. The observations taken in the recovery room are:

Blood pressure

Ideally this should compare favourably with the patient's preoperative blood pressure. However, after major surgery one would expect it to be low, although not below 100 mmHg systolic and 70 mmHg diastolic. Blood pressure below these values is indicative of shock with a consequent reduction in tissue perfusion and possible renal failure; it necessitates immediate treatment with fluid and/or blood and specific drugs. (See Chapter 11.)

Pulse

The pulse is observed for rate, rhythm and volume. It should compare favourably with preoperative levels, however there will usually be a mild tachycardia and a reduction in pulse volume following major surgery. The pulse rhythm should remain regular.

Any significant tachycardia or bradycardia should be reported immediately and treatment instituted to correct this arrhythmia. Tachycardia is very frequently one of the first signs of reactionary haemorrhage.

Ventilation

Ventilation should be observed for rate, rhythm and depth. The patient's ventilations should be between 16 and 20 per minute, of normal depth and without effort. There should be no movement of the chin, glottis or neck; the alae nasac should not be moving and there should be no rib retraction. Ventilation should be silent, however snoring may be normal if the patient is soundly sleeping.

Any disturbance in ventilation should be reported immediately, as ventilatory difficulty may lead to respiratory failure or respiratory arrest if left unattended.

It should be remembered that the patient has usually been paralysed with one of the curare type drugs during the anaesthetic and his paralysis may not be completely reversed. Incomplete reversion can cause respiratory paralysis, respiratory failure and death; therefore close, accurate observation is essential. If the patient is unable to cough and/or is producing excessive secretions he may require aspiration. The patient may also require an additional dose of neostigmine to adequately reverse the respiratory paralysis.

Temperature

The patient's temperature should be taken in the recovery room and if normal 4–6 hourly for the next 24 hours. Temperature should be normal but low temperatures are not uncommon due mainly to mild hypothermia from prolonged exposure in the OR and the use of halothane (see Chapter 5). Hypothermia occurs despite the fact that most operating rooms are kept at 22°C (72°F) and the OR lights give off quite a lot of heat. Low temperatures may also be the result of shock and should be monitored frequently until corrected.

Mental state and general appearance

The patient's state of consciousness should be observed and should be seen to be improving. Deterioration in the state of the patient's consciousness is usually indicative of hypoxia or electrolyte or chemical imbalance, and the cause should be sought and corrected as quickly as possible. The patient will almost certainly be pale, but excessive pallor, especially when accompanied by sweating, is indicative of haemorrhage and impending shock. Conversely, the patient may be flushed and hot to touch, which may indicate carbon dioxide retention. Both these complications can be diagnosed by the measurement of arterial blood gases. Hypoxia or hypercapnia are both indicative of respiratory failure.

Wound dressing

At this stage the operative dressing should be clean and dry with no obvious exudate or bleeding from the wound. The dressing should be reinforced if blood has extravasated, as a wet dressing provides bacteria with a direct portal of entry into the wound.

Equipment

Monitoring and life support machinery must be available at all times. It is the responsibility of the nurse to ensure that he/she is able to operate the equipment necessary for the management of his/her patient.

Drainage systems

Drain tubes which have been inserted into the patient may be connected to one of a variety of drainage apparatus, some of which may be low pressure aspiration devices. The nurse must understand how the particular device functions, and ensure that any drain tubes remain patent at all times.

Analgesia

The prescribed analgesic should be administered if the patient is in pain; however, many anaesthetists give an analgesic just prior to the patient leaving the OR so that his return to the ward may be relatively pain free.

Records

A precise and correct record of all observations, all drugs administered and all treatment carried out must be made on the appropriate forms, prior to the patient leaving the recovery room.

TRANSFER OF THE PATIENT TO THE WARD OR UNIT

In most hospitals the patient is not transferred until he is completely awake and alert, has regained his cough reflex, and his condition has stabilized. During transfer to the ward he is accompanied either by a nurse from the recovery room whose special responsibility it is to transfer patients, or by a nurse from the ward who goes to the recovery room to collect the patient. In either case the recovery room staff and ward staff must meet, and the care of the patient must be handed over from one staff member to the other. The recovery room nurse explains in detail the patient's condition, the surgery he has just undergone, the care he has received in the recovery room, observations that have been taken and any abnormality in these observations. He/she should also check the patient's history with the ward nurse to ensure that sufficient intravenous and analgesic orders exist for at least the next 24 hours. If the ward nurse is dissatisfied with any part of this handover he/she should question the recovery room nurse at this time, as the ward nurse then becomes morally and legally responsible for the patient's safety and well-being.

POSTOPERATIVE NURSING MANAGEMENT

On return to the ward or unit the following patient care should be instituted:

Position, comfort and warmth of the patient

The patient is lifted gently into bed, the lifting aids are removed. The patient is made comfortable, supported on one or two pillows, and covered with blankets to make him feel warm and secure. Often the patient will be very cold and perhaps shivering as he has been disturbed from the relative peace of the recovery room, wheeled through corridors on a trolley, and placed in a bed with fresh, and therefore cold, linen. Ideally, the large cotton operating room blanket which has accompanied the patient from the recovery room and which is already warm should be kept next to his skin under the upper bedclothes. All efforts must be made to stop the patient shivering as this is unnecessarily exhausting; however, care must be taken not to dilate his peripheral blood vessels too quickly as this may cause hypotension. Shivering may follow the administration of halothane during the anaesthetic, and is not the patient's response to cold.

Obese patients should be observed carefully during this stage as the curare type muscle relaxants used during the anaesthesia are stored in fat cells. Rough or too extensive handling of the patient can 'massage' this relaxant back into the bloodstream, and a patient who was apparently completely reverted can quite suddenly be in obvious respiratory distress due to the fact that his ventilatory muscles have been partially reparalysed.

During the first two hours that the patient is back in the ward he should be raised slowly to an upright position with one pillow being added at approximately 30 minute intervals to ensure against a hypotensive episode. It is important that the patient be nursed upright as much as possible until he is ambulant in order to reduce the risk of postoperative chest complications.

Physiotherapy

Almost immediately on return from the OR it is important to have the patient take deep breaths and cough to prevent the collection of secretions in the lungs leading to atelectasis and chest infection. A good analgesic cover and support of the wound, is essential if the patient is to do this effectively.

Leg exercises should also be commenced to prevent thrombosis of the deep veins of the calf. The patient should never cross his legs in bed as this causes mechanical pressure on the calf muscles and predisposes to venous thrombosis. The patient should be taught to dorsi and plantar flex his feet, bend his knees and contract his hamstring and quadricep muscles. These exercises may be supervised once or twice each day by a physiotherapist, and should be supervised hourly by the nurse until the patient becomes ambulant or can move freely in bed.

Any specific postoperative exercises may also be carried out during these physiotherapy sessions. If the patient is unable to perform the leg exercises the nurse should take responsibility for exercising the patient's limbs.

Analgesia

After major surgery all patients will have pain; certainly some are more stoic than others, but that is not a reason for poor analgesic usage. Narcotic analgesia should be given regularly every 3–4 for the first 24 to 72 hours (depending on the extent of the surgery). This can usually then be withdrawn and a minor analgesic used. It is unreasonable to wait for a patient to be in pain before administering the next dose of analgesic; rather, it should be administered knowing that it will be required in the next half hour or so. The patient will be unable to co-operate fully if he is in pain; this is especially true of his physiotherapy, as deep breathing, coughing, and leg exercises are almost impossible if he is in pain. Patients who are sleeping should not be presumed to be pain free and should still have analgesia administered regularly for the first 24 to 72 hours.

Once routine narcotic analgesia has ceased and the patient has commenced minor analgesics, it is often an excellent regime to use a narcotic analgesic to settle the patient at night. This regime should continue according to the patient's progress and the discretion of the nursing staff.

Hygiene

On return to the ward the patient's hands and face should be washed, and his mouth cleaned. If he is alert and would feel more comfortable, his dentures may be replaced. When the analgesic has taken effect the patient's pressure areas should be examined and treated; this is particularly important if the surgery has been lengthy.

Observations

Vital signs

All recovery room observations should be continued. The monitoring and recording of vital signs should continue for 4 hours from the time the patient leaves the OR, as it takes approximately 4 hours for the body to excrete the anaesthetic agents. At the completion of this period the charge nurse will then decide whether to continue the taking of vital signs. When these observations cease, the chart is filed in the patient's history.

Urinary output

In addition, the patient's ability to produce urine should be observed. If the patient has a urinary catheter in situ, hourly measurements of urine may be undertaken and charted. If the patient is not catheterized, his bladder should be palpated on return from the OR, and again in 2 hours; if there is no obvious increase in bladder size it may be necessary to increase the patient's fluid intake, as he is almost certainly in some degree of shock. This is commonly due to insufficient postoperative fluid replacement which has lead to oliguria.

Ideally the patient should void within 4 hours of return from the OR. All urine passed should be collected and measured and the amount recorded on the appropriate chart. Occasionally the patient may have urine retention, which may be due to the use of narcotics such as morphine, or to pain, and less frequently because muscles or nerves have been transiently damaged during the surgery. The patient can usually be induced to void by simple nursing measures, but if these fail a urinary catheter can be inserted if the patient is becoming uncomfortable due to bladder disten-sion. Sometimes changing the analgesic from morphine to pethidine will induce voiding. Uncomplicated urinary retention, however, usually corrects itself within 8 to 12 hours.

Wound checks

The wound should be checked at half hourly to hourly intervals for the first 24 hours. Although reinforcing the dressing is reasonable on one occasion, it should not be reinforced over and over again. If drainage from the wound is prolific the dressing should be taken down, the amount of serous fluid or blood estimated as accurately as possible, and the wound redressed. As the patient's blood pressure returns to normal, a small amount of capillary bleeding is expected, directly proportional to the extent of the surgery under-gone. However, large amounts of blood in the early postoperative phase would be considered abnormal and would require removal of the dressing to allow inspection of the operative site. The nurse should take the opportunity to check for the presence of overt arterial bleeding and

subcutaneous or deep haematoma by gently palpating the area around the wound. Soft doughy distension near an abdominal wound may indicate deep intra-abdominal bleeding. Continued bleeding may necessitate return to the OR to find and seal the bleeding point.

If the wound is dry it should not be touched, and providing the patient does not complain of undue soreness or show other signs of infection, the dressing should remain closed until it is time to remove the sutures. Sutures are usually removed 5–10 days postoperatively.

It has become fashionable in some hospitals to remove the operative dressing after 24 hours and then dress the wound 2 or 3 times a day. This is an unnecessary and dangerous practice as each time the wound is subjected to handling the chances of it becoming infected are increased.

Food and fluid requirements

Fluids via an intravenous infusion are usually administered to the patient. Fluid should be administered at a rate high enough to maintain a urine output of approximately 60 ml per hour (1500 ml per day) and this usually requires a fluid regime of 3 litres in 24 hours. All blood lost during surgery should be replaced whilst the patient is in the OR. Occasionally, further blood transfusions will be administered on return to the ward. It is a common misconception to include blood replacement as part of the patient's general fluid replacement postoperatively. Blood is not part of the fluid regime but rather is a substance that the patient normally would not have lost if he had not undergone surgery. His fluid require-ments must therefore be seen as separate from his blood replacement.

Oral fluids must not be given until the patient's cough reflex has returned. The cough reflex returns very quickly following modern techniques of anaesthesia, and the traditional idea of waiting for a fixed four hour period after surgery before the patient is allowed fluid is without foundation.

On return of the cough reflex the patient may be given ice to suck, then small sips of fluid, and if these are tolerated without the patient feeling nauseated or vomiting he may have clear fluid to drink and then proceed to a normal diet.

In general, where gastrointestinal surgery has been performed the patient may not have oral fluid until bowel sounds have returned and he has passed flatus. This may take several days. The regime for return to a normal diet usually begins with ice to suck, progressing to 30 ml of water hourly for approximately four hours and if this is tolerated the volume of fluid may be slowly increased to a normal volume and variety of fluids. The patient may then commence very small soft meals, eventually building up to a normal diet.

Following some types of surgery, parenteral or enteral nutrition may be necessary. The aim of parenteral or enteral nutrition is to supply the body's daily requirements of protein, carbohydrate, fat, vitamins, and minerals in order to cater to the patient's particular condition, and maintain satisfactory body weight. Problems often associated with this type of nutrition are dehydration and diarrhoea. Intelligent nursing and medical management can prevent both of these complications.

Antibiotics

Antibiotics are given to most patients with known infections. The infecting organism is identified from swabs and/or samples sent for microscopic examination and culture. Studies for antibiotic sensitivity are also undertaken and the appropriate antibiotic is then administered. Antibiotics may be given in the following situations:

- Preoperatively and then continued postoperatively where a known infection exists
- As an antibiotic cover where the type of surgery may put the patient at risk. This is classic of endoscopic procedures and most urinary tract surgery. The antibiotic may be given as a full course or simply one large statim dose, usually given with the premedication
- Antibiotics may be administered topically at operation into the peritoneum or an abscess cavity or sinus. Where it is known that the bowel is to be opened, the patient may have been ordered to take a preoperative course of a non-metabolized antibiotic in order to reduce bowel flora
- A course of antibiotics may be administered postoperatively as a general prophylactic measure, or more specifically to treat a postoperative complication such as a wound or chest infection.

Psychological care

Patients may often be emotionally labile after major surgery and require tactful, gentle and understanding nursing. Where the surgery has caused an alteration to body image the patient will often experience complex psychological problems similar to those experienced by a person who has lost a close relative or friend (see Chapter 2). The patient and his relatives will require strong emotional support from nursing staff during both the immediate and subsequent postoperative periods.

Some patients may be disorientated to place and time following anaesthesia, but this will usually self-correct within a short time. Patients who are accustomed to consuming large amounts of alcohol or addictive drugs may develop delerium tremens, or demonstrate other signs of withdrawal from the drug. The nurse should be aware of the patients to whom this may happen, or be quick to recognize the signs and symptoms of these conditions, should the patient's excessive drug or alcohol useage not have been discovered preoperatively. Although both these conditions have a definite physiological basis, the patient may still present significant psychological problems which the nurse must deal with in a skilled and sensitive manner.

Ambulation

Early ambulation is extremely important as it greatly reduces the likelihood of postoperative complications and the patient's length of hospitalization.

REFERENCES AND FURTHER READING

Texts

Carey K W (ed) 1984 Caring for surgical patients: nursing photobook. Springhouse, Pennsylvania
Luckmann J. Sorensen K C 1980 Medical-surgical nursing: a psychophysiologic approach, 2nd edn. Saunders, Philadelphia.
Urosevich P R (ed) 1984 Providing early mobility: nursing photobook. Springhouse, Pennsylvania.

Journals

Brozenec S 1985 Caring for the postoperative patient with an abdominal drain. Nursing 85 15 : 4 : 54–57
Burton F, Salminen C A 1984 Back to basics: controlling postoperative infection. Nursing 84 14 : 9 : 43
Caramanica L et al 1981 Postoperative complications: how to help the patient when everything goes wrong. Nursing 81 11 : 3 : 50–53
Croushore T M 1979 Postoperative assessment: the key to avoiding the most common nursing mistakes. Nursing 79 9 : 4 : 46–51
D'Agostino J 1983 Set your mind at ease on oxygen toxicity. Nursing 83 13 : 7 : 54–56
Drain C B 1984 Managing postop pain: it's a matter of sighs. Nursing 84 14 : 8 : 52–55
Fraulini K E, Gorski D W 1983 Don't let perioperative medications put you in a spin. Nursing 83 13 : 12 : 26–30
Fraulini K E, Murphy P 1984 R.E.A.C.T.: a new system for measuring postanaesthesia recovery. Nursing 84 14 : 4 : 12–13
Fuchs P 1983 Before & after surgery stay right on respiratory care. Nursing 83 13 : 5 : 46–50
Greenwood B S 1982 The before and after of good postop pulmonary care. Nursing 82 12 : 12 : 26–27
Mangieri D 1983 Looking at the tube . . . and we don't mean TV. Nursing' 83 13 : 4 : 47–49
McConnell E A 1983 After surgery: how you can avoid the obvious . . . and the not so obvious . . . hazards. Nursing 83 13 : 3 : 8–15
Montanari J 1985 Documenting your postop assessment findings. Nursing 85 15 : 8 : 31–35
Patras A Z 1982 The operation's over, but the danger's not. Nursing 82 12 : 9 : 50–56
Seaman D J 1983 Shortcuts to a more complete postanaesthesia room transfer summary. Nursing 83 13 : 9 : 47–49

7

Factors effecting wound union and healing

Chris Game

INTRODUCTION

The traditional concept of the nurse ministering to the sick and injured has always included the ability to tend efficiently to the physical wounds of his/her patients. With improvements in operative and anaesthetic techniques, many postoperative nursing problems of the past have been eliminated. However, the increasingly complex nature of surgery, anaesthesia, and physical needs of postoperative patients have produced different problems that the nurse must now prepare to manage and overcome in the postoperative phase.

In the early days of invasive major surgery, a patient's postoperative progress was considered stormy at best. This was due to the use of less sophisticated instruments, anaesthesia, and surgical techniques that usually resulted in the patient returning from the operating room with large wounds that had experienced extensive tissue trauma intra-operatively. Nowadays, with the use of increasingly complex surgical techniques and instrumentation, the surgeon is able to perform invasive surgery that is both extensive and protracted and yet, with respect to body tissue injury, is less traumatic than the surgery of the past. Dressing techniques have varied considerably with the result that some wounds (for example, dry wounds) are never redressed prior to suture removal, others are redressed tri-daily from the second postoperative day, and the remainder are variations between these two extremes. Yet at the same time hospitals, and in particular surgical units within hospitals, are noted for harbouring pathogenic microorganisms (including those that are antibiotic resistant) that have the potential to cause wound infections if meticulous care is not afforded the patient either pre-, intra- or postoperatively. Whenever a person's normal body defence mechanisms are compromised by surgery (no matter how minor the surgery), other injurious states, or metabolic disorders, the potential for wound malunion and/or infection arises.

In order to enhance patient recovery and to minimize this potential for wound malunion and/or infection, it is essential that the nurse applies knowledge of how wounds heal naturally and the factors that effect good healing to his/her daily management of all patient care.

This chapter will review wound healing and management and highlight those factors which enhance or adversely affect wound union and healing. The focus is the nurse's role in promoting optimal recovery in all patients with tissue injury. However, before addressing those factors which directly influence wound union and healing, it is necessary to review normal body defence mechanisms, inflammation and the inflammatory response, and patterns of wound repair.

NORMAL BODY DEFENCE MECHANISMS

Basically, the human body has three mechanisms of innate defence that protect it from the effects of disease and trauma. They can be functionally described as:

Mechanical barriers. For example, intact skin and mucous membranes provide a defined depth through which either organisms or objects must penetrate before they can gain access to the internal environment and cause injury.

55

Chemical barriers. For example, saliva, gastric acid and skin perspiration provide a second line of defence should organisms penetrate surface cells.

Humoral barriers. For example, the inflammatory response, immunoglobulins and hormone secretions, provide cell-mediated responses should organisms or objects gain access beyond skin and mucous membranes.

INFLAMMATION AND THE INFLAMMATORY RESPONSE

The most important concept with respect to cell/tissue injury and wound repair is that of inflammation and the inflammatory response. The term 'inflammatory response' describes the sequence of events that occur as a result of tissue damage or injury and 'inflammation' refers to the resulting acute or chronic reaction. Any tissue injury will result in a degree of inflammation. Table 7.1 lists the range of typical causative agents and the type of inflammatory response elicited.

If the injury is mild then the corresponding inflammatory response is also usually mild. However, should the injury persist, for example in the event of certain persistent bacterial or viral infections, then the inflammatory response may continue for months or years. Leucocytosis usually accompanies a moderate to severe inflammatory response and heralds the onset of a systemic response to the injury. Leucocytosis

Table 7.1 Causative agents and inflammatory responses

Agent	Inflammatory response
Excessive heat or cold	Burns or frostbite
Mechanical or physical trauma	Lacerations, surface grazes, surgical wounds, gangrene
Radiation or X-ray therapy	Sunburn or radiation reactions
Chemicals	Corrosive injuries, cell destruction
Bacterial infestations	Carbuncles, boils, abscesses
Viral infections	Influenza, pneumonia, gastroenteritis
Hypersensitivity reactions (antigen/immunoglobulin)	Hay fever, asthma

abates with the discontinuance of the inflammatory response.

Acute inflammation

Acute inflammation is a response to tissue injury resulting in characteristic changes in the injured area of dolor, rubor, tumour, (pain, redness and heat, oedema) and full or partial loss of function of the affected part.

Acute inflammation is further described as being exudative because the effect of these characteristic changes is the formation of an exudate. The small vessels in close proximity to the injured tissue engorge and dilate with blood, resulting in oedema and rubor. The selectively permeable capillary membranes allow the escape of protein-rich serum into the tissue spaces, together with erythrocytes which flow passively through the membrane, thus increasing further the oedema and rubor. Polymorphonuclear leucocytes actively enter the tissue spaces ready to engulf and ingest (by phagocytosis) the harmful foreign substances that are causing or extending the injury. This process further increases the oedema and temperature of the area, resulting in further pain and loss of function.

The inflammatory exudate is filtered from the area via the lymph nodes of the lymphatic system. This process results in a reduced likelihood of spread of the inflammatory agent to the blood stream, as well as resulting in a localized inflammatory response of the lymph nodes; for example, swollen, tender and painful lymph nodes of the inguinal canal following drainage of exudate from an infection of the leg or foot.

Acute inflammation will result in complete resolution to normal tissue structure and function, progression to a suppurative stage, or progression to a state of chronic inflammation. Complete resolution with normal restoration of tissue function will occur when the inflammatory process subsides with minimal tissue damage having occurred during the acute response. The inflammatory process reverses, and the affected tissue resumes its normal size, colour, function and no pain persists. Normally, acute inflammation is highly localized. However occasionally, due to failure of the body's ability to contain the infection, the inflammatory response may extend, as seen in cellulitis. Examples of inflammatory responses that commonly result in complete resolution include such situations as small lacerations of the skin and mucous membranes, sunburn, minor wound infections, pharyngitis, tonsillitis, erysipelas and cellulitis.

Should suppuration occur, then most commonly this will be represented by the development of an abscess: the localized collection of pus developing from a suppurative source in inflamed tissue, due usually to infection from pyogenic bacteria. Pus is inflammatory exudate that contains phagocytic polymorphonuclear leucocytes, ingested bacteria, necrotic tissue, cell debris, and fibrin. Pus is contained within the abscess cavity which is itself lined with granulation tissue. Ultimate healing is by scar/fibrous tissue formation as a complete resolution is not possible due to the extent of tissue destruction. Boils and carbuncles are examples of abscesses in surface and subcutaneous tissue.

Abscesses of deeper tissue tend to discharge their contents of pus by forming either a sinus or, in the case of an abscess in an organ, fistula.

Alternatively, abscesses may burst within body cavities and spread their pus content to other internal structures. Any suppurative inflammation that does not thus resolve, will progress to a chronic stage.

Chronic inflammation

Chronic inflammation is characterized by the formation of new scar/fibrous tissue rather than an exudate, and is therefore described as a productive or formative inflammatory response. Unlike in acute inflammation, complete resolution is not possible in the chronic stage as tissue necrosis has occurred, with or without suppuration, and there is permanent disruption to body tissue structure. Early in this stage the developing scar tissue is highly vascular and delicate but as time progresses the scar tissue becomes more collagenous and tough and less liable to tearing injuries.

It is to be stressed that fibrous tissue is a nonfunctioning replacement of destroyed normal tissue and the effects of chronic inflammation will largely be determined by the prior function of the tissue involved. For example, orifices and tubes will stenose, as in salpingitis, valvular endocarditis, and oesophagitis. Similarly, the cells of organs undergoing chronic inflammatory changes will be replaced wholly or in part by granulating scar tissue and the organ will cease to function at its optimum level as in cirrhosis of the liver, chronic nephritis, and pancreatitis. As a result of the sloughing away of necrotic surface tissue that has undergone chronic inflammatory change organs or tissues may develop ulcers, for example, gastric and duodenal ulcers and the varicose ulcers that occur on the legs of persons with poor peripheral vascular function (see also Chapter 32).

WOUND REPAIR

Patterns of wound repair

Complete healing of injured tissue entails the reformation of the tissue by new cells of the same structure and function as those destroyed. This process is called regeneration, but not all cells possess the ability to completely regenerate following injury. Perfect regeneration of epithelial cells occurs when the basement membrane of epithelial tissue remains intact, for example in the epidermis, alimentary and urinary tracts, vascular system, and haemopoietic bone marrow. Cells that may retain a partial ability to regenerate tend to be those that make up the renal tubules, some endocrine glands, the liver and pancreas.

Cells believed to be incapable of regeneration following extensive trauma or inflammation include neurones, renal glomeruli, and striated, cardiac and smooth muscle. In this instance healing occurs by way of the production of scar tissue that is unable to restore the normal physiological function of the injured tissues.

Types of skin wound healing

Should injury/surgery take place, then healing of the resultant wound or tissue damage/defect occurs by one of the following:

- First intention healing (primary union)
- Second intention healing (secondary union)

• Third intention healing (tertiary union/delayed primary closure).

First intention healing is achievable only in clean surgical wounds or in contaminated wounds that have been debrided to provide clean wound edges through all layers, and which can be approximated readily with the use of sutures. First intention healing is characterized by the minimal development of granulating fibrous tissue in the scar and suture tracks, thus achieving regeneration (Fig. 7.1).

Second intention healing occurs in those wounds which were either too contaminated to close even after debridement, that is were incapable of being converted to a tidy wound for primary closure, or became grossly infected following closure. In this type of wound healing, granulation tissue grows from the base of the wound and epithelial cells migrate inwardly from the skin edges to fill the defect. Healing by second intention takes longer to complete than regeneration due to a greater loss of original tissue, and a greater production of granulation tissue which forms the resultant scar (Fig. 7.2). Large tissue surfaces may require skin grafting.

Third intention healing is otherwise known as delayed primary closure. It is the method adopted for the treatment of some wounds that although considered capable of first intention healing are far too contaminated to undergo immediate closure. In this instance the original wound is cleaned and debrided and allowed to remain open for some 4–6 days. After granulation has commenced, providing the wound is without infection, the wound edges may then be approximated with sutures and primary healing will then result (Fig. 7.3).

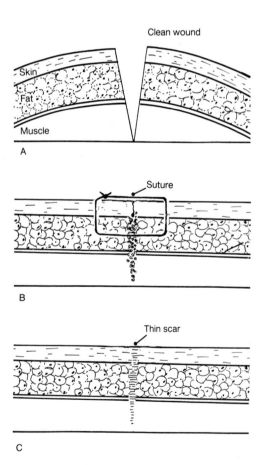

Fig. 7.1 First intention healing. The clean wound (**A**) is sutured, and heals with little granulation tissue developing (**B**). A thin scar results (**C**).

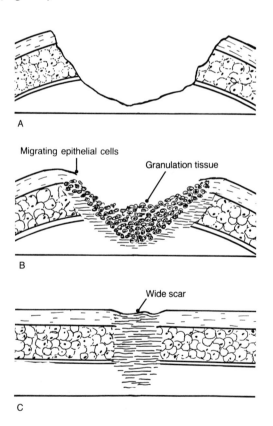

Fig. 7.2 Second intention healing. The wound remains open (**A**), is filled with granulation tissue and covered by migrating epithelial cells (**B**). A wide scar results (**C**).

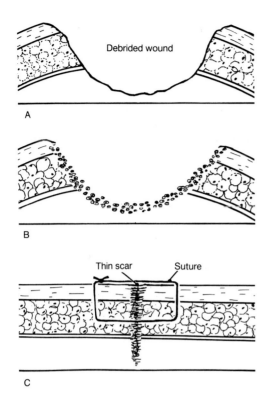

A

B

Thin scar   Suture

C

Fig. 7.3 Third intention healing (delayed primary closure).
The wound remains open (**A**) until granulation tissue begins
to form (**B**). It is then sutured and heals with little scar
formation (**C**).

Factors which influence wound healing/tissue repair

The following factors are discussed in order that
they may serve as a guide for the nurse when
assessing and managing the wound care of the
patients assigned to his/her care.

Types of wounds

Injuries are broadly classified as open or closed
wounds. Open wounds include compound fractures, surgical incisions, penetrating injuries,
lacerations and some crushing injuries. Closed
wounds include simple fractures, ruptured organs
and the remainder of the crushing injuries.

Chemical corrosion from acids or alkalis either
applied directly to the skin surface, injected, or
inhaled will cause tissue necrosis with subsequent
slow healing. Thermal injuries cause trauma
through dry heat, friction burns, scalds, or frost-

bite. The greater the depth of tissue damaged the
larger the wound and the longer the time required
for healing. Electrical burns are caused when a
current passes through tissue, usually leaving a
small surface injury but extensive internal trauma.
Ionizing radiation has the capacity to produce
varying degrees of cell damage and ultimate death.
The tissue damage caused by ionizing radiation
forms the basis of the use of X-rays in cancer
therapy and the nurse should always anticipate
degrees of tissue inflammation or trauma in the
patient undergoing radiotherapy (see Chapter 13).

Obviously, there is a greater potential for
wound malunion and/or infection in the case of
'dirty', contaminated or infected wounds. Tissues
that have a poor blood supply due to the degree
of trauma, the site of the trauma, the prior existence of arterial disease, or the development of
postoperative haematoma or oedema will take
longer to heal. They are less likely to heal by first
intention and are more prone to infection.

Similarly, wound edges that are approximated
under great tension receive minimal blood supply
and will quickly become ischaemic. This will lead
to wound edge necrosis which, if the tension is not
observed and reported so that surgical action can
be taken, will lead to wound dehiscence.

If there is extensive loss of tissue at the time of
injury or as a result of necrotic sloughing and the
defect is allowed to heal by second intention, the
resultant scar will most probably be extremely
thin and weak; it is therefore likely to tear easily
and bleed profusely. Healed varicose ulcers
display this defect (see Chapter 32).

Poorly nourished tissue is more prone to wound
breakdown and is more likely to occur in patients
who have diets deficient in vitamins and minerals.
Vitamins C and K are essential for tissue growth,
as is zinc. Anaemia caused by dietary deficiency
may compound other nutritional deficits, and poor
vascularity.

Presence of bacterial contamination

With modern operative techniques the patient is
less likely to develop an infection introduced intra-
operatively. Improved operative techniques include:
more effective skin disinfectant preparations;
improved hand preparation techniques; disposable

adherent skin drapes that prevent bacterial migration into the wound; reverse-cycle airconditioning; laminar air flow environments for orthopaedic surgery; improved education regarding the use and disposal of masks, gowns, gloves and contaminated articles from the operating room; improved designs and controls on the movement of personnel within the operating room and suite as a whole.

The presence of bacteria will not necessarily mean that infection will ensue. However, should bacterial contamination occur either pre-, intra- or postoperatively, the degree of infection that will result will depend upon all of the following factors:

1. The number of bacteria present (inoculum). Obviously, the more bacteria and the greater their variety the less likely it will be that the patient will easily overcome their presence. The more contaminated the presenting wound, the greater the inoculum factor; for example, victims of motor vehicle accidents who have been in contact with the road surface or patients who have had bowel contents spill into the peritoneum have large inoculum factors.

2. The virulence of the bacteria. That is, the ability of the microbes to remain in the host and produce tissue damage at the site of the wound, or spread to distant targets; for example, *Staphylococcus aureus* and the Clostridia group are both extremely virulent. Virulence depends upon the bacteria being able to withstand the onslaughts of the patient's inflammatory response. The bacteria must therefore be able to resist phagocytosis, as well as to resist the effect of antibiotics that may be employed to treat the resultant infection. Medical and nursing administrations in Australian hospitals are increasingly vigilant to isolate those patients who have developed MRSA (methicillin resistant *Staphylococcus aureus*) wound infections, an example of a virulent microorganism that has been the cause of much suffering and death in postoperative patients in large surgical units in New South Wales and Victoria especially.

3. A nidus for growth. This occurs when either fluid or a retained foreign body allows the bacteria to grow, protected from the body's normal mechanisms of defence and destruction. Most such situations develop further to the abscess stage (refer

page 57) and healing ultimately takes place by second intention.

4. Development of opportunistic infection. Extensive antibiotic use can so suppress or destroy pathogenic microorganisms that protective normal flora are destroyed, or allowed access to areas of the body in which they themselves become pathogenic. This most commonly occurs in the alimentary tract and requires vigilant observation by the nurse to recognize such infections so that treatment can be instituted immediately in order to prevent further damage and tissue injury to the patient.

Overall medical status

The presence of other disease states will affect a patient's ability to overcome acute illness and tissue trauma. Patients whose healing ability is potentially compromised by other disease states will require careful nursing management and diligent observation in order to maximize their healing potential; special groups at risk include those patients with diabetes mellitus, renal insufficiency, or a neoplastic condition. Prolonged steroid therapy or radiotherapy will diminish the body's ability to create an adequate inflammatory response and the necessity for these therapies should alert the nurse to the fact that healing will be delayed to an extent dependent upon the nature and dosage of the treatment.

A patient's immune status will also affect his ability to create an adequate inflammatory response; the patients at greatest risk are those who are undergoing immunosuppression (see Chapter 42).

Other factors

Age. It is recognized that young, healthy persons are more capable of overcoming the effects of injury, inflammatory responses, bacterial infection, and other physical stressors than are the elderly in our society. Ageing brings with it arteriosclerosis and worn out body tissues, organs, and systems.

Economic and social status. Patients who come from a well-knit family group with strong psychosocial supports are potentially more capable of overcoming the stress of injury and disease than are lonely, isolated persons living on the fringe of society. Economically and/or socially disadvantaged groups may not be able to withstand the stressors of acute illness, due to poor nutrition, inadequate housing and hygiene, diminished emotional support, and the additional economic disruption that occurs.

Cultural factors. It is to be emphasized that when assessing patient strengths, the nurse needs to identify those patients whose culture traditionally provides support through a large family network. It is essential to maximize the involvement and input of such support groups as they will increase the likelihood of the patient being able to withstand the effects of acute illness. (See also Chapter 2.)

PRINCIPLES OF NURSING MANAGEMENT

• The type of wound will largely determine the approach that the nurse will take when planning nursing management and instituting nursing care.
• Prior to the institution of specific wound care the patient's general condition should be medically stabilized, the surgeon consulted regarding special areas for consideration, and the patient assessed as to his physical and psychological requirements for nursing management.
• Primary nursing responsibilities in wound care are:
  – observation of the wound to detect early tissue deterioration
  – promotion of a good blood supply

– maintenance of healthy tissue in and around the wound
– and provision of an adequate diet to meet the regenerative needs of the patient's tissues.
• The nurse needs to ensure that the care given to clean wounds does not render them susceptible to contamination and infection, and that the care given to 'dirty' wounds aims at reducing further contamination, minimizing spread of infection to other patients and maximizing tissue regeneration and/or granulation.
• Stereotyping of wound care is to be avoided: what appears to work in the treatment of one patient may not necessarily work in the case of another, regardless of the number of similarities that their conditions may present.

SUMMARY

Each patient must be assessed individually with respect to his nursing care needs and problems. To minimize the potential risk for wound malunion and/or infection, the nurse must apply knowledge of how wounds heal and maximize those factors which effect good healing in his/her daily care of all patients.

Primarily, the nurse must regularly observe the status of the patient's wound and his overall physical and psychological condition, so that appropriate nursing management is effected at all stages of surgical recovery.

Protection of healing tissues from further trauma will reduce the effects of scarring and skin defects, and enhance both the emotional and physical recovery of the patient.

REFERENCES AND FURTHER READING

Texts

Anderson J R (ed) 1976 Muir's textbook of pathology, 10th edn. Edward Arnold, London
Freidin J. Marshall V 1984 Illustrated guide to surgical practice. Churchill Livingstone, Melbourne
Groer M E, Shekleton M E 1979 Basic pathophysiology: a conceptual approach. Mosby, St Louis
Luckmann J, Sorensen K C 1980 Medical-surgical nursing: a psychophysiologic approach, 2nd edn. Saunders, Philadelphia

Roper N (ed) 1978 Nurses dictionary, 15th edn. Churchill Livingstone, Edinburgh
Urosevich P R (ed) 1984 Controlling infection: nursing photobook. Springhouse, Pennsylvania

Journals

Arnell I 1983 Treating decubitus ulcers. Nursing 83 13 : 6 : 50–55

Burton F, Salminew C A 1984 Controlling postoperative infection. Nursing 84 14 : 9 : 43

Brozenec S 1985 Caring for the postoperative patient with an abdominal drain. Nursing 85 15 : 4 : 54–57

Castle M, Watkins J 1979 Fever: understanding a sinister sign. Nursing 79 9 : 2 : 26–33

Doyle J E 1983 All leg ulcers are not alike: managing and preventing arterial and venous ulcers. Nursing 83 13 : 1 : 58–63

Gardner J R 1985 Wound healing in the elderly. Australian Nurses Journal 14 : 11 : 51–54

Gedrose J 1980 When cold can be a killer: prevention and treatment of hypothermia & frostbite. Nursing 80 10 : 2 : 34–36

Humphreys P T 1983 Power spray cleaning for those hard-to-clean wounds. Nursing 83 13 : 4 : 42–43

Jones I 1985 You can drive back infection . . . if you know where to make your stand. Nursing 85 15 : 4 : 50–52

Mackey C, Hopefl A W 1980 Keeping infections down when risks go up. Nursing 80 10 : 6 : 17–21

Mangieri D 1982 Saving your elderly patient's skin. Nursing 82 12 : 10 : 44–45

McHugh M K 1982 Deciphering diagnostic studies: white blood cell tests. Nursing 82 12 : 1 : 10–15

Montanari 1986 Wound dehiscence. Nursing 86 16 : 2 : 33

Neuberger G B, Reckling J B 1985 A new look at wound care. Nursing 85 15 : 2 : 34–42

Neuberger G B, Reckling J B 1985 Wound care: what's clear what's not. Nursing 87 17 : 2 : 34–37

O'Malley P 1979 Managing the difficult draining wound. Nursing 79 9 : 12 : 40–41

Patras A Z 1982 The operation's over, but the danger's not. Nursing 82 12 : 9 : 50–56

Schumann D 1980 How to help wound healing in your abdominal surgery patient. Nursing 80 10 : 4 : 34–40

Shannon M L 1984 5 famous fallacies about pressure sores. Nursing 84 14 : 10 : 34–41

Stark J L, Hunt V 1985 Don't let nosocomial infections get your patient down. Nursing 85 15 : 1 : 10–11

Taylor D L 1983 Inflammation: physiology, signs, and symptoms. Nursing 83 13 : 1 : 52–53

Taylor D L 1983 Wound healing: physiology, signs, and symptoms. Nursing 83 13 : 5 : 44–45

Taylor V 1980 Meeting the challenge of fistulas & draining wounds. Nursing 80 10 : 6 : 45–51

Tinckler L 1983 A significant advance. Nursing Mirror 156(7): 36–39

Wiley L (ed) 1979 Wound management: how teamwork and innovation met a dying patient's needs. Nursing 79 9 : 6 : 38–43

8

Rehabilitation and habilitation

Mary (Errey) Snell

INTRODUCTION

Philosophy of rehabilitation

> The fundamental idea in all rehabilitation care is that man is a total being – that he is composed of physical, mental, and spiritual entities, which taken together constitute a whole person.
>
> Rusk, 1971

Definition of rehabilitation

Rehabilitation is a dynamic process, concerned with the restoration of the disabled individual to live as full a life as is possible within the limitations of his disability. There are, however, many different definitions given for rehabilitation, each one placing the emphasis on a different aspect. The National Council on Rehabilitation in the United States (Terry et al, 1961) state:

> Rehabilitation means the restoration of the handicapped to the fullest physical, mental, social, vocational and economic usefulness of which they are capable.

This very broad definition covers all aspects of an individual's life. Rusk (1971) emphasizes the habilitative element of rehabilitation:

> Rehabilitation is a program designed to enable the individual who is physically disabled, chronically ill or convalescing to live and to work to the utmost of his capacity. It is the integral part of clinical, non-institutional and community responsibility in meeting the problems of chronic illness.

Creativity and individuality are two facets emphasized by Krusen (1971) who also brings the team concept into his definition:

> Rehabilitation is a creative procedure which includes the cooperative efforts of various medical specialists and their associates in the health fields, to improve the mental, physical, social, and vocational aptitude of persons who are handicapped, with the objective of preserving their ability to live happily and productively, on the same level, and with the same opportunities as their neighbours.

The feelings, and the emotions of the patient are very clearly considered by Switzer (1961):

> Rehabilitation is a bridge spanning the gap between useless-ness and usefulness, between hopelessness and hopefulness, between despair and happiness.

Stryker (1977) emphasizes the relevant fact that rehabilitation must commence at the very onset of illness:

> Rehabilitation is a creative process that begins with immediate care in the first stage of the accident or illness. It is continued throughout the restorative phase of care and involves the adaption of the whole being to a new life.

Rehabilitation is therefore concerned with every aspect of the disabled individual, with his restoration to an optimal level of function, and with the preservation of this level. This involves a team of health professionals, working together with the patient and his family to meet these ends.

It must be noted that the term rehabilitation should not be restricted ·only to the physically disabled, but relates also to a wide range of health problems including mental disturbances, mental retardation, and drug and alcohol dependency. Three other terms used widely in rehabilitation also require definition. Wood (1980) quotes the World Health Organization in defining these terms.

Impairment: 'any loss or abnormality of psychological, physiological, or anatomical structure or function'.

Disability: 'any restriction or lack (resulting from an impairment) of ability to perform an activity in the manner, or within the range considered normal for a human being'.

Handicap: 'a disadvantage for a given individual resulting from an impairment or a disability, that limits or prevents the fulfilment of a role that is normal (depending on age, sex, and social and cultural factors)'.

HISTORICAL ASPECTS OF REHABILITATION IN AUSTRALIA

From the dawn of civilization, the welfare of the group depended on the ability of every member to both work and fight. A disabled person who could not fulfil these responsibilities threatened the survival of all, and so was often driven away from the group and left to die.

Attitudes in the early convict days in New South Wales were no different. Dickey (1980) comments that there was no recognition of the disabled; they, together with the chronically ill, the blind, and the insane, were part of a group who were known as 'the poor'.

In 1813, with the forming of the Benevolent Society of New South Wales, the destitute were able to receive handouts of food and clothing; and in 1821 shelter became available with the opening of the Benevolent Asylum in Sydney. However, those receiving assistance were first required to give evidence of their religious beliefs and moral standards. The immoral or alcoholics were left for the Government to look after.

In 1840 a hospital for invalids was built at New Norfolk, and Brown (1972) writes of the 450 invalids who lived in a 'most wretched physical condition: blind, maimed, infirmed and debilitated from age, accident or disease.'

As the Benevolent Society was unable to survive on charitable donations alone, the Government assisted with subsidy. Funds were handled inefficiently, and by the 1850s the Government was forced to take over some of the Society's facilities, and to supervise it more closely. This marked the beginning of a Voluntary Agency, subsidized and supervised by the Government, to assist the disabled in Australia.

When the transportation of convicts ceased in 1840, emphasis was placed on free trade. Institutions such as hospitals, asylums, and workhouses sprang up, but all were selective about whom they admitted. Those who could return quickly to the workforce on discharge were readily accepted, but the disabled or infirm, who were unable to work, were often refused admittance.

Around this time society began to recognize different groups within the disabled, and realized that some were able to contribute to their own keep. Sheltered workshops were set up. The Royal Victorian Institute for the Blind was established in 1868 and the Sydney Industrial Blind Institution in 1879. This identification of groups or clusters of disabled people and their families continues today. It is usually based on medical diagnosis, and so we have institutions such as the Spastic Society and the Multiple Sclerosis Society. In 1900 the old age and invalid pensions were introduced in Australia.

As a result of two World Wars there was a marked increase in the number of disabled persons. It was during this period that the concept of rehabilitation developed, based initially only on physical medicine and exercise then gradually extending to the full rehabilitation programmes we know today.

The United Nations declared a Bill of Human Rights in 1948, and in 1975 a Declaration of Rights of Disabled Persons. 1981 was declared the International Year of the Disabled Person.

Over the years since the early settlers, much has been achieved in breaking down prejudices and suspicions regarding the disabled. In recent years throughout Australia there has been a gradual development and growth of many organizations catering for a wide variety of needs – not only of the disabled, but also of the chronically ill, the elderly, and the lonely. Community Health Centres, Day Hospitals, Day Centres, Drop-in Centres, Elderly Citizens Clubs, Self-help Groups, Home Nursing Services, Meals-on-Wheels, and Life-Line play a great part in helping not only the client but also the family.

CONCEPTS OF REHABILITATION

By definition, rehabilitation is concerned with:

1. The restoring of abilities and functions to an individual who has suffered illness or accident
2. The maintaining of these existing abilities
3. The prevention of any further impairments.

Boroch (1976) stresses the importance of recognizing the habilitative aspects of care that 'assist the individual in maximizing capabilities and in coping with varied current and anticipated situations, to provide a meaningful life within the boundaries to be established by an altered level of health'.

Rehabilitation is concerned with the whole person, and attends to his physical, emotional, social, educational, vocational, spiritual, and cultural needs. It affects every aspect of the person's life: his home and family, housing, income, work, recreation, sexuality, friends, hobbies, and sport. In taking this holistic approach, it must be remembered that each individual is unique, and so a programme must be established to meet each person's specific individual needs. How the individual will cope with his present situation will depend on his cultural background, social status, spiritual beliefs, family support, and pre-morbid characteristics, as well as any previous experiences he may have had with illness, medical or hospital care, or disability.

Rehabilitation is seen as a continuous process, which may extend over a period ranging from a few weeks to many months or even years. During this time changes will take place within the individual himself, as he gradually adapts to an altered lifestyle.

An illness or accident is usually sudden in onset, catching the patient and his family unawares; often it is the first experience the patient has had of hospitalization. Although the concept of rehabilitation begins at the onset of illness or accident, there may be a great deal of anxiety on the part of the patient; therefore it is not always possible for him to participate effectively in the management of his illness at this early stage. This anxiety should respond readily to empathetic reassurance by all staff.

During this early acute stage, the patient, and/or his family, may either deny or be unable to accept the seriousness of the illness or injury, and little or no thought is given to the future outcome. Blame for hospitalization may well be placed onto someone else, especially if an accident has caused the injury.

Once the acute stage has passed, the patient is able to commence the rehabilitation programme in earnest and may possibly be transferred to a rehabilitation hospital or centre. Boroch (1976) emphasizes that not all clients choose to accept rehabilitation and stresses that 'co-operation, or at least lack of resistance' is a prerequisite for rehabilitation.

THE REHABILITATION TEAM

In the rehabilitation setting the chronically ill or disabled person may have only one disability, but associated with this one disability are many and varied problems. To meet these problems and to assess, teach, and care for the patient, a multidisciplinary team is required. This team comprises a group of individuals representing a variety of disciplines. Ford (1979) lists these health professionals as: medical practitioners, nurses, physiotherapists, occupational therapists, speech therapists, music therapists, psychologists, podiatrists, social workers, rehabilitation counsellors, dietitians, prosthetists and orthotists, optometrists, audiologists, and pharmacists. The team members, who each contribute a special expertise and each of whom has a vital role to play, work together towards a common goal: the rehabilitation of the patient to his optimal level of function. Boroch (1976) points out that while each member of the team accepts the responsibility for his professional role, each one must also assume some responsibility for the effectiveness of the team as a whole.

Regular team meetings are held where the patient's medical, functional, psychological, and social problems are identified, discussed, assessed, and evaluated. Short- and long-term goals or objectives are set. This ensures that the whole team is aware of what they are trying to achieve. Goals must be realistic and within the capabilities of the patient.

The rehabilitation process is patient- and family-oriented, so both the patient and his family are involved with the team's decision-making process and goal setting. It is to be remembered that without the patient there would be no rehabilitation, so all team members need to be fully aware of the patient's concept of himself: how he sees his illness and/or disability, what he sees as his problems, and what his future expectations are. His problems and expectations may be very different from those of the team.

Safilios-Rothschild (1970) points out: 'When goals are determined by the rehabilitation team, there is a greater chance that they will not coincide with the rehabilitants' expectations and goals'. She goes on to say that the disabled patients who take an active part in planning their goals are 'generally more motivated to fulfill goals which tend to reflect their own needs and wishes rather than externally imposed ones'.

So the rehabilitation programme is discussed fully with the patient, and his family, taking care to stress the patient's abilities (or strengths), rather than his disabilities (or weaknesses). What the patient can do is emphasized, rather than what he cannot do. While the team members give intelligent, realistic hope to the patient, along with rational alternatives, care must be taken at all times neither to give, nor to imply, false hope.

Roles of some team members

The family

From the onset of illness or accident, the patient's family has been under considerable stress. Home routines have been disrupted, there may have been financial difficulties, and the spouse is exhausted, isolated, and lonely. Friends who were supportive in the early days dwindle away as the period of rehabilitation extends. This may be partly due to an element of embarrassment, as many people find great difficulty relating to a disabled person.

As the rehabilitation programme progresses it may also become apparent that in the future the patient is going to require considerable, or even full time, care. Personal relationships prior to hospitalization have much bearing and influence on the family's reactions. If there has been tension and friction in the past, the spouse may well find the idea of full time care impossible, and so request permanent institutional care. This may lead to guilt feelings on the part of the spouse, and an angry reaction from the patient. Counselling, understanding, and nonjudgemental guidance are required from the social worker and all team members.

For the patient with brain damage there may be behavioural problems, changes in personality, loss of memory, loss of speech, and incontinence. These changes place an immense strain on the whole family. There may be a change in roles where the husband and/or father is no longer able to cope with the simple things which, prior to the accident or illness, were considered to be his task or duty. Scott (1980) points out that the person who comes out of hospital has changed, and often his psychological trauma is untreated. The spouse and family have also undergone psychological trauma; with little or no outside help the situation can slowly destroy their relationship.

The cultural background of the patient can play a major part in his rehabilitation programme. In cultures where the male is the head of the family, he is routinely waited on and pampered by his relatives. The family encourages dependency and is reluctant to allow the patient to do anything for himself. This tends to make rehabilitation a difficult process, and patience and constant education by the team members does little to resolve the problem. Australia has a large multicultural population, whose customs and traditions are perpetuated by many first generation Australians, so this problem will remain for some time to come.

The physiotherapist

Goldenson (1978) writes that the physiotherapist is 'responsible for evaluation of physical capacities and limitations, and for administering treatments designed to alleviate pain, correct or minimize deformity, increase strength and mobility and improve general health'. He/she is also involved in teaching the patient and his family, and other team members, the correct methods of transferring and positioning and, when appropriate, walking.

The occupational therapist

The occupational therapist is primarily concerned with assisting the patient to achieve the optimal level of function in activities of daily living, for example, bathing, toileting, grooming, dressing, and eating. The ability to adapt and/or relearn skills will often mean the difference between a patient living at home, or going to a nursing home when discharged. Assessment and adaptation of the environment both in hospital and later in the patient's home; the provision of aids such as grab rails, ramps, or bath seats; as well as teaching social and occupational skills, all come within the occupational therapist's role.

The social worker

Of the social worker, Goldenson (1978) writes: 'A social worker is a highly skilled specialist in helping individuals and families deal with personal problems that arise when faced with illness or disability'. Ford (1979) refers to him/her as the 'patient's advocate'. Over all, the social worker attends to the social, domestic, financial, and emotional requirements of the patient and his family. He/she, like all other team members, must have a full understanding of the sick, the disabled, and the elderly, together with their many varied and complex needs. To him/her falls much of the counselling of patient and family, and he/she is involved in discharge planning along with the follow up of the patient after discharge.

The speech pathologist

The speech pathologist is concerned with the diagnosis and treatment of disorders of communication, such as language, voice, cognitive skills, and is involved with psychological assessment. Disorders of eating and swallowing are also a concern of the speech pathologist.

The prosthetist and orthotist

These team members design, supply, modify, fit, and adjust prostheses (for example, artificial limbs) and orthoses (for example, mechanical appliances such as splints and braces which correct deformities).

The podiatrist

Care of the feet is of prime importance in the mobility training of the rehabilitation patient, and in maintaining mobility in the elderly. Podiatry care assists in preventing superficial skin lesions and/or nail disorders and provides palliative treatment of minor foot deformities. The provision of silicone devices and footware advice adds to the total care offered by the podiatrist.

The clinical psychologist

Ford (1979) speaks of the patient who suffers a 'damaged mind'. He writes:

> Sometimes the effect of the damage is so subtle that the changes in behaviour are evident only to those very close to the old person. A well-trained clinical psychologist can pinpoint those aspects of intellectual function which are failing and assist the family and the other therapists to minimize the effects. The most common cause of failure in the rehabilitation of a stroke victim results from the patient's inability to understand the new patterns of movement and the safety measures he must take if he is to move about with sufficient security to make the risk of a fall and a fractured neck of femur worth taking. The failed case is often discovered after weeks of repetitive and frustrating work by the physiotherapist and constant and depressing failure by the stroke patient. A clinical psychologist can often predict the probability of success and so be a cost benefit to the rehabilitation service, in terms of wasted time, staff frustration and disillusioned patients.

The nurse

In looking at the role of the nurse in the rehabilitation team, many authors agree that he/she is in a unique position; the nurse is the only one who sees the patient as a whole being. It is the nurse who is responsible for assessing the patient's physical and psychosocial needs, and for planning his individual care to meet those needs over a 24 hour period.

> Nutrition, rest, mobilization, safety, adequate elimination, fluid balance, communication, emotional expression, teaching-learning, and self identity lie within the scope of the nurse's responsibilities. The nurse coordinates the activities of other therapies that are to be continued outside the specific therapy department.
>
> Boroch, 1976

> Careful observation and clear objective reporting of the patient's progress is a primary responsibility of nursing staff who have greater contact with the patient than any other member of the team. Nursing staff also have more contact with relatives. They must, therefore, be very aware of their supportive function, ensuring the reliability and accuracy of information shared.
>
> Shaw, 1984

The nurse is seen as the coordinator of the team and he/she has an important part to play in the team of health professionals caring for the patient.

PRINCIPLES OF REHABILITATION NURSING

Rehabilitation nursing is often referred to as a speciality area of nursing, concerned with the care of people with long term chronic disabilities. Goldenson (1978) sees rehabilitation nursing as 'goal orientated, personalized care that encompasses preventive, maintenance and restorative aspects of nursing as a form of therapy'. He continues: the rehabilitation nurse requires 'perceptive insight and involvement with the whole person within the environment in which the individual will be functioning'.

Brunner & Suddarth (1980) state: 'Rehabilitation is an integral part of nursing and should begin with the initial contact with the patient'. With illness and accident, there is a threat of disability and disability can be greater if adequate nursing care is not carried out from the onset. Correct positioning of the patient, both in bed and out, along with passive exercises will help prevent muscle weakness and contractures. The provision of adequate nourishment, care of bladder and bowel, and prevention of pressure sores, are principles of nursing which apply from admission.

Due to the length of a patient's stay in the rehabilitation setting, it may well be said that rehabilitation nursing is a long, slow process with no dramatic changes. Therefore frustration on the part of the patient may well be high; he may become depressed, angry, or withdrawn. An understanding, empathetic, and nonjudgemental nurse, who gives quiet support and encouragement, will do a great deal to assist the patient through this difficult period.

Van Maanen (1981) calls rehabilitation the 'core of nursing'. She expects the nurse to ascertain just what the patient knows and anticipates regarding his disability, and to find out 'what he does not know or understand, taking into consideration thoughts and feelings he does not express'. The nurse, van Maanen writes, should know his/her patient well enough to recognize what is disturbing him and 'to co-operate with the patient in gaining an understanding of his situation, thus reducing fear and insecurity to a minimum, and helping him discover his own possibilities and capacities.' Rehabilitation begins only 'when the patient knows what is the matter with him, what he can expect of others, and what others expect of him'.

Many nurses find that the most frustrating aspect of rehabilitation nursing is allowing the patient to do things for himself. It is far quicker to shower, dry, dress, and shave the patient yourself than to stand back and watch him struggle to relearn lost skills.

When moving from dependence to independence it is essential that the patient be allowed to participate actively in this struggle from dependence to independence, and to take responsibility for his own personal care within the limits of his capabilities. The nurse works with the patient, not for or on behalf of him, gradually withdrawing assistance as he gains more independence.

McDaniel (1976) states that the attitudes of health professionals towards their patients 'are probably more important in determining the individual's response to treatment and rehabilitation planning than any other single force'. He goes on to say that these professionals 'are typically trained only to perform certain technical duties and have little attention called to the subtleties of the situations in which they work'. It is to be hoped that, with careful guidance, nurses in rehabilitation centres in Australia no longer fit into this category.

Martos (1983) talks of the patient's spiritual needs. He believes that with a holistic approach to health care it is impossible to look at the patient's physical needs without also looking at his spiritual needs – what affects one, affects the other. He says that 'spiritual needs', covers the emotional, social, intellectual, and religious needs of the patient.

Luckmann & Sorensen (1980) recognize the loneliness that illness and hospitalization brings. This is particularly true in the rehabilitation setting where the patient may spend many months. Added to this is the presence of a disability. Separated from family and friends, the patient may not only experience loneliness, but also feelings of rejection, guilt, and worthlessness. No longer able to fulfil his main role of husband, father, or breadwinner, and uncertain about the future, his life lacks meaning and purpose. Due to his disability, a part of his life has changed; he may never be able to use again those talents and abilities which he has always taken for granted. Authors agree that any contact with illness and/or accident changes a person so he will never again be the person he was previously.

The rehabilitation nurse develops his/her own skills and sensitivity to enable him/her to care for, support, and comfort the patient through these difficult periods.

Listening skills are important. Listen actively to the patient, letting him know that you have both heard and understood what he is saying, or trying to say. Allow him to express his fears and anxieties regarding his sickness, his disability, his suffering, his future, his death. While listening to his verbalizing, be also aware of his nonverbal language (see also Chapter 2).

A good understanding of the psychological effects of disability, and of long term illness, is required by the rehabilitation nurse. By both knowing and understanding his/her patient, the nurse will know when to encourage him, when to pressure him to achieve a goal, and when to slow him down if he has been pushing himself too quickly. Praise for effort is as important as praise

for achievement, as it may be many weeks or even months before a goal is achieved.

The rehabilitation nurse requires knowledge in caring for patients with specific problems; for example, communication disorders in patients who have suffered a cerebrovascular accident, the erratic and often uninhibited behaviour of the brain damaged, the needs of amputees and of those patients in long term institutional care. By applying the principles of rehabilitation nursing he/she will be able to plan care for all patients.

Stryker (1977) sums up rehabilitation nursing by saying:

> . . . a rehabilitation attitude along with certain knowledge and skills must be basic to all phases of patient care, whether one works in a hospital for acute diseases, in a nursing home or in a patient's own home. Rehabilitation must be infused into general care, and the maintenance and preventive aspects of rehabilitation must be ongoing throughout a patient's life. It is a part of health care, not a phase of it.

With education, skill, and experience the nurse can hold his/her place as a professional working in a health team aimed at improving the quality of life of the acutely ill, the disabled, the chronically ill, and the aged.

REFERENCES AND FURTHER READING

Texts

Bitter J A 1977 Introduction to rehabilitation. Mosby, St Louis
Boroch R M 1976 Rehabilitation nursing. Kimpton, London, ch 1, p 6–7, ch 4, p 28–36
Brown J C 1972 Poverty is not a crime. The development of social services in Tasmania. Tasmanian Historical Research Association, Hobart
Brunner L S, Suddarth D S 1980 Textbook of medical-surgical nursing, 4th edn. Saunders, Philadelphia, ch 4, p 179–205
Christopherson V A, Coulter P P, Wolanin M O 1974 Rehabilitation nursing perspectives and applications. McGraw-Hill, New York
Dickey B 1980 No charity there: a short history of social welfare in Australia. Nelson, Melbourne
Ford B 1979 The elderly Australian. Penguin, Melbourne, ch 5, p 104–125
Goldenson R M 1978 Disability and rehabilitation handbook. McGraw-Hill, New York, p 724
Krusen F H 1971 Handbook of physical medicine and rehabilitation, 2nd edn. Saunders, Philadelphia
Luckmann J, Sorensen K C 1980 Medical-surgical nursing: a psychophysiologic approach, 2nd edn. Saunders, Philadelphia

McDaniel J W 1976 Physical disability and human behaviour, 2nd edn. Pergamon Press, New York, ch 3, p 51
Rusk H A 1971 Rehabilitation medicine, 3rd edn. Mosby, St Louis
Safilios-Rothschild C 1970 The sociology and social psychology of disability and rehabilitation. Random House, New York, p 154
Shaw M W (ed) 1984 The challenge of ageing. Churchill Livingstone, Melbourne, ch 11, p 109
Stryker R 1977 Rehabilitative aspects of acute and chronic nursing care, 2nd edn. Saunders, Toronto, ch 2, p 13–15
Switzer M 1961 In: Terry et al, op. cit.
Terry F J, Benz G S, Mereness D, Kleffner F R, Jensen D M (eds) 1961 Principles and techniques of rehabilitation nursing, 2nd edn. Mosby, St Louis
Urosevich P R (ed) 1984 Providing early mobility: nursing photobook. Springhouse, Pennsylvania

Journals

Brill C, Hill L 1985 Giving the help that goes on giving. Nursing 85 15 : 5 : 44–47
Cave L, Johnson J M, Komar R, Korth C, Meaker C, Patton R M 1985 When families get together. Nursing 85 15 : 2 : 58–61

DeHoff V 1983 Motivating patients to do what's good for them: the exercise contest. Nursing 83 13 : 12 : 31

Downing P 1985 I am brain damaged. The Australian Nurses Journal 15 : 1 : 44–45

Dugan J S 1984 Winning the battle against incontinence. Nursing 84 14 : 6 : 59

Gutierrez K 1985 Home is where the care is. Nursing 85 15 : 11 : 48–49

Jackson S 1985 The touching process in rehabilitation. The Australian Nurses Journal 14 : 11 : 43–45

Kruse H 1987 Jumping hurdles in geriatric rehabilitation. The Australian Nurses Journal. 17 : 1 : 45–47, 60

Malcolm J D 1985 Battle cry for Mr MacDonald. Nursing 85 15 : 6 : 44–46

Meissner J E 1980 Evaluate your patient's level of independence. Nursing 80 10 : 9 : 22–23

Rankin S H, Duffy K L 1984 15 Problems in patient education and their solutions. Nursing 84 14 : 4 : 17–22

Reeder J M 1984 Help your disabled patient be more independent. Nursing 84 14 : 11 : 53

Scott A 1980 Finishing rehabilitation. National Rehabilitation Digest 4 : 2 : 26–32

Sigmon H D 1984 Helping your long-term trauma patient travel the road to recovery. Nursing 84 14 : 1 : 58–63

van Maanen H M T 1981 Rehabilitation: core of nursing. International Nursing Review 28 : 1 : 9–14

Wells M I 1983 Discharge planning: closing the gaps in continuity of care. Nursing 83 13 : 11 : 45

Williams N O 1984 Listen to me. Nursing 84 14 : 4 : 28

Wood P H N 1980 Appreciating the consequences of disease: the international classification of impairments, disabilities and handicaps. World Health Organisation Chronicle 34 : 376–380

Ziegler J C 1980 Physical reconditioning – Rx for the convalescent patient. Nursing 80 10 : 8 : 67–69

Audiovisual material

Martos J 1983 The ministry of spiritual care. National Catholic Reporter, Missouri, A/V cassettes.

NOTE: the Hospitals and Health Services Yearbook, published by Peter Isaacson Publications Pty Ltd in association with The School of Health Administration University of New South Wales, provides a useful listing of sources of information relating to State-specific social welfare services and agencies.

2

9

Homeostasis – normal and disturbed

Michael Drake

CONCEPTS OF INTERNAL ENVIRONMENT AND HOMEOSTASIS

It is the fixity of the *milieu interieur* which is the condition of free and independent life and all the vital mechanisms, however varied they may be, have only one object, that of preserving constant the conditions of life in the internal environment.

Claude Bernard

No more pregnant sentence was ever framed by a physiologist.

G. S. Haldane

It was Claude Bernard who pointed out that the external environment of the organism as a whole, atmospheric air in the case of man, is not the external environment of the individual cells of the body. He called the interstitial fluid, which bathes the cell, and the plasma with which it carries out continuous exchanges, the internal environment (*milieu interieur*).

All the various systems, which are individually designated as though they existed for their own sake, serve in a subsidiary role to fulfil the biological requirements of the cell by maintaining the correct physical and chemical conditions essential to the life of the cell. This set of essential conditions is the internal environment. Thus the respiratory system, usually described with the emphasis on the lungs and the passages leading to them from the outside, is of significance only in that it brings the oxygen necessary for metabolism to the cells, and removes from the tissues the accumulating carbon dioxide which is toxic in high concentrations. The digestive system is of value to us in that it transforms the appetizing, yet non-utilizable, gross food particles into the smaller and simpler molecules which can penetrate through the walls of the digestive system and pass by means of the blood to the tissues to be ultimately used by the cell for energy or for structure. The finely adjusted activity of the cells of the kidney tubules is responsible for the constancy of the composition of blood, and thereby for the internal environment of all the cells of the body. The autonomic nervous system is particularly important. It controls the glands and muscles of the gut, the body temperature, the blood glucose, the blood pressure, and a host of other things in the face of changes in the external environment.

This leads logically to an integrated study of the ways in which the constancy of the components of the immediate environment of the cell may be maintained. It was Cannon who first used the term 'homeostasis', which differs from the concept of the constant internal environment only in that the latter describes a condition, the former the active processes by which this condition is achieved.

The way in which the constancy of the internal environment is maintained with respect, for example, to acid-base equilibrium, osmotic pressure, concentration of individual solutes (sugar) or of ions (Na^+, Ca^{++}), and temperature is one of the most important problems of physiology. The constancy of the internal environment is not absolute; under normal conditions slight 'permissible' variations occur as with all so-called physiological 'constants'. If the stresses on the system become too great, the composition of the internal environment may alter significantly, often with disastrous effects. Claude Bernard pointed out that the constancy of the composition of the *milieu interieur* is the condition of free and independent life. If by a free life is meant the vigorous and effective activity of the organism as a whole, the aphorism is extremely apt. Thus a disturbance in the volume or composition of the body fluids, relatively minor changes in the acid–base balance of the blood, significant disturbances in the availability of oxygen for cell metabolism or the ability of the body to rid itself of carbon dioxide, or violent fluctuations in body temperature, will seriously impair body function and may result in death.

FLUID AND ELECTROLYTE BALANCE/IMBALANCE

THE BODY FLUIDS

Volume and distribution

Water is the solvent of many substances in the body, and water with its dissolved solutes comprises the body fluids. Considerable variations occur in the volume of body fluids according, for example, to the age, sex, and build of a person. Thus the water content of the body is relatively high in infancy and falls progressively with age. Fat, or adipose tissue, contains relatively little water and hence a fat person contains, by weight, proportionately less water than a thin one. In general women contain more fat than men, so the water content of women is relatively less than that of men. Measurements of total body water in the adult have ranged from as low as 40% to as high as 70%. The most accurate figure would appear to be about 60% and hence an 'average' 70 kg person contains approximately 40 litres of water.

The body fluids are distributed within 3 'compartments':

– The intravascular compartment, which contains the plasma, is bounded by the walls of the blood vessels, and specifically in the capillaries by a very thin wall composed of the endothelial cells.
– The interstitial, or tissue, fluid compartment which is separated from the intracellular fluid by the cell membrane, and from the plasma by the capillary endothelium.
– The intracellular fluid compartment which is bounded by the membranes of the individual cells.

The total volume of body fluid, and the volume within any specific 'compartment' can be measured by a dilution technique. This involves the introduction of a substance into the compartment, allowing it to disperse throughout the compartment, and then measuring the extent to which the substance has become diluted. Thus, one needs to know:

1. The total quantity of the test substance introduced.
2. The concentration of the test substance in the fluid after mixing or dispersement has occurred. For example:
Amount injected = 10 mg
Concentration in sample after mixing = 0.5 mg/100 ml

$$\text{Volume of compartment} = \frac{10 \times 100}{0.5} = 2000 \text{ ml}$$

The substance used for these determinations depends upon the body compartment being measured. In general the substance must be able to diffuse throughout the whole of the compartment under study, but not beyond the limits of this compartment. Radioactive substances that combine with plasma proteins can be used to measure the plasma volume since plasma proteins remain within the blood vessels. Plasma volume may be measured, for example, by 'labelling' albumin with radioactive iodine. Conversely, if a measurement of the total volume of body fluid is required a substance must be used that will diffuse throughout the whole of the body including, of course, into all cells. 'Heavy' water has been used for this purpose. The measurement of the extracellular fluid volume is the least accurate as it requires an indicator that will diffuse into the most remote water droplets in bone and connective tissue yet must not enter cells at all. No such substance exists, but a reasonably valid estimate is obtained using substances such as insulin, sucrose, or radioactive sodium.

Using techniques such as these, it can be shown that the 40 litres of body fluid are distributed as follows:

- Intracellular fluid – 25 litres
- Extracellular fluid – 15 litres

Extracellular fluid can be subdivided into:

- Tissue or interstitial fluid – 12 litres
- Plasma or intravascular fluid – 3 litres

In addition, there are small amounts of water in lymph, cerebrospinal fluid, and the aqueous humor of the eye.

Composition of body fluids

The three most important constituents of the body fluids are water, proteins, and electrolytes or ions. In addition, the intracellular fluid in particular contains literally hundreds of organic compounds that are responsible for the innumerable chemical reactions that take place within the cells.

Water

Water is the most abundant substance in the body. All chemical reactions that take place in the body do so in an aqueous medium, and usually the water molecules are actually involved in the reaction. The principal function, therefore, of water in the body is to act as a solvent for the body constituents and to provide a suitable medium for chemical reactions. Because water is a poor conductor of heat it acts as an insulator, making it possible for the heat regulating mechanisms to adjust gradually to changes in the environmental temperature. The water content of animal tissues prevents heat from being absorbed or lost too rapidly. In addition, the evaporation of water in the form of sweat is an important mechanism in the lowering of body temperature.

Water acts as a fluid medium for the removal of excreted wastes. Metabolic wastes excreted via the kidneys are dissolved in water and thus water is essential for excretion.

Many mechanical processes are lubricated by water fluids. Thus saliva in the mouth aids chewing and swallowing, whilst synovial fluid in the joint space is essential for joint movement.

Water is of importance in maintaining the size and shape of cells and tissues and hence their functional efficiency. Consequently, water excess or water depletion will impair cellular function. The distribution of oxygen nutrients to the tissues and the removal of waste products is dependent partly on water as a mechanical factor in maintaining the volume and thereby the pressure of the circulating blood.

Proteins and other non-electrolytes

Proteins are an important constituent of both intracellular fluid and plasma. The tissue or interstitial fluid contains relatively little protein, since most proteins cannot cross capillary and cell walls. Many non-electrolytes, such as phospholipids, cholesterol, glucose, urea, and bilirubin, are found in all body compartments. The protein molecules and some of the non-electrolyte molecules are extremely large in comparison to the more numerous but smaller ions. Therefore, in terms of mass, proteins and non-electrolytes comprise about 90% of the dissolved constituents in plasma, about 60% of those in interstitial fluid, and about 97% of those in intracellular fluid.

Plasma proteins comprise the major solid component of plasma, the total protein content being about 70–75 g/l. (Traditionally, protein content has been expressed as grams per decilitre – g/dl – but correct SI usage dictates that it be expressed as grams per litre. One decilitre is 10^{-1} litre, or 100 ml.) The two major groups of plasma proteins are albumin and globulin, the normal concentration of albumin being approximately 48 g/l whilst that of globulin is 23 g/l. Thus albumin has the highest mass concentration in plasma and since it also has the lowest molecular weight it is the largest contributor to the intravascular colloid osmotic pressure. In addition, albumin acts as a carrier molecule for bilirubin, fatty acids, trace elements, and many drugs. Albumin is synthesized in the liver.

The serum globulins are a heterogeneous mixture of protein molecules. They are frequently subdivided into alpha-, beta-, and gammaglobulins, sometimes with number designations as well, this subdivision being based on their electrophoretic mobility. A more rational classification is based on their structure or function.

Nearly all known immune globulins are found in the gamma fraction and nearly all gammaglobulins are antibodies. However, some antibodies do occur in other globulin fractions and hence the globulins concerned with immunity are collectively referred to as the immunoglobulins. Five immunoglobulin classes are recognized, IgG, IgA, IgM, IgD, and IgE. All are synthesized in B lymphocytes or their derivatives, plasma cells.

The third major plasma protein group is fibrinogen. This is a soluble plasma glycoprotein which is synthesized in the liver. It is the precursor of fibrin and hence is of paramount importance in the process of blood coagulation.

Electrolytes and ions

Atoms that carry an electrical charge due to the gain or loss of an electron are called ions. They are named according to their behaviour in an electrical field. Thus positively charged ions are attracted towards the negative pole (or cathode) and hence are called cations. Conversely, negatively charged ions would move to the positive pole (or anode) and these particles are referred to as anions. Compounds which give rise to ions in solution are called electrolytes.

Extracellular fluid, both the blood plasma and the interstitial fluid, contains large quantities of sodium and chloride ions, reasonably large quantities of bicarbonate ion, but only small amounts of potassium, calcium, magnesium, phosphate, and sulphate ions. Intracellular fluid contains only small quantities of sodium and chloride ions and almost no calcium ions, but it does contain large quantities of potassium and phosphate, and moderate quantities of magnesium and sulphate ions. In addition, cells contain a large amount of protein.

In summary, sodium is the main cation of extracellular fluid and chloride and bicarbonate the main anions. Potassium is the main cation of intracellular fluid, with phosphate and protein as the main anions.

Measurement of body fluids

In order to study the composition of body fluids it is necessary to define units to express the concentration of the various solutes. Many of the units used in the past, and indeed still used in some areas, for expressing the results of measurements made in medicine developed empirically and became so diverse that there was a danger that results could be misunderstood by those not familiar with the particular scale of units used. This danger can be averted by the universal adoption of a common system of units in all branches of science and medicine. The system recommended is the International System of Units (SI) which is based on the metric system. The SI system incorporates two different types of unit concentration: molar concentration, for example, moles per litre (mol/l), millimoles per litre (mmol/l); and mass concentration, for example grams per litre (g/l), milligrams per litre (mg/l). Note that the volume base is one litre not one hundred millilitres (100 ml) as has often been used in the past. The use of mass concentration with a volume base less than a litre (for example mg/100 ml) obscures functional relationships when dealing with metabolic processes. It is preferable to express these substances in terms of molar concentration which describes the patient's true biological status, and allows direct comparison of all the molecules or ions participating.

The term 'mole' refers to a fixed number of any type of particle. The idea that matter is made up of discrete particles has its roots in history, and the mole concept is a consequence of this particular theory of matter. The word is derived from Latin and means a 'pile' or 'heap'. Thus it is used to designate the amount ('pile' or 'heap') of a substance containing a standard number of specified particles, for example, atoms, molecules, or ions. The standard number is Avogadro's number and is the number of carbon atoms in exactly 0.012 kg (12 g) of pure C^{12} (6.02×10^{23}).

- 1 mole of hydrogen atoms is 6.02×10^{23} hydrogen atoms
- 1 mole of water molecules is 6.02×10^{23} water molecules
- 1 mole of elephants is 6.02×10^{23} elephants.

The mass of a mole of a substance is equal to the formula (molecular) weight of the substance expressed in grams.

A mole of C^{12} atoms has, by definition, a mass of exactly 12 grams. A mole of any other element has a smaller or a larger mass depending on the mass of an atom of that element in comparison to C^{12}. In physiology it is more convenient to deal with milligrams and hence the term millimole is used, that is, the atomic or formula weight in milligrams. Thus the concentration of substances in the body fluids is expressed as millimoles per litre.

BIOLOGICAL EXCHANGES

As already indicated, the body may be considered as being divided into three compartments. In addition, it is important to realise that the body as a whole lives and moves in an external environment. In order to appreciate many of the disturbances of composition and distribution of body fluids it is essential to understand the way in which exchanges occur between the various compartments of the body, and between the body and its external environment. These exchanges occur either by passive processes, in which movement of substances takes place according to basic physico-chemical laws, or by active processes, in which energy is expended by the body to bring about, or facilitate, the exchanges.

Passive processes

Filtration – by filtration is meant the passage of water and dissolved substances through a membrane due to a difference of hydrostatic pressure on the two sides of the membrane. The fluid which passes through is called the filtrate, and consists of water and any dissolved substances to which the membrane is permeable.

Diffusion – all matter consists of atoms or molecules, which are in constant motion. This movement ensures that in time all the particles in a given liquid or gas will be distributed evenly throughout the whole volume of the substance. This process is called diffusion. The ultimate result of the to-and-fro movement of particles is that they will move from an area of higher concentration to one of lower concentration. We say, therefore, that diffusion occurs in accordance with a concentration gradient. Whether or not a particular substance will diffuse across a membrane depends on the properties of that membrane and the properties of the substance, for example, the size and electrical properties of its ions.

Osmosis – this term refers to the spontaneous flow of solvent (for example, water) from a more dilute to a more concentrated solution when the two are separated from each other by a suitable membrane. Membranes that allow the passage of water but none, or only some, of the dissolved substances are said to be selectively-permeable. If there is a greater concentration of non-diffusable dissolved substances on one side of the membrane than on the other, there will be a net movement of water across the membrane to the side where there is a greater concentration of non-diffusable material. This movement of water is referrred to as osmosis. The force necessary to oppose this attraction, that is, the force necessary to prevent the flow of water molecules from the dilute to the more concentrated solution, is referred to as the osmotic pressure.

The magnitude of the osmotic pressure in any system is determined by the total number of particles in solution. The total osmotic pressure of plasma is over 5000 mmHg, but this is not effective within the body as all the body water compartments contain much the same concentration of osmotically active particles. However, whereas the capillary wall is freely permeable to water and the dissolved electrolytes it is impermeable to the larger protein molecules. Thus the proteins exert an osmotic effect across the capillary membrane. The effective osmotic pressure of plasma, due to plasma proteins, is referred to as the colloid osmotic pressure.

Active processes

Carrier-mediated or facilitated diffusion

As already indicated, the concentrations of various ions inside and outside the cell vary widely and hence movements of these ions cannot depend entirely on passive processes relying, as they do, upon concentration gradients. The importance of the problem is illustrated by the fact that cells contain in their cytoplasm much more potassium than sodium and yet must exist in a medium in which the ratio between these two ions is reversed. The maintenance of this differential concentration depends upon a pump mechanism within the cell membrane, the energy for this pump being derived from cell metabolism.

Many substances such as glucose, amino acids, and fatty acids, are believed to utilize carrier-molecules to facilitate their passage across the cell membrane. The carrier forms a compound with the ions on one face of the membrane. The compound then passes through the membrane to be destroyed, releasing the ion at the other face. The movement of the compound, as distinct from the ion, thus follows a chemical concentration gradient. When the transport is with, rather than against, a concentration gradient it is referred to as carrier-mediated or -facilitated diffusion.

Many of the transport mechanisms are at least partially under hormonal control. Thus insulin, for example, increases glucose entry into cells.

In certain situations proteins can enter cells, and a number of hormones secreted by endocrine cells are proteins or large polypeptides. Special cell activities effect these transfers.

Phagocytosis – is the process whereby a cell ingests large particulate matter. It is the process used by the polymorphonuclear leucocyte to engulf bacteria and dead tissue, but it can also be used to transfer protein across the cell membrane.

Pinocytosis – is essentially the same process, the only difference being that the substances ingested are in solution.

Emeiocytosis – is reverse pinocytosis. The membrane around a vacuole or secretion granule fuses with the cell membrane and the region of fusion then breaks down, leaving the contents of the vacuole or secretion granule outside the cell with the cell membrane intact. Emeiocytosis is the mechanism used by a number of endocrine glands to secrete their hormones.

Exchanges between intracellular and interstitial fluids

These exchanges involve the movement of water and solutes, and occur by both active and passive transport. Most cell membranes are freely permeable to water, and the two fluid compartments are in osmotic equilibrium with each other. Thus the concentration of osmotically effective particles in each fluid is the same, although as already indicated the nature of the particles differ. Movement of water across cell membranes is probably always a passive exchange, secondary to the active transport of ions across the membrane, or to changes in ionic concentration inside or outside the cells.

Exchanges between interstitial fluid and plasma

These exchanges occur across the wall of the capillary which may be regarded as a passive filter.

As the blood traverses the capillary, water molecules and dissolved substances diffuse back and forth through the capillary wall. The capillary pores are too narrow, under normal circumstances, to permit the passage of plasma proteins.

There is a continual exchange of water across the walls of the blood capillaries, this exchange being referred to as the 'tissue fluid cycle'. This exchange is an entirely passive one, depending upon the processes of filtration and osmosis, and is due to the separation of two fluids of differing composition and at different hydrostatic pressures, by a selectively permeable membrane – the capillary walls. The factors favouring the passage of fluid out of the capillaries are:

- The hydrostatic pressure of the blood
- The colloidal osmotic pressure of the tissue fluid.

The forces opposing this transudation are:

- The colloidal osmotic pressure of the plasma
- The hydrostatic pressure of the tissue fluid.

As already indicated, the colloidal or effective osmotic pressure of the plasma is due almost entirely to the plasma proteins, particularly the albumin fraction.

As a result of these opposing forces the amount of fluid that escapes from the capillaries into the tissue spaces over a period of time is more or less balanced by the amount of fluid that re-enters the capillaries. A small surplus of fluid does escape, but this excess is drained from the tissues by the lymphatic system.

Exchanges between the organism and the external environment

Water. There are four normal routes of water loss – the skin, lungs, alimentary tract, and kidneys. Loss of water through the skin and lungs is uncontrolled – it depends only upon the humidity and temperature of the surrounding air and on the body's need to regulate its temperature.

In contrast, the amount of water lost through the kidneys is strictly regulated according to the body's needs. In the normal person approximately 99% of the water filtered through the renal glomeruli is re-absorbed in the renal tubules.

Much of this re-absorption is by osmosis and is secondary to the re-absorption of sodium that also occurs in the proximal tubules. Thus, as the sodium is actively re-absorbed the fluid in the tubules becomes hypotonic relative to the plasma, and hence water passes from the tubules into the blood. The re-absorption of sodium is primary, the water following passively. This phase of water re-absorption is sometimes referred to as obligatory re-absorption.

In contrast with this obligatory re-absorption of water, the further re-absorption that occurs in the distal renal tubules is under the control of the antidiuretic hormone (ADH) which is secreted by the posterior lobe of the pituitary gland in response to impulses from the osmoreceptors in the hypothalamus. The secretion of ADH is determined by the tonicity of the plasma and the extracellular fluids, and the hormone acts by increasing the permeability to water of the cells of the distal renal tubules. If the extracellular fluids are diluted, for example, by the intake of a large quantity of water, secretion of ADH by the pituitary gland is repressed, the distal tubular epithelial cells become impermeable to water and, as a consequence, a large quantity of dilute urine is excreted. The end result is to lose water from the body, thus restoring the tonicity of the body fluids to normal. Conversely, concentration of body fluids promotes the secretion of ADH thus leading to increased water re-absorption in the renal tubules and consequent water conservation by the body.

The volume of the body fluids, or the body's water balance, depends essentially on the equilibrium between the amount of water ingested and that lost from the body. The volume of water obtained from food and drink and metabolic reactions is fairly constant in each individual, although it varies over short periods of time. The variation in the volume of water ingested is usually mediated by the sensation of thirst and is adjusted according to the needs of the body. The sensation of thirst is due to the activity of a centre in the hypothalamus which responds to excessive concentration of the body fluids. It must be appreciated that body fluid volume is intimately related to body sodium, because of osmotic factors. (See Fig. 9.1.)

Electrolytes and ions. Much of the excretion of electrolytes and ions is carried out by the kidney in accordance with the needs of the body. The excretion of sodium, for example, is controlled by multiple regulatory mechanisms including the action of the hormone aldosterone. Sodium is filtered freely through the renal glomeruli but the bulk of it is re-absorbed in the renal tubules. This re-absorption is an active process that is regulated by the hormone aldosterone which is secreted by the suprarenal cortex and has a direct action on the renal tubules. The rate of secretion of aldosterone by the suprarenal glands is controlled by the sodium concentration of the extracellular fluids. If the sodium level falls, aldosterone secretion is increased, thus favouring increased re-absorption of sodium by the renal tubules with a consequent conservation of sodium.

Conversely, if the sodium level of the extracellular fluids is excessive, aldosterone secretion is reduced, thus favouring elimination of sodium from the body in the urine. Potassium also passes through the glomerular filter and much of the filtered potassium is re-absorbed in the proximal renal tubule by an active process. The ion is then secreted into the distal tubules, the rate of potassium secretion being influenced by the rate of flow of tubular fluid. Under normal circumstances the amount secreted is approximately equal to the potassium intake, and potassium balance is maintained.

In the final analysis, the availability of the various constituents of the body fluids depends upon a balance between the amount ingested and the amount lost by excretion or by metabolic activities. The amount ingested is regulated to a large extent by the sensation of appetite, a sensation which, like thirst, is mediated by the hypothalamus. The concentration of body fluid constituents does not depend only on the total body content of the particular constituent, but also upon its availability to the body fluids. Thus, for example, most body calcium is 'stored' in the bones, being released to the body fluids as required. This release is controlled by the hormone parathormone. Similarly, glucose is stored as glycogen but is made available to the body fluids in response to complex hormonal mechanisms.

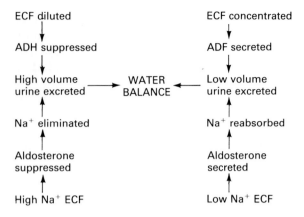

Fig. 9.1 Maintenance of water balance.

FLUID AND ELECTROLYTE IMBALANCE

It is apparent from this brief outline of the normal regulatory mechanisms that the body fluids may be disturbed in three ways. Thus there may be abnormalities of: volume; composition; distribution.

ABNORMALITIES OF VOLUME

Water depletion or dehydration

Water is continually being lost from the body in urine, expired air, and insensible sweating. By these means the irreducible minimum water loss is about 1200 ml daily, representing 2.5% of the total body water. If corresponding amounts of water are not taken in, water depletion will develop. Similarly, water depletion or dehydration may result from excessive sweating, diarrhoea and vomiting, renal disease, or hormonal disturbances.

The initial effect is a reduction in volume of the extracellular fluid with a consequent rise in its crystalloid concentration and osmotic pressure. As a result, water is drawn out of the cells, thus disturbing their metabolism. Ultimately all the fluid compartments lose water and gain in crystalloid content and all end up with the same, slightly elevated, osmotic pressure.

The volume of urine is decreased to a minimum by increased secretion of ADH. The excretion of electrolytes is increased in an attempt to preserve the tonicity of the extracellular fluid but this does,

of course, result in electrolyte depletion. It should be emphasized that in so-called simple water deprivation there is not only obvious water loss but also an additional loss of electrolytes. In correcting dehydration, therefore, both water and electrolytes must be given.

As the plasma volume falls, the osmotic pressure of the plasma protein rises whilst the venous and capillary pressures fall. Acting through the tissue fluid cycle these two factors tend to keep up plasma volume at the expense of the interstitial fluid. Thus the plasma volume changes last and least, its maintenance being vital in order to maintain cardiac output. It is important to appreciate this since the usual estimates of plasma volume, haemoglobin concentration, or plasma protein concentration are not reliable guides to the degree of water deprivation. When changes in plasma volume or composition are obvious, the clinical state is grave.

The patient will present clinically in a state of profound collapse, with a loss of tissue turgor; grey, dry skin and mucous membranes; a rapid pulse and ventilatory rate; and a very low blood pressure. He will be extremely restless and irritable, and may even lapse into unconsciousness.

The effects of water deprivation are particularly important in infants because of the peculiarities of their renal function. Since in utero much of the work of the kidney is carried out by the placenta, the kidney in early life may not be fully developed in a functional sense. An excessive volume of fluid, by adult standards, is needed to eliminate waste products. Water deprivation or excess fluid loss rapidly induces renal failure with retention of urea, electrolyte disturbances and early death.

Water retention or water intoxication

Normally the total water which is ingested is in excess of the volume required to make good the obligatory water losses via the skin, respiratory tract, and kidneys. Normal kidneys have no difficulty in excreting the excess water even when the water intake is considerable. However if the rate of water ingestion exceeds the normal kidney's excretion ability, water intoxication will occur. More frequently this condition occurs when there is some disturbance of renal function or of secretion of the appropriate hormones. The latter may occur, for example, in the postoperative period when there may be excessive secretion of antiduretic hormone or vasopressin.

When water is retained it eventually becomes distributed throughout all the fluid compartments of the body. Initially the extracellular fluids become hypotonic and then water is drawn by osmosis into the cells. The initial relative fall in sodium level, due to water dilution, may be first manifested by nausea and vomiting. With the movement of water into the brain cells, neurological symptoms appear: confusion, irritability, headaches and dizziness, and (later) convulsions, coma, and death. Simple restriction of water is the safest treatment but it may be necessary to give hypertonic saline intravenously. This increases the osmolarity of the extracellular fluid and, as a result, the excess water is drawn from the cells.

ABNORMALITIES OF COMPOSITION

Sodium depletion (hyponatraemia)

Sodium depletion may be seen in severe vomiting, diarrhoea, sweating, haemorrhage, or burns, all of which cause an excessive loss of salt and water from the body. Whilst the water deficit may be made good by drinking, these conditions usually produce a depletion of both salt and water. Sodium depletion may also occur in renal disorders, such as the diuretic phase of acute renal failure, in certain hormonal disturbances, and as the result of various drugs, particularly diuretics.

The reaction of the body is to secrete increased amounts of aldosterone thus ensuring that all the sodium in the glomerular filtrate is re-absorbed. If this is unsuccessful the extracellular fluid becomes hypotonic and water tends to move into the cells. This produces intracellular oedema with disturbance of cell function.

In addition, because of the lowered plasma osmotic pressure, ADH secretion falls and excess fluid is lost by the kidney. The resultant decrease in plasma volume leads to a decreased cardiac output and a fall in arterial blood pressure. The body will initially compensate by a generalized vasoconstriction, but unless hyponatraemia is corrected this compensatory mechanism will ultimately fail and circulatory collapse will ensue.

Sodium retention (hypernatraemia)

Dietary sodium chloride is normally in excess of that required by the body and the excess is excreted by the kidneys. Normal kidneys have no difficulty in eliminating very large dietary intakes of sodium. However, many patients with renal disease retain sodium, a variety of mechanisms being involved. Sodium retention is also seen in congestive cardiac failure and in conditions where excessive aldosterone is secreted. The retention of sodium, with a consequent retention of chloride and water, leads to an increase in the volume of extracellular fluid. This increase is manifested clinically by the condition of oedema. The expansion of the blood volume results in a rise in venous pressure, increased cardiac output, and elevated arterial blood pressure.

Potassium depletion (hypokalaemia)

Potassium depletion occurs when losses from the body exceed the intake. However, a fall in serum potassium can occur if there is excessive uptake of extracellular potassium by the cells. The causes of hypokalaemia, therefore, are complex but the condition may be seen when there is increased secretion of adrenal cortical hormones, when the blood hydrogen ion concentration is decreased, or when renal re-absorption of sodium is impaired. The latter may be seen in association with certain diuretics. The uptake of extracellular potassium by the cells may be increased by the administration of insulin and glucose. Severe vomiting or diarrhoea may also lead to potassium depletion.

Hypokalaemia may produce neurological disorders, including drowsiness, apathy, confusion and coma, muscular weakness, disturbed renal function, and interference with cardiac action which may result in sudden death.

Potassium excess (hyperkalaemia)

This condition is most commonly seen in renal failure but may also be associated with inadequate secretion of aldosterone by the suprarenal glands.

It is sometimes a complication of intravenous therapy and blood transfusion.

The most common manifestation of hyperkalaemia is muscle weakness and, as with the condition of hypokalaemia, high levels of serum potassium may interfere with cardiac function leading to sudden death.

ABNORMALITIES OF DISTRIBUTION

As has been indicated, disturbances of both volume of water and sodium concentration, particularly the latter, will lead to an inappropriate distribution of body fluids. The most common clinical manifestation of an abnormal distribution of body fluids is oedema (excessive accumulation of fluid within the interstitial tissues). From the earlier discussion of the normal tissue fluid cycle, it is apparent that oedema may occur in the following circumstances:

1. When the intracapillary blood pressure is raised
2. When the plasma protein concentration is reduced with a consequent reduction in intravascular osmotic pressure
3. When there is a general expansion of the extracellular fluid volume, secondary to sodium retention.

A localized form of oedema may also be seen when capillary permeability is increased or lymphatic drainage is impaired.

ACID-BASE BALANCE/IMBALANCE

In the previous section the volume and composition of the body fluids, both normal and abnormal, was considered. However, another extremely important aspect of body fluids is their relative acidity or alkalinity – the so-called acid–base balance.

It has been traditional to express this property of body fluids in terms of the pH of the fluid. This term, introduced by Sorensen, is based on the dissociation of water into hydrogen ions and hydroxyl ions. Pure water is ordinarily split up or dissociated to a very slight extent into hydrogen ions (H^+) and hydroxyl ions (OH^-) as follows:

$$H_2O \leftrightharpoons H^+ + OH^-$$

Because the dissociation is so very slight the actual concentration of each of these ions is extremely low. Thus the concentration of each ion is only 10^{-7} mol/litre. The product of the two remains constant at 10^{-14} and hence the concentration of one ion automatically fixes the concentration of the other. The acidity or alkalinity of a solution is a direct function of the concentration of its hydrogen ions. If there are more than 10^{-7} hydrogen ions, the solution is acid; if less, the solution is alkaline.

For convenience, hydrogen ion concentration is expressed as the pH, which is a logarithmic function of the concentration. In this way the pH of a solution can be described as varying between 0 and +14. It is essential to realize that the use of this mathematical manipulation produces a numerical change, in that the lower the pH, the higher the hydrogen ion concentration, and thus the greater the acidity. Conversely, the higher the pH, the lower the hydrogen ion concentration and thus the greater the alkalinity. It is also important to realize that a small change in pH represents a large change in hydrogen ion concentration; for example, a change in the pH of the blood from 7.4 to 7.3 represents an actual increase in hydrogen ion concentration of 26%.

It is also possible to consider and express the concentration of hydrogen ions in the body fluids in absolute terms, that is, as moles per litre. However, because the concentration of hydrogen ions in the body fluids is extremely low, a very small unit is used. The unit, a nanomole, is equal to one thousand millionth (10^{-9}) of a mole.

The body fluids normally have a hydrogen ion concentration of 35 to 45 nanomoles per litre, their pH being 7.45 to 7.35. The maintenance of a stable hydrogen ion concentration is essential to life, as many of the chemical reactions that occur within the body are very sensitive to the level of hydrogen ion. There are two great systems of regulation of hydrogen ion equilibrium, one of a physico-chemical nature and residing in the cells, whilst the other is physiological and depends on the function of the lungs and kidneys. Physico-chemical regulation is immediate, its effects beginning as soon as there is any deviation in the pH of the plasma, whilst the physiological mechanisms are slower in action.

Physico-chemical mechanisms – the buffer system

Buffers are substances which maintain a solution at a relatively constant pH despite the addition of strong acids or bases. A buffer system is usually formed by a mixture of a weak acid and one of its salts. Within the body the principal buffers are haemoglobin, protein, phosphate, and bicarbonate-carbonic acid. Quantitatively, the bicarbonate-carbonic acid is the most important and its action illustrates the general properties of buffers. When a strong acid, such as hydrochloric acid, is added to such a system the reaction is as follows:

$$NCl + NaHCO_3 \leftrightharpoons NaCl + H_2CO_3$$
$$H_2CO_3 \leftrightharpoons H^+ + HCO_3^-$$

The result is a decrease in the amount of sodium bicarbonate and an increase in carbonic acid, but the increase in hydrogen ion concentration is much smaller than if hydrochloric acid had become dissociated in the absence of a buffer system, since carbonic acid is a weak acid and most of its hydrogen ions remain undissociated.

The buffer systems thus provide an immediate mechanism for minimizing the effect of the continual addition, as a result of metabolic processes, of hydrogen ion to the body fluids. The physiological mechanisms are designed to eliminate excess hydrogen ion from the body and thus regenerate the buffer systems.

Physiological mechanisms – the lungs and kidneys

One of the major end products of cell metabolism is carbon dioxide which is rapidly converted to carbonic acid. This dissociates and releases hydrogen ion in accordance with the following equation:

$$H_2CO_3 \leftrightharpoons H^+ + HCO_3^-$$

As already indicated, the hydrogen ion is buffered by the various body fluid constituents but the main outlet for the large quantities of carbon dioxide produced by cell metabolism is the respiratory tract. Since the respiratory centre is highly sensitive to the level of both carbon dioxide and hydrogen ions within the blood, the lungs are ideally suited to carry out the regulation of hydrogen ion concentration. Thus, when the level of carbon dioxide rises the respiratory centre is stimulated. As a result breathing becomes deeper and more rapid, and consequently a greater quantity of carbon dioxide is discharged from the body.

The kidneys have the capacity to excrete both hydrogen ions and bicarbonate ions as required to restore the acid–base balance of the body fluids to normal and to regenerate the buffer systems. Bicarbonate re-absorption is accomplished by the active secretion of hydrogen ion. Thus, the secretion of hydrogen ion (H^+) by the renal tubular cell into the urine results in the formation of an hydroxyl ion (OH^-) within the cell. This immediately combines with carbon dioxide (CO_2) to form bicarbonate ion (HCO_3^-), the combination being aided by the enzyme carbonic anhydrase. The bicarbonate ion thus formed diffuses back into the blood stream.

The excretion of hydrogen ion by the kidney is aided by two important mechanisms:

1. The presence of phosphate ions in the glomerular filtrate that are capable of combining with excess hydrogen ion:
$$HPO_4^- + H^+ \leftrightharpoons H_2PO_4$$
2. The formation of ammonia (NH_3) by the tubular epithelial cells which can combine with excess hydrogen ion to form ammonium:
$$NH_3^- + H^+ \leftrightharpoons NH_4^+$$

These reactions, by 'mopping up' excess hydrogen ion allow the kidneys to overcome the concentration gradient that would otherwise limit hydrogen ion excretion.

DISTURBANCES OF ACID–BASE BALANCE

Hydrogen ion depletion (alkalosis)

As already indicated, the mean hydrogen ion concentration in arterial blood is about 40 nanomoles per litre (pH 7.4) with a range of normal extending from about 35 to 45 nanomoles per litre (pH 7.45–7.35). Hydrogen ion depletion exists when the concentration falls below the lower limit of normal and the condition thus produced is referred to as alkalosis. As with many other electrolyte disturbances the symptoms may be quite non-specific, including such manifestations as anorexia, nausea, vomiting, headache, and dizziness. An associated disturbance of calcium metabolism may lead to tetany whilst, depending on the type of alkalosis, there will be changes in respiratory and urinary function.

Two types of alkalosis are recognized: respiratory and metabolic.

Respiratory alkalosis. Here, there is an excessive loss of carbon dioxide due to hyperventilation. It may be the result of strong central stimulation of ventilation such as may occur in fevers or in association with intracranial neoplasms. It may also occur in hysterical patients, or is occasionally the result of over-enthusiastic artificial ventilation.

The primary problem is a fall in the concentration of carbonic acid in the blood. Compensation in this condition must be by renal action, the main mechanism being an increased elimination of bicarbonate by the kidneys which, if allowed to persist, will produce reflex metabolic acidosis.

First aid management of hysterical hyperventilation and any associated tetany must be immediate and consists simply of placing a paper bag (or other suitable substitute) over the patient's nose and mouth, causing him to re-breathe expired carbon dioxide.

Metabolic alkalosis. Here the problem is a rise in the plasma bicarbonate level. Metabolic alkalosis may be due to the ingestion of large quantities of sodium bicarbonate, milk, or other antacids (excepting those from the magnesium and aluminium groups which are not readily absorbed through the gut) in the treatment of dyspepsia. It may also result from severe and prolonged vomiting with a consequent loss of gastric acid, or as the result of prolonged nasogastric aspiration. Once metabolic alkalosis is established, complicating factors may perpetuate the condition. For example, hydrogen ions normally compete with potassium ions for secretion in the sodium-potassium exchange system in the distal renal tubules. The reduction of hydrogen ion secretion in alkalosis will increase potassium ion secretion and lead to potassium depletion.

In metabolic alkalosis compensatory hypoventilation occurs, leading to carbon dioxide retention in an effort to raise the pH. In addition, renal elimination of sodium bicarbonate is increased.

Hydrogen ion excess (acidosis)

This is the condition that exists when the hydrogen ion concentration of the arterial plasma exceeds the upper limit of normal, namely 45 nanomoles per litre or pH 7.35.

The elevated hydrogen ion concentration of the body fluids interferes with many cellular activities particularly with its effect on enzyme activity. The effect on the brain cells is early and profound, with apathy, drowsiness and, ultimately, coma. Again, both respiratory and metabolic forms are recognized.

Respiratory acidosis. This form of acidosis is caused by a failure of the respiratory system to eliminate sufficient carbon dioxide. It is seen in the following conditions:

– Emphysema and pneumonia, or any other significant respiratory disease
– Chest and/or diaphragmatic trauma
– Pain, causing improper ventilation
– Exhaustion, resulting in respiratory failure
– Depression of the respiratory centre resulting from narcotic usage, or improper reversion from anaesthesia.

Compensating mechanisms are, of necessity, mainly renal with considerable retention of bicarbonate and increased elimination of hydrogen ions.

Metabolic acidosis. This is the result of either the accumulation of too much acid, and/or the body's inability to excrete it. Common examples of excessive accumulation are seen in untrolled Type 1 diabetes mellitus (where there is an excessive production of keto-acids) and overwhelming sepsis or hypovolaemic shock. In these cases compensation is mainly renal, with conservation of bicarbonate and increased elimination of hydrogen ion utilizing the phosphate and ammonia mechanisms.

Hyperventilation also occurs immediately to increase the loss of plasma carbon dioxide and if allowed to persist, may produce respiratory alkalosis. This hyperventilatory state resolves when the underlying pathophysiology is corrected. Metabolic acidosis may also occur in renal failure/disease due to an inability of the kidney to eliminate hydrogen ions. Compensation, therefore, in this case must be ventilatory but this is relatively inefficient. Because of the nature of the acids retained the elimination of carbon dioxide is of limited value and treatment of the acidosis is by treatment of the renal disease.

TISSUE OXYGENATION AND BLOOD GASES

The maintenance of normal levels of the blood or respiratory gases, oxygen and carbon dioxide, is primarily the responsibility of the respiratory system but is dependent upon a number of other body activities. Oxygen is essential for virtually all cellular metabolic activities, whilst carbon dioxide is the major by-product of cellular metabolism. A depleted supply of oxygen to the cells (hypoxia) and an increased level of carbon dioxide (hypercapnia) will each have a profound effect on body function and will cause death if not corrected. In order to understand the conditions of hypoxia and hypercapnia it is essential to have an appreciation of how the body handles oxygen and carbon dioxide. This involves some knowledge of how the gases are exchanged, both in the lungs and in the tissues, and how they are transported between the lungs and tissues.

The exchange of the gases, oxygen and carbon dioxide, occurs both in the lungs and tissues by a process of diffusion. As already discussed, this is a movement of molecules from an area of high concentration to an area of lower concentration. The molecular concentration of gases can be considered in terms of the pressure the gas exerts since the pressure is directly related to the number of molecules present. And since air is a mixture of gases the concept of partial pressure must also be considered. Thus, in a mixture of gases each gas exerts a pressure that depends on the percentage of that gas in the mixture (Dalton's Law). The pressure exerted by each gas is referred to as its partial pressure. The partial pressure of a particular gas in a mixture can be calculated by multiplying the total pressure of the gas mixture by the fraction of the mixture that the particular gas represents.

For example, dry air at sea level is under a pressure of 760 mmHg and contains 21% oxygen. Therefore the partial pressure of oxygen (pO_2) in dry air at 760 mmHg is:

$$\frac{760 \times 21}{100} = 160 \text{ mmHg}$$

When gases are dissolved in a liquid each gas goes into solution independently of the other, in accordance with its own solubility and its partial pressure. The partial pressure of a gas in a liquid, usually referred to as the tension of the gas, is the pressure of the dry gas with which the dissolved gas would be in equilibrium.

The partial pressure exerted by each gas, both within the alveoli of the lungs and in the body fluids, is of great importance in determining the rate and efficiency with which the gas will diffuse through the cell membranes, because it represents the number of molecules per unit area, or concentration, of that gas – it is a measure of the total force that each gas exerts against the walls surrounding it. Thus the 'penetrating power' of the gas is directly proportional to its partial pressure.

GASEOUS EXCHANGE IN THE LUNGS

The efficiency with which oxygen and carbon dioxide are exchanged in the lungs depends upon:

1. The diffusion concentration gradient
2. The properties of the pulmonary membrane
3. The diffusion coefficient of the particular gas.

The concentration gradient

This is represented by the difference in the partial pressures of the gases in the alveoli and in the pulmonary capillary plasma.

The partial pressure of oxygen (pO_2) of non-aerated blood entering the pulmonary capillaries is only 40 mmHg in comparison with the alveolar pressure of 101 mmHg. The diffusion gradient, therefore, is 61 mmHg causing an extremely rapid flow of oxygen from the alveoli into the plasma.

The partial pressure of carbon dioxide (pCO_2) in the blood entering the lungs is approximately 45 mmHg. A pressure gradient of about 5 mmHg exists between the pulmonary capillary plasma and the alveolar air, causing carbon dioxide to diffuse out of the plasma into the alveolus.

The diffusion membrane

The exchange of gases must occur across the pulmonary membrane and hence the properties of this membrane are of importance. Two factors must be considered:

1. The area for exchange – it has been calculated that the 60 ml of blood that are present in the pulmonary vascular bed at any one time, are spread over 60 square metres of pulmonary membrane. This ensures a very adequate exposure of the capillary blood to the alveolar air.
2. The thickness of the membrane – the pulmonary membrane is very thin, being composed of extremely flattened alveolar lining cells, capillary endothelial cells, and their fused basement membranes. In addition, the gases must negotiate the very thin film of alveolar fluid. Although the barrier separating the blood from the alveolar air is a complex one, its total thickness is less than one micron.

The diffusion coefficient of the gas

The ease with which a gas will diffuse across a membrane depends upon the molecular weight of the gas and its solubility in the membrane. These factors are expressed as the diffusion coefficient of the gas. The diffusion coefficient of oxygen is 1, whilst that of carbon dioxide is 20.3, that is, other things being equal, carbon dioxide will diffuse 20 times more rapidly than oxygen. The reason for this is that carbon dioxide is much more soluble in the pulmonary membrane.

The interdependence of these three factors results in an equilibrium of gaseous exchange.

GASEOUS EXCHANGE IN THE TISSUES

In the tissues the gaseous exchanges again occur by means of diffusion, and similar factors are involved.

Concentration gradient

The oxygen pressure in the tissue cells is always very low, rarely rising above 20 mmHg. This is so because the metabolic activities of the cell rapidly use up the available oxygen. The blood in the tissue capillaries has a pO_2 of 100 mmHg and hence oxygen will diffuse out of the blood according to a concentration gradient of over 80 mmHg.

The carbon dioxide pressure of the tissues in the resting state is about 46 mmHg. Arterial blood reaches the tissues with a pCO_2 of 40 mmHg and hence carbon dioxide will diffuse into the blood according to a concentration gradient of 6 mmHg.

Diffusion membrane

In this case the gases must diffuse through the erythrocyte membrane, the plasma, the capillary endothelium with its basement membrane, the tissue fluid, and the tissue cell membrane. Again the barrier is a complex one but very thin.

Diffusion coefficient of gases

These are as described above.

CARRIAGE OF GASES IN THE BLOOD

When oxygen diffuses from the lungs into the blood a small proportion of it becomes dissolved in the fluids of the plasma and erythrocytes, but approximately 60 times as much combines immediately with the haemoglobin of the erythrocytes and is carried in this combination to the tissues. The haemoglobin, which acts as a carrier for the oxygen, is a conjugated protein made up of an iron containing pigment (haem) and protein. It has the capacity to combine with oxygen in the molecular rather than the ionic form and to transport the oxygen in this way. This unusual combination is termed oxygenation rather than oxidation. The most important property of the haemoglobin molecule is its ability to form a loose and reversible combination with oxygen, associating with oxygen in the capillaries of the lung and dissociating with oxygen in the capillaries of the tissues. This reversible reaction of the combination of haemoglobin with oxygen and its subsequent dissociation is usually written:

$$Hb + O_2 \leftrightharpoons HbO_2$$

The amount of oxygen which a given amount of haemoglobin will take up, that is, its percentage saturation, is a function of the partial pressure of the oxygen in the atmosphere with which it is in contact. Thus at the normal oxygen tension (pO_2) that exists in arterial blood (100 mmHg) the haemoglobin is 95–98% saturated. A further increase in oxygen tension has only a slight effect on the saturation of haemoglobin (Fig. 9.2).

As the oxygen tension falls, the saturation of haemoglobin declines slowly until the pO_2 drops to about 50 mmHg at which point a rapid release of oxygen from the haemoglobin takes place. This initial lag in dissociation of oxyhaemoglobin provides a fairly wide margin of safety which permits the pO_2 in the pulmonary capillaries to fall as low as 80 mmHg before any significant decrease in the oxygenation of haemoglobin occurs.

A number of factors, such as temperature and the presence of certain electrolytes, affect the dissociation of oxyhaemoglobin, but most important is the effect of carbon dioxide: the presence of carbon dioxide renders the oxyhaemoglobin more liable to dissociate. It is probable that this influence of carbon dioxide is due to the formation of carbonic acid with a consequent lowering of the pH of the environment, this increase in acidity facilitating the dissociation of oxyhaemoglobin. The importance of this effect is that the raised carbon dioxide level in the tissues facilitates the liberation of oxygen from the blood; conversely, the lower carbon dixoide level in the alveolar capillaries assists the uptake of oxygen by the blood.

The conversion of reduced haemoglobin to oxyhaemoglobin normally takes place very rapidly. Under resting conditions the pO_2 in the pulmonary capillary blood is equal to that in the alveolus before the blood has reached the midpoint of the capillary. During strenuous exercise, therefore, there is a wide safety margin that allows for the more rapid passage of blood through the pulmonary capillaries.

The reduction of haemoglobin, and therefore the release of oxygen, also occurs with great rapidity. In addition, those factors that increase the extent of dissociation of oxyhaemoglobin (raised temperature and increased pCO_2) also increase its rate of dissociation. These influences are present, of course, in active tissues.

Oxygen utilization

Each 100 ml of arterial blood leaves the lungs carrying about 0.3 ml of oxygen in solution, and about 19 ml in combination with haemoglobin. The pO_2 is about 100 mmHg. When the blood reaches the tissues where the oxygen tension at rest is about 40 mmHg the oxyhaemoglobin dissociates and approximately 5–6 ml of oxygen per 100 ml of blood (or 30% of the available oxygen) is liberated. As a result the venous blood as it leaves the tissues has an oxygen tension of 40 mmHg and an oxygen content of about 14 ml per 100 ml of blood. The proportion of haemoglobin that loses its oxygen to the tissues during each passage through the capillaries is called the utilization coefficient. When the tissues are at rest this utilization coefficient is 26%.

When the tissues are in extreme need of oxygen, such as may occur in skeletal muscle during vigorous exercise, the oxygen pressure in the tissues may fall to extremely low levels, allowing oxygen to diffuse from the capillary blood much more rapidly than usual. The oxyhaemoglobin

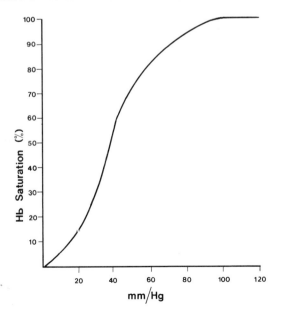

Fig. 9.2 Oxyhaemoglobin dissociation curve.

dissociates more completely and this increased dissociation is further aided by increased temperature, carbon dioxide tension, and the presence of other acid metabolites.

These factors may enable three times the volume of oxygen to be extracted from the same volume of blood compared with the resting utilization; that is, the oxygen utilization coefficient may rise to as high as 78%. Since the cardiac output can increase as much as six-fold then the combination of increased blood flow and increased oxygen utilization provides a potent mechanism for ensuring that the tissues are oxygenated in times of need.

Arterial blood gas analysis

Arterial blood gas analysis gives a measure of the blood's pH, and the levels of oxygen and carbon dioxide expressed as pressure (pO_2, pCO_2).

Normal arterial blood gas values at sea level are:

pH   7.35–7.45
pO_2 90–100 mmHg
pCO_2 35–45 mmHg

The best possible pO_2 a person can have while breathing sea-level air is a little over 100 mmHg:

760 mmHg (air pressure) × 20% (proportion of oxygen in air) = 152 mmHg − 47 mmHg (water vapour) = 105 mmHg.

While blood gas analysis gives a measure of the amount of oxygen dissolved in the plasma, it is not a measurement of the amount of oxygen in the haemoglobin, but does allow an indirect assessment of this. A blood gas analysis demonstrates the lungs' ability to facilitate gaseous exchange, in that if the lungs are working efficiently, oxygen will diffuse across onto the haemoglobin and into the plasma.

The test has clinical use by reference to the oxyhaemoglobin curve (see Fig. 9.2, page 87), which shows that a pO_2 of 90–100 mmHg gives 100% saturation of haemoglobin, and that as pO_2 falls so does saturation.

However, a good level of pO_2 does not necessarily mean that satisfactory tissue oxygenation is taking place. For example, a patient with a pO_2 of 100 mmHg can die from hypoxia if his haemoglobin level is low.

Factors which must be taken into account when assessing the results of a blood gas analysis are:

- The level and functional status of the patient's haemoglobin
- His blood volume
- His cardiac status
- The presence of respiratory disease
- The concentration of oxygen in the inspired air.

Transport of carbon dioxide

The carbon dioxide formed during cell metabolism passes from the cytoplasm of the tissue cells into the interstitial or tissue fluid, and then from the tissue fluid into the blood by a process of simple diffusion. Within the blood the carbon dioxide is carried in three ways:

1. In solution within the plasma.
2. In association with haemoglobin as a compound called carbamino-haemoglobin. Carbon dioxide associates with, and dissociates from, haemoglobin in a manner similar to that of oxygen. When the blood is exposed to the lower carbon dioxide tension in the lungs the carbamino-haemoglobin rapidly dissociates to release carbon dioxide. This dissociation is aided by the fact that the affinity of haemoglobin for oxygen is much higher than its affinity for carbon dioxide.
3. As bicarbonate. As the carbon dioxide enters the erythrocyte it combines with water to form carbonic acid, this combination being facilitated by the enzyme carbonic anhydrase. The carbonic acid thus formed immediately dissociates into hydrogen ion and bicarbonate:

$$H_2O + CO_2 \leftrightharpoons H_2CO_3$$
$$H_2CO_3 \leftrightharpoons H^+ + HCO_3^-$$

Some of the bicarbonate remains within the erythrocyte but most passes out of the cell into the plasma. The hydrogen ions liberated in the erythrocyte by this series of reactions are buffered by the haemoglobin.

PULMONARY FUNCTION – NORMAL AND ABNORMAL

The primary function of the lungs is to 'arterialize' the venous blood. This involves the addition of adequate amounts of oxygen and the elimination of sufficient quantities of carbon dioxide. The achievement of this function involves three processes:

1. *Ventilation.* A large volume of inspired air must reach the alveoli and this air must be distributed evenly throughout the lungs.
2. *Diffusion.* The oxygen and carbon dioxide must pass freely across the alveolo-capillary membranes.
3. *Perfusion.* The pulmonary capillary blood flow must be adequate in volume and all the mixed venous blood must be distributed evenly to all the ventilated alveoli. It is essential that this gas exchange be achieved with a minimal expenditure of energy by the respiratory and circulatory systems. The most important factor here is the work involved in the mechanism of pulmonary ventilation.

Ventilation, diffusion, and perfusion are dynamic processes which have as their aim the maintenance of normal pressures of oxygen and carbon dioxide in the alveolar gas and pulmonary capillary blood flow. Any one or a combination of these processes may be impaired in a variety of diseases, and tests are available to demonstrate impairment of pulmonary function as a whole and to localize the area or process that is at fault.

The diagnosis and treatment of most respiratory disorders depends to a large extent on an understanding of the basic physiological principles involved. In general the abnormalities that lead to respiratory insufficiency can be considered in three broad categories:

1. Those that cause inadequate ventilation of the lungs
2. Those that reduce gaseous diffusion through the respiratory membrane
3. Those that decrease oxygen transport from the lungs to the tissues.

Inadequate ventilation of pulmonary alveoli

Paralysis of respiratory muscles

Paralysis of the respiratory muscles will impair ventilation, although considerable compensation is possible by overactivity of the muscles not affected.

Diseases that increase the work of ventilation

Many pulmonary diseases increase the work required to move air into and out of the lungs. Three different types of abnormality are seen:

Increased airways resistance – the respiratory passages can be obstructed in a number of ways. Airways resistance is particularly increased in bronchial asthma and in emphysema wherein air flow is impeded in the smaller bronchioles.

Increased tissue resistance – many diseases of the lungs often destroy much of the elasticity of the lungs so that little recoil occurs. As a result effort must be expended by the respiratory muscles to deflate the lungs as well as to inflate them.

Decreased compliance of the lungs and chest wall – during inhalation, active muscular contraction is employed to enlarge the thoracic cage. One of the major forces that must be overcome is the elasticity of the lungs and thorax, that is, their tendency to recoil when stretched. The expansibility or 'stretchability' of the lungs and thorax is referred to as their compliance. This is expressed as the volume increase in the lungs for each unit increase in intra-alveolar pressure. A useful analogy is to consider the work involved in blowing up a balloon.

Any disease which makes the tissue of the lungs or of the chest wall less distensible than usual reduces the compliance and therefore increases the work that must be expended by the respiratory muscles to expand the lungs. A reduction in compliance may occur in diseases such as silicosis and sarcoidosis.

Decreased pulmonary diffusing capacity

This may be due to: decreased area of the respiratory membrane – perhaps the best example of this is pulmonary emphysema, where there is progressive destruction of the alveoli walls. However, a similar effect will be produced by removal or destruction of part or the whole of a lung; increased thickness of the respiratory membrane – the most common acute cause of this (an alveolo-capillary block) is pulmonary oedema, resulting from left heart failure, or pneumonia. However, a number of diseases can cause progressive deposition of fibrous tissue in the interstitial spaces between the alveolar membrane and the pulmonary capillary membrane, therefore increasing the thickness of the respiratory membrane. Since the rate of gaseous diffusion through the respiratory membrane is inversely proportional to the distance that the gas must diffuse, it follows that any alveolo-capillary block will reduce the diffusing capacity of the lung.

Abnormalities of oxygen transport from lungs to tissues

Conditions that reduce oxygen transport from the lungs to the tissues include:

Anaemia – in which the total amount of haemoglobin available to transport the oxygen is reduced.

Carbon monoxide – poisoning in which a large proportion of the haemoglobin becomes bound to carbon monoxide and hence is not available for oxygen transport.

Decreased blood flow to tissues – which may be due to low cardiac output or to localized tissue ischaemia.

The various factors listed above that may lead to respiratory insufficiency presuppose that the air being inspired is of normal composition. The inhalation of air deficient in oxygen, such as may occur at high altitude or during anaesthesia, will, of course, lead to a reduction of the partial pressure of oxygen in the alveolar air. As a result the diffusion gradient for oxygen will be reduced and there may be a consequent diminution in the oxygenation of the pulmonary capillary blood.

MANIFESTATIONS OF RESPIRATORY INSUFFICIENCY

Hypoxia

The term hypoxia refers to a diminished availability of oxygen to the cells of the body – a state that is often incorrectly referred to as anoxia. Traditionally four types of hypoxia are described and although many other classifications have been proposed the original categories remain the most useful. Thus hypoxia may be classified as:

Hypoxic hypoxia – here the pO_2 is lower than normal, and consequently the haemoglobin is not saturated with oxygen to the normal content. It is a most serious form of hypoxia and may be due to a number of causes. Most of these causes are discussed when considering inadequate ventilation of the alveoli and decreased pulmonary diffusion capacity (page 92). This type of hypoxia is also associated with decreased atmospheric oxygen, such as may occur at high altitude, and hence it is of importance in aviation medicine.

Anaemic hypoxia – here the pO_2 is normal, but the quantity of functioning haemoglobin is reduced. This is less serious in its effects than the hypoxic form. Of the 19 ml of oxygen normally present per 100 ml of arterial blood, only 5 ml of oxygen are used under resting conditions. Since a person with a haemoglobin of only 50% of normal can carry 9.5 ml of oxygen per 100 ml of blood, his resting requirements are readily satisfied. However, his capacity for increased activity is greatly diminished as he does not have the normal reserves of blood oxygen to call upon. Anaemic hypoxia may occur in:

• Anaemia – where there is reduced haemoglobin.
• Carbon monoxide poisoning – where the haemoglobin becomes firmly united with the carbon monoxide and hence is not available for oxygen transport.

Stagnant hypoxia – the pO_2 and saturation of haemoglobin are both normal, but oxygen is supplied to the tissues in insufficient amounts because of a decrease in the blood flow. This is seen when the cardiac output is impaired such as may occur, for example, in cardiac failure or shock. It may also occur as a local phenomenon. Thus in chronic venous congestion of the liver, for example, hypoxic damage may be evident in the parenchymal cells.

Histotoxic hypoxia – the tissue cells are poisoned and cannot make effective use of the oxygen supplied to them. An example is cyanide poisoning, which interferes with cellular oxidative processes, and it may also be seen in association with certain narcotics.

Clinical manifestations

Hypoxia, if severe enough, can cause death of cells. Sudden hypoxia, such as may occur as a result of de-pressurization of an aeroplane at high altitude, will cause almost immediate loss of consciousness and, if the condition is not relieved, death will occur within 5 minutes or less. Less severe hypoxia will produce a variety of mental aberrations such as drowsiness, impaired judgement, excitability, and disorientation. Headaches may occur, as may nausea and vomiting. Two manifestations of considerable clinical importance are:

Cyanosis – due to the presence of an excessive amount of reduced (that is, deoxygenated) haemoglobin in the blood. About 5 g per 100 ml of blood of reduced haemoglobin is necessary to produce recognizable cyanosis. In polycythaemia, cyanosis is very common because of the large amount of haemoglobin in the blood, whereas in severe anaemia cyanosis is rare because it is difficult for there to be enough deoxygenated haemoglobin to produce the blue colour. Cyanosis is common in all diseases that produce hypoxic hypoxia.

Dyspnoea. Dyspnoea has been defined as a 'consciousness of the necessity for increased ventilatory effort'. It may be physiological, such as occurs after violent exertion, or pathological such as may be seen in a variety of diseases. Thus pathological dyspnoea may occur:

- Where there is mechanical interference with ventilation, for example as in bronchial asthma
- In cardiac conditions which are associated with pulmonary oedema
- In metabolic acidosis such as occurs in diabetes mellitus. The raised hydrogen ion concentration of the body fluids 'drives' the respiratory centre excessively.
- In the presence of carbon dioxide excess.

The first effect is increased depth of pulmonary ventilation, and later actual dyspnoea appears. Then, as the carbon dioxide increases, ventilations become not only deeper but more rapid. Finally, cardiac and respiratory functions are depressed, confusion and headache occur, and then loss of consciousness and death. In many circumstances, conditions of lack of oxygen are associated with excess carbon dioxide.

Oxygen therapy

Oxygen therapy is of great value in certain types of hypoxia but of almost no value in other types. A consideration of the physiological principles outlined above will indicate the relative value of oxygen therapy in various conditions:

- In atmospheric hypoxia, oxygen therapy can obviously completely correct the depressed oxygen level in the inspired gases and therefore provide a totally effective therapy.
- In hypoventilation hypoxia, a person breathing 100% oxygen can move five times as much oxygen into the alveoli with each breath as he can when breathing normal air. Thus the available oxygen can be increased to as much as 400% above normal.
- In hypoxia caused by impaired diffusion, oxygen therapy can increase the pO_2 in the lungs from a normal value of about 100 mgHg to as high as 600 mmHg. This causes a greatly increased diffusion gradient for oxygen.
- In hypoxia caused by anaemia or carbon monoxide poisoning, oxygen therapy is of some value. Thus an increase in alveolar pO_2 from a normal of 100 mmHg to 600 mmHg increases the total oxygen in the blood by some 30% – often the difference between life and death. This increase is due partly to complete saturation of the haemoglobin (from 97% to 100%) but more importantly to increased solution of oxygen in the plasma.
- In hypoxia caused by circulatory deficiency ('stagnant hypoxia') the value of oxygen therapy is slight, as the problem is one of sluggish flow of blood and not insufficient oxygen.
- In hypoxia due to inadequate tissue use of oxygen ('histotoxic hypoxia') oxygen therapy is usually of no benefit.

Oxygen toxicity

Unlike hypoxia, excessive oxygen levels are seldom a problem in clinical medicine. However oxygen toxicity has been noted following prolonged therapeutic administration of oxygen. Initially there may be irritation of the air passages but ultimately lung damage will occur. Thus prolonged exposure to concentrations of oxygen in inspired gases in excess of 40% may result in permanent damage to the lung. Initially there is a swelling of the alveolar lining cells, an exudation of fluid into the alveolar walls, and ultimately the formation of dense membranes over the inner walls of the alveoli. These changes cause serious interference to the processes of gas exchange.

Prolonged administration of oxygen to infants, particularly if premature, may cause damage to the retina with resultant visual defects – a condition known as retrolental fibroplasia.

Hypercapnia

Although one might expect hypercapnia to invariably accompany hypoxia, this is by no means true. However, hypercapnia will be seen in association with hypoxia when the latter is caused by inadequate ventilation. When hypoxia is due to poor diffusion through the pulmonary membrane, serious hypercapnia is seldom present since carbon dioxide diffuses 20 times more efficiently than oxygen.

In the clinical situation hypercapnia may be seen when the muscles of ventilation are weakened or paralysed as, for example, in bulbar poliomyelitis; when airways obstruction is present, as in bronchial asthma; or when there is a gross disturbance of alveolar structure and blood flow, as in pulmonary emphysema.

The carbon dioxide retention results in respiratory acidosis since the gas combines with water to form carbonic acid. In an attempt to correct the acidosis, bicarbonate is reabsorbed from the renal tubules and the blood bicarbonate level rises.

The main clinical manifestations of hypercapnia are due to vasodilation. The patient has an increased skin temperature, and a full bounding pulse. Confusion is usual, followed by coma, with respiratory depression and death.

Hypocapnia

Hypocapnia results from voluntary or involuntary hyperventilation. As a result of the excessive loss of carbon dioxide from the body, a respiratory alkalosis develops.

Prolonged hypocapnia may produce neurological symptoms such as dizziness, and because of associated disturbances of plasma calcium levels, signs of tetany may develop.

BODY TEMPERATURE

NORMAL BODY TEMPERATURE

Animals which are able to maintain a relatively constant body temperature in spite of great variations of external temperature are said to be homeothermal, in contrast to poikilothermal animals whose body temperature varies with that of the external environment. Humans are homeothermal in that they are able to maintain a constant body temperature, achieving this by regulatory mechanisms which continually balance the heat gained by the body against that which is lost by the body. By these mechanisms the body temperature is normally maintained between 36.1–37.4°C.

The control of normal body temperature can best be considered in the form of a simple equation:

$$\text{BODY TEMPERATURE} = \text{HEAT GAIN} - \text{HEAT LOSS}$$

Heat gain

The heat gained by the body is that due to heat produced within the body, plus that gained from the external environment.

Heat production

Heat is produced by the metabolic activities of the body. In some organs, such as the liver and heart, heat production is relatively constant. Skeletal muscle, on the other hand, makes a variable contribution to heat production, producing very little heat at rest but a great deal during vigorous exercise.

The heat produced under resting or 'basal' conditions is 155–167 kJ (37–40 kcal) per square metre of body surface per hour. The average man at rest produces about 7100 kJ per day whilst the average woman at rest produces 6300 kJ per day. Moderate physical activity may double this heat production, whilst with very heavy work production may be increased four-fold or more.

Gain from external environment

The body can take in heat from objects hotter than itself by the process of radiation. The direct heat of the sun is an example. In addition, when the environmental temperature exceeds that of the skin, the body surface takes up heat directly from its immediate surroundings by the process of conduction.

Heat loss

Heat is lost from the body in several ways:

By radiation from the body to cooler objects at a distance. The amount of heat lost in this way depends on the surface area of skin and the temperature difference between the skin and surrounding objects.

By conduction and convection to the surrounding atmosphere if its temperature is lower than that of the skin. The air in immediate contact with the skin is warmed, the heated molecules move away, and cooler ones come in to take their place. These in turn are warmed and so the process goes on. The actual warming of the air is by a process of direct conduction of heat from body to air, whilst the movements of the air constitute convection currents.

The loss of heat by conduction, convection, and radiation is greatly influenced by environmental conditions; it is much greater, for example, when the weather is cool and windy. It also depends on the amount of heat at the surface of the body, this being governed by the state of the blood vessels in the skin and subcutaneous tissues. Vasodilation in these areas aids the loss of heat, whilst vasoconstriction retards this loss. A layer of 'trapped' air will lessen heat loss. Birds achieve this by fluffing their feathers and animals by erecting their hair. Humans, to a large extent, are denied these mechanisms, although 'goose-pimples', due to contraction of the pilo-erector muscles, represent an attempt to reduce heat loss. Both animals and, to a lesser extent humans, decrease heat loss by

'curling-up', thus reducing the body surface area exposed to the environment.

Humans, of course, exercise a great deal of control over these heat loss mechanisms both by artificially altering the environment (heating and cooling devices) and by covering, or partially covering, the body surface with clothing.

By evaporation of water. The essential fact to remember is that when water is converted to water vapour, heat is required, and this heat is taken from the immediate environment. Thus the evaporation of one litre of water from the body surface requires nearly 2500 kJ of heat. Evaporation of water takes place from the lungs and from the skin, the most important site in humans being the skin. Water is lost from the skin both by insensible loss and by sweating.

Insensible loss consists of the passage of water by diffusion through the skin surface. It is called insensible because it cannot be seen or felt. The fluid is not produced by the glands. It is lost over the whole body surface at a fairly uniform rate and is largely independent of environmental conditions.

Sweating is the process whereby a secretion from the sweat glands in the skin occurs in response to a variety of stimuli, for example a rise of external or body temperature, emotional stress, or in association with nausea, vomiting, fainting, and hypoglycaemia.

By far the most important type of sweating, in relation to the control of body temperature, is the so-called thermal sweating – that which occurs in response to a rise of external or body temperature. By means of thermal sweating, up to 12 litres of sweat may be poured out over a period of 24 hours. Since to vaporize 1 litre of sweat requires almost 2500 kJ of heat, it is apparent that the sweating mechanism is an efficient way of reducing body temperature. It is important to realize that if the sweat does not evaporate from the skin but is merely wiped away, no heat loss occurs. By varying the amount of sweat secreted, the body can vary its heat loss.

When the external temperature exceeds that of the body, evaporation of sweat is the only method of heat loss available. Heavy sweating involves a rapid loss of water, together with salt, from the body; hence dehydration and also salt deprivation will occur unless enough water and salt is replaced. This is particularly important since the body gives temperature regulation priority over the maintenance of water and salt balance. Sweating will thus continue, even though it produces severe dehydration and marked salt loss. As the water content of sweat comes from the blood, rapid sweating demands a large cutaneous blood flow and therefore dilatation of the blood vessels of the skin. This is brought about by the regulatory mechanisms described below.

Regulation of body temperature

The overall regulation of body temperature is mediated by the hypothalamus which acts as a thermostat set at approximately 37°C. Two mechanisms, peripheral and central, are involved.

Peripheral

Stimulation of the temperature receptors in the skin reflexly sets up appropriate body responses such as sweating, vasomotor responses such as dilatation or constriction of blood vessels, or shivering.

Central

The hypothalamus is directly affected by the temperature of the blood and reacts by initiating appropriate body responses. Thus if the temperature of the blood is high, the hypothalamus responds by bringing about cutaneous vasodilatation and sweating. Both these responses will, of course, tend to lower body temperature. Conversely, if the hypothalamus is cooled by blood at a low temperature, it initiates heat conservation reactions such as cutaneous vasoconstriction, inhibition of sweating, and (if necessary) shivering to increase heat production. These various effects of the hypothalamus are mediated by the autonomic nervous system.

ABNORMAL BODY TEMPERATURE

Variations beyond the narrow range of normal body temperature will alter cell functions, whilst extremes of temperature may result in cell and tissue destruction.

Hyperthermia (pyrexia)

An abnormal elevation of body temperature due to a disturbance of the temperature regulating mechanisms is referred to as pyrexia. It is most frequently seen in association with bacterial or viral infections, but also accompanies a number of other disease states or injuries. The common factor is tissue destruction.

The elevated temperature is due to a direct effect of chemical substances on the temperature controlling centres in the hypothalamus. It would appear that these centres, which may be likened to a thermostat, are 'set' at a higher level so that the mechanisms for dissipating heat are not initiated until the body temperature has reached a higher level than normal. Thus at the onset of the illness the patient often feels cold despite a normal temperature, with heat production being increased and heat loss being minimized. The skin is pale because of peripheral vasoconstriction and shivering occurs. Usually the heat controlling mechanisms remain in control, with heat loss again balancing heat gain, but set to maintain temperature at a higher level than normal. The fever frequently terminates with a resetting of the temperature controlling centres. The patient now feels extremely hot, sweating is profuse, and the temperature is consequently reduced.

Pyrexia is due to chemical substances known as pyrogens. These substances are present in the microorganisms responsible for an infection, but are also liberated by dead tissue. They may act directly upon the heat regulating centres but more usually cause the inflammatory cells of the body to release similar substances known as endogenous pyrogens. These in turn act upon the hypothalamic centres.

It is generally assumed that pyrexia is a beneficial reaction designed to aid the body's defences against infection. It has been suggested, for example, that the high temperatures inhibit bacterial proliferation or make the microorganisms more vulnerable to other defence mechanisms. In addition, the increased cell metabolism that occurs at higher temperatures could help cells repair damage more rapidly. However, there is very little evidence to support these suggestions and, at the moment at least, we must regard fever as being, at best, of no value and possibly harmful to the patient.

For example, a rise in body temperature interferes with the normal functioning of the central nervous system, the cells of which are very sensitive to any change in their immediate environment. Thus as the temperature rises the patient becomes incapable of concentration and logical thought, may become confused and delirious with incoherent speech and, ultimately, stupor and coma may supervene. In infants and young children heat regulatory mechanisms sometimes fail to reduce temperature and may result in the development of 'febrile convulsions'. The pyrexia and convulsion have usually followed a mild to moderate febrile illness and the child is brought into the emergency department by an extremely anxious and distraught parent. It is not unusual to see the child swathed in clothing – this only increases the likelihood of a convulsion or further convulsions occurring.

Prompt removal of clothing and tepid sponging by wrapping the child in a wet towel will usually lower temperature to prevent the onset of convulsions.

Hyperpyrexia (heat stroke)

In the circumstances described above, the temperature controlling centres, although 'set' at a higher level than normal, continue to function with heat loss again balancing heat gain. Occasionally, however, the thermoregulatory mechanisms fail and the body temperature continues to rise. The abnormally high body temperature further depresses the heat controlling centres of the brain which in turn further raise the body temperature still higher. A vicious circle is then established. Unless treated promptly the patient dies or, even if he survives, may suffer permanent brain damage. Hyperpyrexia is due to a failure of the heat loss mechanisms with, in particular, a cessation of sweating.

Hyperpyrexia is most commonly seen in people who indulge in excessive activity in hot weather, particularly when humidity is high. The growing popularity of extraordinarily demanding sports, such as long

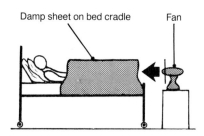

Fig. 9.3 'Wind tunnel', using a bed cradle covered by a damp sheet, and a fan.

distance running, has been accompanied by an increase in the incidence of sport-related hyperpyrexia. It may also occur during the course of an infection where fever is prominent. Occasionally it is seen during general anaesthesia, or it may occur following severe head injuries.

The management of any patient with an elevated body temperature is aimed at treatment of the symptoms. It may range from the removal of excess clothing and the provision of cool drinks, through regular tepid sponging, to the application of ice packs and the use of a wind tunnel (Fig. 9.3). Despite the need to reduce a patient's temperature as quickly as possible, it is imperative that the patient not be allowed to shiver; shivering is the body's method of producing heat, is a form of violent exercise, and will quickly produce exhaustion which may lead to death. Antipyretic drugs may be used to reduce temperature by producing peripheral dilatation and therefore heat loss across the skin surface.

Hypothermia

The body can be harmed by cold in two main ways. Firstly, excessive cooling of tissues in one area may cause local tissue damage (frostbite, see page 110). Secondly, if the whole body is cooled, the normal temperature controlling mechanisms may be overwhelmed and the body temperature will fall. This condition is referred to as hypothermia and is said to be present when the body core temperature falls below 35°C.

Initially the body reacts vigorously to chilling by invoking the mechanisms to increase heat production and decrease heat loss. Violent shivering occurs and this is associated with peripheral vasoconstriction. If cooling continues despite these measures, tissue metabolism throughout the body is depressed with a progressive decrease in heart rate, blood pressure, and respiratory function. (Controlled hypothermia is sometimes utilized as an aid to surgical procedures, particularly those involving the heart and brain.) Finally the temperature regulating centre ceases to function altogether and heat is lost from the body as from an inanimate object. Perhaps the most dangerous effect of hypothermia is the disturbance of cardiac rhythm that it produces. Atrial arrhythmias may occur quite early, whilst death is frequently due to ventricular fibrillation. Hypothermia is most commonly due to exposure to abnormally cold environmental conditions, particularly when the usual protective devices are not available. It is seen, for example, in shipwrecked sailors, marooned climbers, or lost hikers. Elderly people are particularly liable to hypothermia due to inadequate food and clothing, inactivity, and, possibly, less efficient thermoregulatory mechanisms. Infants also are vulnerable as they have a relatively large surface area to body volume, very little subcutaneous fat, and relatively insensitive temperature controlling mechanisms. This is particularly true of premature infants who are virtually poikilothermic.

Early signs are confusion, drowsiness and lethargy, progressing through behavioural changes, coma, and eventual death unless further heat loss is prevented.

When this condition occurs in isolated places, the management is to seek shelter, raise the air temperature without directly heating the patient (as this will cause peripheral vasodilation with a consequent hypotension), insulate the patient (in a sleeping bag or similar device), and provide heat donation by direct body contact. The heat donor's compensatory thermoregulatory mechanism is under pressure to supply heat for two bodies and the donor must therefore be supplied with carbohydrate that can be rapidly converted to energy. Despite popular myth, under no circumstances should the patient be given any form of alcohol, as this too will cause peripheral vasodilation.

REFERENCES AND FURTHER READING

Texts

Brunner L S, Suddarth D S 1984 Textbook of medical-surgical nursing, 5th edn. Lippincott, Philadelphia
Ganong W F 1985 Review of medical physiology, 12th edn. Lange Medical Publication, California
Guyton A C 1982 Physiology and mechanisms of disease, 3rd edn. W B Saunders, Philadelphia
Kaufman E E, Papper S 1983 Review of pathophysiology. Little Brown, Toronto
Long B C, Phipps W J (eds) 1985 Essentials of medical-surgical nursing. Mosby, St Louis.
Moore F D 1981 Homeostasis: bodily changes in trauma and surgery. In: Sabiston C C (ed) Textbook of surgery. The biological basis of modern surgical practice, 12th edn. W B Saunders Company, Philadelphia
Walter J B, Israel M C 1979 General pathology, 5th edn. Churchill Livingstone, London

Journals

Barnes A, Bell J 1984 Prevent shivering during hypothermia treatment. Nursing 84 14 : 8 : 60–61

Folk-Lighty M 1984 Solving the puzzles of patients' fluid imbalances. Nursing 84 14 : 2 : 34–41
Glass L B, Jenkins C A 1983 The ups and downs of serum pH. Nursing 83 13 : 1 : 57
Griffin J P 1986 Fever: when to leave it alone. Nursing 86 16 : 2 : 58–61
Janusek L W 1984 Metabolic acidosis: physiology, signs, and symptoms. Nursing 84 14 : 7 : 44–45
Janusek L W 1984 Metabolic alkalosis: physiology, signs, and symptoms. Nursing 84 14 : 8 : 60–61
Lipsky J G 1984 Saving the elderly from the killing cold. Nursing 84 14 : 2 : 42–43
Palmer L 1984 Arterial blood gas analysis. Nursing 84 14 : 1 : 24–25
Perkins C, Bralley H K 1983 Metabolic alkalosis. Nursing 83 13 : 1 : 57
Romanski S O 1986 Interpreting ABG's in four easy steps. Nursing 86 16 : 9 : 58–63
Stark J L, Hunt V 1984 Managing electrolyte imbalances. Nursing 84 14 : 7 : 57–59

10

The mechanisms of disease

Michael Drake

In order to recognize disturbances in structure and function it is essential to be fully aware of what constitutes normal anatomy and physiology. It is the recognition of the outward manifestations of disturbances and the application of such measures as are necessary to restore the organism to normal, that comprises clinical medicine.

The study of pathology can be systemized in a number of ways. One can simply define a list of disease processes or mechanisms; this list would include such entities as inflammatory, neoplastic, and circulatory disorders. A more useful approach is to classify aetiological agents, and then consider the basic ways in which the body, or its individual cells and tissues, may react to these agents.

AETIOLOGICAL FACTORS IN DISEASE

The many causes of disease may be considered in two main categories: genetic or inherited, and abnormal environmental factors.

Genetic or inherited causes

Genetic abnormalities are the sole or main cause of a variety of diseases, although quantitatively few are of importance in clinical medicine. Examples of genetically determined diseases are haemophilia, neurofibromatosis and polyposis coli. In addition, genetic factors may be of considerable importance in rendering a patient more vulnerable to a disease or predisposing him to react in a particular way to an environmental stimulus.

Abnormal environmental factors

1. Physical injuries or trauma – mechanical, thermal, electrical, and radiational.
2. Harmful inanimate substances – chemicals, toxins, or poisons.
3. Nutritional abnormalities – inadequate food intake or, more commonly, deficiency of specific nutritional factors. The effects of excessive intake of certain foodstuffs, for example, lipids, could also be placed in this category.
4. Microorganisms – viruses, rickettsiae, spirochaetes, bacteria, fungi, protozoa, and metazoa.

DISEASE PROCESSES RESULTING IN CELL AND TISSUE DAMAGE

The diseases encountered commonly in clinical practice are those which result from harmful environmental factors. Many such factors damage cells and tissues in a direct and obvious way; the effects of mechanical trauma and excessive heat or burning being examples of these. However, sometimes cell and tissue damage occurs as part of a more complex process involving a host reaction to a variety of factors.

Infection

The way in which microorganisms cause disease is by invasion of the body and multiplication within the living tissues of the host. This process is referred to as an infection and is discussed in greater detail in Chapter 11. However, the infec-

97

tive process may cause considerable destruction of cells and tissues at a local level, and may also produce systemic manifestations.

Hypersensitivity

One of the fundamental and most important defence mechanisms of the organism is its ability to produce substances that destroy or neutralize foreign materials that may gain access to the body. These protective substances are referred to as antibodies and the foreign materials, usually proteins, that stimulate their formation are called antigens. The best known antibodies are the immunoglobins found in the plasma, but antibodies are also found attached to cells. However, the combination of antibody with antigen is not always beneficial to the organism – sometimes it is responsible for severe and extensive cell damage. These antigen–antibody reactions that are detrimental to the organism are known as hypersensitivity or allergic reactions. The way in which cell damage occurs is complex and not fully understood. It would appear that the process is initiated by the interaction of antigen with antibody with a consequent release of pharmacologically reactive compounds, some of which are directly toxic to cells.

In addition to causing local tissue damage, abnormal immune reactions are also responsible for a variety of disease processes, such as bronchial asthma, and the rather poorly defined group of disorders known collectively as the autoimmune diseases.

Thrombosis, embolism and infarction

Although less clearly a response to abnormal environmental stimuli than the two disease processes already considered, the consequences of tissue ischaemia are considered here as they are of considerable importance in clinical medicine. In addition, the vascular disorders leading to tissue damage are due, in part at least, to nutritional factors, and to the indirect effects of mechanical trauma.

In general and simplistic terms a blood vessel may 'burst', 'bulge', or 'block'. The former two events will lead respectively to haemorrhage and an aneurysm, whilst blockage of a blood vessel, with consequent diminution or cessation of blood flow, may lead to considerable damage to the tissues supplied by that vessel. The tissues may undergo necrosis and the area so affected is known as an infarction. Infarctions may occur in a variety of organs, but those of the heart, brain, and lung are probably of greatest significance. There are many ways in which a blood vessel may be occluded but the most common are by a thrombus or an embolus. A thrombus is a solid mass which forms within the vessels. It may be atheromatous (comprised of fatty plaque) or may be formed from constituents of the blood, and hence consists of platelets and fibrin in which the erythrocytes and leucocytes become enmeshed. The thrombus may remain at its site of formation causing partial or complete occlusion of the vessel at that site or, alternatively, part of it may break away and be carried elsewhere within the circulation to impact ultimately within a vessel and occlude that vessel. This mass, which is transported within the circulation and occludes a vessel by impaction in its lumen, is known as an embolus. There are other forms of emboli but a mass of thrombus material is by far the most common.

It can be seen that in most cases of infarction the primary event is the formation of a thrombus. The causes of thrombosis are complex but in general three factors are concerned. Known as Virchow's triad these comprise:

1. Abnormalities of the vessel wall, particularly of its endothelial lining.
2. Abnormalities in the flow of blood.
3. Abnormalities in the blood constituents, notably the platelets and clotting factors.

Most frequently the damage to the vessel wall and its endothelial lining is caused by the so-called 'degenerative' disorder, atheroma or atherosclerosis. The aetiology of this disorder remains obscure but it is by far the commonest cause of arterial thrombosis. The most important change in the blood flow is a slowing or stasis, such as may occur when a patient is immobilized in bed. Finally, an elevation of platelet count, such as may occur after childbirth or surgical trauma, may favour the development of a thrombus. (See Chapter 32 for further discussion of blood vessel disorders.)

RESPONSE OF CELLS AND TISSUES TO INJURY

The abnormal environmental factors, either directly or by way of the disease mechanisms just discussed, damage or destroy the tissues of the body. However, despite the many ways this damage may be brought about, the ways in which the tissues may respond to such damage are very limited. The most important of these responses are:

1. Inflammation
2. Degeneration and necrosis – usually followed by repair and/or regeneration
3. Disturbances of growth and differentiation.

Inflammation

The process of inflammation is a fundamental reaction on the part of the body and is commonly encountered in the practice of clinical medicine. It has been defined as: 'the local reaction of living vascular connective tissues to injury' or, alternatively, as 'the process by which cells and fluid accumulate in damaged tissues and tend to protect them from further injury'.

The latter definition introduces the concept of protection, or defence against further injury, although it must be appreciated that, in certain circumstances, the inflammatory reaction itself may cause considerable damage to tissues.

When the tissues are damaged by bacterial toxins, mechanical trauma, burning, or indeed by any other means, the damaged cells release substances that bring about the inflammatory reaction. A number of such substances have now been identified but perhaps the best known is the chemical histamine. The most striking effect of these substances is to alter the permeability of the blood vessels in the injured area. Normally the walls of the blood vessels are impermeable to plasma proteins and the blood cells, and hence these substances remain within the blood stream. Conversely, there is a free movement of water and dissolved substances across the walls of the smallest blood vessels or capillaries. This movement of water is controlled by the hydrostatic pressure of the blood opposed by the osmotic pressure of the plasma proteins. The resultant to and fro movement of fluid across the capillary

walls is known as the tissue fluid cycle, a process that has been discussed in Chapter 9. The movement is finely balanced to ensure that the amount of fluid escaping from the blood vessels in any one area is approximately equal to that which re-enters the blood vessel.

This balance, however, is completely dependent on the continued impermeability of the vessels' walls to plasma proteins. The substances released at the site of tissue injury break down this impermeability, allowing the protein to escape into the surrounding tissues. This disturbs the tissue fluid cycle and hence fluid, in considerable quantities, also flows into the tissues. In addition, the leucocytes are induced to migrate from the blood vessels and they also accumulate in the area of injury. This migration is an active process whereby the leucocytes force their way between the cells which form the capillary wall. Sometimes a small number of erythrocytes escape from the blood vessel also. The first cells to migrate are the neutrophils or polymorphonuclear leucocytes, but subsequently the monocytes also move out of the blood vessels. In addition, the wandering tissue macrophages are attracted to the area.

The protein-rich fluid and the blood cells which have accumulated at the site of injury form what is known as the inflammatory exudate. The leucocytes may be particularly numerous and, in association with liquifying dead tissue, form pus, a common manifestation of certain infections. This process of pus formation is referred to as suppuration and if the pus accumulates in one area it is called an abscess. The inflammatory exudate is one of the most striking features of tissue damage, particularly if the damage is due to an infective agent. Examples are the purulent discharge from infected wounds, and the pus cells in the urine of a patient with a urinary tract infection and in the cerebrospinal fluid in bacterial meningitis. The inflammatory exudate may also have important functional effects. In acute pneumonia, for example, inflammatory exudate pours out of the blood vessels in the alveolar walls to fill the alveolar spaces. As the air spaces become filled with exudate the lungs become solid, this change being referred to as pneumonic consolidation. The filling of the air spaces with inflammatory exudate prevents the normal exchange of gases and hence the patient becomes dyspnoeic and cyanosed.

The value of the inflammatory reaction is three-fold. Firstly, the fluid itself may dilute whatever it is that is causing the tissue injury. Secondly, if the injurious agents are microorganisms or their toxins, the host may produce antibodies to these agents. These antibodies, which are proteins, will pass out of the blood vessels as part of the inflammatory exudate, and thus will be brought into contact with the microorganisms or toxins. Finally, the leucocytes which have migrated into the area, have the ability to ingest foreign material, including microorganisms, thus tending to protect the tissues from further injury. This process of ingestion of foreign material is referred to as phagocytosis.

The local signs of the inflammatory reaction are well known. The inflamed area is red, hot, swollen, and painful, and there is also frequently loss of function of the part. There may also be general or systemic manifestations. Many inflammatory reactions, particularly if of infective origin, are accompanied by a rise in temperature and an increased pulse rate.

If the inflammatory process is of short duration it is referred to as acute inflammation. Sometimes, however, the process becomes more protracted and it is then described as chronic inflammation. Chronicity of inflammation may be due to the organism involved – some organisms such as the tubercle bacillus characteristically produce a chronic reaction. Alternatively it may be due to host factors such as diminished resistance to infection, local obstruction to drainage, or local impairment of blood supply. Finally, the presence of a foreign body, such as suture material, in the area of tissue damage may cause a prolongation of the inflammatory reaction.

Degeneration and necrosis

The inflammatory reaction involves mainly the connective or supporting tissues and may be associated with considerable damage to these tissues. More vulnerable, however, are the more highly organized or specialized cells which respond to injury in a passive fashion known as degeneration. According to the nature of the damaging agent, its intensity and duration of action, and the type of cell involved, the degenerative changes may be slight and reversible or, alternatively, they may go on to cell death or necrosis. Cell degeneration and cell death may be due to the direct action of damaging agents (such as bacterial toxins or mechanical trauma) or may result from deprivation of the cell of substances (such as oxygen) which are vital for its metabolic processes. This is the mode of injury when tissue is deprived of its blood supply with resultant infarction.

Repair and regeneration

Tissue may be destroyed in a variety of ways. The damage may result from the direct action of the injurious agent, or the inflammatory response to such injury may itself cause extensive damage to tissues. If tissue is lost it may be replaced in two ways. Firstly, it may be replaced by fibrous connective tissue, the result being known as a scar. To this process the term repair is applied. Secondly, the lost tissues may be replaced by tissue similar to that which was destroyed, this being accomplished by the proliferation of surrounding undamaged specialized cells. This process is called regeneration. In general the latter process is preferable as it results in a complete restoration of normal tissue function. However, for a variety of reasons, regeneration may not be possible and then the tissue defect is filled by scar tissue (see Figures 7.1–3, pp 58, 59).

DISORDERS OF GROWTH AND DIFFERENTIATION

The term 'growth' refers simply to an increase in the mass of protoplasm or body substance, whereas the term differentiation describes the process whereby specialized cells develop from a more primitive stem cell. An example of the latter process is the development, or differentiation, of erythrocytes and leucocytes from more primitive cells in the bone marrow. Disturbances of growth or differentiation, or both processes, in a group of cells give rise to a variety of disorders of profound importance in clinical medicine. Undoubtedly the most important disturbance of growth and differentiation is that of neoplasia. The word neoplasia literally means new growth or new formation, and the resultant mass of tissue is referred to as a neoplasm or tumour. Neoplasms may occur in virtually any organ of the body and many types are described. However, the one of greatest clinical importance is the malignant neoplasm commonly referred to as a 'cancer'.

It is important to realise that the living cell is the essential unit of a tumour, as it is of any normal tissue of the body. The component cells of a tumour are not alien to the body but are actually descendants of normal cells. Hence a tumour cell is a modified normal cell; a cell that has undergone some permanent change, this change being transmitted to successive generations of cells. The reason the cells undergo this change is not yet fully understood but the evidence would indicate that most human tumours are due to abnormal environmental agents which act on the surface of the body or enter the body in the air we inhale or the food we ingest.

In summary, therefore, the vast range of human diseases lend themselves to a systematic approach. The rational management of a patient suffering from a disease requires a knowledge of the cause of that disease and an understanding of the way in which the body or the individual cells and tissues are reacting to the causal factors. In general, an attempt is made to establish both an anatomic and a pathologic diagnosis so that the most effective treatment can be given. A patient presenting, for example, with fever, cough and haemoptysis may be found to have clinical and radiological evidence of an abnormality in his lung. It is important to determine the pathologic nature of the abnormality which in this case would probably be inflammatory (for example, pneumonia), neoplastic (for example, a carcinoma) or circulatory (for example, an infarction).

DISEASE AS A DISTURBANCE OF HOMEOSTASIS

It is fitting to conclude this chapter on disease and the body's response by returning to the concept of homeostasis and disturbed homeostasis, discussed in Chapter 9. Thus, as already indicated, slight or permissible variations in the internal environment may occur without damage to the organism. However, if the stresses on the bodily system become too great the internal environment may alter significantly, often with disastrous effects. Accordingly a new concept of disease has emerged, a concept that disease is essentially a state of imbalance. Under conditions of health the person is in balance with the antagonistic forces of his environment. In disease the patient is out of balance, and the functions of his cells and tissues are disturbed because of this. Thus disease is not an entity in itself but rather it is the expression of conflict between the individual and an adverse environment.

> . . . disease, as all other manifestations of living beings, is life itself and nothing more.
>
> (Perez-Tamayo)

REFERENCES AND FURTHER READING

Texts

Brunner L S, Suddarth D S 1984 Textbook of medical/surgical nursing, 5th edn. Lippincott, Philadelphia
Ganong W F 1985 Review of medical physiology, 12th edn. Lange Medical Publication, California
Guyton A S 1982 Physiology and mechanisms of disease, 3rd edn. Saunders, Philadelphia
Long B C, Phipps W J (eds) 1985 Essentials of medical-surgical nursing. Mosby, St Louis
Perez-Tamayo R 1985 Mechanisms of disease. An introduction to pathology, 2nd edn. Year Book Medical Publishers, Chicago
Walter J B, Israel M S 1979 General pathology, 5th edn. Churchill Livingstone, London

Journals

Burton F, Salminen C A 1984 Back to basics: controlling postoperative infection. Nursing 84 14 : 9 : 43
Jones I 1985 You can drive back infection . . . if you know where to make your stand. Nursing 85 15 : 4 : 50–52
Stark J L, Hunt V 1985 Don't let nosocomial infections get your patients down. Nursing 85 15 : 1 : 10–11
Taylor D L 1983 Inflammation: physiology, signs and symptoms. Nursing 83 13 : 1 : 52–53
Veldman B 1983 Reversing life-threatening sepsis. Nursing 83 13 : 2 : 18–23

11

Infection, shock and trauma

Michael Drake   *Jenny Kidd*

INFECTION

Infectious agents, such as bacteria, viruses, fungi and protozoa are the most frequent causes of acute illnesses and, despite enormous therapeutic advances, are still a significant cause of death. These so-called infectious diseases occur as a result of invasion of the body by the infectious agents, or microorganisms, or the action of their products, or both. The clinical manifestations are due to disturbances of function, and/or injury or destruction of host cells and tissues – events that are usually accompanied by alterations in the body's homeostatic mechanisms. The injuries or functional disturbances may be due directly to the microbes or their products or, indirectly, to host defence mechanisms.

An infectious disease may be viewed as the unfavourable outcome of a battle:

Host defences *v.* organism's virulence

where virulence refers to the organism's capacity to cause disease. In order to produce a disease, most microorganisms must gain entry to the host, multiply locally in host tissues, spread from the site of entry, and overcome host immune systems. At each stage of the infectious process, specific microbial and host factors determine the ultimate outcome of the illness. An understanding of this process is essential for effective management of infectious diseases.

Defence mechanisms

The mechanisms adopted by the body against infection can be considered in two broad categories. Firstly, there are the local mechanisms which are designed to prevent the entry of pathogenic organisms into the body and hence are found in those areas where the body comes into direct contact with the external environment, for example, the skin, and the gastrointestinal, respiratory, and genital tracts. Secondly, there are the general or systemic mechanisms the purpose of which is to eliminate pathogenic organisms should they gain entry to the body, and to combat the toxins elaborated by these organisms.

Local defence mechanisms

Mechanical or physical. All surfaces that come into contact with the external environment are covered by an epithelial layer. By far the most effective of these is the so-called keratinized stratified squamous epithelium which constitutes the skin. This is made up of multiple layers of cells, the surface of which is covered by the hard horn-like material, keratin. Even where this horny layer is absent, as in the mouth, oesophagus and vagina, the squamous epithelium offers considerable resistance to the entry of microorganisms. The integrity of this barrier is, of course, of paramount importance. Thus any breach in the epithelium such as, for example, a cut in the skin, will act as a portal of entry for potentially dangerous microorganisms.

Other physical factors are also important in local defence mechanisms. Thus in the respiratory tract, for example, inhaled microorganisms may become entrapped by the tenacious mucus that covers the lining of the air passages. This mucus is continually being swept proximally by the beating action of the cilia. Ultimately the cough reflex is stimulated and the mucus, with entrapped microorganisms, is expelled.

Biochemical mechanisms. In some areas the pH of the secretions may inhibit the growth of pathogenic microorganisms. Perhaps the best example of this is the hydrochloric acid secreted by the gastric mucosa which, under normal circumstances, prevents bacterial growth in the stomach. However, there are other areas in the body where chemical defences operate. In the vagina, for example, the natural flora, a bacterium known as a lactobaccilus, metabolises the glycogen that is present normally in the vaginal epithelium; a by-product of this metabolism is lactic acid. The consequent acidity of the vaginal secretions inhibit the proliferation of most pathogens.

Biological mechanisms. A number of body secretions contain biological agents that inhibit the growth of microorganisms. In the tears, for example, a substance known as lysozome destroys bacteria and this helps to maintain sterility of the conjunctiva and the sclera.

Although the local defence mechanisms are extremely effective they may be overwhelmed by the infective agent. This is most likely to occur when the mechanisms are impaired. Thus the action of the cilia in the respiratory tract may be inhibited by cold or by the inhalation of tobacco smoke. Alternatively the local mechanisms may be rendered less effective by alterations in the biologic status of the host. In the female genital tract, for example, the stratified squamous epithelium is dependent for its development on circulating oestrogen. Thus the epithelium that protects the vagina and outer cervix is thin before puberty and becomes thin again after the menopause. The deposition of glycogen in the vaginal epithelium is also dependent on oestrogen. When the oestrogen level is low, the vaginal cells become glycogen depleted and the natural vaginal flora are unable to produce lactic acid. As a consequence the pH of the vaginal secretions rises and this may favour the proliferation of pathogenic microorganisms. For these two reasons infections of the lower female genital tract occur commonly in young girls and in post-menopausal women. Even during a woman's reproductive life an infection may flare up around the time of menstruation – the phase of the menstrual cycle when oestrogen secretion is lowest.

The inflammatory reaction as a local defence mechanism. As described in Chapter 10, the inflammatory reaction is essentially a protective response although, in certain circumstances, the reaction itself may cause considerable tissue damage. Should microorganisms gain access to and begin to proliferate in the body tissues, the resultant damage to cells and tissues will lead to an inflammatory reaction with an accumulation of inflammatory exudate in the damaged tissues. This exudate is rich in phagocytic leucocytes, initially polymorphonuclear leucocytes and subsequently large mononuclear cells – the so called macrophages. Both these cell types have the capacity to ingest microorganisms by phagocytosis, and frequently the ingested microorganism is destroyed by enzymes within the phagocytic cell. The inflammatory reaction is of considerable importance in localizing infections and indeed an ability to manufacture sufficient leucocytes, and therefore mount an efficient inflammatory response, renders a patient very vulnerable to infectious diseases.

General or systemic defence mechanisms – humoral factors

Non-specific substances. It has been known for some time that blood and serum are bactericidal. This capacity to destroy microorganisms is due to a number of substances, the most important and best understood of which is known as complement or, preferably, the complement system. This is a group of plasma proteins that play a crucial role in dealing with microorganisms that invade the blood stream. They have the capacity to aid the process of phagocytosis, to assist the action of specific antibodies and, acting alone, to bring about the destruction of microorganisms and of infected cells. Whilst they are complementary to the antibodies they are of particular importance in that they are available for immediate activation and they are also relatively non-selective in their actions. Conversely, antibodies may take days to develop and are highly specific in their functions.

Antibodies. All antibodies are complex glycoproteins known collectively as the immunoglobulins. These proteins are produced by lymphocytes and plasma cells and are present in plasma and all other body fluids. Their production is in direct response to microorganisms and their products and, in general, they act to destroy the microorganisms and to neutralize their toxins. In these actions they show considerable specificity.

Cellular factors

Cellular immune mechanisms are particularly important in dealing with organisms that are usually resistant to phagocytosis. These include bacteria, such as the tubercle bacilli, and many viruses. Cellular immunity is based on a coordinated function of one type of lymphocyte, the so-called T lymphocyte, and the macrophages. The various reactions involved in this type of immunity are not fully understood but they facilitate the eradication of microorganisms that are normally resistant to destruction by phagocytosis or to lysis by complement (see Chapter 77).

In addition to these fairly clearly defined body defence mechanisms it should be appreciated that a number of non-specific factors are important in the prevention of infection. The physiological condition of the host at the time that he is exposed to a particular microorganism is of considerable importance in determining whether infection will occur and, if so, the subsequent course of the disease. Factors such as nutritional state, fatigue, and exposure may be of significance in determining the outcome.

Virulence of organism

The term 'pathogenicity' denotes the ability of a specific microorganism to produce disease, such organisms being referred to as pathogenic. Virulence is a measure of the degree of this ability to produce disease. Whilst virulence is an inherent feature of each microorganism it is also subject to a number of factors including the number of organisms, their route of entry to the body, the susceptibility of a particular host, and environmental conditions such as temperature and humidity. Virulence is a dynamic concept and the term implies a degree of pathogenicity. Thus a strain of bacteria able to produce disease in certain conditions with a small number of organisms is said to be more virulent than another strain that requires a larger number of organisms under the

same conditions. As with the defence mechanisms of the host, the virulence of the organism is a function of a variety of structural and biochemical features that favour adaptation of the organism to the environmental conditions of the host. Essentially there are three requirements that must be met for a microorganism to produce disease. These are:

1. Communicability. The organism must be capable of being transferred from a source of infection to the surface of a new host and of surviving, at least temporarily, on that surface.
2. Invasiveness. The organism must be able to penetrate into the host tissues and to proliferate within these tissues, the latter implying an ability to resist the host defence mechanisms.
3. Pathogenicity. The organism must be capable of damaging the host tissues. The mere presence of microorganisms in body tissues is not necessarily harmful. Disease is the manifestation of some chemical activity of the organism, usually by the action of substances called toxins of which there are two types:
• Extoxins are chemical poisons released by living organisms into the body, and which frequently act at some distance from the focus of infection.
• Endotoxins are structural components of the organism and, although they may escape in small amounts to surrounding body fluids, their release requires the disintegration of the microorganism. Pathogenic organisms may also injure the host less directly by inducing a state of hypersensitivity with consequent tissue damage.

An understanding of these factors involved in host defences and an organism's virulence enables us to influence the battle between the two. In this way infectious disease may be entirely prevented or, if it does occur, the duration and extent of the disease may be modified and a favourable outcome ensured. Thus a person's general resistance may be increased by measures such as adequate nutrition and other measures designed to ensure general fitness, whilst specific immunity may be achieved by measures such as immunization. The organism's ability to cause infection may be diminished by: eliminating reservoirs of infection; minimizing the number of organisms that attack the body, by means such as adequate ventilation;

and preventing entry of organisms by maintaining integrity of body surfaces or, where these are breached deliberately, adopting sterile techniques.

Inevitably, infectious diseases will occur and in these circumstances two different types of clinical manifestations will be observed. Firstly, there are those related to disturbed defence mechanisms and other metabolic changes in the host. These are generally non-specific, occur in most infections, and include such symptoms and signs as fever, anorexia, and leucocytosis. The second group of clinical manifestations are those due to the aggressive properties of the particular microorganism, and these are frequently specific to that organism. The specificity of these manifestations usually facilitates a clinical diagnosis which is subsequently validated by microbiological investigations.

When microorganisms, in particular bacteria, invade the blood stream in large numbers and overwhelm the body's defence systems a devastating constellation of symptoms and signs develop. Known as septicaemia, the condition is a potent cause of the condition of shock, which is often fatal despite vigorous management.

Undoubtedly one of the major advances in medical sciences has been the development of specific antibacterial agents. Unfortunately, microorganisms have the ability to adapt themselves to antimicrobial drugs and become resistant to their effects. This resistance is the result of a change in the DNA of the bacteria due either to a chromosomal mutation or the acquisition of extrachromosomal DNA through genetic exchange. In either case the result is the formation of enzymes or other proteins that inactivate drugs or block access to their site of action. Despite this emergence of resistant strains of bacteria, the advent of antibiotics and the continued production of new types has revolutionized the management of infectious diseases. They are no longer a major cause of death – at least within the so-called developed countries.

SHOCK

Shock is a state of progressive circulatory failure in which the cardiac output is insufficient to meet the body's requirements of nutrition, oxidation, and excretion.

Adequate circulation to the body tissues depends on three components:

1. Blood volume
2. Cardiac pump
3. Vascular tone.

Shock occurs when an effective combination of the triad cannot be maintained.

Classification and aetiology of shock

Shock can be classified according to four pathophysiologic mechanisms:

1. Hypovolaemic shock
2. Cardiogenic shock
3. Neurogenic shock
4. Septic shock.

Hypovolaemic shock

Hypovolaemic shock results from loss of circulating blood volume (hypovolaemia). Sub-classifications include haemorrhagic shock, burn shock (see page 778), wound/surgical shock, and traumatic shock.

Common causes of hypovolaemia include haemorrhage, burns, peritonitis, diabetic ketoacidosis, septicaemia, acute pancreatitis, Addisonian crisis, and severe dehydration from vomiting and diarrhoea.

Cardiogenic shock – pump failure

The most common cause of cardiogenic shock is myocardial infarction where more than 40% of the left ventricle is affected.

Neurogenic shock

Fright causes a degree of hypovolaemia, which is produced by central or peripheral vasomotor activity associated with a change in the contractility and capacity of the vessels. Neural control mechanisms which maintain vascular tone are interrupted and peripheral resistance is lowered resulting in peripheral pooling of blood. In anaphylaxis, the hypovolaemia results from increased permeability of vessels due to histamine release from most cells and dilation of vessels, particularly the microcirculation.

Other causes of neurogenic shock include head injury, deep general anaesthesia, overdose of drugs, spinal cord trauma, hypoglycaemia, and severe pain. Causes of anaphylaxis include transfused blood or blood products, insect stings or bites, allergic drug reactions, and dye injected as a diagnostic agent.

Septic shock (Gram-negative or endotoxic shock)

This is usually caused by an uncontrolled bloodborne infection due to gram negative organisms. Less frequently it follows a gram-positive infection (exotoxic shock). Common causes include urinary tract infection and septicaemia.

Pathophysiology and clinical manfestations

The process and presentation of shock is individual. However, three basic patterns of pathophysiology can be identified:

1. Hypovolaemia – which initiates innate compensatory mechanisms.
2. Cardiac failure – which may be a cause or result of the shock process.
3. Microcirculatory derangements – which initate decompensatory changes.

Hypovolaemia and compensatory mechanisms

In the early stages of shock, compensatory mechanisms are initiated by the body in an attempt to prevent deterioration of the circulation.

Firstly, with the loss of blood volume, the reduced blood flow and therefore the drop in pressure is noticed by the baroreceptors. In response to this, alpha cells, found in skin, muscle, gut, and kidneys, constrict arterioles to these areas under the influence of epinephrine, thereby shunting blood to the central circulation in order to raise the blood pressure. This is referred to as centralization of the circulation. It is an extremely effective mechanism and a shocked patient may initially present with a normal or even slightly raised blood pressure.

It has been demonstrated that in this early stage of compensation there is no restriction to blood flow to the brain and heart. This is due to the action of beta receptors.

This massive peripheral constriction manifests clinically in ashen grey pallor, slightly cyanosed nail beds, and cold and clammy skin due to the stimulation of the sympathetic nervous system. However, patients with septic shock initially present with warm flushed skin; increased levels of epinephrine also cause anxiety and restlessness.

Tachycardia and tachypnoea are always two of the early signs of shock. The tachycardia is usually weak and thready, due to either loss of circulating volume or loss of cardiac muscle activity. Tachypnoea due to hypoxia is often described as 'air hunger'. It is an attempt by the body to maximize erythrocyte oxygen saturation. It is also a response to metabolic acidosis (see page 84). In septic shock, fever and circulating endotoxins also contribute to tachypnoea.

The second compensatory mechanism is a fluid shift. Reduced blood flow in the peripheral circulation results in decreased hydrostatic pressure in the vessels. Fluid is moved from the interstitial space to the vessels thereby increasing overall circulating blood volume. Fluid is freed from the extravascular compartment at rates of up to 1 litre per hour.

These major compensatory mechanisms are supported by the activation of the vasomotor centre in the medulla. Inhibited vagal activity and augmented sympathetic activity simultaneously increase the rate and force of cardiac contraction and increase the constriction of vessels. There is an increase in the secretion of aldosterone and ADH, and an activation of the renin angiotensin system, all of which assist in conserving fluid and supporting the blood pressure.

However, shock is a state of progressive circulatory failure and unless the patient receives treatment to arrest the shock process the body will begin to decompensate.

Microcompensatory derangements and decompensation

Principal decompensatory manifestations include the development of a metabolic acidosis, and the reverse fluid shift due to abnormal permeability of capillaries, pooling of blood in the periphery, and the development of disseminated intravascular coagulation (DIC).

A 'maintenance flow' of blood left in the capillaries following peripheral vasoconstriction rapidly releases its oxygen to the tissues which then revert to anaerobic metabolism. The end product is the formation of pyruvic and lactic acid resulting in a metabolic acidosis. This intercellular acidosis results in considerable damage to the cells and is responsible for many of the changes to be described. Vasoconstriction cannot continue indefinitely, especially in an acidic environment. It is subsequently followed by fatigue of the arterioles, particularly the precapillary sphincter, resulting in dilation of the microcirculation. It appears that the postcapillary sphincter controlling venous outflow is less sensitive to the metabolic acidosis and may remain constricted. Blood then flows from the central circulation into the periphery where it pools, producing a stagnant hypoxia and an substantially reduced venous return to the heart.

During this phase, increased filtration pressure in the capillaries results in a reverse fluid shift from the circulation into the interstitial space, intensifying the hypovolaemia. There is an influx of sodium and water into the cells and the sodium pump fails to function due to lack of ATP, and simultaneously potassium escapes, resulting in hyperkalaemia.

The entire process is exacerbated by the increasing metabolic acidosis and the release of vasodilator substances such as histamine and bradykinin.

Clinically, this phase is characterized by a low pH, increasing tachypnoea in an attempt by the patient to 'blow off' carbon dioxide, a rapidly falling blood pressure, oedema, cardiac arrythmias, severely cyanosed peripheries, marked tachycardia and a deterioration in conscious state. The patient is usually drowsy, vague and confused.

A major consquence of the peripheral vasoconstriction and fall in blood pressure is the impairment of renal function. The renal cortex is deprived of blood flow because of the redistribution mechanism and glomerular filtration is reduced. This results in oliguria or anuria. Urine output is an extremely reliable parameter indicative of the depth and severity of the circulatory collapse.

Cardiogenic shock – pump failure

Cardiogenic shock is characterized by the clinical syndrome encountered in hypovolaemia. However, the differences in the haemodynamics are that this form of shock results from massive myocardial damage which leads to reduced cardiac output, reduced coronary artery perfusion, increased myocardial hypoxia and myocardial damage and a consequent fall in blood pressure. The clinical presentation is that of hypovolaemic shock and severe myocardial insufficiency often with associated pulmonary oedema. Cardiogenic shock has an 80–85% mortality rate.

Anaphylactic shock presents with a similar clinical picture with the addition of dyspnoea, a feeling of asphyxiation, urticaria, pruritis, erythema, oedema of the hands, eyelids, lips, tongue and larynx.

Septic shock

Septic shock is divided into three stages – warm, cool, and cold stages. The cool and cold stages are clinically similar to hypovolaemic shock, however patient generally presents in the warm stage. Signs are: low peripheral resistance, warm flushed moist skin, fever, and chills. It is often difficult to differentiate the onset of shock at this stage from a normal response to a high temperature. The patient with endotoxic shock may initially be confused and has a full, bounding pulse. This stage may last from 1–16 hours. It is not clear as to the exact effect of gram-negative endotoxins on the microcirculation.

Whatever the shock-inducing events, in the late stages changes are always seen in the coagulation status. These changes comprise deposition of hyaline thrombi consisting of fibrin and platelets, and a resultant overall bleeding tendency and tissue necrosis. This condition is referred to as disseminated intravascular coagulation (DIC). The formation of thrombi is probably due to the slowing of the blood flow through the smaller vessels. Clinically, DIC is characterized by the development of purpura, classically across the chest, and widespread haemorrhage.

Tissue damage

Most of the tissue damage seen in shock is due to impaired perfusion and hypoxia. Although all tissues are affected the principle organs involved are the lungs, kidneys, heart, brain, and gastrointestinal tract.

Lung. Pulmonary changes play a central role in the pathophysiology of shock. When shock has persisted for periods ranging from 12–72 hours, pulmonary changes develop to produce what is usually referred to as the 'shock lung'. Breathing becomes rapid and shallow, X-rays show increasing evidence of oedema, and arterial oxygen levels become low – this lowered arterial pO_2 being refractory to oxygen therapy. The respiratory insufficiency caused by the changes is commonly referred to as the adult respiratory distress syndrome, although the changes within the lung are somewhat different to those seen in association with the infant respiratory distress syndrome. At post-mortem examination the lungs are enlarged, with a 'boggy' consistency and evidence of congestion, oedema and diffuse haemorrhage. Microscopic examination reveals extensive changes to the alveolar lining membranes. DIC-caused microthrombi may be found within the alveolar circulation.

Kidneys. Renal failure develops in many patients with severe shock, even when the shock is brief in duration. It is due to a massive death or necrosis of the renal tubular cells, this necrosis being a direct result of impaired renal blood flow. Should the patient survive, he may be maintained by means of dialysis and in many patients there will ultimately be a complete regeneration of the normal tubular structure with recovery of function.

Heart. The cardiac lesions in shock vary from individual muscle fibre necrosis to quite massive infarcts. Of course the state of shock might have been initiated by a myocardial infarct but even those patients suffering from cardiogenic shock may develop additional lesions due to inadequate perfusion, and a cycle of shock–necrosis–shock may be induced with fatal results.

Gastrointestinal tract. In shock, the gut suffers patchy areas of mucosal haemorrhage and necrosis known as 'haemorrhagic gastroenteropathy'. The lesions most commonly occur in the small intestine but can occur throughout the entire tract (see Curlings ulcer page 781).

Brain. The brain is extremely vulnerable to hypoxia and may develop hypoxic encephalopathy.

The concept of 'irreversible' shock

Whatever the cause of shock, unless the haemodynamic and metabolic disturbance can be corrected, a stage is reached when the patient's condition deteriorates catastrophically and then, despite all efforts, death will ensue. The early stages of shock are sometimes referred to as compensated, non-progressive or reversible whilst the late stages are known as decompensated, terminal, refractory or irreversible. The reason that shock becomes refractory to treatment is the development of the lesions already described. Thus every patient dying in refractory shock has recognizable pathologic changes to account for the failure of treatment. The commonest cause of failure to respond to treatment is myocardial damage but lesions in the lung are also extremely common. The latter tend to become progressive even after the shock state has been brought under control, and a patient who has survived myocardial damage may ultimately die from respiratory failure.

The realization that shock may become refractory or irreversible must be borne in mind at all times when treating the shocked patient. Every effort must be made to correct the condition before this stage is reached and hence vigorous therapy is mandatory. However, it is important to realize that there are no known clinical, biochemical or metabolic parameters that enable us to determine unequivocally that the patient has passed the point of no return. As emphasized by Robbins, 'the term irreversibility should never be put on the patient's chart until death writes it'.

The pathogenesis of shock is extremely complex in that several mechanisms often overlap in bringing about the haemodynamic deterioration. For example:

● A patient with an overwhelming infection not only suffers the microcirculatory changes described but may also suffer a degree of cardiac failure and loss of circulatory fluid due to the inflammatory response.

● Extreme haemorrhage and hypoxia may result in myocardial damage and cardiac failure.

● Intracellular electrolyte imbalances in the shocked state are exacerbated by renal failure effecting both fluid and electrolyte imbalance.

The complexity of the pathogenesis creates a therapeutic nightmare.

Medical and nursing management

Shock is a progressive state of circulatory failure: the body's compensatory mechanisms will only operate for a certain period of time before decompensation begins. Once the patient enters the stage of decompensation, reversibility of the shock process becomes increasingly more difficult. Therefore medical intervention must be instituted as soon as possible.

This is directed towards restabilizing blood volume, correcting metabolic disturbances and creating a diuresis. The responsibility of the nurse is to monitor, interpret and report the response of the patient to treatment. On admission to hospital, arterial blood gases are taken to assess the degree of acidosis and tissue oxygenation. O_2 at a concentration of 40% or greater is administered immediately via an intranasal cannula or face mask at a flow rate of approximately 4–6 litres per minute. Blood gas values may be repeated throughout the phase of treatment. The patient's haemoglobin and haematocrit is also assessed to estimate blood loss and plasma loss, respectively, and to enable assessment of O_2 saturation of haemoglobin (see page 87). Blood is taken for group and cross-typing. An intravenous line is inserted for blood and fluid replacement. If shock is profound a CV line may be inserted which will also enable central venous pressure to be assessed. It is not unusual for a severely shocked patient to have several IV lines in situ for rapid fluid replacement.

If blood was lost then whole blood must be replaced. Until blood is available for transfusion, plasma expanders such as stable plasma protein solution (SPPS) and haemocel are used. Once blood is available it is replaced as quickly as possible.

In mild hypovolaemia, fluid replacement with solutions such as compound lactate solution may be sufficient. In more severe hypovolaemia plasma expanders may also be required. However, in overwhelming hypovolaemia where blood has been lost it is necessary to administer fluid as well as blood. It must be remembered that blood is not considered as 'fluid' replacement. When large volumes of blood are to be replaced a blood warmer must be used. The patient should be warmed slowly so as not to cause peripheral vasodilation. During this period of rapid fluid infusion (fluid load) the patient must be observed for early signs of pulmonary oedema. Urinary catheterization is mandatory to assess renal function. It is vital to create and maintain an effective diuresis as soon as possible, as the kidneys are extremely vulnerable in shock.

A burette is attached to enable a constant watch on urine output which is recorded on a 0.5–1 hourly basis. Diuretics such as frusemide may be given to stress the kidneys to produce urine. Mannitol may be given initially but is not repreated unless there is a favourable response. Mannitol is an osmotic diuretic and therefore has the potential to cause fluid retention and overload. Hourly estimations of serum electrolytes should be performed and any abnormalities treated immediately.

In septic shock intravenous antibiotics are given in large doses.

The patient is nursed lying flat. As a first aid measure during the very early stages, the patient's legs may be elevated to enable blood to flow into the central circulation. At no stage should the foot of the bed be elevated in an attempt to raise the blood pressure, as the gravitational flow of blood away from the already compensated kidneys will compound the difficulty of maintaining adequate renal perfusion.

The parameters used to assess the success of medical management include:

● An overall improvement in the patient's clinical presentation, including conscious state and colour.
● A rise in blood pressure and/or CVP
● A slowing of the pulse with improved volume and strength
● An increased urinary output and an increased body temperature

● Normal blood gas, serum electrolyte, haemo-globin and haematocrit values.

Ideally, a severely shocked patient is nursed in an intensive or special care unit, and it is the nurse's responsibility to intelligently observe and report the patient's progress and response to treatment.

Readings of CVP, blood pressure and tempera-ture may need to be taken half hourly to hourly. It is usual to insert a rectal thermometer for immediate assessment of the patient's temperature in order to enable a close watch on the speed at which the patient is being warmed. A monitor attached to the patient's thumb is used to assess peripheral circulation. No food or fluid will be given by mouth until bowel sounds return.

A cardiac monitor will be used to detect arryth-mias due to potassium redistributions. It is also the nurse's responsibility to keep an accurate record of all fluids and drugs administered to the patient during the acute management.

Severe shock is a medical emergency and treat-ment must be rapid to avoid complications and to preserve the patient's life.

TRAUMA

The word 'trauma' simply means injury. It is used sometimes in a very restrictive way to describe only those injuries due to mechanical damage. However there are other ways in which cells and tissues may be injured or traumatized: by extremes of heat or cold, by electrical currents, and by radiant energy. Conversely, the word trauma should be restricted to physical agents and not broadened to include chemical insults and damage due to microorganisms and their toxins.

Mechanical injury

The effects of mechanical violence are seen commonly in clinical practice. A variety of lesions may be produced and distinctive terms such as abrasion, laceration, contusion and incision, are used for them.

In all these various types of wounds or injuries the common factor is destruction of cells and tissues. The effects, however, may differ consider-ably. Thus, an abrasion is unlikely to cause significant haemorrhage but it may act as a portal for infection. Conversely an incision or laceration may result in considerable blood loss. Incisions are usually relatively painless, at least in the short term, whereas a contusion may cause considerable pain. This is particularly so if the transmitted force causes fracture of a bone. It is important to remember that one of the commonest examples of physical violence that the nurse will encounter in the acute care setting is that due to surgery.

Thermal trauma

Cells and tissues may be damaged both by extremes of heat and of cold. Cold damages the endothelial or lining cells of the capillaries causing them to become excessively permeable. The loss of plasma and the slowing of the circulation may result in the smaller blood vessels becoming blocked by solid masses of red blood cells. Cells will then die because of a failure of their blood supply. When tissue is frozen the formation of ice crystals causes extensive cell damage. If the area of exposure is large, the body temperature may be lowered sufficiently to cause death from circula-tory failure without a local injury being sustained.

Much more commonly, tissue injury results from a local increase in heat. Thus local hyper-thermia causes cell and tissue death by damaging or denaturing cell protein. The resultant lesion, known usually as a burn, will vary in depth and extent according to the magnitude of the heat applied and the duration for which it acts.

Electrical trauma

Much of the damage caused by electrical energy is due to the production of heat. The amount of heat produced is influenced by the duration of exposure, the resistance of the tissues, and the intensity of the current. The skin is the tissue of highest resistance in the body and therefore develops the highest levels of heat. Thus the most common local manifestations of electrical injury are skin burns. The passage of an electrical current of sufficient intensity throughout the body may cause death due to a disturbance of nervous conduction and a consequent interference with cardiac and ventilatory activity. In deaths of this sort the maximal local injuries are seen in the skin at the sites of entry and exit of the current.

Radiant energy

The ever increasing use of radioactive substances both in industry and medicine has made the study of radiation damage of great practical importance. On the body its effects vary from local tissue necrosis to genetic damage, cancer, and death. The way in which radiant energy causes tissue damage is extremely complex and still not fully understood but essentially it is due to a disruption of the molecular structure of cells. Cells vary considerably in their sensitivity to radiant energy, the more rapidly dividing cells, such as those in the blood forming tissues, being particularly susceptible. This vulnerability of rapidly dividing cells is utilized in the treatment of malignant tumours by radiant energy.

See Chapter 76 for the nursing management of the patient with burns.

Local effects of trauma

It is apparent that a variety of physical agents can cause damage to cells and tissues. At a local level such damage will lead to a number of cell and tissue reactions.

Inflammation

Inflammation may be defined as the local reaction of vascular connective tissues to injury. It is one of the most frequent and important pathologic processes encountered. As has been discussed it manifests clinically by local heat, swelling, redness, and pain – familiar signs at the site of tissue injury whether that injury be due to excessive heat, excessive cold, or mechanical trauma, the latter including that due to surgical procedures. Although sometimes responsible for considerable tissue destruction, the inflammatory process is considered to be essentially protective in nature. It is due to the liberation of chemical substances from injured cells, many such substances now being recognized.

Degeneration and necrosis

When an injury is such that the cell cannot respond to it in a positive way there occurs a negative reaction referred to as 'degeneration'. Degeneration is essentially a process of progressive deterioration in cell structure and function. Frequently, the degenerative process is reversed and the cells recover, but if the process continues beyond a point of no return the result is cell death or necrosis.

General or systemic effects of trauma

Circulatory responses

Trauma initiates a complex sequence of events which involve virtually every organ and tissue in the body. The earliest, and possibly the most dramatic, of these are the circulatory adjustments which are designed to maintain an adequate blood supply to the vital organs. Cardiac output is increased or maintained by an increased heart rate whilst peripheral vasoconstriction aids in the maintenance of blood pressure. These changes are brought about by reflex mechanisms, acting by way of the vasomotor centre, and also by hormonal activity, notably from the suprarenal glands. Arteriolar constriction is selective, ensuring that the vital organs such as the brain and heart receive adequate blood, often at the expense of other organs and tissues including the skin, kidneys and intestines.

Should these compensatory mechanisms fail to maintain adequate tissue perfusion the clinical state of shock ensues.

Metabolic responses

In recent years there has been a considerable increase in knowledge regarding the metabolic responses to trauma. This knowledge is of great importance in managing the severely injured patient and is of particular significance in planning major surgery and ensuring the recovery of the patient after such surgery. The endocrine and metabolic changes that occur are common to all types of injury and collectively constitute the body's reaction to trauma. The responses may be greatly modified by a number of factors, such as the intensity of the injury, the occurrence of complications such as shock or infection, the nutritional state of the patient, and the immediate post-trauma management. Thus, for example, the end result of injuries sustained in a road accident may be entirely different to that of identical injuries inflicted in a planned elective surgical procedure. Nevertheless any significant injury will affect all phases of body metabolism and the resultant responses can be summarized as:

Carbohydrate metabolism. Most injuries are followed by an elevation of blood glucose level. This hyperglycaemia provides a ready source of energy and also increases the osmolarity of the serum. The resultant attraction of fluid into the vascular spaces helps to maintain circulating blood volume.

Protein metabolism. Protein catabolism is probably the most conspicuous metabolic consequence of trauma. Shortly after the injury is sustained there is an excessive breakdown of protein and a negative nitrogen balance. Protein nitrogen is lost in the urine and as much as 20 g of nitrogen, in the form of urea, may be lost daily. The duration of this loss varies according to the severity of the trauma. It may last for a day or so only after relatively minor surgery whereas severe burns may be associated with nitrogen loss of ten days duration or more. The loss is prolonged by superimposed infection. Since the body contains virtually no excess protein this post-traumatic loss occurs at the expense of body tissues, particularly skeletal muscle. This extreme catabolism is complicated by diminished nutritional intake and hence severe injury is usually characterized by marked tissue wasting and weight loss.

Fat metabolism. Fat is the major source of energy following trauma. Storage fat is mobilized and hydrolysed to produce glycerol and fatty acids. The free fatty acids thus produced replace glucose as the primary energy source whilst the glycerol takes part in glucose production.

Water and electrolytes. The immediate response to trauma is a conservation of water and sodium with a consequent oliguria. Water and sodium chloride retention is one of the primary responses to injury. The usual result is hypotonicity of body fluids, since the retention of water exceeds that of sodium. In addition a considerable amount of water is derived from intracellular fluids and as a result of the oxidation of fats and proteins. Thus a surgical patient may catabolize 500 g of protein and 500 g of fat daily, resulting in a daily production of 1 litre of water. Commonly, following major surgery, a brisk diuresis occurs on the third or fourth postoperative day.

The conservation of water and sodium is accompanied by an increased urinary loss of potassium, a negative potassium balance being particularly prominent during the first postoperative or post-injury day. As potassium is largely intracellular it is presumed to be liberated at the same time as the protein is metabolized.

The general or systemic responses to trauma are thus extremely complex and are as yet not fully explained. However, most would appear to be due to a combination of nervous and endocrine activity and conform to basic physiological principles. The initiation of many of the endocrine changes that follow injury is due to afferent nerve stimuli from the injured area. However hypovolaemia, which characterizes most significant injuries, is also a potent factor. The initial reactions designed to stabilize the cardiovascular system are largely nervous in type and depend upon a reflex increase in sympathetic activity. This activity is augmented by hormonal influences and the latter are responsible for many of the metabolic responses described.

The hyperglycaemia that follows most injuries is the result of breakdown of glycogen, particularly from the liver, associated with an increased synthesis of glucose from other sources – the so-called glucogenesis. These activities are mediated by various hormones; notably by catecholamines and, to a lesser extent, glucagon, cortisol and growth hormone. The same hormones are also responsible for the mobilization and splitting of fat, or lipolysis.

The complex changes in protein metabolism are difficult to explain. They appear to result from increased suprarenal cortical activity but observations and experimental evidence would suggest that other, as yet unexplained, factors are of importance.

The conservation of water and sodium, with the concomitant increased potassium excretion are the result of an increased secretion of vasopressin, or antidiuretic hormone, and aldosterone – mainly as a result of hypovolaemia. Impaired renal function may also be important.

By the mechanisms outlined above, the body has a remarkable ability to compensate for injury. Most of the metabolic changes that occur in response to trauma can be reproduced by the administration of ACTH or cortisone. Accordingly, virtually all hypotheses regard the suprarenal gland as the critical organ. Whilst this may be so, the recovery phase in particular is extremely

complex, and a complete and satisfactory explanation of the changes that comprise this phase is not yet available. Presumably the complex series of reactions have evolved, by a process of selection, to maximize the chances of recovery from injury. Thus John Hunter, in a treatise on the blood, inflammation, and gun-shot wounds, published in 1794 states: 'there is a circumstance attending accidental injury which does not belong to disease, viz., that the injury done has in all cases a tendency to produce both the disposition and the means of cure'.

REFERENCES AND FURTHER READING

Texts

Brunner L S, Suddarth D S 1984 Textbook of medical-surgical nursing, 5th edn. Lippincott, Philadelphia

Ganong W F 1985 Review of medical physiology, 12th edn. Lange Medical Publication, California

Guyton A S 1982 Physiology and mechanisms of disease, 3rd edn. Saunders, Philadelphia

Long B C, Phipps W J (eds) 1985 Essentials of medical-surgical nursing. Mosby, St Louis

Moore F D 1981 Homeostasis: bodily changes in trauma and surgery. In: Sabiston D C (ed) Textbook of surgery. The biological basis of modern surgical practice, 12th edn. Saunders, Philadelphia

Perez-Tamayo R 1985 Mechanisms of disease. In: An introduction of pathology 2nd edn. Year Book Medical Publishers, Chicago

Schwartz S I, Shires G T, Spencer F C, Storer E H (eds) 1984 Principles of surgery, 4th edn. McGraw-Hill Book Company, New York

Smith L H, Thier S O 1985 Pathophysiology 2nd edn. W. B. Saunders Company, Philadelphia

Thomas C G A 1983 Medical microbiology 5th edn. Bailliere-Tindall, London

Tortora G J, Funke B R, Case C L 1982 Microbiology – an introduction. Benjamin/Cunningham, California

Walter J B, Israel M S 1979 General pathology, 5th edn. Churchill Livingstone, Edinburgh

Journals

Bauman E C 1985 Code drugs. Nursing 85 15 : 12 : 50–55

Benson M L, Benson D M 1985 Autotransfusion is here – are you ready? Nursing 85 15 : 3 : 46–49

Foster C A 1984 The pregnant trauma patient. Nursing 84 14 : 11 : 58–63

Griffin J P 1986 Be prepared for the bleeding patient. Nursing 86 16 : 6 : 34–40

Klein D M 1984 Shock: physiology, signs, and symptoms. Nursing 84 14 : 9 : 44–46

Murphy P 1986 When a non-death death occurs. Nursing 86 16 : 7 : 34–39

Nursing Now 1984 Caring for the patient in hypovolemic shock. Nursing 84 14 : 3 : 24–27

Querin J J, Stahl L D 1983 12 simple, sensible steps for successful blood transfusions. Nursing 83 13 : 11 : 34–43

Sigmon H D 1983 Trauma: this patient needs your expert help. Nursing 83 13 : 1 : 33–41

Siskind J 1984 Handling hemorrhage wisely. Nursing 84 14 : 1 : 34–41

Sumner S M 1985 Electric shock. Nursing 85 15 : 7 : 43

Veldman B 1985 Determining priorities for the multiple trauma patient. Nursing 85 15 : 1 : 42–45

12

Pain – its management and therapy

John Sullivan   Chris Game

Pain has never been satisfactorily defined. It may be contrasted with pleasure, as suggested by Aristotle. Or, it may be thought of as a useful or beneficial sensation, as it brings the patient to the physician, however this is a physiological assumption and does not provide an acceptable explanation for the pain of cancer.

Lieutenant Colonel Henry K. Beecher, as triage officer on the beaches of Anzio in 1944 observed that the severity of the pain was not necessarily correlated with the severity of the wound. Those soldiers who were severely wounded but alive and would have to fight no further, suffered less pain than those who suffered minor wounds and would have to return to battle in due course (Beecher, 1956). Emotional factors were important in the pain of the patient and these required treatment in addition to the use of standard analgesics. He explained this by considering that what he saw was suffering, which he equated with the pain sensation plus its psychological modifications. Keele, working on experimental animals and human volunteers, developed a similar concept – the total pain reaction is a product of the pain sensation and the pain experience (Keele & Smith, 1982).

'Don't let me suffer' is one of the commonest requests made by patients and their relatives. Less commonly, the request will be phrased 'Don't let me suffer pain'. Pain is that element of suffering that requires an analgesic and it is important to look beyond the patient's complaint of pain to see the need for total relief of suffering. In the treatment and management of any patient with pain, it is important to consider the suffering of the patient. This includes the pain sensation, any psychological modifications such as depression, past pain experience and, often, iatrogenic contributions.

PAIN SENSATION

The pain sensation component is determined by the pain stimulus. This stimulus is usually peripheral in origin, but may be psychogenic or central as in thalamic pain which occurs with some tumours and after cerebrovascular accidents.

1. Peripheral pain

The peripheral pain stimulus may be divided into superficial pain, intermediate pain, and deep visceral pain.

a. Superficial pain

Superficial pain commonly arises from the skin, and the mucosa of the nose and mouth, although it may arise from any surface stimulus. It is burning or hot or prickling in quality, well demarcated, and does not radiate. It may be surrounded by an area of hyperaesthesia, or increased sensation, usually described as soreness. There is no associated muscle spasm unless the involved area is over a joint and the patient voluntarily restricts movement of the part to reduce this soreness. Autonomic effects such as nausea, vomiting, sweating, or changes in pulse or blood pressure are not present. The nonparenteral treatment of choice is aspirin. Nonsteroidal anti-inflammatory compounds such as paracetamol, indomethacin, phenylbutazone, ibuprofen may be substituted but aspirin is usually the most effective.

Nursing care for superficial pain includes regular dressings, soothing lotions, application of heat, cold, or local anaesthetics. The application of adequate irrigation and frequent dressing changes are an important part in the treatment of superficial pain induced by ulceration. Nursing assessment will determine the frequency of individual dressing changes. Factors influencing the assessment include: the nature of the wound and its dressing; the prevention of infection; the comfort of the patient; and the aesthetic appearance of the wound. The pain of an ulcer, malignant or otherwise, is due to the accumulation of kinins on the exposed surface. Kinins are produced as a consequence of local necrosis, or slough, due to the impairment of blood supply by tumour, previous surgery, and/or radiotherapy. Infection is common and escalates the process of kinin production. Removal of these kinins by frequent dressing of the wound, including irrigation, may lead to a marked or complete reduction in the pain stimulus. Malignant ulceration is often not painful if the tissues are clean and healthy. Wounds should be dressed with a frequency assessed to anticipate the onset of pain and not on an occasional basis. Attention to the detail of wound dressing will reap good dividends in controlling pain.

On a few occasions, with very extensive lesions, it may be found necessary to continually irrigate the ulcer to achieve control of pain. With modern impervious plastic dressings and low pressure pumps, continuous irrigation is easier to achieve than with previous methods. Despite its acceptance in the treatment of burns, we are yet to see widespread acceptance of total immersion of the patient with malignant ulceration using a plunge bath. It is a very effective means of irrigation and many patients experience relief and control of superficial pain. Resistance to the use of a plunge bath is based on the risk of cross infection, the difficulties of sterilization, and the presumed repugnance of subsequent users of the bath. Equally effective and often more acceptable is a shower bath.

Removal of necrotic infected tissue can usually be achieved by frequent dressings, sometimes with the addition of sodium hypochlorite solution. Occasionally, hydrogen peroxide may be used with good effect.

Superficial pain may also arise from the mucosa of the gut, as in gastritis, and the submucosa, as in shallow peptic ulceration and linitis plastica. The pain can be relieved according to the principles of treatment outlined above, using antacids as a soothing lotion, local anaesthetics as in mucaine, and aspirin. There is usually a too rapid desire to change from aspirin to other nonsteroidal anti-inflammatory agents to avoid the possible risk of gastric bleeding. Because the pain of peptic ulceration is dependent upon acid secretion, H_2 antihistamine blockers (such as cimetidine) may be very effective in the treatment of the pain associated with gastric carcinoma. Presumably they act by abolishing the small residual acid secretion in a condition which is usually associated with hypoacidity. As in many situations in the management of the patient with persistent cancer, a cost–benefit analysis is required and certain risks may have to be taken in order to employ the superior pain relieving properties of aspirin.

It is therefore important that the nursing assessment includes: the patient's reaction to the degree of pain relief and/or control achieved by the use of aspirin; the need for increasing dosages to achieve adequate control; and observation for the early signs of gastric bleeding.

b. Intermediate pain

Intermediate pain arises from bone, joints, ligaments, and the capsules of solid or hollow organs such as the liver, lung, bowel, and peritoneum. It may radiate to well recognized sites such as in the association of knee pain with hip pathology, or back pain which may mimic colic. It is a constant pain. There may be associated muscle spasm, usually different from that associated with superficial pain, in that intermediate pain leads to muscle spasm, whereas superficial pain is only associated with muscle spasm of joint movement. There are no associated autonomic effects. Treatment is with aspirin or other nonsteroidal derivatives.

Nursing assessment should therefore include observations to elicit: the presence or absence of muscle spasm; the site of the pain and any radiation of the pain stimulus; the patient's response to the analgesia used; and the need for increasing dosages to achieve adequate control.

c. Deep visceral pain

Deep visceral pain arises from solid and hollow organs as well as from a mass of damaged or injured muscle. It may radiate occasionally and if so, usually in a peculiar or bizarre fashion without apparent anatomical explanation. This is the cause of part of the difficulty in the diagnosis of right upper quadrant abdominal pain associated with pathology of the bowel, liver, gall bladder, or kidney. There is often associated autonomic phenomena such as loss of appetite, nausea and vomiting, pulse and blood pressure changes, and sweating. The treatment is with a narcotic analgesic. Nursing problems are resolved as they arise from the associated autonomic phenomena, and there should be emphasis on emotional support.

2. Central pain

Central pain arises in lesions of the central nervous system which may be induced by trauma (for example, gunshot wound to the skull, paraplegia), vascular obstruction, tumour (usually primary), or infection (for example, post herpetic neuralgia). The pain is expressed by a variety of symptoms more commonly recognized as parasthesiae, such as burning, itching, pins-and-needles; and hyperaesthesiae, which are provoked by light touch and relieved by firm pressure. It is the constancy rather than the severity of these symptoms which causes the patient to interpret them as pain rather than as parasthaesiae. The usual analgesics are ineffective. Hydroxytriptamine blocking agents such as tricyclic antidepressants are often effective.

3. Psychogenic pain

Somatization is common in many types of mental disorders, of which the commonest is depression. It is now recognized that up to 30% of patients admitted to a geriatric unit will be suffering from depression which may be of long duration. As a distinct clinical entity, depression can be seen in 8–15% of cases seen in primary care. The depression which is the primary abnormality is often not diagnosed and the pain which results is accepted as of organic origin rather than as an expression of psychogenic pain. Whenever there is an apparently inappropriate response to analgesia, the patient's mood must be considered. In psychogenic pain, the patient suffers real pain and it is of no value to tell him that it is in his mind. Both the underlying psychological problem and the pain require treatment. This is classically seen in the tension headache due to anxiety, in which the prevention of the pain may ultimately be achieved by treating the anxiety. Meanwhile, the patient needs analgesics for the headache and will take this medication. Psychogenic pain is in contrast to the following condition – malingering.

Malingering

Malingering occurs when the patient falsely claims to have pain symptoms or claims a severity of pain which he knows he does not have. This is done either for profit or as a cry for help.

PSYCHOLOGICAL MODIFICATIONS OF PAIN

Present psychic modification

The patient's mood may alter the pain threshold. The psychological changes induced by the pain include anxiety with acute pain, and depression with chronic pain: anxiety and depression lower the threshold. The pain precedes the mental change or occurs concurrently, rather than the mental change preceding the pain, as is the case with psychogenic pain. In many patients, modification of the present psychological state may be of great help in controlling the total pain reaction or suffering.

Analgesics, particularly morphine, have a significant action in elevating mood, although this effect is usually rather shorter (of the order of 1–2 hours) than the analgesic effect (which is of 4–6 hours duration). This is one explanation for the frequent requirement for morphine in some cancer patients. This need can be obviated by the use of a mood altering drug, such as a short acting antidepressant like amethylphenindate, often combining with a long acting antidepressant of the tricyclic group.

It is therefore essential that nursing assessment includes the observation of the patient's mood status as well as his response to the analgesic effect of a narcotic drug. It is not uncommon for a patient to express the fact that his pain is well controlled, however his state of anxiety in anticipation of the pain's return contradicts the degree of analgesia achieved.

Past psychic modification

Past pain experience may modify patients' interpretation of their present symptoms. This may be related to previous experiences of a relative or friend who died of cancer with pain, or a life-long fear of a mutilating illness. Awareness of these factors may enable the health professional to help the patient minimize these fears (and hence the pain).

IATROGENIC CONTRIBUTIONS

Physician-caused errors in pain management may be errors of omission or commission. Aspirin may be omitted from a pain regime when a patient clearly has superficial pain as well as deep pain. Conversely, morphine may be given in excessive doses when attention to present or past psychic factors using more appropriate drugs may be more efficient and effective.

Nursing contributions to iatrogenic pain usually stem from errors in interpretation of drug orders, or from strict adherence to hospital drug routines in the face of individual patient responses to pain. As well, inappropriate positioning of a patient in bed and the encouragement of ambulation or the performance of nursing procedures without adequate analgesic cover can frequently lead to the patient needlessly suffering a pain stimulus. Intelligent assessment of patient analgesia requirements should reduce nursing-induced iatrogenic pain.

ASSESSMENT OF PAIN

The assessment of pain involves analysis of the pain stimulus, consideration of the past and present psychological influences, and awareness of any iatrogenic contributions. In short, it is a total assessment of the suffering of the patient. It should be appreciated that very commonly there may be more than one type of pain stimulus so that one may see (simultaneously or at various stages of the illness) deep, superficial, intermediate, and psychogenic pain. Malingering may co-exist and, very rarely, central pain occurs.

Pain is severe in proportion to the extent to which it prevents normal body and mental functioning. It is therefore important when assessing patients not simply to ask how bad is the pain, but to determine the alteration in normal function by asking questions concerning alteration of sleep patterns, changes in appetite, loss of concentration (such as inability to read), associated irritability or anxiety, and depression or crying. The observant nurse will note behavioural or physical manifestations of acute or chronic pain. It is important to assess whether the patient has such pain that normal attention to detail has been omitted. One should enquire from a significant other what normal functions have been maintained. For instance, can the patient get out of bed, shower, and attend to personal hygiene? Only by asking a range of such questions can one build up a picture of the extent to which bodily and mental function has been disturbed by pain.

TREATMENT OF PAIN

Mild to moderate pain is often relieved by combination analgesics which include a weak narcotic, such as codeine, to combat deep visceral pain; and aspirin or paracetamol, which affect intermediate and superficial pain. Such combinations have the advantage of affecting all three peripherally derived pains; superficial, intermediate and deep. When the pain is more severe it is common for one of the types to become dominant so that the other less painful sensations will not be appreciated until the greatest pain is relieved. Therefore, it is not unusual for the patient to complain of headache following the administration of morphine for visceral pain. The nurse should realize that on relief of the visceral pain the more superficial pain has manifested, and aspirin for the headache should not be withheld.

The most important factor in the treatment of pain, having selected the correct analgesic, is the method of administration. Each dose of analgesic administered should be considered as an experiment because the degree of pain may vary and the patient's physiology may alter with time. Some patients require enormous doses of narcotics to control pain. The initial dose is certainly an experiment for each patient. With morphine the usual dose is 10 mg unless a higher or lower dose is suggested by the weight of the patient, previous or current exposure to narcotics, or the presence of severe respiratory or hepatic dysfunction. Equianalgesic doses of other narcotics may be used. If there is relief of pain for 6 hours following administration of the drug, then it is considered that the right drug and the right dosage have been determined. If the relief of pain lasts only 4 hours then the drug dosage should be increased by 50%. If the pain relief is less than 4 hours then the dosage increase should be 100%. If the patient experiences only partial relief from pain for the whole 6 hours following administration of the drug, then it should be considered that there may be 2 types of pain present and increase in dosage of that particular analgesic may not necessarily give pain relief. Another class of analgesic, such as aspirin, to combat a superimposed superficial or intermediate pain, may have to be added. This is a common situation in oncology patients. In some patients there is no relief of pain at all. The situation should then be analysed to determine if the correct diagnosis of the type of pain has been made. Some patients suffer from brain pain where every abnormal sensation is interpreted as pain. Some patients may have pain relief on the analgesic regime during the day, but suffer pain at night. Pain relieved during the day with analgesia should be relieved with the same dosage of analgesia during the night. What one usually finds is that the patient is suffering, with the pain sensation being only a part of his overall experience.

The frequency of administration of the drug, unfortunately, is too often left to the nursing staff and can account for the patient suffering unnecessary pain. The order 'p.r.n.' (Pro re nata) is translated 'on behalf of the thing being born'. In practice it means awaiting the return of the pain before administration of the next dose of drug. Drugs ordered as p.r.n. can result in a Pavlovian response, in that pain is followed by relief, which is followed by pain, which in turn is relieved by administration of the drug (see Fig. 12.1A). It takes only 3 days for a Pavlovian reflex to be established and the patient becomes conditioned to the pain relief. This may lead to addiction. After conditioning has been established, it may take 10–14 days to resolve so that the patient, following discharge from hospital, then attends a general practitioner who administers an analgesic and continues the conditioned state. Decondi-

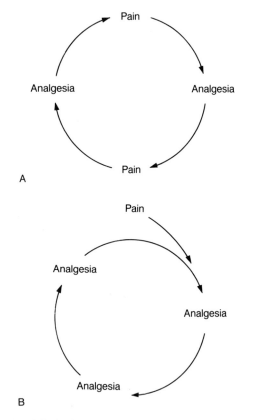

Fig. 12.1 A Pavlovian response to pain and analgesia (**A**) can be avoided if analgesia is given before pain occurs (**B**).

tioning, in the Pavlovian model, takes 7 days and in some patients a lot longer.

To avoid conditioning, the nurse should aim for a situation of uninterrupted absence of pain (Fig. 12.1B) so that the conditioned reflex is not created. Only when the pain stimulus is judged to have resolved, should the analgesia be stopped. In patients with chronic pain, the dosage of the drug should be reduced by 50% after one month, as the cause or severity of the pain may have decreased and the treatment may not be necessary. This is often not appropriate in oncology patients, but the possibility that the pain stimulus has decreased or resolved should always be considered, particularly when analgesic side effects suddenly appear, vomiting being the principal manifestation. Because cancer patients suffer from chronic pain, usually present 24 hours of the day, 7 days a week, it is imperative that the drug be administered, not p.r.n. but in anticipation of the time of the return of the pain irrespective of the length of time between administration of the drug.

Nursing assessment must include objective observation of the patient and his response to analgesic therapy. It is not uncommon for a nurse responsible for analagesic administration to make a subjective observation that a patient is becoming dependent upon his analgesia. Signs perceived as indicating dependence include frequent requests for pain relief, and enquiries regarding the due time for the next pain relief administration. This reaction is most likely the result of the patient equating his pain with the pain relief used. To withhold pain relief until such time as the patient is in extreme pain, or meets the perceived requirements of the health institution's policy on narcotic administration, is to increase the likelihood that addiction will develop. The sensible administration of pain relief in anticipation of the return of pain should be the nursing objective in all instances of pain control management.

ANALGESICS

1. Non-narcotic analgesics

Aspirin is the most effective agent and is used for both superficial and intermediate pain. Because the duration of action is short, usually 3–4 hours, dosages of this frequency are essential. It is often extraordinarily difficult to achieve regular dosages of an apparently innocuous drug such as aspirin or paracetamol. It is a vital nursing responsibility to record the administration of the aspirin. On occasions, the drug may be given 3 or 2 hourly, often as a ploy to obtain administration of sufficient quantity of the drug to have an adequate analgesic effect. The word 'strictly' in a specific drug order should have special meaning for the nurse. Too often nurses fail to comply with such an order due to ignorance of the value of regular drug administration in the fight to achieve pain control. It is difficult to provide adequate aspirin at night and occasionally 1.2–1.5 g may be given as a single dose in an attempt to achieve sleep of 4–6 hours. More often, the patient is woken by pain in the early morning and must take further aspirin. Aspirin suppositories are a useful alternative route of administration in 1 g dosages. They are particularly effective in patients who have recently undergone surgery, or who are otherwise unable to take medications orally. The importance of assessing dosage over 24 hours is nowhere more significant than in the use of aspirin.

2. Narcotic analgesics

Morphine is the preferred agent. Equianalgesic doses of the other narcotics are available, but it is important to understand the other narcotic analgesics, to avoid errors in pain control.

Pentazocine has a 1.5 hour action. Administration results in a less than expected analgesic effect; the equianalgesic dose to 10 mg of morphine is 50 mg. It should never be combined with morphine because of its antagonist activity in addition to being a weak narcotic.

Pethidine has a 2.5 hour action when given in a 100 mg equianalgesic dose. For only 10% of patients will it last longer than 3 hours, although the common method of administration is 4 hourly. If the physician wishes to give the drug on this basis, then doses of up to 400 mg are required.

Methadone has an equianalgesic dose of 10 mg and an analgesic effect lasting 6 hours. Because it is retained in the body for 28–36 hours it prevents withdrawal effect which accounts for its use in the treatment of drug dependence. If used as an analgesic it must be administered no more frequently than 6 hourly.

Dextromoramide (Palfium) has an equianalgesic dose of 5–10 mg of morphine. Tolerance is developed more rapidly than with any other narcotic (after 24 hours), so that more and more tablets are required at shorter intervals. It is effective, but difficult because of the tolerance and dependency problems. Its useage is not recommended.

Heroin. The equianalgesic dose of heroin is 5 mg. It is much more bio-available than morphine and, therefore, can be used orally. In this respect it is similar to methadone, but because of lack of availability of parenteral dosage it is not used extensively.

SIDE-EFFECTS OF ANALGESICS

Morphine and other narcotics

a. Respiratory depression

Narcotic analgesia normally depresses the respiratory and cough centres. However, in the presence of pain the respiratory depressing effect of morphine is decreased, that is, pain is a natural and powerful antidote to the respiratory depression of narcotics. Often the patient is so tired from lack of sleep that normal sleep supervenes upon the relief of pain. This should not be confused with narcotic narcosis or respiratory narcosis (see pages 42 & 45).

In the usual postoperative situation, that is in the patient with normal respiratory function who is receiving postoperative narcotic analgesia, the side effect of respiratory depression is to be expected. This must not be a reason for withholding narcotic analgesia as a patient with a low ventilatory rate during sleep can be roused, which in itself will raise the ventilatory rate. More importantly, the patient will be able to cough more effectively during this period of arousal because of the narcotic analgesic cover. Respiratory depression only becomes a complication when the patient's ventilatory rate is considered to be inadequate to maintain effective gaseous exchange. Should this occur the patient's narcosis can be reversed very easily and instantly by the administration of naloxone, a narcotic antagonist. *Therefore, as long as the patient with a reduced ventilatory rate is able to be roused, the nurse should not be worried about the respiratory depression side-effects of the analgesia administered. Narcotic analgesia should continue to be given for control of the patient's pain.*

The nurse should be aware that a patient with a compromised respiratory system will usually receive a smaller dose of narcotic so as to avoid depressing respiratory function. THA (tacrine) is very effective in increasing ventilatory rate as well as reversing narcosis without altering analgesic effect; hence morphine with tacrine (Mortha) is often the pain relieving drug of choice for patients with poor respiratory function.

b. Constipation

Narcotics often cause coprostasis. To determine whether the patient is constipated, it is important to enquire about the consistency of the stool rather than the periodicity. Coprostasis may be treated by regular small doses of paraffin oil which acts as a lubricant and results in the increased frequency of passage of stool. If the stool is hard, then a wetting agent such as dioctyl sodium sulphosuccinate may be required.

c. Nausea and vomiting

Many patients who complain of nausea and vomiting with opiates relate this to their last experience with morphine. Very commonly, the narcotic has been given as premedication for elective surgery, at which time the patient was relatively pain free. Experimentation has shown that volunteers without pain who are given morphine 20 mg intravenously will vomit in approximately 60% of cases. Patients with pain given 20 mg of morphine will vomit in only 3–5% of cases. This exemplifies the observation that pain is an antidote to many of the side effects of morphine including nausea and vomiting, hence the preferred use of morphine in the postoperative phase regardless of the type of surgery performed.

Therefore, the nursing assessment of the patient who vomits persistently with the use of narcotic analgesia must include not only an examination of the frequency of administration of the narcotic, but also an assessment of the patient's emotional status.

d. Cardiac depression

The ill-effects of pain on the cardiovascular system far outweigh any adverse cardiac effects of narcotics. However, when they do occur, the most common manifestations of adverse cardiac effect are bradycardia and hypotension.

e. Narcosis

This is the state of depressed cerebral function due to the administration of high dose narcotic analgesia, and pain is the antidote. Tacrine or the narcotic antagonist naloxone overcome the narcosis, and the former is used with morphine in the combination called Mortha.

f. Drug dependency

The concept of addiction has been replaced by that of drug dependency, albeit iatrogenic. The commonly held fear of producing dependency remains prevalent but is frequently associated only with opiates. However, drug dependency can occur with a variety of other agents including stimulants, barbiturates, nonbarbiturate hypnotics, sedatives, narcotics, narcotic antagonists, alcohol, and hallucinogens.

Physical drug dependency is a characteristic of the drug involved; after a period of use abrupt withdrawal of the drug is accompanied by characteristic symptoms, and the patient feels compelled to use the drug to prevent these symptoms. Emotional drug dependency is largely due to the patient's personality and how the benefits of the effects of the drugs are viewed. The patient may be given morphine to relieve pain, but it is associated with relief of anxiety. It is this latter effect of the narcotic which the patient desires to be prolonged as he no longer suffers pain.

The nurse's assessment of the patient's psycho-physiological status should lead to an appropriate drug administration regime. The aim is to ensure adequate narcotic usage to achieve pain control and peace of mind, without exposing the patient to the dangers of drug dependency.

PAIN ASSESSMENT SCALES

Of increasing importance to clinical nurses has been the use of Pain Assessment Scales to assist in the accurate and objective assessment of a patient's pain. Many such scales exist as proforma questionnaires, but the common features include a basic nursing history, notation of the type and dosage of the analgesia ordered, and patient-centred questions aimed at having the patient describe the exact site of his pain, what the pain feels like, how the pain changes with time, and how strong the pain is. These assessment scales have been developed in an attempt to determine the totality of a patient's pain experience – not just an assessment of the pain stimulus and its intensity. In this way the effectiveness of a variety of nursing and medical procedures can be assessed with respect to their pain relieving abilities.

CONCLUSION

Control of pain can be easily and simply achieved provided there is knowledge and analysis of the type of pain and the contribution of mood disturbances to patient suffering. Awareness of the modes and duration of action of the common analgesics allows sensible and effective planning of a treatment schedule. Accurate nursing assessment of the patient in pain should lead to enhanced treatment schedules in that pain can be anticipated and the correct relief given before the patient is allowed to experience pain.

REFERENCES AND FURTHER READING

Texts

Brunner L S, Suddarth D S 1984 Textbook of medical-surgical nursing, 5th edn. Lippincott, Philadelphia

Havard M 1986 A nursing guide to drugs, 2nd edn. Churchill Livingstone, Melbourne

Keele C A, Smith R (eds) 1962 The assessment of pain in man and animals. Churchill Livingstone, Edinburgh

Long B C, Phipps W J (eds) 1985 Essentials of medical-surgical nursing. C V Mosby, St Louis

Society of Hospital Pharmacists of Australia 1985 Pharmacology and drug information for nurses, 2nd edn. Saunders, Sydney

Journals

Bast C, Hayes P 1986 Patient-controlled analgesia. Nursing 86 16 : 1 : 25

Beecher H K 1956 Relationship of the significance of a wound to pain experienced. Journal of American Medical Assessment 161, 1609–1613

Drain C B 1984 Managing postoperative pain . . . it's a matter of sighs. Nursing 84 14 : 8 : 52–55

Fagerhaugh S Y, Strauss A 1980 How to manage your patient's pain . . . and how not to. Nursing 80 10 : 2 : 44–47

Haight K 1987 Epidural analgesia. Nursing 87 17 : 9 : 58–59

Harding J E 1984 Chronic pain – a disease in itself. The Australian Nurses Journal 14 : 4 : 50–52, 67

Marcus J 1983 Al wanted just one thing – pain relief. Nursing 83 13 : 8 : 50–51

McCaffery M 1980 Understanding your patient's pain. Nursing 80 10 : 9 : 26–31

McCaffery M 1980 Patients shouldn't have to suffer – relieve their pain with injectable narcotics. Nursing 80 10 : 10 : 34–39

McCaffery M 1980 Relieve your patients' pain fast and effectively with oral analgesics. Nursing 80 10 : 11 : 58–63

McCaffery M 1980 Relieving pain with noninvasive techniques. Nursing 80 10 : 12 : 54–57

McGuire L, Wright A 1984 Continuous narcotic infusion: it's not just for cancer patients. Nursing 84 14 : 12 : 50–55

Meissner J E 1980 McGill-Melzack pain questionnaire. Nursing 80 10 : 1 : 50–51

Nursing Update 1983 Narcotic and opioid analgesics. Nursing 83 13 : 10 : 17–18

Olsson G, Parker G 1987 A model approach to pain assessment. Nursing 87 17 : 5 : 52–57

Pageau M G, Mroz W T, Coombs D W 1985 New analgesic therapy relieves cancer pain without oversedation. Nursing 85 15 : 4 : 46–49

Parish K, Thompson G 1987 Epidural 'port-a-cath' – an analgesic find. The Australian Nurses Journal. 17 : 3 : 44–47

Warbinek E (ed) 1985 Managing intractable pain with methadone. Nursing 85 15 : 5 : 32–37

Wiley L (ed) 1979 Achieving pain control in the patient with multiple myeloma: a team approach. Nursing 79 9 : 11 : 34–39

13

Human malignancy – the basis for treatment

John Sullivan   Chris Game   Graham Joyson

The care of the patient suffering from malignant disease presents a unique challenge to the nurse in its assessment, planning and implementation. The broad spectrum of diseases under this heading, the complexities of the medical approaches to their treatment, and the psychological problems of newly diagnosed patients provide the nurse with almost unlimited opportunities to apply both artistic and scientific skills in the formulation of care plans for the management of each individual.

Problem solving is of paramount importance for the nurse facing the complexity of diseases, therapeutic approaches, side effects of such therapies, and not least their outcomes. It is well to consider at the outset that the treatment can be more debilitating than the disease itself, and to emphasize the importance of a team approach to the treatment and holistic care of patients.

PATHOPHYSIOLOGY

To understand the basis for treatment it is essential to have an outline of the scientific background to the nature and scope of cancer and allied diseases.

The human body is made up of various specific cells which aggregate into structures designated either as tissue (for example muscle or nerve), or as organs (such as lung or liver). Cancer is a pernicious proliferation of these cells. It is progressive and uncontrolled, and spreads by direct infiltration of adjacent structures, or by permeation of both the lymphatic vessels and blood stream. As cancer cells multiply they form a swelling or tumour. A secondary deposit, derived from the primary site, is termed a metastasis. A typical cancer in a solid organ, such as the breast, begins as a mobile mass; as it extends it may involve the overlying skin by infiltration and ultimately ulceration, or the deeper structures of the chest wall with tumour fixation. Spread is to neighbouring lymph glands; spread via the blood to the liver and the lungs may occur directly from the primary tumour or from its metastases. A cancer in a hollow organ, such as the stomach, begins in the mucosa and in most cases causes early ulceration; metastases occur via spread to neighbouring lymph nodes and progressively via the blood stream to major distant organs such as liver, lungs, and brain. In addition, the cancer may have access to a body cavity such as the peritoneal cavity of the abdomen, spreading across it to another organ, as in the Krukenberg tumour of the ovary or in peritoneal seedings. Certain tumours of the central nervous system may spread similarly in the subarachnoid space.

Cancers vary in their growth characteristics – some having rapid increases in cell number and hence in mass, whereas others increase very slowly resulting in great differences in natural history. However, the rate of cell division in cancers is no greater than in some normal growing tissues in children, or in the reparative process following surgery in adults.

Cancers are classified on the basis of their histological appearance. The arrangement of the cells and the degree to which they mimic the normal tissue from which the cancer arises allows a classification which infers growth rate characteristics and probable pattern of spread. Thus one can consider: small cell lung cancer, with a high propensity to spread widely and a short patient survival time; squamous cell lung cancer, which tends to remain localized and has a relatively long patient survival time; and large cell lung cancer, which has intermediate properties.

Carcinomas develop from epithelial cells lining surfaces such as skin, mucosa of gut, urethra, vagina, and the ducts of glands such as the pancreas.

Sarcomas similarly arise from the non-epithelial tissues such as bone, cartilage, or muscle. Certain cells in specialized organs can undergo malignant change, such as islet cell tumours of the pancreas and granuloma cells of the ovary. Rarely, germ cells in the testis and ovary may become malignant, producing teratomas.

DECIDING ON A TREATMENT POLICY

Before a policy of treatment can be logically determined, the presence (by biopsy), nature (by morphology), extent (by examination and investigation – see page 130 for an explanation of cancer staging), and tempo (by history) of the cancer in the individual patient should be known. In addition, we must know the natural history of the type of cancer – the way that particular cancer behaves in most patients. And we must know our percentage chances of varying this natural history by any proposed treatment, and its costs in terms of potential disability due to acute and chronic side effects that the patient may suffer. Only with this knowledge are we in a position to answer, with the patient, the first and most important question: is it in the patient's best interests that he should be treated now; or should we elect not to treat at present, keeping close observation to initiate treatment whenever indicated?

If treatment is indicated the principles that apply are best illustrated by reference to carcinoma of the breast. Local disease requires local treatment. Mastectomy may be carried out with a view to potential cure by removal of the primary tumour and adjacent involved lymph nodes. A palliative mastectomy may be performed, with or without removal of involved lymph nodes, to provide the best means of controlling an ulcerated infected tumour or simply as a means of reducing the possibility of local skin recurrence. Similarly, radiotherapy may be given with curative intent by the use of implants and external beam therapy to the primary tumour. Radiotherapy may be given in addition to primary surgical treatment to reduce the incidence of local recurrence, and perhaps to increase the cure rate in cases in which there is involvement of lymph nodes along the internal mammary artery.

Generalized disease requires general treatment, such as with hormones in the first instance and subsequently chemotherapy – particularly if there is liver involvement. Failed local treatment is an indication for general systemic therapy. In the case of breast cancer, this may be an indication for the institution of hormone therapy with tamoxifen or medroxyprogesterone (Provera), or another form of chemotherapy.

A local complication, or potential local complication, of general disease may need local treatment – such as the use of surgery to internally fix a fracture, or decompress the spinal cord; or the use of radiotherapy to relieve a superior mediastinal obstruction syndrome.

Adjuvant cytotoxic chemotherapy and hormone therapy have been devised with a view to reducing the chance of development of subsequent general disease following apparently successful local treatment with surgery or radiotherapy. This treatment is not always effective. It is still used in the treatment of breast cancer and may exert its effects by induction of ovarian failure and the subsequent indirect hormone withdrawal.

It must be appreciated that a combined modality approach to the treatment of cancer has gained considerable interest and acceptance in medicine today. However, it is vital to understand that the initial approaches by single modality treatments were based on individual professional judgements, of great worth in many instances, but with little thought to an optimum outcome.

The following discussion of the individual modalities and their development will give some appreciation of how the present combined approach has emerged.

SURGERY

The first attempts to cure cancer were by surgery. It was found that removal of the tumour mass would result in cure in some cases, but not all. Either the removal was incomplete, and the patient died by progression of the disease at the primary site; or metastases developed and death occurred due to failure of organs (such as the liver) infiltrated with secondary tumour. Development of surgical and anaesthetic techniques allowed earlier diagnosis, removal of larger amounts of tissue, and improved results. There has been little change in the rate of surgical cure of cancer since the 1950s. Some tumours, such as skin cancer, have high rates of cure. Other tumours, such as bowel and uterine cancer, can be cured in large numbers of patients. For many other cancers surgery offers a chance to remove the primary tumour, but the patients still may die subsequently of metastases.

Nursing care during the postoperative phase employs all the principles discussed in Chapter 6, along with specific care of the operative site. However, one cannot underestimate the psychological support needed in the preoperative and postoperative phases.

The old adage that illness is an act of God, and survival the will of God, was alive and well in the early days of treatment. Patients were condemned variously as unclean, infectious, social lepers, and often were rejected by family and friends. This fear of the disease, repugnance, and denial, are attributable to inherited social stigmata, and emphasize the importance of the extra psychological support required by patients, and their families, when aware of their diagnosis (see Chapter 2).

RADIOTHERAPY

The aim of radiotherapy is to kill the cancerous tissue and cause as little destruction as possible to surrounding healthy tissues. There are a variety of approaches with radiation. Radiotherapy tends to have the most sinister implications for the patient with cancer. Essentially it involves the bombardment of the tumour with radiation.

The sources can be direct, external radiation from powerful X-ray, for example superficial or deep X-ray therapy (SXRT or DXRT) or internal solid source application with radioactive nuclides,

for example, radium or caesium. In the case of the former, precautions apply during treatment, which is normally of short duration, as are applied in normal X-ray diagnostic approaches. In the case of solid sources, precautions are considerable and involve time and distance factors, ensuring minimum nursing and family contact during treatment. In radio-isotope therapy, for example with radioactive iodine, the problem of disposal of body waste is an added consideration.

Radiotherapy has a role in curing cancer, particularly at primary sites where surgery would result in unacceptable deformity or loss of function. In principle, these include carcinoma of the cervix, carcinoma of the head and neck, and Hodgkin's disease. A common use of radiotherapy is for palliation to control the symptoms of cancer, resulting in improved quality of life, and hence possibly a prolonged life while producing minimal side effects. Radiotherapy suffers the same limitations as surgery in that it is unable to eliminate cancer cells outside the field of operation or administration of the therapy.

Refinements in technical approaches by radiotherapists have minimized the side-effects suffered previously by patients in the developmental phases of this therapeutic approach. Again, one cannot over-emphasize the need for psychological support in planning the care of the patient undergoing radiotherapy. This is especially significant in the early stages of planning the therapy, as the machinery itself can be a daunting sight for the patient, and is one factor often overlooked in assessing the support required.

Nursing management of the patient undergoing radiotherapy

With external X-ray therapy (deep or superficial) the patient should be fully advised as to what is expected of him during therapy. Such advice includes informing him that he will be required to lie still on the X-ray table during each session, which may last for up to 30 minutes at a time. However, he will receive radiation for only a maximum of 5 minutes during the session. The area to be radiated will be marked on his skin with a water-soluble blue dye and he will be asked to not wash the markings off during the entire period of treatment; this ensures that exactly the same area is treated at each session.

The patient should be reassured that special lead shields will be provided to protect other areas of his body, and especially organs, from any exposure to the radiation source. Remaining still during the therapy session will ensure that the radiation will be directed to the target area. Most patients need to be reassured that radiotherapy is a painless procedure and that it does not make them radioactive. The patient should also be realistically appraised of the likely reactions that he will have to the radiation therapy, and he should be reassured that these reactions will cease and are reversible on discontinuation of the therapy.

Radiation affects the normal cells through which it must travel on its way to the target area. Any radiation therapy will cause a skin reaction and this will be greatest at the entry site of the radiation beam and only minimal at the exit site; the first sign is localized erythema over the area irradiated. With repeated therapy dry desquamation occurs and the patient will complain of pruritus. He should be advised against exposing the irradiated area to sunlight or direct heat as this will intensify the reaction. Where possible he should avoid covering the area, or rubbing or scratching as friction will also intensify the reaction. Unless advised otherwise he should wash the area as normal but using only luke-warm water and a very mild soap. The area should be patted dry with a soft towel. If the area must be shaved (as in facial radiation areas), only an electric razor should be used. A bland ointment may be applied to reduce dryness and pruritus but only ointments provided by the radiotherapy unit may be used. Any ointment with a metal base must not be used as this will increase the radiation reaction.

The radiation reaction may progress to blistering and this will peak approximately 2 weeks after therapy has ceased. The radiotherapy unit will supply a dusting powder which can be used to absorb moisture, and if ulcers or crusts form the area should be gently bathed in a mild saline solution and then cold cream applied. If a dressing must be used, cold cream must be applied first to prevent the dressing from adhering to the area. Finally, the patient should be advised that epilation will most likely result if hair is present in the treatment area. He should be reassured that the hair will grow back once treatment has ceased. During treatment he should wash his hair gently using a very mild shampoo and avoid excessive brushing and combing. He should also cover his scalp when out in the sun.

Radiotherapy also produces internal side-effects dependent upon the area of the body being irradiated. These effects also occur as a result of the administration of cytoxic chemotherapy agents and the nursing management for either cause is similar. The patient may develop extreme fatigue, muscle aches or pain, with weakness, numbness, or tingling; headaches; nausea and vomiting; indigestion; diarrhoea or constipation; localized mucositis, for example mouth ulcers; and an increased susceptibility to infection.

The patient should be advised to regulate rest and activity and to plan frequent rest periods during the day; he should avoid any activity that aggravates his condition. Mild analgesia will be prescribed to control headaches and pain, and locally applied heat will assist in relieving muscle soreness. The patient will be ordered an antiemetic and the nurse should ensure that he understands the need to take the medication regularly. The eating of small, frequent meals should be encouraged along with the frequent taking of fluids such as fruit juices to aid in overcoming nausea and vomiting. If vomiting persists he must seek medical advice immediately.

Where possible he should clean his teeth with a soft tooth-brush both before and after eating and until mouth ulcers heal he should avoid foods that are hard to chew or are chemically irritant. Extremes of temperature of food and fluid should also be avoided. Nursing measures to control either diarrhoea or constipation should be instituted (see Chapter 49). He should be advised to avoid contact with persons who have colds or other infections and he should see his physician immediately if he develops a sore throat, fever, chills, or any signs of bleeding.

Internal radiation therapy involves the implantation of radioactive material into a body cavity or directly into the tumour mass. This form of radiotherapy is commonly used in head and neck tumours, and in cancer of the female reproductive tract. The aim is to maximize the radiation effect at the target with minimal effect on the surrounding normal tissue. The patient will be hospitalized and in most instances isolated, either within a single room or behind a shield. As well, visitors and hospital staff will only be permitted to spend short time intervals with the patient to minimize radiation exposure. Care must be taken with the disposal of the patient's body wastes, and if the implant is permanent he should be advised that the radioactivity lessens each day and that he will not be discharged until the implant has reached acceptable limits of radioactivity.

CHEMOTHERAPY

Chemotherapy is the treatment of cancer by 'chemical warfare' using chemical substances in both solid and liquid form. There is a broad range of therapeutic agents under this heading which include hormones and antibiotics (see page 128). The principle is to present to the system a toxic substance which mimics closely the natural requirements of a cell and its growth. The cell in taking up the 'bait' is unable to reproduce and subsequently dies. The cell's ability to discriminate quickly causes a problem and a challenge and has necessitated the development of multi-drug protocols to keep the cell either 'fooled' or 'guessing'.

Cancer chemotherapy was developed principally for the treatment of malignancies for which surgery and radiotherapy have little effect, such as leukaemia, and subsequently in an attempt to control tumours which may have spread beyond the surgical or radiotherapeutic treatment sites. The drugs for this so-called systemic therapy are administered intravenously or occasionally orally. Analysis has shown that drugs are much less effective when there is a large bulk of tumour and many experiments have subsequently shown the successful drug treatment of animal cancers occurs when the tumour cell mass is small.

Studies of animal cancers, such as mouse leukaemia L1210, show that after innoculation of the leukaemia from one animal to another, death occurs after an interval required to achieve a cell population growth of about one billion cells (10^{12}). Cancer chemotherapeutic agents, such as cytosine arabinoside, can reduce the cell number to the stage at which no tumour can be detected in the animal, and a complete remission has occurred. In most cases the leukaemia rapidly recurs; this observation in animals is the explanation for the phenomenon seen in humans, that complete remission is usually not followed by cure, although it is a prerequisite for cure. Cancer chemotherapeutic drugs which kill large numbers of cancer cells (high cell kill) often also achieve a high cell kill in tissues of the host animal with similar growth characteristics to that of the cancer. Thus, tissues which grow rapidly, such as the bone marrow, skin and its hair follicles, and the stomach and bowel, are very susceptible to the effects of these drugs. In humans the consequences are: loss of hair; failure of production of all elements of the blood including erythrocytes, leucocytes, and thrombocytes; and loss of lining cells in the mouth and gut, producing mouth ulcers, nausea, vomiting, and diarrhoea. The principal reasons for cessation of treatment are these host toxicities and the development of resistance to the drugs. It is impossible to predict sensitivity to treatment in any individual and a trial of therapy is necessary to determine the effect of each agent.

Responses to chemotherapy have been defined to include complete remission and partial remission. Partial remission is defined as a reduction by 50% or greater in the product of two diameters of the tumour mass without the appearance of new tumour masses. This has led to the expectation that if a partial remission can be obtained with one agent, then combination with a second agent may result in complete remission.

The era of combination chemotherapy began with the treatment of leukaemia and lymphoma, and has now extended to the treatment of most malignancies. Combinations are probably more effective because they provide maximum cell kill while reducing toxicity, and they prevent or slow the development of resistant cells.

Chemotherapeutic agents

The earliest human cancer chemotherapeutic agent was nitrogen mustard, a derivitive of sulphur mustard gas first used in the trenches in the First World War as a form of chemical warfare; it is still in use. This alkylating agent and a subsequent series of drugs including busulphan, chlorambucil, melphalan, and cyclophosphamide, as well as the class of agents termed nitrosoureas, were found to be active in a variety of tumours, particularly lymphoma, leukaemia, and breast and ovarian cancer. Cyclophosphamide requires conversion in the liver to its active form.

Antimetabolite cytotoxic drugs block a specific enzyme or enzymes in the metabolic pathway of all human cells, tending to have a greater effect on human cancer cells. Methotrexate and subsequently mercaptopurine (6-mercaptopurine) and thioguanine (6-thioguanine) were found to be effective in acute leukaemia. Subsequently, other antimetabolites, fluorouracil (5-fluorouracil) and cytarabine (cytosine arabinoside), were synthesized.

The development of cancer chemotherapy has many parallels in the development of chemotherapy for the treatment of infectious disease. An antibiotic is a substance which is synthesized by one organism and is toxic to other organisms. Although most antibiotics are active against micro-organisms such as bacteria and fungi, some have anticancer effects in humans. These include actinomycin D, mitomycin (mitomycin C), mithramycin, daunorubicin, doxorubicin (adriamycin) and bleomycin. All of these agents act by inhibiting cell replication (reduplication).

Vinblastine, vincristine, vindesine, etoposide (VP16) and teniposide (VM26) are used in the treatment of lymphoma, leukaemia and lung cancer and inhibit the so-called M phase of the cell cycle.

Corticosteroids (prednisolone, dexamethasone) are effective in the treatment of breast cancer, acute lymphoma, and leukaemia. Their effectiveness as anticancer agents occurs when they are used in quantities far in excess of those normally present in the body – so called 'pharmacological' doses rather than physiological doses. Side effects include changes in body shape, euphoria, diabetes mellitus, and hirsuitism. There are analogies of this phenomenon demonstrated in human tumours, such as breast cancer and prostate cancer, where pharmacological doses of other hormones such as tamoxifen, aminoglutethimide, androgens and

progesterone are effective anticancer agents. The enzyme, L-asparaginase destroys the essential aminoacid asparagine and slows the growth of human lymphatic leukaemia. Organometal compounds such as cis-platinum, although extremely toxic, have been found to have an anti-tumour action in humans, particularly in testicular and ovarian tumours.

The synthesis of new agents has resulted in the development of a series of dimethyltriazeno compounds, particularly procarbazine, and dacarbazine DTIC (imidazole carboxamide) an alkylating agent used for Hodgkin's disease, melanoma, and sarcoma.

Effective combinations include the MOPP regime (nitrogen mustard, vincristine, procarbazine and prednisolone) for the treatment of Hodgkin's disease; cis-platinum, vinblastine and bleomycin (CVB) for testicular tumours; and cyclophosphamide, vincristine and prednisolone (CVP) for non-Hodgkin's lymphoma. The combination of cyclophosphamide, methotrexate and fluorouracil (5-fluorouracil) (CMF) has proved particularly effective in controlling the effects of extensive breast cancer, although cure has not been achieved. Other combinations have been tried without success in most other tumours.

Nursing responsibilities for the safe handling and/or administration of cytotoxic drugs

A discussion of the agents used in cancer chemotherapy would be incomplete without consideration of the nursing responsibilities when both handling and administering such cytotoxic agents. In particular the administration of parenteral cytotoxic drugs is not without considerable risks, both legal and physical, for the registered nurse (RN).

Cytotoxic drugs may be administered only by a suitably qualified oncology RN under the direct or indirect supervision of a medical practitioner. The degree of supervision required varies between the State Registration Boards and RNs are advised to acquaint themselves with their individual state legislation. Hospital policies regarding the handling and administration of cytotoxic drugs also vary widely both between and within states, and

RNs are further advised to ensure that they are operating within the legal requirements of their hospital's policy, when dealing with any aspect of cytotoxic chemotherapy. Under no circumstances should undergraduate nursing students be involved in the handling, preparation or administration of parenteral forms of cytotoxic drugs.

Any cytotoxic agent in its reconstituted form for parenteral administration has the potential for cell destruction in both the recipient and the preparer/administrator of the agent. Many of the cytotoxic agents mentioned in this chapter have the potential to create mutagenic and carcinogenic effects should they be mishandled during preparation for, and during, administration. In particular some agents are capable of inducing sterility and/or producing teratogenic effects in persons who are exposed topically or parenterally to the agents either during preparation or injection.

The RN should be aware of the need to ensure a separate and adequate area for drug preparation, particularly when the agents are prepared and administered in general hospital wards. He/she should ensure: the correct wearing of protective clothing by all personnel when such agents are being prepared; the correct and safe disposal of sharps/needles, the equipment used in preparation and administration and of any wastes; the correct terminal cleaning of any nondisposable articles used; and that the correct procedures are followed in the event of any spillage.

The suitably qualified oncology RN is also cognizant of the potential problems for the patient during administration of parenteral forms of cytotoxic chemotherapy, and is prepared to observe for and intervene to minimize situations which include: extravasation of the drug; dermal and subcutaneous tissue necrosis due to the use of an intravenous site with poor blood supply; the development of proximal thrombophlebitis in a limb, and its consequences of impaired venous drainage; the administration of cytotoxic drugs via peripheral veins previously involved with thrombophlebotic episodes. The nursing management of the patient with side-effects from cytotoxic chemotherapy is symptomatic and the principles are as for the patient undergoing radiotherapy (see page 126). For the management of the immune suppressed patient, see page 400. The nurse should note that in almost all instances of cytotoxic chemotherapy generalized epilation will occur.

It cannot be overemphasized that RNs owe a duty of care to their oncology patients to ensure that at all times nursing care is assessed, planned, implemented and evaluated by personnel specifically prepared to care for the needs of this specialist group.

CONCLUSION

Human malignancy remains one of the most baffling and challenging areas of health care. The combined efforts of medical practitioners, nurse practitioners, and researchers have made considerable progress in the knowledge and treatment of the wide spectrum of insidious diseases. A medical combined modality approach to decision making in regard to treatment has improved the quality of life for many patients. There has been increasing emphasis on the psychological support required in caring for the patients and recognition of the need for a multidisciplinary approach to care.

The nurse has an integral part to play in this team and often will become the focus of the patient because of the continuity provided in the care situation. Nursing problems are numerous and not easy to resolve, and emotional support for staff becomes a prerequisite in many units. The variety of diseases and approaches to treatment are best handled by a qualified oncology team who jointly consider the question 'Is it in this patient's best interests that he should be treated now, or should we elect not to treat at present, keeping close observations to initiate treatment whenever indicated?'

The patient's contribution to planning care should not be underestimated as the potential for decision making rests largely with him. Options should be presented and considered carefully, especially when the outcome might be severe disability or disfigurement.

NOTE: **Staging of tumours**

Staging of tumours

The extent or stage of a malignancy is an important factor in determining treatment options. The TNM classification is the internationally recognized staging system, although other systems are used for some specific disease, for example the Ann Arbor staging of Hodgkin's disease and the Duke classification of carcinomas of the rectum.

In the TNM system, T refers to the primary tumour, N to regional lymph node involvement, and M to the presence (M1) or absence (M0) of metastases. For example, the stage grouping of lung cancer is:

Stage Ia	T1	N0	M0
	T2	N0	M0
Stage Ib	T1	N1	M0
Stage II	T2	N1	M0
Stage III	T3	N0N1	M0
	Any T	N2	M0
Stage IV	Any T	Any N	M1

The numbers added to the T and N refer to the extent of involvement, which is defined precisely for the different sites of tumours. In the case of lung cancer, T2 refers to a primary tumour greater than 3 cm, with or without extension to the hilar region, and N1 means that there is hilar node involvement. Whereas in bladder tumours, for example, T2 refers to a primary tumour which has invaded the superficial muscle, and N1 means that there is single regional (i.e. pelvic) lymph node involvement of less than or equal to 2 cm.

REFERENCES AND FURTHER READING

Texts

Chaney P S (ed) 1982 Helping cancer patients effectively, 2nd edn. Intermed Communications, Pennsylvania

Cline M J, Haskell C M 1980 Cancer chemotherapy, 3rd edn. Saunders, Philadelphia

Cochet D (ed) 1985 Neoplastic disorders: nurse's clinical library. Springhouse, Pennsylvania

Fawkes B (ed) 1984 Cancer nursing in the 80's. The Cancer Institute/The Royal Melbourne Hospital, Melbourne

Havard M 1986 A nursing guide to drugs, 2nd edn. Churchill Livingstone, Melbourne

Leahy I M, St Germain J M, Varricchio C G 1979 The nurse and radiotherapy: a manual for daily care. Mosby, St Louis

Oppenheimer S B 1982 Cancer: a biological and clinical introduction. Allyn and Bacon, Boston

Society of Hospital Pharmacists of Australia 1985 Pharmacology and drug information for nurses, 2nd edn. Saunders, Sydney

Walter J 1977 Cancer and radiotherapy, 2nd edn. Churchill Livingstone, Edinburgh

Journals

Ballentine R 1983 Nursing implications of cancer chemotherapy Nursing 83 13 : 4 : 50–55

Beaudoin K, Goodemote F, Blendowski C, Downs D 1983 Going the distance with the patient who's a real fighter. Nursing 83 13 : 4 : 6–11

Carley L 1985 Drawing Robbie into a circle of love – just in time Nursing 85 14 : 8 : 58–59

de Ramon P B 1983 The final task: life review for the dying patient. Nursing 83 13 : 2 : 44–49

Dolan M B 1983 If your patient wants to die at home. Nursing 83 13 : 4 : 50–55

Elbaum N 1984 With cancer patients, be alert for hypercalcemia. Nursing 84 14 : 8 : 58–59

Hagan S J 1983 Bring help and hope to the patient with Hodgkin's disease. Nursing 83 13 : 8 : 58–64

Kearney D, Greany L 1983 Death with dignity in a terminal situation. The Australian Nurses Journal 13 : 3 : 40–43

Lyons F 1985 Malignant melanoma: the sunburnt country's dilemma. The Australian Nurses Journal 14 : 10 : 48–50

McCallum L, Carr-Gregg M 1987 Adolescents with cancer. The Australian Nurses Journal. 16 : 7 : 39–42

Ostchega Y 1980 Preventing . . . and treating . . . cancer. Chemotherapy's oral complications. Nursing 80 10 : 8 : 47–52

Ostchega Y, Jacob J G 1984 Providing "safe conduct": helping your patient cope with cancer. Nursing 84 14 : 4 : 42–47

Ostchega Y, Culnane M 1985 Tumor markers: key pieces to your cancer patient's clinical picture. Nursing 85 15 : 9 : 48–51

Pagean M G, Mroz W T, Coombs D W 1985 New analgesic therapy relieves cancer pain without oversedation. Nursing 85 15 : 4 : 46–49

Petton S 1984 Easing the complications of chemotherapy: a matter of little victories. Nursing 84 14 : 2 : 58–63

Rovere R H 1984 Thoughts while dying. Nursing 84 14 : 11 : 17–18

Shoemaker C A, Schaefer K 1985 In planning Mr Bowen's care, one picture was worth a thousand words. Nursing 85 15 : 12 : 44–46

Speciale J L, Kaalaas J 1985 Infuse-a-port: new path for IV chemotherapy. Nursing 85 15 : 10 : 40–43

Warbinck E 1985 Managing intractable pain with methadone. Nursing 85 15 : 4 : 46–49

Welch-McCaffrey D 1983 When it comes to cancer, think family. Nursing 83 13 : 12 : 32–35

Zerwekh J V 1983 The dehydration question. Nursing 83 13 : 1 : 47–51

14

The process of ageing

R. B. Lefroy

With a nursing commentary by Chris Game

GENERAL ASPECTS

Ageing and disease – a dual process

The process of ageing is one of several essential developmental changes. It is already operative by the third decade in some body systems, and becomes increasingly important with the progression of chronological age. But it would be wrong to assume that the changes we observe in old people, and in particular their alteration in functional capacity, are all due to the ageing process. People who survive to old age bring with them the marks and scars of a lifetime. The diseases which these changes represent – arthritis, bronchitis, anaemia, cancer and many others – together with the process of ageing are responsible for the differences between young and old. When studying a particular individual our difficulty is to determine which factor – disease or ageing – has brought about the change. There is an essential difference between disorders in old age (caused by the combined effect of the ageing process and acquired disease) and disorders of old age (caused by the ageing process alone). Examples of the former are common but it is rarely possible to label a particular disorder as being entirely due to the process of ageing.

Nevertheless, the two are often confused, to the detriment of the old person. Age and disease are frequently regarded as synonymous, with a hopeless prognosis. The 'aged and infirm' have been lumped together with the chronic sick and denied the benefits of diagnosis and treatment which are regarded as essential for a young person who presents with an illness. In order to change this habit we need to understand the difference between the processes of ageing and disease.

In our society a person is declared 'old' at a certain time, usually on retirement at 60–65 years of age. Too often, when this 'old' person is admitted to hospital, certain assumptions are made that are in most instances totally erroneous. It is assumed that because he is old he will be unintelligent or senile and needs to be 'protected'; that he will be compliant in all aspects of his health care management; that he is 'too old' to learn or work; that he is ill because he is 'old' and therefore does not warrant aggressive and active treatment beyond control of symptoms, so that he will not 'complain'; and that he is no longer capable of 'normal' emotional and sexual expression and therefore does not require elementary privacy.

In fact, many health workers are unable to accept being confronted by an aware, coping, and productive elderly person. The aged person who asks questions about his care is viewed with suspicion; if he refuses treatment or insists on knowing why procedures are planned he is classed as being 'difficult'; and if he demonstrates 'normal' emotional and/or sexual feelings he is categorized as a 'dirty, old man'.

Influence of the ageing process

One of the difficulties is in understanding how the process of ageing has its effect. There are a number of theories but at present there are no certain conclusions as to the cause. It is, however, possible to make some general statements with regard to what takes place and how people are affected by the process.

Ageing is wear and tear without repair, ultimately leading to death. It is part of the evolutionary process. All body systems are affected, at varying rates and in different ways. It would be responsible for 'natural' death – occurring predictably but at different times in the lives of the various animals and in humans – if there were such a phenomenon in a society which is influenced to such a degree by heart disease, stroke, cancer and traffic accidents. These other events tend to intervene before the process of ageing can complete its series of changes. However, the influence of the former, particularly that of infectious disease, is much less than it used to be.

At the beginning of this century the life expectancy at birth for a man in Australia was not much beyond 40 years. His expectation is now beyond 70 years; a woman's is a little longer. In what we refer to as 'developed' countries death now belongs much more to old age. Not only does the process of ageing have more influence on the event of death but also on those years immediately preceding death. More people survive to old age, and for the first time we are witnessing the phenomenon of the 'survival of the unfittest' (Isaacs, 1972). These are some of the reasons for attempting to understand the process of ageing, as well as the numerous diseases discussed elsewhere in this book.

Ageing or disease?

By studying the changes which take place in individuals over a number of years, it becomes possible to sort out which of those changes are due to ageing and which are due to diseases, either hereditary or environmental. Disease should be regarded as a pathological process occurring occasionally in the young and not universally in the old. Ageing can be defined as a progression of adult changes occurring in all individuals if they live long enough (Libow, 1963).

GENERAL MANIFESTATIONS OF AGEING

The effect of the ageing process can be reduced to two words – increased vulnerability. An old person's illness, whether it is acute influenza or a more chronic disabling disorder such as a stroke or heart disease, is not merely the result of being old; it is a combination of the ageing process and disease. The former makes him more predisposed

to illness and increases both morbidity and mortality; consequently there are several clinical manifestations more commonly found in the old than in the young.

An old person's impairments are likely to be multiple and their effects more difficult to disentangle. Unlike the young, it is the exception for the old person to issue a single 'presenting complaint'. Commonly there is no 'complaint' from the old person with a long-standing disorder.

A number of homeostatic systems are adversely affected by the ageing process; they respond less efficiently and within a smaller range of tolerance. Prominent among them are:

- Control of blood pressure
- Control of temperature
- Stability of posture
- Perception of pain
- Immunity.

Nurses, when initially assessing their aged patients, need to make 'normal' adjustments to 'normal' ageing patients. The assessment phase of nursing care management will take longer with an elderly patient, and the nurse must allow for this factor. Due to slower mental function, history taking will need more time; however, the older person's tolerance for questioning is usually reduced and the assessment of the elderly patient may have to be conducted in stages. If the patient has had information withheld by either his physician or significant others, for whatever reasons, he may be totally unaware of why he has been hospitalized and may seek information that the nurse is either unable or unwilling to give. His attempts at gaining this information may jeopardize the therapeutic relationship between the nurse and patient.

Ageing also produces changes in the structure, and consequently in the function, of several organs and systems – cardiovascular, respiratory, renal, nervous and others. These changes will be further considered.

There is another important variation from illness in a young or middle aged person. All people have three 'territories' – physical, mental and social. In later life it is not uncommon to find that inroads have been made into at least two if not three of these territories. Consequently, in addition to a number of physical impairments, the older person's function is frequently altered by mental and social disabilities. It becomes impossible, therefore, to make a diagnosis or to assess needs with any degree of accuracy unless all these factors are considered – impingement by the process of ageing on a number of systems, the probability of multiple impairments and the likelihood that not one but three 'territories' are affected by the phenomenon of increased vulnerability.

It is not surprising that iatrogenic disease is commonly seen in old people who have multiple disorders, are susceptible to changes in their internal environment, and have a lower threshold of tolerance to the effect of drugs. They constitute an important factor in the predisposition to illness in an old person.

These manifestations necessitate a special approach to the elderly disabled person. In particular we need to question repeatedly whether a person's functional capacity has been altered by ageing or by disease. Although treatment cannot hope to change the former, there are many instances where it can influence the latter. Unnecessary disability will be prevented by making this differentiation, and refusing to accept the common conclusion that old age is solely responsible for illness.

The difficulty of separating the two causes – disease and ageing – will become apparent in the following descriptions, and will influence markedly the selection of problem areas to be considered by the nurse when developing a nursing care plan with and for the elderly patient. Especially, the effects of ageing will influence the potential for nursing problems to develop and even more so for the elderly patient undergoing surgery.

PHYSICAL CHANGES

Skin

Skin changes account for much of the characteristic appearance of an older person; they are, however, not as important as less obvious changes elsewhere, for example, in mental function. Loss of subcutaneous fat and elastic tissue lead to change in facial expression; but this does not necessarily represent a mental change. There is a tendency to skin dryness as a result of atrophy of sweat glands. Malignancies, though they are age-related, cannot be ascribed to ageing.

Of significance to the nurse is the problem of temperature control. The older patient is more apt to feel the cold. Nursing assessment of the elderly patient requires that their needs in this area be met with warmer clothing during the day and more appropriate bed clothing at night. In many agencies the use of continental quilts has overcome the problem of providing adequate warmth without the weight difficulties of excessive layers of blankets.

Skin dryness, along with decreased peripheral arterial blood supply and poor venous return will retard normal wound healing in the elderly. These factors, compounded by increased friability of surface tissues, pose a further threat to the elderly, bed-confined patient in that decubitus ulcers are more likely to occur. Unrelieved pressure or trauma to surface tissue from inadequate position changes, weight and friction from bed clothing, or inappropriate use of equipment (for example, bed cradles, air cushions, adhesive skin plasters, unpadded Thomas splints or bed rails), can quickly lead to the development of pressure areas in the elderly or infirm. Decubitus ulcers can be largely prevented if the nurse, realizing that the elderly no longer possess normal wound healing reserves, implements a programme of regular position changes and care to any potential pressure areas.

Skeleton

Arthritis of joints is a constant change by the fifth decade. Changes in intervertebral discs lead to loss of height and the characteristic stoop of an old person. These are certainly age-related but trauma and perhaps other factors as well as the ageing process are responsible.

Osteoporosis (thinning of bone) is common in late life and is associated with the high incidence of fracture of the femur. Its aetiology is uncertain but the proven relationship with physical inactivity, lack of vitamin D, and hormonal changes of menopause strongly suggest that factors other than ageing are responsible.

Not only are the elderly more vulnerable to fractures, but the fractures are more likely to heal slowly. As muscle wasting generally accompanies limb immobilization following fracture the elderly patient is further compromised in the attempt to regain full range of movement.

The extent of skeletal degeneration will determine the degree of mobility that the patient has, and nursing measures may include:

- *The use of a lower bed (or a bed capable of being lowered) so that the patient can maintain his independence of movement.*
- *The provision of ambulation aids to ensure safety of movement. Disordered ambulatory function increases the risk of injury and the nurse needs to be vigilant at all times to ensure that the patient's safety is not compromised.*
- *A bed positioned closer to the nurse's station, amenities or recreational area so that the patient's ambulatory ability is not extended unnecessarily.*

Poor or disordered posture increases the need for the nurse to handle the patient with care. Rough handling or poor lifting techniques can place strain on the patient's limbs or skeleton, resulting in pain and/or trauma. When it is necessary to perform passive exercise and limb movements (for example, on a patient's hemiplegic limbs following a cerebrovascular accident) it is essential that the nurse assesses the limited range of movement through which the joints can be extended or rotated. Forced passive exercise will lead to joint and/or muscle trauma which will only further increase the recovery phase.

Muscle

Reduction in muscle mass is a feature of old age. Cellular changes are consistently found in muscle, and are related to neuronal atrophy in the nervous system. But relative inactivity must account for some of the diminution of muscle bulk; for example, muscle bulk in the left hand is likely to be less in a right-handed person.

These factors, along with degenerative skeletal changes, mean that the elderly patient will by definition be 'slower' to move and increased time to achieve ambulatory-based goals must be allowed. Specifically, muscle mass reduction will increase the postoperative recovery time. Rehabilitation measures requiring exercise as a therapy will need to be programmed according to the patient's individual needs and abilities. Gentle and regular exercise is preferable to highly active exercise, either regular or intermittent.

Nervous system

Diminishing brain weight due to constant fallout of neurones from the third decade onwards has long been regarded as an example of ageing. The extent and significance of neuronal loss is now being questioned since much of the evidence came from observations on brains affected by age-related disease. Decrease in nerve cell numbers does occur but it takes place in specific areas of the brain, and is not a process which affects the whole nervous system. Nor can it be assumed that there is a direct relationship between loss of neurones and a person's functional capacity (Brody, 1982). On the credit side is the recent evidence that proliferation of nerve processes has been found to occur in the ageing brain (Buell & Coleman, 1979).

An important change is observed in neuronal function. Nerve conduction is appreciably slower; this is a constant change in the ageing nervous system irrespective of disease. As well as being reflected in function of the musculoskeletal system – particularly in gait and general stability of the body – it is related to mental function and behaviour to be described later.

The elderly patient will require more time for analysis and synthesis of information both given and received. Patient teaching will need to be broken down into component parts practised often, rather than attempts made at learning an entire task in one session.

The implication for the nurse is that increased time must be allowed when involving the patient in his care.

Eye

The lens stiffens in old age and can alter shape only with difficulty. Focusing is not as easily performed, resulting in farsightedness or presbyopia. Therefore the majority of elderly patients will use corrective lenses at least for reading, if not for everyday use.

It is not enough just to determine that the patient has his spectacles in his possession; the nurse must ensure that he wears them so that he can see. Too often lack of this simple intervention has resulted in patient frustration and an inability to maintain his independence, his safety, and his dignity.

Glaucoma, on the other hand, is an age–related disorder, associated with an inherited factor in its primary form. In the secondary form, trauma or sometimes disease may precipitate the rise in pressure. Evidence that the process of ageing is an aetiological factor is not clear.

When planning for discharge it is imperative that the nurse ensures that the patient can actually read the dosage instructions on medication containers. For the glaucoma patient it may even be necessary to arrange for labels with larger print. An inability to remember medication instructions, reinforced by an inability to read medication labels, is a significant factor in patient noncompliance and medication errors amongst the elderly.

Ear

Hearing disability is so common that most people manifest a loss, particularly in the higher range of frequency, by the age of 50 years. The fact that it is more common in males, particularly those who have been engaged in noisy industrial work, strongly suggests that the environment as well as the ageing process plays an important part. Some drugs can also adversely affect hearing.

Infection in the middle ear can disturb conduction of sound to the cochlea. The presence of wax must always be suspected when an old person is deaf. Such disorders cannot be ascribed to the ageing process, even though there is little doubt that loss of cells in the organ of Corti is an ageing phenomenon; it is the commonest cause of presbycusis (deafness in old age).

The nurse aware of these factors will utilize strategies aimed at increasing effective communication with elderly patients. These may include: maintaining eye contact when speaking; speaking louder as appropriate; enunciating clearly and using exaggerated lip movements; lowering background noise; making certain that if a hearing aid is normally used that it is correctly fitted and in working order; and referring for investigation any patient in whom deafness is suspected. Additionally the nurse should ensure that the patient is able to socialize effectively by making

certain that he is appropriately positioned in relation to other patients and radio or television receivers. It should be noted that on many occasions patients thought to be deaf simply do not understand what is said, either because they do not understand and speak the same language or because of disease or disability, for example, auditory agnosia following CVA. No amount of shouting is going to increase the likelihood that the patient will 'hear' what is said. Skilled nursing assessment and appropriate referral is required in these instances.

Gastrointestinal tract

Loss of teeth, affecting not only mastication but speech and appearance, is common in old age. The incidence of edentulousness has been reported as high as 75% in people over the age of 75 living in an industrial society (Kart, 1978). On the other hand, elderly Australian Aborigines, living within their traditional culture, show little evidence of the two common forms of oral disease – caries and peridontal disease – but their teeth do show evidence of considerable wear on account of their high fibre diet (Murphy, 1959). In the United States it has been found that there is a strong correlation between edentulousness, low income, and less than nine years' schooling. These findings suggest that neither loss of teeth nor oral disease are inevitable sequelae to the ageing process, but depend to a large extent on the environment we live in and on our behaviour.

The nurse must ensure that prior to each meal the patient with false teeth has them in place and that they fit securely. Poorly fitting teeth, due to denture design, age, or soft tissue and gum disease, or shrinkage, is a significant contributing factor in malnutrition of the aged. If the patient appears to be anorexic it may be largely due to ill-fitting dentures that prevent him from masticating food effectively; a dietician referral for a modified diet may overcome the problem of inadequate nutrition in the short term. In the long term either new dentures or a weight gain will rectify the problem of poorly fitting teeth.

Diminution of taste as well as smell is said to occur with age; therefore, the provision of palatable, tasty foods may increase appetite in the elderly. Catering departments in many health agencies are constantly attempting new approaches to overcome the apparent bland, tasteless fare usually associated with such agencies. The dietary aspects of culture must be considered, and where appropriate home cooked meals may also encourage appetite.

It is likely that the tendency towards achlorhydria, and to diminished motility in the gastrointestinal tract are consequences of ageing. Constipation may be a feature but this may also be due to the development of a 'lazy bowel' as a result of aperient abuse. Disease processes such as carcinoma, hiatus hernia, ulcerations, or diverticulitis are much more likely to produce symptoms than is the process of ageing. Even in the absence of disease an elderly person who is introspective and comparatively inactive, can also display symptoms of gastrointestinal disturbance; the ageing process is, therefore, only indirectly involved.

Health education should be directed towards establishing satisfactory bowel habits by encouraging a diet high in natural fibre and accompanied by an adequate fluid intake. The use of over-the-counter aperients should be discouraged and the value of regular exercise, especially walking, should be stressed.

Nutrition

Faulty nutrition is held responsible for many diseases and also demands consideration with regard to the origin of the process of ageing. Sodium and saturated fatty acids have been connected with the aetiology of cardiovascular disease; lack of fibre with lower gastrointestinal disorders; lack of fluoride with tooth decay. Although these are referred to as degenerative diseases, they are not due to ageing. On the other hand, it has been postulated that abnormalities of protein synthesis – possibly of dietary origin – are primary factors in the cause of ageing.

An older person needs less food because tissue mass and metabolic activity are reduced. Resting metabolic rate is about 10% less than in someone in his twenties. These changes consistently accompany ageing and are not due to disease. In contrast, the quality of food – minerals and vitamins, as well as protein and other ingredients – needs to be at the same level as for younger people.

Nevertheless, deficiencies are commonly found in iron (where there is ulceration associated with hiatus hernia, diverticulitis, or aspirin ingestion), in sodium and potassium (with diuretic therapy), and in folate (after surgery or with anticonvulsant therapy). Elderly people who are seldom exposed to sunlight may suffer from vitamin D deficiency. Vitamin B_{12} deficiency may make its first appearance in late life as Addisonian anaemia; a normal old person does not have a deficiency of this vitamin. These are examples where either some environmental agent or some process independent of ageing, for example, Addisonian anaemia, causes disease; merely being 'old' cannot be held responsible.

The aim should therefore be to provide a diet high in quality whilst being small in quantity. It should be palatable, containing a majority of patient preferred foods; be served attractively; and contain sufficient fibre to prevent faecal incontinence. Whenever possible, and appropriate, the patient should be allowed and encouraged to sit and ambulate outside. Adequate protection must be given so that direct exposure to the sun does not produce unnecessary skin problems.

Liver function

Normal physiologic changes in the liver that accompany ageing include a reduction in liver weight and regenerative capacity, and a decreased blood flow. The functional ability of the liver decreases with age and, consequently, its ability to effectively metabolize lipid soluble drugs is also diminished.

Slower metabolism of some drugs, for example barbiturates, may give rise to the problem of reactional confusion; the patient is administered a 'normal' nocte dose of a sedative and when its effects are not evident within the expected reaction time, a further dose is administered. This leads to the patient being oversedated and difficult to rouse the following day. Thus he suffers a reactive confusional state because he is awake most of the night and asleep most of the day.

There also exists the possibility that slower drug metabolism may lead to accumulation and toxicity of some drugs in the presence of continued administration of 'normal' adult doses. The half-life of drugs must be considered and it is for this reason that many drugs are now presented in a lower dose format specifically for use by the aged patient. An intelligent knowledge *of drugs, including their anticipated and side effects, and the symptoms and signs of toxicity, is required by the nurse responsible for the care of the aged.*

Cardiovascular system

Loss of elasticity resulting in rigid vessel walls is part of the ageing process, whereas atherosclerosis which leads to narrowing of the lumen, though age-related, has an independent cause. Although the former process (arteriosclerosis) contributes to a change in function it is the latter disease which is responsible for a high proportion of deaths in late life. Change in cardiac function, measured as a progressive decline in the cardiac index beginning in middle age, is a constant result of the ageing process.

When nursing the elderly patient it must be anticipated that there will be variations in vital signs due to arteriosclerotic changes in vessels and the decreased response rate of the CVS to changes in the internal environment and the body's position. The effects of ageing, as well as disease, may result in the patient's decreased ability to recover quickly from a disabling illness. Poor vascularity of the extremeties increases the healing time of varicose and decubitus ulcers, and wound healing in general is usually extended in the elderly. The general fragility of the aged person's haemopoietic system and oestrogen deficits in postmenopausal women, may lead to extensive bruising and compound the problem of poor wound healing. As well the body's cellular response to infection and inflammation may be slower, thus increasing any recovery and/or treatment phase.

Respiratory system

Loss of elastic tissue due to ageing leads to changes both in the airways and the air sacs. Breathing is less efficient and fatigue more easily experienced, but if lifestyle changes accordingly these are not of great significance. However, should the person be immobilized for any length of time due to disability, disease, or trauma, then there is a greater tendency to develop atelectasis and/or pneumonia.

Health teaching regarding postoperative breathing exercises and for any patient on restricted ambulation is imperative to prevent secondary respiratory disorders developing.

Lung cancer is an age-related disease and cigarette smoking is the principal factor responsible. Death rates for this disease increase with age; this is evident even in non-smokers. But this does not prove the influence of the ageing process; the increase may well be due to prolonged environmental exposure to carcinogens such as tobacco smoke or industrial pollutants.

Renal system

Loss of nephrons in later life occurs independently of disease. This does not normally lead to significant functional change, but because many drugs depend on renal function for their elimination, it can be a factor in drug toxicity – particularly when disease has already lead to decompensation. Digitalis toxicity, for instance, is dependent on the level of serum creatinine as well as on the dose of digitalis.

Therefore a knowledge of the desired effects and likely side effects of any drug therapy is especially necessary when nursing elderly patients. Any sudden or unexpected changes in behaviour, accompanied by poor renal output and/or changes in fluid balance, should alert the nurse to suspect drug toxicity in those patients whose therapy includes drugs dependent upon renal excretion.

Bladder capacity may be reduced considerably in an older person even though no disease is present, resulting in more frequent micturition. Incontinence of urine is one of the most important problems in disabled elderly people. Some of the many predisposing factors are bladder infection, obstruction to outflow (for example, prostatic hypertrophy or stricture of the urethra), structural changes to the pelvic floor, and neurological disease. In addition to these disorders the process of ageing has a definite influence; bladder contraction can normally be inhibited, thereby maintaining continence, by impulses arising in the cerebral cortex. Ageing results in this mechanism being less efficient; bladder control becomes unstable and incontinence may occur. Alzheimer's disease, age-related but not caused by the ageing process, is one of the commonest causes of incontinence.

It is important that the nurse be aware that old age may be accompanied by more frequent micturition, as a common nursing response to frequent requests for panning is anger directed at the patient. It is not the intention of the patient to be demanding, but enforced bedrest has the effect of increasing the frequency of micturition, so the elderly patient confined to bed is even more prone to urinary incontinence. The nurse should anticipate the needs of the patient and increase the frequency of toileting, or panning, in an attempt to prevent urinary incontinence, thereby safeguarding the patient against embarrassment.

Incontinence may also occur when changes in loco-motion ability result in the ambulant patient being unable to reach the toilet in time. The nurse should teach elderly patients to attempt to void at regular intervals and especially within 1 hour of any fluid intake.

BEHAVIOURAL CHANGES

Intellect

One of the myths about elderly people is that the faculty of knowing and reasoning, and the possession of insight, are subject to inevitable decline. The word 'senile', which strictly means 'old', is often used to describe deficient intellectual function. One of the reasons for this ill-informed conclusion is that when comparison is made between the intellectual function of young and old, no allowance is made for the influence of the different cultural and social patterns experienced by the two groups. Another reason is the difficulty of precise measurement, compared with, say, testing cardiac or renal function. Perhaps the main reason for our state of confusion is similar to our dilemma over physical disorders: are the apparent changes which we observe due to acquired disease or to ageing?

Because the response in mental testing is initiated by external stimulation involving sight and sound, performance may be marred by diminished sensory acuity. The subsequent action may itself be reduced by disorders of the musculoskeletal or nervous systems. All these factors need to be considered before conclusions regarding intellectual change in old people are accepted.

Following peripheral sensory input a compli-

cated central process takes place; the meaning and usefulness of the information are considered; and its appropriateness to what is already known, and particularly concerning possible future action, is determined. These are then integrated in the form of instructions for action. Finally, a response is made. The central phase of integration is more subject to change with ageing than either the sensory input or the motor output. The process is slower so that there is an increase in reaction-time; the entire task becomes more complicated. This alteration in sensory-motor performance is an important change, but should not be over-emphasized or regarded as a serious progressive disease. Making a decision may be more difficult, allowing less choice than in former years because thought processes will be more patterned, but this may result in actions which are more effective and reliable.

When testing intellectual function it is necessary to take into account the use of words, as well as the performance of various tasks. It is found that although some tasks might be performed less efficiently, the verbal skills of older people are often superior to those in younger age groups.

Another common misapprehension is that learning becomes impossible in later life. Impaired short-term memory does create difficulty for an older person when he attempts to reproduce recently acquired information. But if proper attention is given to ways and means of handling new information – in small amounts and with repetition – learning is indeed possible. Significant increments in intellectual performance have been made by these methods.

Neither learning nor general intellectual performance can take place without environmental stimuli. Social and cultural factors are of considerable importance. It is inevitable that these will change during a person's life. When appropriate allowances are made for these changes in mental testing, apparent deterioration in intellectual performance often disappears. And when an old person lives in a society which is capable of reinforcing and supporting his actions, intellectual performance might well be found to improve. Ageing thus becomes a successful process, not dominated by losses in cognitive function; these losses undoubtedly occur, but to a lesser degree than is frequently supposed.

Personality

What changes take place in the sum of characteristics that make up a person's identity? It is commonly thought that there is a stereotype personality moulded by the ageing process. But this is contrary to what has been found by careful study of the developmental changes in an old person; changes in emphasis of one facet or another are overshadowed by the continuity of personality from youth to old age.

It has been argued that 'disengagement' is an inherent part of the ageing process (Cumming & Henry, 1961); both the individual and society disengage from each other with mutual agreement and satisfaction; there is withdrawal both of expectations and obligations. Loss of position in society and change in status resulting from retirement cannot be denied, but others have questioned whether disengagement is inevitable. In contrast, the 'activity' theory has been proposed; successful ageing, it is claimed, is achieved not so much in preoccupation with oneself, but by making a number of adjustments involving interaction with other people (Havighurst, 1963). These adjustments take the form of developmental changes with regard to health, a new level of income, leisure, relationship to other people (including family) following retirement from one's formal occupation, and finding a satisfactory place to live.

With regard to the development of personality, the theories of both disengagement and activity need to be considered. In contrast to more extroverted behaviour during a time when physical activity is at its peak, introversion is common with age; ambition is less obvious, and a different level of achievement is accepted. But these changes should not be thought of in terms of inevitable decline. Contrary to popular opinion there is not one stereotype, not even for successful ageing; one's basic personality is responsible in large measure for the type of old person one becomes. Conversely, active intervention by making adjustments, by modifying behaviour, and by continuing to exploit intellectual ability, can influence the development of personality in old age.

Therefore, it is totally inappropriate to justify the treatment of elderly patients as children, as being 'senile', or as persons devoid of any rights. Nurses should accord respect to patients who happen to be less young than themselves. Consequently patients have the right to expect that appropriate forms of address will not be denied them and that they will have a say in how they wish to be known and by whom they will be seen.

Considerable insight into the expectations of old age has been provided by regarding ageing as a skill (Welford, 1978), defined as the use of refined strategies to improve performance. This is not a matter of passive acceptance, but a positive reaction to changing demands, capacities, and social circumstances, which occur along with alterations in physical and intellectual function. Ageing is seen as a continuum, with changes beginning in the second and third decades, fashioned by forces outside as well as within the person, ending in death but certainly not confined to this final event.

Mental disease

A discussion on mental disease is not in order here except to reiterate the distinction between disorders of old age and disorders in old age. Alzheimer's disease (see Chapter 22), the most common neurological disease in old people, is age-related, occurring in 20% of people over the age of 80 years, but is not considered as part of the process of ageing. Other forms of dementia, particularly associated with cerebrovascular disease, are also common. Elderly people are prone to delirium – an acute and *reversible* change in mental state – from a number of causes. Depression and other psychotic conditions are not infrequent. It is, however, important to regard this group of illnesses as age-related, influenced by the particular circumstances in which elderly people live, but not an inherent part of the ageing process.

SUMMARY

This book is concerned with the various physical disturbances which give rise to illness. This chapter is an attempt to show that ageing, though not itself an illness, leads to certain changes and in particular predisposes the old person to disorders found in late life. It has been noted that many of these disorders are commonly experienced in earlier life. Because of changes in homeostatic mechanisms the process of ageing makes the old person more vulnerable to illness and slower to recover, as well as being more susceptible to the adverse effect of treatment by drugs.

The manifestation of disease in an old person is generally more complex and varied than that encountered in the young; firstly, because it is a combination of the effect of the environment – and at times of heredity – with the influence of the ageing process; secondly, becauses diseases in late life frequently involve a person's mental and social as well as physical 'territories'; thirdly, because the passage of years has resulted in multiple impairments. The disorders found in an old person cannot be accounted for by the process of ageing alone.

The physical changes of ageing are frequently only of comparatively minor importance; behavioural changes are more likely to be in the form of minimal intellectual decline and a shift of emphasis rather than the development of a stereotype personality. But when these are combined with physical or mental disease and compounded by psychosocial changes, serious disorders can arise in old people.

It is incumbent upon the nurse to involve and consult with the elderly patient in all aspects of his care to the same degree that one would with a younger person. The elderly patient has the right to be consulted and allowed to express his opinions. As well, he has every right to be angry when he is 'acted upon' rather than involved in decisions regarding his care.

Failure by the health care team to distinguish between the effect of disease and the influence of the ageing process leads to misunderstanding, incomplete diagnosis, faulty prognosis, and therapeutic neglect.

Conversely, an understanding of the effects of the ageing process coupled with informed and sensitive approaches to care, will accord the elderly person the opportunity of maintaining optimal independence and dignity.

REFERENCES AND FURTHER READING

Texts

Brocklehurst J C (ed) 1978 Textbook of geriatric medicine and gerontology, 2nd edn. Churchill Livingstone, Edinburgh

Brody H 1982 Ageing changes in the nervous system. In: Caird F I (ed) Neurological disorders in the elderly. Wright PSG, Bristol

Cumming E, Henry W E 1961 Growing old: the process of disengagement. Basic Books, New York

Havighurst R J 1963 Successful ageing. In: Williams R G (ed) Process of ageing, volume 1. Longmans Green, New York

Isaacs B 1982 Survival of the unfittest. Routledge & Kegan Paul, London

Lawson P K (ed) 1985 Helping geriatric patients: nursing photobook. Springhouse, Pennsylvania

Levy R, Post F (eds) 1982 The psychiatry of late life. Blackwell, Oxford

Libow L S 1963 Medical investigation of the process of aging. In: Biren J (ed) Human ageing: a biological and behavioural study. Department of Health, Education & Welfare publication (PHS), Washington, p 986

Shaw M W (ed) 1984 The challenge of ageing. Churchill Livingstone, Melbourne

Welford A T 1978 Ageing as a skill. In: Evans L (ed) Psychogeriatrics. Geigy Psychiatric Symposium, University of Queensland

Journals

Belchamber R 1985 Signposts to better psychogeriatric behaviour. The Australian Nurses Journal 15 : 5 : 44–45

Brighton R M 1985 Doing Mrs Angelo a favour. Nursing 85 15 : 2 : 44–46

Buell S J, Coleman P D 1979 Science 206 : 854

Christopher M A 1986 Home care for the elderly. Nursing 86 16 : 7 : 50–55

Corliss J, Kennedy K A, Smith M G 1987 Meeting the needs of geriatric patients on an acute care unit. Nursing 87 17 : 9 : 609–61

Davis L 1984 The coming of age. The Australian Nurses Journal 14 : 6 : 14–16

DeLapp T D 1983 Helping the elderly live longer – and better. Nursing 83 13 : 11 : 61–62

Dolan M B 1980 Being old is not the same as being ill. Nursing 80 10 : 4 : 41–42

Dolan M B 1983 If your patient wants to die at home. Nursing 83 13 : 4 : 50–55

Dolan M B 1985 An eternal flame. Nursing 85 15 : 1 : 20

Dugan J S 1984 Winning the battle against incontinence. Nursing 84 14 : 6 : 59

Fenwick D 1984 Ageism: an introduction. The Australian Nurses Journal. 14 : 6 : 8–10

Gasek G 1980 How to handle the crotchety, elderly patient. Nursing 80 10 : 3 : 46–48

Gray-Vickrey M 1987 Color them special. Nursing 87 17 : 5 : 59–62

Hope A 1983 The relief of constipation in the elderly. The Australian Nurses Journal 12 : 10 : 45–48

Hudson M F 1983 Safeguard your elderly patient's health through accurate physical assessment. Nursing 83 13 : 11 : 58–64

Hudson M F 1984 Drugs and the older adult take special care. Nursing 84 14 : 8 : 46–51

Lipsky J G 1984 Saving the elderly from the killing cold. Nursing 84 14 : 2 : 42–43

Meissner J E 1980 Assessing a geriatric patient's need for institutional care. Nursing 80 10 : 3 : 8–9

Meissner J E 1980 Evaluate your patient's level of independence. Nursing 80 10 : 9 : 22–23

Murphy T R 1959 Compensatory mechanisms in facial height adjustment to functional tooth attrition. Australian Dental Journal 4 : 312–323

Paterson J 1984 The elderly confused patient. The Australian Nurses Journal 14 : 3 : 42–44, 59

Piano L A 1986 Adult day care: a new ambulatory care alternative. Nursing 86 16 : 8 : 60–62

Prinsley D M 1986 Music therapy in geriatric care. The Australian Nurses Journal. 15 : 9 : 48–49

Ramsay K, Wright A, Bak S 1984 Widening horizons at Perry Park. The Australian Nurses Journal 14 : 6 : 11–13

Reynolds B J 1979 Suddenly blind at 80. Nursing 79 9 : 7 : 46–49

Ryan R 1983 Gerontic nursing – a new impetus in nursing care. The Australian Nurses Journal 12 : 10 : 43–44

Williams E J 1980 Food for thought: meeting the nutritional needs of the elderly. Nursing 80 10 : 9 : 60–63

Wysocki M R 1983 Life review for the elderly patient. Nursing 83 13 : 2 : 47–48

Wysocki R M 1983 Urinary incontinence and the older adult. The Australian Nurses Journal 12 : 11 : 49–52

A

The nervous system

15

Introduction to the nervous system and cephalalgia

Jenny Kidd   Chris Game

An understanding of neuroanatomy and physiology of the nervous system is crucial to the understanding of disease processes that affect it, as the pathology of the nervous system is exceptionally complex. The nervous system provides sophisticated communication which, together with the endocrine system, integrates and controls the body's activities. It is this sophistication which complicates diagnosis of dysfunction; for example, a tumour of the brain or spinal cord can provide both local and systemic manifestations ranging from loss of taste to loss of sphincter control.

The nervous system is anatomically divided into two major parts: the central nervous system (CNS), consisting of brain, brain stem, and spinal cord; and the peripheral nervous system, consisting of cranial and spinal nerves. The CNS is the controlling centre and communicates with the body as a whole via the peripheral nervous system. The peripheral nervous system incorporates the autonomic nervous system which consists of sympathetic and parasympathetic nerve fibres responsible for the fine, involuntary regulation of organs and body systems.

The central nervous system

The structures of the CNS are completely surrounded, and protected, by the meninges. The meningeal membranes comprise: the pia mater, the visceral membrane which is closely adherent to the underlying structures; the arachnoid mater, which is separated from the pia mater by a space in which circulates cerebrospinal fluid (CSF); and the dura mater, the parietal layer which is closely adherent to the skull and spinal column and is separated from the arachnoid mater by a potential space only microns in diameter.

Brain

The brain is a soft vulnerable organ which is encased and protected by the rigid vault of the skull and comprises the cerebrum, the diencephalon, the cerebellum, and also includes the neural ventricular system.

Cerebrum. The cerebrum is made up of 2 matched hemispheres divided longitudinally by a fissure but connected deep within this fissure by the corpus callosum, a collection of nerve fibres allowing each specialized area in one hemisphere to communicate with its complementary area in the other hemisphere. The cerebrum is responsible for initiating movement (motor centre), interpreting sensory information (sensory centre), formulating mental functions, and initiating and controlling specialized behaviours (for example, speech, hearing, and sight centres).

The cerebrum has both grey matter (cortical neuron cell bodies and basal ganglia) and white matter (neuron axonal tracts). The basal ganglia, although regarded as grey matter, are neuronal cell bodies in the subcortical (white) area of the cerebrum responsible for the control of fine movement and include the caudate nucleus, the putamen, the globus pallidus, the claustrum and the amygdala. Association and projection neural fibres link the cerebrum with other neural structures. Association fibres link different areas of the cortex in a hemisphere whereas projection fibres link the cortex with subcortical structures, the brain stem, and the spinal cord.

The diencephalon is of importance in that it contains the hypothalamus and thalamus, both of which are groups of specialized nerve cells responsible for control of most body functions. The hypothalamus sits anterior to the brain stem, connected to the pituitary gland by the pituitary stalk and regulates temperature, water balance, pituitary function, appetite, and emotions – especially the emotions of anger and rage. The thalamus sits adjacent to the hypothalamus and relays almost all motor and sensory nerve impulses. It also is the major regulator of primitive responses (for example, the 'fight or flight' reaction).

Cerebellum. The cerebellum, lying at the base of the brain, is primarily responsible for the regulation of balance, the maintenance of muscle tone, and the co-ordination of muscle movement with sensory input.

Neural ventricular system. The third and fourth neural ventricles are located within the centre of the brain and are bordered by 2 lateral ventricles. Within the ventricles are the choroid plexuses formed by invaginations of pia and arachnoid mater. The choroid is responsible for the production of CSF.

Because the brain is both soft and manoeuvrable it is vulnerable to injury, which may range from bruising to complete shearing. Also, inflammation, oedema, haemorrhage and space-occupying lesions increase the size of the brain and cause obstruction of CSF and venous drainage. Because the brain is encased in the skull, this increase of size and build-up of pressure can cause distortion and compression of the brain and brain stem.

Brain stem

The brain stem comprises the midbrain, pons and medulla oblongata and is responsible for the relay of all nerve impulses between the brain and spinal cord. The brain stem, in addition to the thalamus and hypothalamus, forms the reticular formation which is responsible for providing constant muscle stimulus which results in muscle tone. This reticular formation is a vital component of the reticular activating system which is responsible for maintaining consciousness, sleep–wake patterns and mental concentration. The brain stem houses the respiratory, cardiac, and vasomotor control centres, and the centre for control of pharyngeal reflexes: gagging, sneezing, coughing, swallowing, and vomiting. Cranial nerves III–XII arise from the brain stem.

Spinal cord

The spinal cord is a continuation of the brain stem and comprises both grey and white matter with the grey matter forming a characteristic H-shape. The anterior horn cells of the grey matter are responsible for relaying efferent (motor) impulses and the posterior horn cells are responsible for relaying afferent (sensory) impulses. The white matter comprises sensory and motor myelinated axons in ascending and descending tracts which communicate with the brain (corticospinal tracts). The spinal cord is capable of mediating a reflex arc, that is a nerve impulse used in a protective reflex action. The cord is enclosed and protected by the spinal column and gives rise to 31 pairs of spinal nerves exiting between the vertebrae of C_1 and L_5.

Peripheral nervous system

The peripheral nervous system is the means by which nerve impulses are transmitted to muscles of the skeleton and organ systems. Stimuli from the periphery and organs are also transmitted back to the brain via spinal and cranial nerves.

Sympathetic and parasympathetic nerve fibres of the autonomic nervous system innervate the smooth muscle of the body systems and are responsible for the fine regulation of these organ systems.

Cellular structure and function

The nervous system is composed of billions of cells which are either neurons or neuroglial cells.

Neurons

Neurons are the functional units of the nervous system and each neuron is a large cell comprising a nerve cell body, dendrites, and an axon. The nerve cell bodies form the grey matter of the cortex of the brain and of the spinal cord; in clumps neuronal cell bodies are referred to as ganglia. There are basically 3 types of neurons: sensory (afferent) neurons transmit impulses from organs and from the periphery to the CNS; motor (efferent) neurons transmit impulses from the CNS to organs and to the periphery; and association (intercalary) neurons transmit impulses within the CNS between nerve cells. Neurons are critically dependent upon stable blood levels of oxygen and glucose for their cellular function and even small variations, or extreme variations over very short periods, can cause neuronal death. Blood flow to the brain comprises approximately one-fifth of the total cardiac output. Despite wide fluctuations in systemic pressure this blood flow is kept relatively constant by baroreceptors and autoregulation. As neurons cannot replicate, primary tumours in neurons cannot occur and neuronal death, regardless of cause (for example head injury, ischaemia, intoxication), is irreversible.

Dendrites and axons collectively comprise the white matter of the CNS. Dendrites are fairly short fibres and are usually present as multiple branches. Their function is to receive nerve impulses from the axons of other neurons and to conduct these impulses to the nerve cell body.

The axon carries nerve impulses from the cell body and transmits these impulses to other nerve cells, via a synapse, within the CNS or to muscle fibres outside the CNS. Although each neuron normally has only one axon, an axon may divide and form collateral branches thereby increasing the impulse transmission ability of the neuron. Transmission of an impulse occurs at the foot of the axon which has multiple small branches at its tip. Each of these branches is referred to as a presynaptic terminal and the synaptic junction is formed when the axon is in contact with the dendrites of another neuron or the postsynaptic membrane of skin or other tissue, for example the motor end plate of a muscle fibre. Axons within the CNS are normally found in groups sharing similar nerve impulse function (for example sensory axons, motor axons) and if they share a common origin, termination, and direction they form tracts (for example corticospinal tract).

Within the CNS the axons are protected and insulated by neuroglial cells called oligodendroglia; outside the CNS protection and insulation is provided by myelin which is produced in segments by Schwann cells, each segment being produced between two nodes of Ranvier. Neurilemma is the protective and insulating sheath surrounding peripheral nerve fibres and although its formation is unclear it is known to be important in the regeneration of damaged peripheral nerves.

Neuroglia

Neuroglial cells are the structural units of the CNS and although they outnumber neurons by 9 : 1, they are extremely small comprising only 50% of the brain mass by weight. Neuroglia are incapable of nerve transmission but completely surround and support neurons and are of 4 types: astroglia, microglia, oligodendroglia, and ependymal cells. Neuroglial cells are capable of replication and therefore can be replaced should injury or inflammation lead to their destruction; CNS tumours arise from these cells.

Astroglia comprise astrocytes which are responsible for supplying the neuron with its nutrients and help maintain the electrical potential of the nerve cell body. Astrocytes are situated on capillary walls and control the exchanges between the blood and neurons and as such form part of the blood-brain barrier. Microglia are phagocytic cells found throughout the CNS and are responsible for the removal of cellular wastes and for destroying invading microorganisms. Oligodendroglia provide protection and insulation for CNS neural axons by producing myelin. Ependymal cells line each of the 4 neural ventricles and their choroid plexuses; these cells assist in the formation of CSF.

Blood–brain barrier

The blood–brain barrier is formed by astrocytes lying over the endothelial blood capillaries and their basement membranes, thus preventing direct contact between plasma and neurons. This barrier serves as protection for the neurons by minimizing entry of microorganisms, toxins, hormones, and drugs, and controls their entry by selective diffusion. Substances which diffuse readily across the barrier include water, carbon dioxide, oxygen, glucose, amino acids, and lipid soluble anaesthetic agents. Substances which diffuse slowly include sodium, potassium, and drugs including sedatives and hypnotics. Antibiotics, cytotoxic drugs, and other large molecular drugs diffuse either poorly or not at all and therefore require intrathecal injection, or IV administration in extremely high doses, to be effective. The blood–brain barrier breaks down at the site of tumours, therefore it is possible to use IV radio-isotopes to isolate and treat CNS tumours. Injury to the brain causing trauma and inflammation results in increased permeability of the blood–brain barrier, with a resultant disturbance in fluid, protein, and electrolyte concentration of the intra- and extracellular fluid.

Neural transmission

Nerve transmission is aided by chemical neurotransmitters which are secreted by nerve cells, actively carried along the axon, and stored in synaptic vesicles. A nerve impulse travels along the axon under the influence of an action potential which is realized through the stages of axonal segmental depolarization and repolarization. Once the impulse reaches the presynaptic terminal at the tip of the axon, extracellular calcium ions enter the terminal membrane and stimulate the release of the neurotransmitter substance. Once released, the neurotransmitter substance crosses the synapse and binds with the postsynaptic receptor, thus selectively increasing the receptor membrane's permeability to an impulse transmission. The neurotransmitter substance is then neutralized by enzymes. Extracellular chloride ions regulate the intensity and duration of nerve transmission and increase excitability of the neuron.

So far, more than 30 different neurotransmitter substances have been identified in various parts of the body and they usually produce either an excitatory or inhibitory effect. Excitatory neurotransmitters include: acetylcholine, substance P, and glutamic acid. Inhibitory neurotransmitters include: norepinephrine, dopamine, gamma aminobutyric acid (GABA), acetylcholine-5-hydroxytryptamine (serotonin), and glycine.

The exact mechanism of action of these neurotransmitters is not clearly understood, however, this is of increasing importance as drugs are now available which are able to neutralize or enhance these effects.

ASSESSMENT OF NEUROLOGICAL STATUS

Steps in enabling a neurological diagnosis involve obtaining a detailed patient history, containing information about the onset and development of symptoms, and performing a full neurological examination.

The aim of a neurological assessment is to determine the nature and location of disease or trauma, and to recognize deviations from the norm, and warning signs of cerebral deterioration. Accurate assessment is enhanced by the full co-operation of the patient, but unfortunately neurological disorders often make this difficult to obtain.

The routine neurological examination should be preceded by a complete physical examination which includes examination of the cranium and neck. The size and shape of the head are noted and the scalp and skull are inspected and palpated to detect any scars, deformities or tenderness. Auscultation over the skull and mastoid areas, and the carotid and subclavian arteries is important when vascular tumour or anomalies are suspected.

The neurological examination includes an evaluation of:

1. Mental state
2. Motor function (tests of co-ordination, muscle strength, gait and reflexes)
3. Sensory function (senses, perception and proprioception)
4. Cranial nerve function
5. Autonomic function.

Evaluation of mental state

Mental state assessment includes an evaluation of the patient's level of consciousness, his orientation in space and time, his memory and mental calculation skills, his general knowledge, and his comprehension of abstract relations and judgement. It is usual to ask the patient his name and to check that he knows the day of the week. Is he alert or confused and is his memory capable of eliciting recent versus remote past events? He should be asked questions of general knowledge covering current affairs, and be asked to perform a simple arithmetic skill without using a pen and paper. Have the patient describe the meaning of a proverb, for example 'A rolling stone gathers no moss' and give him a simple problem to solve, for example 'If you've lost your keys, how do you get into your house?'

When formulating questions and evaluating responses the nurse must take into account the age of the patient, his ability to understand and speak English, and any other cultural influences.

Evaluation of motor function

Notation is made of contractures, abnormally large muscle masses or evidence of wasting, muscular tone, co-ordination, muscular movement, station, gait, posture, and muscle strength. Grip is commonly tested and abnormal movements and muscle spasms are also noted. Motor signs (that is, indications of motor damage) include restlessness, tremor, and involuntary movements such as clonus – rapidly alternating contraction and relaxation of a muscle in response to a sudden stretch.

Evaluation of reflex activity

The evaluation of a patient's reflexes is part of the diagnostic examination as well as of the on-going assessment, as it can provide information about the nature, location and progression of neurological disorders.

A wide variety of reflexes may be evaluated, but 4 major groups are:

1. Superficial or cutaneous reflexes
2. Deep or tendon reflexes
3. Special reflexes, such as the light reflex in the pupil of the eye
4. Pathological reflex.

Superficial reflex. The abdomen is stroked in its upper and lower quadrant with an implement such as applicator, a match-end, or the pointed end of the patella hammer. The normal response is contraction of the muscles in the area stimulated, which indicates that the spinal nerves to that area are functioning.

Deep or tendon reflexes. When the patella tendon is tapped with the knee flexed and relaxed there is involuntary extension of the leg. This also tests the function of the quadriceps muscle.

Light reflex of the pupil of the eye. When a bright light is shone into the eye, the pupil contracts. This indicates that the oculomotor nerve is functioning normally. Other reflexes of the eye, such as blinking when an object approaches close to the eye, and convergence and divergence of the eyes are easily tested.

Pathological reflex. When the outer side of the sole of the foot, from heel to toes, is stroked with an applicator there is normally downward (plantar) flexion of the great toe. The pathological response is upward movement of the great toe and this is described as a positive Babinski's reflex.

Evaluation of sensory function

The complete sensory examination can be performed only on the conscious patient, as he must be able to focus his attention on the stimuli and cooperate with the examiner.

Routinely during the examination, tests are carried out for awareness of touch, pressure, movement, discrimination, proprioception, vibration, and pain. When there is loss of the sense of pain, tests for temperature awareness are performed.

Evaluation of cranial nerve function

Each of the 12 cranial nerves is tested, as described in Table 15.1.

Evaluation of autonomic function

Many diseases that are not primarily of the nervous system have symptoms of impaired autonomic function, for example, postural hypotension and Raynaud's disease. The physical examination may identify some general symptoms of autonomic dysfunction which include:

1. Alterations in patterns of perspiration
2. Faulty body temperature regulation
3. Abnormal pulse rate

Table 15.1 Functional testing of cranial nerves

Name	No.	Type	Equipment	Procedure
Olfactory	I	Sensory to nose	Volatile oils such as oil of cloves	Pinch one nostril closed. Have patient sniff and identify
Optic	II	Sensory to eye	Ophthalmoscope Snellen chart	Examine optic nerve with ophthalmoscope; visualize fundus; have patient read from Snellen chart. Peripheral vision checked with patient stating the point at which he sees an object brought toward his eye from the side.
Oculomotor Trochlear Abducens	III IV VI	These 3 nerves are motor to the eye	Flashlight	Observe pupillary response to light. Observe convergence and pupillary changes when objects are brought from a distance up close
Trigeminal	V	Motor and sensory. Has three dimensions: – ophthalmic – mandibular – maxillary	Test tubes of hot and cold water Wisp of cotton Pin	Test for sensation to pain, heat and cold. Observe ability to bite. Brush wisp of cotton over cornea and observe reflex. Normal eye will close
Facial	VII	Motor and sensory	Solutions that are sweet, salty, sour, and bitter with four medicine droppers	Ask patient to perform facial movements (raise eyebrows, smile, show teeth, close eyes), facial symmetry. Test taste to anterior 2/3 of tongue by holding tip of tongue with gauze and dropping solutions on it. Patient tastes and identifies substance. Rinse mouth between substances
Acoustic	VIII	Sensory to ear for hearing and balance	Tuning fork Wristwatch	Observe if patient can hear sounds made by tuning fork, wristwatch, whisper. Observe whether patient can maintain balance when standing with eyes closed
Glossopharyngeal Vagus	IX X	Sensory and motor. These two nerves are tested together	Cotton applicator Tongue depressor Sweet, salty, sour and bitter solutions	Test for taste to posterior 1/3 of tongue; hold tongue depressor and touch posterior pharynx with applicator. Observe patient swallowing, coughing, speaking. Speech tests, larynx, which is controlled by vagus nerve. Note hoarseness, ineffective cough
Spinal accessory	XI	Motor to sternocleidomastoid and trapezius muscles in neck and shoulder		Inspect for muscle atrophy. Ask patient to rotate head and elevate shoulders against resistance
Hypoglossal	XII	Motor to tongue		Observe tongue movements, atrophy. Ask patient to stick tongue out and move it from side to side

4. Polyuria
5. Abnormal motility of gastrointestinal tract
6. Urinary and faecal incontinence
7. Changes in thirst, energy, libido, weight and appetite.

The patient's skin, mucous membranes, hair and nails will be examined for obvious trophic changes.

The responsibilities of the nurse in neurological examinations are:
– To conduct all or part of these tests
– To prepare the patient correctly for each test so that optimum results may be obtained
– To care for the patient during the test.

CEPHALALGIA

Cephalalgia (headache) is one of the most common types of pain and is a common feature of neurological and other disorders. The majority of headaches are benign, however chronic recurrent headache or acute severe headache should be investigated. Trigeminal neuralgia (tic douloureux), a common disorder of the fifth cranial nerve leads to severe head and face pain in the distribution of the nerve and its branches.

Headache can be categorized as benign, recurrent or persistent or as secondary to intracranial, extracranial, or systemic causes.

Types of benign headache are:

- Tension
- Tension vascular
- Migraine
- Cluster migraine

Common pathological causes of headache are:

1. Intracranial headache
- Tumour
- Haemorrhage
- Infection
- Disturbances in CSF
2. Extracranial headache
- Eyes – glaucoma, convergence difficulties, optic neuritis
- Ears – otitis externa
- Scalp – infection, for example, herpes zoster
- Skull – tumour or osteomyelitis
- Arteries – temporal arteritis
- Dentition – dental caries, malaligned jaw
- Sinuses – sinusitis
3. Systemic headache
- Hypertension
- Pheochromocytoma
- Influenza

This chapter will address the medical and nursing management of benign, recurrent or persistent forms of headache. The management of headache secondary to other causes is covered where the cause is discussed; for example, headache of meningitis (see page 219). Trigeminal neuralgia and its medical, surgical and nursing management will also be studied.

Clinical manifestations

Headache can be a crippling disorder due to the nature of the pain, which if untreated is gnawing, persistent, and distracting. The pain of headache is often described by the patient as being sharp and/or throbbing, or dull and consistent. Some patients describe their pain as being characteristic of a tight head-band and it may be accompanied by neck stiffness. Symptoms and signs that commonly accompany a headache are painful eye movements, a feeling of a heavy head, and an inability to concentrate. Other features may include dizziness and photophobia, and a generalized 'soreness' over the affected area, including the scalp.

Tension headache

This type of headache usually consists of a feeling of tightness which may be localized to the front or back of the head, or may be circumferential. This may be accompanied by stiffness or ache in the neck and shoulder muscles. There is no accompanying nausea or photophobia and it is usually not so severe as to cause an interruption to normal activities. It is often continuous in its pattern, beginning shortly after waking and lasting most or all of the day, and fluctuating in intensity. Low-grade chronic tension or stress is often responsible for this type of headache.

Tension vascular headache

The pain of this form of headache may be identical to that of tension headache, but at maximum intensity the pain may take on an intense throbbing quality.

This type of headache is often associated with nausea and photophobia and can be precipitated by alcohol, exercise, menses, or use of the contraceptive pill. Attacks may last hours to days, with intermittent pain-free episodes.

It is not unusual for the migraine sufferer to have these types of headaches in addition to migraine. In general, tension vascular headaches respond better to therapeutic regimes used to treat migraine than those used to treat tension headaches.

Migraine headache

This type of head pain is frequently lateralized, often affecting the temporal frontal and periorbital regions. Head pain may be the only manifestation of the disorder, and it gradually spreads to the whole of the affected side and sometimes involves the whole head. The throbbing pain, sometimes described as being of 'ice-pick' intensity, increases and is exacerbated by physical exertion and stooping. The most important diagnostic feature of migraine is its paroxysmal nature and the episodic recurrence of attacks despite wide variations in the clinical presentation.

Common migraine

This accounts for up to 90% of patients suffering vascular headaches.

A proportion of patients will experience a trigger factor which may precipitate an attack, for example, stress or relaxation from stress, glare, menses and certain foods. Others may experience accompanying systemic manifestations such as dizziness, fainting and cold extremities.

Common symptoms include photophobia, nausea, vomiting in 50% of cases, and an intolerance to noise and strong odours. Common migraine can be a very disabling condition.

Treatment of common migraine relies upon a detailed medical history with specific attention to any trigger factors which can then be either avoided or controlled.

Classic migraine

Classic migraine differs from common migraine in that the headache is preceded or accompanied by transient visual, motor, sensory or other focal cerebral symptoms.

Classic migraine accounts for only 10–15% of cases of migraine headache. Environmental triggers play less of a role, and the frequency of attacks is lower than in common migraine.

Visual symptoms. Visual disturbances are the most common aura preceding a classic migraine. They last for approximately 10–30 minutes and usually abate prior to the headache. The patient may see stars, flashing lights, spots, or geometrical patterns in one or both eyes. This is thought to be the result of mild ischaemia of the visual pathway.

Focal sensory symptoms. These include paraesthesia and numbness, commonly affecting the fingers of one or both hands, sometimes ascending up the arm; and sometimes involving the lips and tongue. These occur in one- to two-thirds of attacks of classic migraine.

Disorders of movement. These do not occur as frequently as visual or sensory symptoms and present as a feeling of heaviness or weakness in a limb, often associated with numbness.

Difficulties with speech. These symptoms usually only last for an hour or two. The patient may complain of expressive dysphasia or slow halting speech. It may be associated also with a slowing of thought processes.

Complicated migraine

The effects of complicated migraine are thought to be due to more prolonged and more severe ischaemia. These include ophthalmoplegia, and ocular palsy lasting 1–6 weeks, usually with complete recovery, but cumulative damage may result in permanent visual defects. Paralysis of an arm or leg can occur, also with complete recovery. The patient may also suffer mental aberrations such as severe mental confusion, agitation, amnesia and hallucinations.

Cluster migraine

This is a rare form of migraine which, when it occurs, commonly affects older males. The pain is usually unilateral, is of sudden onset, and is described as being intense, piercing, stabbing pain. Profuse conjunctival watering and redness accompanies the pain. The duration is commonly 30–90 minutes and the migraine is normally precipitated by a vasodilator such as alcohol, histamines, or nitrites.

Pathophysiology of migraine

There are a variety of theories of causation in migraine headache and researchers are unable to agree on the precise pathophysiology. Nevertheless, it is agreed that the majority of migraine sufferers experience 3 distinct phases during the migraine episode, and the following series of events are the most likely whenever migraine occurs.

Prodromal phase. This phase is marked by vasoconstriction of the intracranial arteries and in particular the retinal vessels and those supplying the cerebrum, which show a markedly reduced blood flow. A visual, sensory, or motor aura is commonly described by migraine sufferers and is believed to be a result of this intense vasoconstriction. At this stage there is no headache, however the person may describe a feeling of light headedness accompanied by the onset of a feeling of tightness – as if a rubber band were being applied to the skull. Possibly as a result of the vasoconstriction, there is an increase in thrombocyte aggregation resulting in the release of 5-hydroxytryptamine (serotonin); this is a vasoactive substance which increases capillary permeability and is thought to play a role in the onset of the second phase.

Second phase. This phase is marked by vasodilation of all intracranial and extracranial arteries, resulting in the onset of acute, severe headache that is classically described as throbbing or pulsating in nature. Sodium levels increase and, in some persons, overt oedema may manifest – swelling of the fingers and face being the most common. The vessel walls are also oedematous during this stage and are thought to release bradykinins which lower the person's threshold to pain. Anorexia, nausea and vomiting commonly occur and are believed to be a result of cerebral oedema and/or irritation stimulating the vomiting centre in the medulla oblongata.

Third phase. This phase is marked by rigidity of the vessels and muscular tension of the skeletal muscle of the head and neck. The intense vessel rigidity results in a constant, excruciating headache which is no longer pulsating in nature. Scalp and neck muscle contraction results in constant tension and severe pain which persists for some time after the headache subsides.

Differential diagnosis of headache

The differentiation of headache type is based on the clinical presentation of the patient, and the history of events that led up to the headache. Regardless of the type of headache, the patient is usually able to pinpoint the exact location of the pain.

Most causes of headache produce symptoms, not signs, and even the most exhaustive investigations are of little use. When diagnosing headache the physician is almost totally dependent upon a detailed history from the patient and symptom pattern recognition. The chronological description of a typical attack usually reveals the diagnosis. The overwhelming majority of headaches belong to the benign recurrent or persistent group.

Investigative procedures

Investigations are infrequent in the diagnosis of headache when the clinical features outlined by the patient satisfy the usual characteristics of one of the benign recurrent headaches and the physical examination reveals no neurological abnormalities.

Specific investigations to exclude pathological causes of cephalalgia may include:

- Full neurological and physical examination
- Skull X-ray series
- Lumbar puncture
- Brain CT scan
- Carotid angiogram
- Electoencephalogram
- Psychological testing.

Medical management

The aim of treatment is to:

1. Identify and treat precipitating factors
2. Reduce the frequency, duration, and intensity of attacks.

Most self-medication of over-the-counter analgesics in Australia is due to headache. In the majority of cases, self-medication with simple analgesics such as aspirin, codeine, or paracetamol compounds will successfully relieve the symptoms. If the headache is identified as being stress-related, then steps should be taken to modify the stressful situation. Should eyestrain prove to be the primary cause, an optical consultation should be sought.

It bears mentioning that there has been some recent success in alleviating migraine headache by manipulation of the temporomandibular joint. Some dental surgeons are currently involved in research of this procedure and its long-term effects on migraine sufferers, but to date there has been little published of these research findings.

A chronic headache sufferer should be investigated when the headaches are persistent, fail to respond to the administration of simple analgesics, or are accompanied by signs of other neurological or systemic deficits or manifestations.

Acute migraine attacks are treated by the use of analgesics or ergotamine, a powerful central and peripheral vasoconstrictive drug. Aspirin, paracetamol, and codeine preparations may give pain relief if taken early in the attack. In extreme cases, pethidine may be the analgesic of choice.

Ergotamine, an alpha-adrenoreceptor blocker, is the drug of choice in the treatment of migraine. It causes vasoconstriction and is given to forestall the vasodilatory phase, and is used alone or in combination with other drugs such as caffeine to potentiate its effect. Ergotamine is also a serotonin antagonist, and is most effective if taken early in the attack, either when prodromal symptoms occur, or, if there are none, when the headache starts. Due to its vasoconstrictive properties, care must be taken to ensure that the correct dosage is not exceeded. Ergotamine is poorly and erratically absorbed from the gut, and for this reason it is administered by the sub-lingual route and more recently (and preferably) by inhalation.

The use of an antiemetic assists in reducing or preventing nausea and vomiting. Antiemetics from the phenothiazine group such as prochlorperazine should be used as nausea and vomiting originate from stimulation of the vomiting centre and these drugs act directly on that centre. Metoclopramide is relatively useless as its dominant function is to cause emptying of the stomach; however, in this role it may be of use to promote better absorption of other oral drugs.

Antihistamines may be used to reduce nausea, and sedatives may be prescribed to reduce anxiety.

Prophylactic drug therapy may be prescribed for migraine if more than 2 acute attacks are experienced in a month. The drugs prescribed are not for use during an acute headache but are used to reduce the number and severity of headaches.

These drugs act centrally by modifying vasodilation and inhibiting the action of serotonin, and their dosage is individualized depending upon response to the medication. There are risks in using some of these drugs and medical supervision is necessary, particularly upon commencement of therapy.

Diet

Certain foods may be implicated in precipitating migraine attacks in some individuals. Tyramine-containing foods (such as cheese, broad beans, red wine, and chocolates) and preservatives containing nitrite are some of those implicated. Precipitating foods should be avoided or their intake decreased. As hypoglycaemia may precipitate an attack, fasting should be avoided.

Nursing management

Nursing care needs to be supportive and symptomatic as migraine varies in intensity, duration, and symptomatology, depending upon the individual. The prime responsibility of the nurse is one of patient education. Care is aimed at involving the patient in understanding the problem and how specific interventions may reduce headache and related symptoms. It is the patient who will be implementing these interventions when headache occurs.

Pain relief occurs in response to chemotherapy, provided appropriate medication is taken as ordered. However, individual response to drug therapy will vary, and the physician may have to experiment with several drugs before the right one is found. The patient must learn to carry medication at all times.

Rest in a quiet darkened environment is usually beneficial and ice packs may be of help to some people.

Nausea and vomiting may be avoided or diminished by the administration of antiemetics and avoidance of unpleasant stimuli.

If stress is a precipitating factor, the individual may be encouraged to examine his lifestyle and look at ways to reduce stressors. Relaxation or biofeedback techniques may be useful and appropriate members of the health care team may be involved to teach these techniques.

The patient needs to identify specific precipitating factors. This may involve a food trial to identify those substances which produce the adverse reaction. A carefully structured clinical history is taken to identify other precipitating events and stimuli. Treatment and prevention are then largely by avoidance.

It is also important that the patient reports any increase in the number, severity or symptoms associated with the headaches, or failure to respond to the prescribed therapy. The anticipated side effects and recognition of adverse effects of therapy must also be part of the patient's education.

Trigeminal neuralgia (tic douloureux)

Trigeminal neuralgia is a localized disorder of the Vth cranial nerve. It is characterized by sudden paroxysms of severe, stabbing pain and muscle spasm lasting for up to 1 minute in the distribution of one or more branches of the trigeminal nerve – usually the 2nd division or 2nd and 3rd divisions. Attacks may be precipitated by stimulation of a 'trigger point' by mechanical stimuli, such as chewing, smiling, cleaning teeth, or washing the face. Trigeminal pain may be secondary to sinus or dental pathology, trauma, posterior fossa tumour, multiple sclerosis, and vascular compression; idiopathic trigeminal neuralgia also occurs.

Trigeminal neuralgia usually occurs in adults in the fifth decade of life and affects women twice as often as men. It occurs more often on the right side of the face than on the left.

During the initial stages attacks may be intermittent but will increase with time and the person may experience a dull, aching pain between attacks. Pain may be so intense that patients contemplate suicide unless relief can be obtained.

Diagnosis

Diagnosis is based on the patient's history and the observation of an attack. During an attack it is common for the patient to 'splint' the affected side and, if talking is a common trigger, he may hold his face still with his hands whilst talking so as to prevent an attack. X-ray and CT scan may be performed to exclude possible secondary causes.

Medical and surgical management

Management is aimed at reducing the frequency and intensity of attacks by the use of drug therapy. Anticonvulsants, such as phenytoin, may be prescribed, and carbamazepine inhibits sensory impulse conduction in the Vth cranial nerve. Pain relief is extremely difficult to achieve and even narcotics have only a minimal effect during an acute attack.

Surgical techniques utilized in the treatment of trigeminal neuralgia include:

1. Local injection of alcohol into the trigeminal ganglion
2. Glycerol injection into the trigeminal cistern
3. Rhizotomy
4. Microvascular decompression
5. Division of the sensory nerve root
6. Wrapping the nerve in a piece of fascia.

Injection of the nerve may provide relief for about 12–18 months. Procedures that involve cutting of the nerve cause loss of sensation in the division of the nerve severed, for example, loss of corneal reflex following division of the ophthalmic nerve. However, modern microsurgical techniques now allow a greater accuracy when nerve dissection or division is performed. This results in more selective treatment and pain relief.

Nursing management

Nursing management is related to assisting the patient during an attack, caring for the patient following surgical intervention, and/or providing health education in the areas of pain avoidance and protection of deinnervated tissue. During an attack the nurse should observe and record the sequence of events, the patient's responses including any efforts at splinting, and the effect of any pain relief agents administered. If the patient is prescribed anticonvulsants the nurse should observe for the expected effects of drug therapy and advise the patient regarding any anticipated side effects or toxic reactions (see page 185). Male patients should also avoid shaving during episodes of facial pain.

Following surgery the nurse will be responsible for the care of the patient's wound and for minimizing the risks of infection. Facial wounds heal quickly and sutures are usually removed within 5 days.

Division of the first branch of the trigeminal nerve will result in poor lacrimation and the nurse should advise the patient to wear glasses or avoid cold wind on the face when outside, avoid touching or rubbing the eye, and to develop a habit of frequent blinking to prevent corneal dryness. As sensation to the face and mouth is lost following division of the second or third branches, the patient should be taught to avoid hot food in the mouth, to eat foods that can be chewed easily, to chew on the unaffected side, and to perform regular oral hygiene using a soft toothbrush. In some cases a mouthwash may be preferable.

Patients with unremitting recalcitrant pain should be referred to a specialist pain clinic for long-term management.

16

Head and spinal injuries

Chris Game   Jenny Kidd

HEAD INJURY

Head injury is a cause of death and disability across the age spectrum. Trauma may occur due to motor vehicle accidents, falls, assault, industrial accidents, and sporting injury. Approximately 35% of all head injuries are due to motor vehicle accidents and 80% of cerebral trauma is due to an external blow to the head. Approximately 65% of persons with head injury are male, and injury is commonest in the 15–24 year age group.

Head injury rarely presents as an isolated injury but frequently occurs in, and often complicates, multiple trauma. Hypoxia and blood loss attributable to associated injuries can further exacerbate the specific effects of head injury. Injuries frequently associated with head injury include: faciomaxillary fractures, fractures of the cervical spine, thoracic and abdominal injuries, and multiple limb fractures.

Injury to the head may result in trauma to the scalp, skull and brain, singly or in conjunction. The extent of injury depends on the primary tissue damage, the magnitude, type and direction of the force, the site of injury, brain movement on impact, and the incidence of secondary events such as haemorrhage and cerebral oedema. Cerebral trauma also results from spontaneous haemorrhage, as in rupture of a vessel or aneurysm.

Pathophysiology and mechanisms of injury

In almost all cases of head injury some nerve cells are rendered hypoxic due to an interruption to their blood supply. Head injury, irrespective of cause, may also result in cerebral oedema and/or death of neurons. The capacity of a person to recover from head injury depends upon the number of neurons involved in the injury, the capacity of those neurons to recover either completely or partially, the site of the damage, and the degree of associated structural damage.

Injury is due to a sudden external force applied to the head. Injuries are broadly classified as penetrating or nonpenetrating (commonly referred to as blunt trauma).

Penetrating injuries result from foreign bodies such as bullets, knives, and bony fragments. The degree of damage will largely depend upon the velocity and nature of impact of the projectile; for example, a high velocity projectile such as a bullet may cause diffuse neuronal damage, whereas a lower velocity projectile such as bone fragments from a depressed skull fracture may cause local neuronal injury due to laceration and bruising.

Blunt trauma frequently results in acceleration/deceleration injuries. These injuries occur when the head is freely moveable at the time of impact and damage will reflect the movement of the brain within the skull, for example as seen in motorcycle accidents or brawls. The brain is a soft, freely moveable organ cushioned and protected from the skull's internal bony prominences and ridges by cerebrospinal fluid. Its only point of fixation is the brainstem. A blow to the skull may be mild and cause slight bruising and therefore concussion, or be so severe as to result in twisting or severing of the brainstem and/or a swirling or shearing of the cerebral hemispheres across the bony prominences of the skull. This gives rise to gross neuronal and blood vessel damage resulting in multiple petechiae, large vessel haemorrhage, bruising and laceration of brain tissue, and cerebral oedema which will increase the intracranial pressure and often exacerbates the original injury. A serious head injury may therefore result in instant death or the comatose patient who may or may not be classified as 'brain dead'.

Injuries to the scalp

Scalp injuries usually comprise bruising, lacerations and foreign bodies. The scalp is highly vascular and will readily bruise and bleed. It is not uncommon for a person to require blood replacement following a severe scalp laceration. Foreign bodies may include glass, dirt, gravel, wood, insects, or scalp hair. Most scalp injuries are treated in emergency departments on an outpatient basis.

Assessment and treatment of any scalp laceration or injury is impossible until the injured area has been thoroughly cleansed and trimmed of hair. Patient education must include prevention of infection, care of the wound, and advice on when to return for follow-up. Scalp wounds heal quickly and hair regrowth is fairly rapid.

Industrial accidents involving the scalp are common, as hair may be caught in machinery causing a complete or partial scalping. The exposed bone must be covered with an appropriate moist dressing and the patient transferred to hospital immediately. The scalp should be wrapped in plastic and transported in ice, if possible, as microsurgery will be required for its reimplantation.

Injuries to the skull

The principle injuries to the skull are fractures, which may be linear, comminuted, or depressed. Linear fractures are are hairline breaks without displacement, and are common; comminuted fractures involve splintered bone which may lacerate the scalp and/or brain; and depressed fractures suppress underlying brain tissue. The presence of a skull fracture does not necessarily indicate that brain damage has occurred.

Fractured base of skull. A fracture of the base of the skull is a serious injury because of the vital positioning of the nerve pathways and control centres, and also because of the proximity of the meninges to the bone. Should a basal fracture occur, the patient is at risk of developing either meningitis (see page 218) or brain abscess (see page 221).

Oedema formation associated with the trauma may also obstruct the flow of cerebrospinal fluid resulting in an increase in intracranial pressure thereby complicating the injury.

If the fracture has caused direct communication between the cavities of the sinuses or middle ear it will result in rhinorrhoea and otorrhoea respectively. Part of the nurse's observations of a patient suffering cerebral trauma is to observe for either of the above manifestations which are strongly suggestive of a basal fracture.

Injuries to the brain

Concussion and contusion. Concussion results from a blow to the head which is severe enough to jostle the brain inside the skull, but not so severe as to cause contusion.

A contusion is a structural alteration resulting from extravasation of blood, without associated tearing of tissues. Contusion can occur directly at the site of the injury or on the opposite side. A concussion or contusion site may be classified as a coup (at the site of injury) or contrecoup (opposite the site of injury).

Concussion and contusion are the most common of all head injuries and cause temporary neuronal dysfunction which clinically manifests as mild headache and vomiting, but may be so severe as to cause transient loss of consciousness with or without associated memory loss (retrograde amnesia). Most persons who suffer concussion and/or contusion recover completely within 24–48 hours. However, repeated concussions, such as those commonly seen in boxers, will result in progressive neuronal death.

In association with the trauma caused by a blow to the head, cerebral oedema causes brain swelling but the brain is held within the confines of an inexpandable vault. As a consequence many deaths from head injury are often due to cerebral oedema and the associated raised intracranial pressure (see page 161) rather than from the injury itself.

The structural damage that can be demonstrated in brain injuries is often in disproportion to the functional incapacity.

Postconcussional syndrome. Although most patients recover completely from a concussion, there are 3 symptoms which may persist and can be quite disabling: headache, giddiness, and mental disturbances.

The headaches are severe and tend to occur in paroxysms brought on by coughing, sneezing, bending over, excitement, and loud noise.

Giddiness is precipitated by sudden head movement and change of posture.

The most common mental disturbances are impaired memory, inability to concentrate, tiredness, degrees of nervousness and anxiety, and intolerance to alcohol.

These may take from 1–3 years to resolve and appear to be directly proportional to the extent and duration of the concussion.

Traumatic delerium (cerebral irritation). In less severe cases of head injury the patient may pass into a state of stupor or confusion. He may lie with his body flexed or extended, resenting interference of any kind, and be restless and often aggressive. When roused the patient may become noisy and violent.

This may last for days to weeks, and should the patient recover he will return to normal cerebration with an associated retrograde amnesia corresponding to the degree and length of cerebral irritation. In less favourable situations the patient may remain stuporose for many months. Any recovery from this stupor will be accompanied by a degree of permanent brain damage.

Differential diagnosis

It is important to establish whether the injury is isolated to the scalp, the skull, or the brain, or whether it involves a combination of these structures.

An injury to the scalp will present in an overt and dramatic form, but it is vital to appreciate that covert brain injury has the potential to become life threatening. Therefore, the nurse must observe for and be alert to the significance of any deterioration in the conscious state or increase in the degree of restlessness of a head injured patient. Immediate investigation is mandatory.

Physical examination will identify specific diagnostic signs such as otorrhoea or rhinorrhoea and any other signs of physical injury. Diagnosis of the cause of loss of consciousness is assisted by a history of events surrounding the incident.

A neurological examination is of more assistance when the patient is conscious. A skull X-ray may demonstrate the position and type of a fracture. CT scan may identify soft tissue damage and the position of a haemorrhage; and a lumbar puncture may show blood, indicating trauma to the meninges.

Medical, surgical, and nursing management

Most head injuries are uncomplicated, and therefore medical and nursing management is largely symptomatic. It involves discharging the patient to the care of a responsible adult, resting the patient in bed, controlling headache, and minimizing irritating stimuli (such as bright lights and loud noises).

However, if the patient sustained (or is suspected of having sustained) a period of unconsciousness, he should be observed in an emergency room for at least 4 hours. It is during this period of time that any life threatening complication will manifest. Observation involves physical and neurological assessment (see page 149), for which the patient must be completely roused. It is wise not to allow a patient with a head injury to sleep during this 4-hour period so that any alteration to conscious state, no matter how slight, can be accurately observed and reported. This is of special importance if the patient is away from an acute care setting as detection of early changes to conscious state provides adequate time for transport of the patient to an acute care setting.

If the person is allowed to go home after the observation period, a parent, spouse, or significant other must be prepared to take responsibility for his continued observation for a further 24 hours. The observer should be instructed to rouse the patient hourly and establish the person's spatial and time orientation, using a simple conversation. In the event of any vomiting, increasing headache, or deterioration in conscious state, the person must be immediately transported to hospital.

The patient with a head injury who requires further care will be suffering associated complications.

COMPLICATIONS OF HEAD INJURIES

Haemorrhage

Haemorrhage is a severe and potentially life threatening complication of craniocerebral trauma. Patients with haemorrhage associated with raised intracranial pressure require careful and continuing observation (see below). Common types of haemorrhage are:

- Scalp
- Epidural
- Subdural
- Subarachnoid (see page 175)
- Intracerebral
- Intraventricular.

Scalp wounds usually bleed prolifically but, following suturing, heal quickly. If a piece of scalp is missing, treatment will involve microsurgery and skin grafting.

Epidural haematoma is a collection of blood between the dura and the skull, and is commonly caused by laceration of the middle meningeal artery. In such cases bleeding is prolific and produces rapid and large clot formation resulting in equally rapid deterioration in conscious state because of raised intracranial pressure. Other epidural haemorrhage is associated with basal and temporal skull fractures.

Subdural haematoma is a collection of venous blood beneath the dural surface. Haematoma formation is relatively slow and if not evacuated results in pressure on the brain, causing its displacement and the associated clinical sequelae of raised intracranial pressure.

The seriousness of the haematoma is associated with its locality and compression of vital centres, and the focal neurological signs of the haematoma formation can also be related to its site. If a patient has been conscious for several days or weeks after a head injury and begins to show marked deterioration in conscious state, a chronic subdural haematoma should be suspected.

Intracerebral and intraventricular haemorrhage may occur as the result of severe trauma to the head, and contribute to fatal head injury. The symptoms and signs are similar to those associated with a cerebrovascular accident (see page 221). Should the patient survive, permanent brain damage is likely.

Raised intracranial pressure

The rigid vault of the skull and the dura protect the brain from injury. However, their restrictive nature poses problems in times of increased intracranial pressure (ICP).

The causes of raised intracranial pressure include: epidural and subdural haematomas, bleeding or infarction in brain substance, cerebral oedema, space occupying lesions such as tumours (see Chapter 19), or an intracranial abscess (see page 221), and an increase in cerebrospinal fluid.

Clinical manifestations

These reflect pressure and/or displacement of the brain and have a wide degree of severity and speed of onset.

The diagnosis of the onset of increased intracranial pressure is assisted greatly if the patient is conscious, as this allows a baseline comparison of conscious level and a comparison of verbal responsiveness of the patient.

In an unconscious patient the nurse must rely on recognizing a deepening of unconsciousness, and any subsequent alteration in vital signs. It must be stressed, however, that *if action is delayed until changes occur in vital signs, permanent brain damage or death may result.* The most significant signs and symptoms indicative of raised intracranial pressure are:

1. Increasing restlessness and irritability.
2. Headache. This is a leading symptom not necessarily significant on its own. Increasing headache however could suggest a rise in ICP.
3. Deterioration in conscious state. This is the most significant of all signs. To wait for a complete comatosed state is to wait for death.

4. Pupils. Changes in the pupil are due to pressure on the occulomotor nerve. The first effect of pressure on this nerve is stimulation, causing the pupil to constrict. This is a transitory phase, frequently occurring before the patient reaches hospital. It therefore may be, and often is, missed. Paralysis then occurs and the pupil progressively dilates and ceases to react to light, resulting in a fixed, dilated pupil. The affected pupil is almost invariably on the side of the lesion and if the pressure progresses, bilateral fixed dilated pupils will occur, indicating an extremely poor prognosis.

5. Vital signs. Ventilation, circulation, and temperature control are likely to be disturbed. The first effect of rising pressure upon the vasomotor and respiratory centres is one of stimulation. This later gives way to depression, which progresses to paralysis and death if untreated.

Ventilation. Stimulation of the respiratory centre results in deepening of ventilation without a change in rate; this is known as stertorous ventilation. Later, the ventilatory rate may increase, but usually ventilatory depression intervenes and results in progressive slowing, and Cheyne Stokes ventilation.

Circulation. The vasomotor centre has two main functions – vagal cardioinhibition and sympathetic vasoconstriction. Stimulation increases the effects of these so that the pulse slows and the blood pressure rises. Bradycardia may become extreme, with the pulse rate as slow as 35 beats per minute, and the blood pressure rises. The systolic pressure is affected much more than the diastolic pressure, so that pulse pressure increases, sometimes to the extent that the bed rocks with each heart beat.

6. If these signs do not occur or are ignored, the next changes seen will be tachycardia and hypotension, which are late signs and circulatory collapse may be imminent. They indicate the need for immediate surgical intervention to relieve the pressure.

7. The effect of rising ICP on the hypothalamus causes alteration in temperature regulation, and may lead to hyperpyrexia (see page 95).

8. Decerebrate rigidity may ultimately occur. This manifests as tonic spasm of all skeletal muscle, with associated tetanic spasm of hands and feet. Ventilatory ability may be severely impaired.

As the pressure increases, the cerebrum displaces and causes distortion of the midbrain at the level of the tentorium cerebelli and the medulla at the level of the foramen magnum. If the pressure is unrelieved, one or more of the cerebella tonsils will herniate into the foramen magnum. If this happens suddenly, the vital centres of ventilation and circulation fail as a result of cerebral compression and death will rapidly ensue. This process of herniation is also known as 'coning'. It sometimes occurs gradually, allowing time for the medulla to compensate but because the area is so sensitive, death can occur at any stage.

Carefully designed neurological observation charts assist the nurse in monitoring a patient's conscious state (Fig. 16.1). When used consistently by medical and nursing staff they will clearly demonstrate an improvement or deterioration in the patient's condition and eliminate subjective interpretation of a patient's response. Interpreting the significance of deterioration in the patient's conscious state and vital signs will enable the nurse to detect early an increase in ICP and therefore prevent the devastating consequences of herniation. The full classical picture described above is rare, therefore the nurse must act on a much less complete clinical picture to prevent irreversible morbidity and death.

Medical, surgical, and nursing management

In cases of mounting pressure, burr holes are created in the skull to relieve pressure, release any haematoma, or to ligate bleeding vessels.

Raised ICP caused by cerebral oedema is treated conservatively, usually with osmotic diuretics and/or steroids, the major steroid being dexamethasone.

Short- or long-term unconsciousness

In the event of either short- or long-term unconsciousness the priority of first aid is to maintain a patent airway. The patient's mouth must be cleared of blood, vomitus and/or any foreign bodies, such as broken teeth or glass. He must be moved away from danger and placed in lateral position with the neck extended and the angle of

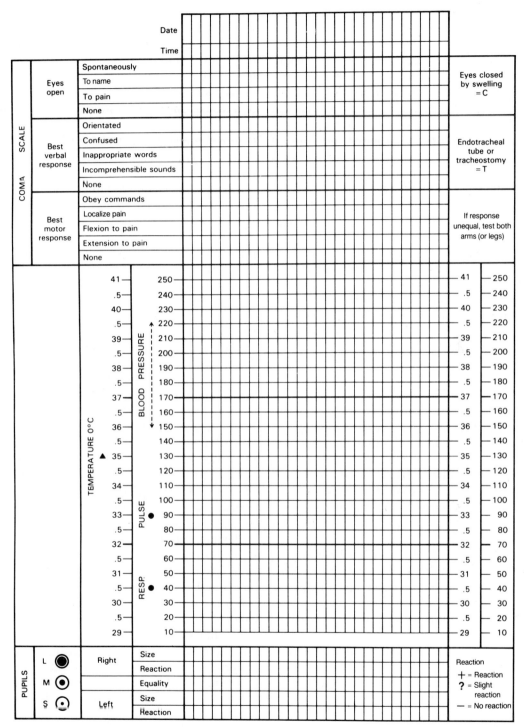

Fig. 16.1 Glasgow coma scale. (Modified from Boore J, Champion R, Ferguson M 1987 *Nursing the Physically Ill Adult.* Churchill Livingstone, Edinburgh).

the jaw supported in order to prevent the tongue from falling backwards and obstructing the oropharynx. Tight clothing should be loosened.

Any obvious bleeding points in the mouth should be treated with direct pressure. Any further overt bleeding on other parts of the body should be treated with direct pressure and/or firm bandaging. If there are penetrating foreign bodies in situ they should not be removed, just padded and supported. Any exposed brain tissue is covered with a clean, moist dressing.

It is important to observe for leaks of cerebrospinal fluid from either the nose or ears, incontinence, fitting, and spasticity or flaccidity of limbs.

In hospital, oropharyngeal aspiration, oxygen, intubation and assisted ventilation may be applied, where necessary. The patient's wounds should be appropriately cleaned, dressed and sutured if required, and investigative procedures can begin. The patient may be stabilized with intravenous fluids and antibiotics and tetanus toxoid given if necessary.

Nursing management

The aim of nursing management of the unconscious patient is the prevention of complications. Common complications of unconsciousness are: airway obstruction, pneumonia, contractures, muscle wasting, diarrhoea and weight loss, skin breakdown, urinary tract infection, hyperthermia, and corneal ulceration. Less common complications include epilepsy, meningitis, and cerebral abscess.

Airway maintenance. A Guedel's airway may be of assistance in maintaining a patent airway. This should not prevent oral hygiene and the airway should be changed at least three times a day. Oropharyngeal aspiration may be performed to assist in the removal of pooled secretions and also to stimulate coughing. A plastic nasal implant may be inserted into the patient's nostril to allow nasopharyngeal aspiration to be performed with a reduced amount of trauma.

Position and movement. The unconscious patient is nursed in lateral position with his neck extended. Normal body alignment is maintained and supported by pillows. The patient's fingers should be extended in order to assist in the prevention of contractures. Two to four hourly position changes help prevent tissue breakdown and encourage coughing and drainage of lung secretions. During turning, the nurse must perform a complete range of passive exercises on the patient, involving all the joints. This need not be a tedious and time-consuming exercise. Two or three movements per joint every time the patient is turned are sufficient to keep joints supple and prevent contractures. Splints and bandages to maintain digital extension may be used for the hands and fingers but tend to prevent the ongoing exercises required to prevent contractures and should therefore be avoided.

Nutrition and hydration. A nasoenteric tube (see page 470) connected to an intermittent or continuous infusion of a complete liquid diet is the preferred method of nutrition. If the flow rate is adjusted to the patient's individual physiological response then he should not develop diarrhoea. However, should this occur it must be reported and treated rapidly to prevent nutritional loss, dehydration and skin breakdown.

The patient should also receive water via the nasoenteric tube during the day to prevent dehydration, constipation, and urinary tract infection. Where possible, catheterization of the patient should be avoided to maintain bladder tone and to reduce the risk of urinary tract infection; rather, bed linen must be changed each time the patient voids. A skilful application of a condom drainage system will provide a dry environment for the male patient.

Should a patient require catheterization a closed system of drainage must be in operation together with adequate hydration and fastidious genital care in order to reduce the risk of infection.

Hygiene and skin care. This is one of the most basic of all nursing procedures and one of the most important and most neglected areas of nursing practice. Meticulous general hygiene is required for the unconscious patient to maintain optimum physical presentation. This will preserve his dignity and ease the distress of the patient's significant others who spend time at the bedside.

Patients who have been comatosed for a long time may be washed in a bath. Those patients who are sponged require thorough wet washes in order to remove the build up of skin cells normally lost through daily movement and showering. Creams and/or oils should be applied liberally to the patient's skin twice weekly to prevent dryness and cracking. His hair should be washed and his nails kept clean, neat and short.

The patient's teeth should be cleaned 3 times per day and water syringed into the mouth and aspirated immediately to remove toothpaste and oral secretions; this procedure may require 2 nurses. Mouth toilets should be performed 2-hourly to keep the buccal mucosa moist. Aerosol breath fresheners may also be used to reduce the patient's halitosis, particularly prior to visiting hours. If the patient has lost blink reflex, artificial tears may be used to keep the cornea moist, and the eyelids must be taped closed.

Safety. Side rails should be kept up at all times and if the patient is restless, they should be padded. Care must be taken to support the patient's limbs during turning to prevent damage, dislocation or overextension of the joints. It should be remembered that the unconscious patient may be able to hear and see. Therefore conversation should be appropriate in the presence of the patient and directed towards him as often as possible. The patient's significant others should also be encouraged to chat to him, thus creating as normal an environment as possible.

Rehabilitation

The patient's capacity for rehabilitation will be determined by his physical and mental state. To maximize his chance of returning to a normal lifestyle rehabilitation must begin from the first day of hospitalization. His progress should not be restricted due to complications which arise as a result of poor nursing management during the unconscious phase.

The rehabilitation programme can be extremely detailed involving input from many members of the health team (see Chapter 8).

SPINAL INJURY

Patients who sustain multiple trauma or head injury carry a high risk of spinal cord trauma at the time of the accident. Trauma to the spinal cord itself may be irreversible and if so is associated with disastrous physical, social, and economic consequences. The direction of many patients' lives turns from one of independence to one of at least partial dependence.

There are varying types of spinal cord injury and nearly all are severe, as damage to a small portion of the spinal cord has widespread motor and sensory consequences.

Aetiology and incidence

Sixty-five percent of people who suffer acute spinal cord trauma are younger than 35 years, with the greatest incidence amongst the ages of 16–25 years.

Males are affected more than females in a ratio of 3 : 1, and injuries tend to occur more frequently during the summer months, holidays, and weekends. The most common cause of injury is motor vehicle accident, with other causes including injuries sustained from diving into shallow water, sporting injuries, stabbing, gunshot wounds, and birth injuries resulting from hyperextension of the cervical spine.

The most frequent mechanism of spinal cord injury is an indirect force applied to the spinal column. This can be due to sudden flexion or hyperextension; rotation of the vertebral column; or vertebral compression resulting in a fracture dislocation of the vertebral bodies, splinting of the vertebrae or herniation of the disc. The damage to the cord may be compression, concussion, contusion, stretching, crushing, or laceration (transection). Damage can be complete or incomplete.

Spinal cord compression

The causes of spinal cord compression are divided into extradural and intradural, the latter being inter- or extramedullary. The principle extradural causes of compression are cervical spondylosis with protusion of intervertebral discs (see page 723) and secondary carcinoma. Less frequent causes include primary neoplasms arising from the vertebrae, such as sarcoma and osteoma; osteitis from tuberculosis or Paget's disease (see page 746); and abscess formation (see page 736). Intradural causes include spinal tumour, meningioma, neurofibroma, and subdural haematoma. Direct pressure on the cord itself interferes with nerve conduction, pressure on the spinal veins leads to oedema of the cord below the compression, and compression of the spinal arteries leads to ischaemia of the cord.

Clinical manifestations

The clinical manifestations of compression of the spinal cord differ according to the segmental level, the degree of compression and whether the lesion is extradural or intradural.

The onset of symptoms is gradual and progressive when due to a spinal tumour, but more rapid in cases of acute compression from causes such as abscess or secondary carcinoma. The first symptoms are usually sensory, characteristic of a nerve root lesion; therefore resulting in nerve root pain which can be unilateral or bilateral. This is classic in distribution, according to the area of skin, muscle, and bone which is supplied by the dorsal nerve root, and results in severe pain, exacerbated by coughing, sneezing and changes in position.

The patient may also complain of paraesthesia, numbness, coldness, anaesthesia, and a feeling of heavy, tight limbs. He may be unable to distinguish light touch, and the sensations of cold and heat. Motor symptoms usually follow rapidly and, in a minority of cases, these may be first to appear. Such symptoms include weakness, unsteadiness, dragging of limbs, wasting of limbs, and fasciculation of muscles. Reflexes may also be reduced or even lost; sphincter disturbances are usually late in onset. In the patient with secondary carcinoma of the vertebral column the onset of symptoms is usually rapid, accompanied by acute pain.

Investigations and diagnosis

Firstly, other lesions which give rise to similar symptoms must be excluded, the level of the compression established, the pathology of the lesion determined and whether it is extradural or intradural.

On examination, the spine may be tender, painful on movement and may show some deformity. A thorough neurological examination will localize the pain to the nervous system and exclude pain from visceral organs. CT scanning and/or myelography to exclude diseases such as motor neuron disease and multiple sclerosis will be undertaken.

Cerebrospinal fluid analysis is of great diagnostic value. A marked rise in protein is typical of extramedullary spinal compression, and a decreased level is common with an intramedullary tumour. The protein content tends to be lower in cases of cervical compression irrespective of the cause.

Management of spinal cord compression

The management of compression of the spinal cord involves specific treatment of the compressive lesion, and care of the paralysed patient if paraplegia is present (see page 171).

Cervical spondylosis (see page 732). Immobilization of the neck by means of a cervical collar is helpful in controlling the symptoms in rapidly progressive cases. Surgical intervention is usually contraindicated if 3 or more discs are involved, but consists of either anterior removal of the discs with spinal fusion or posterior decompression by laminectomy (see page 725).

Tubercular spinal disease. Chemotherapy has reduced the rate of mortality from tuberculosis, and 70% of patients with paraparesis recover completely. Orthopaedic treatment in the form of immobilization in a plaster bed is used in conjunction with the anti-tubercular chemotherapy.

Secondary carcinoma. Treatment is palliative. Few patients survive for longer than 12 months following diagnosis of metastatic involvement of the vertebrae. In some cases, surgical decompression followed by chemotherapy and/or radiotherapy will assist in the reduction of pain and increase longevity.

Spinal tumour. Extradural and extramedullary spinal tumours may be treated by laminectomy and removal of the tumour. The use of lasers and ultrasonic scalpels has reduced the risk of complications. Most intramedullary tumours are inoperable and are therefore treated by radiotherapy. A palliative laminectomy may be performed to relieve pressure on the cord.

Concussion and contusion of the spinal cord

These terms can be used synonymously to mean bruising of the spinal cord (without rupture of the pia mater) resulting from a compression or displacement injury. The contused cord is swollen and may show small haemorrhages, which may ultimately cause necrosis and softening of the cord.

In non-severe cases of spinal cord concussion, the neurologic symptoms are transient, lasting only minutes to hours. However, a severe contusion may give rise to severe disturbance of function, and symptoms may increase in severity for several days. Paralysis is rarely a feature of spinal cord concussion or contusion.

Transection of the spinal cord

Transection (laceration) of the spinal cord is usually due to a penetrating injury. The agents of penetration are most commonly fragments of bones from the spine itself, or foreign objects such as a bullet or knife. Bone fragments may lacerate the cord following fracture, dislocation, or fracture dislocation following forcible extension or flexion of the vertebrae. The most common site for transection of the cord is the lower cervical region.

Any trauma which causes a forcible extension of the neck can fracture the odontoid process and/or contuse the spinal cord, but most spinal cord trauma is due to forcible flexion. The sorts of injuries which cause flexion of the spinal column may be sustained from diving into shallow water; sports such as rugby or trampolining; severe 'whiplash'; heavy objects falling on the shoulders; landing on the feet or buttocks from a fall; and lifting heavy weights, causing a prolapse of intervertebral discs.

Spontaneous fracture dislocation can also result directly from disease of the spinal column such as tuberculosis or spondylitis; also these can exacerbate the extent of damage to the spinal cord from any of the above causes. Laceration of the cord is a much more severe injury than contusion as it involves rupture of the pia mater and complete or partial transection of the cord.

Complete transection

Complete transection of the cord results in the total loss of all voluntary motor and sensory function below the level of the lesion. It also results in a temporary loss of autonomic, reflex, and sexual function, as well as bladder and bowel control. This temporary loss is referred to as the phase of spinal shock.

Quadriplegia (tetraplegia) results from damage to cervical segments of the cord. When damage to the thoracic, lumbar and, to a lesser extent, the sacral cord is complete the patient suffers paraplegia.

Incomplete transection

Incomplete transection of the cord results in partial loss of voluntary motor and/or sensory function below the level of the lesion. The nature of the loss depends upon whether the ascending or descending neural tracts are severed, and to what degree. Preservation of ascending tracts results in the retention of sensory function, and when descending tracts are preserved motor function is retained. Spinal shock is also a feature. Patients commonly preserve a mixture of motor and sensory function, for example, retention of the sensations of discrimination and position but with reduced motor function, along with the loss of the sensation of pain, touch and temperature.

The long-term prognosis for the overall return of normal function is better than for the patient with complete transection of the spinal cord. If neurological recovery is likely to occur, the signs should appear fairly early. Any patient who experiences a total neurological loss below the level of the lesion can expect the loss to be permanent unless return of some function begins within 24 hours. In many cases a number of weeks must pass before it is possible to determine exactly the extent of the loss, and some lower motor neuron lesions may take up to 3–6 months to resolve.

Spinal shock

Spinal shock occurs after any complete or incomplete transection of the spinal cord. There is immediate, complete, flaccid paralysis (hypotonia), anaesthesia, areflexia, and loss of plantar responses below the level of the lesion. Spinal shock may last from weeks to months and as such prevents accurate early forecasting of the degree of recovery the patient may expect.

Clinical manifestations and sequelae of spinal cord injury

It is estimated that 40% of all patients with spinal cord injury die within 24 hours of the accident. An injury to the cervical cord above C4 is rapidly if not immediately fatal, as it causes paralysis of the diaphragm and intercostal muscles.

All patients who suffer complete or incomplete transection of the cord will experience some degree of motor, sensory, and autonomic nerve dysfunction, respiratory embarrassment, and loss of bladder and bowel control. Additionally, some patients will also experience metabolic disturbances and gastrointestinal dysfunction such as paralytic ileus, or acute peptic ulceration. Although sensory loss occurs, patients still feel pain, and paralysis and prolonged immobilization will produce a degree of osteoporosis.

Motor deficit

Injuries to the spinal cord result in upper and/or lower motor neuron dysfunction, which results in paralysis of skeletal muscle below the level of the lesion. Upper motor neuron dysfunction is found in lesions above the L1 vertebra and is characterized by hyperreflexia and loss of voluntary control. Lower motor neuron dysfunction is found in lesions below L1 and is characterized by loss of voluntary control and loss of muscle tone reflexes resulting in flaccidity.

Following resolution of spinal shock, patients with upper motor neuron lesions may develop increased tone and involuntary movement of paralysed muscles. This hyperreflexia, or spasticity, is associated with almost all cervical injuries and 75% of thoracic injuries. It occurs 6 weeks after a cervical lesion is sustained, and approximately 10 weeks after a thoracic lesion. It usually lasts for 2 years then gradually subsides; this should not be mistaken for return of function. Excessive and/or untreated muscle spasm can result in the development of contractures and can also lead to limb injury.

Sensory deficit

Complete lesions usually result in loss of sensations such as position, pain, touch, and temperature below the level of the lesion. There is also loss of visceral sensation. Sometimes, however, the patient suffers abnormally increased sensation, and occasionally phantom pain, which subsides within days.

Autonomic deficit

Complete lesions involving cervical and high thoracic segments of the cord can cause hypotension because of interruption to the sympathetic splanchnic control. Also, during the first few days following cervical cord trauma, the vasomotor system is extremely unstable and there is risk of cardiac arrest during routine turning of the patient. Temperature control is also altered as the autonomic mechanism of vasoconstriction and vasodilation to alter body heat is inoperative. Patients are unable to shiver or sweat and this is of major significance to the quadraplegic, who will assume the temperature of his environment.

Neurogenic bladder

This occurs when the nerve supply to the bladder has been damaged. The interruption to bladder function depends on the level of the lesion and the degree of damage to the cord. In both upper and lower motor neuron lesions the patient suffers incontinence of urine, with no sensation of bladder fullness or desire to void. A cystogram is performed after spinal shock has resolved to assess the degree of functional bladder capacity.

Neurogenic bowel

In the presence of upper motor neuron lesions the external sphincter is hypertonic or spastic, and automatic defaecation of semi-formed stools from the rectum will occur as the normal voluntary control of the external sphincter is lost. In the presence of lower motor neuron lesions, the external sphincter is open and the smooth muscle of the bowel retains some contractile response, producing frequent passage of loose stools.

Ventilatory embarrassment

A cervical cord lesion below C4 results in paralysis of the intercostal muscles, which account for 60% of effective ventilation. Injuries above C4 will involve the diaphragm and the patient will require immediate assisted ventilation.

Paralytic ileus

The cause of paralytic ileus in acute paralysis following a spinal cord lesion is unknown. It occurs in both upper and lower motor neuron lesions. It lasts approximately 7 days but can last for several weeks. Paralytic ileus may cause death, due to inhalation of vomitus. The severity of paralytic ileus increases in cervical and/or complete lesions of the cord.

Acute peptic ulceration

Approximately 5% of patients with acute spinal cord injury develop peptic ulceration, which is thought to be due to an endogenous release of steroids. It occurs approximately 7–10 days after injury and commonly presents as acute gastrointestinal haemorrhage. The ulcer is treated conservatively (see Chapter 52).

Metabolic disturbances

Enhanced mineralocorticoid activity can initially result in hypernatraemia. Therefore IV sodium solutions should be avoided, and diuretics may be required to prevent fluid overload and hypokalaemia due to urinary loss of potassium. Potassium supplements in the acute stages will prevent complications such as prolonged paralytic ileus and cardiac arrythmias.

The patient must be observed for a post traumatic diuresis which may occur within the first 10 days, and requires appropriate fluid and electrolyte replacement.

Chronic pain

It is extremely rare for a paralysed patient to experience a complete lack of sensation. Rather, patients suffer many sensations below the level of the lesion, some of which are painful. There is no obvious cause for this and the pain is diffuse in nature. Most patients can tolerate the pain but a minority find it disabling. Codeine compounds provide effective relief.

Osteoporosis

Osteoporosis (see page 744) occurs rapidly in paralysed limbs. Immediately following spinal trauma, calcium is lost from the bone and excreted in the urine, which accounts for the high incidence of bladder and renal calculi in patients with paralysed limbs. Patients are thus prone to pathological fractures during physiotherapy or as the result of a fall from their wheelchair. These fractures heal quickly and are managed conservatively (see page 700).

First aid management of a patient with suspected spinal cord damage

The symptoms and signs indicative of cord damage are an inability to move or to feel areas of the body, a feeling of 'pins and needles' in the vertebral column and/or extremities, and the presence of intercostal paralysis with diaphragmatic breathing.

Initial management

The patient should not be moved but supported and made comfortable in the exact position in which he has been found. However, if the patient must be moved because of further danger, or because he has life threatening complications which require attention, then the following principles must be observed.

The patient should be lifted as a whole, with a straight spinal column maintained. This will require a lifting team of at least 4 people. One of the team should be at the head maintaining the patient's chin in straight alignment to his body; this person should be the supervisor of the lift. Ideally the patient should be lifted with the aid of a frame which will ensure minimum movement of the vertebral column.

The patient should be placed in a supine position with his neck supported by, for example, a rolled towel or newspaper. Should the patient vomit or otherwise suffer airway obstruction, he must be log rolled with his spine in alignment and the airway cleared. If the patient is wearing a helmet it must only be removed whilst the patient is on his side, to avoid flexion of the neck. Any objects in the patient's pockets which could cause pressure must be removed as they could predispose to the early development of decubitus ulcers during the transit period.

Management in the emergency room

The patient is given oxygen via an intranasal catheter or mask. Intravenous fluid therapy is commenced immediately and the patient is allowed nothing by mouth. A nasogastric tube is inserted to decompress the stomach so as to prevent vomiting and its aspiration, and to minimize the effects of a paralytic ileus.

An indwelling urinary catheter is inserted to drain residual urine as the patient will have a neurogenic bladder. If respiratory embarrassment is present, assisted ventilation will be required. All precautions should be taken against the development of decubitus ulcers during this early management and transfer period. The patient should be nursed on a sheepskin as soon as practicable.

It must be remembered that the spinal patient is poikilothermic below the level of the lesion and will tend to assume the temperature of the environment. Therefore the patient's body temperature must not be allowed to become overheated in warm weather and must be preserved in cold weather. This is of special importance in patients with quadriplegia.

Patients may also present with hypotension and bradycardia. This is not due to blood loss but results from spinal shock which causes paralytic vasodilation below the level of the lesion. The condition is usually self-limiting and only requires medical intervention if the systolic blood pressure falls below 80 mmHg.

Respiratory depressants such as morphine must be used with caution in patients with quadriplegia. If necessary, fracture sites must be reduced and immobilized until body and ligamentous healing takes place.

Medical and surgical management

Treatment is directed towards protection of the spinal cord from further injury and provision of an optimum environment for maximum neurological recovery. Wherever possible, following stabilization the patient is transferred to a specialized spinal unit for long term care and rehabilitation.

Cervical spine

A stable cervical injury can be immobilized with a cervical collar which is considered to be sufficient treatment.

Cervical dislocations and fractures are reduced and immobilized by the insertion of skull tongs and the application of traction for approximately 6–8 weeks to enable bone healing. Following removal of traction the patient wears a cervical collar to prevent extremes of motion until muscle tone and strength is sufficiently developed to support the weight of the patient's head.

Thoracic and lumbar spine

Most of these injuries can be managed conservatively by postural reduction for approximately 6–8 weeks using a pillow placed under the fracture site. Perfect anatomical reduction is impossible and is not necessary to achieve good functional results. If a fracture site fails to achieve good bone union after 6–8 weeks of bedrest it may be necessary to perform a fusion of adjacent vertebrae.

Lumbar fractures are occasionally reduced surgically and stabilized by either fusion of vertebrae, or insertion of rods or plates.

Hydrotherapy is useful in controlling muscle spasm, as is the application of heat or cold; the effects of such therapy varies amongst individuals. Diazepam may be of use in some patients as are nerve blocks of peripheral nerves. Surgical intervention for severe muscle spasm consists of neurotomy, myelotomy, and rhizotomy.

Nursing management of the paralysed patient

The nursing management of a paralysed patient requires a great deal of skill, care, and time, as these patients are prone to complications which have the potential to severely retard progress and may even prove fatal. Such specialist nursing care can only be provided in a dedicated spinal unit.

Psychological support

Transection of the cord with resultant paralysis is a devastating diagnosis for the patient and his significant others. Even when the symptoms and signs are insidious in onset, as in spinal tumour or spinal cord compression due to chronic disease, the eventual paralysis is no less devastating in its effects on the patient and the adjustments that must be made by his significant others. The onset of sudden paralysis evokes coping mechanisms in the patient that are akin to those which occur after a diagnosis of inoperable cancer. You must anticipate the patient exhibiting the stages of denial, awareness and anger, adjustment and anxiety or despair, before he can reach the position whereby he can accept his altered physical state and self-image. Only then can the patient and his significant others effectively work towards making the necessary readjustments that will enable him to realize his full potential and maximize his independence.

Skin care

Decubitus ulcers are complications which must be avoided. They are most likely to occur over bony prominences such as hips, shoulders, and sacrum. Factors which lead to their development in the spinal patient are loss of sensation and mobility, initial shock at the time of the injury, poor blood vessel tone and sluggish peripheral circulation.

The major principle of prevention is constant relief of pressure, and this is achieved by a 2-hourly change of position. Patients with cervical tongs in situ are preferably nursed on a Stryker frame which enables safe turning in normal body alignment. All other patients are lifted and their pillows are adjusted to protect bony prominences.

Eventually the patient will become responsible for his own pressure area care. Paraplegic patients must perform chairlifts (raising and repositioning) every 15–20 minutes; and the nurse must reposition quadriplegic patients hourly.

Various aids can also be used to assist in relief and distribution of pressure. Such aids include pillows, foam overlays, sheepskins, water and ripple mattresses, and wheelchair cushions. Aids should be used carefully to ensure that they do relieve, rather than cause, pressure.

In general, the patient's skin must be kept clean and dry. Brisk but gentle drying helps keep the skin supple; drying agents such as methylated spirits should be avoided, as should creams which can keep the skin too moist. Bed linen should be dry and free of wrinkles and foreign bodies, such as crumbs. Tight footwear should be avoided and the patient's nails kept short to prevent scratching.

The paralysed patient should be taught to inspect his body daily with the aid of mirrors for signs of pressure areas. He must realize that he must be vigilant in avoiding pressure areas for the rest of his life. Should a decubitus ulcer develop, the patient will most likely require hospitalization for regular and adequate dressing; some ulcers may even require a split skin graft (see page 780). Healing may take months of careful nursing attention.

Respiratory management

Arterial blood gas analysis may be taken to assess tissue oxygenation, and hypoventilation must be observed for and reported. Patients with diaphragmatic paralysis and/or a severe chest injury will require assisted ventilation.

Due to a significantly reduced cough reflex, the paralysed patient will require vigorous chest physiotherapy and postural drainage to assist in establishing effective coughing.

Diet

The patient must receive a highly nutritious diet and a large volume of fluid to promote tissue healing, retain bladder tone, and minimize osteoporosis, renal calculi and muscle wasting. Initially, fluids, kilojoules and nutrients are provided by intravenous therapy. Once bowel sounds return, gastrointestinal feeding is commenced by either the nasoenteric or oral route. The patient will require a daily intake of at least 14 500 kJ including 125 g of protein, 3.5–4 litres of fluid, adequate fibre, and vitamin supplementation.

Bladder management

The long-term aim of bladder management is to establish continence, and thus remove the need for an indwelling catheter. The short-term aims are to maintain bladder tone, effect regular and complete bladder emptying, and to prevent urinary tract infection. In the acute stages, depending on the existence of other injuries and general condition of the patient, continuous bladder drainage or intermittent catheterization is used. In general, the indwelling catheter is removed within a 2–7 day period.

Following this, the patient is catheterized 4–6 hourly or at such intervals as will prevent spontaneous voiding. The length of time between catheterization is increased until the patient's bladder is conditioned into a voiding pattern, that is, the bladder will hold at least 350 ml of urine, and will not release that urine spontaneously. The aim is to have the patient catheter free, although once-daily catheterization may be necessary to remove any residual urine.

The success of establishing continence depends on the level of the lesion, and the attitude and motivation of the patient. Drugs such as phenoxybenzamine and distigmine may be used to assist the detrusor muscle of the bladder to contract.

The female quadriplegic patient who is unable to transfer to the toilet may require a suprapubic catheter. Male patients are able to use a condom drainage apparatus. All paraplegics and quadriplegics must have an annual intravenous pyelogram to check the structure and function of the kidney, and 3-monthly blood analysis for urea and electrolytes and a urine specimen for microscopy and culture.

With correct and meticulous attention to personal hygiene, asepsis during catheterization, adequate fluid intake and regular check ups, the paralysed patient should remain free of bladder infection.

Bowel care

During the phase of spinal shock, manual removal of faeces from the rectum is performed every 2–3 days to keep the rectum empty. Bowel training begins once spinal shock has resolved.

The aims of bowel training are to establish continence and a regular pattern of defaecation, and to prevent complications such as diarrhoea or constipation. The usual pattern is evacuation every second day using suppositories or enemas. This may be preceded on the previous night by oral administration of faecal softeners.

A diet containing adequate fibre is encouraged. Bowel training is by trial and error but the aim is to establish the time, method and laxative that suit the individual. Most paraplegics and quadriplegics can transfer, or be transferred, to a toilet.

Allied paramedical care

Physiotherapy

The aim of physiotherapy is to obtain and maintain the maximum potential of all muscles which have some remaining voluntary power. Special attention with the use of slings is given to the muscles of the trunk, and passive movements are carried out on the limbs at least twice daily.

The risk of deep vein thrombosis in the spinal patient is high. There is considerable stasis in the venous system due to lack of movement, prolonged immobilization, and the constant pressure of the mattress on the patient's calves and thighs. The patient has diminished pain sensation, therefore the thrombosis is clinically significant before it is recognized, perhaps presenting as a pulmonary embolus.

The risk of development of deep vein thrombosis can be greatly reduced by performing a full range of passive movements of the lower limbs at least 2-hourly. Such exercises will also assist in controlling the problem of gravitational oedema, as will the elevation of the legs and the wearing of elastic stockings.

Patients are encouraged to sit in a wheelchair as soon as flaccid paralysis has resolved and they are also encouraged to exercise to improve trunkal and upper limb strength. Most paraplegic patients will become wheelchair-independent and some eventually may learn to walk. At first, parallel bars are used to support the patient until he can manage elbow crutches. Some patients can attempt walking under the supervision of a physiotherapist, with the help of full length calipers with knee locks and toe springs, and a spinal brace if trunkal muscles are involved.

Sexual counselling

Sexual function and expression in the paralysed patient differs greatly between individuals. Despite paralysis, the patient's sexuality remains intact although functional ability may vary. The male patient may be totally unable to achieve erection and/or ejaculation or he may have function ranging to normal. Males who are unable to function sexually often consider that their masculinity is at risk and that they are inadequate and incompetent as life partners.

Similarly, females may be unable to achieve orgasm or they may have a range of residual sexual function. It is important that patients, and their significant others, understand that paralysis does not cause infertility.

Any sexual dysfunction or anxieties require referral of the patient and significant other for sensitive counselling. Various sex aids can be employed and in general if a realistic and frank approach is adopted towards the problem, some suitable and satisfying sexual practice will be found.

Rehabilitation and habilitation

The task of assisting the patient to adjust to a new way of life and a new future is challenging and must begin from the day of trauma. Some patients find it more difficult than others to see life in terms of normality and to understand that activity is still possible. Psychological states such as anxiety, anger, depression, and denial are natural reactions and occur in the early stages of hospitalization.

The patient's family and significant others should be involved in the rehabilitation programme. Advice will be necessary regarding alterations to the patient's home to accommodate a wheelchair; ramps replace steps, doorways are widened, sinks are lowered, and appropriate bathing and toileting facilities are installed.

Part of the patient's rehabilitation programme may be the training for a change of employment. There is no reason why a paraplegic capable of holding employment and earning income should not do so.

Social workers are heavily involved in the patient's transition from hospital to home and in settling the patient back into the home and community.

17

Other lesions of the central nervous system

Jenny Kidd Chris Game

Vascular lesions of the central nervous system (CNS) are the second most common cause of neural dysfunction, after trauma. Lesions occurring due to infection (see Chapter 24), tumour (see Chapter 19), and toxic agents although less common, may cause dysfunction ranging from localized tissue ischaemia to widespread neuronal death and these lesions can affect all brain structures and the cranial nerves.

In this chapter cerebrovascular lesions will be studied in the context of cerebrovascular accident – the most common presentation of a vascular cerebral lesion.

CEREBROVASCULAR ACCIDENT

Cerebrovascular accident (CVA) or 'stroke' are terms used to refer to any disturbance of cerebral blood flow, although 'stroke' generally refers to a sudden onset of neurological deficit.

Cerebrovascular disease is one of the three major causes of death in Australia and 1 person in 5 will experience some form of cerebrovascular disturbance. Those in the over–50 age group are particularly at risk. A large number of people surviving a cerebrovascular accident are left with a residual disability. People suffering hypertension and/or heart disease or diabetes mellitus, those with a family history of CVA, cigarette smokers, and the obese are especially at risk. Women on long-term oral contraceptives, with associated cigarette smoking, are more likely to suffer a CVA at a younger age.

Aetiology and pathophysiology

The three major causes of CVA are thrombosis, embolism, and haemorrhage; these are frequently associated with factors present in cardiac and renal disease, diabetes mellitus and hypertension. Less commonly, compression of cerebral vessels leading to infarction may be caused by cerebral neoplasms or cerebral oedema, as seen in acute infections of the central nervous system (see page 218).

The brain is dependent upon an adequate blood supply to gain oxygen and glucose which enable neuronal function to continue. Any interruption to this supply will cause ischaemia and, if prolonged, cerebral infarction will occur. Cerebral oedema appears at the site of the lesion within 8–24 hours, peaks within 5–7 days, and then gradually resolves. Softening and necrosis of the brain tissue occurs about 7 days following the infarction, and phagocytic removal of the debris results in cavitation and subsequent scarring at the site of injury.

Depending on the area of the brain affected, the person who sustains a CVA may have any of the following deficits: impaired motor control, perceptual difficulties, aphasia or dysphasia (if the dominant hemisphere is involved), sensory deficits, poor memory, altered emotions, loss of balance, spasticity, paralysis, or altered consciousness. In CVA involving cerebral vessels (as opposed to vertebral/basilar arteries) the motor and sensory deficits will manifest on the side of the body opposite to the lesion; hence left hemispherical CVA produces right side dysfunction. Damage to cranial nerves will, of course, be manifest as cranial nerve dysfunction on the same side as the lesion. The degree of damage depends upon many factors, not least of which is the adequacy of collateral circulation.

Cerebral thrombosis

Cerebral thrombosis is a frequent cause of CVA, especially in the older patient, and the major cause of this is atherosclerosis, which is often associated with diabetes mellitus or hypertension. Most persons with cerebral thrombosis had premonitory episodes prior to their completed 'stroke', for example, transient slurring of speech, unilateral weakness, or paraesthesia. Symptoms of cerebral thrombosis tend to occur during sleep or soon after waking and the symptoms may be progressive for the initial 24–48 hours.

Cerebral embolism

Cerebral embolism is seen more frequently in younger persons and symptoms occur suddenly and at any time of the day. The embolus lodges at the bifurcation of a narrow lumen in the cerebral circulation. The most common cause of a cerebral embolism is cardiac disease, such as atrial fibrillation, myocardial infarction, or mitral stenosis, where there is thrombus formation from which the emboli originate. An embolus can also comprise atheroma, vegetation as a result of bacterial overgrowth, or air. Untreated valvular disease, bacterial endocarditis, or complications of cardiac surgery also act as foci for emboli, as does atherosclerotic disease of the carotid artery.

Cerebral haemorrhage

Cerebral haemorrhage results in blood escaping from a ruptured artery. This blood may then invade the brain tissue or surrounding spaces. Arterial rupture results from either a degenerative change in the integrity of the arterial wall or from an anatomical defect, either an aneurysm or an arteriovenous malformation. Haemorrhage will be either intracerebral or subarachnoid.

Intracerebral haemorrhage involves bleeding into the brain tissue, causing dissection and displacement of the brain, which is ultimately compressed outwards against the rigid skull. If the haemorrhage is large then raised intracranial pressure may cause midline displacement, with the risk of brain herniation and brain stem compression. Blood may also leak into the ventricles and/or cerebrospinal fluid.

The most common cause is hypertension, and the small penetrating arteries deep within the brain tissue are most likely to be involved. Blood normally supplied to the area by the ruptured artery is lost and tissue damage results from the combination of the effects of compression and tissue ischaemia. Intracerebral haemorrhage has a high mortality rate.

Subarachnoid haemorrhage results from the rupture of a cerebral aneurysm, or of an arteriovenous malformation, with leakage of blood into the subarachnoid space and cerebrospinal fluid. 80% of aneurysms occur on the Circle of Willis and the most common site is the junction of the internal carotid and posterior communicating arteries. Decreased collagen at the bifurcation of cerebral arteries is thought to be responsible for the aneurysm formation. Mycotic aneurysms are due to partial destruction of the artery wall due to infective emboli and subsequent aneurysm formation.

Aneurysms are 50% more common in women and the peak incidence of rupture is between 30–60 years of age. The rupture of the aneurysm causes a sudden, high-pressure haemorrhage into the subarachnoid space with resultant severe meningeal irritation. This manifests as an explosive headache with nuchal rigidity and severe photophobia. The brain tissue supplied by the vessel becomes ischaemic, and as there is a concurrent release of vasoactive substances which may cause arterial spasm, the degree of cerebral ischaemia is further increased. Blood may also collect within the tissues and form an intracerebral haematoma which will give rise to a further increase in intracranial pressure. It is fairly common for a subarachnoid haemorrhage to recur when natural lysis of the blood clot occurs after 7–10 days. Intracranial aneurysms account for 25% of deaths due to cerebrovascular disease.

Clinical manifestations

Cerebrovascular disease may manifest in a variety of ways:

1. Transient ischaemic attacks (TIAs)
2. Reversible ischaemic neurologic deficits (RINDs)
3. Evolving 'stroke'
4. Completed 'stroke'.

TIAs are episodes of temporary neurological disturbance varying from minutes to hours in duration, and complete recovery occurs within 24 hours. They are thrombotic in origin and in 30% of cases are followed by a CVA within 3–5 years. The neurological disturbance may be focal, and manifestations depend upon the area of the brain involved. Common manifestations are limb weakness, and disturbances in speech, vision, gait, and sensation. RINDs are TIAs that take more than 24 hours for complete recovery.

An evolving 'stroke' is one where symptoms of neurological deficit develop slowly over the course of several hours to days, culminating in a completed 'stroke'. Recovery in this instance may occur once the pathophysiological process is complete and cerebral oedema has subsided.

Despite the above manifestations, the majority of patients who suffer a CVA fail to recognize these preliminary signs and symptoms, and present with the sudden onset of neurological deficits. The deficits may range from mild to severe and the type will be dependent upon the artery involved. For example:

• Middle cerebral artery CVAs result in hemiplegia, hemiparaesthesia, aphasia, homonymous hemianopia, paralysed side neglect, and apraxia.
• Internal carotid artery CVAs commonly cause unconsciousness and seizures may also occur. These CVAs also result in hemiplegia, hemiparaesthesia, aphasia, paralysed side neglect, apraxia, homonymous hemianopia, and transient ipsilateral blindness.
• Anterior cerebral artery CVAs are the least common and may be complete or partial. They cause hemiplegia and hemiparaesthesia which is more pronounced in the legs than the arms, urinary incontinence, and depressed cognition and emotional affect.

• Vertebral and basilar artery CVAs cause hemiplegia and hemiparaesthesia either on the same side as the lesion or in all limbs, and if the brain stem is involved to a large degree, unconsciousness occurs. They also result in nystagmus, vertigo, diplopia with lateral and vertical gaze palsies, visual field deficits, ataxia, dysphagia, and dysarthria.
• Posterior cerebral artery CVAs result in hemiparaesthesia, blindness (if involvement is bilateral) or visual field deficits.

The degree of permanent neuronal damage, and hence potential neurological deficit, depends upon the extent of the pathological process and the adequacy of any collateral circulation. Following resolution of the acute episode, some neurons will recover, the extent of this recovery varying greatly between patients. The time of resolution is also individual, but generally it can be expected that if the patient demonstrates marked improvement within the first week following the onset of the CVA, then minimal deficit will result. Conversely, little or no improvement shown in the first week is usually indicative of a poor prognosis and/or a severe and permanent disability.

Investigative procedures

The diagnosis of a CVA is primarily based upon the observation of the clinical features; the patient's history, including known or observed risk factors; the report of any witness to the sequence of onset of the symptoms; and the result of a thorough physical examination which includes full neurological testing. Additionally, the following procedures may be performed to assist in determining the extent of neuronal damage:

• CT scan may determine the location and type of CVA or confirm an alternative intracranial pathology, for example tumour or abscess. CT scan is invaluable in determining the 'mass effect' (or extent) of haemorrhage or oedema compression by revealing areas of distortion of brain tissue.
• Lumbar puncture may be performed; bloody cerebrospinal fluid with an accompanying rise in pressure is found with subarachnoid haemorrhage and the majority of intracerebral haemorrhages.

- EEG by differentiating seizure activity can assist in the location of the lesion should these occur with the CVA.
- An ECG is commonly performed to exclude or confirm any cardiac causes, for example, myocardial infarction and atrial fibrillation.
- Cerebral angiography permits detection of arterial plaque formation, occlusion, or stenosis, and can locate arterial aneurysms.
- Serum and blood analysis is usually undertaken to determine a baseline for future comparison of the patient's progress.

Medical, surgical, and nursing management

The results of cerebrovascular dysfunction can vary widely from mild and transient symptoms through to severe, devastating disability and even death. Unfortunately, the majority of patients experience sufficient neuronal damage to suffer permanent neurological deficits. These deficits may range from mild memory loss, speech impairment, or muscle weakness, through to severe hemiplegia and loss of speech. The long-term effects of cerebrovascular disease and the patient's eventual prognosis depend upon the site of the arterial occlusion or rupture; the degree and extent of the ischaemia and/or haemorrhage; the effectiveness of medical and nursing management; and the response of the patient to rehabilitation.

Therefore the aims of management are to:

1. Prevent further brain damage or stroke
2. Reduce risk factors
3. Give supportive care
4. Regain functional independence.

Conservative management may include the use of drug therapy, for example anticoagulants, to reduce the risk of further thrombosis or emboli, corticosteroids to reduce cerebral oedema, anticonvulsants if seizures co-exist, analgesics to relieve headache, and treatment of pre-existing conditions (for example hypertension with antihypertensive agents and diuretics).

Heparin is the anticoagulant of choice. It prevents the conversion of prothrombin to thrombin and warfarin inhibits vitamin K synthesis, thereby interfering with the clotting cascade (see page 379). Aspirin may also be used for its anticoagulant properties.

Antithrombotic agents, for example dipyridamole, may be ordered to depress thrombocyte aggregation and therefore prevent further thrombosis or embolism. The use of these drugs is controversial as they increase the risk of haemorrhage from other sites.

Antifibrinolytics, for example aminocaproic acid, reduce the rate of clot breakdown at the aneurysm site by inhibiting substances normally involved in fibrinolysis. They are also used to prevent recurrent subarachnoid haemorrhage.

If an aneurysm cannot be treated surgically then conservative management will consist largely of bed rest for a minimum of 4 weeks; activities will be resumed progressively following this period.

Aggressive management may include surgery, which is usually performed only in the case of the patient with atherosclerotic disease of the carotid arteries or in the patient with an aneurysm. The types of surgery that may be performed include:

1. Carotid endarterectomy (see page 295).
2. Revascularization of affected tissue by the anastomosis of vessels, for example, superficial temporal artery to a cortical vessel.
3. Craniotomy to evacuate an intracerebral haematoma.
4. Clipping the neck of an aneurysm. If clipping of the aneurysm is impossible and there is adequate collateral blood supply, common carotid artery ligation may be performed.
5. Thrombosing of the aneurysm. This procedure is best performed when vasospasm is decreasing so that surgery itself does not result in severe neurological damage.

Diet

Specialist dietary therapy is aimed at reducing risk factors such as obesity and hyperlipidaemia, and maintaining diabetic and antihypertensive control.

Specific nursing care

Nursing care will depend upon the individual needs of the patient in relation to both his CVA and any pre-existing disease. The ultimate outcome for the patient will depend largely upon the success of rehabilitative techniques and methods aimed at preventing residual deformity or dysfunction. The earlier rehabilitation is commenced the more likely a return to normal function is achieved. For example, the immediate commencement of passive and full range of motion exercises to the paralysed limbs will, in many instances, minimize or prevent joint stiffness and muscle contracture. Therefore the nurse responsible for the care of a patient diagnosed as having suffered a CVA must establish a database from which a comprehensive nursing care plan can be developed.

Nursing care should be aimed at maximizing the potential for a return to independence in self-care and will include measures to:

1. Ensure a patent airway
2. Maintain patient safety and comfort
3. Provide for nutrition and hydration needs
4. Maintain elimination patterns
5. Ensure effective alternative methods of communication
6. Maintain emotional support and ensure that expectations are realistic.

Ensure a patent airway. In the majority of cases of CVA patients will have an alteration to their level of consciousness and have some degree of interruption to their cough and gag reflexes. Associated inadequate lung expansion puts the patient at risk of ventilatory complications, for example, hypoxia, respiratory distress, hypostatic and aspiration pneumonias.

On admission to the emergency room, an unconscious patient must be placed in a lateral position, with an oral airway inserted, and oropharyngeal suction applied as necessary. In some instances the patient may have been alone and unconscious for several hours or days so the amount and nature of secretions will vary. Oxygen will be administered by either mask or intranasal catheter; in only a minority of cases will the patient require intubation and/or assisted ventilation.

The patient should be turned frequently and where possible the head of his bed should be raised with his head positioned to one side. These measures assist in maintaining a patent airway,

assist in preventing pooling of secretions in the base of his lungs, and minimize the risk of aspiration. The conscious patient should be sat upright to assist with normal lung expansion; oxygen may be required and is best administered by face mask. Oropharyngeal suction may be necessary to relieve excessive dribbling if the swallow reflex has been impaired.

The administration of humidified oxygen or air will prevent secretions becoming thick, tenacious, and difficult for the patient to expectorate. If the patient regains control over his swallow and other reflexes, coughing and deep breathing exercises should be commenced.

Maintain patient safety and comfort. Until consciousness is regained care must include special attention to the paralysed limbs: the patient should be nursed in a position of comfort with the paralysed limbs well supported and protected from accidental injury or pressure. Nursing observation of the patient's neurological status must be undertaken frequently (see page 161) and any signs of increasing intracranial pressure should be recorded and reported immediately (see page 161). If necessary, bed rails should be padded to prevent self-injury and suction equipment must be ready at all times.

Once consciousness is regained constant reassurance must be provided by the nurse because in most instances the patient is unsure of what has happened, is frightened and confused, and may be extremely frustrated by a variety of motor, speech, or perception disorders. Speech disorders can result in the patient being unable to verbalize his needs and therefore compromise his independence even further. The nurse is responsible for protecting the patient from the hazards of immobility should he be confined to bed. In particular, the risks of venous stasis and skin breakdown should be minimized. The motor abilities retained by the patient will determine the degree of independence, with or without nursing supervision, that the patient can be allowed.

The ambulatory patient's environment should be kept free of clutter and any obstacles removed or padded. Any patient unsteady on his feet should not be left unattended or allowed to ambulate at will as ataxia may cause him to lose balance and suffer falls. Paralysed side neglect will result in the patient experiencing trauma to a part of his body that he just does not know exists, for example hitting door frames with his hemiplegic limbs.

In most cases of hemiplegia the patient cannot feel his hemiplegic side. Therefore, the nurse must take care to minimize pressure on the limbs by ensuring that the patient has frequent position changes and is not forced to lie on abnormally placed limbs for long periods. All baths and showers should be supervised until the patient can safely regulate water temperatures so as to prevent burns of the limbs. Gait training for ambulation will be commenced as soon as possible but usually only when the patient has regained his balance, with or without the aid of a walking frame or stick. The nurse should continue physiotherapy instructions for gait retraining, weight bearing, and proper body mechanics and alignment.

Paralysis may resolve gradually or remain as a permanent deficit. A full range of passive and active exercises, performed frequently on limbs and all joints, will assist in maintaining optimal function and preventing venous stasis. Correct positioning of limbs will further assist in preventing deformities, reducing spasticity, and minimizing skin breakdown; limbs should be supported in a functional position and the patient repositioned 2-hourly. Care must be taken not to extend any joint forcefully beyond its limits as traumatic subluxation or fracture may occur. Splints may be useful in the prevention of hand and arm contractures and foot drop; these are usually applied only at night.

Any oedematous limbs (a common condition in hemiplegia due to interruption to autonomic regulation of fluid dynamics in the vessels) should be elevated and supported. Where possible, intramuscular injections, blood pressure readings, and intravenous lines should be avoided on hemiplegic limbs.

The patient's skin should be kept clean and free from excessive perspiration and any soiling by urine and/or faeces, and supervision with bathing is essential to ensure adequate cleansing of skin folds, under nails, and around the genital and perianal areas.

Wherever possible the patient should be approached from his intact side and all objects kept within easy reach and within his field of vision. When approaching the patient from his deficient side remember that you are outside his field of vision. Speaking to him as you approach will assist in reorienting him and minimizing paralysed side neglect.

Provide for nutrition and hydration needs. Initially the patient will receive fluids and nutrients via IV infusion and the nurse is responsible for ensuring that the infusion is maintained as ordered, so as to prevent circulatory overload and possible cerebral oedema. Once the patient's physical condition has stabilized either nasogastric or nasoenteric feeds may be commenced, and as soon as his swallow reflex is re-established he may recommence oral food and fluids. The patient will require assistance with meals and this may vary from feeding him to providing him with adapted equipment that will enable him to feed himself. Soft foods should be provided initially and the patient taught to place food in the nonparalysed side of the mouth and to chew it well. Sips of fluid will aid in swallowing and iced fluids will aid in heightening perception in the mouth. Meals should not be rushed and the patient should be given abundant encouragement to perservere.

Maintain elimination patterns. Initially, urinary incontinence is usually the result of unconsciousness or disturbed neurological function. Unless it is absolutely essential for maintaining an accurate record of fluid balance, urinary catheterization should be avoided to prevent the development of urinary tract infection. Wherever possible measures should be taken to increase bladder tone. For example, regular panning of female patients and regular offering of a urinal plus support to stand for the male, should assist in the return to continence. Additionally, taking the patient to the toilet, regulating fluid intake, and using condom drainage with males will assist in continence training. In the majority of cases the patient will regain independent control of micturition.

If the patient is incontinent of faeces, steps should be taken to help bring this under control by increasing dietary fibre and bulk, maintaining an adequate intake of fluids, allowing the patient to use a commode or toilet to heighten his sense of control, and where necessary treating diarrhoea or constipation.

Ensure effective alternative methods of communication. As soon as possible the patient is referred to a speech pathologist so that the speech deficit can be identified and measures instituted early to effect return of optimal speech. Between sessions with the speech pathologist, the patient will be reliant upon the nurse to continue with speech therapy exercises so that learning can be continued. Whilst the patient is relearning basic speech patterns, communication tools such as flip charts, alphabet boards, cue cards, and the use of closed-ended questions may facilitate in minimizing communication difficulties and frustration in the patient. Exercises of the facial muscles will not only assist in the return of locomotion of speech but will also help in the return to normal swallowing and control of salivation.

Maintain emotional support and ensure that expectations are realistic. Initially, the patient will be either indifferent to his condition or will be extremely angry, frustrated, or frightened. Frustration leading to depression commonly arises due to his lack of independence and/or his inability to make himself understood (naming and/or motor aphasia). Being unable to chew and swallow food results in the lowering of self-concept at each meal, due to constant dribbling, coughing, and spilling of food. It is during these frustrating times that the patient is tempted to give up and will therefore require maximum understanding and reassurance from the nurse and his significant others. Any forms of stress should be avoided in the initial phase and positive reinforcement should be used at all times and praise given for any achievement, no matter how slight. It is important for the nurse to constantly observe the patient's mental status for any early signs of depression and/or anxiety and to report these immediately.

Care must be taken to ensure that the frustration and/or depression being felt by the patient's significant others, and members of the health team, does not compound that which is being felt by the patient. The patient's significant others must be involved in as much of the rehabilitation programme as possible and be encouraged to accompany the patient to his therapy sessions, providing that this is not to the detriment of the patient's progress in that they take over functions

in which the patient should be becoming self sufficient.

Rehabilitation and habilitation

Once the physical effects of the CVA have been identified, nursing and other health team measures are aimed at restoring maximal function in the patient and preventing any complications of the CVA. All measures are geared towards maintaining the patient's ideal body weight and nutrition, and his being able to function independently at his optimum level. Therefore the nursing care as outlined above is continued until the patient's discharge, and assistance with activities of daily living is continued if necessary after the patient returns home or is discharged to a rehabilitation facility.

Allied paramedical care

Prior to discharge the patient's total welfare must be considered and the expertise of other health team members must be enlisted. The social worker and the occupational therapist are of paramount importance in providing assistance in the areas of employment, life style, activities of daily living and domestic modifications. The physiotherapist will establish the physical programme for the patient and ensure that this is maintained through to discharge and in the post-acute care setting. The community health nurse will be involved in the provision of home visits, follow up care and organisation of community resources, for example, home help and Meals-on-Wheels.

Health education

In many instances the patient with readily identifiable risk factors does not present until such time as the CVA occurs. In other patients the risk factors are identified but not controlled adequately and CVA results. It is important to identify risk factors in all patients and to institute health education to minimize further occurrence of CVA. Measures may include; dietary advice to control obesity, hypercholesterolaemia, and/or diabetes mellitus; education regarding the need to continue established drug therapy and its known side and toxic effects; and advice regarding the need for regular physical examinations.

Anticipated outcome

Occurrence of further cerebrovascular accidents is not uncommon, although identification and control of risk factors may reduce this incidence; some patients may recover from their CVA and never experience a recurrence. Complications associated with a CVA are those related to immobility and spasticity (for example, pneumonia or contractures), and any cerebral injury resulting in permanent neurological deficit.

The outcome for the patient depends upon the severity and area of damage, and recovery may be complete or partial. If surgery has been performed, the patient may suffer a neurological deficit if an ischaemic episode or cerebral oedema occurred in the postoperative phase.

The resultant lifestyle varies with individuals, and the patient and his significant others may need to make many adjustments to his altered state. The ultimate aim is that the patient can achieve maximum independence within the limit of his disabilities.

18

The epilepsies

Chris Game   Jenny Kidd

'Seizure' is the term used to describe a diverse group of behavioural and muscular changes which occur in response to abnormal electrical activity in the cerebrum. These may be abrupt in onset, of varying duration, preceded by an 'aura', and mild or severe in nature. A seizure may render the patient unconscious. Seizures are described, and present clinically, as being generalized, partial (focal) and unilateral or bilateral. The term 'epilepsy', or more correctly 'the epilepsies', is used to describe those neurological conditions of which recurrent seizures are a manifestation.

Epilepsy has been recognized historically and descriptions of this disorder can be found in the Bible and in the writings of early Greek physicians such as Hippocrates.

Pathophysiology and incidence

Epileptic seizures are due to episodes of abnormal or excessive paroxysmal electrical discharge occurring in the cerebrum. This activity may be confined to a specific area or may spread in a generalized manner. Seizure manifestations vary and may present as alterations in motor, sensory, or autonomic functioning or behaviour, with or without loss of consciousness. Alteration to motor function may present as tonic or clonic muscular activity. Tonus describes a state of continuous muscle contraction without a refractory stage; clonus describes a series of intermittent muscle contractions and relaxations which are usually rhythmic in nature.

Presentation depends on the area of the brain in which the electrical discharge originates. In generalized seizures the electrical activity spreads throughout the cortex bilaterally, while focal activity is localized in one or both cerebral hemispheres.

Epilepsy affects approximately 1 in 200 persons and the majority of seizures begin before 20 years of age. The role heredity plays is not completely clear, however there is some evidence that a predisposition to epilepsy may be transmitted in the form of a tendency to cerebral dysrhythmia. The likelihood of a familial tendency is greater if the condition manifests itself in early childhood.

The epilepsies are classified as primary or secondary. Primary, or idiopathic, epilepsy occurs in approximately 80% of cases; no organic cause for the seizures is identified but they are thought to be due to a biochemical imbalance. Primary epilepsy usually manifests during the first two decades of life, often in response to an identifiable external trigger factor.

Secondary epilepsies occur due to any of 4 factors:

1. Pathologic disorders. For example, brain abscess, tumour, haematoma, cerebral oedema, vascular malformation, or neuronal hypoxia
2. Metabolic disorders. For example, electrolyte imbalance, uraemia, or advanced hepatic failure
3. Ingestion of toxic substances. For example, alcohol, lead, or drugs.
4. Fever. For example, febrile convulsions or uncontrolled hyperthermia following severe head injury.

Seizures that develop during the first 6 months of life are usually due to birth injury, infection, or fever. Onset of epilepsy after the first 2 decades should be investigated for secondary causes.

Clinical manifestations

Epileptic seizures are broadly divided into generalized and partial seizures, which can be distinguished by their clinical and electroencephalographic (EEG) manifestations.

Generalized seizures begin bilaterally without any local onset and have diffuse EEG abnormalities; they may be grand mal, petit mal, or minor motor seizures.

Partial seizures, also known as focal epilepsy, are confined to one (unilateral) area of the cortex and therefore show localized changes on an EEG. Partial seizures constitute approximately 60% of all cases of epilepsy and they may present as motor or sensory manifestations, or a combination of both.

Generalized seizures

Grand mal (generalized tonic–clonic seizures). These are characterized by a sudden loss of consciousness, with or without an aura, associated with tonic and clonic motor activity. If an aura precedes the seizure it is usually of a sensory nature and is peculiar to the individual, for example, identifiable smells, noises, or changes in light. Initially there is stiffening of the body, the person falls to the floor (if standing or sitting prior to onset), and a cry may be heard as muscular contraction forces air through the glottis. Ventilation ceases temporarily and cyanosis usually occurs. The jaw is firmly shut, hands are clenched into fists, and the eyes may be wide open with fixed and dilated pupils. This tonic phase may last 30–60 seconds.

The clonic phase involves generalized jerky and rhythmic contractions of all limbs accompanied by noisy, shallow ventilation and frothing at the mouth due to an increased amount of saliva being produced and blown out. The person may bite the sides of his tongue, his lips, or the inside of his mouth. Urinary and/or faecal incontinence may also occur due to loss of sphincter control. This phase may last up to 3 minutes and no attempt should be made to restrain the person as such measures will usually intensify the clonic contractions.

On cessation of the clonic phase, muscular relaxation and the return of normal ventilation occurs. The person is usually unresponsive for a short time and then may rouse briefly and lapse into a postictal (post seizure) sleep which may last from seconds to hours. A period of confusion may exist on wakening and the person may complain of headache and generalized muscle soreness. It is not unusual for the epileptic to have complete amnesia of the period preceding, during, and immediately after the seizure. Physical recovery is normally complete; however, because the person cannot protect himself during the seizure, he may show evidence of injuries on wakening. The period of hypoxia may, however, produce minor neurological damage which can have a cumulative effect after years of seizures.

This sequence of events is to be expected in any person experiencing a grand mal seizure and apart from ensuring the safety of the person and observing the events that take place, there is nothing that the nurse can do to prevent or stop the seizure episode and the respiratory embarrassment, or to relieve the cyanosis. Grand mal seizures vary in their frequency with each individual and may be as rare as 1 or 2 a year, or as common as a number per day. EEG manifestations will be found only during a seizure.

Status epilepticus. This is the occurrence of serial, generalized, tonic–clonic seizures without consciousness being regained between seizure activity. This condition has a high mortality due to extreme exhaustion, cerebral anoxia, or cardiorespiratory failure. Its usual cause is the sudden withdrawal of established anticonvulsant drug therapy, often due to patient noncompliance.

Petit mal (absence). These seizures have their onset during childhood and may continue into early adolescence. Petit mal seizures diminish or disappear after puberty but the person may be susceptible to grand mal or focal seizures later in life. This type of seizure classically presents as a period of 'absence' with cessation of activity accompanied by blinking of the eyes, a fixed gaze, and sometimes slight mouth movements. This may last from 5–30 seconds; the person will retain his posture and after the episode resume pre-seizure activity, often being unaware of the event.

Characteristic EEG changes are found on examination.

This type of epilepsy usually becomes less frequent as the child grows and many children are not diagnosed until they are at school, when repeated seizures interrupt attention spans and lead to learning difficulties. If this disorder is unrecognized or untreated up to 100 episodes may occur over a 24-hour period.

Minor motor seizures. Minor motor seizures are generalized seizures that may be myoclonic, akinetic, or atonic in manifestation. Myoclonic epilepsy is characterized by brief, involuntary muscular contractions of the body or extremities which may occur in a random fashion. There is no loss of consciousness but contractions may be of sufficient intensity to throw the person to the floor. This type of epilepsy usually commences within the first 2 years of life.

Akinetic seizures are manifested by the momentary loss of all muscle movement. Atonic seizures are characterized by loss of muscle tone resulting in the person falling to the ground.

Partial seizures

Partial or focal epilepsy is characterized by electrical activity originating in an area of the cortex and remaining localized to that cerebral hemisphere. Manifestations correspond to the location of the focus and are motor, sensory, or psychomotor in presentation; there may even be a combination of these manifestations (complex partial seizures). It is common for partial seizures to be preceded by an aura, and if so a description of the aura may assist in the diagnosis of the affected area of the cortex. Partial seizures are indicative of focal brain dysfunction and should be investigated to rule out a cerebral lesion.

Jacksonian seizure occurs when electrical activity spreads from the focus to other areas of the cortex, and thus involves other muscles. A Jacksonian seizure typically presents with a stiffening or jerking in one extremity, for example, the seizure may begin in the thumb and spread to involve the hand and entire arm. In some cases a Jacksonian seizure can progress to a grand mal seizure.

Psychomotor seizures (temporal lobe epilepsy) are characterized by changes in awareness, distortions of memory, or affective and cognitive dysfunction, accompanied by automatic nonpurposeful motor activity. This may take the form of continuous chewing movements, lip smacking, undressing, or episodes of violent behaviour. Communication with the person during the seizure reveals that he is out of contact with reality, but cessation of the seizure restores normal physical and mental activity.

Investigative procedures

The overt presentation of a seizure is clinically obvious and is either witnessed by, or described to, the physician. Confirmatory diagnosis is made by:

- Supporting past history. Antenatal, birth and developmental information along with family history, age at seizure onset and a description of the seizure, and details of all past illness and trauma must be included. Any known precipitating factors or postictal symptoms should also be identified.
- Physical examination with emphasis on a complete neurological examination to exclude any organic lesions, and blood analysis to exclude electrolyte or metabolic imbalance.
- Skull X-ray and CT brain scan. These may identify any structural abnormality or degenerative disease.
- EEG. This may demonstrate the presence of abnormal electrical activity.
- Lumbar puncture, cerebral angiography, or pneumoencephalography. These may be performed to exclude secondary causes.

Medical, surgical, and nursing management

The aim of management is to reduce the number and severity of seizures, and this is usually accomplished by the prescription of anticonvulsant drug therapy or surgical intervention. The aims of nursing management of the hospitalized patient are to care for the person during any seizure episode; to educate him regarding his drug therapy and measures that he, and his significant others, can institute to minimize trauma during any future seizures; and to assist the person and his significant others in their psychological adjustment to this condition.

Related pharmacology

Anticonvulsant drugs act by either depressing the cerebral cortex and reticular system, or by inhibiting the spread of seizure discharge through the cortex. Seizures may be controlled by the administration of one or more anticonvulsant. Therapeutic drug level is said to have been achieved when the person, receiving the lowest dose possible of the drug, is experiencing few, if any, seizures. Once the person is established on a drug regime, it is necessary to ensure that he receives regular follow up, including the monitoring of serum drug levels, to prevent toxic side effects.

Phenytoin is the most widely used drug for all types of epilepsy except petit mal seizures (which are commonly treated with succinamides, for example ethosuximide). Carbamazepine may also be used as first line management in the treatment of grand mal epilepsy, or may be given in combination with other drugs for people who have previously been resistant to treatment. Benzodiazepines, for example diazepam and clonazepam, are particularly useful in controlling status epilepticus. Sodium valproate is effective in controlling most seizures but there have been reports of severe liver damage, particularly in children; the Australian Drug Evaluation Committee (ADEC) strongly recommends that alternative drug therapy should be utilized. Barbiturates, for example phemitone and primidone, may be used for treating major seizures and for febrile convulsions, where sedation is a desired outcome. Anticonvulsant therapy should never be withdrawn suddenly, as status epilepticus may result.

Side-effects of drug therapy. Most side-effects are mild but overdosage may lead to unpleasant effects. Drowsiness is one of the most common effects of anticonvulsants and may occur at the start of therapy and resolve within a week or so. If the seizures cannot be controlled without using doses producing drowsiness then alternative medication may be prescribed.

Ataxia, diplopia, and nystagmus occur with high levels of phenytoin and there is a possibility of bone marrow depression. Excessive hair growth and gingival hyperplasia are also associated with phenytoin use, and skin rashes may occur with any of the anticonvulsant medications.

Gastrointestinal disturbances can be minimized by taking phenytoin with food, and stringent oral hygiene and dental care assist in minimizing gingival hyperplasia. Liver function tests are performed to monitor the effects of sodium valproate.

Anticonvulsant medications increase the metabolism of oral contraceptive agents thus making them less effective. Women prescribed anticonvulsants should consult their physician when contemplating pregnancy as fetal hydantoin syndrome can occur.

Surgical management

Surgical intervention for epilepsy, usually cortical resection, is carried out if the patient has a demonstrable epileptic focus involving an area of the cerebrum that if excised, will not produce neurological deficit; or if seizure activity is not controlled by drug therapy and is interfering with the person's normal daily living. In order to establish the validity of such surgical intervention, a preoperative evaluation consisting of a thorough medical, neurological, and psychological profile must be obtained to isolate the focus. Continuous complex EEG or telemetry is performed. Approximately 5% of all persons with epilepsy may appear to be candidates for cortical resection but the intensive preoperative evaluation procedure decreases this figure. It is frequently the case that resection would involve such a wide area of the cortex that severe dysfunction would result, or that the focus cannot be isolated.

Surgical intervention will normally take place if the causative factor is a cerebral space-occupying lesion such as a cerebral abscess or tumour.

Nursing management during a seizure episode

The primary objectives are to protect the patient from injury and observe the seizure pattern. If an 'aura' gives warning of an impending seizure, the person should be laid flat, and if time permits a small padded object should be placed between his teeth. This will allow access to the oropharynx and enable the insertion of an oral airway and the commencement of oropharyngeal aspiration. Tight clothing should be loosened and if possible something soft (such as a jacket or pillow) placed under the person's head. Any objects likely to cause injury to the person should be either moved or padded. Unless the patient is in immediate danger no attempt should be made to restrain his movements or to move him, as these will accentuate the seizure episode.

Due to both the sudden onset of the tonic phase and the degree of muscle spasm of the jaw, it is often impossible to insert an object such as a padded spoon, or to remove dentures. To attempt this forcibly will cause trauma to the person's teeth and gums. At no stage should the nurse use his/her fingers in an attempt to keep the jaws apart; to do so could result in traumatic amputation of the nurse's fingers.

The nurse should record any specific events and/or behaviour that occured prior to the onset, of the seizure and once the tonic phase has begun note the time of onset, the extent of cyanosis, the duration of ineffective ventilation and fixed and dilated pupils, and the location of any muscle contraction or twitching.

Once the clonic phase begins the nurse should again note the time of onset and its subsequent duration, the location and extent of the jerky movements, the quality of ventilation, and whether any incontinence occurred. During this phase oropharyngeal aspiration will usually be required to remove excess saliva and maintain a patent airway should vomiting occur. An oral airway can be inserted if required.

Following the seizure the nurse should attend to the patient's hygiene needs, place him in a position of comfort and safety, provide reassurance that the seizure has ended, and allow him to sleep. A clear and concise record must be made of the seizure and its events and should include a note of the return of normal mental function. If the patient is having a number of seizures, precautions such as use of padded bed rails, provision of an oral airway at the bedside, and supervision with some activities, may be indicated.

Status epilepticus. The priorities of care are to: bring about the cessation of seizure activity; establish and maintain a patent airway; provide adequate hydration and energy replacement; and to ensure patient safety.

Usually the patient is intubated during one of the clonic phases and oxygen therapy is commenced. If intubation is not possible then oxygen is administered via a nasal catheter. Due to the nature and duration of the seizure activity exhaustion and dehydration could rapidly ensue; therefore an attempt is made to insert an intravenous line to provide fluids and energy replacement and a route for drug administration.

Intravenous sedation will be prescribed in an attempt to depress the excessive cortical activity and the drug of choice is diazepam; phenytoin administered IV will be necessary to prevent recurrence of the seizures. Nursing care to ensure patient safety is as for any patient experiencing a seizure.

Health education

Education is of primary importance in the care of an epileptic in order to assist him and his significant others to understand the dysfunction and to deal with any lifestyle alterations. They must understand the disorder and the medication used in its control, and that compliance with drug therapy is mandatory in order to prevent further seizures.

The patient should be reassurred that there are very few major alterations required to lifestyle provided that the seizures are well controlled. However, the patient must be aware of: the need to balance rest and activity; the need to avoid excessive stress or fatigue; the importance of having someone to accompany him when swimming or driving; the importance of maintaining good oral hygiene if on phenytoin; and the necessity to carry identification and a health warning such as 'Medi Alert'.

The patient should be cautioned regarding the potential dangers of swimming in cold water, which may stimulate a seizure; climbing ladders, which, if it results in vertigo, may also stimulate a seizure; and strobe and/or flickering lighting experienced by driving on a road with reflected sunlight shining through the trees.

The patient and his significant others must thoroughly understand the extreme dangers of the ingestion of alcohol and the withdrawal from anticonvulsant drug therapy.

If an aura is identified for the person, education is directed towards having him place himself in a position of safety as soon as he experiences the aura. The seizure cannot be stopped but aura identification will decrease the likelihood that the person will suffer injury during the episode.

Its unpredictability, and the frightening features of a frank seizure have generated unwarranted societal attitudes towards epilepsy and epileptics. Thus the person's adjustment to and acceptance of his own condition may be hindered by the stigma that accompanies this condition. Fortunately, there are epilepsy support groups which can assist the epileptic and his significant others with any problems they may experience.

Allied paramedical care

The social worker or rehabilitation counsellor can give advice and assistance with any social and occupational problems.

Psychotherapeutic measures, for example biofeedback and relaxation techniques, may be of value if stress or emotional triggers are identified.

Complications

Complications are not common but when they do occur result from the seizures themselves and/or from the related drug therapy. Seizure related complications include status epilepticus, hypoxic brain damage, respiratory arrest, inhalational pneumonia, and physical injury.

Anticipated outcome

Persons with epilepsy should be able to live normal lives as long as their seizures are well controlled and they remain compliant with their medication regime.

19

Oncological disorders of the nervous system

Jenny Kidd

There is a great variety of nervous system neoplasia arising from cells of the brain or of the spinal cord (see page 165), or from neural structures outside the central nervous system. They may be primary or secondary. Tumours arising in neural structures outside the CNS are generally either benign or occur as metastases from tumours in adjacent tissues (for example, malignant melanoma) and are therefore treated along with the primary neoplasm. In the cranium they compete for space with the brain; they are therefore termed space-occupying lesions.

Intracranial tumours are primarily benign or malignant neoplasms of the cerebrum. Intracranial tumours account for 10% of all human malignant neoplasms and generally affect both sexes equally. The cause of these tumours is not well understood as there is no convincing evidence that viruses, trauma, or chemical carcinogens play a significant role in the pathogenesis of primary intracranial neoplasia.

Pathophysiology and incidence

Tumours may occur at any age, with childhood and the fifth decade being periods of peak incidence. The severity of a tumour depends upon its type, growth pattern and effect on neural structures.

Primary tumours arise from cells of neural tissues whereas secondary or metastatic tumours originate from structures outside the nervous system.

Subtentorial tumours are more common in children, whereas in adults most tumours occur above the tentorium.

CNS tumours may be classified as:

1. Glioma. The most common are: astrocytoma, medulloblastoma, and glioblastoma multiforme. Less common forms include oligodendroglioma, ependymoma, neuroblastoma, ganglioglioma, and gangliocytoma
2. Meningioma
3. Blood vessel tumours
4. Schwannoma
5. Tumours related to the hypophysis and third ventricle
6. Intraspinal tumours
7. Tumours of infective origin
8. Metastatic tumours
9. Neurofibroma.

Gliomas

Gliomas constitute 40–45% of all intracranial neoplasia. These tumours arise from giant glial cells, are invasive and are extremely difficult to completely remove at surgery.

Astrocytoma. A tumour involving the astrocytes is relatively benign, slow growing and occurs in the white matter of one of the cerebral hemispheres. This tumour occurs at any age and is prone to cystic formation.

Medulloblastoma. This rapidly growing tumour is most frequently found in the cerebellum of children, occurring in the fourth ventricle. It is rarely seen in adults. The tumour is composed of masses of round undifferentiated cells which disseminate into the subarachnoid space surrounding the brain and spinal cord. It is one of the more malignant gliomas and, following surgical removal and radiotherapy, 40% of patients can expect a five year survival rate and 35% a ten year survival rate.

Glioblastoma multiforme. This highly vascular tumour appears in the middle decades of life and is an extremely malignant glioma. It occurs in the cerebral hemispheres, and infiltrates the brain, involving undifferentiated round or oval cells. The survival rate is approximately 12 months.

Oligodendroglioma. This is a rare, slow growing tumour occurring in the cerebral hemispheres of young adults. It is relatively benign and shows a tendency to calcify. A rarer, more malignant form is the oligodendroblastoma.

Ependymoma. Such tumours are derived from the cells of the lining of the ventricular system and most commonly arise from the floor of the fourth ventricle. They present in children and young adults.

Neuroblastoma, ganglioglioma, and gangliocytoma. These tumours are rare and principally contain ganglion cells.

Meningioma

This is an extracerebral tumour arising from the arachnoid cells of the arachnoid villi. It occurs mainly in the areas of the dural venous sinuses, the parasagittal area, the splenoid ridge, and anterior fossa. Posterior fossa meningiomas originate near the tentorium. A meningioma tends to invade overlying bone due to its close relationship to the skull. It is slow growing and usually benign, and occurs more commonly in women than in men.

Blood vessel tumours

The two principal blood vessel tumours are the angioblastoma and the angioma.

Angioblastoma is composed of angioblasts and forms cysts in the surrounding nerve tissue. It chiefly involves the cerebellum. Angioma is a congenital abnormality involving capillary, venous or arteriovenous malformations, occurring in the region of the middle cerebral artery. The tumour consists of large masses of tortuous vessels.

Schwannoma

These tumours are derived from Schwann cells, are usually unilateral and may be intracranial, intraspinal or peripheral. Intracranial sites include the auditory nerve (acoustic neuroma) and the trigeminal nerve, the first symptoms being those of VIIIth or Vth cranial nerve dysfunction. When Schwannoma occur bilaterally they are usually of peripheral nerves and are often associated with neurofibromatosis (von Recklinghausen's disease).

Tumours related to the hypophysis and third ventricle

Most tumours arising from the hypophysis itself are adenomas. The most common of these is the chromophobe adenoma. If it occurs prior to puberty it causes gigantism and after puberty, acromegally (see page 235).

Intraspinal tumours

Primary: these may be either extramedullary or intramedullary. Secondary: these are metastatic tumours which may also involve the vertebrae, meninges, and spinal cord.

Tumours of infective origin

The most common space-occupying lesion of infective origin is a tuberculoma. Others include abscesses (see page 221) and parasitic cysts.

Metastatic tumours

Secondary cerebral tumours grow rapidly and usually arise from carcinoma of the lung, breast, stomach, thyroid, kidney, and prostate. Approximately 1 in 5 cerebral neoplasms are metastatic in origin.

Neurofibroma

Benign tumours may arise in peripheral nerves and a group of nerves or a nerve plexus may be involved. The sciatic nerve is a common site. Neurofibromatosis is manifested by the appearance of hundreds of varying sized nodules along branches of nerves. They are most commonly found on the skin but can occur on nerve branches of the viscera. Because of their diffuse nature they are usually not amenable to treatment.

INTRACRANIAL TUMOURS

Clinical manifestations

An intracranial tumour will increase the mass effect of the brain, eventually giving rise to symptoms of increased intracranial pressure and tumours which embarrass cranial circulation result in oedema. Others cause the cerebrospinal fluid pressure to rise, and direct obstruction in either of the third or fourth ventricles will also cause a rise in intracranial pressure. Symptoms of raised intracranial pressure, however, may be slight or absent for long periods in the case of a slow growing tumour. The mode of onset of symptoms of a cerebral tumour is variable and depends upon the nature and site of the lesion. Symptoms are slower to occur in the astrocytomas, oligodendrogliomas, pituitary adenomas, and acoustic neuromas. Symptoms arise more rapidly with metastasis and glioblastomas.

The 4 most common patterns of onset are:

1. Progressive focal symptoms such as epilepsy, hemiplegia, paraesthesia, monoplegia, paralysis, and aphasia, coupled with symptoms of increased intracranial pressure. Local symptoms such as unilateral exophthalmos may accompany a retro-orbital meningioma
2. Symptoms of increased intracranial pressure alone
3. Focal symptoms alone
4. A long history of epilepsy preceding the onset of other symptoms by many years.

The manifestations of an intracranial tumour can be divided into those caused by the increase in pressure and those caused by the local effects of the lesion.

Increased intracranial pressure

The clinical effects of raised intracranial pressure (ICP) due to tumour growth are similar to those

seen in trauma (see page 161). However, the symptoms and signs will occur more slowly and over a greater period of time, due to the nature of tumour growth. Thus, some manifestations of depressed brain stem activity seen in the oncology patient are seldom, if ever, witnessed in the acute head injured patient.

The classic triad of symptoms of raised ICP in the patient with an intracranial tumour are headache, papilloedema, and vomiting. However they do not all necessarily occur together and usually appear prior to the onset of any local symptoms.

Headache. The headache is mainly due to compression and/or distortion of the dura and blood vessels.

The pain is described as a bursting, throbbing pain and initially is paroxysmal in nature. The patient usually wakes with the headache which may last minutes to hours before subsiding. It is exacerbated by stooping, lying on one side, exertion, coitus, straining at stool, coughing, sneezing, and vomiting, and may be relieved by sitting upright. As the tumour enlarges, the headache increases in severity and becomes constant.

Headache, due to its diffuse nature, is not of benefit in localizing the site of the tumour. Pain, however, may be unilateral with associated tenderness of the skull.

Papilloedema. This usually develops in tumours of the cerebellum, temporal lobes, and fourth ventricle, and is often more severe in extracerebral rather than intracerebral lesions. It is most severe in tumours of the cerebellum. Papilloedema is not always associated with visual disturbances but in severe cases it is not uncommon for a patient to suffer transient episodes of unilateral or bilateral blurring of vision or blindness.

Vomiting. This usually occurs in the early morning in association with a severe headache.

Most patients with increased ICP due to a space occupying lesion complain of dizziness and unsteadiness. However, true vertigo is rare even in patients with an acoustic neuroma. Other manifestations of raised ICP include:

Pulse rate and blood pressure alterations. An acute or subacute rise in ICP causes a slowing of the pulse rate to between 40–50 beats per minute. The pulse may be regular or irregular. If the pressure is not relieved, the rate will alter to become extremely rapid. A slow onset of raised ICP does not cause a bradycardia. A rapid onset due to haemorrhage will result in an increase in blood pressure occurring simultaneously with the reduction in pulse rate (see page 162).

Ventilation rate disturbances. A rapid rise in ICP in association with unconsciousness results in slow, deep, snoring ventilation known as stertorous ventilation. This may become Cheyne-Stokes in type, and in the terminal stages becomes rapid and shallow. These alterations in ventilation are due to compression or distortion, or from haemorrhage or infarction of the medulla oblongata. The latter usually results from tentorial herniation and causes irreversible coma.

Hypopituitarism. Chronic increased ICP in association with hydrocephalus may produce symptoms of hypopituitarism. This is due to the downward pressure on the hypothalamic nuclei in the floor of the enlarged third ventricle, or compression of the pituitary gland itself. It is most often seen in children with tumours of the cerebellum.

Mental symptoms. These are many and varied. A rapid rise in ICP leads to confusion prior to the onset of coma. Chronic raised ICP may cause dementia, a reduction in intellect, apathy, impairment of memory, irritability, and an inability to concentrate.

Local effects

Local effects will depend on the type, size, and site of the tumour, for example:

- Visual field defects – pituitary tumours
- Ataxia – posterior fossa tumours
- Deafness – acoustic neuroma
- Dysphasia – hemisphere lesion
- Personality disturbances – frontal lobe lesion
- Simple partial motor seizures – prefrontal gyrus lesion
- Motor and sensory deficits – extramedullary spinal cord tumour.

Epilepsy and somnolence are normally directly attributable to a tumour rather than to raised intracranial pressure. Epileptic seizures are usually due to the direct effect of the neoplasm on the surrounding brain tissue. 10% of patients who present with epilepsy over the age of 20 years are shown to have intracranial tumours. Approximately two-thirds of patients with slow-growing meningiomas or astrocytomas suffer seizures at some stage and these are more likely to occur when the tumour involves the cortex.

True narcolepsy is rare, but hypersomnia occurs with some tumours and severe hydrocephalus.

Investigative procedures

Examination of the patient's head may demonstrate:

- Generalized enlargement, in cases of hydrocephalus
- Separation of the sutures in young children
- Local tenderness of the skull over the tumour
- Dilated and tortuous scalp arteries, in particular the superficial temporal artery.
- Congested veins of the scalp.

An EEG may demonstrate the size of the tumour and any displacement of the ventricles. It may indicate a lesion in one of the cerebral hemispheres, but a negative result does not rule out the presence of a tumour.

CT scanning is the investigation of choice as it is the most effective method of imaging the brain. It is non-invasive, accurate in localizing neoplasms, and supplies information which in many cases enables conclusions to be made regarding the pathology of the lesion. The CT scan is more effective when combined with isotope scanning in emission tomography.

Magnetic resonance imaging (MRI) is likely to become more popular than CT scanning as it is more accurate in diagnosing some tumours and gives more information regarding the chemical changes in nervous tissue whilst producing images of lesions.

Lumbar puncture is best avoided in cases of raised intracranial pressure due to the risk of herniation ('coning') when the pressure is suddenly relieved. However it is useful in detecting malignant cells.

Full series skull X-ray, carotid and vertebral angiography, pneumoencephalography, and ventriculography may also be performed.

Medical and surgical management

Without intervention most cerebral tumours will continue to grow and produce increasing symptoms, and eventually result in death due to destruction of brain tissue and increasing intracranial pressure.

Improvements in neurosurgical and anaesthetic techniques have reduced the risk and improved the outcome of surgical procedures in many patients. The immediate mortality rate of patients undergoing surgical removal of a cerebral tumour is under 10%.

Removal of any cerebral tumour necessitates considerable cerebral trauma, with risk of permanent disability. Additional hazards are created by encroachment of the tumour on cranial nerves and major blood vessels.

Extracranial and extracerebral tumours can often be removed without damage to the underlying brain, but adjacent structures can still be damaged, for example the VIIth cranial nerve in the removal of an acoustic neuroma. The more malignant the tumour the greater the likelihood of its regrowth following removal.

In cases of obstructive hydrocephalus a shunt operation may give temporary relief of symptoms.

In cases where total removal of the intracranial tumour is surgically impossible, decompression or debulking can be performed by removal of some of the mass of the tumour. As well, craniectomy or craniotomy (see page 222), by interrupting the confines of the skull, will reduce intracranial pressure and papilloedema. In such cases steroids are given postoperatively to reduce cerebral oedema. Dexamethasone is the drug of choice. In some situations, following a significant reduction in cerebral oedema, surgery may be possible. Maintenance management with steroids improves the quality of life of the patient with terminal disease.

Radiotherapy combined with surgery and high dose steroid therapy can produce excellent results. Radiotherapy alone has produced encouraging results in cases of cerebral metastases and in some cases has proven curative. However radiotherapy can produce dysfunction in healthy neuronal cells and it should be remembered that the objective of radiotherapy is to improve the quality not just the quantity of the patient's life.

The same objective must also apply to the use of cytotoxic chemotherapeutic agents (see Chapter 13) which are administered systemically in the case of nervous system tumours. Such drugs include lomustine (CCNU) somustine (methyl CCNU) and carmustine (BCNU), and the latter combined with surgery and radiotherapy seems to produce the most successful results. Intrathecal methotrexate combined with radiotherapy is the treatment of choice in meningeal carcinomatosis and central nervous system leukaemia.

Nursing management

The nurse must remember that a diagnosis of brain tumour will instill fear in both the patient and his significant others and that they will have ahead of them many weeks or months of emotional strain as the patient undergoes treatment. Prognosis for the majority of brain tumour patients is poor, especially those with medulloblastomas or glioblastomas, and the uncertainty of success of any therapy available increases the emotional vulnerability of the patient and his significant others. Surgery and/or radiotherapy may result in alterations to the patient's self-image and his ability to relate with the health team or his significant others. The nurse will be required to provide support during the therapy period and to institute measures to assist in maintaining the patient's self-concept and emotional well-being.

The nurse must assess the presentation of the patient's headache and plan to maintain his comfort and to keep him pain free. Accurate assessment of the headache will enable the nurse to administer the ordered pain relief before the headache recurs. If the effects of the tumour prevent the patient reporting any pain the nurse must observe him for any irritability, restlessness or distress so that pain relief can be given and a pain free state maintained. Observe the patient for the effect of the analgesic and report any signs that the dosage or schedule is no longer controlling the pain. Also note the effect of any other measures to relieve pain, for example massage, quiet or dark environment.

Nursing measures should aim to prevent any further elevation of ICP. For example: elevate the head of the bed to assist in venous return, institute measures to prevent constipation and straining at stool, keep secretions moist and avoid suctioning wherever possible, and reduce the need for the patient to bend or assume a head low position.

Should seizures be a feature of the tumour presentation the nurse must ensure patient safety and education to prevent injury (see Chapter 18). Speech, motor, and sensory deficits may occur and nursing care must aim to promote effective communication, perception, and motor function (see page 177). Those patients undergoing surgery for removal of a tumour will require nursing management as for any patient undergoing a craniotomy (see page 222). Patients who are treated with radiotherapy and/or chemotherapy will require the specific nursing management of any

patient receiving this type of treatment (see Chapter 13).

Anticipated outcome

Some intracranial tumours can be removed completely with an excellent prognosis, providing that irreversible damage to nerve and other structures has not occurred. Others can be managed with a combination of surgery, steroid therapy, radiotherapy, and chemotherapy to provide improved prognosis and quality of life.

However, the majority of intracranial tumours will progress relentlessly and the patient will experience progressive cerebral degeneration. Death usually occurs within 18 months of diagnosis and is commonly the result of cerebral haemorrhage due to tumour invasion of a major vessel.

20

Disorders of movement

Jenny Kidd

Movement disorders occur as a result of dysfunction of the basal ganglia, a particular grouping of differentiated neurons appearing as an area of grey matter within each hemisphere below the level of the cortex. A motor nerve impulse, which will produce movement, originates in the motor area of the cortex and travels along efferent fibres to the target muscle. The basal ganglia is responsible for the fine regulation of the impulse as it passes through the subcortical layer of the cerebrum. Dysfunction of these groups of control neurons may result from trauma, infection, chemical toxins or, more commonly, for reasons unknown.

The basal ganglia comprise a variety of neuronal structures with each specialized area requiring a specific neurotransmitter to effect its form of control over movement. Deficiencies of these neurotransmitters or damage to these areas interfere with control of voluntary movement and are manifested by alterations in muscle tone, involuntary movements and abnormal posture.

PARKINSON'S DISEASE

Parkinson's disease (paralysis agitans) is a progressive neuromotor disease of the basal ganglia of unknown aetiology, especially effecting the substantia nigra and the corpus striatum. It is a relatively common disease of late middle life, occurring from the age of 50 years, with males being affected more often than females. There is little evidence that it is hereditary or familial. As Parkinson's disease occurs in later life, it has been suggested that it could be related to the pathology of the ageing process of neuronal cells.

Pathophysiology

The disease causes degeneration of neurons in the substantia nigra of the basal ganglia. The substantia nigra extends fibres to the corpus striatum at the base of the forebrain, and these fibres secrete dopamine, which is a neurotransmitter. It appears that the corpus striatum cannot carry out its task of initiating and controlling certain movements without a constant supply of dopamine from the substantia nigra. In Parkinson's disease there is an almost total loss of cells that produce dopamine, which cripples the corpus striatum.

Other disorders have Parkinsonian features but they are distinguishable from paralysis agitans. These include: encephalitis lethargica and arteriosclerotic Parkinsonism, carbon monoxide poisoning, pseudobulbar palsy, encephalitis, and high dosages of drugs such as antidepressants, reserpine, and phenothiazides, all of which deplete tissue of catecholamines. Catecholamines, for example adrenalin and noradrenaline, are chemicals resulting from the breakdown of dopamine.

Clinical manifestations

The triad of symptoms of Parkinson's disease is composed of tremor, rigidity, and dyskinesia. Early symptoms are usually subtle and often go unrecognized for a period of years. These include loss of agility, a general slowness, and a slight tremor; all of which could be attributable to the effects of normal ageing. Early diagnostic signs, often present for years, consist of lack of mobility of facial expression, infrequent blinking, and a general slowness, with a tendency to stay in the one position for long periods, hesitancy in rising from a chair to the upright position, and difficulty in sitting down. On questioning, a patient can usually recall at least one of these symptoms being present for many years prior to the onset of the clinical disease state.

Tremor may be the first presenting symptom and may precede rigidity by many months. The tremor is most pronounced in the hand, and finger movements combined with thumb movements create what is classically described as a 'pill-rolling tremor'. The tremor usually begins on one side, involving the hand and arm and later the leg. Spread to involve the other side may take months or years.

Tremor occurs at rest but can become markedly worse when the patient performs a task such as writing or eating; tremor is also increased by emotional excitement. In the early stages the tremor can be voluntarily controlled by conscious effort and disappears during sleep. In the lower limbs, the ankle is the most affected. When the head is involved it is a rotatory or flexion and extension tremor, and if the mandible is involved the patient opens and closes his mouth rhythmically.

Rigidity. Posture and mobility are principally affected and the patient takes small shuffling steps, leaning forward. He often finds difficulty in getting out of a chair and, prior to walking, marks time on the spot before taking a few shuffling steps. There is also lack of arm swing when walking. Initially, the rigidity may be in only one limb and only noticeable on passive flexion and extension of the wrist; eventually rigidity progresses to marked resistance to passive movement in all joints. The patient has a typical stoop with a flexed spine, the arms are moderately flexed at the elbows and adducted, and the thumbs are usually adducted and slightly extended (Fig. 20.1).

Dyskinesia. In general the smaller skeletal muscles are most greatly affected. There is weakness of the muscles of the eyes with characteristic tremor of the eyelids upon closure. There is also a loss of the blinking reflex, and reduced facial mobility specifically related to mastication, speaking, and swallowing; the latter leads to drooling of saliva.

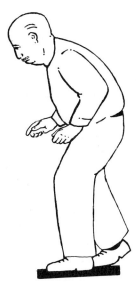

Fig. 20.1 Parkinson's disease.

Dyskinesia and bradykinesia are the most disabling features of Parkinson's disease and have a severely limiting effect on daily activities. A meal normally eaten in 15–20 minutes may take one hour or more to consume, and washing and dressing may take the best part of a morning. When walking, a patient may come to a standstill, being 'frozen' to the spot for varying lengths of time. His voice is monotonal and he develops a mask-like, staring, facial expression.

Other symptoms of Parkinson's disease, not yet fully explained physiologically, include: flushing of the skin together with marked diaphoresis and greasiness of the face. Parkinsonian patients prefer a cool environment which, combined with their immobility, makes them susceptible to hypothermia. In the late stages the patient may become restless and complain of pain in the arms, legs, and back due to rigidity and altered posture.

Diagnosis

Diagnosis of Parkinson's disease is primarily based on the patient's history and clinical signs and should be distinguished from other diseases which cause the Parkinsonian syndrome, the classical features of which are tremor and rigidity.

Other causes of tremor which must be excluded are senility, hyperthyroidism, multiple sclerosis, hysteria, and drug or toxin withdrawal. Other causes of rigidity include rheumatoid arthritis, hysteria, and lesions of the corticospinal tract.

Medical and surgical management

There is no cure for Parkinson's disease, however the patient can lead a normal life when the symptoms are well controlled on a satisfactory drug regime.

Levodopa is the drug of choice as it significantly increases cerebral dopamine. It is rarely given alone but is combined with a decarboxylase inhibitor (for example carbidopa) which makes the dopamine more readily available to nerve cells of the brain. Combination therapy significantly reduces the side effects of involuntary movement.

Bromocriptine is also used as a dopamine antagonist which allows the production of endogenous dopamine. Doses are given alone or in combination with levodopa and carbidopa or benserazide. In general bromocriptine is reserved for the patient who responds poorly to the levodopa combined therapies.

Surgery involves exposing the thalamus via a craniotomy to achieve destruction of part of the thalamus using chemical agents (chemopallidectomy), or freezing as in a cryothalamectomy. Since the introduction of levodopa, surgery is now only indicated in the minority of patients who have severe tremor which is poorly controlled by drug therapy.

Nursing management

Nursing care must be planned on an individual basis as each patient will have varying degrees of problems and his own specific needs.

Aims of care are to:

1. Assist in reduction of muscle spasticity, incoordination and tremor. Warm baths or showers, maintenance of passive and active exercise programmes and correct positioning of the patient will assist in overcoming these problems. The nurse is responsible for administering the ordered drug therapy and monitoring for desired/undesired effects (see above).
2. Ensure adequate nutritional status. If there is pronounced muscle rigidity the patient may have difficulty in maintaining an adequate nutritional intake due to slowness in chewing and social embarrassment. A well balanced diet is essential, and heated plates to keep food from cooling, and food of a consistency that the patient can manage will assist him in maintaining an adequate intake. Often patients require assistance with meal preparation and eating.
3. Prevent constipation, which may occur due to weakness of trunk muscles and anticholinergic drug therapy. Adequate fluids and dietary fibre are given; and faecal softeners as necessary.
4. Prevent skin irritation, which may occur if drooling is present. Cleanliness of the chin and use of a protective skin cream will help prevent excessive irritation and excoriation.
5. Promote independence. Encourage the patient to achieve maximum self-care. Assist the patient with activities of daily living as necessary. It is helpful if patients can wear clothing which has few buttons and zips, and can wear slip-on type shoes. This avoids unnecessary frustration and fumbling.
6. Minimize social isolation. Encourage socialization, and explain the need for the patient to socialize to his significant others, as mental activity helps slow the course of the disorder. They should spend time with the patient encouraging him to verbalize his feelings and thus maintain social interaction. The nurse must also ensure that plenty of time is set aside for the patient to perform his assisted activities of daily living and this time should also be used to maintain his ability to interact at a social level. Positive reinforcement will often be necessary to encourage the patient to interact in a social setting.
7. Provide health education. The patient and his significant others should understand the disorder and the importance of chemotherapy and exercise programmes in alleviating its manifestations. They should be taught: the need for a balanced rest and exercise regime; to observe for undesired effects of chemotherapeutic agents; that it is necessary to avoid stress and temperature extremes which exacerbate symptoms; to recognize that depression may occur in response to the manifestations of the disorder; the importance of adequate dietary and fluid intake; and the safety factors related to problems of gait. The importance of maintaining a healthy life style, as near to 'normal' as the disorder allows, should be stressed.

Persons who are close to the patient need a complete understanding of the progressive nature of this disease. It is inevitable that the patient will become bedridden and require institutionalized care. An understanding of the eventual social and physical circumstances can assist significant others in helping the patient to make the adjustments that will eventually be necessary.

Allied paramedical care

The physiotherapist and occupational therapist play an important role in planning exercise programmes to maintain function and minimize gait and muscle rigidity, and muscle wasting problems. Patients with severe dyskinesia will often require the assistance of a walking stick or walking frame. Other aids such as chairs which can be mechanically or electrically elevated are also useful. The occupational therapist will assist in activities of daily living and speech pathology may improve voice volume and assist in the management of problems with eating.

Inherent problems associated with treatment

Most problems inherent in treatment are due to the unpleasant effects of drug therapy. Levodopa commonly causes anorexia, nausea and vomiting, which should decrease once the dosage is stabilized. These effects can be reduced by giving the drug with food, but antiemetics may be required.

Orthostatic hypotension may appear during the initial stages of chemotherapy; it can be reduced by teaching the patient to change position slowly, and the monitoring of lying and standing blood pressure, pulse rate and response to treatment is important. These effects are less when a levodopa-decarboxylase compound is prescribed.

Confusion, cardiac arrythmias, sleep disturbances, and drug exacerbated dyskinesia can also occur and are controlled by reduction of dosage. Anticholinergics are usually introduced slowly to minimize their effects such as dry mouth, blurred vision, constipation, and urinary retention.

Anticipated outcome

With a proper medication regime and supportive/assistive therapy, the patient's quality of life is improved. Progression of the disease is variable, with some patients having little or gradual progression and others rapid, marked deterioration.

Patients with well managed Parkinson's disease can live from 5–20 years following diagnosis. It is, however, a progressive disease and death usually results from problems relating to immobility, such as infective thromboembolism, malnutrition, or failure of a major body system. Respiratory infection exacerbated by the rigidity of the respiratory musculature is commonly seen as a cause of death.

MISCELLANEOUS MANIFESTATIONS OF MOVEMENT DISORDER

Tremors

- Dyskinetic tremor – a rhythmic involuntary oscillation
- Rest tremor – occurs at rest as in Parkinson's disease
- Postural tremor – occurs when the hands are held out palms down.
- Essential familial tremor – a benign hereditary tremor, aggravated by stress or fatigue. This tremor may be quite disabling and propranolol or primidone may be prescribed in an attempt at gaining control.
- Intention tremor – occurs when performing a voluntary action. Examples of this tremor are seen in multiple sclerosis, alcohol ingestion and following cerebrovascular accident.
- Tremor may also be due to excessive caffeine intake, and cerebellar disease.

Chorea

Chorea is a disease manifested by irregular and spasmodic muscular movement that is beyond the patient's control. Even voluntary movement by the patient becomes jerky and ungainly. Childhood chorea is known otherwise as rheumatic chorea or 'St Vitus' Dance'; adult chorea is the movement disorder that occurs most commonly in Huntington's disease and this form is known as 'Huntington's chorea' (see page 207).

Choreiform movements may also manifest in thyrotoxicosis, drug intoxication, for example with phenothiazines and levodopa, and may also be a manifestation of old age. Drug therapy which inhibits dopamine function may be of help in controlling chorea.

Other movement forms

• Ballism – violent involuntary flinging movements of a limb, commonly due to vascular lesions of the subthalmic area.
• Dystonia – slow involuntary torsion movement of a muscle group. It may be idiopathic or drug induced and can occur symptomatically following a hypoxic episode.
• Athetosis – slow, irregular, writhing movements, usually of the distal muscle groups. The cause of athetosis is usually the same as the causes of dystonia.
• Myoclonus – irregular jerking of muscle which occurs with epilepsy and metabolic disorders, such as renal and hepatic failure.

Drug induced movement disorders

Drug induced movement disorders occur due to the inhibition of dopamine when reserpine, phenothiazines, tetrabenazine or metoclopramide are prescribed. Movement disorders can appear within 4–5 days of commencing the drug or following a dosage increase. Parkinson's syndrome begins 2 weeks to 3 months after commencing therapy. Anticholinergic agents or diazepam may relieve the signs, but on withdrawal of the drug causing the movement disorder not all patients recover completely, and in this case anticholinergic agents need to be continued.

Tardive dyskinesias occur following long term (6 months or more) chemotherapy and are often a persistent problem. Lip smacking, chewing and grimacing actions are commonly seen, and the condition responds poorly to therapy. Treatment is by withdrawing or reducing the dosage of the causative drug. Dyskinesia due to levodopa can be reversed by reduction of the dosage.

21

Multiple sclerosis and the neuropathies

Chris Game

MULTIPLE SCLEROSIS

Multiple sclerosis (MS) is a primary demyelinating disease occurring in the white matter (myelin) of the central nervous system. It is a chronic degenerative disorder characterized by exacerbations and remissions. MS is a leading cause of chronic disablement in young adults.

Aetiology and pathophysiology

Demyelination results in patchy degeneration of the myelin within the central nervous system, with axonal sparing. Inflammation and oedema are initially present at the site of demyelination and tissue repair takes place with subsequent cellular proliferation occurring – this gives rise to scar tissue formation, or sclerosis. Because myelin increases the speed of nerve impulse conduction, demyelination results in disrupted motor and sensory nerve activity as nerve impulse transmission is slowed.

The demyelination process tends to have a predeliction for the optic nerve, brain stem, spinal cord and cerebrum. Peripheral nerves are not affected. Likewise nerve cell bodies are not affected and should muscle wasting occur, it is mostly due to muscle disuse rather than to neuronal damage. Effects tend to be diffuse due to the varied areas which may be affected by the demyelination process. There is a cumulative effect with subsequent episodes leading to repeated scarring and thus permanent damage. Remissions may vary in length from months to years; some persons only have one episode, others develop a progressive form of the disorder. Approximately 15% of those afflicted will have

slight disability and 15% severe disability, 10–15 years following onset.

There have been many theories as to the cause of MS but its aetiology is still unknown. Theories include an abnormality of lipid metabolism; an autoimmune response in which there is a defect in self-cell recognition (see Chapter 77); a deficiency of trace elements or minerals; a defect in enzyme production; and environmental hazards. However, the belief that MS is due to a slow-acting viral infection that may have been initially acquired during childhood and triggers an autoimmune response in later life, is currently supported by many researchers.

Incidence

MS is more common in women than in men by a ratio of 3 : 2, with the onset of clinical manifestations occurring between 20–40 years of age; 10% of these people will demonstrate a progressive course. The disorder is more common in northern, temperate climates such as North America and Europe (50–80 per 100 000). In southern temperate areas such as New Zealand and southern Australia there are approximately 20–27 cases per 100 000, these persons usually being of European descent and therefore indicating a genetic rather than a geographical theory of aetiology. The risk is further increased (12–20-fold) if a primary relative has the disorder which supports a familial tendency or genetic susceptibility.

Clinical manifestations

The symptoms that cause the patient to seek assistance depend upon the site and extent of the demyelination and episodes of myelin destruction. Early manifestations may be vague, transitory, and variable. At the onset of the disorder 80% of persons may be monosymptomatic; this increases the difficulty of a correct diagnosis.

Common presenting manifestations are unilateral or bilateral retrobulbar neuritis, and a history of eye pain with associated visual disturbance such as blurred vision is common. Improvement usually occurs over 2–3 weeks following onset of these symptoms.

Spinal cord involvement may manifest as sudden or gradual muscle weakness of one or more limbs with or without sensory disturbances; the patient may describe band-like sensations around the limbs. Urinary frequency or urgency may occur and the patient may also be troubled by impotence.

Brain stem involvement may manifest as vertigo, ataxia, tremor, or problems with coordination.

An intention tremor is a common early feature of MS; it occurs with voluntary movement and subsides when the person rests. Slurred speech is not uncommon but is usually only transitory in the early stages.

Late symptoms of MS include mood swings, euphoria or depression, irritability, intellectual deterioration, gait ataxia, severe dysarthria, and failing vision. Acute episodes of MS can be exacerbated by factors such as: physical and psychological stress; fatigue; poor nutrition; pregnancy; infections, especially of the urinary or upper respiratory tracts; and alterations in temperature.

Investigative procedures

There is no definitive diagnostic test for MS. A complete clinical history and neurological examination to differentiate the disorder from other conditions, such as sub-acute degeneration of the spinal cord, are necessary. A definitive diagnosis of MS is usually not possible until the characteristic pattern of remission and exacerbation is exhibited. The following procedures are usually performed to confirm the initial diagnosis:

● Lumbar puncture. An elevated CSF IgG has been found to occur in 80–90% of persons with MS; there may also be an increase in CSF protein and leucocytes.

● Evoked potential responses. Measurement of visual, auditory, or somatosensory evoked responses will demonstrate that there is disruption of nerve impulse transmission.

● CT scan. Plaques may be demonstrated at the sites of demyelination.

● Electroencephalogram. Nonspecific abnormal EEG readings occur in approximately 50% of all persons with MS.

Medical, surgical, and nursing management

Management is aimed at:

1. Relieving neurological deficits
2. Maintaining general physical and psychological health
3. Shortening exacerbations and minimizing long-term disability
4. Preventing complications.

Medical and surgical intervention is concerned with reducing the inflammatory process present during an exacerbation of the disorder and reducing symptomatic problems such as spasticity. Procedures such as cordotomy, rhizotomy or intrathecal injection of phenol may be indicated if spasticity or pain are a problem.

Anti-inflammatory drugs are usually prescribed during the acute attack. The use of steroids is controversial but as MS is thought to have allergic, autoimmune, or inflammatory causes, it is believed that steroid action reduces inflammation and oedema, reduces the length of exacerbation, and assists in the healing process. Parenteral adrenocorticotrophic hormone (ACTH), oral prednisolone, or dexamethazone are commonly prescribed.

If muscle spasticity is present, medication may be indicated to reduce disability, pain, and potential deformity. Baclofen has been found to be most effective although diazepam and dantrolene may be prescribed. The dosage levels of these drugs are gradually increased until the patient's maximum tolerance and response is reached, the aim being to avoid causing flaccidity which will be as disabling as the initial spasticity. Immunosuppressive therapy, for example cyclophosphamide, may be utilized as it is thought to reduce the length of an acute attack.

Various alternative dietary regimes have been advocated in MS and the theory behind such diets is based on individual beliefs or causative theories. The use of unsaturated fat in the diet, based on the belief that MS is due to abnormal lipid metabolism, is one such example. Other diets which have been advocated for patients with MS include those concentrating on: raw, gluten free, high magnesium, high vitamin, and allergen free food. Provided that the diet is not potentially harmful there is no need to dissuade the patient from following a regime he feels is helpful.

Nursing management depends largely upon the severity of the disease and whether the patient is being managed in an acute care facility or within the community. The major aims of nursing management for the MS patient are to provide maximum support and relief of symptoms.

It is important to demonstrate empathy and give the patient the emotional support he requires. The use of good communication techniques and allowing the patient to express himself is an important factor in enabling him to resolve his feelings; emotional lability can be a factor in many patients. Sexual counselling may be required, and it is important to assess the need for such counselling early in the presentation of the disorder.

The promotion of a healthy lifestyle is important and the patient should be educated in the correct balance of exercise and rest. He should also know the benefits of a balanced nutritional intake and how to prevent or reduce the effects of infection. The importance of avoiding temperature extremes or hot baths should be stressed as a rise in temperature of as little as 1°C has been found to disrupt a nerve impulse transmission and lead to an exacerbation of symptoms.

The distress of diplopia can be alleviated by the application of an eye-patch. Maintenance of skin integrity is of paramount importance in the patient with any form of paralysis (see page 179).

Bladder training programmes may need to be initiated to overcome neurological bladder problems. The nurse may also need to administer drugs as ordered, for example propantheline bromide to reduce bladder spasticity, and/or urinary antiseptics to prevent and treat urinary infection. Urinary catheterization should only be necessary if bladder training is unsuccessful and skin integrity is compromised. Constipation or diarrhoea may occur and the addition of bran in the diet and bowel training regimes may also be indicated. The incontinent patient will require advice as to the appliances available to both maintain skin integrity and prevent social embarrassment.

During the acute phase the patient will be required to rest. Passive and active exercises to prevent the complications of immobility should be continued during this phase. Nursing assistance with gait training, the use of supportive appliances, and the performance of exercise is required during the later phases.

As MS is a degenerative disorder that affects younger people, it is likely to frustrate the patient. The nurse must therefore be prepared to educate him, and his significant others, about the disease, its likely pattern of progress, and the measures that can be taken to minimize the effects of the symptoms.

For the patient who is to be managed in the community, an assessment should be made of his need for support services prior to his discharge from acute care. An inspection should be made of his house, so that arrangements may be made for the installation of equipment to increase his degree of independence and mobility, for example handrails, shower chairs, ramps. The patient and/or his significant others should also be encouraged to make contact with the Multiple Sclerosis Society which provides a wide range of support services.

Allied paramedical care

The patient with MS may require a variety of paramedical services. Physiotherapy needs will vary according to the individual's disease pattern. The aim of physiotherapy is to keep the person active without fatigue, and to give specific therapy if spasticity or gait problems are present. Swimming assists in maintaining muscle tone and range of movement. The physiotherapist also assists in the selection and teaching of the use of supportive appliances as required.

Optometrical services, speech therapy, social welfare, and occupational therapy may be required depending upon the individual needs of the patient.

Should bladder problems remain unresolved, the patient should be referred to an incontinence advisor and may need referral to a urologist so that the correct management approach can be determined.

Psychological counselling may be required if the patient and/or his significant others are finding difficulty in coming to terms with the disorder.

Inherent problems associated with treatment

The use of steroidal anti-inflammatory drugs can give rise to side-effects and the patient should be informed of these and urged to seek medical advice should they occur. If drugs are prescribed to reduce muscle spasticity it is important to balance the dosage so that the person does not lose useful movement due to muscle flaccidity.

Emphasis should also be placed on the importance of balanced rest and activity as attempts to maintain independence by exercising vigorously are counter productive and likely to result in exacerbation of the disease.

Complications

The incidence and effects of complications increase in relation to the progression of the disorder. Decubitus ulcers and contractures occur if immobility and spasticity are present and are poorly managed. Urinary and respiratory tract infections can develop, particularly in patients with a more progressive disease, and it is the effect of such infections that may place the patient at greater risk. Complications of immobility and systemic infection are more likely to have serious consequences than MS itself.

Anticipated outcome

Because MS is a disease with a variable pathology and presentation, the prognosis for patients is equally variable. The site and extent of the demyelination process will determine the degree and extent of any exacerbations and remissions. In nearly 70% of all cases patients lead a fairly active and productive life with minimal changes to their lifestyle. Prolonged remissions in these instances are common and life expectancy is fairly normal. In the remainder of patients the disorder is rapidly progressive and produces severe disablement in early adult life; death may even occur within months of onset of the disease.

NEUROPATHY/POLYNEUROPATHY

Neuropathy or polyneuropathy describes those pathological conditions of the peripheral nerves that are not due primarily to inflammation (neuritis and polyneuritis are covered in Chapter 24).

There are many presentations of peripheral neuropathy, however 3 major categories have been identified: primary degeneration of the nerve cell (parenchymatous neuropathy); Schwann cell dysfunction neuropathy; and vascular induced neuropathy. Acute, inflammatory polyneuropathy (Guillain-Barré Syndrome) is considered a true polyneuritis and is therefore discussed in Chapter 24. The nursing management of the patient with a neuropathy occurring as a manifestation of another disorder, for example as seen in herpes zoster, sarcoidosis, and leprosy is outlined elsewhere in the text, with the respective disorders.

Focal and multifocal neuropathy (mononeuropathy) is a neuropathy resulting in one peripheral nerve being affected. The most common cause is trauma. In some persons, a familial tendency to neuropathy development has been demonstrated, as in upper motor neuron disease.

Parenchymatous neuropathy

This disorder is manifested by the symmetrical degeneration of the nerve cell body and axon (distal axonopathy) resulting in damage and/or death of the cell body and axonal degeneration. If the attack is severe the nerve cell will die, resulting in severe motor and sensory impairment. Distal axonopathy in which the degeneration extends proximally ('dying-back' neuropathy) is the most common pathological process of the peripheral nervous system. The axonal degeneration is slow, as is the often incomplete regeneration.

The most common cause of parenchymatous neuropathy is a nutritional deficiency of vitamin B_1 (thiamine), nicotinic acid, or vitamin B_{12} and this neuropathy is commonly seen in persons suffering chronic alcoholism with or without Wernicke-Korsakoff syndrome. Toxic chemicals can also produce this disorder as can the accumulation of metabolic toxins as seen in uraemia and carcinoma. Motor neuron disease has also been implicated as a cause.

Schwann cell dysfunction neuropathy

Segmental demyelination, that is demyelination between 2 nodes of Ranvier, occurs and this process predominates in many neuropathies resulting in demyelination in multiple sites. The axon is usually left intact. The onset is rapid and recovery (if it occurs) is also rapid but incomplete. This is because, although remyelination can occur, the new sheath is much thinner than the original myelin and the formation of extra nodes of Ranvier cause disturbances to stimulus transmission. The predominant clinical features are generalized weakness and loss of reflexes.

This form of neuropathy is most commonly seen with diabetes mellitus, lead poisoning, or following post-diphtheria paralysis.

Vascular induced neuropathy

This usually presents as a local, asymmetrical disorder although many nerves may be involved. The degree of nerve dysfunction is directly related to the extent of the ischaemia and most commonly presents as a peripheral neuropathy accompanying peripheral vascular disease due to atheroma. Unrelieved pressure as seen in 'crutch palsy', crush injury, and carpel tunnel syndrome may also cause this form of neuropathy. Vascular induced neuropathy may also result from generalized disorders including autoimmune diseases, such as systemic lupus erythematosus, rheumatoid arthritis, and polyarteritis nodosa.

Clinical manifestations and diagnosis

The clinical manifestations of traumatic neuropathy vary depending on the site and severity of the injury. Manifestations of non-traumatic neuropathy also vary considerably, according to type. In general, numbness and paraesthesia of the hands and feet are common. The patient often complains of severe cramping pain in the calves at night and this progresses to weakness. Symptoms are more noticeable in the lower limbs.

In advanced cases of non-traumatic neuropathy, wrist drop and foot drop may occur. Sometimes the patient has little or no movement in his limbs, and ataxia is common. Cutaneous anaesthesia extending to the elbows and knees may present, as may severe pain in the calf muscles when pressure is applied. Reduction in, or loss of, tendon reflexes may also occur – especially of the ankle and knee. The patient's extremities may become oedematous and sweaty and they may develop muscle contractures.

Polyneuropathy is not difficult to diagnose due to its clinical presentation of peripheral, symmetrical muscle weakness and atrophy, pain, calf tenderness (particularly associated with pressure), and varying degrees of sensory loss. Rare forms of polyneuropathy may be diagnosed with the assistance of electromyography or, sometimes, nerve biopsy.

When attempting to isolate the cause of neuropathy the following should be considered:

- The mode of development – acute, sub-acute, progressive or recurrent.
- The distribution – proximal, distal, isolated or diffuse.
- Any associated hypertrophy.

Classic neuropathies, such as those caused by diabetes or alcoholism, have obvious clinical manifestations related to the patient's overall physical condition.

General management of the neuropathic patient

During the severe presentation of neuropathy the patient should rest in bed because of muscle weakness. A specific physiotherapy regime should be instigated to prevent muscle contractions and to reduce muscle wasting in legs and arms. Foot drop and wrist drop can be prevented by correct application and wearing of splints. Aluminium night shoes can replace splints eventually – muscles can also be stimulated electrically.

Because of the severe pain of neuropathy, active and/or passive exercises may not be possible, or the patient may only be able to perform during the peak of analgesic cover. Splints may be too painful to wear, in which case sandbags can be used for support of the weakened hands and feet, and bed cradles should be used to bear the weight of the bedclothes.

THE DIABETIC NEUROPATHIES

The peripheral nerve disorders that occur in diabetes take several forms and reflect the multiple causes of nerve degeneration seen in this disorder. Diabetic neuropathies are classified as symmetrical polyneuropathies and mononeuropathies.

Symmetrical polyneuropathies (distal primary sensory neuropathy)

This is the most common form of diabetic neuropathy and occurs in approximately 40% of patients with diabetes of over 25 years duration. It affects the lower limbs and usually presents with a variety of symptoms, the classic symptom being burning pain in the legs. Paraesthesia of the legs, insensitivity to light touch and temperature changes, dull aching pains, loss of ankle jerks and trophic lesions of the skin are also common.

Medical and nursing management

This neuropathy, like all diabetic neuropathies, will recover with better control of the diabetes and a more supervised metabolic state.

The treatment is symptomatic and consists largely of simple analgesics for pain control. Because of reduced sensitivity to pressure, sharp objects, and temperature changes, the hands and feet are prone to injury that can then develop into

ulcers, cellulitis, or even lymphangitis and osteomyelitis. The principle of management of such patients therefore is to prevent the occurrence of, or rapidly treat, the injury.

Repeated inspection of the hands and feet for any damage, avoidance of hot water, avoidance of manual labour that could cause injury, the wearing of well-fitting and possibly orthotically designed shoes, avoidance of walking in bare feet, and professional manicuring of nails are all essential measures. Skin care in the form of mild moisturizers helps maintain skin integrity.

Cranial nerve neuropathy in the diabetic patient

Isolated cranial nerve neuropathies are often the first presenting symptoms in a previously asymptomatic adult diabetic. The IIIrd cranial nerve is most frequently affected and the patient presents with sudden onset of a severe retro-orbital ache – diabetic third nerve palsy. Recovery usually occurs within several weeks of initial treatment of the diabetic condition.

Isolated peripheral nerve lesions in the diabetic patient

Any peripheral nerve can be affected by diabetic mononeuropathy but the most common are the radial, ulna, peroneal, sciatic, tibial and the lateral cutaneous nerves. Lesions frequently present at these sites causing compression of these vulnerable nerves. The onset is acute and painful, and the more distal the lesion, the greater the success of treatment.

Treatment consists of physiotherapy and orthopaedic supports where necessary.

Proximal lower extremity motor neuropathy (diabetic amyotrophy)

This neuropathy occurs in middle-aged and older diabetics, and presents progressively, causing pain often restricted to the proximal leg muscles, with associated loss of tendon reflexes and weakness of thigh muscles. Recovery is slow and treatment consists of strong analgesia, and physiotherapy involving the hip and thigh muscles.

22

Chronic neurological dysfunction

Chris Game   Jenny Kidd

CHRONIC BRAIN SYNDROME (DEMENTIA)

Dementia is the diffuse, irreversible deterioration in intellectual function due to chronic, progressive degeneration of the brain. The term 'chronic brain syndrome' more accurately describes the disorders of progressive dementia and delirium and is more highly favoured in texts discussing chronic neurological dysfunction. It presents with failing memory, intellectual deterioration and retrograde changes in personality and behaviour. Chronic brain syndrome is probably one of the most feared conditions of the elderly.

In Australia it is estimated that over 100 000 people are incapacitated by chronic brain syndrome and approximately 50% of these suffer from Alzheimer's disease. Most dementing diseases occur from the sixth decade of life onwards, with increased incidence with age, but can occur at an earlier age.

Aetiology

Chronic brain syndrome may follow progressive cerebral atrophy; be caused by systemic disease, many of which can be treated successfully; or more rarely follow chemical or mechanical injury.

The presenile and senile neurological disorders which lead to chronic brain syndrome are Alzheimer's disease, Huntington's chorea and Pick's disease. Cerebral atherosclerosis may result in cerebrovascular accident and multi-infarct dementia. Organic disorders (such as syphilis, encephalitis, meningitis, sarcoidosis and intracranial abscess) and metabolic disturbances (as seen in alcoholism, carbon monoxide and heavy metal poisoning, Wernicke's encephalopathy, myxoedema and Vitamin B_{12} deficiency) may all contribute to progressive cerebral deterioration. As many of these conditions respond to treatment, early recognition and medical intervention may prevent irreversible progression into dementia.

Demyelinating diseases such as multiple sclerosis, and head injury with brain damage have also been known to lead to the development of chronic brain syndrome.

Clinical manifestations

Initial deterioration may be observed in the person's mood, memory, and judgement, and changes are usually noticed by his family and friends.

Some people become apathetic and/or depressed, while others become irritable and anxious, sometimes even paranoid. Forgetfulness or loss of memory, particularly the short term memory, is very common and manifests as impaired ability to concentrate. A typical example is when a person writes several shopping lists, having forgotten the whereabouts and/or the existence of the previous ones. Conversations or questions are often repeated with no insight. Orientation is often affected, and past life often takes priority over present events. In later stages of chronic brain syndrome, the person becomes disoriented in previously familiar surroundings, and this often results in wandering away from home.

Meals are often served cold, uncooked or half-cooked and the patient may be found eating foods prepared in an inappropriate manner. Forgetting to eat is also common. Interest in reading and television slowly decreases. Speech may become affected, with the correct words or names proving elusive; this may result in extreme frustration. Ultimately the person's speech becomes incoherent and confused.

As the dementia progresses the manifestations worsen. Physical deterioration resulting from malnutrition and emaciation and a disregard for personal hygiene is common; the patient's appearance is dishevelled and he may even be in a filthy state. Co-ordination is poor, making eating and walking difficult. Incontinence eventually results and ultimately the patient is bedridden. Death usually results from an infection such as pneumonia.

This whole process may evolve rapidly over a period of months. More commonly it may develop more slowly over a number of years with the patient's condition remaining stable between periods of further decline.

Alzheimer's disease

This is the most common cause of progressive dementia in the elderly. It affects the sexes equally and occurs in approximately 5% of persons over the age of 65 years and progresses to involve 20% of persons over the age of 80 years. Rarely it has been diagnosed in persons 20 years and younger.

The terms 'pre-senile dementia' and 'senile dementia' were used to describe the condition in persons under and over 65 years, respectively, and embraced a variety of different diseases. However the terms are now recognized as describing Alzheimer's disease specifically, irrespective of age.

Aetiology and pathophysiology

The cause of Alzheimer's disease is unknown. There is a family history in approximately 25% of cases and almost all patients over the age of 30 years with Down syndrome develop the brain degeneration seen in Alzheimer's disease, suggesting a genetic factor.

The principle pathological changes are a progressive neuronal degeneration in the cerebral cortex, affecting memory and association.

At autopsy, a number of characteristic changes are seen in the brain. It is found to be smaller than is usual, due to loss of neurons, and the cortical neurons are found to be clumped together in neurofibrilliary tangles, predominantly in the basal nuclei and the thalamus. There is also a profusion of senile plaques throughout the cerebral cortex. The neurons of the hippocampus show a cytoplasmic degeneration characterized by the presence of argyrophil granules inside small vacuoles.

Clinical manifestations

The symptoms are those of chronic brain syndrome: progressive dementia and delerium. Classically, the first symptom is loss of short-term memory. In the early stages there may be no other symptoms, and the disease may be confused with the benign memory loss common in old age. Social graces are preserved and the patient dresses normally. Loss of interest in daily activities could be the first indication of Alzheimer's disease. The patient experiences difficulty in managing motor skills and spatial relationships. It is not uncommon for the patient to set out from home on a particular errand, for example to buy milk, and to become suddenly lost and terrified. Alternatively, the patient may be unable to manage routine household tasks; teapots may be stored in the refrigerator, salt may be added to the sugar bowl, and a significant other's preference for tea or coffee may be forgotten. Such episodes are often the first clear sign significant others cannot ignore, that the patient is suffering from this disorder.

As the disease progresses the patient becomes careless in dress and often dresses inappropriately. Basic hygiene is often neglected as are household chores, meal preparations and eating. Eventually there is complete disorientation and a tendency to become restless and wander away. Speech eventually becomes totally incoherent and the patient becomes frail, requiring full-time supervision and care. Incontinence, due to loss of sphincter control, and severe dementia (manifesting as total loss of rational, cognitive function) are extremely late changes. The duration of the disease can range between 1.5 and 15 years.

Diagnosis

Diagnosis is made largely on clinical grounds, and exclusion of other causes of chronic brain syndrome, many of them treatable.

Within weeks or months of the clinical progression diagnosis becomes accurate in 90% of cases, as sometimes time is required to distinguish the clinical difference between Alzheimer's and the rare Pick's disease.

The brunt of the care and responsibility for the patient suffering from Alzheimer's disease falls on the shoulders of family members and friends. Often the spouse of the patient is elderly and is himself incapacitated and unable to care for a partner. The greatest difficulty arises in the early stages when the partner is unsafe to leave unattended and yet has not reached the stage of being institutionalized.

The emotional dilemma facing relatives and/or spouse when this occurs can be quite draining. It is not uncommon for family members, particularly the spouse, to suffer a great sense of guilt, loss and grief when the patient must ultimately be placed in an institution.

These very real problems, shared by many people in the community and exacerbated by a lack of suitable long-term health care facilities, have lead to the founding of support groups such as The Alzheimer's Disease and Related Disorders Society (ADARDS), for the relatives and significant others of sufferers.

Pick's disease

This condition is much less common than Alzheimer's disease and is characterized by atrophy of the cerebral cortex, confined to the frontal and temporal areas including the hippocampus. It is of unknown cause and develops insidiously over a period of 3 to 12 years. Females are affected more frequently than males, and the age incidence is that of Alzheimer's disease.

Pathologically there is neuronal loss and there are characteristic swollen pear-shaped cells called 'pick bodies'. Unlike in Alzheimer's disease there is usually an absence of plaques and neurofibrilliary tangles.

Pick's disease is characterized by progressive mental deterioration, predominently in memory.

Patients are often restless and lack normal inhibition, but this gives way to apathetic hypoactive behaviour. Unlike in Alzheimer's disease, patients retain spatial orientation and direction. Another difference is that incontinence develops early and speech is reduced to one or two phrases. The patient becomes emaciated, bedridden, and often develops contractures. There is no specific treatment for Pick's disease and nursing management involves providing care for the frail bedridden patient.

Huntington's disease

Huntington's disease is characterized by chorea and chronic progressive dementia, and is inherited as an autosomal dominant trait. Both sexes are affected and genetically transmit the disease equally. The disease occurs worldwide and in some countries many seemingly isolated sufferers can be traced back to a common forebear. There is a 50% chance that the offspring of an affected parent will inherit the disorder. It can occur in children (St Vitus' dance) or adults.

Huntington's disease is characterized pathologically by atrophy of the cerebral cortex and basal ganglia, and is associated with a deficiency of the neurotransmitters acetylcholine and gamma-aminobutyric acid (GABA); this deficiency results in an imbalance of dopamine.

It is a progressive disease manifesting in approximately the third to fourth decade of life but may occur later or earlier; it usually causes death within 15 years of onset of symptoms.

Clinical manifestations

Both physical and mental symptoms and signs vary in occurrence and severity, and early signs may be as vague as general restlessness and personality or mood changes.

The first clinically recognizable symptom is usually that of chorea. Chorea is a condition manifested by irregular and spasmodic muscular movement that is beyond the patient's control; even voluntary movement becomes jerky and ungainly.

The choreiform movements occur in the face, head, trunk, and upper limbs and lead to the development of a shuffling and clumsy gait. Mental changes can be quite diverse and specific alterations develop insidiously, usually a few years after the movement disorder. They may manifest as irritability, aggression, delusions, paranoia, outbursts of excitement, depression, hallucinations and apathy. However, the full clinical picture does not always occur and sometimes the mental changes may precede the chorea or the chorea may never manifest.

Classically though, there is progressive mental deterioration which leads to dementia and depression. The disease will progress relentlessly and the patient will become unable to perform the activities of daily living. Thought disorder becomes disabling and eventually severe dysarthria and ataxia results. The patient becomes bedridden, requiring total nursing care.

Diagnosis

In cases of previous family history, the diagnosis is obvious. In cases without known family history, progressive dementia associated with choreiform movements (the latter rarely seen in other presenile dementias) is indicative of Huntington's disease.

Medical management

Medical therapy aims to control involuntary movements, and to provide genetic counselling and psychological support for the family.

Drug therapy with neuroleptic agents, for example haloperidol or tetrabenazine, acts by blocking dopamine in the globus pallidus and corpus striatum, thereby correcting the neurotransmitter imbalance and controlling chorea. Anxiolytics, for example the benzodiazepines, may be prescribed.

It is possible to eradicate Huntington's disease but this is highly improbable. As each sufferer can be clearly identified, should they not produce, Huntington's disease could be eradicated within a generation. One of the difficulties in controlling the morbidity of this disease is that the symptoms do not usually appear until middle life, that is, after the affected person has reproduced. Each offspring has a 50% chance of inheriting the disorder and research is concentrated on being able to identify before puberty the offspring who can transmit Huntington's disease.

Nursing management

Nursing management will depend upon the severity of symptoms and is aimed at assessing each patient and providing care that will alleviate individual problems.

● The ataxic patient should be assisted with ambulation and protected from injury, especially if choreiform movements are severe.
● Dysphagia may be overcome by providing a soft or liquid diet consisting of foods of one texture only which should also be high in protein and have added vitamins and minerals to prevent tissue wasting. Fluid intake of 3 litres per day is necessary, as are increased calories to prevent weight loss.
● The patient will need assistance with feeding himself and care must be taken to prevent airway obstruction.
● Urinary incontinence should be managed with special attention given to the protection of skin and the maintenance of the patient's self-concept.
● Constipation is common and can be controlled by including fibre and fluids in the diet.
● Nursing staff will need to encourage independence to minimize depression and where possible psychological support should be provided for the patient and his significant others.
● The patient and his significant others need to understand the disease's progression, its hereditary aspects, the medication regime, and the need for regular medical checkups.
● The patient will require support from his significant others and health care workers in order to cope with the psychological stress and lifestyle disruption that this disorder creates.

Anticipated outcome

Chemotherapy may reduce chorea, resulting in an improved self-concept and the ability to perform self-care. The main complications, malnutrition and aspiration pneumonia, are related to swallowing difficulties. Other complications may occur due to injury as a result of involuntary movement.

However, the disorder is progressive and death usually occurs within 15 years of diagnosis.

Multi-infarct dementia

This condition results from cerebrovascular disease. Multi-focal infarcts of cerebral arteries and arterioles result in diffuse cerebral dysfunction and are most often seen in association with diabetes and widespread hypertensive vascular disease. The areas of the brain most affected are those supplied by the middle and anterior cerebral arteries, affecting sensorimotor areas as well as the patient's cognitive function. As a result of the diffuse disease, the patient's memory, thought processes, speech, moods, motor function, and gait are often affected, resulting in dysarthria, apraxia, aphasia, and epilepsy in some cases. Pseudobulbar palsy (see page 216) is common in a slowly progressing syndrome and manifests as abnormal motor reflexes and abnormal bouts of crying or laughing. Many patients develop urinary incontinence. The disease tends to progress in a step-like manner in that each infarct leaves more evidence of mental and physical deterioration. The presence of abnormal motor reflexes differentiates the condition from Alzheimer's disease and on investigation, there is evidence of widespread cerebrovascular disease and often associated systemic vascular disease.

The patient ultimately progresses to the stage of being bedridden and requiring institutionalized total nursing care.

NUTRITIONAL AND METABOLIC DISORDERS

Wernicke-Korsakoff syndrome

This is an acute or subacute disorder affecting the midbrain and hypothalamus, due to a thiamine deficiency, which usually results from chronic alcohol abuse.

Pathologically, there are two syndromes – the Wernicke syndrome, and the Korsakoff syndrome. At postmortem these syndromes are indistinguishable, however the clinical manifestations are quite distinct. The Korsakoff syndrome rarely occurs without a background of the Wernicke syndrome.

Aetiology and pathophysiology

Wernicke-Korsakoff syndrome causes lesions within the central nervous system: capillary proliferation and congestion, and petechiae. These may result in neuronal loss from extensive axonal and myelin destruction. However, damage to nerve cells may be slight despite the extensive myelin destruction and gliosis. Lesions affect the thalamus, hypothalamus, midbrain, pons, and medulla.

The thiamine deficiency may be due to many causes, such as inadequate diet, persistent vomiting, anorexia nervosa, and gastrointestinal disorders. It was a disease common in prisoners of war, and it is now most commonly seen in chronic alcoholics.

There appears to be a genetic association in the syndrome's development, as not all alcoholic and malnourished people suffer Wernicke-Korsakoff syndrome and Caucasians appear to be more susceptible.

Clinical manifestations

It is useful for the nurse to consider Wernicke-Korsakoff as separate syndromes in order to understand the clinical manifestations.

Wernicke syndrome. In acute Wernicke syndrome the onset of symptoms is often insidious, developing over a period of days or weeks. Mental symptoms consist of global confusion, a sense of unreality, impaired memory, lethargy, confusion, and disorientation.

As an example of his altered perception, a patient may perceive his hospital room as his lounge room at home. It is rare for stupor or coma to occur, and patients often have difficulty sleeping.

Abnormal eye movements such as nystagmus are common, progressing to complete ophthalmoplegia. Ataxia occurs in most cases and, if severe, will prevent the patient from walking or standing. This is often accompanied by polyneuropathy. Patients with Wernicke syndrome will often have associated manifestations of nutritional deficiencies, such as a red swollen tongue, and skin rashes and bruising. Other general signs of debility such as acute tachycardia, postural hypotension, and dyspnoea on exertion are common. In the acute phase, the patient becomes anorexic and is unable to maintain an adequate diet. He does, however, have extreme thirst, which may put him at risk of drinking harmful liquids.

Korsakoff syndrome. The symptoms of Korsakoff syndrome tend to emerge as those of Wernicke syndrome are treated. The most characteristic Korsakoff symptom is a specific form of amnesia. Typically, the patient is unable to learn and retain new information and has an inability to recall information or situations of the past, even as recent as the previous half hour. Behaviour is relatively normal, and there is a tendency for the patient to make up stories to fill in the gaps – this is referred to as 'confabulation'. On occasions the patient may be disorientated and confused.

This form of psychosis can be caused by other disorders, such as posterior artery cerebrovascular accident, head trauma, encephalitis, ruptured anterior communicating artery aneurysm, cerebral atherosclerosis, cerebral tumour, carbon monoxide poisoning, and epilepsy. It is seen typically in chronic alcoholism and invariably occurs with an encephalopathy. Korsakoff syndrome is incurable when associated with alcoholism.

Medical and nursing management

Wernicke-Korsakoff syndrome is a progressive syndrome which, untreated, is fatal. Treatment may halt the progression, but cannot reverse the course of the disease. Even with treatment the mortality rate is still approximately 10%.

The treatment of choice is thiamine, 50–100 mg daily, until the patient can tolerate an adequate diet. Thiamine should be administered IM or IV, as oral thyamine is poorly absorbed in chronic alcoholism. The complete range of vitamins and minerals is also administered, and consideration is given to protein restriction, according to the patient's liver function.

Thiamine is necessary for the normal metabolism of carbohydrate, and if carbohydrates are administered to a thiamine deficient patient, Wernicke encephalopathy will result. Therefore when administering glucose to an alcoholic or undiagnosed comatosed patient, thiamine should also be administered.

With thiamine treatment ocular abnormalities disappear within hours. Global confusion may disappear within hours or may take days to a month. However the Korsakoff amnesia persists in over 80% of patients, only 25% of whom will recover their memory function. Ataxia usually improves over a period of days but recovery is incomplete in approximately 50% of patients. No overall improvement is seen in 35% of patients. Wernicke syndrome responds to thiamine better than does Korsakoff syndrome.

Many patients present with acute alcoholic withdrawal and emergency medical therapy will usually include the IV infusion of chlormethiazole. The nurse will be responsible for ensuring that the IV infusion is maintained until the patient's behaviour settles. This may take considerable creative effort.

Specific nursing care

Bizarre behaviour patterns and total non-compliance with therapy are to be expected in these patients, as is an inability to achieve satisfactory personal hygiene. As these patients are not inhibited by any physical disability, their behaviour can prove to be a constant source of frustration to the nurse responsible for their care. Any form of restraint to ensure patient safety will only increase the bizarre behaviour and may also promote violent actions. The nurse may experience anger towards patients with Wernicke-Korsakoff syndrome, and this is not uncommon. Support services for nursing staff working with these patients is mandatory.

The aims of nursing care are to achieve

- Patient/staff safety
- Improved patient reality orientation
- Compliance with therapy.

Patient/staff safety. The patient should be allowed to move freely about the ward, and all staff have a responsibility to ensure that he is supervised at all times. Potentially harmful objects (including liquids) should be kept out of his reach. He should be clearly identified so that he can be returned to the ward if necessary. Patients rarely initiate violence; but nurses should implement nursing care with caution, since physical contact may provoke a violent reaction.

Improved patient reality orientation. The nurse should endeavour to answer all the patient's questions and to repeatedly orient him in both space and time. It is useful to attempt to develop a pattern of care; for example, meals at the same times each day, interspersed with hygiene activities.

Compliance with therapy. The major form of therapy is avoidance of further ingestion of alcohol. However, as most patients are alcoholics, this aim is often frustrated. It is also essential that thiamine therapy is maintained, and in the long term this may only be achievable with weekly injections.

23

Disorders of nerve transmission

Jenny Kidd   Chris Game

When an electrical impulse passes from a nerve across the motor end plate of a muscle fibre, the muscle is stimulated to contract. Dysfunction or degeneration of the nerve cell or muscle fibre will interupt or prevent the normal transmission of electrical stimulus and the muscle will either not contract or contract ineffectively. The presence of calcium ions at the motor junction is essential for normal nerve transmission as is the presence and effective utilization of the neurotransmitter acetylcholine and the enzyme cholinesterase.

Myasthenia gravis is a disorder involving the utilization of acetylcholine characterized by the inability of skeletal muscle groups to maintain continuous or repeated contraction, resulting in muscle fatigability. Motor neuron disease affects both upper and lower motor neurons and degeneration results in muscle wasting and atrophy, and disordered muscle function.

MYASTHENIA GRAVIS

Myasthenia gravis is a chronic neuromotor disease which is thought to be of autoimmune origin. It is characterized by abnormal susceptibility of skeletal muscle to fatigue. Muscles most affected are facial, oculomotor, pharyngeal, laryngeal, and intercostal muscles. It is a progressive disease, often resulting in respiratory failure and death.

Approximately 75% of patients with myasthenia gravis have thymic abnormalities which manifest as either thymoma or thymic hyperplasia.

Myasthenia gravis manifests most frequently in the third or fourth decade of life, and women are affected three times more often than men. Men and women are equally affected over the age of 50

years. It often arises without any apparent cause and occasionally follows pregnancy, a febrile illness, or physical and emotional stress. Remissions tend to occur within the first 5 years, as do most deaths.

Aetiology and pathophysiology

Myasthenia gravis is thought to be of immunological origin because of its association with thymic disorders, and the known importance of the thymus to the immune system. Also, myasthenia gravis is associated with other autoimmune diseases, including thyroid disorders, SLE, sarcoidosis, and diabetes. However the trigger for the autoimmune reaction is still unknown.

Current thinking suggests that acetylcholine (necessary for depolarization of muscle receptor plates) is produced normally but that acetylcholine receptor (AChR) antibodies clog the post synaptic receptor sites of the muscle plate, thereby preventing acetylcholine making effective contact. The person is able to initiate a muscle contraction but the presence of the AChR antibodies prevents effective utilization of acetylcholine and muscle contraction cannot be maintained. Attempts at sustaining contraction (for example carrying a moderate weight or combing hair) result in muscle fatigue which can be extreme. Eventually the antibodies also damage the receptor sites and reduce their number leading to their progressive disability and death.

There is evidence that AChR antibody is present in all four IgG subclasses, occasionally in IgM, and also in sensitized T cells from the thymus. Therefore it appears that cellular immunity, mediated by T lymphocytes and humoral factors, play a major role in the pathogenesis of myasthenia gravis.

Clinical manifestations

The outstanding clinical manifestation is the onset of abnormal muscular fatigability to the point of exhaustion. The weakness first becomes evident in the muscles most frequently used: the extra-ocular muscles, those of the face and tongue, and those of upper extremities, such as arm and ventilatory muscles. Ptosis of one or both upper eyelids is often the first symptom. Patients may report having noticed the weakness while showering or combing their hair, or when an attempted smile became a snarl. It may be difficult for the patient to keep his eyelids open and his mouth closed, and he may find chewing, swallowing and speaking difficult. Patients may have difficulty in finishing a meal because of fatigue in the muscles of mastication. The patient supporting his jaw in his cupped hand is a common sign of weakened jaw muscles. Weakened neck muscles may produce an inability to hold the head up for even a short time; lolling may occur.

Fatigability of muscles of speech can be demonstrated by asking the patient to count up to 30. As the patient counts, speech becomes progressively more difficult and indistinct.

However, the principle danger is the development of weakness in the intercostal muscles leading to inadequate ventilation and, at worst, respiratory failure.

The disease runs a chronic course with punctuations of exacerbation and remission. Some remissions can be as long as five years, making a prognosis difficult.

Diagnosis

Diagnosis is supported by identification of immunoglobulins against the acetylcholine receptor and by electromyographic tests confirming impaired transmission of neuromuscular impulses.

Investigative procedures

These consist of history and physical examination, and:

- Anti-receptor (anti-AChR) antibody titre. This is the most sensitive diagnostic test
- Chest X-ray to detect thymoma
- Electromyography to demonstrate abnormalities of neuromuscular function
- Tensilon test. The administration of up to 10 mg of endrophonium chloride (Tensilon) will provide rapid relief of symptoms. This test virtually confirms the diagnosis as myasthenia gravis, rather than other causes of ptosis and general muscle weakness and fatigue.

Medical and surgical management

The administration of anticholinesterase drugs, such as neostigmine, has produced encouraging results. These drugs block the action of cholinesterase (neutralization of acetylcholine) at the myoneural junction and thus allow the accumulation of acetylcholine to enable transmission of impulses to the muscles. As anticholinesterase drugs produce cholinergic side effects, atropine is usually administered concurrently.

Many patients with mild myasthenia gravis, whose symptoms are restricted to only a few muscles, manage well on anticholinesterase therapy.

Neostigmine greatly improves the power of the muscles still capable of responding to it, but the response is poorer later in the disease when degeneration has occurred. It is usually given orally in divided doses of 15 mg one hour before meals. (When given before meals the effect of the drug enhances the capacity of the patient to chew and swallow without excessive fatigue.) In severe cases it is given intramuscularly 3–4 times per day in doses of 0.5–2.5 mg. Additionally, pyridostigmine (a long-acting form of neostigmine) may be given and its dosage is steadily increased until therapeutic levels are obtained.

However, treatment with steroids and immunosuppressives has become increasingly more popular as it is now believed that prolonged use of anticholinesterase drugs may actually potentiate AChR destruction. Prednisilone given daily or on alternate days in a double dose reducing to a lower maintenance dose, has been found to be an equally if not more effective form of treatment. However, some patients may require anticholinesterase drugs as well but in reduced dosages.

Immunosuppressive drugs such as cyclophosphamide either alone or with prednisilone are used by some physicians. Plasmapheresis may also be used in an emergency or before thymectomy to remove circulating antibodies. Rarely is this form of treatment used in the long term.

Patients on anticholinesterase therapy must be observed at all times for the onset of a cholinergic crisis. This may manifest as a sudden and rapid increase in muscular weakness and ventilatory insufficiency which is life threatening. In order to distinguish whether this is due to the myasthenia itself or the anticholinesterase therapy an IV injection of endrophonium chloride (Tensilon) is given. If this increases muscle power then the weakness is due to the myasthenia and the patient will require a larger dose of current drug therapy. However, if muscle power is reduced the weakness is probably cholinergic and drug therapy must be decreased. Unfortunately, on occasions anticholesterase therapy can be selective in that it can cause improved power in limb muscles and paralysis of the diaphragm. Signs of ventilatory insufficiency usually indicate the need to stop all treatment and to begin assisted ventilation via a tracheostomy; in some cases plasmapheresis may also be indicated.

Thymectomy

Although the exact role of the thymus gland in this disease is not clear, it is an established fact that thymectomy in some patients can lead to great improvement. Women appear to respond better than men, particularly young women with a short history of myasthenia. If thymectomy is contraindicated, the patient is stabilized on drug therapy. The place of thymectomy is still controversial because of the effects on the patient's immune system. However, it is obligatory in patients with histological evidence of thymoma.

Nursing management

Newly diagnosed myasthenics and regulated myasthenics with a few symptoms are often admitted to hospital for medication adjustment. The nurse should always be prepared for a cholinergic crisis and ventilatory equipment to deal with this should be readily available. A baseline of muscular strength must be established and any changes closely monitored.

The nurse should observe and record the results of tests of the patient's muscle strength, such as the number of times he can blink, and cross or raise his arms; the strength of his grip; what he can swallow and how many swallows he can perform; and how many times and to what level he can pump a sphygmomanometer.

It is not unusual for a patient to feel anxious, frightened, and stressed by his disease and his need for reassurance cannot be over-emphasized. His significant others must be involved in learning how to manage at home, and where to go, who to contact, and what to do in an emergency.

The nurse should encourage the patient to develop a regular schedule which will help him plan and space activities during the day to avoid fatigue, maximise efficiency, and enable him to lead as normal a life as possible. Alternating activities with rest periods, pacing himself carefully towards the end of the day, and getting a good night's sleep are strategies the patient should be taught. Taking medication one hour prior to eating a meal enables him to maximize chewing and swallowing. He must be taught to maintain optimum health, and to avoid infection and fatigue. Menstruation may temporarily worsen the condition, however pregnancy is not contraindicated. The patient must never alter his medication without consulting his physician, and he must know that many drugs should be avoided or used cautiously. These include morphine, quinidine, procainamide, antibiotics which act at the neuromuscular junction such as streptomycin and neomycin, and steroids (unless prescribed as treatment for myasthenia gravis). Sedatives and narcotics, when prescribed, should be given in reduced doses.

The patient must understand that overdosage of drug therapy can be as dangerous as underdosage, and that even the optimum dosage may not restore his full strength.

The patient should be warned of the dangers of upper respiratory tract infection. The inability to cough adequately can lead to pneumonia, so assistance with removal of secretions may be necessary in the form of an expectorant or, in severe cases, oropharyngeal aspiration (see page 164).

In advanced cases of myasthenia gravis, assistance with eating and drinking may be necessary. In situations where it is too dangerous for a patient to eat or drink, a nasoenteric tube may be required (see page 466). Where ventilatory muscles are involved, a close observation and recording of ventilation rate and depth, and tidal volume is necessary. Assisted ventilation may be required via a tracheostomy, which may be permanent (see page 338).

MOTOR NEURON DISEASE

Motor neuron disease is a triad of disease states which cause a degeneration of the corticospinal pathways, and the motor nerve cells of the brain stem and spinal cord. Motor neuron disease is unrelentingly progressive and, depending upon the type, is invariably fatal within 2–10 years of onset of symptoms.

The disease states are: amyotrophic lateral sclerosis, progressive muscular atrophy, and progressive bulbar palsy.

Aetiology and pathophysiology

Motor neuron disease affects males more commonly than females in a ratio of 2 : 1, and symptoms usually begin between the ages of 50–70 years. The disease occurs worldwide and in all races. The cause of motor neuron disease is unknown, but in some cases it is thought to be either hereditary or of an autoimmune origin.

The disease may occur in association with other diseases of the nervous system of a progressive degenerative nature and of unknown origin, for example Parkinson's disease and Pick's disease. There is also a familial incidence of a rare variety of motor neuron disease endemic among the Chamono tribe on the island of Guam.

The degenerative changes are most marked in the anterior horn cells of the spinal cord, and the motor nuclei of the brain stem, cortex, and corticospinal tract.

Clinical manifestations

Motor neuron disease is chronic. The onset is often insidious, although it can be sub-acute.

The clinical manifestations depend upon whether there is a predominance of upper or lower motor neuron involvement, or a distribution of both.

1. Amyotrophic lateral sclerosis (ALS; Lou Gehrig's disease)

This, the most common form of motor neuron disease, is an organ specific disorder characterized by both lower and upper motor neuron degeneration. The signs of lower motor neuron disease are seen in the upper limbs and signs of upper motor neuron degeneration are seen in the lower limbs. It is thought to be caused in part by autoimmune responses. In approximately 10% of patients, ALS is inherited as an autosomal dominant trait.

The small muscles become wasted and disproportionately severe weakness usually presents as an inability to hold objects or to feed oneself. Since atrophy beginning in the lower limbs is relatively uncommon, the legs present an uncomplicated picture of corticospinal tract degeneration, with weakness and spasticity.

Muscle wasting and fasciculation spread proximally to involve the upper arms and legs. Degeneration of the lower motor neurons causes impairment and loss of tendon reflexes; however corticospinal tract degeneration exaggerates them, leading to a tonic muscular atrophy.

2. Progressive muscular atrophy

The initial symptoms are those associated with lower motor neuron lesions and symptoms of upper motor neuron involvement do not occur for some years after onset. Muscle wasting may begin in the hands. Sometimes one hand will begin to waste months ahead of the other; in other cases wasting is symmetrical. The patient may complain of weak and stiff fingers, leading to clumsiness of finger movement, and twitching. Cramp like pains are not uncommon. Muscle wasting progresses to the muscles of the forearm. Less often the muscles of the upper arm and shoulders are affected first. Lower motor neuron lesions involving the legs initially present as asymmetrical foot drop which ultimately becomes bilateral.

In the terminal stages there is weakness in the muscles of the trunk and finally in those of ventilation. Fasciculation, either local or widespread, is a prominent symptom, and is indicative of the distribution of the degenerative process.

3. Progressive bulbar palsy

This occurs when the lower motor neuron degeneration spreads to involve the bulbar muscles. The tongue becomes shrunken and wasted and shows marked fasciculation; the palate then becomes involved together with the muscles of the pharynx and larynx. The patient suffers paresis of the lips and the tongue protrudes, making swallowing and talking increasingly difficult. Food tends to get caught in the patient's throat and often regurgitates through the nose. The facial muscles, including those of the eyes, are affected later and in a less severe form. However, it is in the muscles innervated from the medulla that the effects of corticospinal tract degeneration are of the greatest importance.

Pseudo-bulbar palsy, that is, upper motor neuron degeneration involving cortico-bulbar fibres may occur in isolation or, more commonly, in combination with progressive bulbar palsy. In pseudo-bulbar palsy, the lesion involves both corticospinal tracts above the medulla and causes weakness of the bulbar muscles resulting in a dysarthria and dysphagia. The weakened muscles are not wasted as seen in progressive bulbar palsy, but spastic. The tongue is not wrinkled and does not fasciculate. The patient's jaw jerks and the reflexes of the pharyngeal muscles are exaggerated, leading to abnormal excitability of sneezing and coughing. Pseudo-bulbar palsy also leads to a degree of loss of voluntary control of emotions resulting in inappropriate paroxysms of laughter or crying, unrelated to the patient's emotional state. In the late stages there is often loss of subcutaneous fat with an associated muscle wasting resulting in marked emaciation.

Diagnosis

Motor neuron disease must be distinguished from other conditions leading to muscular wasting and from other causes of bulbar palsy. Groups of symptoms mimicking motor neuron disease can occur in other situations such as:

- Carcinoma, especially of the bronchus
- Certain metabolic disorders, for example diabetic amyotrophy, and uraemia
- Central nervous system infection, especially meningovascular syphilis
- Degenerative disorders, especially cervical spondylosis
- Following trauma to a limb
- Chronic poisoning with mercury, lead, or manganese.

Diagnosis of motor neuron disease depends upon the exclusion of these causes.

Medical and nursing management

Because motor neuron disease is progressive and fatal within 10 years of diagnosis, management of the patient is basically symptomatic with emphasis on avoiding stress and activities which result in excessive muscle fatigue. He should be encouraged to continue independent activities for as long as possible. He should be advised to avoid undue fatigue and where possible to perform regular, moderate exercise to maintain muscle power.

Motor neuron disease is rapidly debilitating and therefore causes despair and frustration for the patient and his significant others. The nurse must be prepared to provide psychological support and referral to specialist counsellors so that the patient and his significant others can make the adjustments necessary in their lifestyle.

In the patient with ventilatory insufficiency, portable ventilatory support equipment is of assistance, especially for the patient in whom mobility is reasonably preserved. Deep breathing and coughing exercises will assist him in maximizing his ventilatory effort whilst minimizing the risk of him developing a chest infection.

Muscle weakness and/or spasticity may increase the risk of injury to the patient and he must be taught to protect his extremeties and to adapt his physical environment where necessary. The patient will progressively become immobile and will require nursing care to minimize the effects of immobility. If he develops foot drop, calipers or toe springs can help maintain ambulation;

however, the disease will usually progress to the stage where a wheelchair will be required.

Neostigmine and atropine may be prescribed to assist speech and swallowing in the patient with bulbar palsy, but these drugs are transient in benefit. Antibiotics are useful in combatting respiratory and urinary tract infections resulting from dysfunction of muscle groups and/or progressive immobility and, when dysphagia occurs, soft foods are required. Only in severe situations may a nasoenteric tube be necessary to maintain an adequate nutritional intake.

Prognosis

Motor neuron disease is a progressive disease but its effects vary from person to person. In some cases the patient's condition deteriorates rapidly and death may occur within months to a year of diagnosis. Following the onset of symptoms, most patients with progressive bulbar palsy survive for 2–3 years; those with amyotrophic lateral sclerosis 3–5 years; and those with progressive muscular atrophy 8–10 years.

24

Inflammatory disorders of the nervous system

Chris Game

Infection of the brain and spinal cord is not uncommon and may involve the meninges, brain tissue, and blood vessels. Meningitis usually occurs as a result of bacterial infection, whilst encephalitis is most commonly due to a viral infection. Intracranial abscess and thrombophlebitis of cranial vessels are usually the result of secondary spread from a focus of infection either inside or outside the skull.

Infection may follow an open head injury, spread from an infected middle ear, from nasal sinuses, or infected bone, or be introduced during lumbar puncture or cranial or spinal surgery. Secondary spread from a pneumococcal pneumonia is not uncommon.

Peripheral nerves are also susceptible to inflammation and the terms neuritis and peripheral neuritis have previously been incorrectly used to describe virtually any disorder of peripheral nerves (neuropathy). True peripheral neuritis, that is inflammation within the neuron (including Bell's palsy), and acute infective polyneuritis (Guillain-Barré syndrome) will be considered in this chapter whereas the neuropathies can be found in Chapter 21.

Nervous system infection can present a dramatic picture as seen in meningitis or encephalitis, which are accompanied by raised intracranial pressure; or as seen in Guillain-Barré syndrome, which is accompanied by ventilatory paralysis. Some infections of the central nervous system are associated with a high mortality, for example intracranial abscess and some forms of meningitis, and severe infection invariably results in some degree of permanent brain dysfunction.

MENINGITIS

In meningitis there is an acute inflammation of the meninges which may be pyogenic or aseptic (viral).

Pyogenic meningitis

In almost all cases pyogenic meningitis occurs as a complication of a bacterial infection. The primary infection may occur elsewhere in the body (for example pneumonia, osteomyelitis, otitis media, severe sinusitis, encephalitis, or intracranial abscess) or it may follow a skull fracture. Alternatively, the causative organism may be introduced at lumbar puncture or via any contaminated needle.

Meningococcal meningitis is an airborne, droplet infection more commonly seen in people living in overcrowded conditions with poor hygiene measures. The pneumococcus is usually the responsible organism in meningitis secondary to pneumonia or otitis media. *Haemophilus influenzae*, the streptococcus, or *Escherichia coli* commonly cause meningitis in small children or the elderly. Aseptic meningitis is usually the result of a viral infection.

All three meningeal membranes may be inflamed and there may be associated pus covering the dura mater. The infection may spread to involve the ventricles or brain substance, and cerebral oedema with a resultant increase in intracranial pressure may occur. The flow of CSF may be impeded due to thickening of the pia mater.

Clinical manifestations

The cardinal symptoms and signs of meningitis reflect infection and rising intracranial pressure.

Therefore the patient will complain of fever, chills, general malaise, headache, vomiting, constant drowsiness, and photophobia. On examination the patient will be found to have tachycardia, nuchal rigidity and, in cases of meningococcal meningitis, a skin rash. The patient's significant others may also indicate that he has become increasingly irritable and confused and, in the case of children, seizures may have occurred.

Investigative procedures

Diagnosis is confirmed by culture and sensitivity of CSF. CSF pressure is usually elevated due to an obstruction to flow, the protein level is high and the glucose level is decreased. The CSF may appear cloudy and the degree of cloudiness is dependent upon the number of leucocytes present.

Positive Kernig's and Brudzinski's signs confirm the CSF findings. Kernig's sign is tested for with the patient in a supine position. The nurse flexes the patient's leg at the hip and knee to 90° and then extends the leg at the knee. Kernig's sign is positive if the patient experiences headache, neck, back or leg pain when leg extension occurs. The pain results from irritation of meningeal and spinal nerve root inflammation. Brudzinski's sign is also tested for with the patient in a supine position. The nurse places his/her hand behind the patient's neck and draws the patient's head forward towards the chest. The sign is positive if the patient responds by flexing both his hips and knees. The flexion is in response to stretching of inflamed meninges.

The primary site of infection may be established following cultures of blood, urine, sputum, and nose and throat swabs. A complete physical examination is performed with special attention paid to skin, ears, and sinuses. A chest X-ray should be performed to exclude or confirm pulmonary infection.

Medical and nursing management

The major aims of management are to eradicate the infection, prevent complications, and provide supportive care. The blood–brain barrier causes difficulty in getting sufficient quantities of antibiotics to the site of the infection, so antibiotic therapy is usually aggressive. High-dose penicillin will be administered initially and replaced with the specific broad-spectrum antibiotic as soon as culture and sensitivity results are available. It is common for an intrathecal dose of penicillin to be administered during diagnostic lumbar puncture. The nurse is responsible for managing the IV infusion of high-dose antibiotics usually administered via a central venous line. IV therapy may continue for as long as 2 weeks and then be replaced by high-dose oral antibiotics.

Associated cerebral oedema may be controlled by mannitol and dexamethasone. Convulsions are controlled by phenytoin, and aspirin is usually sufficient to control headache and fever. Sedation is used with caution as it may mask neurological signs of deterioration of the patient's condition.

Observation of the patient, his neurological function, and his vital signs is of paramount importance. Any alteration to conscious state, or other signs of increasing intracranial pressure, must be recorded accurately and reported immediately in order to prevent complications from occurring (see page 161). Observation for side-effects of the high-dose antibiotics must be maintained and the central venous line managed according to the hospital's policy.

The patient's fluid balance must be monitored closely and fluid intake should be sufficient to prevent dehydration or avoid fluid overload which could lead to increasing cerebral oedema. A balanced diet is essential to hasten recovery, and small, frequent meals will usually prevent nausea. Added fibre in the diet will assist in the prevention of constipation which is to be avoided because of the danger of a rise in intracranial pressure caused by straining at stool.

The patient should be nursed in a quiet, darkened room until photophobia and cerebral irritation subside and his significant others should be reassurred that the period of delerium and behavioural changes will diminish and disappear on resolution of the infection. He should be encouraged to adopt a position of comfort and nursing procedures should be planned so as to avoid sudden movement which may aggravate headache or neck pain. Active and passive limb exercises will be required to prevent muscle wasting and joint stiffness. Aspirin should be administered to control the patient's headache and fever.

If meningococcus is the causative organism, the patient must be isolated to prevent spread of the infection.

Aseptic meningitis

When compared with pyogenic meningitis this is a fairly benign disorder which results from a viral infection; it is most commonly termed viral meningitis. The enteroviruses are the most common cause along with herpes simplex virus and infectious mononucleosis.

It is characterized by the sudden onset of headache, fever, vomiting, nuchal rigidity, and photophobia. The patient is usually able to describe a recent viral illness with sore throat, abdominal pain, and upper respiratory tract infection. There are usually no focal neurological signs.

Lumbar puncture usually reveals a crystal-clear CSF under normal pressure. Microscopic analysis of CSF reveals only a slight elevation in protein, the presence of a lymphocytic pleocytosis, and a sterile bacterial culture. The diagnosis is confirmed by isolating the virus in the CSF but, as this takes considerable time, the patient has usually fully recovered by the time confirmation is received.

Antibiotics are obviously not required in the treatment of aseptic meningitis. Isolation is not necessary and most patients are managed at home and make a complete and uncomplicated recovery. However, patients should be warned to expect fatigue for some weeks after recovery and should be advised to take plenty of rest.

Complications

Complications of meningitis are not common as most patients respond quickly to high-dose antibiotic therapy. However, should the organism prove resistant to antibiotics, or the infection spread quickly to involve the brain and/or cranial blood vessels, then residual neurological deficits may occur.

ENCEPHALITIS

Encephalitis is a severe inflammation of the brain tissue and meninges which results most commonly from a viral infection transmitted by a mosquito or tick. It can also be produced by bacterial infection as an extension of pyogenic meningitis or secondary to intracranial abscess formation. Viral encephalitis can occur as a complication of measles, chickenpox, mumps, or following vaccination, but is most commonly caused by enteroviruses or the herpes simplex virus.

There is an intense inflammation of the brain parenchyma and the meninges and this causes cerebral congestion and oedema. Cerebral ganglion cells degenerate and there is diffuse nerve cell destruction; herpes simplex encephalitis also causes haemorrhagic necrosis of brain tissue.

Clinical manifestations

The patient will normally present with the acute onset of headache, fever, malaise, and vomiting. Meningeal irritation, demonstrated by for example nuchal rigidity, occurs and the evidence of neuronal damage may develop, for example altered consciousness, paralysis, and convulsions. Following the acute phase the patient may remain unconscious for days or weeks and on recovery may exhibit mild to severe neurological deficits. The course and extent of the disease will be dependent upon the type of virus implicated and its virulence.

Investigative procedures

Encephalitis is difficult to distinguish from meningitis or other febrile illnesses by clinical history and/or general physical examination. Lumbar puncture for examination of CSF is performed with caution in patients with severe infection and elevated intracranial pressure, as herniation ('coning') of the brain is a distinct possibility. When performed, lumbar puncture reveals CSF under increased pressure and there is usually no turbidity. Microscopic examination reveals slightly elevated protein and leucocyte levels, but glucose remains normal. Isolation of the virus from CSF or blood confirms the diagnosis.

CT scan is usually performed on patients with a severe presentation to exclude other intracranial pathology and to determine the extent of neuronal damage. EEG may demonstrate classic slow-wave abnormalities. Brain biopsy may also be performed to identify the cause of a fungal or parasitic infection and may be the only way of confirming infection by the herpes simplex virus.

Medical and nursing management

The aims of medical and nursing care are the same as for the patient with meningitis, that is: to eradicate the infection, prevent complications, and provide supportive care.

Antiviral agents may be prescribed but these are useful only against the effects of the herpes simplex virus. Associated cerebral oedema may be controlled by mannitol and dexamethasone. Convulsions are controlled by phenytoin, and aspirin is usually sufficient to control headache and fever. Sedation is used with caution as it may mask neurological signs of deterioration of the patient's condition.

Specific nursing care is the same as for the patient with meningitis (page 218). Observation of the patient, his neurological function, and his vital signs is of paramount importance. Any alteration to conscious state or other signs of increasing intracranial pressure, must be recorded accurately and reported immediately (see page 161).

Should unconsciousness be a feature, then nursing care will involve the management of the unconscious patient (see page 162).

Anticipated outcome

For patients with mild encephalitis the prognosis is good and the majority make a complete recovery. Only a small percentage of those patients with mild disease are left with any permanent neurological deficit. Herpes simplex encephalitis has a high mortality and morbidity rate and any survivors are usually left with severe, permanent brain damage.

INTRACRANIAL ABSCESS

Intracranial abscess formation usually occurs within the substance of the brain and is more commonly referred to as brain abscess. It is a free or encapsulated collection of pus and usually occurs secondary to an infective focus elsewhere in the body, especially from otitis media, mastoiditis, dental abscesses, sinusitis, or an embolic vegetation from an infected cardiac valve.

Common abscess sites are the frontal lobe, cerebellum, or temporal lobes. Extradural abscesses are usually associated with chronic sinusitis causing localized osteomyelitis of the skull, middle ear infection, and infected skull fractures, for example of the cribiform plate. Untreated intracranial abscess is, in almost all cases, fatal and many survivors of treated abscess are left with mild to severe neurological deficits.

Causative organisms are usually *Staphylococcus aureus*, *Streptococcus viridans* or *haemolyticus*, the pneumococcus and klebsiella.

There is usually an initial, localized inflammation, necrosis, and oedema of brain tissue which extends to a septic thrombosis of the surrounding cerebral vessels. Suppurative encephalitis results in a thick encapsulation of the accumulating pus by a proliferation of fibroblasts and microglia. Surrounding meningeal linings are infiltrated by lymphocytes, neutrophils, and plasma cells.

Clinical manifestations and investigative procedures

The patient can usually describe a history of a previous extracranial infection, for example severe mastoiditis. This history, in conjunction with a full neurological examination to elicit the cardinal signs of raised intracranial pressure, are normally indicative of an intracranial abscess. There may also be manifestations of a focal neurological lesion, for example epileptoid seizures.

CT scan, EEG, and cerebral arteriography assist in isolating the site of the abscess. A full series skull X-ray to visualize the sinuses and mastoid area may be ordered, and microbiological culture of any suspected focus is undertaken to isolate the causative organism. Lumbar puncture is rarely performed as the risk of 'coning' of the patient's brain due to the raised intracranial pressure is extremely high.

Medical, surgical and nursing management

The aims of medical management are to eradicate the underlying infection and to surgically excise or drain the abscess (craniotomy). It should be noted that surgical intervention will not take place until such time as the abscess is encapsulated; this will minimize the likelihood of spreading infection during surgery.

Broad spectrum antibiotic therapy specific to the causative organism will be ordered to treat both the abscess and the primary focus. Otherwise, medical and nursing care is as for the patient with meningitis (see page 218). Observation for both the expected and side-effects of the administered drugs must be maintained and recorded. Intubation and mechanical ventilation of the patient may be necessary during the acute phase to ensure an adequate airway.

Nursing management of the patient undergoing craniotomy

Prior to surgery the patient and his significant others should be warned that he will have his head shaved and that initially his head will be swathed in a large bandage. He should also be informed that periorbital oedema and haematoma commonly occur following craniotomy and they may be found on the affected side or be bilateral.

Following surgery the patient should be nursed in a quiet room until cerebral irritation subsides. Elevation of the head of the bed will assist in preventing a rise in intracranial pressure. The patient should be observed closely for any signs of developing meningitis, for example nuchal rigidity or photophobia and half-hourly neurological observations will be necessary until his condition is stable. He should be encouraged to adopt a position of comfort and, to promote drainage of the abscess, he should be nursed on the operative side.

The wound will normally contain at least one, and more commonly two, thin, flexible, glove drain tubes which will ensure drainage of purulent material and any haemoserous fluid. The wound dressing should be checked and changed frequently to prevent the development of another focus for infection. The wound dressing is normally removed after 24–48 hours when the drain tubes are also removed. The wound is then either redressed as necessary or left open. As scalp wounds heal quickly, sutures are usually removed after 6–7 days.

The use of ice packs to the eyelids will assist in reducing periorbital oedema; haematoma usually resolve within 2 weeks. Lubrication of the eyelids may be necessary and frequent eye care will minimize any conjunctival irritation.

Nursing procedures should be planned so as to avoid sudden movement which may aggravate any headache. Active and passive limb exercises will be required to prevent muscle wasting and joint stiffness.

Should the patient remain unconscious following surgery then the nurse must be prepared to care for this patient with special attention to the complications of prolonged immobility and unconsciousness (see page 162).

Anticipated outcome

If drainage of the abscess is successful and infection is controlled without neurological deficits occurring, then the prognosis for the patient is very good. However, epilepsy is a common complication of intracranial abscess and if it occurs life-long anticonvulsant therapy must be maintained.

Prevention of intracranial abscess includes adequate antibiotic cover for any extracranial infection, especially of the ear, mastoid, sinuses, and pulmonary system and such cover should be mandatory for any person who has previously experienced an intracranial abscess.

The mortality rate for intracranial abscess is approximately 35% when the patient presents with a rapid progression of symptoms or if the organism is resistant to antimicrobial therapy. Unfortunately, many surviving patients are left with severe neurological deficits on resolution of the abscess and may require intensive rehabilitation and long-term supportive care.

GUILLAIN-BARRÉ SYNDROME

Guillain-Barré syndrome is also known as acute infective polyneuritis, acute post-infective polyneuritis, and febrile polyneuritis. It is an acute post-infective, rapidly evolving paralyzing illness involving the spinal nerves. It is the most common inflammatory demyelinating nerve disorder. Guillain-Barré syndrome is thought to be due to an autoimmune reaction of the peripheral nervous system.

The aetiology of Guillain-Barré syndrome is unknown, however there is strong evidence to suggest a recent association with an infective agent. The attack often follows an acute illness which may be viral, such as influenza, herpes simplex or mumps. In many cases no infective agent can be identified, but 60% of cases follow an upper respiratory tract infection or gastrointestinal illness within one month of onset. Other predisposing factors include surgery, pregnancy, lymphoma, and vaccination.

Any age group is affected but most patients are young to middle-aged adults.

Clinical manifestations

The disease is rapidly fulminating and often febrile. When an acute illness precedes the disease, symptoms usually do not appear until the fever has subsided. Unexplained deep pain especially in the back and legs is an early feature in 50% of patients. The pain is described as unremitting, and cannot be controlled by either mild analgesics or position changes.

Neurological symptoms may manifest initially as tingling in the periphery which advances proximally, and if the cranial nerves are affected tingling of the tongue and face may also occur. This paraesthesia usually resolves quickly. Muscle weakness is a feature in over 50% of patients and may range from mild weakness to severe prostration.

Unlike peripheral neuropathies, Guillain-Barré syndrome affects proximal and distal muscles equally. Muscle weakness occurs so rapidly that muscle atrophy is not a feature. It usually presents in the legs, often involving proximal rather than distal muscles, and is more severe than associated sensory problems.

Limb weakness is usually symmetrical and tendon reflexes are absent. This weakness will in almost all cases progress to paralysis, the degree and extent varying from mild foot drop to flaccid quadriplegia and inability to speak, swallow and breathe: Guillain-Barré syndrome can be life-threatening and the mortality rate is approximately 5%.

The paralysis is ascending although the patient may present with weakness of the proximal upper limbs and face. Usually the patient is not systemically ill.

Involvement of autonomic nerve pathways may occur as associated orthostatic hypotension or hypertension. Such involvement is not uncommon and complicates the management of the condition. Patients can die suddenly from cardiac arrythmias or extreme fluctuations in blood pressure. There is occasional involvement of cranial nerves. Involvement of the optic nerve can cause papilloedema and involvement of the VIIIth cranial nerve can cause deafness.

In 80% of cases, the paralysis is rapidly progressive and it may last for anything from a week to a month, the latter being more common; and in some instances it may last for up to 8 weeks. Recovery from paralysis usually begins 2–4 weeks after the peak and is usually steady and complete. Within 6 months, most patients are ambulatory.

Diagnosis

Rapid progression of the weakness and paralysis is characteristic of Guillain-Barré syndrome.

The CSF often has a greatly raised protein content (20–30 g/l or more), may be yellow in colour, and has slightly increased opening pressure.

Poliomyelitis must be discounted, as must diphtheria, tick paralysis, cervical spine fracture, botulism, and acute myelitis.

Electromyography shows decreased velocity in nerve conduction.

Respiratory function tests show reduced vital capacity if there is respiratory involvement.

Medical and nursing management

All patients suspected of Guillain-Barré syndrome must be admitted to hospital because of the progressive and unpredictable nature of the disease. The sudden onset of total inability to move not unnaturally produces fear, helplessness, uncertainty, and frustration. The patient will be dependent upon life support systems and skilled nursing care for an indeterminate period of time. It is not possible to predict when, or how completely, a patient will recover. Such dependence strips the patient of self-concept, dignity, and control.

The nurse must constantly involve the patient in all decisions about care and will need to exercise exceptional creativity in anticipating the patient's needs. The creation of a stimulating environment (with the assistance of the patient's family and friends) will maximize patient optimism and reality orientation. In addition nursing care is directed towards alleviating the difficulties and avoiding the dangers of paralysis. For the patient with severe symptoms, care is as for the paralysed patient (see page 171).

However, the nurse must appreciate that the patient severely affected by Guillain-Barré syndrome, although fully conscious, will most likely be unable to speak due either to the need for assisted ventilation or the involvement of the muscles of speech. Communication problems may be further compounded if the patient is so completely paralysed that he is unable to use mechanical speech aids. The nurse and the patient will need to develop appropriate codes and cues to minimize the extreme frustration of an almost total verbal isolation, and to enable the patient to communicate even the most basic needs.

The patient's ability to cough, swallow and breathe effectively must be monitored closely. Blood gas analysis may be helpful in predicting the onset of respiratory failure and, if this is anticipated, the patient must receive assisted mechanical ventilation immediately.

Some patients with progressive bulbar weakness will be unable to swallow or cough and will require nourishment via a nasoenteric tube (see page 466). Oropharyngeal aspiration may be required to maintain a comfortable oropharynx, free of secretions. Hypotension may need to be treated with pressor drugs but, due to the fluctuating nature of the blood pressure, pharmacological interference can be dangerous and should be avoided if possible.

It is not uncommon for these patients to experience intense and prolonged diaphoresis. Frequent bedbaths and washing of hair will assist in maintaining patient comfort and in alleviating psychological distress. Wherever possible, as soon as the patient's physical condition is stabilized, daily bathing should be performed.

Acute polyneuritis results in highly sensitive peripheral nerve endings. Therefore, the patient is intolerant of heat, changes in pressure, and movement. Nursing procedures and passive exercises must be performed carefully and gently (and under the cover of narcotic analgesics or hypnotic sedation if necessary) to avoid the generation of extreme pain. Highly sensitive nerve endings can also be easily irritated by any external stimulus, therefore the nurse must be aware of the pain that can be generated by noise, light, or odours.

Anticipated outcome

In the majority of patients with Guillain-Barré syndrome complete recovery occurs. However, some 5% of patients are left with a degree of permanent residual weakness, according to the extent of nerve damage. Children who contract Guillain-Barré syndrome are more likely than adults to be left with a permanent disability.

Although complete recovery is the normal outcome in some patients this is achieved only after a period of prolonged and painstaking rehabilitation.

PERIPHERAL NEURITIS

True peripheral neuritis, that is inflammation of the nerve cell body and fibres, rarely occurs; however, inflammation may involve the interstitial tissue of the neuron and hence the term interstitial neuritis is more correct. Interstitial neuritis is usually the result of spread of a local adjacent tissue inflammation and if acute results from, for example, surgical wound infection, abscess, boil, arthritis, cellulitis, or from an infected, deep decubitus ulcer. The most dramatic form of acute neuritis is seen in Bell's palsy.

Chronic neuritis is characteristically seen in the person with leprosy (see page 764) or tertiary syphilis (see page 667). Meningitis may lead to chronic neuritis and chronic arterial disease commonly causes interstitial neuron sclerosis and hence chronic neuritis.

IDIOPATHIC FACIAL PARALYSIS (BELL'S PALSY)

This condition presents as an acute onset of facial paralysis which may or may not be accompanied by pain, and is due to a non-suppurative inflammation of the facial nerve. In most cases the cause is unknown but it has occurred following an infection of the nasopharynx, following exposure to draughts, and herpes zoster virus.

Males are affected more often than females and although occurring across the age spectrum, it most commonly occurs in young adults.

Clinical manifestations

The onset is acute and the patient often wakes with unilateral facial paralysis. At the onset there is often pain in the angle of the jaw and inside the ear. On the affected side the eyebrow droops and the mouth is drawn to one side, closure of the eye is impossible. The tongue deviates to one side and the patient is unable to purse his lips, as in whistling. The cheek is puffed out during exhalation and food tends to catch between the cheek and the teeth. Only when the chorda tympani nerve is involved does the patient also suffer loss of the sensation of taste.

Diagnosis

Diagnosis is relatively easy when an otherwise well person presents with the sudden onset of facial paralysis as an isolated symptom. The only other conditions which simulate Bell's palsy are disseminated sclerosis and poliomyelitis.

Medical and nursing management

This is basically symptomatic and consists of mild analgesia and the administration of eye drops until the ability to blink returns. If paralysis persists after 5 days, a 10 day course of steroids is helpful in reducing the swelling of the facial nerve. Surgical decompression is not indicated as most persons recover spontaneously in a period ranging from weeks to months. If complete denervation occurs, paralysis will be permanent; fortunately this is rare.

Nursing intervention is aimed at protecting the patient from injury until the paralysis resolves and he must be given a clear understanding of the disorder. Health teaching, concentrating on the maintenance of oral hygiene and the avoidance of temperature extremes must be given. The patient should be encouraged to eat foods that can be chewed easily.

Facial spasm may occur but 90% of persons will recover without therapy. Persons older than 60 years, or those who have hypertension or diabetes mellitus, may be left with a residual deficit due to underlying generalized neuropathy resulting from chronic arterial, small vessel disease.

DISORDERS OF CRANIAL NERVES

Disorders of the cranial nerves are not common but may be caused by injury to the cerebrum due either to trauma of the cranium or infection, or by the effects of intracranial tumours. Table 24.1 lists the cranial nerves and their common dysfunctional features.

Table 24.1 Cranial nerve dysfunction

Nerve		Causes of dysfunction	Dysfunction
I	Olfactory	Fracture of cribiform plate	Anosmia
II	Optic	Orbital trauma or pressure on optic tracts from meningioma or aneurysm	Loss of pupil constriction Visual field defect Proptosis
III	Oculomotor	Cavernous sinus thrombosis Pressure on nerve from pituitary tumour or aneurysm Multiple sclerosis, poliomyelitis Viral infection, eg herpes zoster	Loss of pupillary reflexes Proptosis Unable to turn eye medially Ptosis
IV	Trochlear	Injury to nerve with fracture of orbit or As for III	Eye cannot move down and out As for III
V	Trigeminal	Injury to nerve branches Otitis media ⎫ Meningioma ⎬ Aneurysm ⎭	Loss of pain and touch Difficulty in chewing Pain
VI	Abducens	Fracture of orbit Otitis media ⎫ Meningioma ⎬ Aneurysm ⎭	Eye will not move laterally Diplopia Proptosis; pain
VII	Facial	Fracture of temporal bone Acoustic neuroma Meningioma	Paralysis of facial muscle Loss of taste ipsilateral side of tongue
VIII	Acoustic	Fracture of petrous bone Acoustic neuroma Meningioma	Deafness in affected ear
IX	Glossopharyngeal	Brainstem damage as in skull fracture Tumours of the nasopharynx	Loss of taste posterior third of tongue Loss of sensation affected side of palate
X	Vagus	Brainstem damage as in skull fracture Tumours of the nasopharynx	Deviation of uvula to unaffected side Paralysis of vocal cords
XI	Spinal accessory	Laceration of neck Skull fracture Tumour	Trapezius and sternocleidomastoid muscles fail to contract
XII	Hypoglossal	Tumour Skull fracture	Dysarthria Tongue protrudes toward affected side

SECTION A – REFERENCES AND FURTHER READING

Texts

Adams R D, Victor M 1985 Principles of Neurology, 3rd edn. McGraw-Hill, New York

Anderson J R (ed) 1976 Muir's textbook of pathology, 10th edn. Edward Arnold, London

Anthony C P 1984 Structure and function of the body. Mosby, St Louis

Ashworth B 1985 Management of neurological disorders, 2nd edn. Butterworths, London

Barnett H J M et al (eds) 1986 Stroke: pathophysiology, diagnosis, and management. Churchill Livingstone, New York

Bannister R 1985 Brain's clinical neurology, 6th edn. Oxford University Press, London

Bickerton J 1981 Neurology for nurses. Heinemann, London

Boore J, Champion R, Ferguson M 1987 Care of the physically ill adult. Churchill Livingstone, Edinburgh

Cahill M (ed) 1984 Neurologic disorders: nurse's clinical library. Springhouse, Pennsylvania

Creager J G 1982 Human anatomy and physiology. Wadsworth, California

Diamond S, Dalessio D J (eds) 1986 The practicing physician's approach to headache, 4th edn. Williams & Wilkins, Baltimore

Dinning T A R, Connelley T J (ed) 1981 Head injury. An integrated approach. John Wiley & Sons Brisbane

Dyck P J et al (eds) 1984 Peripheral neuropathy, 2nd edn. Saunders, Philadelphia

Havard M 1986 A nursing guide to drugs, 2nd edn. Churchill Livingstone, Melbourne

Hickey J V 1981 The clinical practice of neurological and neurosurgical nursing. Lippincott, Philadelphia

Hickey J V 1984 Quick reference to neurological nursing. Lippincott, Philadelphia

Luckmann J, Sorensen K C 1980 Medical-surgical nursing: a psychophysiologic approach, 2nd edn. Saunders, Philadelphia

Macleod J 1987 Davidson's principles and practice of medicine, 15th edn. Churchill Livingstone, Edinburgh

McLeod J G 1983 Introductory neurology. Blackwell Scientific, Melbourne

Mohr J P (ed) 1984 Manual of clinical problems in neurology: with annotated key references. Little, Brown & Co, Boston

Pallett P J 1985 Textbook of neurological nursing. Little, Brown & Co, Boston

Purchese G 1984 Neuromedical and neurosurgical nursing. Bailliere Tindall, London

Read A E, Barritt D W, Langton Hewer R 1986 Modern medicine, 3rd edn. Churchill Livingstone, Edinburgh

Scheinberg L (ed) 1983 MS A guide for patients and their families. Raven Press, New York

Selecki B R et al 1977 Injuries to the head, spine and peripheral nerves. Epidemiology of neurotrauma in NSW, SA, and ACT. Neurosurgical Society of Australia.

Snyder M (ed) 1983 A guide to neurological and neurosurgical nursing. Wiley, New York

Society of Hospital Pharmacists of Australia 1985 Pharmacology and drug information for nurses, 2nd edn. Saunders, Sydney

Storlie F J (ed) 1984 Diseases: nurse's reference lilbrary, 2nd edn. Springhouse, Pennsylvania

Sugarman G 1984 Epilepsy Handbook – a guide to understanding seizure disorders. C.V. Mosby, St Louis

Urosevich P R (ed) 1984 Coping with neurologic disorders: nursing photobook. Springhouse, Pennsylvania

Walton J N 1985 Brain's diseases of the nervous system, 9th edn. Oxford University Press, London

Journals

Anderson M 1984 Assessment under pressure: when your patient says 'my head hurts'. Nursing 84 14 : 9 : 34–41

Arnold B 1984 Brain death. The Australian Nurses Journal 14 : 5 : 46–47, 58

Barrett-Griesemer et al 1981 A guide to headaches – and how to relieve their pain. Nursing 81 11 : 4 : 50–57

Baum P L 1983 Carotid endarterectomy: one strike against stroke. Nursing 83 13 : 3 : 50–59

Book R 1986 Nursing Parkinsonism. The Australian Nurses Journal 15 : 11 : 45, 61

Callahan M E 1984 Caring for a stroke patient – like me. Nursing 84 14 : 5 : 25–27

Cameron-Barry J 1984 Overcoming acute complications in the unconscious patient. Nursing 84 14 : 5 : 42–45

Dalgas P 1985 Understanding drugs that affect the autonomic nervous system. Nursing 85 15 : 10 : 58–63

Downing P 1985 I am brain damaged. The Australian Nurses Journal 15 : 1 : 44–45

Ensuring intensive care 1984 Caring for the patient with elevated intracranial pressure. Nursing 84 14 : 3 : 12

Fagerness A, David J B 1985 Helping your patient survive the perils of C.N.S. infection. Nursing 85 15 : 5 : 11–13

Field K L 1984 Alcoholism: helping the patient off the not-so-merry-go-round. Nursing 84 14 : 8 : 13–14

Fowler S 1986 Small hopes: care of the patient with head trauma. Nursing 86 16 : 5 : 52–55

Fritz C P 1983 Spinal injuries (without cord damage). Nursing 83 13 : 11 : 14–15

Gresh C 1980 Helpful tips you can give your patient with Parkinson's disease. Nursing 80 10 : 1 : 26–33

Hahn K 1987 Left vs right: what a difference the side makes in stroke. Nursing 87 17 : 9 : 44–47

Herzberg L 1986 The diagnosis of Parkinson's disease. The Australian Nurses Journal 15 : 11 : 44, 61

Hylands J 1970 The Wernicke-Korsakoff syndrome. Nursing 70 9 : 7 : 26–29

Ingersoll G 1985 Caring for the quadriplegic patient with ankylosing spondylitis. Nursing 85 15 : 10 : 44–48

Jess L W 1987 Assessing your patient for increased I.C.P. Nursing 87 17 : 6 : 34–41

Johnson L K 1983 If your patient has increased intracranial pressure, your goal should be: no surprises. Nursing 83 13 : 6 : 58–63

McGaffin J F 1984 Basic cerebral trauma care. Journal of Neurosurgical Nursing. 15 : 4 189–193

Minion B J 1985 Truly caring for the patient who's an alcoholic. Nusring 85 15 : 8 : 55–56

O'Dea K, Peers E, Tuffin P 1986 Successful behaviour modification in a CVA patient. The Australian Nurses Journal 15 : 8 : 34–35, 53

Pluckhan M L 1986 Alzheimer's disease: helping the patient's family. Nursing 86 16 : 11 : 63–63

Rabin D 1986 Practical tips for patients with ALS. Nursing 86 16 : 2 : 47–49

Rich J 1986 Generalized motor seizure. Nursing 86 16 : 4 : 33

Robinson J (ed) 1982 Coping with neurologic problems proficiently, 2nd edn. Springhouse, Pennsylvania

Samonds R J, Cammermeyer M 1985 The patient with multiple sclerosis. Nursing 85 15 : 9 : 60–64

Speers I 1981 Cerebral oedema. Journal of Neurosurgical Nursing 13 : 2 102–114

Swift N 1979 Why the MS patient needs your help. Nursing 79 9 : 9 : 57–61

Taylor D L 1983 Increased I.C.P.: physiology, signs, and symptoms. Nursing 83 13 : 4 : 44–45

B

The endocrine system

25

Introduction to the endocrine system and disorders of the pituitary gland

Jenny Kidd

THE ENDOCRINE SYSTEM

The endocrine system is an integrated chemical communication system which helps regulate the basic metabolic functions of the body. The endocrine system works in harmony with the nervous system, and the biofeedback that ensures that all metabolic functions are integrated is extremely complex. Disturbances in endocrine function can represent a considerable threat to homeostasis.

The endocrine system comprises the body's ductless glands and other structures which secrete hormones directly into the circulation. A hormone is a complex protein which acts as a chemical messenger and stimulates either a target gland or target tissues. The major, and controlling, endocrine gland is the pituitary (hypophysis cerebri). Other glands include thyroid, parathyroid, adrenals, the islet cells of Langerhans in the pancreas, testes and ovaries. Although the pineal and thymus glands are ductless glands and secrete hormones, their precise endocrine function is not clearly understood; neither is their role in the maintenance of homeostasis, although thymus activity is essential for control of immune responses.

Structures which secrete hormones include the gastrointestinal mucosa which secretes hormones that aid in the control of digestive processes, and during pregnancy the placenta, which secretes hormones that maintain the pregnancy and promote embryonic growth in utero.

The hypothalamus, although part of the nervous system, lies superiorly to the pituitary gland and is connected via the pituitary stalk. The hypothalamus co-ordinates the function of the pituitary gland via neural and venous pathways.

Hormones may be classified according to their protein structure: peptides, steroids, or amino acid analogues. Peptide hormones are secreted by the pituitary, parathyroids, and pancreas. Steroid hormones are secreted by the adrenal cortex and testes or ovaries. Amino acid analogues are secreted by the thyroid and adrenal medulla. Prostaglandins (see also page 278) are chemical substances with hormone-like properties that affect many body functions; however, their precise origin and chemical effect is not yet fully understood.

Biofeedback controls all hormone secretion in the body via complex biofeedback loops. Basically a gland secretes a hormone which is primarily responsible for stimulating a target gland or tissues to produce another hormone which is responsible for controlling or regulating a body function. The circulating levels of the target gland or tissue's hormone either stimulates or inhibits the primary gland's function. For example, the pituitary secretes thyroid-stimulating hormone (TSH) which stimulates the thyroid to produce its hormone, thyroxine. (Thyroxine increases the metabolic activity of all body tissue.) As serum levels of thyroxine rise the pituitary is inhibited from secreting TSH, therefore thyroxine levels fall. When the serum concentration of thyroxine is low the pituitary is stimulated once again to secrete TSH and serum thyroxine levels rise.

Disorders of the endocrine system

Disruption in the endocrine system can occur at a variety of levels which include the endocrine glands themselves, the target glands or tissues, and the feedback loops which link the two together. Disorders of endocrine function in general can be characterized broadly as either disturbances in hormone production, or as alterations in the body's response to particular hormones. Causes of endocrine disorders include: congenital abnormalities, hyperplasia which can be an adenoma or a malignancy and, in some cases, trauma to a gland.

An endocrine disorder will result from a hormonal imbalance and all endocrine disorders can be classified as: primary or secondary hypofunction or hyperfunction; failure of the target gland or end-organ to respond; a functional disorder caused by nonendocrine disease; iatrogenic disorders; or abnormal or ectopic hormone production.

Hypofunction resulting in decreased hormone production is most commonly primary and develops slowly over a long period. Causes include congenital abnormalities, infarction or infection of a gland, autoimmune disease involving a gland, or tumours. Secondary hypofunction most commonly results from reduced hypothalamic and/or pituitary stimulation. Hyperfunction resulting in excessive hormone secretion is usually primary and results from hyperplasia of a gland which, in most circumstances, is benign. Hyperplasia may occur in the form of tumour growth or be in response to a hormone-secreting tumour of another gland.

The target gland or end-organ may fail to respond to hormonal stimulation or may develop hormone resistance due to genetic or acquired disease. Nonendocrine disease (for example, cirrhosis of the liver) can affect glandular secretions and cause endocrine disturbance. Iatrogenic endocrine disorders can occur due to the administration of drugs, especially high dose corticosteroids and the use of cytotoxic chemotherapy, radiation and surgical ablation of a gland. An inborn error of metabolism may result in abnormal hormone production and ectopic hormone production is most commonly caused by a malignant tumour, especially tumours of endodermal cellular origin, for example, oat cell carcinoma of the lung.

Management of endocrine disorders

The management of the patient with an endocrine disorder can be extremely complex and in most instances the patient is treated on an outpatient basis, is under the care of a specialist endocrinologist, and does not require hospitalization. Nursing intervention is usually only required should the patient be hospitalized for treatment of symptoms or for surgery to correct hypo- or hyperfunction. The nursing management of the patient following surgery for pituitary dysfunction is as for the patient following craniotomy (see page 222). The nursing management of the patient with thyrotoxicosis and following thyroidectomy will be discussed later in this section, as will the nursing management of the patient diagnosed with diabetes mellitus.

Hypothalamic co-ordination

The hypothalamus (see also page 147) co-ordinates activities of the endocrine and nervous systems by way of hormonal control of the pituitary gland mediated through neural or venous pathways and, as such, can be considered as having endocrine function. The hypothalamus sits anterior to the brain stem, connected to the pituitary gland by the pituitary stalk and regulates temperature, water balance, appetite, and emotions, as well as pituitary function.

The hypothalamus produces 2 hormones – antidiuretic hormone (ADH) and oxytocin – and these hormones are transferred via neural pathways to the posterior lobe of the pituitary where they are stored and, when needed, secreted into the circulation.

The hypothalamus also secretes specific releasing and inhibiting hormones which help in the complex biofeedback regulation of pituitary anterior lobe function; these releasing and inhibiting hormones reach the anterior pituitary via venous pathways. These hormones include: thyrotrophin-releasing hormone (TRH) which stimulates the secretion of TSH; luteinizing hormone releasing hormone (LH-RH) which stimulates the release of follicle stimulating hormone (FSH) and luteinizing hormone (LH) and, in many texts, is referred to as gonadotrophin-releasing hormone (GNRH); growth hormone releasing hormone (GH-RH); and growth hormone inhibitory hormone (GHIH). There are other hypothalamic secretions that are thought to influence hormones released by the anterior pituitary gland, and because they have not yet been identified as hormones they are termed factors. These are corticotrophin-releasing factor (CRF), somatotrophin-releasing factor (SRF) and prolactin-inhibitory factor (PIF).

These releasing hormones enter the anterior pituitary gland via the pituitary portal system, which is the major blood supply of the anterior pituitary gland. It is also believed that blood may travel in a retrograde flow from the pituitary to the hypothalamus. The control of anterior pituitary hormones, therefore, is through a feedback inhibition mechanism by target hormones, as previously described for thyroxine, and by hypothalamic regulation. For example, a slight rise in the secretion of thyroxine will block the release of thyroid stimulating hormone from the anterior pituitary in response to TRH. However some hormones, for example growth hormone, may act directly on the hypothalamus, thus regulating their own secretion. The blood supply to the hypothalamus is important with regard to this feedback mechanism, as the blood–brain barrier is incomplete at the origin of the major plexus of the pituitary portal system. Therefore large molecules, such as hormones, can cross the blood–brain barrier and gain access to both the hypothalamus and the pituitary gland in order to provide this feedback mechanism.

Disorders of the hypothalamus are rarely seen in isolation and are often concomitant with abnormalities of the pituitary gland, due to the close anatomical and physiological relationship of the two glands. For example a pituitary tumour may cause hypothalamic compression with resultant disturbance in temperature regulation, sleep patterns, and emotions. Manifestations of hypothalamic or pituitary lesions include enlargement of the sella turcica and visual field defects due to their close anatomical position to the optic chiasma.

PITUITARY GLAND (HYPOPHYSIS CEREBRI)

This small gland lies in the bony cavity of the sella turcica (pituitary fossa) at the base of the brain.

The gland is divided into anterior and posterior lobes.

The posterior pituitary lobe (neurohypophysis) develops as a downward projection of the hypothalamus. Two hormones are secreted, vasopressin or antidiuretic hormone (ADH) and oxytocin, which are produced and synthesized in the hypothalamus and transported to the posterior pituitary for secretion into the systemic circulation. The neurohypophysis is mainly concerned with the regulation of fluid balance through its secretion of ADH.

The anterior lobe of the pituitary (adenohypophysis) develops from completely separate tissue and has no direct neural connection with the hypothalamus. The adenohypophysis synthesizes and secretes 7 hormones under the control of the hypothalamus. These are:

1. Thyroid stimulating hormone (TSH), which stimulates the synthesis of thyroid hormones.
2. Growth hormone (GH), which has a general affect on somatic growth.
3. Adrenocorticotrophic hormone (ACTH), which acts on the adrenocortical cells.
4. Luteinizing hormone (LH), which in the male stimulates the testes which are responsible for male hormone secretion, and in the female initiates ovulation.
5. Follicle stimulating hormone (FSH), which stimulates growth of the Graafian follicle, oestrogen secretion in the female and spermatogenesis in the male.
6. Prolactin, which is responsible for lactation.
7. Melanocyte stimulating hormone (MSH), a pigment-metabolizing hormone responsible for the dispersal of melanocytes in the fetus.

There are two basic hormonal mechanisms which regulate pituitary functions. The first is a primary effect on target tissues directly, and the second is to stimulate other endocrine glands to secrete their hormones. The pituitary gland has a large functioning reserve and it is estimated that well over half of the gland can be destroyed without causing noticeable dysfunction.

Enlarged lesions (hyperplasia) may produce both destructive changes in the sella turcica and/or pressure symptoms such as visual disturbances, headaches, nausea, vomiting, and elevated CSF pressures, and may mimic those of any brain tumour. Lesions of the pituitary gland will either increase or decrease the production of hormones, which in turn affects the relevant endocrine glands either directly or indirectly. For example, a hyperfunctioning pituitary gland will lead to excessive activity of the thyroid, gonads, and adrenals. Conversely, destructive or degenerative changes in the pituitary gland will result in regressive changes in these glands. These changes will in turn affect the target organs of the respective glands. For example, a pituitary lesion causing the female gonads to regress would result in changes to the target organs of the gonads, such as the uterus and the vagina.

ANTERIOR PITUITARY GLAND (ADENOHYPOPHYSIS) DISORDERS

Hypopituitarism – pituitary insufficiency

In this condition there is a deficiency of one or more pituitary hormones and as a result both the causes and the clinical manifestations are diverse. A deficiency in secretion of all of the pituitary hormones results in a condition known as panhypopituitarism.

Hypopituitarism results in a diminution of secretion of one or more target gland stimulating hormones. The target gland will continue to produce some of its hormone but will not produce sufficient quantities for long-term needs. Therefore, as the primary disorder is of the pituitary, which is responsible for stimulating the target gland, the clinical effects of hyposecretion will take longer to manifest than if the primary disorder was in the target gland. If the primary disorder is in the target gland, the clinical effects of hyposecretion are usually quite graphic.

Aetiology

Hypopituitarism can be caused by damage or destruction of the anterior pituitary, or result from similar damage to the hypothalamus, which itself has a direct affect on the stimulation or inhibition of hormones released by the anterior pituitary. It is often difficult to distinguish whether the cause is primarily pituitary or hypothalmic, as many lesions affect both the hypothalamus and the pituitary gland. The three most common causes of

hypopituitarism are Sheehan's syndrome (necrosis of the pituitary resulting from severe postpartum haemorrhage), chromophobe adenoma, and craniopharyngioma in children. Other causes are:

Infarction. Peripheral vascular collapse (as seen in Sheehan's syndrome), severe anteriolar spasm, ruptured internal carotid artery aneurysm, and small vessel disease can all lead to pituitary ischaemia and infarction. Spontaneous haemorrhage of the pituitary gland is known as pituitary apoplexy.

Tumours. These can be intrasellar tumours such as the chromophobe adenoma, extrasellar tumours such as the craniopharyngioma, or metastatic tumours from breast or lung.

Inflammation. This can be either acute or chronic. The most common causes of chronic inflammation are syphilis, systemic sarcoidosis and tuberculosis. Acute inflammation is usually of bacterial origin and is rare.

Infiltration. This may be due to amyloid or iron deposits in the pituitary gland, as in haemochromatosis, or can be due to an enlargement in the sella turcica causing glandular atrophy.

Trauma. This situation may follow severe head injury especially if a fractured base of skull involves the cribiform plate. In children this is often a result of child abuse, or when an object held in the mouth (such as a pencil) pierces the cribiform plate in a fall.

Iatrogenic. This results from surgical hypophysectomy for pituitary tumours, radiation of the gland, or yttrium implantation.

Idiopathic. In a small percentage of persons presenting with pituitary insufficiency, no cause can be identified.

Clinical manifestations

The onset of signs and symptoms is often insidious and they are often related specifically to the particular hormone(s) that are deficient and their respective target organs. For example, a lack of TSH leads to mild hypothyroidism. Lack of ACTH causes adrenal insufficiency and again the symptoms are not as severe as they would be in primary adrenal insufficiency, but the patient's response to any form of stress is poor. In contrast to the hyperpigmentation that occurs due to an ACTH excess in primary adrenal disease, a deficiency causes a depigmentation and decreased tanning. The only symptom of a prolactin deficiency is failure of postpartum lactation. Lack of FSH and luteinizing hormone results in amenorrhoea in women, and either decreased libido or impotence in men.

On clinical examination the patient with hypopituitarism is often slightly overweight, body and pubic hair may be reduced and there may be atrophy of the genitalia. The skin is pale and smooth with a fine wrinkling, particularly of the face. In severe cases postural hypotension and bradycardia may be present. Hyponatraemia is common and is due to defective water excretion based on deficient levels of thyroid and adrenocortical hormone deficiencies.

In a patient undiagnosed with pituitary insufficiency, stress such as an illness, surgery, or an accident can precipitate a condition known as 'pituitary crisis' where the patient suffers nausea, vomiting, severe dehydration, hypotension and ultimately coma. This is similar to an adrenal crisis (see page 267).

Diagnosis

Sometimes it may be necessary to treat the patient before a conclusive diagnosis can be made. If the patient presents with signs of pituitary crisis this will need treatment before conclusive tests can be performed. These tests include CT brain scan, sellar tomography, air encephalography, and radioimmunoassays of hormone levels.

Medical and nursing management

Depending on the cause of the pituitary insufficiency management of the patient may be conservative or surgical. Medical treatment consists of replacement of the specific hormones related to each deficiency. Consideration is given to the extent of the deficiency, and with the exception of growth hormone, replacement therapy is with synthetic target gland hormones. Observation of the patient during such replacement therapy will be tailored towards monitoring for the effects of the specific hormone(s) being administered. The nurse must remain sensitive to the patient's needs during what can be an emotionally and

physically taxing period. Achieving a delicate and effective balance of hormones can be very tedious for the patient who must undergo numerous tests and experience physical responses to the replacement therapy. If an operable tumour is the cause of the pituitary insufficiency, then nursing care will be as for the patient following craniotomy (see page 222).

Panhypopituitarism

This condition is characterized by an insufficiency in the secretion of all pituitary hormones and, in children, is most graphically demonstrated by growth hormone deficiency.

Clinical manifestations

These will depend on the degree of pituitary failure and to what extent each hormone is involved. Panhypopituitarism in children is usually the result of a congenital abnormality and causes pituitary dwarfism due to a deficiency in growth hormone. Children are normally short in stature but normal in proportion. They often display slow intellectual behaviour and varying degrees of adrenal insufficiency and hypothyroidism. The skin is often pale, due to the absence of melanocyte stimulating hormone (MSH), and fine; and bone and teeth formation is often immature. At adolescence there is failure to develop secondary sex characteristics.

Panhypopituitarism in adults usually results from a slow-growing pituitary tumour and varies from its presentation in children since adults have already completed somatic growth. Clinical manifestations of decreased growth hormones in adults are hypogonadism, impotence, and a decrease in body hair. In women these changes are accompanied by atrophy of the breasts and external genitalia, and amenorrhoea. Both men and women suffer varying degrees of adrenal insufficiencies and hypothyroidism.

Investigative procedures

The clinical features exhibited by the patient will depend upon which of the trophic hormones are deficient. The clinical features of hypopituitarism and dwarfism points strongly towards the diagnosis. X-rays of the skull will enable the identification of a tumour and serum levels of pituitary trophic hormones will be reduced. Random growth hormone sampling is of little value due to the lability of this hormone. If panhypopituitarism is present, then exercising the patient to the point of exhaustion will usually cause an elevated growth hormone level. Inducing hypoglycaemia by the administration of insulin will not produce a rise in the level of growth hormone in the presence of panhypopituitarism.

Medical, surgical, and nursing management

This simply consists of replacement of the deficient hormones. In children, human growth hormone can be administered prior to closure of the epiphyses and is continued until growth is complete. Tumours such as a craniopharyngioma will require surgery and radiation therapy, and nursing management would be the same as for the patient undergoing craniotomy (see page 222) and radiotherapy (see page 125).

Hyperpituitarism

In this condition any or all of the anterior pituitary hormones can be secreted in excess. Hyperplasia of the gland results in hypersecretion of one or more hormones; adenomas are the most common lesions affecting the pituitary gland, and of these the most common are prolactinomas. As prolactin release is under the control of the hypothalamus, and dopamine in particular influences the release of prolactin, the prolactinoma usually causes signs of hypothalamic disturbance as well as pituitary dysfunction.

Prolactinoma

This is a prolactin-producing, pituitary tumour which produces hyperprolactinaemia which results in the signs and symptoms of hypopituitarism as the adenoma replaces normal gland tissue. In women the most common features are galactorrhoea and amenorrhoea, and in men decreased libido and/or impotence.

Aetiology. There are many causes of hyperprolactinaemia and these include hypothalamic/pituitary disorders such as adenoma, drugs such as antidepressants, methyldopa and cimetidine, and primary hypothyroidism. Therefore when diagnosing a prolactinoma other causes of hyperprolactinaemia must be excluded. Information and tests, where appropriate, regarding the patient's fertility, sexual function, any symptoms of hypothyroidism and hypopituitarism, and a history of current and previous drug therapy should be ascertained. When these possible causes have been deleted the most likely cause is then a prolactinoma, particularly if the patient is suffering hypogonadism.

Diagnosis. Basal plasma prolactin levels will be elevated.

Medical, surgical and nursing management. Treatment of prolactinoma can either be medical or surgical. Surgery is either trans-sphenoidal microsurgery or transfrontal craniotomy. Medical treatment is with drugs such as bromocriptine, which is a dopamine antagonist and directly inhibits prolactin secretion by the tumour. Radiation is usually the subsequent form of treatment for those postoperative patients who have persisting prolactinaemia.

Nursing management is as for the patient undergoing craniotomy (see page 222) or radiotherapy (see page 125).

Acromegaly and gigantism

The second most common adenomas are those that secrete growth hormones producing the syndromes known as acromegaly and gigantism. Clinically, these terms refer to an increased production of growth hormone. If this occurs in children before the epiphyses have closed, it results in gigantism. In adults it results in acromegaly. The sexes are affected equally, and the mean age of diagnosis is 40 years. A pituitary adenoma is found to be the cause in 90% of cases.

Clinical manifestations. Hypersecretion of growth hormone stimulates growth of connective tissue, especially cartilage and bone. Overgrowth of skull and facial bone and cartilage causes generalized enlargement of the supra-orbital ridges, nose and ears. The jaw protrudes due to increased length and width of the mandible, and the teeth are often widely spaced. The costal cartilages of the larynx may be affected, causing deepening in the voice. Soft tissue growth leads to an increased size of hands and feet, with fingers and toes becoming thickened, blunt and spade-like. These overall body changes lead to muscle weakness, osteoporosis and eventual osteoarthritis. The increased growth of subcutaneous tissue causes coarse features with a generalized thickening of the skin. This is often accompanied by increased oiliness and sweating, acne, and the formation of skin tags and papillomas. Systemic manifestations may include heat intolerance, weight gain, lethargy, tiredness and an increased sleep requirement. Carpal tunnel syndrome affecting the hands may occur due to compression of nerves by enlarging bones of the wrist, giving rise to troublesome parasthesia. Photophobia may occur in approximately 50% of cases.

Gigantism is identical to acromegaly in its pathophysiology but differs obviously in clinical appearance. An overproduction of growth hormones before closure of the epiphyses causes rapid overgrowth of the long bones. Persons affected commonly attain a height of 2.0–2.5 metres. These people do not develop the overgrowth of peripheries seen in acromegaly, but they do share osteoporosis, muscle weakness and several other clinical aspects.

Both pituitary giants and acromegalics suffer generalized visceromegaly of the liver, spleen, kidneys, myocardium, salivary glands, thyroid and other internal organs. These patients are also prone to coronary atherosclerosis and hypertension, and diabetes mellitus from impaired carbohydrate metabolism as growth hormone is an insulin antagonist. Acromegalics have a carbohydrate intolerance.

Investigative procedures and diagnosis. Both gigantism and acromegaly in their full-blown state are clinically obvious. However, in most cases these conditions run an insidious course over many years and the subtle changes may be missed. For example, a child's excessive growth may be ignored until such time as he has attained a height out of all proportion to his peers. An acromegalic person usually undergoes subtle changes over many years and only by comparison of photo-

graphs taken years apart can the dramatic differences be seen.

Diagnosis of gigantism can be confirmed by elevated levels of growth hormone in the plasma. This, together with the clinical features, strongly suggests the diagnosis in acromegaly. X-rays of the skull may show evidence of a pituitary tumour, enlargement of the paranasal sinuses, prominence of the jaw, and destruction of the sella turcica. CT scanning may show more subtle changes in the pituitary fossa. A glucose tolerance test may be performed. Other conditions which also cause growth hormone hypersecretion must also be excluded. These include diabetes mellitus type 1, cirrhosis of the liver, malnutrition, anorexia nervosa and severe illness.

Medical, surgical and nursing management. The aim of treatment is to restore growth hormone levels to normal and, where possible, to reverse the clinical features by removal or destruction of a tumour, or control of the hypersecretion. Treatment may be conservative or surgical.

Partial or complete trans-sphenoidal hypophysectomy is the treatment of choice and is highly successful resulting in an immediate reduction in growth hormone levels. However, occasionally a craniotomy (see page 222) is required where tumour size prevents a trans-sphenoidal approach. Postoperative patients are reviewed 4–6 weeks post surgery for growth hormone levels and pituitary function. Complications of surgery are rare, but ablation of the gland can result in hypopituitarism.

The response to radiation therapy is slower than that to surgery and is associated with a higher incidence of hypopituitarism. In patients with either small or large tumours, radiation is effective: however, as the response time may take months or even years for reversal of the clinical features of acromegaly, radiotherapy is often secondary to surgery. Trans-sphenoidal implantation of radioactive yttrium seeds is also very effective. Nursing management is as for the patient undergoing radiotherapy (see page 125). Hypopituitarism, visual impairment, oedema and haemorrhage into the pituitary gland, and meningitis are possible complications of therapy.

Medical treatment is usually with a dopamine antagonist such as bromocriptine, which suppresses growth hormone secretion. This treatment is not curative and hypersecretion recurs when treatment ceases, therefore this line of treatment is often secondary to surgery or radiation.

When treatment has been successful bone overgrowth reduces and ultimately ceases, as does tissue overgrowth along with many of the other clinical features. This occurs faster following surgery and can begin within a matter of days postoperatively. Patients who have undergone conservative management often have ongoing twice yearly follow-ups.

POSTERIOR PITUITARY GLAND (NEUROHYPOPHYSIS) DISORDERS

The posterior pituitary gland secretes two hormones, vasopressin and oxytocin.

Vasopressin stimulates the reabsorption of water from the tubular fluid and regulates the concentration of sodium. As its main action is to increase the amount absorbed (which leads to a decreased diuresis), it is often known as the antidiuretic hormone (ADH). It is also a powerful vasoconstrictor. Deficiency of secretion of vasopressin can lead to diabetes insipidus.

Oxytocin, is a hormone which is present in the neurohypophysis of both males and females. Oxytocin stimulates the contraction of smooth muscle, in particular the uterus and breasts. In males, its physiological functions are uncertain. Some evidence suggests that it is released from the neurohypophysis on stimulation of the male genitals and as it is present in increased amounts in the blood on ejaculation it may have a role in maintaining penile erection. An excess of oxytocin has not been described and a deficiency state does not appear to be clinically significant.

Diabetes insipidus

This condition refers to production of excessive amounts of diluted urine in response to an absence of suffcent quantities of vasopressin. It is primarily an endocrine disorder and not a disorder of the kidneys.

Aetiology

Diabetes insipidus can be due to reduced secretions or absence of vasopressin from the posterior pituitary. This occurs in association with surgery to the hypothalamus and pituitary gland, sella tumours, or cerebral trauma or infection. It can also be idiopathic. Nephrogenic diabetes insipidus can occur due to a failure of the kidneys to respond to vasopressin, as in chronic renal failure (see page 595). A clinical state resembling primary diabetes insipidus may occur in the patient prescribed drugs such as lithium carbonate, which reduces the sensitivity of the renal tubule to vasopressin.

Clinical manifestations

The most outstanding sign of diabetes insipidus is polyuria of up to 20 litres per day with an associated insatiable thirst. Life-threatening dehydration can occur, particularly in unconscious patients who are not able to provide their own fluid replacement.

It is important to distinguish this condition from two others which can be confused with primary diabetes insipidus: nephrogenic diabetes insipidus, and psychogenic polydipsia – where the patient is a compulsive water drinker. Inappropriate administration of ADH in the case of the latter condition could lead to circulatory overload and cerebral oedema.

Investigative procedures

Samples of urine and plasma are taken simultaneously to assess osmolarity. In diabetes insipidus the urine will be less concentrated than the plasma, but the plasma osmolarity will be higher than normal. Blood urea will be elevated and hypernatraemia will be a feature.

The patient with primary diabetes insipidus (unlike nephrogenic diabetes insipidus) responds well to the administration of ADH and this confirms the diagnosis.

Medical and nursing management

Rehydration of the patient and correction of electrolyte imbalance is the first goal in the medical management of this condition. The nurse will be responsible for the regulation of the patient's intravenous therapy which will most likely be via the central venous route. Initially large volumes of fluid and added electrolytes will be required until the condition can be chemically controlled by drug therapy.

Diabetes insipidus can be successfully treated with desmopressin acetate (DDAVP: desamino-cys-d-arginine vasopressin) which is an analogue of vasopressin, but has a greater antidiuretic effect and a less vasopressor effect.

DDAVP administered by intranasal spray once or twice daily is usually sufficient to control the symptoms. DDAVP can also be administered parenterally.

26

Disorders of the thyroid gland

Jenny Kidd

The thyroid gland is the largest of all endocrine glands. Microscopically it consists of follicles which are bound together in groups to form lobules. Within each follicle is a substance known as colloid, which is largely made up of proteins, principally thyroglobin. The thyroid gland secretes two types of hormones: thyroxine (T_4) and tri-iodothyronine (T_3), which are involved with iodine metabolism and the regulation of basal metabolic rates; and calcitonin, a hormone which lowers serum calcium and is produced by the parafollicular cells. Thyroxine contains four iodine atoms (T_4) and tri-iodothyronine contains three iodine atoms (T_3), tri-iodothyronine being the more potent of the two hormones. Both T_3 and T_4 are stored in the colloid as part of the thyroglobin molecule and these hormones can be released only when thyroglobin is broken down by specific enzymes.

An adequate dietary intake of iodine is essential as thyroid hormones require large amounts of iodine for their synthesis. Iodine in the diet is largely derived from eggs, sea fish and milk. Iodides are absorbed readily from the stomach and upper small bowel, and as nearly all iodine absorbed is utilized, stored or excreted, only minute quantities are present in the circulation.

The secretion of thyroid hormone is regulated by the hypothalamic–pituitary–thyroid feedback system. In this system, thyroid releasing hormone (TRH) from the hypothalamus controls the release of thyroid stimulating hormone (TSH) from the anterior pituitary gland which in turn regulates the activity of the thyroid gland to produce thyroid hormones, especially thyroxine. The principal functions of the thyroid gland are to concentrate absorbed iodine, and regulate iodine metabolism.

The thyroid gland takes up approximately 10–40% of the body's circulatory iodide and the remainder is excreted in the urine.

All major organs in the body are affected by altered levels of thyroid hormones. Both thyroxine and tri-iodothyronine stimulate growth and regulate the overall basal metabolic rate, lower serum cholesterol, and are involved in normal development of the central nervous system and attainment of sexual maturity.

Disorders of the thyroid gland can be divided into those which relate only to an enlargement of the gland (goitre), and those which cause a change in the amount of thyroid hormone secreted.

GOITRE

The most common disorder of the thyroid gland is enlargement, or goitre. A non-toxic goitre may be caused by iodine insufficiency, congenital defects in hormone synthesis (dyshormonogenesis), certain drugs which cause defects in enzymatic reactions (goitrogens), and autoimmune or chronic thyroiditis (Hashimoto's disease).

When there is iodine insufficiency, there is a reduced output of thyroid hormones, which causes the hypothalamus to prompt the pituitary gland to release relatively large amounts of thyroid stimulating hormone (TSH). The resulting increased activity in the thyroid can lead to hyperplasia of the gland.

Colloid (simple) goitre

This is a benign self-limiting condition often seen during pregnancy or in females during puberty. The condition rarely produces significant neck swelling and does not usually require treatment.

Multinodular goitre

This is usually due to hyperplasia of the gland, and women are more often affected than men. The two most common causes of this type of goitre are iodine deficiency and ingestion of goitrogens such as lithium carbonate. This results in reduced output of thyroid hormone, and thus an increase in the levels of TSH, leading to hyperplasia of the gland. Nodular goitres also occur during puberty and pregnancy when the demand for thyroid hormones is increased.

Endemic goitre

This occurs in those parts of the world where the levels of iodine in the soil are low. In most developed countries this is compensated for by the addition of iodine to table salt or bread. Such areas in Australia are Gippsland and Tasmania.

Familial goitre

This is due to a congenital lack of an enzyme involved in the biosynthesis of thyroid hormone. It may become evident in the newborn or again during puberty or pregnancy when the need for thyroid hormone is increased.

Iatrogenic goitre

This type of goitre can develop through the prolonged administration of iodide and/or thioureas, for example in the management of asthma or chronic bronchitis where iodides are used as expectorants.

Toxic multinodular goitre

This condition arises from a focus within the gland which undergoes hyperfunction and therefore causes the symptoms and signs of thyrotoxicosis (see later).

Clinical manifestations

The gland size increases over a period of months to years and produces neck swelling which is often of a significant size. This may be accompanied by retrosternal spread of the goitre resulting in pressure symptoms: difficulty in swallowing, shortness of breath, and difficulty with speech due to pressure on the recurrent laryngeal nerves.

Most patients presenting with goitres are in fact euthyroid. Enormous goitres can be tolerated with remarkably little disability and often the only problem is cosmetic.

HYPERTHYROIDISM – THYROTOXICOSIS

Hyperthyroidism or thyrotoxicosis results from excessive production of thyroid hormone. It is most frequently seen in women between the ages of 20–40 years. Hyperthyroidism causes an increase in metabolic rate and alterations in body function that are similar to those produced by increased sympathetic nervous system activity. Hyperthyroidism is otherwise known as Graves' disease when hyperthyroidism is accompanied by goitre, and exopthalmus. Less commonly it may be due to toxic multinodular goitre and toxic adenoma of the thyroid. Many of the clinical manifestations of hyperthyroidism are related to increased oxygen consumption and increased utilization of the body's fuels, resulting in an increased metabolic rate and an increase in the activity of the sympathetic nervous system.

Clinical manifestations

The patient often displays restless, irritable, and hyperkinetic behaviour and has difficulty sleeping. Other symptoms include palpitations and tachycardia, increased appetite but accompanying weight loss, diarrhoea and fine tremor of the hands. The patient also suffers heat intolerance, increased skin temperature and sweating. The skin is often thin and soft, the hair fine and silky and the blood cholesterol levels are decreased.

The onset of clinical manifestations of hyperthyroidism are often insidious and the disorder may have been present for some time before a diagnosis is made.

Diagnosis is aided by classical clinical states and a raised sleeping pulse. Diagnosis is confirmed by an elevated T_4 and elevated T_3 resin uptake. Radioactive iodine uptake will also be increased.

Graves' disease

This is an extremely common form of thyrotoxicosis and is thought to affect approximately 1% of the adult population.

Aetiology

Graves' disease is an autoimmune disease. A specific pathological immunoglobulin has been isolated from the lymphocytes both within and outside the thyroid gland in patients with Graves' disease. This immunoglobulin is a long acting thyroid stimulator and antibody to the TSH receptor thereby stimulating the thyroid to produce thyroxine.

The mechanism that causes this to occur is unknown. Some cases have occurred following viral thyroiditis, and patients with Graves' disease often have other associated autoimmune disorders such as pernicious anaemia, Addison's disease, Hashimoto's disease and insulin-dependent diabetes mellitus.

Clinical manifestations

In addition to the state of hyperfunction, patients with Graves' disease demonstrate varying degrees of opthalmic involvement which bears no relationship to the excess levels of T_3 and T_4.

The eye involvement can be unilateral or bilateral. Exopthalmus is the most obvious feature and gives the patient an unfortunate staring or startled appearance.

The exopthalmus is often associated with lid retraction and in severe cases, corneal exposure, optic neuritis due to pressure of the optic nerve, and retinal vascular necrosis which can lead to blindness.

Medical, surgical, and nursing management of the patient with thyrotoxicosis

Management of the patient is largely directed towards controlling the hyperthyroidism. Three avenues of treatment exist: antithyroid drug therapy, radioactive iodine therapy and surgery.

Antithyroid drug therapy

In general this is indicated in young patients with mild disease. Drug therapy is principally from the thiourea derivatives, the most common of which are: carbimazole or methimazole or propylthiouricil.

Initially it may be necessary to give these drugs 6–8 hourly to gain control quickly in view of their short half life. Once the patient is euthyroid, daily doses are sufficient together with appropriate replacement of T_3 or T_4 daily. Drug therapy usually spans a 12–18 month period and relapse occurs in approximately 40–50% of cases.

The side-effects of antithyroid drugs include: skin rashes, drug fever, arthralgia, hypothyroidism and agranulocytosis. This is usually reversible when the drug is ceased but the development of a sore throat in patients receiving antithyroid drug therapy is a classic indication of agranulocytosis, and patients must be informed of the immediate reporting of such an occurrence.

Radioactive iodine therapy

Radioactive iodine (^{131}I or ^{125}I) is the treatment of choice for patients in whom surgery is inappropriate, or where medical treatment has failed. However, there is some risk of mutagenic effects, so its use is often restricted to patients unlikely to bear (more) children.

The therapeutic dose of radio-iodine will render the patient euthyroid in 2–4 weeks. Thyroid replacement must be commenced in 4–6 weeks and continued for life. The only contraindication for the administration of radioactive iodine is pregnancy.

Surgery

A subtotal thyroidectomy is the treatment of choice for patients with very large goitres, multinodular goitres, or malignancy. Preoperatively the patient receives antithyroid drugs for approximately 6 weeks to render them euthyroid.

This may be followed by a 10 day course of Lugol's iodine which reduces the size and vascularity of the gland, thus facilitating surgery and reducing the potential problem of haemorrhage. Lugol's iodine is often more palatable disguised in milk or fruit juice.

An electrocardiogram is taken to assess the patient's cardiac status and blood taken for grouping and cross typing.

An explanation is given to the patient regarding the position of the wound, and any other equipment, such as an IV line, which is likely to be in situ. On return from theatre the patient is nursed in a semi-recumbent position with his head and neck well supported with pillows.

Immediately on return from theatre the patient's neck is assessed for swelling and the position, number and type of drain tubes in situ. This observation of the degree of swelling can then be used as a baseline for future comparison. A full set of vital signs is taken again as a baseline as the main purpose of post anaesthetic observations in these patients is to enable early detection of possible complications, the principle one being reactionary haemorrhage. The patient must receive adequate analgesia to enable him to turn his head. Initially the patient may feel loath to do this due to the pain and uncomfortable position of the wound and dressings. It is helpful if the things the patient requires, such as mouth wash, tissues, and buzzer are within reach and do not require unnecessary strain on the operative area. Return to food and fluids should be gradual and preceded by an antiemetic as vomiting will cause the patient a great deal of pain and discomfort. The drain tubes will usually be removed after a 24–48 hour period, and the sutures in 5–7 days.

The patient can sit out of bed the following day and begin gentle ambulation, and proceed to a complete recovery.

Complications

Reactionary haemorrhage may occur during a 12–24 hour period postoperatively. The haemorrhage may be concealed or overt. Local signs may include increasing neck swelling, difficulty in swallowing, and the patient may complain of a lump in his throat. If the bleeding continues these symptoms will progress to dyspnoea, respiratory stridor, and difficulty with speech. These signs are often accompanied by systemic signs of haemorrhage which include restlessness, pallor, sweating, and tachycardia. It is of vital importance that the nurse be aware of the significance of any of the above signs and symptoms as this situation is life threatening for the patient. Where possible, and where time and circumstances permit, the patient should be transported to the operating room for cautery of bleeding points. However where this is not practical the nurse must take the initiative. This involves cutting the skin, subcutaneous, and muscle sutures and removing the clot. Gentle pressure may need to be applied to any overt bleeding points. This will be life saving and will resolve the problems of respiratory difficulty.

Arrangements are then made for the patient to return to theatre for cautery and resuturing. A tracheostomy tray in some hospitals is routinely kept at the bedside to enable immediate access to equipment that may be needed in such an emergency.

Respiratory obstruction. This complication usually only results when reactionary haemorrhage has been undetected or untreated and the pressure of the blood and clot is sufficient to compress the trachea resulting in respiratory obstruction.

Hoarse voice. If the recurrent laryngeal nerve is severed, damaged or bruised during the surgery this can result in a partial or complete loss of voice. The patient may have a hoarse voice for 24 hours to a few days which will spontaneously return to normal; or if the damage is more severe, the patient may be left with a 'gravelly' voice.

Tetany. This condition is manifest initially by a tingling or paraesthesia of the mouth, fingers and toes and can develop into carpopedal spasm. It can begin with facial twitching and extend to spasm of the muscles of the throat causing laryngeal spasm and extreme dyspnoea in addition to spasm of the hands and feet.

It results from accidental removal or damage to the parathyroid glands during thyroid surgery which causes a lowering of the serum calcium (see Chapter 27). Tetany in its full blown state is an extreme emergency and is treated with intravenous calcium 10 ml 10% solution and subsequent calcium supplements.

Atrial fibrillation. This can occur in a patient who may have had cardiac arrythmias prior to surgery, or whose heart has been affected by the thyrotoxicosis.

Hypothyroidism. This is a long term complication and can occur due to inadequate follow up postoperatively when a large portion of the gland has been excised. It is simply and effectively treated by oral thyroxine for life.

Thyroid crisis – thyroid storm. This is a rare but acute exacerbation of all the symptoms of hyperthyroidism. It may be precipitated by emotional stress, or physical stress such as general surgery, inadequate preparation for the thyroidectomy, following radioactive iodine therapy, poorly controlled thyrotoxicosis during pregnancy, uncontrolled diabetes, myocardial infarction, or severe trauma or infection.

Clinical manifestations of thyroid crisis include extreme hypertension, tachycardia, life threatening arrythmias, atrial fibrillation and eventual vasomotor collapse. Other symptoms include severe gastrointestinal disturbances and dehydration, delirium, agitation, and extreme hyperpyrexia.

Unless the condition is promptly brought under control it will result in coma and death.

Treatment is aimed at control of the severe cardiovascular problems, hormone release and synthesis, and symptomatic relief. Hormone release is retarded by the administration of potassium iodide and hormone synthesis is blocked by administration of propylthiourical.

Symptomatic therapy includes tepid sponging, cooling sheets, and the administration of antipyretic agents such as panadol. Aspirin is contraindicated.

During the management of thyroid crisis it is essential to identify and treat the underlying disease process that caused the exacerbation.

A range of antihypertensive drugs can be used to lower the blood pressure and propranolol is used to control the atrial fibrillation. Oxygen, diuretics, and digoxin are useful for any associated heart failure.

Specific nursing management of the patient with thyrotoxicosis

When admitted to hospital these patients, due to the metabolic nature of their condition, are often anxious and hyperactive.

Rest is of primary importance as the myocardium is already stressed and in a state of permanent tachycardia, and may fail under additional stress.

It is ideal for the patient to rest in bed, and mild sedation may be of use to assist him to rest during the day and sleep at night. A fan and tepid sponging and change of linen may be required to make the patient more comfortable.

Excessive visiting should be restricted in order to maximize the patient's resting time. If he has exopthalmos it may be necessary to instil artificial tears. Minor eye involvement requires no treatment. If the patient is photophobic, a darkened room may be therapeutic and reduce discomfort.

In cases of severe intraocular involvement corticosteroids such as prednisolone can be of benefit, and sometimes treatment consists of surgical orbital decompression via a transantral approach.

HYPOTHYROIDISM

Hypothyroidism exists where the thyroid gland fails to secrete enough thyroid hormone.

Cretinism

Hypothyroidism can occur as a congenital defect known as cretinism caused by lack of thyroid hormone before or after birth. If untreated during the first months of life it will cause mental retardation and severe growth impairment.

The causes of cretinism are thyroid aplasia, a congenital or hereditary deficiency in one of the thyroid enzymes necessary for hormone production, and inadequate intake of iodine during pregnancy.

Clinical manifestations of cretinism become rapidly apparent in the child as he literally fails to thrive both physically and mentally. Due to slow bony development the child cannot sit up unassisted and often has an enlarged head. The neck is short and thick and the tongue enlarged and often protruding. The nose is short and flattened in appearance and the eyes wideset. The child has a protruding abdomen, thickened dry skin, and sparse hair growth.

Diagnosis is made on the typical clinical picture and supporting history. Diagnosis can be confirmed by depressed levels of thyroxine.

When promptly recognized and effectively treated with 1-thyroxine the condition can be reversed and subsequently controlled providing irreparable damage has not occurred.

Myxoedema

Aetiology

When the deficiency of thyroxine occurs later in life it is known as myxoedema and is caused by a variety of pathological processes which destroy the structure and function of the thyroid gland.

It can occur as a result of chronic autoimmune thyroiditis (Hashimoto's disease); destruction of the gland with radioactive iodine, or excessive removal of the gland during thyroidectomy; and ingestion of goitrogens such as para-aminosalacylic acid (PAS) used in the treatment of tuberculosis; lithium, and iodine preparations. It can also be caused by idiopathic atrophy of the gland, iodine deficiency, or extensive amyloid deposits.

Myxoedema affects most organs in the body resulting in a hypometabolic state. There is also an accumulation of a mucopolysaccharide substance in the interstitial spaces which attracts water, causing a mucus type non-pitting oedema that is characteristic of many of the clinical manifestations of myxoedema.

Clinical manifestations

The patient suffers gradual onset of fatigue, with weight gain despite a reduced appetite. There is also a reduced tolerance to cold together with reduced sweating. The skin becomes dry and rough and the hair coarse and dry. Gastrointestinal motility is reduced resulting in increased flatulance, abdominal distension, and constipation occasionally accompanied by faecal impaction.

The patient is mentally slow, with a poor memory and inability to concentrate. The face is often puffy especially around the eyes, due to oedema. The tongue has a swollen appearance and the voice is deepened and sometimes hoarse and husky. There is decreased cardiac output and bradycardia, and blood cholesterol levels are elevated, thus accelerating the development of atherosclerosis, folic acid anaemia, iron deficiency anaemia; pernicious anaemia may also present due to decreased intestinal absorption of vitamin B_{12}.

Diagnosis

Elevated serum TSH, low serum levels of T_4, and low resin T_3 uptake are characteristic of primary hypothyroidism. The clinical picture is usually quite clear.

Medical management

Levothyroxine is the drug of choice in the treatment of hypothyroidism and due to its long half life of approximately 8 days need only be administered once daily. Only 40–60% of the drug is absorbed. Dosage ranges are dependent upon age and body weight.

Blood levels of free thyroxine index and TSH are measured every 4–6 weeks until a suitable balance is reached, and subsequently once a year. Patients receive replacement therapy for life.

Myxoedemic coma

This condition is the result or end stage of untreated hypothyroidism. It occurs most frequently in older patients particularly those with underlying vascular and/or pulmonary disease.

The onset is usually gradual, characterized by progressive lethargy, stupor, severe hypothermia with temperatures as low as 25°C, hypoventilation leading to carbon dioxide retention, and hypoxia, hypoglycaemia, hyponatraemia, water intoxication, shock and death. Patients who develop myxoedemic coma are often obese with other underlying predisposing factors such as heart failure, pulmonary oedema, anaemia, pleural or peritoneal effusions. Myxoedema coma can occur as a result of the administration of sedatives or narcotics.

Medical and nursing management

Myxoedemic coma is an acute medical emergency and as such patients should be admitted to intensive care for intubation and assisted ventilation with regular monitoring of blood gases. Water restriction and sodium replacement is important.

Intravenous fluids should be administered with caution. The patient should be warmed slowly, so as to prevent peripheral vasodilation and increased shock, whilst a constant check is kept on the patient's temperature.

Thyroxine is administered intravenously beginning with an initial loading dose followed by daily intravenous doses until the patient's condition stabilizes.

A loading dose of hydrocortisone is also given, followed by a maintenance dose IV 6 hourly.

Signs of improvement in the general condition of the patient are particularly those of a rise in body temperature and a return to normal cerebral function.

The success of the treatment overall depends upon how well the underlying disease is controlled.

27

Disorders of the parathyroid glands

Jenny Kidd

The parathyroid glands are small, oval shaped, encapsulated glands. Approximately 80% of people have 4 parathyroid glands, with nearly all others having a varying number from 2–6 glands.

The glands are approximately 4–6 mm in length, 2–4 mm in width, 0.5–2 mm in thickness. The parathyroids are situated in pairs, the superior pair at the level of the lower position of the cricoid cartilage and the inferior pair beneath the thyroid gland itself.

The function of the parathyroid glands is to secrete parathormone (PTH), which is the principle regulator of serum calcium levels, and therefore the calcium content of bone. Vitamin D and calcitonin are also involved in the regulation of serum calcium. Parathormone is not stored in the parathyroids but is synthesized and secreted continuously. Its stimulus for synthesis is a decrease in serum calcium levels.

Parathormone elevates the serum calcium levels by causing:

1. Resorption of calcium from the bone
2. Increasing reabsorption of filtered calcium in the renal tubules
3. Increasing the absorption of calcium in the gut
4. Increasing the activation of vitamin D.

The serum levels of calcium are inversely related to the serum phosphate levels and an elevation in one causes a lowering of the other, thereby maintaining a constant balance of the two. The serum level of calcium is controlled by a negative feedback mechanism. Very simply, a decrease in serum calcium stimulates an increase in parathormone and vice versa.

Normal serum calcium depends on regular and adequate dietary intake of calcium, stable para-thyroid function, and levels of vitamin D and calcitonin.

Calcium and phosphate

Calcium and phosphate enter the body through the gastrointestinal tract. Calcium is poorly absorbed and phosphate absorbed extremely well. The kidney controls calcium and phosphate losses by selective reabsorption. The amount of phosphate lost in the urine is directly related to phosphate concentration in the blood. Calcium excretion is inversely related to phosphate excretion.

Vitamin D enhances the absorption of calcium from the gastrointestinal tract by acting directly on the calcium transport mechanism across the intestinal wall, and aids in both the depositing and mobilization of calcium and phosphate into and out of bone.

Calcitonin

This is secreted by the parafollicular cells in the thyroid gland. The secretion of calcitonin is inversely proportional to serum calcium levels. Calcitonin inhibits calcium mobilization from bone, thereby lowering the serum calcium. Its release is stimulated by hypercalcaemia.

Hypocalcaemia

The causes of a low serum calcium include: impaired ability to mobilize calcium from the bone, abnormal loss of calcium by the kidney, and decreased absorption of calcium from the gastrointestinal tract.

The ability to mobilize calcium from bone stores is impaired in hypoparathyroidism due to a parathormone deficiency or surgical removal of the parathyroid glands. Intestinal reabsorption of calcium is decreased when vitamin D is deficient. This can occur in malabsorption syndromes such as coeliac disease (see page 505). Vitamin D is stored in its inactivated form and is activated by the liver and kidneys. Patients with renal failure have problems with the absorption of calcium due to impaired activation of vitamin D.

Altered function of the parathyroid glands can be divided into hyperfunction and hypofunction.

HYPOPARATHYROIDISM

This condition results in decreased levels of parathormone.

Aetiology

The most common cause of hypoparathyroidism is accidental removal of the glands during thyroidectomy or after parathyroid gland surgery, following removal of a functioning parathyroid adenoma. This latter form of parathyroidism is usually transient.

Parathyroid function may also be impaired due to treatment of thyroid disorder with radioactive iodine.

Less commonly, hypoparathyroidism can be ideopathic. It is not clear why the parathyroids may be absent or atrophied, but it may be due to imperfect development of the parathyroids in utero. Transient hypoparathyroidism with symptoms of hypocalaemia may occur in babies who have a high phosphate diet, such as cow's milk, or those born to mothers with hyperparathyroidism where parathyroid activity has been suppressed in utero by the mother's hypercalcaemia. Rarely, it can be due to a congenital absence of the parathyroid glands.

It is thought that acquired ideopathic hypoparathyroidism may result from autoimmune processes, especially as it is sometimes associated with pernicious anaemia, Addison's disease, and chronic thyroiditis all of which are suspected to be autoimmune disorders.

Clinical manifestations

The dominant and most characteristic clinical features are those due to hypocalcaemia and hyperphosphataemia. Hypocalcaemia induces symptoms of tetany, which include increased neuromuscular activity in the form of parasthesiae, such as numbness and tingling of the mouth and extremities, carpopedal spasm (Trousseau's sign), and generalized muscle cramps.

Facial neuromuscular activity can be stimulated by tapping the facial nerve in the parotid gland just above the angle of the jaw, with a resultant twitching of the lips nose or eye. It can involve the whole of one side of the face. This is known as Chvostek's sign.

In an extreme tetanic attack the hyperreflexion and carpopedal spasm can be accompanied by laryngeal spasm, stridor, and convulsions which may result in fatal hypoxia. Other clinical manifestations include psychological disturbances, epilepsy, brittle nails, dry scaly skin, rashes, and cataract formation. These symptoms often accompany mild hypocalcaemia.

Diagnosis

Diagnosis of hypoparathyroidism can be made on the biochemical findings of hypocalcaemia and hyperphosphataemia, and the clinical syndrome of tetany.

Other causes of hypocalcaemia, for example low dietary calcium, must be excluded.

Medical and nursing management

Treatment with parathyroid extract is expensive; therefore, chronic hypoparathyroidism is usually treated by calciferol or one of its analogues.

These compounds are used individually or sometimes with calcium supplementation. The success of this treatment is measured by the serum calcium level.

Oral vitamin D and calcium supplements usually restore the serum calcium to normal. However, a degree of hyperphosphataemia may persist and if so aluminium hydroxide may be given to bind phosphate in the gut. Milk should not be used as a source of calcium due to its high phosphate content.

Management of tetany

An acute attack of tetany is a medical emergency and is best treated by intravenous calcium chloride solution, administered slowly. This may need to be repeated if symptoms do not readily subside.

During the management of hypoparathyroidism signs of hypercalcaemia should be observed for, as overuse of calcium may lead to renal calculi.

Pseudohypoparathyroidism

This condition characteristically presents with the biochemical and clinical features of ideopathic hypoparathyroidism with some additional features.

It is believed to be a familial disorder characterized by an end-organ unresponsiveness to parathormone and therefore an inability to increase serum calcium levels.

The additional somatic features, which may not all present in the one patient, are short stocky stature, obesity with a round face, mental retardation, and short metacarpal and metatarsal bones, particularly the 4th and 5th bones.

Biochemical analysis shows a low serum calcium and an elevated serum phosphate, with normal or elevated serum parathormone levels. Treatment is usually with calciferol.

HYPERPARATHYROIDISM

Hyperparathyroidism may be primary, secondary, or tertiary.

Primary hyperparathyroidism

Hyperparathyroidism is associated with increased levels of parathormone and subsequently an increase in serum calcium.

Aetiology

This condition most commonly results from adenoma of the parathyroid glands (approximately 80%), less commonly from hyperplasia, and rarely from carcinoma. Adenomas are benign tumours which are usually small in size and can occur in either sex at any age. They are difficult to locate surgically due to their small size. In a small percentage of patients with adenoma there is an association with a second endocrine tumour such as phaeochromocytoma or thyroid carcinoma.

Primary hyperplasia usually occurs as a secondary response to chronic hypocalcaemia and the result is an increase in the size of the parathyroid glands. Carcinoma of the parathyroid glands is often difficult to distinguish from adenoma. The diagnosis of parathyroid carcinoma is made if there appears to be local invasion beyond the capsule, evidence of metastasis, or local recurrence of the neoplasm following resection.

Investigative procedures

In primary hyperparathyroidism the serum calcium level is elevated, usually with a low serum phosphate. However the phosphate levels can be normal or even raised, particularly if renal damage has occurred.

Serum alkaline phosphatase can be elevated if there is radiological evidence of bone disease.

Serum parathormone can be measured by radioimmune assay – and raised serum parathormone levels, together with hypercalcaemia is only found in primary hyperparathyroidism.

X-rays of the skeleton may demonstrate demineralization or bony cysts as found in osteitis fibrosa cystica.

Secondary hyperparathyroidism

Chronic hypocalcaemia, irrespective of its cause, will induce parathormone secretion and eventually lead to secondary hyperparathyroidism.

Aetiology

Diseases such as chronic renal failure, chronic glomerulonephritis, and chronic pyelonephritis are common causes. In these conditions there is often a hyperphosphataemia due to the kidneys' inability to excrete phosphate. This results in an associated hypocalcaemia which stimulates parathyroid hyperplasia and hyperfunction and there-fore parathormone secretion is increased.

Hypocalcaemia and secondary hyperparathy-roidism may also result from vitamin D defi-ciency, and malabsorption syndromes preventing adequate absorption of calcium and vitamin D.

Investigative procedures

Classical findings are:

• Low serum calcium, but occasionally it may be normal due to compensatory parathormone secretion.
• Raised or normal serum phosphate
• Raised serum alkaline phosphatase
• Raised serum parathormone which is often quite marked
• Evidence of demineralization and osteomalacia in skeletal X-ray.

In summary, primary and secondary hyperpar-athyroidism present with similar clinical manifes-tations, but biochemically they are quite different.

Primary hyperparathyroidism is classically char-acterized by hypercalcaemia and hypercalciuria. In secondary hyperparathyroidism the serum calcium levels are low and the phosphate levels conversely high or sometimes normal.

It is interesting to note that hyperparathy-roidism is not the most common cause of hyper-calcaemia. The most common cause in adults is metastatic breast carcinoma where the tumour has eroded the bone, causing release of calcium into the blood stream.

Other causes of hypercalcaemia include hyper-thyroidism, milk alkali syndrome, sarcoidosis, and immobilization.

Tertiary hyperparathyroidism

This results from secondary hyperparathyroidism of long standing, leading to continuous stimu-lation of parathormone. It is most commonly seen after long term haemodialysis and post renal transplantation (see page 604). It can be prevented by adequate treatment of secondary hyperparathy-roidism but successful treatment is usually only achieved by total parathyroidectomy.

Clinical manifestations of hyperparathyroidism

Both primary and secondary hyperparathyroidism have virtually the same clinical manifestations, with those of primary disease being more marked. Hypercalcaemia is the most common presentation, but very often the patient is asymptomatic and the condition is discovered during routine blood screening for calcium which is routinely included in laboratory screening of patients. The onset may be insidious with the patient complaining of weak-ness and lethargy and sometimes of accompanying bouts of renal colic and renal calculi. However, the onset may also be very rapid with high levels of calcium accompanied by nausea, vomiting, and lethargy and the patient has brittle bones which are prone to fracture. Clinical manifestations can be viewed according to those produced by the effects of parathormone excess and those produced by the hypercalcaemia.

Effects of parathormone excess

Skeletal involvement. The severity of the para-thormone excess will determine the extent of bony alterations. Progressive calcium loss resulting in demineralization of the bone results in bone pain, and deformities, kyphosis, vertebral collapse, pathological fractures, and osteomalacia.

Continued and severe demineralization results in a condition known as osteitis fibrosa cystica representing extreme skeletal damage.

The magnitude of bony alterations are more pronounced in primary hyperparathyroidism than the bony changes that occur in secondary hyperparathyroidism.

Renal involvement. Due to hypercalciuria, deposits of calcium occur in and around the renal tubules, resulting in the condition nephrocalci-nosis. Renal calculi can also develop with associ-ated renal colic.

Gastrointestinal involvement. Gastric and duodenal ulcers can occur due to an increase in gastric acid secretion. Excess parathormone levels with hyper-calcaemia stimulate gastric acid secretion.

Effects of hypercalcaemia

A raised serum calcium level inhibits the action of antidiuretic hormone on the distal tubules and collecting ducts of the kidneys; this produces a syndrome similar to diabetes insipidus, with polyuria, polydypsia, and eventually dehydration. Atony of skeletal muscles produces weakness and lethargy and cardiac arrythmias are common. Calcium levels of greater than 3 mg/l produce symptoms of a myopathy such as tiredness and muscle weakness. Atony of gut smooth muscle results in nausea, vomiting, and constipation and occasionally paralytic ileus. Calcium levels of greater than 4 mg/l produce drowsiness, confusion, and disorientation which progress to coma and death.

Any of these signs and symptoms can be associated with any other cause of hypercalcaemia.

Medical, surgical, and nursing management of hyperparathyroidism

Surgical removal of the parathyroid glands is indicated when there is renal or bone involvement or when the patient has symptoms related to hypercalcaemia. The surgery is difficult to perform and is often compounded by the number and location of the parathyroid glands. The surgery consists of removal of an adenoma, or subtotal excision or total resection followed by radiotherapy in cases of carcinoma. Excessive serum calcium should be controlled preoperatively to avoid a hypercalcaemic crisis. Postoperatively, the patient usually develops a transient hypocalcaemia, which can be severe. The nurse must observe the patient closely for signs of hypocalcaemia (see page 247) and Trousseau's sign (carpal spasm in response to induced ischaemia of the arm).

Postoperative treatment with IV infusions of calcium may be required, and life-long vitamin D and calcium supplements will be necessary.

In patients in whom surgery is contraindicated, drug therapy may be successful. For example, oestrogens inhibit bone reabsorption influenced by parathormone, and diuretics such as frusemide enhance calcium excretion.

If the patient's calcium level requires lowering, this can be achieved by the administration of phosphate intravenously over a 6–8 hour period. Calcitonin can also be used but is expensive and requires a daily injection.

28

Pancreatic disorders

Jenny Kidd

The pancreas has both endocrine and exocrine functions and the two principle hormones produced by the pancreas are insulin and glucagon.

INSULIN

Insulin is synthesized as a precursor molecule called pro-insulin in the beta cells of the pancreas. The pro-insulin molecules are incorporated into granules and converted to insulin. The insulin is stored within the granules in amounts of up to 10 times that of the average daily requirement.

The release of insulin is principally brought about by a raised blood glucose level. When the blood glucose rises above 4.5 mmol/l, insulin is released and new insulin synthesized. Insulin release also has been shown to require calcium. Substances which increase the response of the beta cells to glucose are gastrointestinal hormones, the release of which is stimulated by the ingestion of food, to the extent that the ingestion of a meal induces a greater insulin response than does intravenous glucose. These hormones include gastrin, cholecystokinin, and secretin. Substances which inhibit insulin release include catecholamines and some drugs such as colchicine and phenytoin sodium.

Action of insulin

Insulin is an anabolic hormone. The principle action of insulin is to decrease the blood concentration of glucose by actively transporting glucose into the cell. It is the only hormone that lowers blood glucose, in contrast to those hormones that raise blood glucose (for example, glucagon, glucocorticoids, adrenalin, and growth hormone).

Insulin is necessary for glycogen formation, glucose conversion to triglycerides, nucleic acid synthesis, and protein synthesis.

Carbohydrate metabolism

Normal blood glucose ranges between 4.2–6.4 mmol/l. Very little glucose moves into cells by simple diffusion. Insulin stimulates the assisted diffusion of glucose both into and out of cells which involves a carrier molecule located in the cell membrane. This process, which accounts for most of the body's uptake of glucose, occurs in skeletal muscle, cardiac muscle, and adipose tissue. The cells of the liver and central nervous system receive their glucose by simple diffusion and therefore rely completely on adequate blood glucose. Erythrocytes, gastrointestinal cells, and cells of the kidney receive their glucose by an active pump mechanism in association with sodium which is also not influenced by insulin.

Protein metabolism

Insulin stimulates both protein synthesis and the active transport of amino acids in the cells. Protein breakdown for energy production is normally inhibited by the fact that insulin causes increased utilization of glucose for energy and therefore has a protein-sparing effect.

Fat metabolism

Insulin increases both the uptake and oxidation of glucose by adipose tissue. It also has a fat-sparing effect as a result of direct stimulation of lipogenesis in adipose tissue, increasing the storage of fats.

Potassium

Insulin is also necessary for the maintenance of extracellular potassium ion concentration.

GLUCAGON

Glucagon is synthesized in the alpha cells of the islets of Langerhans involving an initial precursor molecule called pro-glucagon. The hormone glucagon is actually formed and subsequently stored within the cell granules of the cytoplasm. The mechanism of release is mainly by the process of exocytosis.

Action of glucagon

Glucagon also acts on the metabolism of carbohydrate, protein, and fat. Its main action is to raise the level of blood glucose.

The release of glucagon is stimulated by hypoglycaemia.

Glucagon and insulin appear to work together under the control of the sympathetic nervous system in a 'push–pull' relationship. In order to regulate blood glucose levels, for example, sympathetic stimulation inhibits insulin release but increases glucagon release. Acetylcholine, however, stimulates the release of both insulin and glucagon.

DIABETES MELLITUS

The word 'diabetes' is derived from a Greek word signifying a syphon, which highlights two of the primary symptoms of diabetes – polyuria and polydypsia. Diabetes mellitus is a syndrome representing a multifactorial group of disorders, where both genetic and environmental factors (such as a high carbohydrate diet) play a part in this disordered metabolism. Diabetes mellitus is also thought to be autoimmune in origin (see page 784).

It is characterized by a partial or complete lack of insulin which results in impaired use of carbohydrate, and altered metabolism of fats and protein.

Incidence

Approximately 1.5%–2% of the population of the industrialized world suffers from diabetes, with a higher incidence of up to 15% in some groups such as Jews of middle European origin, Australian Aboriginals, South Pacific Islanders, and North American Indians. A proportion of the 2% of diabetics are undiagnosed.

Diabetes is classified into primary diabetes (which is further divided into Type I – insulin dependent diabetes – and Type II – non insulin dependent diabetes) and secondary diabetes.

Secondary diabetes mellitus

This occurs as a result of altered metabolism which results in hyperglycaemia. These conditions include: growth hormone excess – acromegally; cortisol excess, Cushing's syndrome; and catecholamine excess – phaeochromocytoma. Pancreatitis, haemochromatosis, and carcinoma of the pancreas can also cause secondary diabetes.

Primary diabetes mellitus

Primary diabetes is classified into either Type I and Type II diabetes, due to different genetic factors and differences in clinical manifestations.

Type I – insulin dependent diabetes mellitus. This is a severe form of diabetes which is associated with ketoacidosis in its untreated form. It accounts for approximately 25–35% of all diabetic cases. It has been suggested that genetic influences are less marked in Type I diabetes than in Type II diabetes. This results from studies of monozygotic twins: only 50% of people who have identical twins who suffer from Type I diabetes will develop the disease; this also suggests that environmental influences may contribute towards the diabetes in these cases. In contrast, the identical twin of a Type II diabetic patient will nearly always develop the disease within one year of the onset of diabetes in the sibling.

Type I diabetes is strongly associated with an increased frequency of certain HLA antigens (see page 782). These antigens are found on the surfaces of all cells (except erythrocytes and sperm) and they allow the immune system to recognize homologous tissue and detect foreign antigens. Environmental factors are still not clear, however it is believed that Type I diabetes mellitus can result from damage of a toxic or infectious nature to the beta cells of the pancreas in genetically predisposed persons. Causes include viruses such as Coxsackie B4, variola, rubella, and toxic chemical agents such as some rat poisons.

Circulating islet cell antibodies have been detected in 85% of Type I diabetics during the first weeks of onset, which adds support to the theory that autoimmune mechanisms may contribute to the progressive destruction of the beta cells of the pancreas. Circulating islet cell antibodies are virtually absent in nondiabetics.

Type II – non insulin dependent diabetes mellitus. This represents the majority of all diabetic cases. It occurs predominantly in adults, but can occur in childhood.

It is a nonketotic form of diabetes with no clear HLA genetic markers, no islet cell antibodies, and patients are usually not dependent on synthetic insulin to sustain life, as insulin is produced by the pancreas, but not in quantities to maintain normal glucose transport.

Genetic factors are of much greater importance in Type II diabetes and often a family history of diabetes can be obtained. Obesity, frequently present in Type II diabetics, reduces insulin receptor concentration and diminishes insulin effectiveness in a number of target tissues which together raise the blood glucose level.

Pathophysiology

Due to the partial or complete absence of insulin, blood glucose will rise to a level which exceeds the renal threshold (180 mg per 100 ml blood) which results in glucose being excreted in the urine. Because of the osmotic effect of glucose, this results in polyuria which in turn results in dehydration and polydypsia. There is an overall increase in protein breakdown for energy, which raises the amino acid levels. These amino acids are deaminated and the residues of the glucogenic amino acids contribute to the formation of glucose, which further exacerbates the hyperglycaemia. The protein depletion adds to the weight loss typical of this condition. Fats are also broken down, resulting in raised blood levels of free fatty acids and glycerol, and the level of blood cholesterol may rise. An excess of acetyl co-enzyme A in the liver is converted to acetoacetic acid, which is in turn reduced to form acetone – commonly termed 'ketone bodies'. Some of the accumulated acetyl co-enzyme A is converted to excess synthesis of cholesterol adding to the hypercholesterolaemia. These ketone bodies are produced in excess resulting in a ketometabolic acidosis and ketonuria. This increased utilization of fat also contributes to the overall weight loss in diabetes.

Type I diabetes in its undiagnosed, untreated state can rapidly give rise to a ketoacidosis which can be severe and life threatening. In Type II diabetes ketoacidosis is not prevalent, as there is always some circulating insulin.

Diagnosis

There are several classifications of diabetic patients.

Latent diabetic. A patient who has received therapy such as corticosteriods, which provoked the condition; but the glucose tolerance has subsequently returned to normal.

Potential diabetic. This term is used to describe the children of two diabetic parents where the child has a normal glucose tolerance.

Chemical diabetic. The patient has hyperglycaemia but is asymptomatic.

Clinical diabetic. The patient has hyperglycaemia with symptoms and may have other complications of the disease.

A blood glucose level, taken 2 hours after a meal or the ingestion of 50 g of dextrose, which exceeds 11 mmol/l is diagnostic of diabetes. Only if the blood glucose is between 7–11 mmol/l need a glucose tolerance test be performed.

Diabetes should also be suspected in women who deliver babies heavier than 4.1 kg, and/or who suffer pre-eclampsia, or in persons suffering a high blood cholesterol. Diabetes is often discovered on routine urinalysis.

Clinical manifestations

Onset of symptoms may be abrupt or insidious and patients classically present with polydypsia, polyuria, polypepsia, and weight loss over a period of several days to a week. If the diagnosis of diabetes is missed, or the insulin deficiency is severe, then the above symptoms progress in an accelerated manner, resulting in ketoacidosis. Weakness and lethargy occur due to potassium loss and protein breakdown. Paraesthesias may also be present in Type I diabetes due to the neurotoxicity of prolonged hyperglycaemia. Small vessel disease (see page 292) and peripheral nerve disorders also result from prolonged hyperglycaemia.

Medical and nursing management of the diabetic patient

There are six major components of diabetes therapy:

1. Diet
2. Oral hypoglycaemic drugs
3. Insulin
4. Exercise
5. Education
6. Prevention of complications.

Diet

All diabetics must follow some form of dietary modification, which will vary according to the severity of the disease. A diabetic's diet should, like any other, maintain normal body weight and supply adequate vitamins and minerals. Some obese diabetics may undertake an initial reduction diet. Principles of dietary management are:

1. Avoidance of high carbohydrate foods that contain little, if any, nutritional value. These are classified as 'danger foods'.
2. An even spread of carbohydrate throughout the day. Diabetic diets consist of a specified number of portioned food, with foods containing 15 gm of carbohydrate equalling 1 portion. The number of portions a patient can eat depends upon his age, sex, weight, and exercise level. The patient's daily activities will also determine the spread of food throughout the day. It should be remembered that extra food is required for extra activity. Meals should never be omitted and the portioned foods always eaten. This will prevent the occurrence of hypoglycaemia. Diabetics should always carry glucose in case of the onset of such a reaction.
3. The diet should be sufficient to suppress hunger and provide adequate calories, minerals and vitamins.

Diabetics receive assistance from dietitians who, together with nursing staff, are responsible for patient education about their future dietary management. The patient and significant others receive counselling and advice to help them adjust to the new dietary regime. Literature is available to help patients and relatives learn about the foods that should be eaten in moderation, those that are unrestricted, and those that are totally restricted. Worldwide, the management of diet therapy in diabetic patients varies and the nurse should be aware that different regimens and calculations may be described. In particular the use of 'food exchanges' rather than portion diets is an increasingly popular diet therapy.

In hospital it is important for the nurse to check the patient's meal tray for the correct number of portions and following the meal to ensure that the patient has eaten those portions.

Oral hypoglycaemic drugs

Oral hypoglycaemic agents are indicated for those patients whose diabetes cannot be controlled by diet alone. These drugs act by either stimulating the release of insulin from the beta cells in Type II diabetes or by enhancing the effect of the insulin released.

Sulphonylureas stimulate insulin production from the islets of Langerhans and control the diabetes for as long as the pancreas can produce insulin. When the patient is well controlled with sulphonylureas, blood glucose levels should be within physiological ranges with no glycosuria.

Biguanides are used mainly in conjunction with the sulphonylureas, especially when control with sulphonylureas is inadequate.

The action of biguanides is not fully understood but it is believed that they assist the cellular uptake of available glucose where the patient has become resistant to the function of his own insulin. Their use is associated with gastrointestinal disturbance and they are rarely used as initial therapy and dosages should be strictly controlled and not exceeded.

Insulin

All unstable diabetics, generally all thin diabetics and all diabetics who produce ketones, will be treated with insulin. Insulin is a hormone and cannot therefore be given by the oral route as it would simply be digested along with all other protein. Insulin is prepared in either solution or suspension and presented in multidose vials for injection preparation. Throughout Australia, the UK, the USA and most of Europe the strength of insulin preparation is standardized to 1 unit per 0.01 ml.

The drug is prepared from bovine (cattle) or porcine (pig) sources. 'Human insulin for injection' is not from humans but is an extremely highly purified form of porcine insulin. Bacterially produced insulins are now in limited use, and will become more widely used when testing of these substances (and legislation) allows, as they are the purest form of synthetically produced insulin.

Insulins differ greatly in their duration of action, peak performance time, pH, and degree of purity. The duration of action varies from 4 hours for the soluble and neutral types of insulin to 36 hours for the extremely long acting varieties.

In diabetic emergencies, or when a diabetic patient is under extreme physical stress (for example, surgery), one of the short acting forms of insulin is used to control the patient's blood sugar. The dosage levels of short acting insulin can be readjusted every 4 hours according to the blood sugar level and the amount of sugar and ketones in the urine.

The insulins with medium length of action are given to patients once their diabetes has been stabilized. Ideally, insulin should be given twice daily, however this regime is not met with great enthusiasm from the patient. Therefore, to enable a once-daily injection to be given, short and long acting insulins are mixed to give better and smoother control.

More than with any other drug, patient compliance in the use of insulin is essential. Generally speaking, the patient's way of life cannot be greatly changed and therefore the type of insulin given must be tailored to the requirements of the patient; the patient cannot be changed to fit the insulin.

Diabetics over 5 years of age should be taught to give their own insulin; obviously young children should be supervised by a parent or guardian when administering insulin, but it is imperative that from very early diagnosis the patient be responsible for his own well-being. Teaching aseptic preparation techniques is the responsibility of the nurse, the patient must also be taught how to administer the drug, care for and safely dispose of the equipment, and effectively and safely store his insulin.

During this teaching period many centres allow the patient to experience partial hypoglycaemia so that he may recognize and treat the symptoms should they occur outside a treatment centre.

Patients should also be taught the sites that may be used for administration of insulin and the site of injection should be in a different place each day.

The sites illustrated in Figure 28.1 are the most commonly used, but any area of the body where there is a reasonable amount of subcutaneous tissue may be used. Problems arise when patients are severely restricted in their movements (as in

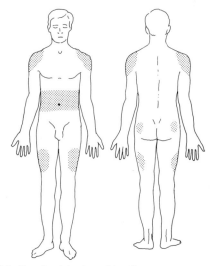

Fig. 28.1 Sites for injection of insulin.

severe rheumatoid arthritis) and can only reach one or two of these sites. Repeated injection into one area can cause atrophy of fatty tissue with consequent depression and hardening of the skin over the site. Eventually there will be little or no absorption of the drug from these areas and it may become necessary for the insulin to be administered by a family member or a domiciliary nurse.

Insulin pumps are becoming more widely used, but are useless in patients with all but the most stable diabetes. However, the time is rapidly approaching where the body's own ion movement will be able to be used as a battery to drive more sophisticated pumps which will be linked to an implanted and transistorized device to measure blood sugar. These pumps will then function exactly as a pancreas, and release precisely the correct amount of insulin for the body's needs.

The problems associated with insulin therapy include:

• The patient will have to learn, basically by trial and error, to administer more insulin and ingest more carbohydrate if he is going to participate in vigorous exercise.
• The patient may require spectacles or a new optical prescription after stabilization on insulin. There is little point in having spectacless made during the stabilization period as blurring of vision is common during this time.
• Skin responses occur only rarely nowadays, as insulin has become more highly purified. When they do occur they appear as local, red, painful swellings around the injection site.
• Hypoglycaemia may occur as a result of too much insulin or the failure to ingest carbohydrate within a reasonable time of administering the insulin. Diabetic patients should always carry processed carbohydrate (sweets or biscuits) in order to be able to respond quickly to the early symptoms of hypoglycaemia and prevent coma occurring.
• Generalized reactions to insulin occur very rarely in the form of anaphylactic reactions. In this case, as in the case of local reactions, the type of insulin used must be changed from bovine to porcine or to human insulin.
• Oral contraceptives can significantly reduce the therapeutic effect of insulin and for this reason the

use of oral contraceptives in diabetic women may be contraindicated.

Exercise

Exercise plays an important part in the overall control of diabetes. In Type I diabetes it would appear that muscular activity assists the entry of glucose into the cells and therefore has a synergistic effect with insulin in lowering blood sugar. The significance of this is that patients who require insulin therapy must increase their carbohydrate intake before exercise. They should continue to maintain an increased carbohydrate intake for several hours after the exercise, particularly if the urine test is negative for sugar, in order to avoid hypoglycaemic reactions. In patients with Type II diabetes, exercise is of primary importance in weight control. Some patients can gain good control of their diabetes with diet and exercise, which may eliminate the need for oral hypoglycaemic drugs.

Education and prevention of complications

A thorough knowledge and understanding of this condition is required by the patient, medical, nursing, and paramedical staff. A very large part of the nurse's responsibility is to assist the patient to accept and manage all aspects of diabetes. Well managed and well controlled diabetes will increase the quality of life and longevity of the diabetic patient.

The education programme begins from the very first day of diagnosis. The patient needs to be taught dietary management, urine testing, insulin storage and administration, care of feet, teeth, and wounds, and prevention and/or management of complications associated with this condition (see below). The patient and his significant others must also be aware of the support available in the community, such as Foundations, Support Associations and Education officers in community health centres.

Psychological counselling is often required to help the patient adjust to this new lifestyle. This can be a more difficult adjustment for children and adolescents who, because of their insulin administration and dietary restrictions, view themselves as 'different'. The majority of diabetics assume a responsible and therefore positive role in the management of their condition and adhere to their diet and insulin regimes assiduously, however, some patients can react in an irresponsible manner by ignoring carbohydrate restrictions and missing meals. This can result in more frequent and unnecessary complications, but may also reflect a period of denial during which time the patient may need psychological support and counselling. The patient should carry and/or wear identification stating the fact that he is a diabetic. This can be of assistance in the event of a hypoglycaemic reaction.

The optimum time to teach urine testing, blood glucose monitoring, and insulin administration is during the patient's hospitalization. Before discharge he should be skilled in these techniques, as insulin dosage should be calculated according to their results. Following discharge, home visits by community nurses and follow-up outpatient appointments enable the continued supervision and habilitation of the patient and his significant others.

Increased community education programmes and improved screening and early detection techniques are proving so effective that some patients do not require hospitalization for stabilization and initial management of their diabetes. The role of the community nurse in ensuring that these patients understand and comply with management techniques cannot be underestimated.

Because of the patient's increased risk of peripheral vascular disease and gangrene it is important that the diabetic, particularly the adult patient, is aware of the need for meticulous care of the feet. Toe nails must be kept short and cut by a podiatrist. The patient should dry between the toes to prevent fungal infections and ulcerations, and should wear protective and well fitting footwear. Where appropriate, assistance with footwear may be sought from a prosthestist/orthotist. Such assistance may include advice on type and size of shoes, construction of specific footwear, and provision of prostheses to be worn within the shoes.

Because the diabetic patient is prone to dental caries, meticulous care of teeth and gums, and regular visits to the dentist are necessary to maintain good oral hygiene.

Should the patient cut himself, great care must be taken to prevent the wound from becoming infected and the patient should expect to heal slowly as wound healing in diabetics is prolonged.

COMPLICATIONS OF DIABETES

Hypoglycaemia

Hypoglycaemia usually occurs when the blood glucose level is 2 mmol/l or less. It can be a complication of Type I or Type II diabetes.

Aetiology

The administration of too much insulin or the failure to eat a meal after insulin administration can cause hypoglycaemia. Increased exercise without an appropriate increase in carbohydrate intake, and illness such as diarrhoea, vomiting, and infection, or trauma such as surgery may also be causes.

Clinical manifestations

These differ greatly in presentation and severity and consist of hunger, sweating, syncope, tremor, confusion and aggression, and ultimately coma. The aggression can often mimic alcohol intoxication and can be misinterpreted by unskilled people. If hypoglycaemia develops rapidly the patient may lose consciousness without any warning signs at all.

Medical and nursing management

This is an emergency situation and treatment must be instituted as quickly as possible before the patient becomes uncooperative and loses consciousness.

The longer the brain is without glucose the greater the neuronal damage. Treatment consists simply of the administration of oral glucose. Glucose is absorbed rapidly through oral and gastric mucosa. The amount should be as much as is necessary to restore the patient to normal. In general 2 portions, that is 30 g, of carbohydrate is sufficient and can be given in a variety of ways. A sweet drink is ideal, such as lemonade, orange juice and sugar, milk and sugar, or Dexal or any other suitable fluid which can be prepared rapidly and can be easily swallowed by an uncooperative patient or a person who is very drowsy. Other forms of glucose enriched foods are glucose lollies, sweet biscuits, and jam, and these are often given subsequent to the sweetened drink when the patient is alert and conscious.

Unconsciousness complicates the treatment. In a first aid situation glucose in the form of honey, Dexal granules, a glucose lollie, or castor sugar can be rubbed around the patient's oral mucosa in an attempt to restore him to a conscious level to enable him to swallow fluid.

In sustained unconsciousness the patient is quickly transported to hospital where an IV infusion of glucose 50% solution is administered until the patient is conscious and can drink. If the cause of unconsciousness is unknown, thiamine should be administered along with the glucose (see Wernicke-Korsakoff's syndrome, page 209).

Glucagon can be administered subcutaneously or by intramuscular injection as an alternative, and many relatives of diabetics are taught to administer this medication in such an acute emergency.

All patients respond rapidly to glucose either orally or intravenously and make a spontaneous recovery.

Hypoglycaemia should not be a frequent complication and usually occurs in newly diagnosed or unstable diabetics; it may also be due to the irresponsible management of diabetes. Patients are encouraged to experience several hypoglycaemic reactions under supervision in hospital to enable them to recognise the early onset of symptoms and treat them accordingly. Therefore, the nurse must respect a patient's ability to recognize hypoglycaemia and must not hesitate to respond immediately to a request for glucose. If hypoglycaemic attacks are occurring frequently the patient may need to be rehospitalized for further assessment and stabilization of the diabetes.

It must be stressed that whenever the nurse is in doubt when treating a diabetic patient – give sugar.

Ketoacidosis

Ketoacidosis occurs as a result of total insulin deficiency and therefore only occurs in Type I diabetics. It is to be noted that some Type II diabetics tend to take on the characteristics of Type I diabetics when subjected to severe physiological stress, for example pregnancy, myocardial infarction, and surgery.

Aetiology

Ketoacidosis is not a condition that occurs suddenly but takes approximately 12 hours or more to develop and may be precipitated by:

1. Untreated or undiagnosed diabetes
2. Too little insulin either by accidental omission or insufficient dosage
3. Ingestion of too much carbohydrate over a period of at least a few days
4. Acute infections which increase the body's need for glucose, and therefore insulin, accompanied by the failure to adjust insulin dosage
5. Use of hyperglycaemic drugs such as corticosteroids and thiazide diuretics.

Clinical manifestations

Initially, the ketoacidotic patient is drowsy, weak, lethargic, anorexic, nauseated, and may vomit. There is excessive glycosuria and ketonuria. The patient's breath smells of ketones, he is polyuric, and his skin feels hot and dry. As the condition worsens he becomes unconscious, dehydrated, and pyrexic; and metabolic acidosis results from increased ketone levels. As a consequence, ventilation becomes slow and deep (Kussmaul ventilation) in an attempt to 'blow off' CO_2, thus transiently raising the pH. However, this often complicates the clinical picture by initiating a reflex respiratory alkalosis.

Death ensues if treatment is not effectively and immediately instituted.

Investigative procedures

Ketoacidosis can be strongly suspected with a supporting history and the classical clinical presentations. The investigations performed to confirm diagnosis include:

• Urinalysis, which will show gross ketouria and glycosuria
• Measurement of blood sugar levels, which will be raised
• Measurement of blood gases, which will indicate a metabolic acidosis and may also reveal a reflex respiratory alkalosis.

Medical and nursing management

This is a medical emergency. The aims of treatment are to correct dehydration and electrolyte imbalance, and restore insulin and glucose levels to normal.

Fluid is replaced by IV infusion of normal saline and Hartmann's solution.

A reasonable fluid regime for the severely ketotic patient would be 10–15 litres in the first 24-hour period. This is monitored clinically by a restoration of tissue turgor and an equal fluid balance. Care must be taken not to overload the patient. Potassium is the major electrolyte which requires careful replacement and close 2-hourly monitoring. In patients with ketoacidosis the combination of a hyperglycaemia and the administration of IV insulin causes a rapid decline in the patient's extracellular potassium levels as cell metabolism is increased by the now available glucose. Potassium rushes into the cells causing a hypokalaemia. (In nondiabetic patients the administration of 50 ml of 50% glucose and 8 units of soluble insulin is the first line management of hyperkalaemia.)

A urinary catheter is inserted to obtain fresh urine samples for glucose testing usually on an hourly basis and to allow accurate measurement of fluid output. Blood glucose is sampled as required and the readings are measured by a portable dextrose manometer.

Soluble insulin is given in IV doses of 20–100 units and repeated 1–2 hourly according to blood glucose levels.

A cardiac monitor is attached to the patient to enable the observation of cardiac arrythmias that may occur due to the potassium shifts and hypokalaemia.

IV infusion of sodium bicarbonate is given to help buffer the acidosis.

These patients require intensive nursing and medical care until their condition is stabilized. If the patient is unconscious, full nursing care of an unconscious patient is instituted (see page 164).

When preparing for the admission of a patient with ketoacidosis it is the nurse's responsibility to ensure that all the above mentioned equipment is available.

The patient's vital signs and/or neurological observations will be taken and recorded during the initial period of therapy until his condition has stabilized. This monitoring of blood glucose and urine glucose will continue less frequently, until the patient has been restabilized on both diet and insulin.

When the patient can eat and drink it is usual to begin with glucose and water, or tea with sugar and then gradually increase to a full portion diet.

Ketoacidosis can be fatal. It is a complication that can be prevented by adequate education of the diabetic patient, his significant others, and the medical and paramedical professions.

It should be noted that, whenever the cause of unconsciousness in a diabetic is unknown, the rule of thumb is: when in doubt give sugar.

Hyperosmolar non-ketotic coma

This condition is associated with hyperglycaemia and clinically mimics ketoacidosis without the ketone formation. It occurs in elderly patients with Type II diabetes and the ketone formation is suppressed, possibly due to the presence of some circulating insulin.

Clinical manifestations

The principal presentation is dehydration due to the osmotic diuresis. This is progressive and can be severe and life threatening. Coma and death will rapidly ensue unless treatment is instigated.

On investigation, the patient will be found to have hyperglycaemia, which is usually at a higher level than that found in ketoacidosis. The patient is not acidotic and therefore has a normal pH and a normal sodium bicarbonate level. Because of the disproportionate loss of water to sodium the patient will be hypernatraemic. His serum osmolarity will be high.

Medical and nursing management

Fluid replacement to rehydrate the patient must be performed slowly and be monitored carefully, as excessive and rapid rehydration can lead to circulatory overload, and pulmonary and cerebral oedema. Initially, the intravenous fluid of choice is normal saline or half-strength saline. Once the glucose level has fallen to normal a dextrose/saline mixture will be continued. Insulin is given to reduce hyperglycaemia, but it is only given in small doses of 2–3 units per hour, as patients with an absence of ketoacidosis are hypersensitive to insulin.

Complications

The mortality rate from this condition is very high – approximately 30% – and it is usually due to dehydration, myocardial infarction, or cerebrovascular accident.

Infection

The physical stress of infection can either precipitate diabetes or destabilize a previously well controlled diabetic. The focus of the infection should be sought and rapidly treated. The hyperglycaemic state normally existing in diabetics makes them prone to infections, particularly those of bacterial and monilial origin. These infections can be, and often are, the presenting feature of diabetes; for example, a chronic monilial vaginal infection, puritis vulvae, a wound that fails to heal, or an inappropriate reaction to what would normally be a minor illness. It is of major importance to maintain a normal blood glucose level during times of infection.

Long-term complications

The diabetic patient has an increased susceptability to generalized vascular disease: atherosclerosis, and small vessel disease known as microangiopathy.

Atherosclerosis

The development of atherosclerosis is accelerated in the diabetic; so much so that after a 10–15 year history of diabetes it is common to find ischaemia of many organs, particularly the brain, heart, and kidneys; and in the peripheral vessels, resulting in gangrene of the extremities. Cerebrovascular accident, myocardial infarction, and renal failure are major causes of death in diabetics.

Small vessel microangiopathy

Diabetics may suffer from microangiopathy in any vessels, but especially those of the feet (see page 292) and eyes. Retinopathy is an extremely common complication in diabetes. It is classified into two types: non proliferative and proliferative.

Non proliferative (background) retinopathy. This represents the earliest stages of the retinal disease and is characterized by microaneurysms, spot haemorrhages, retinal oedema, and exudates due to leakage of protein lipids on red blood cells into the retina. This is not likely to cause visual impairment unless it affects the macula densa which is the area of greatest concentration of visual cells.

Proliferative retinopathy. As a consequence of small vessel occlusion causing retinal hypoxia, there is a corresponding new growth of capillaries which are fragile and bleed easily into the vitreous humour. These vitreous haemorrhages and ultimate retinal detachment will eventually result in blindness within a period of a few years. Once the proliferative changes have been detected treatment consists of laser photocoagulation. This destroys the new retinal tissue which means that the remaining tissue will receive more oxygen. The condition is more successfully treated if diagnosed early.

Cataracts

Cataracts are more common and progress more rapidly in diabetic patients than in others. This is most likely due to an accumulation of sorbitol which is toxic to lens protein. Sorbitol is formed from increased quantities of glucose found in the lens of the non insulin dependent patient.

Diabetic nephropathy

This is a disease affecting the basement membrane of the capillaries of the glomerulus. Proteinuria is the presenting symptom, and may progress to a full blown nephrotic syndrome, or ultimately chronic renal failure. Renal biopsy will show the changes in the microvasculature and treatment may consist of haemodialysis or renal transplantation from a compatible donor.

Diabetic neuropathy

The peripheral nervous system is vulnerable in diabetics (see also page 204). The neuropathy appears to be caused by the formation of neurotoxic sorbitol.

Sensory neuropathy. This is often a late complication and presents with paraesthesia, increasing pain, and foot ulceration. Reversal of the condition is uncommon.

Motor neuropathy. This occurs less frequently than sensory neuropathy and it manifests as nerve palsies of the III, IV, VI and VII cranial nerves, causing lid ptosis, lateral deviation of the eye, inability to move the eye laterally, and facial paralysis, respectively.

Peripheral nerves can also be affected causing, for example, footdrop.

These changes have a good prognosis and are completely reversible. They can also be a presenting sign of the diabetes.

Autonomic neuropathy. Neuropathy of the autonomic nervous system can result in many manifestations in patients with long-standing diabetes. The common features are:

1. Tachycardia at rest
2. Postural hypotension
3. Delayed gastric emptying with alternating constipation and diarrhoea
4. Diabetic diarrhoea, due to bacterial overgrowth from stasis of contents in the small intestine
5. Neurogenic bladder, causing urinary incontinence and large residual volumes of urine predisposing to infection
6. Impotence.

Anticipated outcome of diabetes mellitus

The majority of diabetic persons live normal and active lives with minimal disruption to their activities of daily living. The well controlled diabetic who maintains an ideal body weight, a normal blood sugar, and cares appropriately for his feet and eyes, can expect a normal life span. Rapid and appropriate responses to ill health and/or sudden exercise will help to ensure his continued well being. Brittle, poorly controlled diabetics will almost certainly suffer complications with a resultant shortened life span.

29

Disorders of the adrenal glands

Jenny Kidd

The adrenal glands are small bilateral structures situated on top of the kidneys.

The inner portion known as the medulla secretes epinephrine and norepinephrine and is an extension of the sympathetic nervous system. The bulk of the gland is the cortex and is responsible for the synthesis and secretion of 4 types of adreno-cortical hormones: glucocorticoids, mineralocorticoids, androgens and oestrogens. Aldosterone is the principal mineralocorticoid and cortisol is the principal glucocorticoid. These hormones are all derived from cholesterol.

The adrenal cortex has an enormous functional capacity: up to 90% of the gland can be destroyed before insufficiency is clinically evident. Such insufficiencies are known as hypoadrenalism or hypocorticolism (Addison's disease). However, neoplasia and hyperplasia can lead to hyperadrenalism or hypercorticolism. Major disorders of the adrenal glands are classified into hyper- and hypofunction.

HYPERADRENALISM (HYPERCORTICOLISM)

There are 3 main forms of hyperadrenalism with differing clinical manifestations:

1. Cushing's syndrome – excess production of cortisol
2. Aldosteronism (Conn's syndrome) – excess production of aldosterone
3. The adrenogenital (AG) syndrome – excess production of androgens.

Each of the 3 conditions involves an increased secretion of one or more of the adrenocortical ster-oids. Hyperplasia, adenomona or carcinoma of the cortex are the most common causes. Conn's syndrome is usually caused by an adenoma and the AG syndrome and Cushing's syndrome are often due to hyperplasia of the adrenal gland.

Cushing's syndrome

In 1932 Harvey Cushing documented the presence of basophilic pituitary adenomas in patients suffering the clinical syndrome now known as Cushing's syndrome.

Cushing's syndrome is characterized by chronic elevation in glucocorticoid hormones.

Aetiology

There are 4 major causes of Cushing's syndrome. It can be due to the autonomous production of cortisol by either a benign or malignant tumour of the adrenal cortex. Secondly, it can result from excessive secretion of ACTH from the pituitary gland, which results in excessive production of cortisol; this may be due to an adenoma or hyperplasia of the pituitary gland itself. Thirdly, the ectopic production of ACTH from a non pituitary tumour, such as an oat cell carcinoma of the lung. Fourthly, the condition is commonly iatrogenic, resulting from chronic glucocorticoid therapy in patients suffering asthma, rheumatoid arthritis, or chronic skin disorders where there has been long term treatment with cortisone as an anti-inflammatory agent. Females are more often affected than males and the age at diagnosis is usually between 30–50 years.

Pathophysiology and clinical manifestations

Glucocorticoid excess affects protein and carbohydrate metabolism, electrolytes, gastric secretion, brain function, erythropoiesis and the distribution of adipose tissue. The catabolic effects of glucocorticoids on protein result in a decrease in the ability of protein forming cells to synthesize protein. Consequently, there is a loss of protein from the skin, muscle, bone, and blood vessels. Clinically the skin breaks down easily and wounds heal slowly. Purple striae occur from rupture of elastic fibres and are distributed largely over the abdomen and hips. Muscles become weak and atrophied, and bone is also affected, resulting in osteoporosis which can lead to pathological fractures. This is more common in the vertebrae causing back pain and vertebral collapse. Calcium is mobilized, and this can lead to renal calculi. Altered fat metabolism causes a peculiar deposition of fat causing trunkal obesity, subclavicular fat pads or 'buffalo hump' on the back, and a round, 'moon-shaped' face. Derangement of the glucose metabolism, usually hyperglycaemia, is found in a large percentage of patients, with full blown diabetes mellitus occurring in a few patients. Petechiae, or large areas of echymosis occur due to thinning of blood vessel walls and these can occur even with gentle pressure. There is inhibition of the inflammatory and immune responses, resulting in an increased susceptibility of infection.

Gastric secretory activity is increased by glucocorticoids which may provoke gastric ulceration and bleeding. Psychological changes are frequently seen in glucocorticoid excess, ranging from euphoria to acute depression.

An associated rise in androgen levels causes hirsuitism, mild acne, and irregularities in the menstrual cycle.

Investigative procedures

Diagnosis can be suspected from the clinical picture.

Serum and urine levels of cortisol will be raised.

A skull X-ray may show damage to the sella turcica, which can occur in an ACTH secreting tumour.

Adrenal venous angiography via the right and left adrenal veins can be used to visualize the adrenal glands and show distortion of the venous network, indicative of adrenal hyperplasia or tumour formation.

An IV infusion of radioactive cholesterol is taken up and concentrated by the adrenal cortex, and is followed by a CT scan of the adrenal cortex within 5–10 days. CT scanning of the sella turcica (pituitary fossa) may not show pathological signs due to the small size of the tumours, so a firm biochemical diagnosis is essential.

Medical and surgical management

Treatment of Cushing's syndrome can be surgical, radio-therapeutic or pharmacological and the choice largely depends on the aetiology.

Surgery. In the case of a pituitary macroadenoma, a trans-sphenoidal resection of the ACTH pituitary secreting tumour is the treatment of choice. The operation is extremely successful and has a low mortality rate and a low incidence of postoperative complications. In patients with microadenomas, selective microsurgery is successful in correcting the hypercorticolism. If the tumour is too small to visualize at surgery, and the adult patient is beyond reproductive age, a total hypophysectomy may be performed.

Postoperatively, most patients require glucocorticoid support for several months whilst the hypothalmic pituitary adrenal axis recovers. This therapy is mandatory for the patient who has undergone total hypophysectomy.

In some patients a bilateral adrenalectomy may be performed, usually when other attempts at treatment have failed. This surgery results in permanent hypoadrenalism which requires glucocorticoid and mineralocorticoid replacement therapy for life. In cases of adrenal neoplasia, chemotherapy follows surgery. Adrenal adenomas are successfully treated by unilateral adrenalectomy, with some follow up glucocorticoid support therapy, until the remaining adrenal gland recovers. This is necessary due to the suppression of the hypopituitary axis due to the chronic excess of cortisol. Adrenal surgery can have a high mortality rate due to poor wound healing and generalized infection.

Treatment of ectopic ACTH syndrome consists of surgical removal of the ACTH secreting tumour. Cure is more likely to be achieved if the tumour is benign. If it is malignant the surgery is often difficult and unsuccessful. Metastases are often present, therefore treatment is usually directed towards correcting the hypercortical state.

Complications of surgery are rare, but include haemorrhage, transient or permanent diabetes insipidus and visual disturbances. Hypopituitarism (see page 233) occurs in patients who undergo a total hypophysectomy.

Radiotherapy. When the tumour is not clearly defined, radiotherapy is effective in doses of 4500–5000 rads; particularly so in children. Heavy partical radiation is becoming increasingly more common.

Implantation of radioactive gold or yttrium seeds into the sella turcica is also effective, but the post therapy complication of panhypopituitarism is high.

Pharmacology. Aminoglutethimide is the drug of choice, and causes adrenal atrophy. The response to treatment is slow and is commonly associated with side effects, such as severe nausea, vomiting, diarrhoea, depression, and skin rashes.

Nursing management

The nursing care for the patient with Cushing's syndrome must be tailored to his individual requirements, as the physiological manifestations vary so widely in their severity. Nursing management is required for those patients who are awaiting surgery, or who have been admitted for stabilization of their condition or as a result of a complication such as osteoporosis. Following surgery, the nurse must be especially observant for signs of a developing adrenal crisis (see page 267).

Extreme care must be taken when lifting, turning, washing, and dressing the patient, due to the ease with which skin breakdown and bruising can occur. The patient's bones will also be prone to fracture if osteoporosis is present; he must be guarded from falls. The nurse must be prepared to understand and cope with the patient's mood swings. Any loin pain experienced by the patient must be recorded and reported, as it may be indicative of renal calculi. When this is suspected

the patient's urine will be strained, and tested for haematuria. The patient must be protected from infection. Any wounds are dressed aseptically. Observation should be made for signs of a gastric ulcer, such as dyspepsia and abdominal pain, and the appropriate dietary changes made (see page 492).

See Chapter 13 for the nursing management of the patient receiving cytotoxic therapy.

Aldosteronism

Aldosteronism is a condition resulting from excess production of aldosterone, the major mineralocorticoid from the adrenal cortex. Aldosterone regulates electrolyte and fluid balance by enhancing the reabsorption of sodium and the excretion of potassium in the proximal renal tubule. When aldosterone levels are in excess the result is hypernatraemia and hypokalaemia. There are two types of aldosteronism: primary and secondary.

Primary aldosteronism (Conn's syndrome)

In primary aldosteronism the stimulus for excessive aldosterone secretion lies within the adrenal gland itself. The majority of cases are due to a unilateral adenoma and rarely a carcinoma. Conn's syndrome usually occurs between the ages of 30–50 years and is twice as common in females as males.

Clinical manifestations

The excessive and continual hypersecretion of aldosterone increases the exchange of intratubular sodium for secreted potassium and hydrogen ions, with a progressive depletion of body potassium resulting in hypokalaemia. Potassium depletion results in muscle weakness, fatigue, cardiac arrythmias, and premature ventricular contractions. Patients also suffer hypertension and headaches, probably due to hypernatraemia and an increasing extracellular volume. The hypernatraemia is due to both sodium retention and water loss from polyuria, which results from impairment in concentrating ability. This is often associated with polydipsia.

Investigative procedures

The clinical picture of muscle weakness, hypertension, polydipsia, and polyuria, together with persistent hypokalaemia, elevated serum sodium, alkaline urine, and low serum renin levels strongly suggests primary hyperaldosteronism. Diagnosis is confirmed by elevated serum and urinary aldosterone levels, together with a low plasma renin level and consistently low levels of serum potassium – less than 3.4 mmol/l.

Medical and surgical management

Primary aldosteronism due to an adenoma is treated by surgical excision. However, some patients can be successfully treated conservatively by a dietary restriction of sodium and the administration of an aldosterone antagonist such as spironolactone which is effective in controlling hypertension and hypokalaemia.

Secondary aldosteronism

In this condition the renal cortex is stimulated to produce renin, which stimulates the adrenal gland to produce large quantities of aldosterone. This is due to the activation of the renin–angiotensin feedback system, resulting in a rise in angiotensin II levels due to increased renin release.

Aetiology and pathophysiology

Any cause of reduced renal perfusion will cause a rise in renin levels. These include:

1. Diuretic therapy. The most common cause of secondary aldosteronism is diuretic therapy. This results in renal sodium loss and volume depletion which activates the renin–angiotensin feedback mechanism.
2. Hypovolaemic states due to haemorrhage, dehydration, and oedematous conditions such as cardiac failure and oedema, nephrotic syndrome, cirrhosis, and ascites. The mechanism of increased renin levels involves the changes in renal haemodynamics and the redistribution of fluid to the extravascular compartment. This stimulates the activation of the renin–angiotensin feedback mechanism, which is regarded as a homeostatic mechanism. However, in disease it appears that this mechanism becomes deranged and the increased levels of aldosterone compound the degree of oedema by increasing sodium retention.
3. Oral contraceptives.
4. Obstruction of blood flow to the renal arteries, as in malignant hypertension and atheroma. The intense nephrosclerosis that occurs in these conditions causes a profound hyperreninaemia resulting in extremely high serum levels of aldosterone.
5. Renin secreting tumour.

Clinical manifestations

Unlike primary aldosteronism, where the clinical manifestations are entirely due to elevated levels of aldosterone, secondary hyperaldosteronism presents primarily as the cause of increased renin secretion.

The principal difference between primary and secondary hyperaldosterone is that in primary disease, both angiotensin and renin levels are depressed, whilst in secondary disease they are elevated.

Adrenogenital syndrome

This condition is associated with an adrenal enzyme deficiency which blocks normal steroid production. This results in increased adrenogenic activity leading to virilism. Adults and infants of either sex can be affected. In infants it is thought to be due to a congenital error of metabolism which causes a lack of specific adrenal enzyme, thus inhibiting the normal biosynthesis of cortisol; the result is a loss of feedback inhibition and ACTH is secreted in excess. Congenital adrenal hyperplasia or adrenal carcinoma may also be a cause in infants. In adults the syndrome is usually due to an autonomous hyperfunctioning adenoma or carcinoma.

Clinical manifestations

Because of overproduction of androgenic hormones, virilism is the most outstanding clinical feature. The female infant may present as a pseudohermaphrodite and in the male child there may be an enlargement of the penis. In addition to the virilism there may be accompanying vomiting and dehydration due to what is termed a 'salt losing crisis'. Such a crisis can be confused with a gastroenteritis or pyloric stenosis, and if a diagnosis of adrenogenital syndrome is missed, the crisis may be fatal. The older female child may present with an enlarged clitoris; the older male child with a sexual precocity. Both can develop hirsuitism, increased bone age, and premature closure of the epiphysis. In the adult female, virilism is manifest by hirsuitism, male distribution of hair, baldness of the scalp, an enlarged clitoris and the development of a male physique.

Medical and surgical management

Medical management is aimed at controlling the symptoms and providing counselling for the parents of the infant patient.

Surgical intervention can assist in cosmetic correction, and when the syndrome is caused by adenoma or carcinoma, surgery (with or without cytotoxic therapy) may be undertaken.

HYPOADRENALISM

Adrenal insufficiency may present as an acute adrenal crisis (Addisonian crisis), or, more commonly may present in chronic form – Addison's disease.

Addison's disease

Aetiology

Chronic adrenal insufficiency (Addison's disease) is characterized by the chronic deficiency of hormones concerned with glucogenesis and mineral metabolism. Addison's disease may result from a primary disorder of the adrenal cortex, such as haemorrhage, or inflammation as seen in neonates who suffer delayed and difficult delivery with associated asphyxia and hypoxia. It can also occur due to diphtheria and systemic pneumococcal, streptococcal, and meningiococcal infections.

Atrophy of the gland is the most common cause. One known cause of atrophy is the chronic administration of glucocorticoids, which suppress the adrenohypophyseal axis (iatrogenic atrophy). The steroid deficiency may become evident in patients whose corticoid therapy is omitted for some reason, is inadequate in times of increased stress such as illness or surgery, or is withdrawn too rapidly. Idiopathic atrophy is thought to be an autoimmune disorder with evidence of circulating auto-antibodies against adrenocortical antigens.

Necrosis of the cortex can occur with any form of acute and prolonged stress, such as severe burns and shock, and long standing debilitating illnesses. A decrease in the production of ACTH occurs due to disease of the hypothalamus or pituitary, or suppression of the adrenocortical axis by corticosteroid therapy.

Other less common causes include tuberculosis, fungal infections, amyloidisis and carcinoma. Tuberculosis is the second most common cause and still accounts for some 5–10% of cases of Addison's disease.

Clinical manifestations

These vary in severity depending on the degree of hypofunction, and they are usually insidious in onset. Progressive weakness and constant fatigue is often a key sign. Hyperpigmentation may be present and commonly appears as a diffuse bronze tan of both exposed and unexposed parts of the skin. Other symptoms include weight loss, anorexia, sodium loss and potassium retention, and hypoglycaemia. Hypotension is frequently present and is posturally accentuated. Gastrointestinal symptoms can vary from mild nausea to fulminating vomiting, diarrhoea, and abdominal pain. A decrease in pubic hair is common in females due to a decrease in adrenal androgen production.

Investigative procedures

The diagnosis of adrenal insufficiency should be confirmed by ACTH stimulation tests to ascertain the adrenal capacity for steroid production.

Medical and nursing management

Treatment in severe cases consists of replacement of glucocorticoids, mineralocorticoids, and anabolic steroids. In milder cases, replacement therapy with one or two hormones may be sufficient. Cortisone and hydrocortisone are the drugs of choice and will correct most metabolic disturbances with the addition of dietary salt in some instances. A high carbohydrate, high protein diet will help overcome fatigue and muscle weakness, with small frequent meals being better tolerated than three large ones. Because of the patient's reduced ability to cope with physical and emotional stress, it is wise to protect him from exposure to infection and treat any infection immediately and aggressively with a rise in cortisone dosages. The dose of cortisone should be also raised in cases of trauma, illness, surgery, or in any form of stress that the patient may be experiencing. Such patients should carry information at all times regarding their steroid therapy, as this could be life saving.

Acute adrenal insufficiency; adrenal crisis; Addisonian crisis

Addisonian crisis is a rapid and overwhelming exacerbation of chronic adrenal insufficiency. It most commonly results from the rapid withdrawal of steroids from patients with adrenal atrophy, secondary to chronic steroid administration. These patients are also at risk of an Addisonian crisis if their intake of steroids is not sufficiencly increased in times of stress. Any form of excess physical or mental stress is potentially dangerous.

Inadequate replacement therapy following bilateral adrenalectomy can also cause a crisis.

Clinical manifestations

These include nausea, vomiting and diahorrea leading to dehydration and hyponatraemia, severe abdominal pain, extreme lethargy, and exhaustion. Hypotension and tachycardia may lead to circulatory collapse. If treatment is not instigated then death may result in hours.

Medical and nursing management

Treatment consists of rapid replacement of glucocorticoids together with correction of fluid and electrolyte deficits intravenously until the patient is able to tolerate oral fluids and drugs. Steroid dosage is eventually tapered to maintenance levels. A supplementary mineralocorticoid is given only if necessary.

The nurse should observe the patient for any signs of impending Addisonian crisis, and report these immediately. It is not unusual for the physician to have a standing order of steroids available to meet such a crisis.

ADRENAL MEDULLA

The adrenal medulla constitutes approximately one tenth of the weight of the adrenal gland and is comprised of cells called phaeochromocytes. These cells are responsible for producing the catecholamines epinephrine and norepinephrine. The adrenal medulla is innervated by preganglionic fibres of the sympathetic nervous system which release acetylcholine and activate synapses. The chromatin cells store both epinephrine and norepinephrine, and the conversion of epinephrine to norepinephrine is induced by adrenocortical steroids. Epinephrine is synthesized mainly in the adrenal medulla. Norepinephrine is found in the adrenal medulla, the central and peripheral nervous systems, and the sympathetic system. Dopamine is the precursor of norepinephrine and is also found in the adrenal medulla.

Catecholamines are found in the adrenal medulla and in other areas innervated by the central nervous system, for example, the spleen, heart, brain, liver, gut, and skeletal muscle. Secretion is increased by stressful stimuli such as exercise, severe illness, myocardial infarction, and surgery. Catecholamines play a very important role in the regulation of hormone secretion. Both norepinephrine and dopamine play a major role in the regulation of secretion of anterior pituitary hormones. Catecholamines also influence secretion of renin, increase the release of thyroxine, calcitonin, and parathyroid hormone, and inhibit insulin secretion.

Catecholamines are known to increase blood pressure by their vasoconstrictive action on arterioles, thereby increasing peripheral vasoconstriction and increasing the cardiac output. Secondly, as previously mentioned, they can increase renin secretion which results in increased levels of angiotensin II which also raises the blood pressure.

The most significant pathologic conditions which affect the adrenal medulla are phaeochromocytoma and neuroblastoma.

Phaeochromocytoma

Phaeochromocytomas are tumours arising from phaeochromocytes which secrete epinephrine and norepinephrine. The tumour occurs most often between the ages of 30–50 years and affects males and females equally. It can also occur in children, and it may occur as a familial disease. It is not a common condition and is often associated with other endocrine tumours, for example, thyroid or parathyroid tumours.

Clinical manifestations

In most patients symptoms are paroxysmal and vary in severity. The dominant feature is hypertension which may be either constant or episodic. The attacks occur as a result of a release of catecholamines into the blood stream which cause an increase in the force of the heart beat. The patient experiences a pounding sensation in his chest, not necessarily associated with a tachycardia. This pounding sensation spreads throughout his body and causes a severe headache. Due to the effect of catecholamines on the alpha receptors, peripheral vasoconstriction occurs, causing cooling of the extremities, and pallor. The combined effect of the increased cardiac output and peripheral vasoconstriction causes hypertension. The patient may also suffer sweating, hot flushes, tremors, abdominal or chest pain, nausea, vomiting, visual disturbances, and marked anxiety.

The paroxysms may last minutes to hours and leave the patient feeling lethargic and exhausted. Frequency of attacks vary from several times per day or week or there may be intervals of weeks to months between attacks. The attacks may occur for no apparent reason or can be brought on by activities that aggravate or compress the tumour, such as exercise, eating, defaecation, and emotional anxiety. Phaeochromocytomas may

occur wherever chromatin tissue is found. Most tumours occur in the adrenal glands and other common sites are in the post mediastinal area of the chest. The majority of phaeochromocytomas are not malignant, but if a tumour is malignant, spread is rapid and the patient's prognosis is poor.

Investigative procedures and diagnosis

Diagnosis is made on the clinical picture of paroxysmal symptoms. A diagnosis of phaeochromocytoma should be considered in any child with hypertension, or in any adult with hypertension that does not respond to therapy, particularly those with a familial history of phaeochromocytoma.

Hormone assays of catecholamines in plasma and urine may be normal or increased over a 24-hour period so it may be necessary to take plasma and urine samples during an attack. Paroxysms can be induced for this purpose by the administration of 1 mg of glucagon intravenously. After diagnosis the location of the tumour is established by CT scan.

Medical, surgical, and nursing management

Surgical removal of the tumour is the treatment of choice, however immediately following diagnosis the patient is hospitalized and drug therapy is commenced, with adrenergic antagonists which will lower blood pressure and relieve symptoms. Prolonged drug therapy can be advantageous in stabilizing a patient with severe phaeochromocytoma or one who has had associated complications such as an acute myocardial infarction which prevents immediate surgery. A well prepared patient for surgery will suffer fewer intra- and postoperative complications. A cardiac monitor is attached to the patient and frequent recordings of blood pressure are also taken. Following successful surgery the patient's blood pressure will return to normal.

Neuroblastoma

Neuroblastomas are highly malignant tumours, and approximately 50% occur in the adrenal glands. Children and young adults are most often affected, and approximately 80% of neuroblastomas are found in children under 5 years of age. Males are affected more often than females. Neuroblastoma ranks highly as one of the most common tumours in childhood. The tumour metastasizes rapidly and widely to lymph nodes, liver, lungs, and bone. Prognosis is poor, radiotherapy is relatively ineffective, and few patients live longer than 12 months following diagnosis.

30

Endocrine disorders of the male and female reproductive systems

Jenny Kidd

This chapter discusses common manifestations of hypo- and hyperfunction of the gonads, and common genetic-based disorders. Non endocrine disorders of the male and female reproductive systems are discussed in Section I.

The male reproductive system

The testes have 2 important functions: the first is principally exocrine – the production of gametes (spermatogenesis); and the second is endocrine – the synthesis of male sex hormones (androgens). The androgens are involved in spermatogenesis, and during puberty they are responsible for the growth of long bones, the closure of the epiphyses, the deepening of the voice, the distribution of male hair patterns, and the normal development of the external genitalia. They are also responsible for the normal development of musculature and the maintenance of libido and potency. Testicular function is regulated by pituitary gonadotrophins, luteinizing hormone and follicle stimulating hormone.

The female reproductive system

In the female there are 2 ovaries, which produce the hormones oestrogen, androgen, and progesterone. At puberty oestrogen stimulates growth of the uterus and breasts, and controls the deposition of fat and thus female body shape. Oestrogen also contributes towards the closing of the epiphyses and has important effects on personality and sexual responsiveness.

Hypogonadism results from the decreased function of the gonads, and may be due to: failure of

the pituitary gland and/or hypothalamus, of primary gonadal origin, or of genetic origin with either an excess or absence of X or Y chromosomes.

HYPOGONADISM IN THE MALE

Common causes are:

– Anorchia or atrophy of the testes
– Maldescent of the testes
– Congenital abnormalities
– Injury to the testes, for example that due to surgery, mumps, radiation and any other form of orchitis
– Klinefelter's syndrome.

Clinical manifestations

Hypogonadism usually presents before the onset of puberty. There is failure of the genitalia to develop, deficiency of body hair in general and failure to develop pubic and axilliary hair. The voice remains high pitched, and there is lack of development of adult male musculature. Due to delayed epiphyseal closure the patient often has disproportionately long arms and legs.

Post puberty the patient presents with infertility, and reduction or absence of libido and potency.

Diagnosis

The above signs and symptoms together with normal to high serum gonadotrophin are indicative of primary testicular dysfunction. With low serum gonadotrophin they are indicative of hypo-thalamic/pituitary dysfunction. Serum testosterone levels indicate the degree of androgen production by the testes.

Medical management

Spermatogenesis can sometimes be transiently restored in patients by the administration of oral testosterone.

Klinefelter's syndrome

Klinefelter's syndrome is the most common cause of hypogonadism and occurs in approximately 1 in 500 males. It is genetic in origin and is due to an extra X chromosome.

Clinical manifestations

Usually the symptoms present following puberty. In approximately 50% of patients, the major complaint is gynaecomastia. Other manifestations include small firm testes, reduced facial and body hair, infertility, and reduced libido and potency. These men tend to be taller than average because of the disproportionate length of their legs. Associated abnormalities include diminished thyroid function, an increased risk of mild diabetes, and a tendency towards chronic pulmonary disease and varicose veins. Patients with gynaecomastia have an increased predisposition to cancer of the breast.

It is not uncommon for these men to have violent and aggressive personalities, however such behavioural changes may also have an organic origin.

Diagnosis

Klinefelter's syndrome should be distinguished from other forms of hypogonadism. Chromosomal analysis confirms the diagnosis.

Medical management

The patient with low androgen levels should be prescribed replacement testosterone. A mastectomy may be performed if gynaecomastia is present.

HYPOGONADISM IN THE FEMALE

This may be due to

- Primary ovarian disorder – due to tumour, surgical excision, infection such as tuberculosis, radiation damage, or premature menopause
- Disturbance in gonadotrophin production due to pituitary/hypothalamic disorder.
- Turner's syndrome
- Excess androgen production.

Hypogonadism may also be associated with other endrocrine or metabolic disturbances, for example Cushing's syndrome, thyroid disease, renal failure or diabetes mellitus.

Clinical manifestations

If onset is prior to puberty there is lack of breast and external genitalia development and primary amenorrhoea. Post puberty the patient suffers scanty, irregular menses progressing to secondary amenhorrhoea and infertility, and hot flushes.

Investigative procedures

A skull X-ray is performed to assess the size of the pituitary fossa.

A high serum gonadotrophin is indicative of ovarian lesion, whilst a low serum gonadotrophin is indicative of a pituitary lesion.

Medical management

Secondary causes must be identified and treated appropriately. The patient may also be prescribed oestrogen to assist in the development of secondary sex characteristics, to establish menstruation, and to improve her emotional outlook.

Turner's syndrome

Turner's syndrome is a genetic disorder characterized by gonadal dysgenesis. It is an XO chromosome manifestation. One in 10 000 females has Turners syndrome.

Clinical manifestations

The patient with Turner's syndrome can be diagnosed in infancy due to the characteristic lymphoedema of the feet and hands and loose skin folds over the nape of the neck. Later in life the patient has a short stature, a square, shield-like chest, and a short, webbed neck. Low set ears, a fish-like mouth and ptosis are also characteristic of this disorder, as is sexual infantilism. Associated abnormalities include coarctation of the aorta, pigmented naevi, cubitus valgus, hypertension, and renal abnormalities. There may also be a tendency toward keloid formation, recurrent otitis media, puffiness of the dorsum of the hands, short fourth metacarpals and hypoplastic nails.

Disorders associated with this syndrome include diabetes mellitus, obesity, rheumatoid arthritis, Hashimoto's thyroiditis, inflammatory bowel disease, and congenital heart disease.

Investigative procedures

A buccal smear for sex chromatin and karyotype analysis should be performed on phenotypic females with the following features:

- Short stature
- Somatic anomalies associated with gonadal dysgenesis
- Delayed adolescence and increased concentration of plasma gonadotrophins.

Medical management

Oestrogen is often prescribed to promote the development of secondary sex characteristics and menstruation. Associated disorders are treated.

HYPERGONADISM

Precocious puberty

Sexual development before the age of ten years in boys and eight years in girls is considered abnormal and is termed precocious puberty.

Aetiology

In the majority of female patients the underlying cause cannot be found. In the remainder, and in males, the cause may be either:

1. Increasing concentrations of androgens or oestrogens produced by disease of the adrenals or gonads, or tumours containing gonadal components.
2. Premature secretion of gonadotropins by the hypothalamus or pituitary gland.

Clinical manifestations

Precocious puberty manifests as a deepening of the voice and development of external genitalia in boys, and breast development and the onset of menstruation in girls.

Both sexes experience abnormal growth due to the influence of sex hormones on muscle and bone, but dwarfism eventually results due to the premature closure of the epiphyses.

Medical management

In boys the treatment of choice is cyproterone, an anti-androgen drug. Certain progestational agents can be used to inhibit gonadotrophin secretion in both sexes. In girls these halt menses and breast development. In boys they decrease testicular size, halt penile erections, and modify any tendency to aggressive behaviour. Skeletal development and maturation can also be slowed. In girls, if the underlying cause cannot be identified, treatment is prohibited.

Psychological support is of great importance as the child may become the object of ridicule and amusement by peers. Often there is a tendency for relatives, parents and teachers to treat him as if he was older, not realizing that the social maturation does not match the physical development.

Hirsuitism and virilism

Hirsuitism is the term used to describe excessive body hair, that is, more hair than is cosmetically acceptable to a woman living in a given culture.

Virilism is the syndrome of masculinization of females.

Aetiology

Most cases of hirsuitism have no underlying endocrine disease. It is often familial and strong racial differences exist in the amount of hirsuitism normally found in women. In general, dark haired, pigmented Caucasians from Mediterranean and southern European stock have a tendency to develop coarse hairs on the face, abdomen and thighs. Approximately 50% of hirsuitism is idiopathic.

Endocrinologic disorders associated with hirsuitism without virilism include: Cushing's syndrome; excessive use of glucocorticoids and androgens; and growth hormone excess due to pituitary tumours.

When virilism accompanies hirsuitism it is likely that malignant adrenal tumours, ovarian tumours, congenital adrenal hyperplasia, or polycystic ovarian disease will be present.

Clinical manifestations

Excessive hair is found on the face, breasts, abdomen, thighs and extremities. It is usually coarse and dark in colour. In ideopathic hirsuitism excess hair growth appears at puberty and continues to develop into the third decade.

When hirsuitism occurs with an accompanying endocrine disease, there is accompanying thick oily skin with acne. There is a tendency toward irregular menses and obesity but patients are usually fertile.

If there is an underlying pathology, additional symptoms specific to that endocrine disease will also be present.

The most common of the polycystic ovarian diseases is the Stein-Leventhal syndrome. Patients with this disorder suffer polycystic ovaries, amenorrhoea, obesity and acne. In virilism, the additional features include deepening of the voice, increased muscularity, receding hairline and an enlarged clitoris.

Investigative procedures

Measurement of plasma and/or urinary androgens should be performed. Patients displaying signs of virilism must be fully investigated to establish the underlying cause and they will generally have elevated testosterone levels.

Medical management

Cosmetic measures are usually the only management required if underlying causes have been excluded or treated. Depilatory creams, shaving, or waxing are simple, effective and inexpensive methods of temporary removal of excess hair.

Suppression of androgen production can be instigated with combination oral contraceptives, progestins, or glucocorticoids.

Cyproterone is an excellent anti-androgen and is extremely effective in the management of severe hirsuitism.

HERMAPHRODISM

True hermaphrodites have both ovarian and testicular tissue present in the same or opposite gonads.

Aetiology and diagnosis

Hermaphrodism is a genetic disorder and diagnosis should be considered in children with ambiguous external genetalia. Histological testing of ovarian and testicular tissue should be performed to determine the dominant sex. The finding of an XX/XY karyotype and an ovatestis in the inguinal region or labioscrotal fold establishes diagnosis.

Clinical manifestations

The external genitalia is highly variable and may be those of female or male, or more commonly a combination of both. Cryptorchidism and hypospadias are common and a uterus is present in all cases. The most common gonad found in the hermaphrodite is the ovotestis, followed by the ovary and less often the testis.

In over 50% of cases, menstruation occurs at puberty and in untreated children breast development will occur at this time. The ovary or the ovarian portion of the ovotestis will usually function normally whereas the testicular portion is dysgenetic.

Medical management

This depends largely on the age of the child at diagnosis, and on the assessment of the functional capacity of the gonads, genital ducts and external genitalia. In the majority of cases, feminization is the surgical treatment of choice.

SECTION B – REFERENCES AND FURTHER READING

Texts

Anderson J R (ed) 1976 Muir's textbook of pathology, 10th edn. Edward Arnold, London

Anthony C P 1984 Structure and function of the body. Mosby, St Louis

Cahill M (ed) 1984 Endocrine disorders: nurse's clinical library. Springhouse, Pennsylvania

Chaney M (ed) 1982 Managing diabetes properly, 2nd edn. Springhouse, Pennsylvania

Creager J G 1982 Human anatomy and physiology. Wadsworth, California

Davidson M B 1986 Diabetes mellitus: diagnosis and treatment 2nd edn. Wiley, New York

Felig P et al (eds) 1987 Endocrinology and metabolism 2nd edn. McGraw-Hill, New York

Fletcher R F 1987 Lecture notes on endocrinology. Blackwell, Oxford

Greenspan F S, Forsham P H 1986 Basic and clinical endocrinology 2nd edn. Lange, Los Altos

Havard M 1986 A nursing guide to drugs, 2nd edn. Churchill Livingstone, Melbourne

Kohler P O, Jordan R (eds) 1986 Clinical endocrinology. Wiley, New York

Larkins R G 1985 A practical approach to endocrine disorders. Williams & Wilkins, Sydney

Laycock J 1983 Essential endocrinology. Oxford University Press, Oxford

Lewis J G 1984 The endocrine system. Churchill Livingstone, Edinburgh

Luckmann J, Sorensen K C 1980 Medical-surgical nursing: a psychophysiologic approach, 2nd edn. Saunders, Philadelphia

Macleod J 1987 Davidson's principles and practice of medicine, 15th edn. Churchill Livingstone, Edinburgh

Read A E, Barritt D W, Langton Hewer R 1986 Modern Medicine, 3rd edn. Churchill Livingstone, Edinburgh

Society of Hospital Pharmacists of Australia 1985 Pharmacology and drug information for nurses, 2nd edn. Saunders, Sydney

Storlie F J (ed) 1984 Diseases: nurse's reference library, 2nd edn. Springhouse, Pennsylvania

Taft P 1985 Diabetes mellitus. Adis, Sydney

Tindall G T, Barrow D L 1986 Disorders of the pituitary. Mosby, St Louis

Wilson J D, Foster D W (eds) 1985 Williams textbook of endocrinology 7th edn. Saunders, Philadelphia

Journals

Arcangelo V P 1983 Simple goitre. Nursing 83 13 : 3 : 47

Bille D A 1986 Tailoring your diabetic patient's care plan to fit his life style. Nursing 86 16 : 2 : 54–57

Byrnes C A 1987 What's new in the diabetic diet. Nursing 87 17 : 8 : 58–59

Chambers J K 1983 Save your diabetic patient from early kidney damage. Nursing 83 13 : 5 : 58–63

Childs B P 1983 Insulin infusion pumps: new solution to an old problem. Nursing 83. 13 : 11 : 54–57

Christman C, Bennett J 1987 Diabetes: new names, new test, new diet. Nursing 87 17 : 1 : 34–41

Crigler-Meringola E D 1984 making life sweet again for the elderly diabetic. Nursing 84 14 : 4 : 61–64

Essig M 1983 Update your knowledge of oral antidiabetic agents. Nursing 83 13 : 10 : 58–63

Foubister J K 1985 Diabetes education and management. The Australian Nurses Journal 15 : 4 : 43–45

Knott S P, Herget M J 1984 Teaching self-injection to diabetics: an easier and more effective way. Nursing 84 14 : 1 : 57

Larson C A 1984 The critical path of adrenocortical insufficiency. Nursing 84 14 : 10 : 12–15

Lindsey N M 1983 Coping with Diabetes. Nursing 83 13 : 3 : 48–49

McConnell E A 1985 Assessing the thyroid. Nursing 85 15 : 5 : 60–62

Nurse's Reference Library 1983 Assessing the thyroid gland. Nursing 83 13 : 10 : 5

Robertson C 1984 Clear the exercise hurdles for your diabetic patient. Nursing 84 14 : 10 : 58–63

Robertson C 1986 When an insulin-dependent diabetic must be NPO Nursing 86 16 : 6 : 30–31

Robertson C 1986 Interpreting blood glucose studies. Nursing 86 16 : 8 : 64

Slaytor K 1987 Negotiating diabetes management. The Australian Nurses Journal. 17 : 5 : 47–49

Stock P L 1985 Insulin Shock. Nursing 85 15 : 4 : 53

Stock-Barkman P 1983 Confusing concepts: is it diabetic shock or diabetic coma? Nursing 83 13 : 6 : 33–41

Surr C W 1983 Teaching patients to use the new blood glucose monitoring products. Part 1. Nursing 83 13 : 1 : 42–45

Surr C W 1983 Teaching patients to use the new blood glucose monitoring products. Part 2. Nursing 83 13 : 2 : 58–62

Taylor D L 1983 Hyperglycaemia: physiology, signs, and symptoms. Nursing 83 13 : 2 : 52–54

Taylor D L 1983 Hypoglycaemia: physiology, signs, and symptoms. Nursing 83 13 : 3 : 44–46

White N E, Miller B K 1983 Glycohemoglobin: a new test to help the diabetic stay in control. Nursing 83 13 : 8 : 55–57

C

The cardiovascular system

31

Introduction to the cardiovascular system

Chris Game

The cardiovascular system comprises the heart and blood vessels – the arteries, arterioles, capillaries, venules, and veins. It is a closed circulatory system responsible for the constant circulation of blood throughout the body. Figure 31.1 shows the normal heart. The average person has 6.5 litres of blood and the heart pumps this volume approximately 1200 times per day, that is nearly 8000 litres. It has been estimated that the average person contains the equivalent of 95 000 km of vessels. The circulatory system comprises 2 major divisions: the pulmonary circulation and the systemic circulation.

In the pulmonary circulation, the heart pumps deoxygenated blood to the lungs via the pulmonary artery, where blood is reoxygenated and cellular waste products including carbon dioxide, are removed. The oxygenated blood is returned to the heart via the pulmonary veins and then pumped into the systemic circulation via the aorta.

Systemically, the vessels form a continuous network of blood supply to every living cell in the body. Arteries deliver nutrients in solution and oxygenated blood to the arterial capillary network, where the products necessary for normal cell function are released through the capillary membrane and transported to the cells. Cellular waste products cross back into the venous capillary network along with deoxygenated blood, and are transported back to the heart via the superior and inferior vena cavae. Waste products are also transported to the kidneys, liver, and skin for excretion. The portal circulation, a further division of the systemic circulation, is responsible for transporting nutrients absorbed via the gut to the liver.

The factors that regulate blood flow are complex and interact with each other to ensure that the heart and vessels function in the most efficient manner, regardless of the stress under which the body is operating at any given time. Blood pressure and its neurological and hormonal control

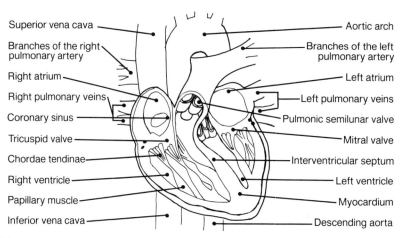

Fig. 31.1 The normal heart.

are the chief determinants of cardiovascular function. Blood pressure (BP) can be expressed as the product of cardiac output (CO) and peripheral resistance (PR).

Cardiac output depends upon stroke volume (SV) and the heart rate (HR). The stroke volume of the heart is the volume of blood that can be pumped from the left ventricle with each beat and in the average person equals 60–70 ml. Cardiac output is the volume of blood that can be pumped from the left ventricle into the aorta in 1 minute. As the average person has a heart rate of approximately 75 beats per minute then, under normal circumstances, the average cardiac output is approximately 5 litres; therefore CO = SV × HR.

Not all blood received by the ventricle is pumped with each beat and normally, at rest, nearly 40% of blood received remains as a residual volume in the ventricle and contributes to the next stroke volume. Under stress the residual volume decreases as the stroke volume increases to 80–90% and it is this residual volume which plays a vital role in enabling the body to increase cardiac output without an excessive increase in heart rate.

Peripheral resistance depends upon 3 factors: the viscosity of the blood; the length of the blood vessel; and the internal diameter of the vessel. The thicker the blood the greater the peripheral resistance and, the shorter and wider the vessel the lower the resistance. Arteries have thicker walls than veins which allows the movement of blood under high pressure and at great speed. Arterioles, although having thinner walls than arteries, are able to constrict and dilate quickly thus allowing fine regulation of blood flow into the capillaries, the walls of which consist of only a single layer of epithelial cells. Venules collect blood from the capillaries and have thinner walls than arterioles as do veins have thinner walls than arteries. However, venules and veins have far wider diameters than arterioles and arteries thus they offer very little resistance to the flow of blood back to the heart. Veins also contain valves which prevent the back flow of blood in response to gravity. (See Fig. 31.2)

Blood flows from areas of high pressure to areas of low pressure therefore blood flows from the heart via the arterial system and returns to the heart via the venous system. Blood will flow from

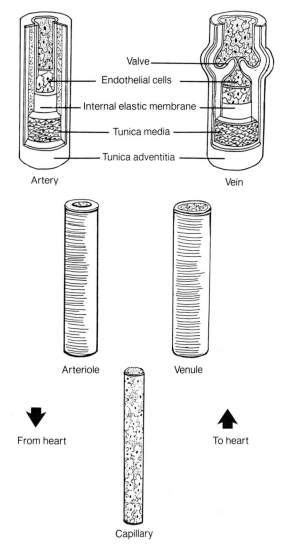

Fig. 31.2 Structure and comparative thickness of blood vessel walls.

the heart under a systolic pressure measuring, for example 120 mmHg in a large artery and progressively this pressure will fall as the blood travels further along the vessel system away from the heart. Capillary blood pressure measures approximately 35 mmHg at the arterial end and 15 mmHg at the venous end and central venous pressure of blood returning to the heart is normally only 1 mmHg.

Neurological control of blood pressure is effected through specialized nerve endings called baroreceptors and chemoreceptors. Baroreceptors are situated in most blood vessel walls but are in greatest numbers in the carotid arteries and the carotid sinuses. An increasing blood volume causes the vessels to dilate and baroreceptors respond to this stretching effect by increasing parasympathetic drive via vagal stimulation and inhibiting the vasomotor centre in the medulla. This results in peripheral vasodilation, a decreased heart rate, and less forceful cardiac contraction; the net result is a fall in arterial blood pressure. In reverse, when blood volume falls the baroreceptors stimulate the vasomotor centre and inhibit vagal stimulation. Thus a sympathetic drive occurs with a resultant rise in arterial blood pressure due to peripheral vasoconstriction, an increased heart rate and force of cardiac contraction.

Chemoreceptors are situated in vessel walls of the carotid arteries, the aorta, and the medulla. These nerve endings measure the levels of oxygen and carbon dioxide in the blood and respond to falling levels of either gas. As the gas concentrations fall, chemoreceptors cause a sympathetic drive and inhibit parasympathetic activity, to increase arterial blood pressure.

Hormonal regulation of blood pressure is effected by: adrenal secretion of epinephrine and norepinephrine; the secretion of the enzyme renin by the juxtaglomerular cells of the kidney resulting in the production of angiotensin; hypothalamic secretion of vasopressin; and general cellular secretion of hormone-like substances called prostaglandins. Epinephrine and norepinephrine secretion causes an increase in sympathetic drive with a resultant increase in arterial blood pressure. Specifically they stimulate alpha and beta receptors in the sympathetic nervous system dependent upon the body's needs; alpha receptor stimulation results in vasoconstriction, beta receptor stimulation results in vasodilation.

If blood pressure to the kidney falls, renin is released into the circulation and effects the conversion of angiotensinogen to the hormone angiotensin I. When blood containing this hormone reaches the lungs, another enzyme is released which converts angiotensin I to angiotensin II. Angiotensin II causes arterioles to constrict and also decreases the excretion of salt and water via the kidney; hence blood volume is

increased and arterial blood pressure rises. Vasopressin (antidiuretic hormone) is secreted in response to a falling blood pressure and acts on the renal tubules to cause water retention. In this way blood volume is increased and therefore blood pressure rises. Prostaglandins are thought to have an effect on blood pressure regulation by causing vascular constriction and dilation according to local cellular needs.

The neural control of cardiac contraction is via the conduction system of the heart. Sympathetic fibres of the cardiac nerves and parasympathetic fibres of the vagus nerve form the cardiac nerve plexus located near the arch of the aorta. Nerve fibres from this plexus form the sinoatrial (SA) and atrioventricular (AV) nodes (Fig. 31.3). Stimulation of the SA node with resultant transference of the stimulus to the AV node causes atrial contraction (systole). Transmission of the electrical impulse from the AV node to the AV bundle and Purkinje fibres results in ventricular systole and atrial relaxation (diastole). The cardiac cycle, that is each complete heart beat consisting of atrial and ventricular systole and diastole, occurs approximately once every 0.8 second. The average person is therefore said to have a heart rate of 70–75 beats/minute. Heart rate and myocardial contractility is increased when sympathetic stimulation of the SA and AV nodes occurs. Parasympathetic stimulation of the SA node results in decreased myocardial contractility and a lowered heart rate. It should be noted that sympathetic stimulation of the heart results in vasodilation of

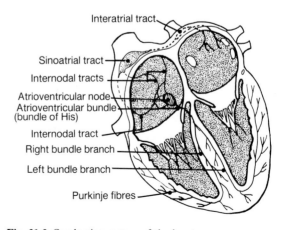

Fig. 31.3 Conduction system of the heart.

the coronary vessels, thus allowing maximum oxygenation of the myocardium whenever it is under an increased load.

Cardiac muscle is characterized physiologically as having excitability, automaticity, conductivity, and contractility. Excitability relates to the myocardial cell's capability to respond to an electrical stimulus; it depolarizes and repolarizes in response to the movement of sodium, potassium, and calcium ions across the cell membrane thus allowing an electrical charge to be transmitted. The period of depolarization to repolarization describes cardiac systole whilst the resting/refractory phase describes cardiac diastole. During the resting phase cardiac muscle will not respond to any stimulus.

Automaticity relates to the myocardial cell's capability to generate an action potential without external stimulation. The cells of the SA node in particular are capable of generating spontaneous action potentials. As a result, in certain circumstances, the heart is capable of independent function without autonomic nervous stimulation. Conductivity refers to the myocardial cell's ability to transmit an electrical stimulus and is closely related to the automaticity function. The SA node is capable of independently transmitting 60–100 beats/minute, the AV node 40–60 beats/minute, and the AV branches and Purkinje fibres 40 beats/minute. Therefore in situations of heart block (see page 329) self-pacing of the heart can occur.

Contractility relates to the ability of myocardial muscle fibres to shorten when stimulated. The presence of calcium ions is essential for cardiac muscle contraction in that calcium controls the degree of lengthening of cardiac muscle fibres. According to Starling's law, the force of a contraction depends upon the length of the myocardial muscle fibres, that is, the more cardiac fibres are stretched during diastole, then the more forcefully they will contract during systole. Therefore cardiac output can be increased by increasing the stroke volume and thus the force of contraction.

32

Disorders of vessels

Chris Game

ARTERIOSCLEROSIS AND ATHEROSCLEROSIS

Pathophysiology

The two most common terms that the nursing student will encounter when studying cardiac and peripheral arterial diseases are arteriosclerosis and atherosclerosis. Some authors fail to differentiate between the two pathologies, using both terms synonymously. By definition arteriosclerosis is 'hardening of the arteries', that is, degenerative arterial change associated with advancing age – primarily a thickening of the media. Atherosclerosis on the other hand is a hardening or thickening of the arteries caused by the deposition of hard yellow atheromatous plaques of lipoid material in the intimal layer of the arteries, thereby narrowing their lumina. Suffice to say that atherosclerosis rarely occurs in the total absence of arteriosclerosis and as the eventual presentation of both conditions is essentially the same, they will be considered together.

The World Health Organization has defined atherosclerosis as a complex intermix of changes in the intima of arteries consisting of 'the focal accumulation of lipids, complex carbohydrates, blood products, fibrous tissue and calcium deposits and associated with medial changes' (in Luckman & Sorensen, 1980). Atherosclerosis can therefore be seen as a generalized, patchy and irregularly occurring disease of arteries, characterized by narrowing of the lumina due to plaques/patches of fatty material and hardening of the walls – a condition both accelerated and aggravated by systemic hypertension (see page 282) and increasing age.

When a vessel is affected by atherosclerosis, the effect of the pathology will be seen in the organ supplied by the artery/arteries. For example, if a small vessel is involved it takes only a very small atheromatous plaque to block the lumen of the vessel completely, sometimes with disastrous results. The coronary arteries are examples of such small vessels wherein an occlusion can lead to extensive myocardial damage and necrosis, or even be fatal.

In larger vessels the atheroma so disturbs the flow of blood that the increased turbidity leads to fractionalization of the blood products and increased deposition of blood fragments, which in turn will increase the size of the atheroma. Turbidity is also increased at vessel bifurcations and lumina of branches, hence the high incidence of atheroma in the lower branches of the aorta. This vicious cycle will continue unabated until such time as the person experiences symptoms of ischaemia, that is, deficient blood supply resulting in reduced oxygenation to the tissues distal to the obstruction. Cerebral ischaemia due to atheroma of the carotid, vertebral, basilar and cerebral arteries, and the vessels of the Circle of Willis, may ultimately lead to a cerebrovascular accident or 'stroke'. In the periphery, due to atheroma of the femoral or popliteal arteries, progressive loss of blood supply to the legs gives rise to the condition of intermittent claudication, that is, pain experienced when exercising calf muscles, for example in walking, and may ultimately lead to the development of gangrene which occurs after total occlusion to the periphery. Gangrene commences in the toes and if untreated progresses proximally up the limb.

It is estimated that close to 2000 Australians die each year from atherosclerosis alone; this represents 1.8% of all deaths. When added to deaths due to other ischaemic disorders, for example hypertension, acute myocardial infarction and cerebrovascular accidents, the toll rises to 48 000 or 45% of all deaths (Cameron, 1983). Ischaemic heart disease is still the most common killer of adult Australians and atherosclerosis has a proven predilection for the coronary arteries. The importance of this knowledge to the nursing student is that if persons at risk of developing atherosclerosis and/or arteriosclerosis can be identified, then health education programmes instituted at an early age may significantly reduce the incidence of the disease in the future.

Risk factors

Although the specific cause(s) of the disease state are unknown, many factors have been identified that are believed to lead to the development of atheroma and hardening of arterial walls. Factors identified in susceptible persons include the following:

1. Age – atheroma increases with advancing age and brittleness of arterial walls occurs in extreme old age.
2. Sex – atheroma development is more severe in males and occurs more commonly in males than in females of pre-menopausal age. Following menopause the incidence of atheroma development in women equals that of men.
3. Systemic hypertension – although atheroma is found in the systemic vessels of persons with 'normal' blood pressure, it is seen to be more intense and widespread in persons with hypertension.
4. Hypercholesteraemia – although many forms of hyperlipoproteinaemia exist, hypercholesteraemia is considered to be the most common of the hyperlipidaemias that predispose grossly to atheroma formation.
5. Cigarette smoking – the mechanism of effect is unknown, but the statistical incidence of cigarette smokers with gross atheroma continues to increase.

6. Physical activity and obesity – people with more physically strenuous jobs and who are of the correct weight for their height, have a lower incidence of atheroma formation.
7. Diabetes mellitus – people in whom diabetes mellitus is diagnosed stand an increased risk from arteriosclerosis, especially those persons who developed adult onset diabetes. It is to be also noted that both clinical conditions have similar symptoms and signs and therefore the diabetic with arteriosclerosis/atherosclerosis is likely to manifest a more severe presentation of the disease condition.
8. Genetic influences – these are definitely important in persons with a family history of diabetes or familial hypercholesteraemia, and population studies based on genetic influences can assist to identify persons at greatest risk of atheroma development.

A person who has a combination of risk factors is more likely to develop atheroma than is the person with only one risk factor identified. Therefore the obese, hypertensive person with hypercholesteraemia is especially at risk.

Clinical manifestations

The clinical manifestation of these pathologies occurs only after vessel occlusion is either complete (resulting in, for example, a myocardial infarction, cerebrovascular accident or gangrene) or when blood flow is severely compromised (resulting in the development of symptoms and signs of ischaemia, for example, angina, intermittent claudication or transient ischaemic attacks affecting the cerebrum).

Discussion of investigative procedures and specific medical and nursing assessment and management will occur in the following chapters, where the specific clinical conditions associated with arteriosclerosis and atherosclerosis are covered.

Health education

The nurse, through his/her involvement in patient care and health education in all areas of the health service, has a major role to play in educating the general public, especially those persons with one or more of the previously identified risk factors.

Early identification of persons with disorders such as systemic hypertension, diabetes mellitus and obesity can lead to prompt and adequate medical and nursing management. This will help to either eliminate adverse factors, prevent further progression of the disease, or to bring under control the patient's physical condition so that optimal health is attained and maintained, and the risks of associated complications from atherosclerosis are minimized. The nurse assumes an important role in recognizing 'at risk persons', teaching them to understand the potential dangers and assisting them to take responsibility for achieving the desired goal of optimal health.

Reduction of weight to normal standards for height and build is advocated in order to reduce cardiac workload and the likelihood of developing systemic hypertension. Treatment of hypercholesteraemia through dietary control has finally been proven to reduce the risk of the development of heart disease, most probably by preventing the development of coronary atherosclerosis. The suspicion of diets high in animal fats and therefore high in cholesterol and triglycerides has been supported, and in Australia the National Heart Foundation advocates dietary reduction in cholesterol and saturated fatty acids, and that saturated fats in the diet be replaced with polyunsaturated fats. However, it must be noted that polyunsaturated fats should also be kept to a minimum wherever possible.

The identified association of cigarette smoking with atheroma formation warrants intensive education of the public to reduce the incidence of smoking in the community. More especially, concentration in school health education programmes is needed to attempt to prevent young people from taking up smoking in the first place.

Regular and controlled exercise is advisable and may help in the prevention of ischaemic heart disease; such exercise is believed to promote the development of collateral circulation. The nurse, either in the community or when planning the discharge of patients from hospital, has a valuable opportunity to assist in the development of, or actually plan, individualized exercise and rest

regimes, and other health programmes. Patients should, especially males and post-menopausal women, also be advised to have regular medical examinations.

HYPERTENSION

Pathophysiology

Blood pressure (BP) is normally described as the sum total of the cardiac output (CO) or blood flow, in relation to the peripheral resistance (PR) or the ability of peripheral vessels to constrict, that is, $BP = CO \times PR$.

In the healthy individual, should cardiac output increase, as in exercise, there is a corresponding resultant decrease in peripheral resistance so that the individual's blood pressure is maintained at a normal level (normotension). The converse of the equation is also true: should a person's cardiac output fall, as in haemorrhage, there is a corresponding increase in the peripheral resistance in an attempt to maintain normotensive blood pressure.

There is debate 'as to whether the initiating lesion in essential hypertension is increased total peripheral resistance (TPR) or a normal TPR in the face of increased cardiac output, for which some evidence does exist' (Groer, 1979). The question remains: is either factor the cause or the result of the disease? 'Sclerosis of many . . . vessels is found in essential hypertension, and it is believed that prolonged exposure to elevated blood pressure *itself* can damage blood vessels, causing them to become thickened and sclerotic and even haemorrhagic and necrotic' (Groer, 1979).

Regardless of the debate over cause and effect, in the hypertensive individual normal reflex reduction in peripheral resistance does not occur due to the inability of the smooth muscle in the arteries and arterioles to relax, and therefore the hypertensive state occurs. Any factors that will increase cardiac output and/or peripheral resistance in the hypertensive person, will maintain his hypertensive state.

The single most common characteristic in the development of hypertension is increased peripheral resistance. This is due to narrowing of the lumina of arterioles in atherosclerosis, and hardening of the artery and arteriolar walls by fibrotic replacement of smooth muscle in arteriosclerosis.

The underlying pathology of hypertension is cyclic in effect. If the arterial system increases its peripheral resistance then the heart has to work harder in order to pump blood into the system against the increased pressure; therefore cardiac workload increases. In order to cope with this increased effort and to prevent eventual heart failure the mass of the left ventricle increases (left ventricular hypertrophy). This in turn causes an increase in cardiac workload.

Therefore it can be seen that the effects of hypertension are paradoxical – if peripheral resistance is allowed to continue to increase then so will cardiac output and the hypertensive state will progress even further.

Systemic hypertension, or 'high blood pressure', is a disease of the arteries that is said to exist when an individual's blood pressure remains consistently above 150 mmHg systolic and/or 90 mmHg diastolic.

Descriptive terms applied to the classification of this disease include primary/essential, secondary, malignant and benign.

Primary/essential hypertension

The specific cause(s) are unknown, although many contributing factors may be identified in the course of the disease. Of all persons with systemic hypertension, 80% fall into this group, that is, 860 000 adult Australians, or approximately 6.1% of the total population (Cameron, 1980) are estimated to suffer from this form of hypertensive disease. In 1981, over 1200 deaths from hypertension were recorded, this figure representing 1.2% of all deaths in that year. When this statistic is considered along with deaths from other cardiovascular and cerebrovascular causes to which systemic hypertension may have contributed (see page 281), it can be seen why community health groups are actively involved in identifying both sufferers of hypertension and persons at risk. The success of such health education programs is demonstrated in the decrease in the number of deaths due to hypertension and atherosclerosis specifically.

Secondary hypertension

In this form the hypertensive state is due to a known cause and therefore is secondary to, or exists as a result of, a known disease state. Common causes of secondary hypertension in Australia are:

- Chronic glomerulonephritis and pyelonephritis (highest incidence)
- Stenosis of a renal artery
- Thyrotoxicosis
- Coarctation of the aorta
- Phaeochromocytoma
- Toxaemia of pregnancy.

Malignant hypertension

This refers to an accelerated form of hypertension that is both severe in degree and rapid in progression. Once established the condition is hard to control by medical or nursing measures and death usually results within 2–3 years. Death occurs as a result of damage to organs from the excessively high blood pressure. Myocardial infarction, congestive heart failure, cerebrovascular accident and renal damage leading to uraemia are common causes of death.

Benign hypertension

This refers to the chronic development of the clinical state of hypertension, in that it describes a more moderate rise in blood pressure over a number of years.

In all, the most common presentation of hypertension in the Australian community is benign and/or primary/essential hypertension. Unfortunately, it is estimated that over 50% of persons with clinical symptoms and signs are undiagnosed and, of those who have been diagnosed, a large number are not receiving adequate treatment due to a variety of reasons (see page 287).

Risk factors

Identified factors which place individuals at risk of developing hypertensive disease are:

- Atherosclerosis (leading risk factor)
- Hypercholesteraemia, leading to the formation of atheromatous plaques

- Age, wherein arteriosclerotic changes decrease the distensible ability of arterioles
- Stimulation of the sympathetic nervous system to release epinephrine and norepinephrine due to environmental stressors, hormones (for example, renin or catecholamines), or other autonomic antagonist activities
- Abnormal sodium metabolism, which leads to increased sodium and water retention, the end result of which is an increased extracellular fluid volume (see page 81)
- Obesity, which increases cardiac workload
- Cigarette smoking, wherein nicotinic acid stimulates vasoconstrictors
- Sex. Women are affected more often than men, a factor sometimes attributed to the prescription of birth control pills and oestrogen compounds
- Familial history of hypertension (there is no proven genetic link)
- Exercise. Persons with a sedentary lifestyle are at a greater risk

Clinical manifestations

Symptoms that usually force the patient to seek medical aid are likely to be some or all of:

- Headache, usually occipital with dizziness
- Blurred vision
- Nausea and vomiting
- Shortness of breath
- Dependent oedema
- Chest pain and/or palpitations
- Lethargy, fatigue
- Increasing tension, anxiety
- Epistaxis.

On clinical examination, the patient will exhibit some or all, depending upon the severity of the disease presentation, of the following:

- Systolic BP > 150 mmHg (consistently)
- Diastolic BP > 90 mmHg (consistently)
- Left ventricular hypertrophy
- Decreased renal perfusion
- Proteinuria and/or haematuria
- Papilloedema and ocular fundal changes
- Cerebral encephalopathy, manifested as a rise in intracranial pressure (see page 161)
- Cerebral haemorrhage
- Angina pectoris and/or myocardial infarction
- Congestive heart failure.

Investigative procedures

- Chest X-ray, and electrocardiogram are used to determine the degree of left ventricular hypertrophy and cardiac failure.
- Blood analysis for full blood count, electrolytes, urea/nitrogen and creatine to both exclude secondary causes and ascertain renal effects of the disease process.
- Urinalysis with microscopy and 24-hour collections for creatinine clearance and vanillylmandelic acid (VMA) estimations are performed.
- Intravenous pyelogram (IVP) assesses renal perfusion.

Medical and surgical management

The aims of treatment are to:

1. Reduce the elevated blood pressure to within 'normal' limits.
2. Maintain the patient's blood pressure at his 'normal' level.
3. Prevent complications both of the disease and its treatment.

Surgical intervention in the treatment of hypertension is restricted to the removal of secondary causes. However, not all secondary causes can be treated surgically, for example, chronic glomerulo- or pyelonephritis. Also if a secondary cause of hypertension has been undiagnosed for a length of time, then surgical intervention may not reduce the hypertensive state or restore a 'normal' blood pressure. For example, if renal artery stenosis is left untreated then renin/angiotensin ratios can become fixed, and despite surgical correction the patient's blood pressure may remain high.

Medical intervention is therefore aimed at controlling the disease process by either eliminating or managing the patient's symptoms and signs. This control is most often accomplished by the use of a variety of drugs aimed at affecting one or more of the three determinants of blood pressure: blood volume, cardiac output, and peripheral resistance.

Diuretics

These reduce the amounts of water, sodium, and chlorine being retained by the body and therefore reduce extracellular fluid volume, especially blood volume. In mild hypertension, diuretics in conjunction with weight reduction diets and restrained sodium intake may be the only form of treatment necessary to control the hypertensive state. In moderate to severe hypertension, diuretics also enhance the effect of antihypertensive agents.

Thiazides are commonly used diuretics that inhibit sodium reabsorption at the diluting segment of the ascending limb of the renal tubule and cause mild potassium depletion. Their action lasts for about 12 hours; they are well tolerated and have few side-effects. These diuretics are also known to have an antihypertensive effect which is independent of their diuretic action. As many as 50% of people with mild hypertension will respond to a thiazide prescribed without an antihypertensive drug.

Frusemide and ethacrynic acid are loop of Henle diuretics that act at most proximal sites and therefore produce an intense diuresis of relatively short duration (4–6 hours). They have the potential to cause severe hypokalaemia and other electrolyte disturbances, and potassium supplements must be prescribed concurrently.

'Potassium-sparing' diuretics are gaining popularity, as they increase patient compliance because only the one drug needs to be taken. Commonly prescribed diuretics from this group include spironolactone, amiloride, triamterene, and mixed hydrochlorothiazide/amiloride.

Antihypertensive agents

These are drugs which lower blood pressure and are used in the treatment of moderate and severe hypertension. They are not free from risk and patients must remain under medical supervision whilst taking these drugs; both these factors may increase patients' anxiety about their condition and lead to the poor compliance generally associated with the drug treatment of hypertension. These drugs are broadly divided into two categories: those which reduce the sympathetic outflow from the autonomic nervous system, and those which act directly as vasodilators.

Drugs reducing sympathetic outflow from the autonomic nervous system fall into several categories:

1. Centrally acting drugs. These reduce sympathetic drive and there is a resultant fall in peripheral blood pressure; clonidine and methyldopa are the commonly prescribed drugs from this group
2. Drugs which block noradrenergic receptors: beta-blocking drugs. These can be either nonselective or cardioselective. The latter have the advantage that they do not significantly stimulate beta-2 receptors in the respiratory tract which cause bronchodilation, unless administered in extremely high doses; however, any patient with a history of asthma or obstructive airways disease should not be administered beta-blocking drugs for fear of developing bronchospasm. The nurse should also note that in order to prevent rapid deterioration of the patient's condition, discontinuance of beta-blockers should be gradual and over a period of days. Nonselective beta-blockers include propranolol, pindolol and oxprenolol. Metoprolol and atenolol are commonly used cardioselective beta-blockers. Labetolol is sometimes prescribed because it is both an alpha- and a beta-blocker.
3. Drugs which deplete autonomic transmitters. Reserpine blocks the release of noradrenaline from post-ganglionic neurones and also has a tranquillizing effect on the patient

Adrenergic neurone-blocking agents, for example, guanethidine and bethanidine, and ganglion blocking agents, such as pentolinium and mecamylamine, are not commonly prescribed nowadays. This is due to the adverse effects associated with their use, for example, orthostatic hypotension and unwanted anticholinergic effects, and the availability of more acceptable therapeutic agents.

Drugs which act directly as vasodilators act by causing relaxation of smooth muscle in the vessel walls, thus resulting in a fall in blood pressure due to vasodilation. Hydralazine is the most commonly prescribed in this group and others include diazoxide, prazosin, and sodium nitroprusside.

Potassium supplements

These may be used when the patient is established on diuretic therapy using nonpotassium-sparing drugs, and certainly if the patient is currently prescribed digoxin (see page 312). Many forms of supplements are available and the sustained-release tablet is the most common type used.

Dosage is controlled by regular serum potassium analysis.

Diet

As each patient is an individual who is reacting individually to his disease state, there is no specifically recognized dietary management for hypertension. The type of diet for any one patient will depend largely upon his individual needs, the severity of the hypertensive state, the degree of sodium restriction ordered, the type and dose of diuretic and other drugs prescribed, the presence or absence of obesity, and any existing cardiac diseases.

It is recommended that a patient with moderate to severe hypertension should restrict his dietary intake of added salt, cholesterol and fats both saturated and polyunsaturated. He should also maintain moderate caloric restriction. Dietary supplements of foods high in potassium may assist in the prevention of hypokalaemia in the patient who is prescribed nonpotassium-sparing diuretics.

Wherever possible the patient's cultural influences regarding diet must be taken into account and specific customary foods incorporated into daily allowances.

Nursing management

Patients react differently to their hypertensive state and will therefore present with individual problems to be overcome and individual needs to be met. Not all patients have the same cause and symptomatology nor do they have the same degree of severity of hypertensive state. Therefore care should be individualized and involve the patient and his significant others in its planning, implementation, and evaluation.

Few patients require hospitalization for reduction and stabilization of blood pressure. Some patients may be hospitalized for investigation as to the cause of the hypertension or, for control of complications including uncontrolled hypertension. Patients must be encouraged to take responsibility for their own health and the nurse may be involved in the education of the patient and his significant others.

Basically this responsibility will involve: adequate rest during the day; promotion of good sleep patterns; management of emotional stress; mild analgesia to control headaches; reduction or cessation of alcohol and/or smoking; improvement in diet in terms of less salt, fats, and cholesterol; and weight reduction.

Health education

The patient must recognize the importance of his drug therapy and the need for strict adherence to the drug regime. This may involve the nurse in developing a teaching plan that will enhance patient compliance with respect to his drug treatment. Appointments for regular medical check-ups will be required, and the patient should be encouraged to keep these appointments. As well, family members should be encouraged to seek regular blood pressure checks.

The patient should be encouraged to seek medical help if symptoms return and/or extend, and the detrimental effects and risks associated with continued cigarette smoking and high alcohol consumption should be stressed, where necessary. Drug therapy and recognition of its toxic and side effects should be completely explained to the patient and his significant others.

Allied paramedical care

In the case of the patient hospitalized for stabilization of uncontrolled hypertension or for treatment of complications the total health team is involved in the return of the patient to his optimal health. Other therapists should be consulted in the planning stage and be encouraged to contribute to the patient's management.

The social worker or welfare officer can give valuable advice and assistance in the reduction of the patient's lifestyle stressors. The physiotherapist assists in planning exercise and rest programmes and the occupational therapist assists in the streamlining of activities of daily living to further reduce stressors. The degree of allied therapy input will be largely determined by the extent of the disease state and the presence of complications.

Inherent problems of treatment

Most problems inherent in treatment stem from:

- Unpleasant side effects of the drug therapy
- Patient noncompliance with drug therapy
- The need to reduce caloric and salt intake
- Disruption to family and work life necessitated by changes to the patient's lifestyle.

Unpleasant side effects of drug therapy. Because most antihypertensive agents block or reduce sympathetic activity, most side effects will be due to a resultant increase in parasympathetic drive or adverse reactions specific to the prescribed agent; these may include transient headaches, depression, drowsiness, nasal stuffiness, muscle cramps, orthostatic hypotension, bronchospasm, dry mouth, gastrointestinal upsets, and sexual impotence. Propranolol and pindolol may cause hallucinations, insomnia, and bizarre dreams.

To minimize the adverse effects of diuretic therapy these drugs should be taken in the early morning, and certainly before the midday meal, so that the patient has his diuresis during his waking hours.

Patient noncompliance with drug therapy. For a patient to accept responsibility for his own treatment and condition he must fully understand the medications that have been prescribed, and the effects that may ensue should he cease treatment. Often patients fail to comply with drug therapy simply because they either don't understand why they need to take the drugs, or do not understand how to take them correctly.

Diet therapy. The need to reduce sodium intake will require the patient's meal to be cooked separately from the family's meal if salt reduction is to be severe. Avoidance of cholesterol and saturated fats as well as a reduction in caloric intake may well mean a change in established dietary habits that the patient may be neither willing nor able to undertake. Close attention to diet may make the patient over-anxious about his condition, and this could cause psychological disruption within the family unit.

Disruption to lifestyle. The patient will require considerable support from both his significant others and the health team if drastic changes are to be made in his home and work environment.

These changes will be another source of socio-economic and psychological stress for the patient and his family.

Complications of hypertension

As mentioned at the beginning of this chapter, complications of hypertension are due to organ damage from the high blood pressure in the vessels supplying the organs. Common presentations of complications from hypertensive disease are:

- Left ventricular heart failure
- Congestive heart failure
- Myocardial infarction
- Cerebrovascular accident
- Hypertensive encephalopathy, manifested as severe raised intracranial pressure
- Papilloedema
- Renal failure and uraemia
- Retinal haemorrhages, infarcts, and blindness.

Left ventricular heart failure and congestive heart failure cause 60% of the known deaths from benign, essential hypertension. Cerebrovascular accidents as a result of cerebral haemorrhage causes 30% of these deaths.

It may be well to re-emphasise at this point that it is estimated that of all hypertensive disease in Australia, only 50% of sufferers are diagnosed and of those only 50% are under treatment; even more alarming is the estimate that only 50% of these individuals being treated are adequately controlled. Therefore many patients may escape either detection or revised treatment until such time as they present with a complication, for example, cerebrovascular accident.

Anticipated outcome

Patients with uncomplicated hypertension should be able to live normal lives without drastic changes to their lifestyle or dietary habits, for as long as their blood pressure remains under control and they are free of complications. Patient compliance in drug therapy will largely determine the degree of control that a patient's condition will manifest.

As far as is practical, the individual patient should be assessed according to his pattern of disease presentation and care should be taken to overcome his own particular problems with a minimum of disruption to his normal living pattern.

With moderate to severe hypertension, care should be taken to minimize the inherent effects of treatment, whilst at the same time maintaining the patient's optimum health and preventing the tragic complications of this disease.

VASCULAR DISORDERS

Vascular disease can affect arteries or veins or present as disorders affecting both forms of vessels simultaneously. It is normally a degenerative process and therefore is seen more commonly in elderly patients. Vascular disease usually presents with arterial aneurysm, as arterial or venous inflammation, or occlusion. With increasing age, it is more likely that vascular disease will co-exist in both veins and arteries. As the aims of nursing management for the patient with either arterial or venous vascular disease are essentially similar, specific nursing care is included where the disorder is discussed; otherwise general nursing care encompasses all vascular disorders outlined.

Amputation as a surgical intervention for lower extremity vascular disease will be studied. As the techniques for the treatment of peripheral gangrene in the patient with diabetes-induced vascular degeneration and the principles for lower limb amputation following trauma are consistent with this intervention, the principles of treatment and nursing management will be covered in detail in this chapter. Amputation as a result of trauma is often associated with a speedier rehabilitation because these patients tend to be younger and are less likely to have associated chronic vascular, or other medical disease.

Risk factors

Many factors have been identified as predisposing an individual to the development of vascular disease, and chief among these are the effects of ageing, obesity, and smoking; diabetes mellitus and/or hypertension commonly co-exists. Medications that a person may have been previously, or is currently, prescribed can contribute to the disease process, and people in whom there is already evidence of other vascular disturbance are more likely to develop a vascular disorder.

In arterial vascular disease, changes within the vessels themselves are most likely to place the person at risk and especially such changes as those seen in atherosclerosis, hypertension, hypercholesteraemia, and hyperlipidaemia. As well, arterial vascular disease occurs more frequently in males; in those persons with an inherited predisposition; or in those with a history of diabetes mellitus (especially adult onset); and in people with a sedentary and/or stressful lifestyle.

The commonest causes of venous vascular disease are thrombi and insufficiency resulting from venous stasis, hypercoagulability, and vein wall trauma. These causes are usually secondary in those persons in whom surgery has injured vessel walls, for example in orthopaedic procedures; those in whom venous stasis is likely, for example persons who are pregnant, immobile, elderly, dehydrated, or who stand for long periods, such as nurses and shop assistants; and those who are in a hypercoagulable state, for example patients with cancer. Venous vascular disease occurs more frequently in females and particularly in women taking oral contraceptives or oestrogen replacement therapy. Diseases such as congestive heart failure and inflammatory responses to lymphoedema and phlebitis are known to predispose to venous vascular disease.

Arterial aneurysm

An aneurysm occurs when the arterial wall is weakened and the weakened area balloons outward. Rupture is a distinct possibility but containment of the ballooning process by surrounding tissue and/or organs normally prevents this occurring before corrective surgery can be performed. Arteriosclerosis is the most common cause of arterial wall weakening, although hypertension, trauma, arterial infection, and arterial occlusion can also lead to aneurysm. The most common site for aneurysm development is the abdominal aorta between the level of the renal arteries and the iliac bifurcation. Other sites include the thoracic aorta, especially involving the arch of the aorta; and peripheral aneurysms involving the femoral and popliteal arteries.

Ballooning of the arterial wall can occur unilaterally, producing a saccular aneurysm or it can involve the entire diameter of the artery producing a fusiform aneurysm (Fig. 32.1A). Initially the degenerative process of arteriosclerosis weakens the wall of the artery. The effect of arterial blood pressure is to increase the tension on the weakened area which finally gives way and the aneurysm results. The stretched and roughened intima of the aneurysm triggers the development of a mural thrombus (Fig. 32.1B) which will ultimately decrease the lumen of the vessel. The combination of effects of weakening of the wall, the presence of the mural thrombus, and the increasing blood pressure required to permit blood flow through the narrowing lumen of the aneurysm predispose it to rupture.

A false aneurysm (Fig. 32.1C) occurs following haematoma development on the tunica adventitia due to either trauma or a leaking anastomosis. As the haematoma increases it pulsates and mimics an aneurysm in its presentation.

A dissecting aneurysm (Fig. 32.1D) occurs when the weakened wall of the aneurysm splits and a false lumen is created between the tunica intima and tunica media. An intimal tear is the usual cause of weakening of the intimal layer and cystic medial necrosis will then produce weakening of the medial layer. The artery will lose elasticity and as blood enters the false lumen the degree of dissection is increased. Acute dissection along the length of the aorta is usually fatal as blood is directed into the false lumen and away from arteries supplying vital organs.

Fusiform aneurysms are the most common and they occur more frequently in the abdominal aorta. Should an aneurysm rupture, the direction of the rupture will determine the fate of the patient. Nearly all abdominal aortic aneurysms rupture extraperitoneally and the kidneys, perirenal fat, and the peritoneum control the degree and rate of haemorrhage by creating a tamponade. Intraperitoneal rupture is almost always fatal as there are no structures to create a tamponade effect. If a large aneurysm is ignored and goes

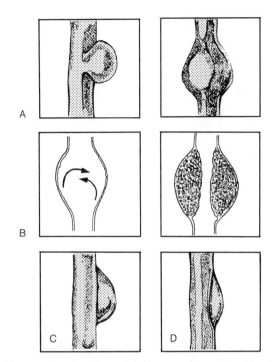

Fig. 32.1 A – Saccular and fusiform aneurysms. **B** – Blood swirls within aneurysm, causing development of mural thrombus and further stretching the arterial wall. **C** – False aneurysm. **D** – Dissecting aneurysm.

untreated it will ultimately progress to fatal rupture.

Clinical manifestations

Unfortunately, the majority of patients with an aneurysm remain asymptomatic until either just prior to rupture or until rupture occurs.

Abdominal aneurysm. Usually impending rupture is signalled by the onset of a dull ache felt in the middle of the left flank region accompanied by a low back pain or 'dragging' feeling. Most patients are able to describe abdominal palpitations on assuming a lying position and the aneurysm may be palpable as a pulsating abdominal mass.

Thoracic aneurysm. Impending rupture is usually signalled by the sudden onset of a 'tearing' chest pain extending to the neck, shoulders, and then proceeding down into the abdomen or lower back. A slowly developing aneurysm may be accidentally discovered on routine chest X-ray in which it is seen distorting other chest structure alignment, for example, midline displacement of the trachea.

Alternatively the patient may present with diffi-culty in swallowing if the aneurysm is compressing the oesophagus.

Angiography is usually performed in combina-tion with an ultrasound. An angiogram will deter-mine the location of the aneurysm and the integrity of the proximal and distal vessels whereas the ultrasound will determine the shape and size of the aneurysm. As angiography only visualizes the lumen of the aneurysm, comparison of the tests will ascertain the size of the mural thrombus.

Medical and surgical management

Acute rupture of an aneurysm is a medical emerg-ency and the patient should be transported to hospital for immediate surgery. The patient will suffer acute circulatory collapse and will be in a profound state of shock (see page 105). The appli-cation of medical antishock trousers (a MAST suit) may prevent total circulatory collapse until the patient can reach the operating room. Alterna-tively, a balloon-tipped catheter may be inserted into the brachial artery and then passed into the aorta until the neck of the aneurysm is reached. The balloon is then inflated and creates a tempo-rary tamponade to control haemorrhage until surgery can be performed (Fig. 32.2).

Surgical repair of an aneurysm consists of resec-tion of the portion of artery containing the aneu-rysm and grafting of a synthetic crimp prosthesis (usually dacron) in the case of fusiform, dissecting, and large saccular aneurysms. Patch grafting of a small saccular aneurysm may be performed although resection is safer; synthetic patches tend to provide an area of arterial wall weakness which may again form an aneurysm some time later. Should a patient be a poor surgical risk for resection and grafting, then a crimp prosthesis may be applied externally to the aneurysm to minimize the likelihood of rupture (Fig. 32.3).

Aneurysm repair is major surgery and places the patient at a grave risk. It is not unusual for the patient to be transfused with blood equivalent to 4 or 5 times their total blood volume, or even more in instances of acute rupture. Complications

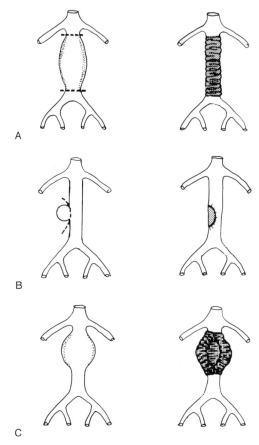

Fig. 32.3 Repair of aneurysms. **A** – artery is resected and replaced with a synthetic crimp prosthesis. **B** – Patch grafting of saccular aneurysms. **C** – Crimp prosthesis applied over unresected artery.

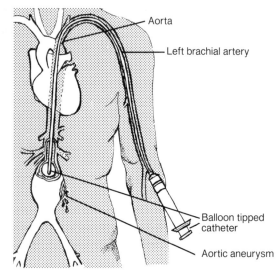

Aorta

Left brachial artery

Balloon tipped catheter

Aortic aneurysm

Fig. 32.2 Temporary control of aortic aneurysm using ballon tipped catheter.

of surgery may be due to either the extreme length of the intraoperative period, which may extend to many hours, or be due to the surgery itself. The former include the development of deep vein thrombosis, decubitus ulcers, infection, respiratory narcosis, and atelectasis; and the effects of poor perfusion of tissues supplied by arteries distal to the aneurysm, for example renal failure, hepatic failure, or peripheral arterial ischaemia. The latter include embolus, either from air or thrombi, usually causing a CVA; leaking of the prosthesis, usually at the anastomosis; and disseminated intravascular coagulation (DIC, see page 107) from the excessive transfusion of blood and blood products.

Nursing management

In nearly all instances of aneurysm repair the patient is nursed in an intensive care unit for at least the first 24–48 hours. Close observation of the patient's condition and vital signs is imperative to detect the early onset of any complications, especially leaking of the prosthesis, peripheral arterial ischaemia, and renal failure.

Regular repositioning of the patient, full range-of-motion, coughing, and deep breathing exercises will assist in reducing the likelihood of postoperative skin breakdown, deep vein thrombosis, atelectasis, and chest infection, which are even more probable following such long surgery. Specific nursing care of the patient undergoing arterial surgery is discussed on page 294 and, depending on the site of the aneurysm, nursing management will include care as for the patient undergoing general abdominal surgery (see page 499) and/or chest surgery (see page 341).

Arterial disorders with an autoimmune basis

Polyarteritis nodosa

Polyarteritis is an inflammatory process in which lesions occur randomly distributed throughout the medial layer of small and medium-sized arteries. This disorder is believed to be autoimmune in that the body fails to recognize the cells of the tunica media as 'self' and produces antibodies to these cells. The lesions may extend through the tunica adventitia and tunica intima, leading to arterial wall weakening and ultimate aneurysm formation.

As well, small pea-like projections may develop along the course of the artery. Lesions may not affect the entire circumference or length of the vessel.

Polyarteritis may present as an acute illness but more commonly has an insidious onset following a previous infection, usually viral in origin. Initially the patient presents with fever, general malaise, weight loss, lethargy, and a leucocytosis. Ultimately clinical features will be those of arterial damage to the organ involved, for example haematuria and proteinuria in kidney involvement; pericarditis, cardiac failure, and chest pain with heart involvement; and nausea, haematemesis, malaena, and anorexia with gastrointestinal involvement. There is no specific clinical test for polyarteritis, however the patient's history and clinical presentation can be confirmed by biopsy of either a lesion or an involved organ.

Medical management is symptomatic as there is no cure for this condition and normally involves the aggressive use of corticosteroids, with prednisone the drug of choice. The patient is usually managed by the physician in the community until such time as hospitalization is required for treatment of chronic organ disease.

Relapses are common and limited results have been achieved with the combined use of immunosuppressive agents. Organ involvement may require treatment, for example dialysis in the case of renal failure, and digitalis and antihypertensive therapy for cardiac disease.

Nursing management is dependent upon the individual needs of each patient and these will be determined by the area of the body affected and the type of organ dysfunction present. The nurse should understand that the patient will be suffering from a chronic disorder for which there is no cure and that support to the patient and his significant others will be a paramount requirement.

Raynaud's disease

Another disorder with strong autoimmune links is Raynaud's disease, in which the person experiences episodic vasospasm in small peripheral arteries and arterioles in response to cold or stress. Raynaud's disease occurs bilaterally and most often affects the hands rather than the feet. Vasospasm causes the fingers to become cold, and they also become either cyanotic or blanched. Raynaud's disease occurs most commonly in women in a ratio of nearly 20 : 1 and immersing hands in cold water, or not wearing gloves in cold weather, most often precipitates an attack. It is usually a benign condition that requires no treatment and produces no long-term effects.

However, these episodic attacks of vasospasm (Raynaud's phenomenon), when found in conjunction with connective tissue disorders such as systemic lupus erythematosus (SLE, see page 786) and systemic sclerosis (scleroderma), may lead ultimately to ischaemia and gangrene of the digits, which will usually require amputation.

As cigarette smoking and beta-blocking agents produce reflex peripheral vasospasm the patient who smokes should be encouraged to quit, and beta-blockers should be used with caution. The patient should be encouraged to avoid exposure to cold and to protect his hands from mechanical injury. Should symptoms cause continued pain or discomfort, the physician may order a course of vasodilators, and sympathectomy (see page 295) may provide relief in severe situations.

PERIPHERAL VASCULAR DISEASE

The most common occlusive disorder, peripheral vascular disease (PVD) affects both arteries and veins and usually presents as 'poor circulation' in the lower limbs. Less commonly involved are the vessels of the upper limbs and therefore discussion will concentrate on the lower limbs. PVD can be either chronic or acute in presentation. Arteriosclerosis obliterans, due to atherosclerosis and/or arteriosclerosis, is the commonest arterial occlusive disorder, resulting ultimately in occlusion by thrombosis or embolism. Venous thrombosis, chronic venous insufficiency, and varicose veins are the commonest causes of occlusive venous disorders.

Occlusive arterial disease

Arteriosclerosis obliterans causes peripheral arterial vessels either to become clogged within their intima by atheroma, or their function to be impaired by calcification of their media. These pathological changes are the most likely cause in the patient who exhibits occlusive arterial disease; and hardening of the arteries prevents normal vessel function and leads to the inability of the circulatory system to meet the body's oxygen demands. The ultimate effects of this disease are the development of ischaemia and gangrene if the arterial passage is narrowed, ulcerated, or occluded by thrombosis or embolus; or the development of an aneurysm due to a weakened and dilated arterial wall. Of significance is that if atherosclerosis is pathologically evident in peripheral vessels, then it is most likely to be also present in either coronary and/or cerebral vessels.

Chronic arterial PVD follows the long-term development of atheroma-induced changes within the vessel walls. The deposition of atheromatous plaques initiates intravascular changes such as intravascular coagulation, minute haemorrhages in, and scarring of, the subintimal layer resulting in further increase in size of the thrombus. The thrombus thus formed may remain stationary and continue to increase in size until such time as vessel occlusion occurs and local tissue necrosis results. During this time the body adapts to decreased distal blood flow by developing local collateral circulation (Fig. 32.4). This is the usual mechanism in the development of small vessel disease, ultimately resulting in chronic ischaemia, such as that seen in diabetes mellitus or thromboangiitis obliterans (Buerger's disease, see later).

In 1984, 3500 deaths were attributed to arterial diseases, of which approximately 75% occurred after the age of 65 years in both sexes, giving

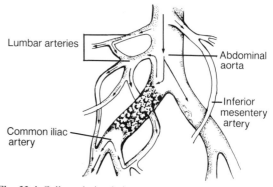

Fig. 32.4 Collateral circulation.

further support to the belief that the effects of ageing predominate in the development of this disorder. Nearly 80% of all lower limb cases present with disease in the femoropopliteal region and 15% present with aorto-iliac disease. As coronary and/or cerebral atherosclerosis is almost always co-existent in these patients, experience has shown that more than 50% of all persons with occlusive peripheral arterial disease ultimately experience either a fatal myocardial infarction or cerebrovascular accident.

Intermittent claudication is the initial symptom and this causes ischaemic pain on exertion, in all patients with occlusive arterial disease. In the leg it is usually described by the patient as pain in the calf muscle, but it can involve the entire limb, hip, and buttocks. (In the arm a similar muscle pain/cramp description is given related to exercise/exertion.) Characteristically, the pain is relieved within 2 minutes of resting the limb; it is not necessary to sit or lie down – just to cease the physical activity that bought on the pain. Initially in the disease process the pain does not occur at rest and is at its worst when the person is walking either up a hill, or quickly. A significant diagnostic characteristic of this symptom is that intermittent claudication is very specific for the individual; it will always occur the same way and to the same intensity each time the same pain-initiating activity is repeated.

As the occlusion becomes complete, arterial pulses in the distal extremity diminish and eventually become absent. The loss of pulses and the location of intermittent claudication are very closely related, for example, femoropopliteal occlusion results in calf pain and absent pulses below the femoral level, small vessel disease results in foot pain and absent foot pulses, and aorto-iliac occlusion results in hip and buttock pain with absent femoral pulses.

Should the condition continue unchecked then the patient will describe a history of increasing pain over shorter distances walked, until the onset of rest pain. Rest pain occurs in the distal part of the limb, increases when the limb is elevated and is usually severe enough to prevent sleep. The patient will describe obtaining relief by either lowering the limb to a dependent position, or sitting out of bed in a chair.

Colour and sensory changes are related to the position of the limb. Characteristically there is elevational pallor, poikilothermia, and paraesthesia when the leg is raised, due to the inability of the arterial circulation to pump against gravity, and rubor of the leg when it is kept in a dependent position. Chronic vasodilation occurring as a secondary effect of accumulating lactic acid in the tissues surrounding the affected vessels is the cause of the colour changes.

Acute arterial occlusion

This presents a dramatic picture of symptoms and signs, with a history of sudden severe pain in the leg, accompanied by coldness, numbness, pallor, and absence of all pulses in the area of ischaemia beyond the obstruction. The onset of acute ischaemia is usually caused by either a local thrombus forming from an ulcerated intima, or an embolized thrombus lodging some place distant from its formation site. The principal sites are the left side of the heart and the arch of the aorta.

Obviously large emboli can be fatal should they lodge in the vessels supplying critical organs and causing an acute ischaemic episode, for example, cerebrovascular accident, myocardial infarction, or pulmonary embolus. These large emboli are also responsible for causing acute ischaemia in the extremeties should they lodge in a peripheral vessel. The vessels most commonly affected are the lower abdominal aorta, or one of its branches, or the femoral or popliteal arteries.

Systemically the patient usually presents in a clinical state of shock, the severity of which is dependent upon the degree of arterial occlusion. Management is the same as for any peripheral occlusive disease except that emergency surgical intervention is almost always inevitable, dependent upon the severity of the occlusion.

Nursing management of the patient undergoing arterial surgery is discussed on page 296 whilst the nursing management of the patient with PVD is discussed on page 302.

Thromboangiitis obliterans (Buerger's disease)

This is an occlusive condition of peripheral arteries (and, sometimes, veins) that is not attributable to the development of atheroma. It is an extremely painful condition that is characterized by the development of acute inflammatory lesions and occlusive thromboses of the vessels. This disease almost exclusively affects males and becomes evident before the age of 40 years. The patient is usually a heavy cigarette smoker. The vessels affected are usually of the lower limbs, but involvement of arteries of the upper limbs is fairly common.

The condition is extremely difficult to manage and control and the thrombosis is usually relentless, leading to the need for multi-limb amputation. Patient compliance with the need to cease smoking is extremely difficult to attain and frequently total denial of his condition is the coping mechanism utilized by the patient. He therefore continues to smoke even after one leg is amputated, knowing that the risks of bilateral amputation are extremely high should he not comply with therapy. Drug therapy with oral vasodilators may provide some relief and delay amputation for a short period of time. It is imperative that the patient, and his significant others, understands the need for him to avoid exposure of his limbs to cold. Protection from any form of mechanical injury and scrupulous care of his feet and legs is necessary to reduce the early onset of ulceration and gangrene.

Clinical manifestations of arterial occlusive disease

Symptoms that usually force the patient to seek medical aid are likely to be a variety of the following:

• Gradual onset of chronic leg pain relieved by rest
• Rest pain relieved only by lowering the leg
• Coldness and numbness of the limb distal to the area of occlusion
• Ulceration of the skin usually on the toes, heel, or over the lateral malleolus
• Development of gangrene in the above ulcer beds.

On clinical examination the patient will exhibit some or all of the following, dependent upon the severity of the disease presentation:

• Absence of pulses distal to the level of occlusion
• Colour changes of the limb. Skin pallor of the extremity occurs when the limb is elevated, and skin rubor occurs when the limb is lowered
• Thin, shiny, dry and scaly skin distal to the area of occlusion
• Diminished hair growth and thickened nails of the extremity
• Reduced tissue mass, leading to atrophy
• Dry gangrene in the absence of venous congestion, or wet gangrene if venous pooling or infection is also present.

Investigative procedures

The physician will conduct a thorough physical examination and document the patient's previous history, especially with respect to identifiable risk factors. The physical examination will include measurement of limb symmetry and inspection for the presence of ulcers, abrasions, and any poorly healed wounds. Should an underlying condition be found or suspected, for example, diabetes mellitus or hypertension, then investigation of that condition will also be included with the following specific procedures:

• Exercise tests to evaluate the degree of intermittent claudication present
• Angiography of the peripheral vascular tree to view any obstructions to blood flow
• Skin temperature studies to determine poor circulation. These tests rely on predominantly subjective data, so they are of limited use in diagnosis
• Oscillometry and plethysmography to detect alterations in pulse volume and limb size
• Doppler ultrasound to measure any obstruction to blood flow velocity
• Lumbar sympathetic block to determine whether or not sympathectomy could improve peripheral circulation.

Surgical management

Conservative medical and nursing management has always been preferred when treating patients with chronic occlusive disease, as the damaged tissues involved render the limb a poor surgical risk due to the likelihood that healing will be incomplete. However, in more and more patients surgical intervention in the form of bypass graft is being indicated and surgery may also include one or more of the following procedures:

- Lumbar sympathectomy
- Embolectomy
- Thromboendarterectomy
- Bypass graft surgery
- Patch grafting
- Amputation.

Lumbar sympathectomy. This surgical procedure involves the severing of the sympathetic nerve fibres of the vertebral ganglia that supply the lower limb, resulting in relaxation of the walls of arterioles and therefore leading to improved circulation. Sympathectomy also provides a measure of relief from ischaemic pain by interrupting the transference of pain stimuli to the central nervous system. Therefore these patients have an increased potential for tissue damage as they are unable to adequately differentiate between the extremes of heat and cold.

It should be noted that in the majority of cases a paramedian abdominal incision is used. Not all patients are likely to benefit from sympathectomy as it will improve blood supply only in arterioles that are still elastic and not yet affected by the calcification process of arteriosclerosis. Consequently, many physicians will first perform a chemical sympathectomy (by injecting the vertebral ganglia with alcohol) to gauge the likelihood of success of the surgical procedure.

Embolectomy. This surgical procedure involves the insertion of a balloon-tipped catheter to remove thrombotic material usually from femoral, popliteal, or mesenteric arteries. The catheter is passed into the artery and threaded past the thrombotic material; the balloon is inflated and then gently withdrawn bringing the debris with it. Obviously this procedure is not without great risk as some of the material may in fact become an embolus and cause acute arterial occlusion and ischaemia.

Thromboendarterectomy. This surgical procedure involves an incision through the wall of the artery and removal of an atheromatous core, or thrombus, from the intima. Prior to this

procedure angiography will have been performed to gauge the exact location and extent of the occlusion. It is commonly performed either in the treatment of carotid artery occlusion, or in combination with bypass graft surgery to improve collateral circulation.

An inherent risk of this surgical technique is that the atheromatous plaque or thrombus may be friable and during extraction a small piece may break off and become an embolus, the size of the embolus determining the degree of residual damage. In a limb this would manifest as acute ischaemia with pallor, poikilothermia, and absence of pulses distal to the embolus occlusion. During carotid endarterectomy the resultant cerebral ischaemia may range from mild to a severe cerebrovascular accident.

Bypass graft surgery. With occlusive arterial disease the commonest surgical procedure performed is either a femoropopliteal bypass graft for lesions in the femoropopliteal area or a coronary artery bypass graft (see page 323) for lesions in the coronary arteries. This procedure is used as an active treatment and, even in elderly patients with well established chronic arterial PVD, the good results from bypass graft surgery have increased its acceptance.

The bypass may be accomplished using an autogenous saphenous vein graft (the preferred option) or a plastic or dacron prosthesis; the latter prostheses are more commonly utilized for grafting in aortic and iliac artery occlusion. The saphenous vein is taken usually from the same leg in which the occlusion has occurred and the graft is carefully checked after removal to ensure that all venous branches have been adequately ligated so that the graft will not leak. One end of the graft is anastomozed to the femoral artery above the level of the occlusion whilst the other end is anastomozed to the popliteal artery, or to the anterior tibial artery, distal to the occlusion. It should be noted that the vein graft is positioned in reverse so that the valves of the vein will not impede arterial blood flow. Blood then flows through the graft and bypasses the thrombosed arterial segment. Figure 32.5 shows the subsequent wound site.

Patch and interposition grafting. In these procedures the thrombosed material is removed

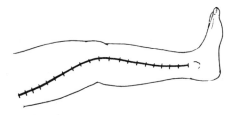

Fig. 32.5 Suture/incision line following femoropopliteal bypass graft.

via an incision in the artery (arteriotomy). If a portion of arterial wall must be removed, the defect is repaired using an autogenous or dacron patch graft to prevent vessel stenosis. If a circumferential segment of artery is removed along with the thrombus then an autogenous or dacron graft is anastomozed into position to replace the arterial segment (see Fig. 32.3, page 290).

Amputation. The surgical removal of a limb or, more commonly, a part of a limb is not an infrequent outcome of PVD, especially of small vessel disease as found in diabetes mellitus. Amputation surgery is necessary when gangrene results and may involve removal of digits, removal of half the foot, disarticulation through the ankle joint (Syme's operation), below knee amputation (BKA), or an above knee amputation (AKA).

Nursing management of the patient following arterial surgery

As the femoropopliteal bypass graft is the most common arterial surgical procedure performed, nursing management of the patient following this procedure will be detailed. The principles of care for the patient following other forms of arterial surgery are similar and, apart from specific points of care, general nursing management will be assumed in this discussion. Amputation surgery and specific nursing care of the amputee is discussed on page 304.

If the surgery performed has not been for an emergency such as a ruptured aneurysm or acute arterial occlusion, then preoperatively the patient will have undergone extensive education to prepare him for the postoperative phase. He must understand the need for co-operation with chest and limb exercises and be reassured that he will be provided with adequate analgesia. The entire length of his leg will be shaved, as will be his groin and pubic areas, and antibacterial skin preparation will also be performed.

Following transfer to the operating room, an IV infusion will be commenced (this may be via a central vein) and generally an arterial line is also established for accurate assessment of arterial pressure during the operative phase. Urinary catheterization is usually performed as it is not unusual for the patient to experience considerable difficulty in voiding during the postoperative phase. Catheterization also minimizes the likelihood of trauma which may occur due to undue strain on the suture lines whilst attempting to void.

Postoperatively the patient is nursed in a recumbent position with one pillow. The grafted limb is enclosed in firmly applied crepe bandages and it is elevated on one pillow to assist venous return. There are usually a minimum of 2 drain tubes attached to low pressure suction and the incision extends from the groin to the ankle (see Fig. 32.5) or from the groin to the mid-calf area.

The nurse will be responsible for the careful monitoring of the IV infusion which, in most instances, will contain heparin in order to minimize the development of postoperative deep vein thrombosis (DVT). Frequent observation of the patient's vital signs and of the neurovascular function of the affected limb must be undertaken (see page 706). Marking the skin over distal pulses with ink facilitates the localization of these for frequent monitoring.

Leg bandages and drain tubes are usually removed after 48 hours and the incision is then left open, or sprayed with plastic dressing material; the drain tube sites are dressed as necessary. Ambulation, for short periods, is normally commenced on the third postoperative day and the patient should be fully ambulant by 6 days post surgery. Whilst he is confined to bed, nursing measures to prevent the development of a DVT are mandatory (see page 299 for nursing management of the patient with PVD).

Complications

Complications following arterial surgery include:

Haemorrhage (reactionary haemorrhage is not uncommon during the first 48 hours) due either to leaking of the graft at the anastomosis or as a result of disturbed coagulation. The wound should be inspected frequently for any swelling or strain on the suture lines. Diminishing peripheral pulses, an increase in patient restlessness, or any complaint by the patient of unrelieved pain should be reported immediately. Following abdominal aneurysm repair haemorrhage may manifest as abdominal distension and rigidity accompanied by the cessation of bowel sounds and diminishing peripheral pulses. Haemorrhage from a thoracic aneurysm repair is likely to be overt, in the form of increased frank blood draining via the basal chest drain tube.

Thrombosis/embolus formation. Although the patient will undergo anticoagulation in an attempt to minimize intra- or postoperative thrombolic episodes it is not uncommon for thrombosis to occur. Thrombus formation may result at the anastomosis, or within the graft (on a valve cusp in an autogenous vein graft or a crimped area of a dacron graft). If an arterial thrombus embolizes it will ultimately lodge in a distal artery that prevents its onward passage. Therefore the patient may manifest the symptoms and signs of acute arterial occlusion, for example, a cerebrovascular accident (see page 174), a coronary occlusion (see page 314), a mesenteric thrombosis, spinal shock (see page 314), or acute peripheral ischaemia due to the interruption of blood supply to these organs or body areas. It should be noted that a pulmonary embolus may also occur due to a concurrent DVT.

Infection of the graft and/or wound. Infection is not uncommon, especially in femoropopliteal bypass surgery from contamination by *S. aureus* or *E. coli* organisms from the perineal area; contamination of the graft may occur during surgery or via wound or systemic infection post surgery. Close attention to skin preparation and patient hygiene both pre- and postoperatively is the responsibility of the nurse. Aseptic wound dressing and close monitoring of the patient for signs of infection must be instituted. Infection may manifest initially as general malaise accompanied by a slight fever. Ultimately purulent wound drainage with graft exposure may result; haemorrhage may also occur and graft occlusion is not uncommon.

Anticipated outcome

Following uncomplicated arterial surgery, the patient can anticipate returning home within approximately 2 weeks. He should understand the need to continue any medications, especially anticoagulant therapy, and to return for regular medical check ups. He should be instructed in follow up wound care and in the need to continue regular inspections of his legs and feet for any early indications of deteriorating peripheral vascular function. Health measures such as a reduction diet and cessation of smoking should be encouraged where applicable.

The majority of patients recover completely and enjoy both an improved quality of life and an increased life span free of debilitating pain. In a few patients arterial reconstructive surgery is performed too late to halt the progression of the disease, and chronic PVD with peripheral ulceration results.

Occlusive venous disease

Chronic venous insufficiency usually caused by varicose veins or venous thrombosis is the most common form of occlusive venous disease. Weakening of the walls of veins and failure of the valves within the veins leads to gravitational pooling of venous blood in the legs. As intravenous pressure rises, fluid migration from the swollen, tortuous, and incompetent veins to the interstitial fluid space occurs. Oedema in the affected leg(s) results and chronic oedema leads to tissue fibrosis and induration. Capillary venous blood also escapes into the tissue space and skin discoloration results; as the condition continues and the blood cells are broken down, the skin discoloration changes from reddish-blue through to a brown. The increased presence of cell metabolites in the fluid spaces causes further tissue damage and discoloration. Ultimately, stasis ulcers form around the ankles.

Many patients do not present to the physician until such time as stasis ulcers have occurred. Varicose veins are extremely common in the community, and not all people seek medical intervention and may ignore their presence until such time as it is too late for surgical treatment. Likewise venous thrombosis (especially that due to untreated varicose veins) may go untreated for many years and the patient first presents with stasis varicose ulcers of the legs.

Varicose veins

These are distended, tortuous superficial veins accompanied by valvular incompetence, usually affecting the saphenous veins of the legs and their branches. As the lateral pressure of blood rises inside the vein, the vein dilates and prevents complete closure by the incompetent valves. A backflow of blood results and further increases the varicosity and, if untreated, will predispose to the development of venous thrombosis and chronic venous insufficiency.

Varicose veins occur most commonly in persons of middle age, and women are affected more often than men; varicose veins tend to occur bilaterally. They can occur as a result of chronic thrombo-phlebitis, or as a result of diseases of the venous system, or congenital weakness of the valves. More commonly, people with varicose veins have a history of a condition that produces long-term venostasis, for example obesity, pregnancy, ascites, or the occupational hazard of prolonged standing. However, not all people with such predisposing factors develop varicose veins and in those persons who do there is an increased inci-dence of haemorrhoids and diverticulosis co-existing. As varicose veins, haemorrhoids, and diverticulosis all have a higher incidence in western societies, they are believed by some researchers to be connected with low fibre diets.

Clinical manifestations. Varicose veins are in many cases asymptomatic until they produce effects of chronic venous insufficiency. When acute symptoms are experienced the patient generally complains of a feeling of heaviness in the legs, leg cramps at rest, especially at night, a persistent dull ache in the legs after walking or prolonged standing, and easy fatigability. Women also complain of dull aching associated with menses.

On examination, the patient will have distended nodules palpable over the varicosities; and mild to severe orthostatic oedema and skin discoloration, seen as stasis pigmentation of the calves and ankles, due to deep vein valve incompetency.

The person with chronic, untreated varicose veins will also have ruptured communicating veins causing leakage of haemosiderin, an insoluble form of storage iron; this classically stains the skin a port-wine discoloration. The person's skin characteristically takes on the texture of candle wax and yet has superficial flaking of cells. Some patients may experience spontaneous rupture of the varicosities on rising from a lying position. This can range from pin prick haemorrhages to substantial subcutaneous blood loss.

Investigative procedure. The Trendelenburg test is used to demonstrate the degree and precise location of the varicosity: the patient is placed in the recumbent position and his leg is elevated above the level of his heart to cause gravitational emptying of the veins. Whilst still elevated the leg is enclosed with a tourniquet bandage to occlude the superficial veins. The patient quickly assumes a standing position and the tourniquet is removed; long saphenous incompetency, for example, is demonstrated by the back flow of blood distending the saphenous vein from the level of the thigh down to the lower leg.

Medical, surgical, and nursing management. In the instance of mild to moderate varicose veins the patient must wear elasticized stockings whenever he is out of bed, to provide external support to the veins, improve circulation, and reduce ankle oedema. He should also be encouraged to under-take moderate exercise; walking increases the muscle pump action of the legs and potentiates venous return and minimizes venous pooling. He should be advised to elevate his legs when sitting as often as possible, and be further advised against prolonged standing or sitting with his legs dependent. The wearing of tight, constrictive clothing, particularly around the upper calf and groin must also be avoided. Additional simple measures include the placement of a brick under the foot of the bed which will encourage venous drainage whilst sleeping.

Varicose veins which produce severe symptoms of pain and discomfort may be treated by injection or by ligation and stripping.

Injection entails the introduction of a sclerosing agent into segments of the varicosed vein; the intima scleroses and effectively prevents venous pooling.

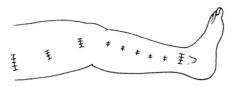

Fig. 32.6 Suture/incision line following stripping of varicose veins.

More commonly, the surgical procedure of mobilizing and ligating the saphenous vein along its entire length is performed. Once all communicating veins have been ligated a stripper is passed down through the saphenous vein and the vein is removed by stripping it from the leg. If varicosities occur bilaterally then usually both legs are operated on at the same time.

Postoperatively the patient will have multiple small skin incisions along the length of the vein with a larger incision in the groin and ankle (Fig. 32.6) and the legs will have firm elastic bandages applied. The nurse must observe the patient closely for signs of reactionary haemorrhage, and inspect the wounds for haematoma formation. The patient will require frequent analgesics for at least the first 24 hours postoperatively. Elevation of the legs will assist in preventing both pain and haematoma development. The feet and toes should be inspected frequently for any impairment to circulation due to the bandages being too tight. Generally the bandages are untouched for the first 24 hours and then are reapplied as necessary in order to maintain constant firm support. When reapplying the bandages the limbs must be elevated and bandaged from ankle to thigh. Some centres prefer the use of full length elasticized stockings.

Any loss of sensation may be caused by saphenous nerve injury; severe calf pain may herald a deep vein thrombosis; and fever and wound redness may indicate infection. When ambulating the patient must be fitted for, and wear, full length elasticized bandages or stockings. These must also be worn following discharge (see also page 302 for nursing management of the patient with PVD).

Venous thrombosis

Thrombophlebitis is an acute inflammation of veins in which there is phlebothrombus formation (venous thrombosis) with a reactionary inflammatory response. Most thrombi begin in the valve cusps due to localized venous stasis allowing activated clotting factors to accumulate. Thrombin combines with thrombocytes to form a thrombus which continues to grow until it either occludes the vein or becomes dislodged. Varicose veins and prolonged immobility are common conditions under which local venous stasis will develop.

Thrombophlebitis may occur in either superficial or deep veins and superficial vein thrombosis is, in the majority of cases, self-limiting and unlikely to lead to long-term complications. Superficial thrombosis occurring in the non-hospitalized person is most commonly a result of either localized trauma or infection, and is increasingly seen as the result of long-term IV drug abuse. In the hospitalized person inflammation secondary to chemical irritation is the most common cause. This may be due to either the long-term use of the IV route for nutrition, or the use of peripheral veins for the administration of high-dose substances, for example highly concentrated antibiotics.

Deep vein thrombosis. Deep vein thrombosis (DVT), when it occurs, most commonly affects the saphenous and femoral veins of the legs, the iliac and subclavian veins, and to a lesser extent the venae cavae. DVT is a life-threatening condition in that a portion of the thrombus may break away and, as an embolus, travel to the lungs, lodge, and result in pulmonary embolism (see page 346). Although DVT may be idiopathic it most commonly results from a combination of the effects of venous stasis, accelerated blood clotting, and local injury to the vein.

Therefore any form of mechanical pressure leading to venous stasis will predispose the patient to the development of a DVT. Examples are prolonged bed rest and immobility, coupled with unrelieved pressure on the calf muscles from the mattress, crossing of legs in bed, a pillow placed between the legs of a patient lying in lateral position, bandages or plaster casts which finish mid-calf, pregnancy, or a tight-fitting ring of a Thomas splint. Accelerated blood clotting is associated with blood dyscrasias such as polycythaemia, the use of oral contraceptives, and the presence of malignancy. Local vein injury may occur through surgery, trauma (especially limb fracture), incompetent valves, and following injection. Other factors include prolonged sitting or standing, varicose veins, obesity, hemiplegia, dehydration, and the presence of cardiac failure.

It should be noted that in the majority of instances of DVT the condition is preventable with the institution of correct nursing care. Part of such nursing care includes education of the patient in his role in the prevention of DVT. Only in a minority of instances is the condition a direct result of the patient's primary disorder.

Clinical manifestations. Superficial vein thrombosis characteristically produces symptoms and signs that are both visible and localized to the vein involved. There is redness, heat, pain, swelling (seen as induration along the length of the affected vein), and, in some instances, lymphadenitis. Diagnosis is made on the clinical examination supported by a patient history of vessel trauma or infection.

Unfortunately, DVT may be asymptomatic until such time as pulmonary embolism occurs; however, in most cases, DVT causes both local and systemic symptoms and signs. The patient's temperature may be raised, he may have general malaise and chills, and the affected limb is mildly or grossly oedematous and painful due to the accumulation of metabolites in the tissues distal to the site of the DVT. The leg may appear normal in colour, it may be red and hot over the site of the DVT, or it may be blue and suffused.

Investigative procedures. Diagnosis is normally made on the clinical examination and can be differentiated from acute arterial occlusion by the presence of distal arterial pulses. Doppler ultrasound will confirm reduced venous blood flow and the presence of valvular incompetence, whilst impedance plethysmography can accurately measure blood flow and therefore indicate the site of the DVT. Venography can detect filling defects and show collateral systems of venous drainage as well as detect the site of the thrombus. However, as venography is an invasive procedure it is not routinely performed as it may increase the risk of further DVT development or indeed precipitate an embolus.

With lower limb DVT the patient may exhibit a positive Homans' sign (pain in the calf region on dorsiflexion of the foot). However, this is not necessarily a reliable indicator of either the presence or absence of a DVT, as pain generated could be musculoskeletal in origin and a small thrombus may not as yet have triggered a strong inflammatory response.

Medical, surgical and nursing management. The aims of therapy are to control the thrombus development, provide pain relief, and prevent any complications. With either a superficial or deep vein thrombosis these aims can be achieved by elevating the affected limb, providing short-term bed rest, applying gentle heat in the form of a moist compress or poultice, and providing pain relief with analgesics, for example aspirin or an anti-inflammatory agent.

The patient is rested in bed for a minimum of 5–10 days so that 'organization' of the thrombus can occur and lessen the likelihood of pulmonary embolus. Organization refers to the adherence of the thrombus to the intima of the vein. Physical activity such as standing out of bed should be reduced to a minimum during this time. During this period of enforced bed rest, the patient should actively exercise his unaffected leg and perform isometric exercises of the affected limb to prevent the formation of further thrombi, and muscle wasting.

The nurse should advise the patient not to massage the affected area of the limb as such action could cause a fragment of the thrombus to embolize. Pillows used to elevate the limb should be placed in such a way as to support the entire length of the limb and not promote further venous stasis and therefore further thrombus formation. Once the acute phase of thrombosis has subsided the patient will be encouraged to ambulate and the nurse should ensure that the patient wears elasticized stockings in the case of superficial thrombosis of lower limb veins, and that he wears antiembolism stockings in the case of a DVT. The patient should continue to wear these stockings following his discharge.

In the case of a large DVT the patient will require either anticoagulant or thrombolytic drug therapy depending upon the severity of the thrombus. If the thrombus has not caused total venous occlusion and is unlikely to fragment into an embolus then anticoagulant therapy will be prescribed in order to prolong the patient's clotting time. It is necessary to stress that anticoagulant therapy will only prevent the likelihood of other thrombi forming, it will not cause the lysis of the thrombus that is present. Initially IV heparin sodium, either as a continuous infusion or intermittently via an IV cannula, will be commenced, and once adequate heparinization of the patient has been achieved, anticoagulation can be maintained by the use of either subcutaneous heparin calcium or by oral warfarin sodium. As oral anticoagulants take approximately 3–5 days to be effective, heparin and warfarin are administered in combination for some days, and heparin is then withdrawn. Heparin is never administered intramuscularly due to the danger of haematoma formation.

Anticoagulant therapy is normally continued for many weeks or months following resolution of the thrombus and the patient will be advised that the oral dose of warfarin will be calibrated in response to regular testing of prothrombin time. The major risk of therapy is haemorrhage and the patient should be advised to report immediately any sign of bleeding, for example, epistaxis, haematuria, or bruising. Heparin overdosage can be controlled by either ceasing the drug, in the case of mild bleeding, or by administering the antidote protamine sulphate, should severe haemorrhage occur. With overdosage of oral warfarin the drug is ceased in the case of mild bleeding, or vitamin K administered IV in the case of more severe bleeding. Aspirin is known to potentiate the effect of heparin. Therefore, non-aspirin based analgesics are usually prescribed for the patient with a large DVT. Oral anticoagulants interact with a variety of other drugs. These can either potentiate the anticoagulant effect, for example diuretics, broad spectrum antibiotics, and nonsteroidal anti-inflammatory agents; or diminish the anticoagulant effect, for example antihistamines, oral contraceptives, and barbiturates.

Only if the thrombus is likely to threaten the viability of the limb, or when a pulmonary embolus has occurred is a thrombolytic agent, for example streptokinase, prescribed. The patient should then be nursed in an intensive care situation, as extremely close monitoring of his condition is mandatory whilst thrombolytics are used. Uncontrollable haemorrhage is always a risk and adequate supplies of the antithrombolytic aminocaproic acid must be available at all times during therapy.

Surgical intervention will only be necessary in the presence of a large thrombus which is life threatening, and even then only if anticoagulant and/or thrombolytic therapy fail. Surgical techniques include plication of the vena cava, which allows normal blood flow but prevents the further movement of emboli, or a thrombectomy. The latter is rarely performed as subsequent thrombus formation at the site of thrombectomy is common.

The nurse will be responsible for observing the patient for any signs of adverse reaction to anticoagulation therapy, for example, haematuria, subcutaneous bruising, or epistaxes. Signs of resolution of the DVT include limb circumference measurement returning to normal as distal oedema subsides, return of skin to normal colour, resolution of fever, and lessening of pain (see also page 302 for nursing management of the patient with PVD).

Prevention of deep vein thrombosis

In the situation when any patient is confined to bed, or is otherwise at risk of DVT development as previously outlined, nursing management must be directed towards prevention of DVT. Such management includes: education of the preoperative patient of the risks of post surgical DVT and the measures for which he is responsible to prevent its occurrence, for example, frequent movement of his feet and legs to minimize venous stasis; the use of calf stimulators during surgery and for the patient with prolonged unconsciousness. Dorsi and plantar flexion must be instituted as soon as the patient regains consciousness, and must be performed each time the patient's vital signs are recorded and until such time as he can assume responsibility for these exercises. Early ambulation, adequate hydration, and the prevention of mechanical pressure such as crossing legs will also assist in preventing DVT development.

Arterial and venous ulcers

The patient who responds poorly to treatment of either occlusive arterial disease or occlusive venous disease will probably develop the hallmark of PVD – arterial or venous leg ulcers. It is important to stress that all leg ulcers are not alike, that the differences between arterial and venous ulcers are characteristic, and that these ulcers require specific nursing and medical management dependent upon their type.

Arterial ulcers

Arterial ulcers develop as a result of chronic arterial ischaemia. As blood supply falls, perfusion of cells decreases, metabolic needs cannot be met, and tissues become increasingly susceptible to trauma. If small vessel disease co-exists, as in diabetes mellitus or Buerger's disease, neuronal damage increases the patient's susceptibility to trauma. Ulcers may appear in areas subject to constant wear and pressure: between the toes, on the tips of toes, over phalangeal heads and the lateral malleolus, on the heel, and on the side or the sole of the foot.

The ulcer has a clearly demarcated edge, is likely to be deep, has a pale base, does not contain any healthy granulation tissue, and is susceptible to necrosis. Depending upon the degree of arterial insufficiency, the surrounding skin may show signs of cellulitis or, more likely, ischaemia: cool, dry, shiny skin, with little or no hair growth, and thickened horny nails. Pain is usually quite severe and ischaemic pain as well as skin pallor occurs when the limb is elevated. Rubor develops when the limb is dependent.

Ulcer healing is largely dependent upon the restoration of blood supply; without an adequate circulation treatment is likely to produce only minimal results. Additionally, a necrotic ulcer bed is an ideal medium for bacterial growth and arterial ulcers are prone to infection. Poor circulation makes treatment with systemic antibiotics difficult as the antibiotic cannot effectively reach the focus of infection. Therefore treatment aims at revascularization, through procedures such as bypass graft or endarterectomy. If revascularization fails and gangrene develops, amputation will be required to prevent the septicaemic effects of the gangrene.

Venous ulcers

Chronic venous insufficiency causes blood to back up in the periphery and as intravenous pressure rises, excess fluid is forced into the tissue spaces. Oedema in the affected leg(s) results and chronic oedema leads to tissue fibrosis and induration. Capillary venous blood also escapes into the tissue space and skin discoloration results; as the condition continues and the blood cells are broken down, the skin discoloration changes from reddish-blue through to brown. The increased presence of cell metabolites in the fluid spaces causes further tissue damage and discoloration. The cells are so fragile that even the slightest injury can result in ulceration.

Ultimately, stasis venous ulcers develop at the ankle usually just above either malleolus or in the pretibial area. There is usually evidence of past healed ulcers. The ulcer will involve superficial tissues, have very uneven edges, be very red, and be characterized by the presence of granulation tissue. They have a tendency to weep serous fluid and although painful rarely cause the equivalence of extreme pain as seen in arterial ulcers.

Surgical treatment of venous ulcers aims at either correcting the defect with split-thickness skin grafts, or increasing the competency of the vascular tree by ligating and stripping incompetent veins or by valvular transposition. Conservative management, however, is more commonly employed and when successful can eliminate the need for surgical intervention.

Nursing management for the patient with peripheral vascular disease

Regardless of whether the patient's chronic PVD is arterial or venous in origin, he will be experiencing problems associated with leg pain, ulceration and/or infection of tissues, and either poor arterial blood flow or increased venous stasis. Nursing management is therefore directed at achieving the following goals of care:

1. Increase arterial blood supply to the periphery whilst at the same time promoting venous return.

2. Prevent the development of further vessel obstruction whilst reducing the obstruction already present.

3. Relieve the pain of ischaemia or of venous pooling.

4. Prevent injury, infection, and further ulcer formation and promote healing of tissues and ulcerated areas.

Increase arterial blood supply and promote venous return

Correct positioning, exercise, and health education of the patient, can achieve this goal. If arterial disease is the cause of the ulcer development ensure that the patient understands that blood flows to dependent parts of the body and therefore he will achieve an increased blood flow to his periphery by keeping his legs dependent. Raising the head of his bed 15–20 cm will ensure adequate blood flow to his legs whilst sleeping and when sitting he should keep his feet flat on the floor and not cross his legs. By contrast, the patient with poor venous return should understand that gravity increases venous pooling and regularly elevating his legs above the level of his heart will aid in overcoming the effects of gravity. Raising the foot of his bed 15–20 cm will promote venous return whilst sleeping and he should be advised against prolonged standing or sitting, and when sitting his legs should be elevated.

Gentle active exercise of the extremities and short periods of walking over a flat surface will assist in improving arterial flow and promoting venous return. It is important that the patient understands the need to intersperse regular periods of rest so that neither ischaemic pain nor venous pooling occurs.

However, exercise should be avoided if leg ulcers, cellulitis, or gangrene are present, as exercise increases the presence of cell metabolites in these conditions. Likewise, exercise is contraindicated if a DVT or arterial thrombus is present as exercise could cause fragmentation of the thrombus or further occlusion.

Patient education should be concentrated on ensuring that he understands that obesity should be avoided as it increases tissue demands and promotes poor venous return. He should avoid prolonged sitting or standing and the wearing of tight or constricting clothing, for example belts, girdles, tight shoes, as these will either prevent adequate blood flow to or from the periphery. He should be further advised not to sit with his legs crossed at the knee as this constricts the popliteal vessels.

Prevent or relieve vessel obstruction

The local application of heat will assist in maintaining vasodilation and the patient should be advised to always wear warm clothing when outside on cold days. He should avoid vasoconstrictors such as nicotine and be given support and encouragement to cease smoking. Stress and extremes of emotion also cause reflex vasoconstriction and therefore relaxation therapy may be indicated. He should be advised against exercising (including walking) outside in cold weather. If he is prescribed a vasodilator the nurse should ensure that he understands the dose and expected effects of the drug. The measures to prevent venous pooling, as outlined, should be stressed as these will also prevent the development of venous thrombosis.

Relief of pain

Any of the measures already outlined to increase circulation to or venous return from the periphery will assist in alleviating pain. Analgesics may be prescribed and their strength will be dependent upon the type and degree of pain present. As pain prevents the patient from sleeping it must be controlled in order to promote rest to allow healing.

Promote tissue healing and prevent complications

The management of arterial and venous ulcers varies widely between institutions, especially in dressing techniques. However, the following broad principles apply in the majority of instances.

Arterial ulcers should be managed with moist dressings to promote the lifting of necrotic areas and regranulation of tissue. If the ulcer bed is infected, a topical antibiotic should be applied only if prescribed by the physician. Adhesive tape should be avoided as this further damages the fragile skin; dressings should be held in place with a loose crepe bandage. The patient should be kept at bed rest to reduce oxygen demand by the body and to ensure adequate oxygenation of the periphery. If ulceration is extremely deep, or if the patient is unable to protect the limb from further damage, an immobilization splint may be utilized.

Venous ulcers require frequent dressing changes using a debriding agent to remove necrotic tissue. Porous dressing material should be used so that exudate can be absorbed; occlusive dressings should not be used on venous ulcers as they will prevent the absorption of the exudate. Adhesive tape should also be avoided and the dressing held in place with a firmly applied crepe bandage. If the patient is ambulatory then elasticized stockings or compression bandages should also be applied to reduce venous stasis. Whenever possible the limb should be elevated and if the ulcer bed is infected, or if cellulitis is present, a systemic antibiotic will probably be prescribed.

Research on ulcer healing has demonstrated the therapeutic benefits in using occlusive methylcellulose dressings for both arterial and venous ulcers. Such dressing technique reduces the frequency of wound disturbance, as well as encouraging rapid tissue regeneration.

The patient should be advised to take care of his legs and feet by: keeping his legs and feet clean, soft, and dry; inspecting his legs and feet every day; avoiding injury and any extremes of temperature; not using any medicated foot preparations unless prescribed by his physician; and not wearing any clothing or footwear that restricts his circulation. If he smokes he should be encouraged to quit. He should be advised to visit a podiatrist for the regular care of his toenails.

Anticipated outcome

Following vascular reconstruction and by heeding advice and education regarding the care of his feet and legs, the patient with arterial ulcers can expect complete healing and minimal likelihood of ulcer recurrence. Likewise the patient with chronic venous ulcers can expect good healing should he heed advice regarding protection of his legs from injury and the wearing of full length elasticized stockings whenever he is out of bed.

However, should vascular ulcers fail to respond to any of the medical and/or nursing management outlined, and peripheral gangrene develop, further surgery in the form of amputation of the gangrenous part will be necessary in order to prevent life-threatening systemic toxicity.

AMPUTATION

The surgical removal of all or part of a limb is psychologically as well as physically traumatic for the person and the nurse will play a large part in assisting him to adjust to the surgery and the resultant alteration to body image. Until recently amputation for the patient with unresponsive PVD was most commonly regarded by health professionals as the final treatment available. Consequently amputation was seen as a last resort and the result of failed medical therapy. When decisions regarding the level and type of amputation and the type of prosthesis were made, there was minimal input by specialist prosthetists. More recently amputation is being viewed as an active form of treatment and decisions made preoperatively are specifically geared towards enhancing the patient's postoperative recovery. For example, aggressive intervention, in the form of a below-knee amputation for gangrene of the toes and foot due to small vessel disease, will result in maximizing the patient's rehabilitation potential and quality of life. Years of repeated operations and disability will be avoided.

Amputation of lower limbs is most commonly performed as the end result of long-standing peripheral vascular disease, and less often because of life-threatening infection, for example gas gangrene or septicaemia; severe crush injuries; or malignant tumours, for example osteosarcoma. Upper limb amputation most often follows severe trauma, for example, burns, explosive accidents, gunshot wounds, or frostbite. Severe and intractable ischaemic limb pain or a useless, deformed extremity may also result in amputation. Trauma and congenital deformities are the major reasons for amputation in children.

The ultimate therapeutic goal for any amputee should be total rehabilitation/habilitation to ensure the maximization of his independence. Amputation as a result of trauma is often associated with a speedier rehabilitation because this patient tends to be younger and is less likely to have associated chronic vascular, or other medical disease. However, the principles of nursing management of the patient undergoing amputation for either chronic limb disease or trauma are similar.

Prior assessment will determine whether amputation is the appropriate treatment and, if so, the type and its level. These decisions will, to a large extent, be based upon the potential for patient rehabilitation.

Whether to amputate depends upon the cause of the limb dysfunction. If PVD is responsible, the decision to amputate will be made only after physical assessment can determine that viability of the stump and wound are assured. The patient's attitude will also influence the decision; the patient who finds he cannot face the mutilation of amputation may suffer greatly in the postoperative period and be unable to reach his full rehabilitation potential. On the other hand the patient with chronic PVD may see amputation as a welcome release from severe ischaemic pain.

Amputation surgery involves either open or closed procedures. The open, or guillotine, method is only ever used in the presence of overwhelming infection that cannot be controlled by systemic antibiotic therapy; it is a method rarely used. The amputation is performed without wound closure; the stump is allowed to drain openly and secondary closure/stump revision is performed when the infection has subsided.

The majority of amputations are closed. Following amputation the stump is covered by a flap containing muscle and skin which is sutured over the bone end of the stump (Fig. 32.7). If delayed fitting of a prosthesis is planned then the wound will contain drain tubes attached to negative suction apparatus to ensure that a haematoma does not develop.

The level of amputation is determined by the condition that has led to the need for the procedure. Amputation through the foot, or by disarticulation at the ankle joint (Syme's oper-

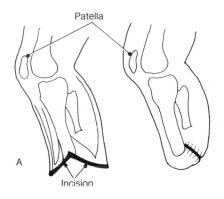
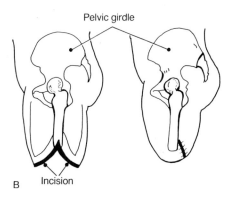

Fig. 32.7 A – Below knee amputation. **B** – Above knee amputation.

ation) is commonly performed for diabetic gangrene of the toes. Other levels for lower limb amputation are below knee (BKA), disarticulation at the knee, above knee (AKA), or disarticulation at the hip. Upper limb amputation levels are finger, disarticulation at the wrist, below elbow, disarticulation at the elbow, above elbow, and very rarely disarticulation at the shoulder. The higher the amputation level the greater the energy that must be expended by the patient to mobilize with a prosthesis. Wherever possible the knee joint is saved in elderly diabetic patients as this increases their rehabilitation potential. Therefore amputation is performed at the lowest level likely to ensure viability of the stump and wound. Adequate circulation at the amputation level is mandatory to ensure wound healing.

In order to effectively use a prosthesis the patient must be able to undergo extensive physiotherapy, have good coordination, and be physically fit as he must expend a large amount of energy. Unfortunately, many patients who undergo amputation are destined to be bedridden or at best wheelchair independent, as chronic disease may prohibit either the fitting of, or effective mobilization with, a prosthesis. The patient with a condition such as a chronic neurological dysfunction, congestive cardiac failure, chronic obstructive airways disease, or progressive diabetic neuropathy will be an unlikely candidate for prosthesis fitting.

The types of prostheses available are the conventional, delayed fitting prosthesis or an immediately fitted prosthesis. In Australia the conventional prosthesis is most commonly used; however, immediate fitting of a prosthesis is being sought by more and more patients and prosthetists, as it increases the patient's acceptance of the artificial limb as well as his rehabilitation potential.

With a delayed fitting the patient's stump is wrapped in bandages until the operative dressing is removed, usually within 48–72 hours, and the drain tubes are also removed. The stump is then redressed and rebandaged at least twice a day until the sutures are removed 10–14 days postoperatively. Once the sutures are removed, moulding of the stump to receive a prosthesis can proceed more effectively, as moulding prior to this is difficult due to the likelihood of wound breakdown. Moulding is effected by the method of stump bandaging (Fig. 32.8) and where possible the patient is taught to perform his own stump bandaging. This assists in helping the patient come to terms with the alteration in body image but usually results in better moulding as the patient can more effectively apply even pressure when bandaging his own stump. A temporary prosthesis is then fitted within 14 days of suture removal and the patient commences weight-bearing and gait re-training under physiotherapy supervision.

Fitting of an immediate prosthesis occurs whilst the patient is still in the operating room. Following amputation the wound flap is sutured, and drain tubes are not used. The stump is dressed and covered with a stump sock, and felt pads are placed at the distal end of the stump to act as cushions. The stump is then covered in a rigid plastic bandage and the prosthetist then

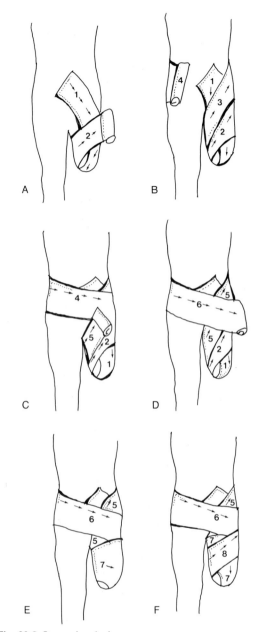

Fig. 32.8 Stump bandaging.

moulds a plaster of Paris prosthesis over the rigid dressing which is attached distally to a steel pylon and artificial foot (Fig. 32.9). The rigid dressing serves as a protection against injury to the stump, prevents any oedema or swelling, and maximizes stump moulding to receive a permanent prosthesis. The cast is removed after 10–14 days when

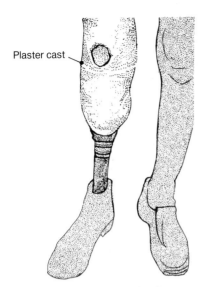

Plaster cast

Fig. 32.9 Prosthesis, fitted immediately after amputation.

sutures are also removed and a new cast and pylon replaced.

Preoperative preparation

The nurse will be responsible for preparing the patient both psychologically and physically for amputation. Ensure that the patient fully understands the procedure planned and if doubt exists, facilitate his seeking clarification and further information from the surgeon. Honest explanations of postoperative events and planned progress must be given, and it is important for the nurse to assist the patient in understanding what will be expected of him in the postoperative phase. He should be warned to expect 'phantom limb sensation', that is the peculiar sensation that the limb is still present after amputation; it may or may not be a painful sensation. Phantom pain, on the other hand, is pain experienced in the area of amputation; this pain is real and although the part is no longer present the pain can be extremely severe. The patient should be reassured that should he experience such pain he will be given analgesics for its control. The nurse should assist the patient to see amputation as an active form of treatment that will increase his well-being and quality of life postoperatively.

The patient should be in the best physical condition possible for surgery and may require a period of hospitalization prior to amputation. If possible the patient should be seen by the prosthetist, physiotherapist, and occupational therapist prior to surgery and given the opportunity to practice weight-bearing, gait-training, and transfer methods. This will increase his compliance with postoperative therapy.

Postoperative nursing management

The nurse must observe the patient and his stump closely for any signs of excessive bleeding and a tourniquet should be readily available for the first 72 hours for use in the event of haemorrhage. Wound management and stump redressing as outlined above is attended. Pain, either from the wound or phantom limb sensation, is controlled by narcotics for at least the first 4–5 days, when oral analgesics should be sufficient. Pain is less severe in the patient with an immediate prosthesis fitted.

The patient is positioned with the stump elevated on a pillow for 24–48 hours to assist in venous drainage and to prevent oedema from occurring. However, the stump should not be elevated for longer than 48 hours as hip contracture may develop. From the first postoperative day the patient should lie for short periods, at least three times per day, in the prone position; this will assist in preventing flexion deformities of the hip or knee. Active range of motion exercises will be commenced early to reduce contractures and the patient with an immediate fitted prosthesis will commence partial weight-bearing from the first day; transfer techniques and crutch-walking will be commenced for the patient with a delayed fitting prosthesis.

Complications

Complications following amputation occur more commonly in the patient with a delayed fitting prosthesis and include: haemorrhage; haematoma formation if wound drainage is not used; stump oedema which is inevitable because of the lack of a rigid dressing; wound malunion or necrosis of the skin edges which may require stump revision; joint contracture; phantom limb sensation and/or phantom pain; and poor or disturbed stump moulding due to inappropriate bandaging techniques.

For the patient following immediate prosthesis fitting these complications are minimal; however, complications may occur as a result of the use of the rigid dressing technique. Skin or wound breakdown may remain undetected for many days as direct visualization of the stump is not possible. The rigid dressing may fall off; therefore, a reflex development of stump oedema may result. Should this occur the stump should be immediately firmly bandaged and elevated until a new cast can be applied. There is a tendency for the patient to undertake too much weight-bearing ambulation in the first few days and this can lead to wound breakdown or skin edge necrosis requiring further stump revision.

With either prosthesis wound infection is a likely complication and the nurse should observe the patient for any symptoms and signs, for example, fever, general malaise, increased incisional pain, or purulent wound drainage.

Anticipated outcome

Following successful recovery from amputation surgery the patient will be transferred as soon as possible to a rehabilitation facility where mobility training can be continued. It is during this phase of care that the patient receives his permanent prosthesis. With improved surgical and prosthetic techniques most patients facing amputation can expect to recover their full independence.

33

Disorders of the heart

Robyn Anderson

CARDIAC FAILURE

Pathophysiology

The causes of cardiac failure can be classified into 3 main areas: mechanical failure; consequences of disease process; and the results of normal ageing.

Mechanical failure

This may be due to:

1. Valvular disease. Stenosis and/or incompetence of the valves on the right side causes right heart failure and on the left side causes left heart failure
2. Obstruction to blood flow. When the heart tries to pump blood against constriction or pressure mechanical failure may ensue. For example, pulmonary artery stenosis and chronic lung disease cause right heart failure (right heart failure secondary to lung disease is called cor pulmonale) and coarction of the aorta causes left heart failure
3. Congenital heart disease, such as septal defects
4. Hypertension
5. Atherosclerosis.

Disease process

The disease processes which can lead to cardiac failure are: myxoedema (see page 244); thyrotoxicosis (see page 240); cardiomyopathies, caused by, for example, viral infection, pregnancy, drug and alcohol abuse, vitamin deficiency, and generalized malnutrition; myocardial infarction (see page 314); severe sepsis; and rheumatic carditis (see page 320).

Old age

It is entirely possible for the heart to simply wear out.

Cardiac failure can be said to exist when the heart can no longer supply the needs of the body and there are degrees of cardiac failure depending on the patient's exercise level. In most patients cardiac failure is a progressive condition and the cardiovascular system is able to maintain circulation by undergoing certain compensatory changes. These, however, can create additional problems.

1. The chambers of the heart dilate to hold more blood
2. The increased stretch of the fibres causes the cardiac muscle to contract more vigorously (Starling's law)
3. Hypertrophy of the myocardium occurs due to the individual fibres thickening because of prolonged overstretching. This occurs more commonly in young patients and in patients in whom the myocardium has a good blood supply. Cardiac failure must be gradual and of long duration in order for the heart to undergo hypertrophy
4. As the body attempts to maintain its blood pressure the juxtaglomerular apparatus of the kidney secretes renin, which activates angiotensin in an effort to maintain perfusion of the glomerulus. As a consequence of this mechanism, systemic blood pressure is raised
5. The pulse rate increases to maintain cardiac output (a prolonged tachycardia may also cause cardiac failure)

6. Prolonged strain leads to excessive dilation of the ventricles, overstretching the muscle fibres and causing permanent damage

7. The renin-angiotensin mechanism eventually fails, blood pressure is not maintained, and the glomerulus is no longer adequately perfused. Consequently the urine output falls and this contributes to the development of generalized oedema

8. Increased hypertrophy requires increased oxygen and nutrients – these are not forthcoming.

Clinical manifestations of cardiac failure

When the heart fails, two major groups of problems arise; those caused by insufficient blood being moved onwards, and those caused by a bank-up of blood behind the ventricle which has failed.

Clinical manifestations of right heart failure (RHF) which cause the patient to seek medical help are breathlessness on exercise, leading eventually to breathlessness at rest; and oedema of the ankles. The pathophysiology of the systems breakdown in RHF is described in Figure 33.1.

Clinical manifestations of left heart failure (LHF) which cause the patient to seek medical help are:

● Breathlessness. This often occurs at night; the patient wakes gasping for breath and will get out of bed to walk to the window, whereupon the attack subsides quickly. (This is because the

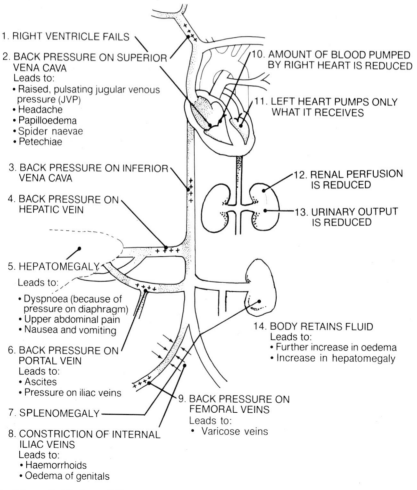

Fig. 33.1 Pathophysiology of right heart failure.

patient is standing and allowing some of the blood to drain into his legs – this condition is called paroxsymal nocturnal dyspnoea)
- Cough. This usually produces clear, thin sputum
- Haemoptysis
- Fatigue.

The pathophysiology of the systems breakdown in LHF is described in Figure 33.2. Failure of one side is rarely seen alone, as this failure inevitably leads to failure of the other side. Hence a patient usually has all the clinical manifestations of right and left heart failure as illustrated in Figures 33.1 and 33.2.

End stage cardiac failure

As total cardiac failure progresses, control of the condition becomes more and more difficult until the patient no longer responds to normal therapy.

The patient at this stage is grossly oedematous and orthopnoeic, massive ascites is present, and the cardiac rhythm is usually severely disturbed. The most common disturbance is an extremely fast atrial fibrillation with a huge pulse deficit.

All other major systems fail as a consequence of the cardiac failure, the patient ceases urine production and potassium, urea and creatinine levels start to rise; these may have been high for some time due to poor perfusion of the kidneys. The liver fails, producing a bleeding tendency and the lungs which have not worked effectively for some time worsen and become completely unable to supply the body's need for oxygen. The patient becomes cerebrally hypoxic and his level of consciousness usually deteriorates or he becomes confused and/or irritable. Slowly, as hypoxia increases, the patient slips into coma and eventually dies.

During the end stages of cardiac failure a variety of palliative measures may be undertaken to produce transient relief of symptoms. These may include: venepuncture, abdominal paracentesis, drainage of the pleural effusion and direct drainage of the oedema of the legs.

The patient may exist in this condition for days or weeks but longer survival is rare.

Investigative procedures

- Chest X-ray. Most commonly an upright antero-posterior view is used. The heart is usually enlarged and often classically described as 'boot-shaped'; the lungs may show some degree of pulmonary oedema.

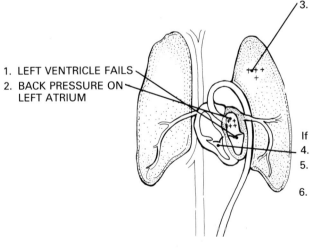

1. LEFT VENTRICLE FAILS
2. BACK PRESSURE ON LEFT ATRIUM

3. BACK PRESSURE ON THE LUNGS
causing 'waterlogged' lungs, leading to:
- Cough
- Paroxysmal nocturnal dyspnoea
  leading to haemoptysis
- Acute pulmonary oedema
- Wet chest sounds
- Production of clear, thin sputum
If untreated, leads to:
4. RIGHT CARDIAC FAILURE
5. REDUCED AMOUNT OF BLOOD PUMPED INTO AORTA
6. REDUCED BLOOD SUPPLY TO WHOLE BODY
- Brain – slowed cerebral activity
- Kidneys – reduction in perfusion leads to reduction in urine output, which results in an increase in retained fluid; therefore oedema
- Bowel – slowing of activity, therefore constipation

Fig. 33.2 Pathophysiology of left heart failure.

- Auscultation reveals a third heart sound (gallop rhythm).
- Electrocardiogram (ECG) is taken to see how much strain there is on the ventricles, and to eliminate as a cause of cardiac failure any of the correctable cardiac diseases, for example, blocking of conduction of the electrical impulse in the Bundle of His, and atrial fibrillation.

Medical management

The treatment of cardiac failure is aimed at supporting the failing heart as much as possible, and at restoring the circulation to its best possible level.

Dyspnoea and hypoxia are the symptoms which cause the patient greatest distress. Oxygen is administered by any suitable means, and a bronchodilating drug may be used to improve the patient's ventilatory status. There are many of these drugs available but most of them contain theophylline which has a great stimulating effect on the myocardium, and by increasing the heart rate can worsen the cardiac failure. Salbutomol is an excellent bronchodilator which has a more selective effect on the lungs, without extreme stimulation of the myocardium.

Related pharmacology

Drug therapy is an important adjunct to the care of the cardiac patient. Their action is to increase the effectiveness of the heart by:

- Decreasing the heart rate and hence allowing ventricular filling
- Increasing the contractility of the myocardium
- Reducing the fluid load in the body, and hence the work load of the heart
- Correcting arrhythmias.

Digitalis group. The functions of digitalis are:

- To act on the atrioventricular node and cause the node to hold the impulse from the sino-atrial node for a longer period before passing the impulse on, thus slowing the heart rate and allowing the ventricle time to fill
- To act directly on the cardiac muscle to strengthen the force of contraction

- To act directly on the sympathetic innervation of the heart to slow the impulse
- To act as a diuretic by increasing renal perfusion.

Diuretics. There are several different groups of these drugs, most of which are quite effective.

Frusemide and ethacrynic acid work on the loop of Henle. They are relatively violent diuretics of short action, and are therefore excellent drugs to cause a quick diuresis, particularly in an emergency situation.

Thiazide diuretics. There are about 6 of these in common use: they work primarily on the distal convoluted tubules. They are relatively mild diuretics and have about a 12-hour period of action. They are therefore excellent drugs to give a patient who is to be discharged.

Both these types of diuretics cause hypokalaemia and must therefore be given with potassium supplements.

Potassium supplements. There are many potassium supplements available. When selecting one, it is important to ensure that the patient can swallow it with ease, and that it does not cause him nausea or gastric irritation. Dosage should be governed by measurement of serum potassium.

Diet

There is no specifically recognized dietary management for cardiac failure. The type of diet for any one patient will largely depend upon his/her individual needs, the severity and extent of cardiac failure, the degree of sodium restriction prescribed, and the presence or absence of obesity. It is generally believed that patients with moderate or severe cardiac failure should restrict their dietary intake of salt, cholesterol, and saturated fats. They should also maintain a moderate caloric restriction.

Nursing management

Emergency treatment of acute left side heart failure

Left side heart failure usually manifests as pulmonary oedema, which is discussed in greater detail in the section on cardiac emergencies on page 330.

Emergency treatment involves the administration of:

1. Frusemide 20–100 mg IV very slowly
2. Morphine 10–15 mg IV or IM
3. Oxygen
4. Emergency measures to stop blood returning to the heart: rotating tourniquets on 3 limbs
5. Digoxin is commenced, or the dosage of digoxin is increased
6. Aminophylline 100–250 mg IV very slowly. (Extreme care must be exercised as this drug can worsen cardiac failure).

Generally pulmonary oedema should not have occurred if the diagnosis and treatment had been effective, therefore a review of the treatment of the patient's cardiac failure is needed promptly.

Nursing management of cardiac failure

The nursing management of cardiac failure is symptomatic and commonsense. It is based on resting the heart, and relieving the unpleasant effects of the congestion. The patient should be confined to bed except for brief periods, for example, when he may need to be taken to the toilet.

The care of each patient must be considered separately and individual nursing care should be planned to cater for that patient's individual and special needs. However, the following measures will apply to most patients.

1. Use a minor analgesic to relieve headache
2. Nurse the patient in an upright position to relieve dyspnoea
3. Gentle chest physiotherapy is essential to prevent sputum retention
4. Give small meals frequently to relieve nausea and vomiting, and to prevent an increase in dyspnoea and upper abdominal pain which may be caused by the overloaded stomach pressing on the diaphragm and liver
5. Fluid intake should be reduced, and a 'no added salt' diet commenced in order to attempt to reduce oedema and ascites
6. Fluid balance must be strictly recorded, the patient kept in balance
7. Weigh the patient daily

8. If the patient has scrotal oedema a scrotal support may be necessary
9. A mild aperient may be necessary to prevent the patient becoming constipated.
10. Leg exercises must be performed whilst the patient is confined to bed to prevent deep vein thrombosis
11. Special care of the patient's skin is necessary as the patient is oedematous, and oedematous skin is easily damaged.

A patient in this type of severe physical distress will need psychological support. The patient requires helpful explanations at a level which he can understand. It should be pointed out that although cardiac failure is debilitating, when his drugs are balanced and he is over the acute episode, he should be able to resume many of his previous activities.

Allied paramedical care

A social worker may be necessary to help the patient overcome any changes in lifestyle (such as moving to a less stressful job) necessitated by his condition.

A physiotherapist should be involved to help plan an exercise regime.

A dietitian is consulted to help plan a diet that meets the patient's nutritional needs, is palatable, and is economically realistic.

Complications of cardiac failure

The main complications are those associated with stasis of the blood: deep vein thrombosis (see page 299), and pulmonary embolus (see page 346). Other complications are renal failure (see page 590), and hepatic failure (see page 435).

Anticipated outcome

With proper diet, drug balance and supportive therapy, many patients are able to live long and active lives with controlled cardiac failure. Although it is not always possible to cure the underlying disease, in many cases it is quite possible to revert the acute cardiac failure to a more manageable form. However, other patients become severely compromised by the disease, become 'cardiac cripples', and as a result lead a very restricted life.

In some patients marked improvement is not attained and the patient will deteriorate until eventually the cardiac failure will cause death.

Habilitation

The patient requires help to learn to live with cardiac failure, to develop his exercise tolerance to its best possible level, and possibly to find employment of a suitable type and of which he is physically capable.

MYOCARDIAL ISCHAEMIA

Myocardial ischaemia occurs when the oxygen need of the cardiac muscle exceeds the amount of oxygen supplied through the coronary arteries. Here, myocardial ischaemia will be discussed under the headings of angina pectoris and acute myocardial infarction.

Myocardial ischaemia is a condition which often presents initially in an acute form, such as in the above conditions. It is caused by atherosclerosis and most commonly presents from the third decade of life onwards. In broad terms, angina pectoris is a symptom of myocardial ischaemia, while acute myocardial infraction is a result of extreme ischaemia.

Both conditions are characterized by severe, crushing, constrictive chest pain, which may be referred to the neck and jaw. It may radiate down the left (and on occasions the right) arm, down as low as the epigastrium, from nipple line to nipple line, into the tip of the left shoulder, and through to the back.

Angina pectoris

Generally, angina pectoris occurs as a result of physical or emotional stress. It is relieved by rest and/or the use of vasodilators, such as glyceryl trinitrate; beta-blocking agents, such as propranolol; or long acting nitrates, such as isosorbide trinitrate.

Unstable angina (occasionally referred to as crescendo angina) can occur with the patient at rest and can even wake the patient from sleep. It is important to stabilize this form of angina as quickly as possible, using sublingual glyceryl trinitrate and glyceryl trinitrate paste (the latter is used in the attempt to prevent further attacks). Beta-blocking drugs are also used in this instance and the patient should be seriously considered for coronary artery surgery, in order to prevent infarction of the ischaemic area.

Prinzmetal's angina is caused by spasm of the coronary arteries and may be responsible for angina associated with stress or emotional disturbance. It can occur in both stenosed and non-stenosed vessels. It occurs more commonly at rest than during effort, and most frequently in women under the age of fifty. Prinzmetal's angina responds well to sublingual glyceryl trinitrate.

Acute myocardial infarction

Acute myocardial infarction occurs when ischaemia is so severe as to completely interrupt the blood flow to part of the heart. This results in necrosis of the area of myocardium that is supplied by the involved artery.

Nearly 25 000 patients die in Australian hospitals from acute myocardial infarctions each year, and almost 10 000 others die from other forms of ischaemic heart disease.

Ischaemic heart disease is responsible for more Australian deaths than any other single cause, accounting for over 30% of all male deaths and nearly as many female deaths.

Pathophysiology

The mechanisms by which the involved artery becomes occluded are:

1. Embolism
2. Thrombus formation on an atherosclerotic plaque
3. Blood forcing its way in between the plaque and the intima, causing a dissecting aneurysm.

Acute myocardial infarction is predominently a condition involving the left ventricle, although

40% of inferior infarctions have some degree of right ventricular involvement. Atrial infarctions are rare and are only diagnosed during cardiac surgery or at post mortem examination.

Acute myocardial infarctions can be broadly divided into two groups: transmural infarction, in which the entire depth of the ventricular wall is involved; and subendocardial infarction, in which the area involved is usually more localized and not as deep.

Within 24 hours of an acute myocardial infarction, the dead tissue has been infiltrated by leucocytes, and lysis of the dead muscle begins. Cardiac glycogen decreases and the blood levels of the various cardiac enzymes rise. These enzymes are creatinine phosphokinase (CPK or CK) serum glutamic oxaloacetic transaminase (SGOT) and lactic dehydrogenase (LDH). By the third day the area is thin, grey, and depressed; and from the third to the 14th day the involved and damaged muscle progressively degenerates and disappears. By about the third week the involved area becomes even thinner, and the laying down of scar tissue commences. An acute myocardial infarction involving 40% or more of the left ventricle is almost always fatal.

Clinical manifestations

Most patients present with sudden, severe, crushing, constrictive chest pain that may or may not occur on exertion. The patient will often discuss his pain while he gently pounds his chest with a clenched fist; this is presumably a subconscious method of emphasizing the crushing and constricting nature of the pain. The pain of acute myocardial infarction is very similar to that of angina pectoris, but it is not relieved by glyceral trinitrate or rest. The pain can also mimic indigestion. The patient may have a feeling of impending death, which is classically described by the Latin words *angor amini*: 'fear for the soul'.

The patient may be either quiet or restless, and will be obviously afraid. He is possibly shocked and will, therefore, appear grey, cold, and clammy; some patients may have a profuse diaphoresis; dyspnoea and cyanosis are not uncommon. Up to 15% of patients with acute myocardial infarction may have essentially no symptoms and sudden collapse may be the only presenting sign.

The extent of the myocardial damage will determine the degree of systemic circulatory insufficiency (shock), which, in turn will determine the severity of any associated hypotension. Where extreme hypotension is associated with acute myocardial infarction, cardiogenic shock should be suspected. It should be remembered that severe chest pain can of its own accord be the direct cause of shock, or a contributing factor towards the overall clinical manifestations of shock (see Chapter 11). The patient may be nauseated, and may vomit; he may also be disorientated and confused.

Pulse rate and rhythm changes may occur at the time of the infarction, particularly if the electrical conductive system of the heart is damaged. The arrhythmias following a myocardial infarction can vary from mild, relatively unimportant changes, to fatal arrhythmias. A variety of these are discussed on page 327.

If the pericardium has been damaged by the infarct there may be an audible pericardial rub.

Diagnosis

Acute myocardial infarction may be strongly suspected by the clinical presentation of the patient and a supporting history of symptoms. Definitive diagnosis includes:

1. Changes in serum cardiac enzyme levels in the ensuing 24 hours
2. Electrocardiographic changes.

Investigative procedures

Leucocyte count will rise to 12 000–15 000 cells/mm^3 within 12–36 hours and blood glucose levels may be raised (particularly in diabetics).

Cardiac enzyme levels:

– CK will rise within 3–6 hours, and remain elevated until the third or fourth day
– SGOT will rise within 6–8 hours and return to normal after 4 days
– LDH will rise within 12–72 hours and return to normal in 10–12 days

Electrocardiogram changes will usually not become evident for 24 hours. These changes are: inversion of the T-wave; elevation of the ST segment; and large Q waves. As these changes may not be seen immediately it is important that a 'baseline' ECG be taken on admission.

Chest X-ray should be taken to assess clarity of lung fields and heart size.

Serum electrolyte levels are monitored daily and particular importance is placed on the levels of sodium and potassium:

- If the patient is retaining sodium, then he will also be retaining fluid, which causes an added workload on the heart.
- Following acute myocardial infarction, the patient's heart is particularly sensitive to changes in potassium. A raised, or more commonly, a low potassium level may precipitate cardiac arrhythmias with possible fatal results. Sodium and potassium levels are corrected intravenously as necessary.

Medical and nursing management

The rationale for treatment of an acute myocardial infarction is to prevent extension of the infarction and to relieve pain, treat shock, relieve anxiety and minimize complications. Complete rest is vital to reduce the load on the heart.

Prompt treatment is essential, and where possible the patient should be admitted to a coronary care unit where monitoring and treatment are instituted simultaneously.

Shock is treated (see Chapter 11) and relief of pain is mandatory. If pain is allowed to continue it may cause extension of the infarction. Morphine is the prescribed drug of choice and is administered in dosages large and frequent enough to keep the patient pain free. All drugs given in the acute phase should be administered intravenously. Due to the state of shock after acute myocardial infarction, the intramuscular circulation is inadequate to ensure complete absorption of the drugs.

Oxygen is given, ideally via an intranasal cannula or by mask. The ultra-short nasal cannulae preferred by some nurses and physicians are useless if the patient is mouth-breathing (as he probably will be due to fear and pain), as most of the oxygen is lost through the mouth (Fig. 33.3).

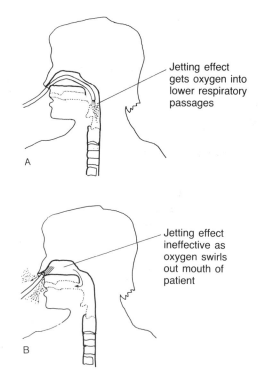

Fig. 33.3 Intranasal cannula (**A**) ensures efficient delivery of oxygen, unlike short nasal cannula (**B**) which results in oxygen being lost if patient is mouth-breathing.

The aim of oxygen therapy is to increase tissue oxygen levels, which will improve oxygenation in the marginally ischaemic areas.

Prevention and treatment of life threatening arrhythmias

The patient's pulse rate and heart beat must be monitored. Pulse should be observed for rate, rhythm, and volume, and a cardiac monitor should be attached to the patient. The pulse rate will probably be normal or above normal but on occasions, especially when the conducting mechanism has been involved in the infarction, the pulse rate may be quite slow. The pulse volume will be weak. Arrhythmias of various types are quite common after acute myocardial infarction; the most common are:

Sinus bradycardia. Following acute myocardial infarction, bradycardias of less than 60 beats per minute are considered treatable. Atropine is the drug usually used to increase the rate of the beat.

Heart block. This can occur if the Bundle of His or its branches are involved in the infarction, and requires the immediate insertion of a pacemaker. In most cases, a temporary transvenous pacemaker is used in the first instance as the conducting mechanism may only be temporarily damaged. If necessary, a permanent pacemaker can be inserted when the patient is well enough.

Premature ventricular contractions (PVCs) or ventricular extrasystoles (VEs). These are common and are considered dangerous in any of the following situations:

1. One ventricular extrasystole in every 4 normal beats.
2. 'R on T' extrasystoles – when the extrasystole occurs on the T-wave of the previous beat.
3. Salvoes or runs of VEs of more than four in a row.
4. Multifocal extrasystoles, where there is more than one area in the heart responsible for causing extrasystoles; this is easily diagnosed by the different shape of the extrasystoles.

The drug of choice in ventricular arrhythmias is lignocaine 100–150 mg intravenously immediately, and then ideally the drug should be infused at a rate that will prevent further arrhythmias occurring. The benefits of controlled infusions are that the patient receives precisely the amount of the drug required at any time to control the particular situation; in this case, if more VEs appear on the cardiac monitor the drip rate is increased, and subsequently slowed when the VEs stop.

Other drugs may be used such as procainamide, quinidine, or propranolol.

Ventricular tachycardia and ventricular fibrillation. These are both life threatening arrhythmias and must be treated immediately with large doses of lignocaine; and in the case of ventricular fibrillation, in which all cardiac output has ceased, by defibrillation. Cardiopulmonary resuscitation (CPR) is instituted in ventricular fibrillation and continues until the patient is either successfully defibrillated or has died.

Atrial arrhythmias. These are paroxysmal atrial tachycardia and atrial fibrillation, both of which respond well to treatment with digoxin. If atrial fibrillation is causing the patient to feel weak and

ill, he may be defibrillated using a special synchronized defibrillator. This ensures that the patient is reverted from atrial fibrillation to a normal sinus rhythm, and not sent into ventricular fibrillation by receiving the impulse from the defibrillator at the wrong time in the cardiac cycle.

Rest

Physical, mental, and emotional rest for the patient is essential. Initially, he is confined to bed and will, therefore, require the fundamentals of basic hygiene to be performed for him. During this time care should be taken by the nurse to maintain as much of the patient's independence and self-esteem as possible. The patient may be able, or indeed may need, to perform much of his own hygiene requirements, and this should be recognized and facilitated by the nursing staff. A commode at the bedside, or gentle assistance for a male patient to stand to void, may be less stressful than attempting to use a urinal or bedpan. Gentle aperients should be used to prevent straining during defaecation, as this can lead to cardiac arrhythmias. All articles the patient may require are placed within easy reach.

The nurse should ensure that the patient and his family have access to nursing and medical support personnel, such as a social worker and a member of the clergy.

Diet and fluid regime

In the early stages the patient will probably be nauseated and not wish to eat; the administration of an anti-nauseant may make him more comfortable. When the patient is ready to eat, a diet moderately low in sodium and potassium is given. Small meals will reduce nausea, and prevent over distension of the stomach, the pressure from which may precipitate cardiac arrhythmias. The patient requires about 4800 kilojoules per day and should have his combined fluid intake restricted to 1000–1500 ml per day. This restriction will be much more rigorous if there are signs of cardiac failure. An intravenous line must be inserted and care taken to ensure that the intravenous infusion is functioning correctly. The cannula site should be dressed according to hospital policy. All intravenous tubing should be changed every 24 hours.

Fluid intake and output should be charted, and care taken to ensure that the patient remains in a slightly negative balance in order to reduce the workload of the heart.

Other observations

Pulse, ventilation, and blood pressure should be measured half-hourly for the first 4 hours or until the patient's condition is stable. Hourly, 10-second ECG monitor strips should be taken, as should tracings of abnormal rhythms; these should be kept in chronological order. Sleep is of paramount importance to the patient, and those in a stable medical condition should not be woken for the taking of these vital signs. Monitor readings can be obtained without disturbing the patient and are a visual warning of life threatening arrhythmias. Blood should be taken for 3 consecutive days for estimation of enzyme levels, and electrolyte and urea levels. Imbalance is corrected on a daily basis. A full 12-lead ECG should also be performed daily for at least 3 days. Urine should be tested on admission for the presence of sugar, as the patient may have underlying diabetes mellitus. Investigations for diabetes mellitus should be performed before the patient is discharged.

Temperature is taken daily. As lysis of the damaged muscle increases, the patient's temperature will rise. However, sudden steep rises in temperature are more probably significant of chest infection; initial decrease in the patient's temperature is probably indicative of shock.

Related pharmacology

Anticoagulation. There are two schools of thought on whether anticoagulants should be used. The reasons for using anticoagulants are, firstly, that the patient is confined to bed and therefore at risk of deep vein thrombosis of the muscles of the calf. This risk is increased by the fact that his blood pressure at this stage is almost always low, and therefore his circulation is extremely poor. Secondly, the damaged, roughened areas of the myocardium can 'snag' platelets and cause a clot to form on the area; this can break free to become an arterial embolus.

The anticoagulant used in the acute phase is heparin and the aim is to increase the patient's clotting time to 2–2.5 times normal. This is usually achieved by giving 5000 units of sodium heparin subcutaneously into the abdomen TDS. Heparinization can also be achieved by using a loading dose of 7500–10 000 units of heparin and then approximately 1000 units per hour intravenously.

Whole blood clotting time is monitored daily and the rate of heparin administration is adjusted in accordance with these results. Sometimes when the patient is well enough (usually within 24 hours) he is commenced on an oral coagulant, for example, warfarin. It takes about 3 days for warfarin to reach therapeutic levels, as it acts by depressing prothrombin formation. As warfarin starts to become effective the patient is weaned from heparin. Alternatively, on discontinuation of the heparin infusion, small doses of aspirin may be used daily instead of warfarin; this reduces platelet stickiness and is preferred by some physicians.

Those physicians who do not use anticoagulants point out that the survival rates in both the anti-coagulated patients and the non-anticoagulated patients are identical.

Cardiac glycosides (digitalis derivatives). These drugs are not routinely used in acute myocardial infarction except where there are indications of cardiac failure.

Sedatives/tranquillizers. Mild sedatives are occasionally used to promote rest and to alleviate anxiety.

The other drugs used in acute myocardial infarction have been discussed earlier in this chapter; they are: morphine for the relief of pain; lignocaine to suppress arrhythmias; antinauseants to suppress nausea.

Complications of acute myocardial infarction

Arrhythmias. These can vary in severity from minor rhythm disturbances to life threatening arrhythmias; the most serious of these have been discussed earlier in this chapter.

Cardiogenic shock. Infarction of more than 40% of the left ventricle will almost always result in cardiogenic shock or death. The mortality rate from cardiogenic shock is over 50%.

Clinical manifestations of cardiogenic shock. The patient is restless and often disoriented. The skin is cold and clammy due to peripheral vasoconstriction, the pulse volume is weak, tachycardia is evident, and the patient may be oliguric due to low cardiac output and severe hypotension. If the patient's mean arterial pressure is less than 75–85 mmHg the myocardium itself cannot be effectively perfused, resulting in left heart failure and pulmonary oedema.

Treatment of cardiogenic shock. The aim of treatment is to restore the integrity of the myocardial muscle and to increase the cardiac output.

1. Ventilation is assisted to prevent, or at least reduce hypoxia – the patient, therefore, requires an endotracheal tube and ventilation with 100% oxygen.
2. Fluids should be given intravenously with great caution and in conjunction with diuretics in order to achieve a urinary output of 50–60 ml/hr.
3. Give ionotropic agents (those that will increase the force of contraction: digoxin, dopamine, glucagon).
4. Correct acid–base balance/imbalance and electrolyte abnormalities.
5. Correct arrhythmias.
6. Give mechanical cardiac assistance with an intra-aortic balloon pump. This will raise the pressure in the first part of the aorta and therefore in the coronary arteries, and also aids ventricular emptying.

Congestive cardiac failure (see page 309).

Conduction defects. These may be minor, but most ultimately require the insertion of a pacemaker

Rupture of the heart. This may occur between the 3rd and 10th day post infarction. It causes sudden death due to the massive haemopericardium. Occasionally rupture occurs in the intraventricular septal wall, causing a huge ventricular defect.

Rupture of a papillary muscle. If the infarct occurs at the base of a papillary muscle, the whole muscle with its attached cordae tendinae can tear free of the wall. This results in the related valve

(usually the mitral valve) becoming totally incompetent.

Ventricular aneurysm. Due to the intraventricular pressure, the weak fibrosed wall may bulge slowly. Where the bulge is of reasonable size it may be the site of thrombus formation due to the swirling motion of the blood, which quite effectively breaks up blood cells, and initiates clotting.

Continued care and rehabilitation

The patient is nursed in a coronary care unit for the first 3–5 days, he is then transferred to a less intensive unit for the next 10 days to 3 weeks. During this time all investigations and observations that had been performed in the intensive care unit will be reduced gradually or ceased completely; however, temperature, pulse, and blood pressure readings should be taken and recorded on at least a daily basis. This is done to watch for late complications, such as a chest infection or incipient cardiac failure. The patient will be encouraged to cease smoking or at least cut down cigarette usage, as forcing patients to stop smoking is now considered unnecessarily stressful.

There are a variety of cardiac ambulation programmes, all of which follow the basic rule of common sense. On the 3rd to the 5th day the patient may sit out of bed for approximately 10 minutes. His exercise tolerance is increased daily until he can produce the effort required to cope at home. For example, if he has to walk up 2 flights of stairs when he gets home, then he will have to be capable of walking up 2 flights of stairs prior to his discharge. An example of a cardiac ambulation program is:

Day 3:	Sit out of bed for 10 minutes
Day 4:	Sit out of bed for 1 hour
Day 5:	Walk around the bed
Day 6:	Walk to shower and shower in warm water whilst seated and supervised
Day 7:	Walk to shower and shower whilst standing and supervised
Day 12:	Continue to walk gently around ward/unit, sit in chair for longer periods

Days 21–28:   Return home with complete understanding of exercise program, diet and medications.

As the patient's heart becomes more stable, medications are ceased, with the exception of warfarin which may be continued for 6–12 months. This is used by some physicians to reduce the likelihood of further thrombus formation in the atherosclerotic arteries or over the area of the infarction. The dosage of warfarin will be controlled by the patient's general practitioner who will use as a guide weekly prothrombin estimations.

Diet. A dietitian will be consulted and the patient established on a diet which will lower, and then maintain at a lower level, his cholesterol and triglyceride levels. These levels will be monitored on a regular basis (approximately monthly). Reduction of cholesterol and triglyceride levels will help to reduce further atherosclerotic vessel changes, and therefore may reduce the chance of further myocardial infarction. The patient should be assisted to obtain and maintain ideal body weight.

Allied paramedical care

A social worker will be consulted in order to allay the patient's stress in relation to financial commitments which he may not be able to meet while in hospital. Occasionally arrangements can be made with employers to reduce some of the stressors relative to the patient's occupation. Suggestions that the patient should change his occupation if it is too stressful are not helpful as it is often physically, emotionally, and sometimes intellectually impossible, especially with the present levels of unemployment. It is more reasonable that the social worker (or the nurse) arrange for the patient to attend classes which can teach him how to cope with stress, and how to utilize his leisure time more effectively.

Home help may be useful in some instances to perform tasks, such as washing and ironing and vacuuming. Heavy groceries should, where possible, be delivered rather than carried home.

An occupational therapist may be able to help by arranging for small structural changes to the patient's home and by helping with anti-stress programmes. The patient and his sexual partner should be advised about the resumption of sexual activity; they may both require counselling aimed at teaching them how sexual activity can still be enjoyed with the patient possibly taking a less vigorous role. Where the initial infarction has been related to intercourse they may both be afraid of further sexual activity. This places a great deal of unnecessary stress on the relationship.

Anticipated outcome

In Australia 70% of all patients who have myocardial infarctions survive, 10% die in hospital, and 20% die before reaching hospital. Those patients who survive should be able to continue their lives with minimal change to their life style or to the life style of those around them.

BACTERIAL ENDOCARDITIS

This is a condition in which bacteria grow on previously damaged areas of the heart. It occasionally also occurs on completely normal cardiac tissue. Classically this damage is caused as a result of rheumatic fever which is a systemic, non-suppurative, inflammatory disease which probably results from an autoimmune reaction to a beta haemolytic streptococcus. Rheumatic fever affects the connective tissue in the heart, and thus the valves are the areas of the heart most affected; the mitral valve is by far the most commonly affected with the aortic valve being the second most commonly damaged.

Bacterial endocarditis is responsible for approximately 1% of all cardiac disease.

The organisms most often responsible for this phenomena are *Streptococcus viridans* and *Staphylococcus albus* which are both inhabitants of skin and mucous membrane. The portal of entry is most frequently through dental caries, dental abscess, or following dental surgery of some type. Minor breaks in other mucous membrane on skin may be responsible for entry of the causative organism.

There are two forms of bacterial endocarditis. In the less severe form often referred to as sub acute bacterial endocarditis, the patient presents with a swinging temperature, night sweats, loss of weight, general malaise and possibly an audible murmur over the heart. The organisms tend to grow in colonies which adhere to the damaged tissue in beads. A colony may break away from the tissue and travel via the bloodstream to the brain where it may form a cerebral embolus and produce the symptoms of CVA. These colonies may progress to brain abscesses.

The more extreme form of the disease is caused by more virulent organisms and can result in septicaemia, destruction of the tissue on which the organism is growing, and total failure of the valve, with a resultant cardiac failure causing imminent death.

Investigative procedures

Investigative procedures are aimed at isolating the organisms and monitoring the degree of cardiac damage.

A series of blood cultures are performed at the height of the fever (the patient is classically febrile in the late afternoon or early evening) until the causative organism is located. A sensitivity test is then performed to ascertain the most appropriate antibiotic.

ECGs are performed at 3–4 daily intervals, as are auditory studies of the heart. These are performed in order to assess increasing valve damage and therefore resultant cardiac failure.

Medical and nursing management

Treatment involves bed rest in an attempt to relieve the work load on the heart and thereby reduce the likelihood of detachment of the bacterial colonies from the valves.

Specific treatment is usually with massive doses of penicillin, to the order of 50–100 million units per day (in divided doses), other antibiotics are sometimes used, but always in high dosages in order to penetrate the bacterial colonies. Antibiotics are given intravenously.

There are no special dietary requirements, but it must be remembered that while these patients are usually anorexic, they still require a normal protein, and raised carbohydrate intake to compensate for the metabolic increase concomitant with the fever.

The patient requires gentle handling and general fever care, as in the acute stages he may have rigors. The condition necessitates long term medical and nursing management which involves bed rest and the administration of antibiotics. Supervised active leg and chest exercises will help to prevent the problems of stasis.

Complications of bacterial endocarditis

These include:

• Cerebrovascular accident (CVA) due to migration of bacterial colonies
• Cerebral abscess due to lodging and subsequent growth of a colony in the brain
• Valvular incompetence due to colonies in situ preventing proper closure of the valves and leaking of blood around and between the colonies
• Cardiac failure
• Unresolved bacterial endocarditis
• Renal insufficiency
• Septicaemia.

Anticipated outcome

Only slightly more than half of all patients with bacterial endocarditis survive; death results from cerebral abscess, CVA, cardiac failure, renal insufficiency or unresolved infection.

Resolved endocarditis allows the patient to return to a completely normal life. An antibiotic cover may however be necessary during periods of risk, such as infections in other family members, or prior to minor surgery and dental procedures.

CARDIAC SURGERY

Cardiac surgery is highly specialized. It often requires very special equipment which is not usually available in an ordinary operating room; it also requires specialist support staff to manage the equipment during surgery. Cardiac surgery is therefore performed only in those hospitals with special units.

The aims of cardiac surgery are: to prevent necrosis or further necrosis of myocardium; to create a better blood supply to the heart; to prevent regurgitation of blood through damaged valves; and to prevent swirling and haemolysis of blood.

Preoperative management

Ideally, the patient is brought into hospital some 4–6 weeks prior to surgery and has a cardiac catheter passed so that the coronary vessels and the aorta may be thoroughly investigated using angiography techniques.

A dental check is carried out and any necessary dental work is completed prior to surgery. (This is important as the bacteria which commonly cause sub-acute bacterial endocarditis may enter the body through dental caries.)

Prior to all cardiac surgery, the patient is shaved from neck to knees anteriorly and posteriorly. If a vein is to be taken from a leg to act as graft material, the legs are shaved to the ankles. All male patients have a facial shave.

The patient should shower using Phisohex or Gamophen soap for several days prior to surgery.

A high dose, broad spectrum antibiotic is given with the premedication. Most patients are transported to the operating room sitting upright on a trolly to ensure normal chest and lung function until just prior to anaesthesia. Glyceryl trinitrate paste may be applied to patients with cardiac disease at the time of premedication in an attempt to prevent angina and a possible acute myocardial infarction on the way to the operating room as, despite the premedication, these patients are usually very frightened. In the past if a patient did have an infarction on the way to the operating room, the operation was cancelled; now, however, the surgeon usually proceeds with the surgery and the infarcted area may be revascularized with a graft.

Surgical management

There are two classic methods by which the heart is approached.

Sternotomy. This is a midline incision from the suprasternal notch to below the xiphoid process

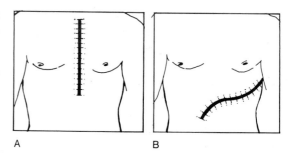

Fig. 33.4 Wound sites following sternotomy (**A**) and thoractomy (**B**).

(Fig. 33.4A) in which the sternum is split lengthwise to allow access to the heart and great vessels. A sternotomy is used whenever it is necessary for the patient's life to be maintained by a cardiopulmonary by-pass (heart–lung) machine during surgery.

Thoracotomy. Involves an incision which is made in the 6th, 7th or 8th intercostal space (Fig. 33.4B) and the chest is opened using a rib spreader. In relation to cardiac surgery a thoracotomy is used only for valvotomy.

To gain access to the heart the pericardium must be opened; this is inelastic fibrous tissue and may be left open, or indeed a small section may be removed before the chest is closed to ensure that cardiac tamponade does not develop.

Patients who have had cardiac surgery through either a sternotomy or a thoracotomy have two drain tubes in situ on return from the operating room. One is in the pericardium along the posterior wall of the heart and the other is a high intercostal catheter draining air from the pleural space via an underwater seal drainage system (see Fig. 36.2 page 343). Both tubes have a negative pressure applied to them.

Following cardiac surgery two ventricular pacing wires are left in the heart; these can, if necessary, be connected to an external pacemaker should the heart's natural pacemaker fail.

Cardiac surgery often involves cardiopulmonary bypass which is the method by which blood is oxygenated and pumped around the body whilst the heart is not beating during the surgical procedure. Oxygenation of blood is achieved by removing venous blood with cannulae inserted into the inferior and superior venae cavae passing it through an oxygenator, removing all air bubbles and returning it via another cannula to the aorta. The major hazards of such a procedure include that of a fall in the patient's core temperature due to the large extracorporeal blood volume. This has largely been coped with by adding a heat exchange to the line returning blood to the aorta. Also, there is a small possibility of either a blood clot embolus or an air embolus. Because of the large extracorporeal blood volume large doses of heparin are necessary to prevent clotting of blood.

Where it is necessary to clamp the aorta for longer than 30 minutes the coronary arteries must be cannulated and the myocardium supplied with blood.

Types of cardiac surgery

Cardiac surgery can be divided into 6 main areas:

1. Repair of congenital defects. This is a huge area of highly specialized cardiac surgery which will not be dealt with in this text book.

2. Surgery of the coronary blood vessels. This type of surgery has completely revolutionized the treatment of patients with coronary heart disease. The procedure involves revascularizing areas of the heart by bypassing one or more of the coronary arteries or the major branches of the arteries (Fig. 33.5). The material used may be a specially woven seamless teflon tube, or more commonly a piece of the patient's own long saphenous vein.

If the long saphenous vein is to be used it is taken from the patient's leg at the time of the cardiac surgery.

3. Repair of wall defects. These may occur in either the atria or the ventricles and are closed by direct suturing or by patching the deficit with teflon. The approach to the heart for these procedures is usually via sternotomy.

4. Valvular surgery. Valvular surgery has become much less common than it was between 1950 and 1970, due to a general improvement in the treatment of minor infections and thus rheumatic fever has decreased in incidence; consequently the valvular damage subsequent to the condition is less common.

There are two major types of valve surgery.

(a) Valvotomy. This is usually only palliative or temporary surgery to allow a valve to open properly. In later years the valve may have to be replaced. Generally, the surgeon either frees the adhering tissue by dissection or simply forces his finger through the valve thereby breaking adhering tissue

(b) Valve replacement. Heart valves are replaced by removing the damaged valve and suturing into its position an artificial valve. These consist of a ring of porous material which will eventually become part of the healing and scarring process as it is invaded by blood cells and eventually fibrous tissue. Attached to the ring are either artificial valve leaflets, a ball and cage type valve (Fig. 33.6) or specially treated pig or calf heart valves. The choice of a valve depends largely on the preference of the surgeon. Artificial heart valves generally function very efficiently. The order of incidence of replacement is most commonly the mitral valve, followed by the aortic and tricuspid valve.

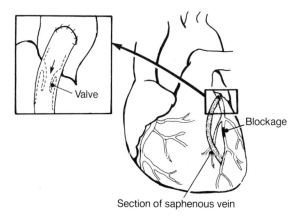

Fig. 33.5 Coronary bypass.

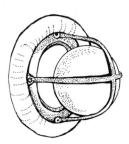

Fig. 33.6 Artificial heart valve.

5. Pacemaker insertion. In an emergency an extracorporeal pacemaker can be attached to wires inserted through the chest wall directly into the ventricular muscle or connected to a wire passed into the ventricle via the brachial vein.

This type of pacemaker functions effectively but is inconvenient and potentially dangerous as infection can easily track along the wires; it is therefore only used for short term pacing of the heart.

Where long-term pacing will be required the pacemaker itself will be implanted into the muscle; either pectoralis major or the muscles of the abdominal wall are used. A wire from the pacemaker may be either passed through the superior vena cava through the left atrium and into the left ventricle or may be sutured along the ventricular wall.

The pacemaker consists of two parts. One measures the rate at which the heart is beating and the other fires the impulse which artificially stimulates the heart to beat. Most pacemakers used these days are 'demand' pacemakers, that is, they are preset at (say) 70 beats per minute. When the cardiac rate falls below the set rate, the device fires the impulse which will keep the rate at no less than 70 beats per minute.

Pacemakers generally function on battery power although there are some atomic pacemakers in use. Battery powered pacemakers have a life of around 5 years and must therefore be changed at approximately 5-yearly intervals.

6. Heart transplant. These are performed in several centres throughout the world. The heart may be transplanted alone or together with the lungs. Technically heart transplantation is quite successful but it is plagued with the problem of the body's rejection of foreign tissue, as is all transplant surgery. Implantation of an artificial heart or a partially artificial heart will probably become more common in the future.

Related pharmacology

Most patients following cardiac surgery are given anticoagulants in order to prevent clot formation on suture sites on new valves and grafts. The drug used is sodium heparin which is given subcutaneously into the abdomen in doses of 5000 units TDS. Whole blood clotting time is monitored

daily and the rate of heparin administration is adjusted in accordance with these results. Patients are prescribed an oral anticoagulant, for example warfarin. It takes about 3 days for warfarin to reach therapeutic levels, as it acts by depressing prothrombin formation. As warfarin starts to become effective the patient is weaned from heparin. Alternatively on discontinuation of the heparin small doses of aspirin may be used daily; this reduces platelet stickiness and is preferred by some surgeons.

Pain relief is mandatory and morphine is the drug of choice. This can be given in bolus intravenous dosages or as a continuous intravenous infusion. The advantage of IV infusions is that the patient can be given additional small boluses whenever painful procedures, such as chest physiotherapy, are to be performed.

Diet

If surgery is required for cardiac disease a dietitian will see the patient in order to assess his personal likes and dislikes in regard to food and a diet will be designed which is low in salt and triglycerides and cholesterol whilst maintaining normal protein and vitamin content. Weight modification may be a pertinent issue in designing the patient's diet.

Nursing management

Post cardiac care is usually performed in a special cardiac surgery unit, the staff of which have undertaken post-graduate education in this area. Nurses who work in these specialized areas must not only be excellent technicians but must also be skilled general nurses, as their patients require gentleness and understanding, while receiving the best nursing care available. The temptation exists in these units for nursing staff to become little more than extremely dextrous technicians. Very often in the critical care situation the nurse is the co-ordinator of all care for the patient.

The special nursing care needed after cardiac surgery is to constantly monitor the patient's condition and to be able to interpret and act upon the information gleaned from these observations. The patient will almost always be artificially ventilated and will have cardiac, blood pressure, and a variety of other monitors attached. Drain tubes must be kept patent and these are removed when they are no longer bubbling, usually within 24–48 hours.

Following either sternotomy or thoracotomy, the patient must not be shoulder-lifted but cradle-lifted up the bed as too great a pressure on the arms can cause the sutures of a thoracotomy to burst or can rupture the sternum.

Patients can be assisted to help themselves and to move much more easily by the nurse tying a strong soft rope to the bottom of the bed. The patient can pull on this in order to sit up without too much difficulty.

Pacing wires are coiled and left on the chest wall under small occlusive dressings. These dressings are usually changed on a daily basis. The wires are usually removed 24–28 hours before the patient is discharged.

Allied paramedical care

Both thoracotomy and sternotomy patients will need chest physiotherapy and the physiotherapist will usually see these patients twice each day. In between visits from the physiotherapist, the nurse must help the patient perform his physiotherapy. Coughing and deep breathing can be made much easier for the patient if the nurse sits behind him on the bed and firmly clasps a soft pillow in front of the patient's chest in order to brace his chest during the exercise. Later, the patient will be able to do this by himself.

Following cardiac surgery most patients have a period of severe depression, or of inexplicable disorientation, variously referred to as 'post cardiac surgery syndrome', 'intensive care syndrome', 'critical care neurosis' and other similar titles. It is presumably due to the fact that these patients have been under a great deal of stress prior to surgery and they are frightened that the degree of change to their lifestyle will be enormous; they have difficulty in foreseeing a complete recovery. They feel that they have lost their competence, and independence, and they are generally worried as to how they will cope when they return home, especially as there will be no full time medical or nursing assistance at home. The methods used to alleviate this effect are to

explain procedures to the patient, and preoperatively to take him to the immediate postoperative unit so that he can see the life support equipment which will be attached to him on his return from the operating room. This should reduce his postoperative disorientation. He should also be introduced to a patient who has undergone the same type of surgery and who is looking forward to being discharged. Added to all these concrete fears is the popular belief that 'the heart is the seat of the soul' and is far more than just a muscular bag which pumps blood.

Most patients return to a normal psychological state within a few days, but some patients may take weeks, and others may require the professional help of a psychologist or psychiatrist.

A social worker is of great value in offering additional explanation to the patient, alleviating financial problems for the period in which the patient may be unable to be responsible for his financial commitments, and in finding accommodation for significant others who may have travelled to a major city in order to be near the patient during the surgery. The social worker can be of further assistance when the patient returns home, in ensuring that council (or other) assistance is available if required for any heavy tasks such as vacuuming or mowing lawns.

Complications of cardiac surgery

These are the same as for any other surgery with the addition of:

1. Rupture of the sternum. Through persistent coughing the sternum can become partially or totally divided, as the suture wires are pulled through the body of the sternum due to pressure. Should this occur the patient will usually be returned to the operating room for resuturing of the sternum. If the sternum is not resutured, malunion may occur.

2. Malunion of the sternum. This also requires rewiring. It is extremely painful and will greatly inhibit coughing and chest physiotherapy as well as general movement.

3. Herniation of the sternal wires. This occasionally happens and requires the patient to be returned to the operating room to have his ster-

num resutured or the wires removed. The great danger is that infection can track down one of the wires.

4. Cardiac tamponade. This occurs when there is bleeding into the pericardium and the pericardial drain tube is blocked and/or the pericardium has been sutured closed. Tamponade is a potentially lethal situation in which pressure increases between the heart and the pericardium. The heart is compressed, the cardiac output falls, the pulse pressure narrows and the patient becomes shocked. One of the classic initial signs of tamponade is pulsus paradoxus in which the pulse rate fluctuates in response to breathing and is classically felt as a decrease in pulse pressure and volume on inspiration. Death will ensue rapidly. A patient with cardiac tamponade must be returned to the operating room immediately in order to have the tamponade drained.

5. Bacterial endocarditis. A variety of bacteria can grow on damaged heart valves, on the leaflets of an artificial valve, or on sutures within the heart. See page 321 for the nursing management of the patient with bacterial endocarditis.

34

Cardiovascular emergencies

Robyn Anderson

CARDIAC ARREST

A cardiac arrest occurs when a person exhibits the sudden and unexpected signs of clinical death.

Clinical manifestations

When cardiac arrest occurs the patient will present in a state of collapse, with no cardiac output and hence no pulse, and with unrecordable blood pressure and hence no tissue perfusion. There will be gross cyanosis, especially of the face, and there will usually be no ventilations. The patient is usually unconscious.

Occasionally, cardiac arrest may be accompanied by vomiting and/or epileptiform seizures. The patient will develop a metabolic acidosis due to the hypoxic metabolism that results from the lack of tissue perfusion. Brain damage or death will ensue within several minutes if immediate treatment is not instituted.

The heart may be in one of two rhythms: ventricular fibrillation, in which there is chaotic electrical activity; or asystole, in which there is no electrical activity. In both rhythms the ventricles fail to contract and therefore do not shift blood. Thus it is impossible to clinically distinguish between the two rhythms. A cardiac monitor must, therefore, be attached to the patient immediately. In more than 80% of cardiac arrests, the heart is fibrillating.

Aetiology

The major cause of cardiac arrest in hospitals is electrolyte imbalance; and in the community most cardiac arrests are caused by myocardial infarction (see page 314). Other causes of cardiac arrest are: generalized massive trauma leading to shock; hypoxia as a result of, for example, drowning or electrocution; and trauma to the heart.

Medical and nursing management

Help is summoned by whatever emergency method is hospital policy; the patient is placed in recumbent position on a firm surface; the airway is checked to ensure that it is clear and dentures, providing they are well-fitting, should remain in situ. The carotid and/or femoral pulses are checked and, if absent, expired air ventilation is commenced immediately. External cardiac compression is commenced immediately. A vein is cannulated and an infusion line established and 50–100 ml of 8.4% sodium bicarbonate is given to reverse acidosis. The heart is monitored to discover whether it is fibrillating or in asystole, and the situation is treated appropriately (see below).

The patient should be intubated as soon as possible with an oral-endotracheal tube, and then ventilated with pure oxygen.

Any known electrolyte imbalance should be corrected. Cardiopulmonary resuscitation (CPR) should be continued until the patient's heart beat is restored and he is breathing spontaneously, or until the decision is made that he is dead.

POTENTIALLY LETHAL CARDIAC RHYTHMS

Ventricular fibrillation

In ventricular fibrillation (VF) individual muscle fibres are depolarizing; there is no proper ventric-

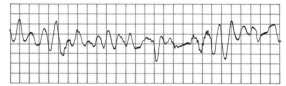

Fig. 34.1 Ventricular fibrillation – coarse. (From Hampton, 1986.)

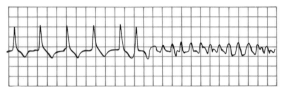

Fig. 34.2 Ventricular fibrillation – fine. (From Hampton, 1986.)

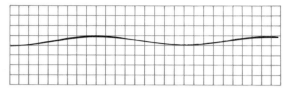

Fig. 34.3 Asystole.

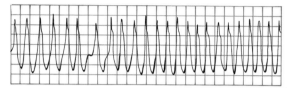

Fig. 34.4 Ventricular tachycardia. (From Hampton, 1986.)

ular contraction, and the heart wriggles and twitches. VF is divided into two types:

- That with a coarse fibrilliary line (Fig. 34.1)
- That with a fine fibrilliary line (Fig. 34.2).

Fine VF responds very poorly to defibrillation and should be converted by drug therapy to coarse fibrillation which responds well. There is no pulse. CPR is instituted and must be maintained until the patient is successfully defibrillated. Defibrillation is first line treatment. If this fails the patient should be given 50–150 mg of lignocaine intravenously (1 mg/kg of body weight) then defibrillated; if there is no response, a second dose of lignocaine is given, along with 0.2 mg isoprenaline and a further attempt is made to defibrillate the patient. If there is still no response 10 ml of 10% calcium chloride is given intravenously in order to sensitize the myocardium to defibrillation and to convert the fine VF to coarse VF; a further defibrillation attempt is made. When the patient has been successfully defibrillated lignocaine may be infused in order to suppress any irritable focus within the heart.

Asystole

In asystole the heart is devoid of electrical activity and ventricular contraction. It is sometimes referred to as cardiac standstill (Fig. 34.3). It is almost always caused by direct vagal stimulation such as: Valsalva's manoeuvre, pressure on the carotid sinus(es), firm pressure on the eyeballs,

vomiting and over-distension of the rectum, or passage of an endotracheal tube.

Treatment involves instituting CPR and administering drugs to excite the myocardium into some electrical activity. The drug of choice is adrenaline; and 0.5–1 ml of adrenaline 1 : 1000 should be given into a large vein or directly into the heart.

CPR is continued until the heart is beating again or the decision is made that the patient is dead.

Other drugs used in asystole are given either after the heart has exhibited electrical activity or, inappropriately, in panic.

Ventricular tachycardia

In ventricular tachycardia (Fig. 34.4) the ventricles are dominated by an irritable focus. There is little, if any, blood being pumped; the pulse may not be detectable and is extremely fast. Ventricular tachycardia can very easily deteriorate into VF.

It should be treated with lignocaine 50–150 mg (1 mg/kg body weight) intravenously as an immediate dosage, followed by lignocaine infusion until the irritable focus is suppressed. Other antiarrhythmic drugs may also be used, such as phenytoin, procainamide and quinidine.

Ventricular ectopic beats or ventricular extrasystoles (VEs)

These are premature contractions which originate from an irritable focus in the ventricle; they are usually followed by a compensatory pause, and for this reason may be felt at a pulse point as 'coupled beats'. They are broad, bizarre-shaped waves, and can be precipitated by: electrolyte imbalance, myocardial ischaemia or infarction, emotional stress, fear, and a variety of other factors. The patient is occasionally aware of these ectopic beats and may describe their feelings variously as: 'rabbit kicks', a 'missing beat', 'my heart turned over', 'palpitations'.

Random VEs are alarming, but not particularly dangerous; however, there are 4 situations in which VEs are extremely dangerous:

1. Salvoes. These are runs of 4 or more VEs in a row which can easily precipitate ventricular tachycardia and fibrillation.
2. One VE in every 4 or less normal beats (Fig. 34.5).
3. R on T ventricular extrasystole. In this situation (Fig. 34.6) the VE occurs on the T wave of the previous beat; this too can precipitate ventricular fibrillation.
4. Multifocal VEs. These are different shaped extrasystoles which originate from different foci in the ventricles and are evidence that there is more than one irritable area (Fig. 34.7).

VEs are generally suppressed with infusion of lignocaine. Occasionally where VEs occur over a long period of time quinidine or a beta-blocker may be the appropriate treatment. VEs are commonly caused by disturbances in potassium levels; this should be rectified as quickly as possible, to prevent a lethal arrhythmia.

Heart block

Following myocardial infarction, first degree heart block is seen in 7–10% of all patients; 5% will have second degree block; and 5–6% will have complete heart block.

First degree heart block (Fig. 34.8) is seen by prolongation of the P–R interval and a mild slowing of the heart rate; it usually does not require treatment.

In second degree heart block (Fig. 34.9), occasional ventricular beats are blocked. This may require treatment which could be with a drug, such as isoprenaline, or more usually by the insertion of a pacemaker.

Complete (third degree) heart block (Fig. 34.10) exists when there is no relationship between the

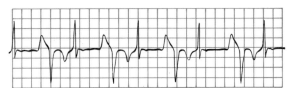

Fig. 34.5 Ventricular extrasystole – occurring every second beat. (From Hampton, 1986.)

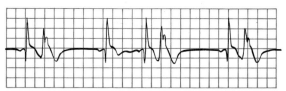

Fig. 34.6 R on T ventricular extrasystoles. (From Hampton, 1986.)

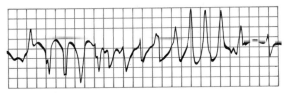

Fig. 34.7 Multifocal ventricular extrasystoles. (From Hampton, 1986.)

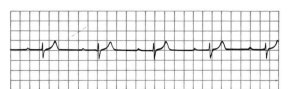

Fig. 34.8 First degree heart block. (From Hampton, 1986.)

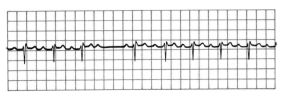

Fig. 34.9 Second degree heart block. (From Hampton, 1986.)

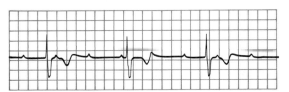

Fig. 34.10 Complete (third degree) heart block. (From Hampton, 1986.)

atrial and the ventricular rates. The ventricles often pace themselves at extremely slow rates at 20–40 beats per minute.

A small number of patients with heart block respond to a long term form of isoprenaline, however most of them require the immediate insertion of a pacemaker.

Atrial arrhythmias

These are rarely lethal, but in the long term may be the cause of cardiac failure which in itself may be fatal. Generally, atrial arrhythmias, such as atrial fibrillation and atrial flutter respond well to cardiac glycosides (digoxin). If the patient feels weak and ill, or is not compensating, he should be defibrillated using a synchronized defibrillator (cardiversion).

A pulse deficit may be detected in these patients; the apex beat of the heart may be quite fast without all the beats being strong enough to get through to the wrist, and the radial pulse is therefore slow and usually irregular. Pulse deficits should be assessed by two nurses who simultaneously count the apex and the radial pulse rates.

PULMONARY OEDEMA

Pulmonary oedema is a sign of left heart failure. There is backlog of blood in the lungs; the hydrostatic pressure within the vessels of the pulmonary system increases greatly, and fluid is extruded into the lung tissue itself. In its minor form it is characterized by a cough which is productive of clear, frothy sputum; this can be accompanied by mild dyspnoea and tachycardia. In its extreme form the patient has pink frothy fluid flowing passively up his trachea and into his mouth. Dyspnoea and tachycardia are extreme. The great danger is that the patient will, quite literally, drown in his own fluid.

Medical and nursing management

The principles of treatment are much the same as they would be for somebody who was drowning:

'Get him out of the water; get the water out of his lungs; and ensure that he can breathe properly'.

In pulmonary oedema, the fluid is removed from the patient's lungs by the following measures:

1. Sit the patient up
2. Aspirate any fluid that enters the mouth or pharynx
3. Prevent any further fluid from entering the lungs. Appropriate methods are:
(a) Use a diuretic, such as frusemide to reduce blood volume. Frusemide is used in dosages from 20–200 mg (or more) in order to create a diuresis; it is also believed that it may have some role in dilating the great veins and thereby reducing the load on the heart
(b) Give morphine 10–20 mg IV to allay anxiety and dilate the great veins
(c) Venous tourniquets are used to trap fluid in the peripheral circulation in the extremities, thereby reducing the amount of blood which must be pumped. If venous tourniquets are used they must be rotated so that no limb has a tourniquet in position for longer than 45 minutes (Fig. 34.11). Care must be taken to occlude the venous return rather than the arterial flow. A record of the movement of the tourniquets should be kept, preferably on the patient's limb. Gradual changing of the tourniquets is essential to prevent a sudden rush of blood to the heart and a rebound overload of the central circulation.

The simple use of tourniquets can be so efficient as to relieve all symptoms until an effective diuresis is produced. Rotating tourniquets can be used for a long as necessary.
(d) Occasionally, an oral endotracheal tube is inserted and the patient is ventilated on 5–10 ml of positive end expiratory pressure (PEEP). This tends to oppose the hydrostatic pressure which is causing the fluid movement and therefore reduces the fluid volume in the lungs. This is usually done only in critical care units.

It is also necessary to ensure that the patient's breathing improves by giving oxygen, ideally by nasal catheter rather than by a mask of any type, as masks increase the patient's sense of suffocation and therefore his degree of panic. A bronchodilator may be used if, after clearing the fluid from

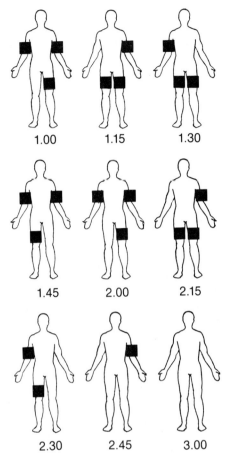

1.00   1.15   1.30

1.45   2.00   2.15

2.30   2.45   3.00

Fig. 34.11 Tourniquet rotation. Tourniquets are rotated clockwise every 15 minutes. In this example, the decision is made at 2.15 to remove the tourniquets. One tourniquet is removed at subsequent rotations until, at 3.00, all have been removed.

the airway, the patient has some degree of bronchospasm. Aminophylline 250–500 mg is still the drug of choice. It is imperative to remember that aminophylline speeds up the heart; this patient is already in cardiac failure and will have a tachycardia, by worsening the tachycardia, the patient will be pushed further into failure. Aminophylline is, therefore, very much a second line drug in this situation as it may do a great deal more harm than good. Salbutamol is an excellent bronchodilator with a high beta-2 bronchodilatory selectivity. It has much less beta-1 selectivity (ionatropic) than aminophylline and may well replace aminophylline in the treatment of patients with cardiac problems.

When the emergency is over, the patient will need a potassium supplement to replace the potassium lost during the diuresis. The underlying left cardiac failure should be treated with cardiac glycosides (digoxin). If the patient is already receiving digoxin, then the dosage almost certainly needs to be increased and the patient restabilized. Pulmonary oedema should not have occurred in a well stabilized patient.

MASSIVE HAEMORRHAGE

Excessive loss of blood may present as either overt or concealed haemorrhage. Overt haemorrhage is dramatic; the visual loss of blood sometimes creates panic. Concealed haemorrhage, as its name suggests, is more difficult to detect. The skilled nurse should suspect a concealed haemorrhage, within the context of the injury, before decompensation occurs, as massive haemorrhage results in profound shock.

Massive haemorrhage occurs as a result of trauma to major blood vessels. It may be the result of:

● Trauma which occurs immediately prior to the haemorrhage
● Reactionary haemorrhage due to rising blood pressure blowing a ligature off an artery
● Secondary haemorrhage where infection has eroded away part of the wall of an artery
● Erosion of an artery by a peptic ulcer, a malignancy, or (rarely) a syphilitic gummata
● Ruptured oesophageal varices.

Medical and nursing management

The principles of treatment of massive haemorrhage are:

1. Control the haemorrhage
2. Replace the blood loss
3. Treat the shock (see Chapter 11).

Control of haemorrhage

Venous bleeding is generally easier to control than is arterial bleeding. Where the bleeding is from large veins the blood will be dark red in colour, and the blood loss will be a continuous flow. The part should be elevated (where this is possible) and a large pad of dressing material bandaged firmly into position directly over the bleeding area. The patient should be placed in recumbent position and transferred to a hospital and, if necessary, to the operating room.

In arterial bleeding, the blood is bright red in colour and the flow will be intermittent in accordance with the pulse. To stop arterial bleeding, the first line of treatment is for the nurse to place her hand or fist into the wound and apply firm pressure to the area of bleeding (however, see page 786 for protocols of managing patients with AIDS). A dressing pad should replace the position of the nurse's hand as soon as possible, and be bandaged firmly into place. The part should be elevated if possible and if necessary pressure should be applied to the major artery where it crosses a single bone proximal to the wound.

The patient should be transferred to the operating room as soon as possible.

Where massive haemorrhage is concealed, there is very little that can be done to control the bleeding. The patient is transferred to the operating room so that the haemorrhage may be controlled.

Replacement of blood loss

The amount of blood lost should be replaced with grouped and cross-matched whole blood, as there is no fluid which will perform the functions of blood. In an extreme emergency group O Rh− low-titre (universal donor) blood may be used. Other solutions, such as stabilized plasma protein solution (SPPS) or Haemacel may be used to help keep the patient's blood pressure at a reasonable level until whole blood is available.

SECTION C – REFERENCES AND FURTHER READING

Texts

Alpert J S 1985 Manual of cardiovascular diagnosis and therapy 2nd edn. Little, Brown & Co, Boston

Anderson J R (ed) 1976 Muir's textbook of pathology, 10th edn. Edward Arnold, London

Anthony C P 1984 Structure and function of the body. Mosby, St Louis

Behrendt D M 1985 Patient care in cardiac surgery 4th edn. Little, Brown & Co, Boston

Berkow R (ed) 1977 The Merck manual of diagnosis and therapy, 13th edn. Merck Sharp & Dohme, New Jersey

Berne R M, Levy M N 1986 Cardiovascular physiology 5th edn. Mosby, St Louis

Brandenburg R O et al (eds) 1987 Cardiology: fundamentals and practice. Chicago Year Book

Chaney P S (ed) 1982 Managing diabetics properly, 2nd edn. Intermed Communications, Pennsylvania, ch 6, p 70–72, ch 10, p 101–114

Creager J G 1982 Human anatomy and physiology. Wadsworth, California

Connor W E, Bristow J D 1985 Coronary heart disease: prevention, complications, and treatment. Lippincott, Philadelphia

Ford R D (ed) 1984 Cardiovascular disorders: nurse's clinical library. Springhouse, Pennsylvania

Groer M E, Shekleton M E 1979 Basic pathophysiology: a conceptual approach. Mosby, St Louis

Guyton A C 1976 Textbook of medical physiology, 5th edn. Saunders, Philadelphia

Guzzetta C E 1984 Cardiovascular nursing: bodymind tapestry. Mosby, St Louis

Hamilton H (ed) 1982 Combatting cardiovascular diseases skillfully, 2nd edn. Intermed Communications, Pennsylvania

Hampton J R 1986A The ECG in practice. Churchill Livingstone, Edinburgh

Hampton J R 1986B The ECG made easy 3rd edn. Churchill Livingstone, Edinburgh

Havard M 1986 A nursing guide to drugs, 2nd edn. Churchill Livingstone, Melbourne

Hojnacki L H 1985 Handbook of cardiac rehabilitation for nurses and other health professionals. Reston, Virginia

James R (ed) 1980 MIMS annual, 4th edn. Intercontinental Medical Statistics, Sydney

Kaplan N M 1986 Clinical hypertension 4th edn. Williams & Wilkins, Baltimore

Laurence D R, Bennett P N 1980 Clinical pharmacology, 5th edn. Churchill Livingstone, Edinburgh

Loustau A, Blair B J 1981 A key to compliance: systematic teaching to help hypertensive patients follow through on treatment. Nursing 81 11(2) : 36–39

Luckmann J, Sorensen K C 1980 Medical-surgical nursing: a psychophysiologic approach, 2nd edn. Saunders, Philadelphia

Macleod J 1987 Davidson's principles and practice of medicine, 15th edn. Churchill Livingstone, Edinburgh

Mandel W J 1987 Cardiac arrhythmias: their mechanisms, diagnosis, and management, 2nd edn. Lippincott, Philadelphia

McCarthy D O 1984 Hypertension. In: Hamilton H K (ed) Diseases, 2nd edn. Springhouse, Pennsylvania, ch 18, p 1109–1111

Phipps W J, Long B C, Woods N F (eds) 1983 Medical-surgical nursing: concepts and clinical practice, 2nd edn. Mosby, St Louis

Potter D O (ed) 1985 Hypertension. In: Emergencies. Springhouse, Pennsylvania

Read A E, Barritt D W, Langton Hewer R 1986 Modern medicine, 3rd edn. Churchill Livingstone, Edinburgh

Robinson J (ed) 1981 Giving cardiovascular drugs safely. Intermed Communications, Pennsylvania

Roper N (ed) 1978 Nurses dictionary, 15th edn. Churchill Livingstone, Edinburgh

Sadler D 1984 Nursing for cardiovascular health. Appleton Century Crofts, Norwalk

Society of Hospital Pharmacists of Australia 1985 Pharmacology and drug information for nurses, 2nd edn. Saunders, Sydney

Storlie F J (ed) 1984 Diseases: nurse's reference library, 2nd edn. Springhouse, Pennsylvania

Turner P P 1985 The cardiovascular system 2nd edn. Churchill Livingstone, Edinburgh

Vinsant M O 1985 Commonsense approach to coronary care: a program 4th edn. Mosby, St Louis

West R S (ed) 1984 Giving cardiac care: nursing photobook, 2nd edn. Springhouse, Pennsylvania

Woods W L (ed) 1983 Cardiovascular critical care nursing. Churchill Livingstone, New York

Journals

Adelman E M 1980 When the patient's blood pressure falls . . . What does it mean? What should you do? Nursing 80 10 : 2 : 26–33

Barrows J J 1984 Turning the tide against acute pulmonary oedema. Nursing 84 14 : 3 : 58–63

Baum P L 1985 Heed the early warning signs of PVD: peripheral vascular disease. Nursing 85 15 : 3 : 50–57

Baum P L 1986 Taking the PVD patient's history. Nursing 86 16 : 5 : 30

Bennett M J, et al 1985 Leg ulcer management at home. The Australian Journal of Advanced Nursing 2 : 4 : 36–44

Burden L L, Atwell K 1983 The treacherous waters of unstable angina pectoris. Nursing 83 13 : 12 : 50–55

Burden L L, Atwell K A, Kupper N S, Duke E S 1984 Bradycardia: the signals of a slowing heart Nursing 84 14 : 9 : 60–63

Buschiazzo L 1986 What's new in CPR? Nursing 86 16 : 1 : 34–37

Cameron R J 1980 Australian health survey 1977–78 chronic conditions. Australian Bureau of Statistics, Canberra

Cameron R J 1983 Causes of death Australia 1981. Australian Bureau of Statistics, Canberra

Dalgas P 1985 Understanding drugs that affect the autonomic nervous system. Nursing 85 15 : 10 : 58–63

Dennison R 1986 Cardiopulmonary assessment: how to do it better in 15 easy steps. Nursing 86 16 : 4 : 34–39

Doyle J E 1981 If your patient's legs hurt, the reason may be arterial insufficiency. Nursing 81 11 : 4 : 74–79

Doyle J E 1983 All leg ulcers are *not* alike: managing & preventing arterial & venous ulcers. Nursing 83 13 : 1 : 58–63

Erickson B A 1986 Detecting abnormal heart sounds. Nursing 86 16 : 1 : 58–63

Fahey V A 1984 An in-depth look at deep vein thrombosis. Nursing 84 14 : 3 : 34–41

Feldstein A 1986 Detect phlebitis and infiltration before they harm your patient. Nursing 86 16 : 1 : 44–47

Forshee T 1986 Track down the what, where, when, and how of chest pain. Nursing 86 16 : 5 : 34–41

Frank-Stromborg M 1981 Managing the patient with hypertension. Nursing 81 11 : 3 : 56–59

Gandy E D, Veigh G 1984 Help the amputee stand on his own again. Nursing 84 14 : 7 : 46–49

Goldstein J M 1986 M.I. the rescue is just the beginning. Nursing 86 16 : 12 : 44–49

Gordon H S 1986 Cardiac tamponade. Nursing 86 16 : 8 : 33

Hackett C 1983 Limbering up your neurovascular assessment technique. Nursing 83 13 : 3 : 40–43

Hartshorn J C 1980 What to do when the patient's in hypertensive crisis. Nursing 80 10 : 7 : 37–45

Hill M, Fink J W 1983 In hypertensive emergencies, act quickly but also act cautiously. Nursing 83 13 : 2 : 34–41

Hill M N, Foster, S B 1982 Seeking and finding all those patients with high blood pressure. Nursing 82 12 : 2 : 12–15

Hussar D A 1979 Your role in patient compliance. Nursing 79 9 : 11 : 48–53

Karnes N J 1984 Premature ventricular contractions: when to sound the alarm. Nursing 84 14 : 6 : 34–39

Kelleher J 1985 Partial hand amputation. Nursing 85 15 : 8 : 25

Kern L S, Gawlinski A 1983 Stage managing coronary artery disease. Nursing 83 13 : 4 : 34–40

Klein D M 1984 Angina: physiology, signs, and symptoms. Nursing 84 14 : 2 : 44–46

Kleinhenz T J 1985 The inside story on preload and afterload. Nursing 85 15 : 5 : 50–55

Koszuta L E, Koszuta J 1986 The ins and outs of measuring cardiac output. Nursing 86 16 : 3 : 54–56

Kupper N S, Duke E S, Burden L L, Atwell K A 1984 Tachycardia: stay a step ahead of your patient's racing heart. Nursing 84 14 : 8 : 34–41

Lamb L S, DiGiacomo B M 1985 What to expect when your patient's scheduled for mitral valve replacement. Nursing 85 15 : 1 : 58–63

Millam D A 1984 Postinfusion phlebitis: physiology, signs, and symptoms. Nursing 84 14 : 12 : 36–37

Miller P G 1985 Assessing C.V.P. Nursing 85 15 : 9 : 44–46

Miracle V A 1986 Anatomy of a murmur. Nursing 86 16 : 7 : 26–31

Moore L C, Pulliam C B 1986 An on-the-spot guide to antihypertensive drugs. Nursing 86 16 : 1 : 54–57

Norsen L H, Fox G B 1985 Understanding cardiac output – and the drugs that affect it. Nursing 85 15 : 4 : 34–41

Norsen L, Telfair M, Wagner A L 1986 Detecting dysrhythmias. Nursing 86 16 : 11 : 34–40

Nurse's Reference Library 1984 A quick guide to chest pain. Nursing 84 14 : 3 : 22–23

Quinless F 1984 P.V.D.: Physiology, signs and symptoms. Nursing 84 14 : 3 : 52–53

Quinless F 1984 Myocardial infarction: physiology, signs, and symptoms. Nursing 84 14 : 4 : 52–54

Rudy S F 1986 Take a reading on your blood pressure techniques. Nursing 86 16 : 8 : 46–49

Slusarczyk S M, Hicks F D 1983 Helping your patient to live with a permanent pacemaker. Nursing 83 13 : 4 : 58–63

Smith C E 1984 "My chest hurts". Nursing 84 14 : 4 : 34–39

Solid R 1984 Give venous leg ulcer the boot. Nursing 84
14 : 11 : 52–53

Spangler R A 1985 Update on pulmonary artery
catheterization. Nursing 85 15 : 8 : 42–45

Strong A 1983 Monitoring central venous pressure. Nursing
83 13 : 10 : 8–10

Taylor D L 1983 Congestive heart failure: physiology, signs,
and symptoms. Nursing 83 13 : 9 : 44–46

Taylor D L 1983 Thrombophlebitis: physiology, signs, and
symptoms. Nursing 83 13 : 7 : 52–53

Taylor D L 1985 Assessing heart sounds. Nursing 85
15 : 1 : 51–53

Tribulski J A 1984 Back from the brink: resuscitating and
rehabilitating the M.I. patient. Nursing 84
14 : 9 : 60–63

Van Every S L, Curwen E H 1985 Combating heart attacks
on the home front. Nursing 85 15 : 10 : 55–57

van Parys E 1987 Assessing the failing state of the heart.
Nursing 87 17 : 2 : 42–49

Wade D W 1982 Teaching patients to live with chronic
orthostatic hypotension. Nursing 82 12 : 7 : 20–21

Youngren D E 1981 Improving patient compliance with a
self-medication teaching program. Nursing 81
11 : 3 : 22–23

SECTION

D

The respiratory system

35

Introduction to the respiratory system and respiratory failure

Jenny Kidd

The lungs are composed of alveoli. These are microscopic grape like structures that are one cell in diameter, and because of their structure, provide the lungs with their enormous capacity for gaseous exchange. Surrounding each alveolus is a network of capillaries which are also one cell in diameter (Fig. 35.1). It is this intimate structural relationship that allows the smooth, uninterrupted diffusion of oxygen and carbon dioxide. Therefore to maintain gaseous exchange, it is of paramount importance that the integrity of the alveolar wall be maintained, together with an adequate blood supply to the lungs themselves.

The respiratory function of the lungs can be divided into two parts: ventilation and gaseous exchange. Ventilation is the movement of air into and out of the alveoli, and gaseous exchange is the diffusion of oxygen into the blood stream and carbon dioxide out of the blood stream and into the alveoli.

Ventilation depends on both the function of the respiratory muscles, the major one being the diaphragm, and volume capacity, that is the ability of the lungs to maintain normal tidal volume and vital capacity. Conditions which will affect ventilation are space-occupying fluid or tumours, thoracic deformities, obstructive diseases such as asthma, neurological diseases, pain, and injuries to the diaphragm.

Gaseous exchange is the second part of respiratory function. All respiratory diseases are either caused by or result in oedema, exudate and/or inflammation, which scar the alveoli, and thus cause an alteration in gaseous exchange, giving rise to certain phenomena. Therefore it is reasonable to say that all respiratory conditions share many clinical manifestations to a greater or a lesser extent, depending upon the severity of the disease. Briefly, these are: breathlessness, dyspnoea, tachypnoea, cyanosis, hypoxia, hypercapnia, cough and sputum production.

In addition to this, many of the organisms responsible for respiratory inflammation can cause a variety of diseases with variation in severity. The diseases commonly termed flu, chest cold, head cold, and bronchitis are all used synonomously by lay people to cover a wide range of respiratory diseases, all of which have similar aetiology and clinical manifestations but differ in severity and pathology.

The importance of lung disease cannot be over-emphasized. Diseases such as coryza, bronchitis and pneumonia are common findings in clinical practice and the incidence of emphysema and malignancy of the lung due to cigarette smoking and a polluted environment appear to be increasing significantly. The lungs are also involved in terminal disease, although in a secondary capacity. For example, bronchopneumonia, pulmonary oedema and atelectasis are

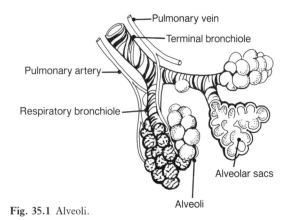

Pulmonary vein

Terminal bronchiole

Pulmonary artery

Respiratory bronchiole

Alveolar sacs

Alveoli

Fig. 35.1 Alveoli.

common findings at postmortem. A wide knowledge of respiratory disease in general will enable the nurse to both recognize and prevent many disease states that can affect the lungs, which are, of course, vital organs.

RESPIRATORY FAILURE

Respiratory failure is diagnosed both clinically and physiologically, and is confirmed by a set of arterial blood gas values. Respiratory failure is said to exist when the pH, pO_2 and pCO_2 levels are outside the normal limits. Respiratory acidosis is a significant indication of respiratory failure where the pH and pO_2 are below normal and the pCO_2 is raised. Clinically, the findings are an increase in ventilatory rate, and ventilations are often laboured and difficult. There is abnormal movement of the diaphragm, the glottis moves up and down, and the ali nasi flare with each breath. The patient will also show signs of confusion, aggression, and restlessness. Impending respiratory failure should be recognized early and the actual state of failure therefore prevented. If respiratory failure is not recognized and treated, the situation will worsen steadily. Exhaustion becomes overwhelming, the patient finds ventilation increasingly difficult, and hypoxia and hypercapnia worsen. The patient will eventually become comatosed and die. Restlessness, confusion and aggression should always be suspected as signs of respiratory failure, particularly if there is pre-existing chest trauma.

It is the nurse's responsibility to ensure that sedation for these patients is withheld until respiratory failure is discounted, as sedation may mask the clinical signs and will further suppress the patient's ventilatory function with a resultant increase in hypoxia and hypercapnia. The general rule of thumb is that one should never sedate a patient in impending or actual respiratory failure unless the patient is intubated and artificially ventilated.

Causes of respiratory failure

Any disease of the lung – acute or chronic – has the potential to cause respiratory failure.

Additionally, improper reversal from an anaesthetic, pain, abdominal binders that restrict diaphragmatic movement, rupture of the diaphragm, and chest injuries such as flail chest or pneumothorax are all potential causes of respiratory failure.

Medical and nursing management

Treatment of respiratory failure is effected by treating the underlying cause, if this is possible. Therefore the nursing management relates to the management of the causative disorder. Skilled observation by the nurse is essential to assess either improvement or continued deterioration in the patient's condition. In nearly all circumstances (excluding terminal disease) the patient with respiratory failure will be nursed in an intensive care unit.

Intubation

Intubation of the trachea refers to the passage of an endotracheal tube via either the nose or mouth, through the vocal cords and into the trachea. The purpose of this is to either create an airway and/or enable manual or mechanical assisted ventilation for the patient. These needs may arise in any of the following: general anaesthesia, cardiac arrest, respiratory arrest, oropharyngeal trauma and/or oedema, and to allow easy access to the lungs for aspiration of sputum. The articles required for intubation are: an endotracheal tube of appropriate size, a laryngoscope, a pair of Magill forceps, a pair of padded artery forceps and a Kigliss syringe.

The patient is in a recumbent position with his neck hyperextended, with the operator standing behind the patient's head. The blade of the laryngoscope is placed in the patient's mouth to lift the tongue and jaw upwards to enable the vocal cords to be viewed. The endotracheal tube is then passed through the vocal cords and into the trachea. Sometimes, especially in the conscious patient, Magill forceps are necessary to assist the smooth passage of the tube through the vocal cords. Once the tube is in situ the cuff is inflated and the padded artery forceps are clamped in position to seal the cuff line.

Manual ventilation

The articles required for manual ventilation are a Magill bag (2 l to 4 l) and an endotracheal adaptor.

Manual ventilation is usually of short duration and is used during anaesthesia, cardiac arrest, and respiratory arrest. Patients who are receiving ventilatory support via mechanical ventilation will also require intermittent manual ventilation, to stimulate coughing and loosen lung secretions, to enable more productive tracheal aspiration, to increase the patient's oxygen levels prior to aspiration, and to compensate for the 'sigh' reflex if it is not already built in to the ventilator's cycle. Intubation via the nose and mouth is usually of short-term duration. If the patient requires long-term ventilation, that is, longer than 48 hours, a tracheostomy is performed.

TRACHEOSTOMY

A tracheostomy is an opening into the trachea for the purpose of creating an airway. A tube is inserted into the trachea which bypasses the larynx and upper airway. Tracheostomies are either permanent or temporary. The reasons for a permanent tracheostomy include total laryngectomy, and severe laryngeal stenosis. A temporary tracheostomy may be used to enable short-term assisted ventilation to allow easy access to the lungs for removal of secretions, and to bypass the upper airway where obstruction is present due to a foreign body, trauma, or oedema.

The operation is generally elective and many patients who require a tracheostomy already have an endotracheal tube in situ. The patient's neck is well extended and a horizontal incision is made approximately 2 cm above the suprasternal notch. The surgeon then uses blunt dissection to expose the upper part of the trachea. A vertical incision is made in the trachea at the level of the second or third cartilagenous ring, and the tracheostomy tube is introduced. The cuff is inflated and the external flanges of the tracheostomy tube are often stitched to the patient's skin for added stability; these sutures are removed when the tube is changed for the first time. The tube is held in position by tapes which are tied securely around the patient's neck and attached to the tube's external flanges. A tracheostomy tube may be

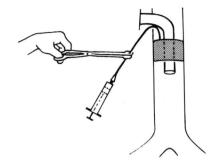

Fig. 35.2 Cuffed tracheostomy tube in situ.

made of metal or plastic. Metal tubes are used for patients with permanent tracheostomies; they are easy to maintain and consist of an inner and outer tube, with the inner tube able to be removed and cleansed of secretions.

Most adult-sized synthetic tubes have an inflatable cuff which is situated at the base of the tracheostomy tube. The cuff is made of a highly refined plastic and usually is of low pressure and high volume. It is prestretched and floppy and, when correctly inflated, pressure is spread over a large area of trachea (Fig. 35.2).

Once the tracheostomy is in situ the cuff is inflated to create a seal between the tube and the trachea. This seal prevents an air leak around the tube and also protects the lungs by preventing the entrance of food and secretions.

In order to prevent overdistention of the cuff, air is slowly introduced into the cuff until the air leak is no longer audible through a stethoscope placed on the patient's neck. Subsequently, it is not usually necessary to deflate the cuff because of its low pressure design; however, some institutions may still deflate the cuff on a regular basis for a stated period of time in order to prevent tracheal ulceration and necrosis which would ultimately result in the complication of tracheal stenosis.

Nursing management of a patient with a tracheostomy

As the majority of tracheostomies performed are elective, preparation of the patient for the reality of the postoperative period is possible and mandatory. However, in a minority of cases (for example, severe trauma, or acute airway obstruction) this is not possible and the nurse must ensure that all care is explained fully on return of the patient to the ward.

Because of the communication difficulties this procedure produces, care of the patient with a tracheostomy requires considerable preoperative planning in conjunction with the patient. It is essential to provide prior explanation and education; the patient must know what to expect on return from surgery and should be assured that a nurse will be with him at all times for at least the first 24 hours. The nurse should agree with, and teach, the patient the use of a few simple signals by which he will communicate basic needs; and the patient should be introduced to and allowed to become familiar with the more elaborate communication tools that will be used. Communication aids will range from the use of pen and paper, buzzers or bells, to simple or sophisticated flip charts.

The non-English speaking patient will experience special problems, and the assistance (both pre- and postoperatively) of an interpreter will be essential. Flip charts in various languages are available, and their use will greatly facilitate postoperative communication and nursing management. It should be noted that the patient whose first language is not English may, under the stress of the situation, revert to the mother tongue for some time following surgery.

On return from the operating room, the patient is usually nursed in a semi-upright position to facilitate breathing. For the first 24--48 hours tracheal aspiration will be required on an hourly basis, and more frequently if necessary, to keep the trachea free of secretions. Often these aspirations follow manual ventilation.

The need for tracheal aspiration is usually indicated by the sound of the air passing in and out of the tube. Bubbling, gurgling, or other sounds of increasing secretions, require attention. Alternatively, the patient may be able to indicate his need for aspiration. Chest physiotherapy is always an indication for tracheal aspiration. It should be noted that the patient who is able to cough and expectorate secretions through the tube will require less frequent aspiration. A patient with a tracheostomy must receive nebulized oxygen, especially for the first few days postoperatively, as his upper airways, which normally filter and moisten the air, have been bypassed.

Emergency articles which must be kept at the bedside include a spare tracheostomy tube, and tracheal hooks and dilators in case of respiratory obstruction or collapse of the airway following accidental removal of the tube. The tube is changed for the first time on approximately the 3rd to 5th postoperative day, and subsequently weekly. After a three day period the stoma will be firm enough to enable the safe removal of the old tube and replacement with a new one. The patient may be reluctant to move his head and neck during the initial postoperative period, therefore effective analgesia is mandatory and articles the patient may require should be within easy reach. To be effective, analgesic dosage must suppress pain but not depress the respiratory centre.

Initial nourishment is usually provided via the intravenous route and adequate hydration is essential to keep secretions moist. Those patients who do not have a nasogastric tube inserted receive fluids orally from the first postoperative day. Many patients are afraid to eat as they have a fear of choking, but once they realize it is possible to swallow with a tracheostomy tube in situ, thicker fluids, leading to a soft and ultimately a full diet, may be introduced.

When a patient has a nasogastric tube inserted, fluid is usually introduced following the initial postoperative fasting period, and once this is tolerated the equivalent of a normal diet can be administered enterally. Patients with a nasogastric tube usually have a permanent tracheostomy and the reason for the surgery (and its nature) will dictate the length of time that enteral feeding must continue. For some patients this could be up to 3 months.

Food and fluids should be administered with caution as vomiting causes unnecessary strain and pain to the patient's neck. The ease with which patients return to oral diet depends on the nature of the surgery and the support and reassurance they receive when foods are introduced. At all stages during the patient's return to a normal oral diet, close nursing supervision is essential.

Chest physiotherapy is of great importance due to the patient's increased risk of developing a chest infection. This is due to the fact that both his upper airway and his primary cough reflex have been bypassed, and he must rely on a secondary cough reflex from the carina. Direct entrance into the trachea without filtration permits the inhalation of dust and microorganisms into the lungs, and the regular passage of a suction catheter into the trachea, although an aseptic procedure, also carries with it an increased risk of introducing infection.

Frequent observations and recording of vital signs are taken, noting in particular the patient's colour and rate and depth of ventilations. The tube is checked for patency and the tapes must be tied securely around the patient's neck. The wound is observed for bleeding which should be minimal and should rapidly subside. The wound is cleansed with sterile normal saline and the stoma dressed with sterile, non-adhering, split gauze. This must be kept clean and dry, and changed as necessary. In the event of the tube becoming dislodged due to vigorous coughing, carelessly tied tapes, or the patient pulling it out, tracheal dilators should be placed immediately into the wound in order to maintain an airway, whilst the spare tube is prepared for insertion. When the walls of the stoma are firm, (in the later postoperative days) this is not so much of an emergency.

In the event of respiratory obstruction due to a blocked tube, tracheal aspiration should be attempted in order to relieve the obstruction. If this fails, 5 ml of normal saline can be introduced rapidly into the tube to dislodge the obstruction, followed by tracheal aspiration. If all else fails, the tube is removed and a new one inserted.

In most situations the patient with a tracheostomy tube in situ is both conscious and alert. In the main, the major problem for the patient is that he feels isolated and extremely frustrated because he has lost (either temporarily or permanently) the use of a major organ of communication. His frustration and isolation can be largely diminished by the nurse who will be anticipating his needs and providing him with the alternative communication tools already described. The nurse should also ensure that all health professionals and the patient's significant others, employ the following communication techniques:

• Speak distinctly, but at normal volume and maintain eye contact with the patient
• Communicate using closed-ended questions, that is, those which require only a yes/no response, and therefore a nod of the head by the patient
• Separate communication into small, manageable units and allow time for the patient to respond.

Once the need for the tracheostomy tube is resolved and prior to its removal, the patient is usually enabled to speak by the nurse deflating the cuff of the tube and teaching him to place his finger over its lumen. The patient thus breathes normally and speech (although quite husky and indistinct) will be possible.

Following removal of the tube a sterile dry dressing (changed as necessary) is placed over the stoma site until healing occurs. During healing, the patient ensures occlusion of the stoma by applying gentle pressure to the dressing whenever he is speaking or coughing.

Permanent tracheostomy care

A patient with a permanent tracheostomy should not be discharged until his ventilatory capacity is at its optimum, and he can cough effectively. Secretions will be expelled to the opening of the trachea at which point they can be wiped away with tissues.

In general no tube is left in situ as a fistula has been created from the trachea to the skin. On occasions however the development of the fistula may not be complete and a fenestrated tracheostomy tube will be placed in situ until this occurs. These tubes are made of teflon which may be silastic coated, or occasionally, silver. The tube is removed and cleaned by the patient every 2–3 weeks or as necessary. Silver tubes have an inner and an outer lumen. The inner lumen must be removed and cleaned every 4 hours. People with permanent tracheostomies need to protect themselves from upper respiratory tract infections, and protective filters or scarves should be worn in dusty environments.

Electronic voice stimulation can be used to augment faint vocal sounds in post laryngectomy patients, which greatly assists communication. Persons with a permanent tracheostomy can lead a normal life; even swimming may be possible with 'snorkel' attachments to the tracheostomy.

36

Respiratory emergencies

Jenny Kidd

CHEST INJURIES

Any injury to the thoracic cavity can potentially result in a reduction in the vital capacity, tidal volume, and gaseous exchange of the lungs; and ultimately, generalized tissue perfusion. Cardiac output may also be adversely affected. Because of the intimate association of the lung parenchyma with the ribs, intercostal muscles, and pleura, any injury to these structures will result in an immediate compromise of lung expansion. Abnormal collections of blood and air, or a reduction in negative intrapleural pressures, or just simply the restriction of chest movement due to pain, will result in varying degrees of hypoxia and hypercapnia. Traditionally, chest injuries have been broadly classified into two groups: penetrating (open), or non-penetrating (closed) injuries.

Penetrating chest injuries

These result from any object which causes a wound and subsequent hole in the chest wall; knives, bullets, or foreign objects may penetrate the chest as a result of trauma.

Non-penetrating chest injuries

These may be caused by blunt trauma such as a solid blow to the chest, or by a crushing injury, and usually result in fractured ribs and associated contusion of the lungs. Commonly, other organs and structures suffer simultaneous damage or rupture; the diaphragm, trachea, oesophagus, heart, aorta, and sternum may be involved. This naturally complicates the chest injury. When the diaphragm is significantly traumatized, ventilatory paralysis and subsequent paroxysmal breathing may ensue. Abdominal organs may also herniate into the thoracic cavity with a further reduction in lung vital capacity. The normal bellows action of the lungs is not possible without a functional diaphragm, and it is likely that patients with a traumatized diaphragm will require assisted ventilation and, possibly, surgical repair.

Clinical manifestations

These will depend on the extent of the lung or airway trauma involved. General signs and symptoms shared by all chest injuries include dyspnoea, cyanosis, hypoxia, tachycardia, chest pain, and haemoptysis.

In the event of a tear in the trachea, surgical emphysema will result. This refers to air in the tissues and gives the patient a puffy appearance. The skin feels crackly to gentle pressure.

Diagnosis

Diagnosis is confirmed by chest X-ray. If respiratory embarrassment is severe, blood gas analysis may be undertaken.

Medical and nursing management of chest injuries

If there is a wound this should be covered with a clean or sterile dressing and pressure applied to bleeding sites. The patient should be sat up and transported to hospital as soon as possible. Most patients with chest injuries will require oxygen therapy.

Flail chest

This occurs when several successive ribs are fractured and disassociate completely from the rib cage. As the chest moves upwards and outwards on inhalation, the disassociated section of the rib is drawn in by a less than atmospheric pressure which prevents the expansion of the underlying lung (Fig. 36.1). This type of breathing is termed paradoxical and is so typical of a flail chest that diagnosis can be made on evidence of paradoxical breathing alone.

Flail chest may result from a penetrating or non-penetrating injury.

Medical and nursing management of the patient with a flail chest

The intercostal muscles will usually stabilize the flailing segment and the patient maintains bed rest until union of the fractured ribs occurs. The shunting of air from the affected lung to the unaffected lung will cease when the fracture has stabilized.

Morphine is used to relieve the chest pain and make ventilation easier and more relaxed.

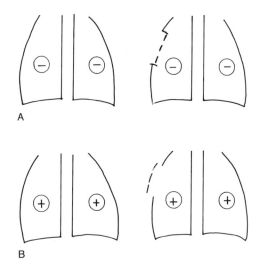

Fig. 36.1 Paradoxial breathing. **A** – On inhalation, the rib-cage expands to create a negative pressure in the lungs and thus suck in air. This negative pressure also draws in the disassociated ribs. **B** – On exhalation, the rib-cage contracts to expel air from the lungs, but the resultant positive pressure also forces out the disassociated ribs.

Fractured ribs

This is a common injury and results from trauma to the chest wall or from chronic coughing. Most fractured ribs are stable and do not require any treatment. The patient suffers chest pain on either inhalation and/or exhalation which is exacerbated by sneezing, coughing and laughing.

It is possible sometimes to feel the crepitations of the fractured area by placing a hand on the chest wall over the injured area. Overt bruising may occur on the chest wall. Treatment consists of rest, avoiding heavy physical activity, and analgesia. Healing takes place rapidly and the patient makes a complete recovery.

Compound fractured ribs are more serious and usually cause greater respiratory embarrassment and sometimes pneumothorax. The wound must be cleaned and the patient taken to the operating room for realignment of the ribs and debridement of the wound. Antibiotic and tetanus cover is given.

COMPLICATIONS OF CHEST INJURIES

- Pneumothorax – air in the pleural cavity.
- Haemopneumothorax – the presence of blood and air in the pleural cavity.

A pneumothorax or haemopneumothorax is, in most cases, unilateral and in both of these conditions there is partial or complete collapse of the lung. Both may progress to tension pneumothorax – a life threatening condition (see page 344). Pneumothorax can be caused by either open or closed chest trauma.

An open pneumothorax is often referred to as a 'sucking chest wound'. This occurs where there is an opening through the chest wall of sufficient size as to allow the free movement of air in and out of the pleural space.

Causes of closed trauma include fractured rib or ribs, or rupture of a bleb as seen in asthma. When the latter occurs it is termed spontaneous pneumothorax. Ideopathic spontaneous pneumothorax also accounts for one of the forms of pneumothorax. It appears to occur in relatively young persons with no evidence of pulmonary pathology.

Diagnosis

In a closed pneumothorax there is little or no movement of the affected side of the chest. Air entry into the affected lung is poor and often inaudible. An open pneumothorax is clinically obvious. Diagnosis of the deflated lung in either condition is confirmed by chest X-ray.

Clinical manifestations

The patient suffers sudden onset of dyspnoea, tachypnoea, often with associated chest pain. Haemoptysis may occur and the patient suffers tachycardia due to hypoxia and anxiety. Cyanosis may also be evident. An open pneumothorax may have additional signs of overt haemorrhage or even that of a foreign body in situ in the chest wall.

Medical and nursing management

Immediate first aid treatment consists of sitting the patient in an upright position or laying him on the affected side, thus splinting and supporting the injury. If it is an open pneumothorax it is advisable to put a clean occlusive dressing (such as a towel, handkerchief, or plastic wrap) over the wound to prevent entry of dirt and microorganisms and to assist in control of bleeding. However, one must suspect the onset of a tension pneumothorax (see page 344) and release pressure as necessary by removal of the dressing to allow escape of air. It is not advisable to remove a foreign body for fear of uncontrollable haemorrhage; the object is merely supported whilst awaiting and during transport of the patient to hospital. The patient will require a great deal of reassurance particularly in reducing anxiety which may be contributing towards the tachypnoea. Arrangement must be made for transport to hospital as soon as possible.

On admission to the emergency department, and following chest X-ray, the patient will have an apical intercostal catheter inserted in the pleural cavity which is connected to underwater-seal drainage apparatus (Fig. 36.2). If the patient has a haemopneumothorax, 2 intercostal catheters will be required to drain both blood and air and

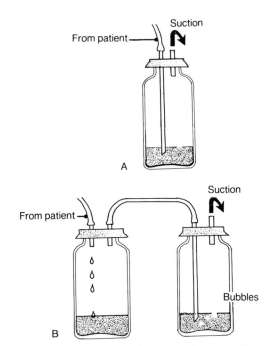

Fig. 36.2 Underwater-seal drainage. **A** – One-bottle. **B** – Two-bottle.

will therefore be placed at the basal and apical levels of the chest wall respectively. The purpose of the underwater-seal drainage is to allow the escape of air and to prevent its re-entry.

Insertion of an intercostal catheter

Due to the frightening nature of the condition the patient may require a narcotic analgesic which will both relax him and alleviate his chest pain. This results in slower, deeper and more effective ventilation.

The patient must be realistically informed of the procedure as it entails insertion of a wide bore, fairly rigid plastic tube through the anterior chest wall. He must understand the position in which he will be placed for the procedure, and be advised against any undue movement whilst the catheter is being inserted. Although the procedure is potentially painful, due to the force needed to insert the catheter, the patient must be reassured that both analgesic and local anaesthetic cover will prevent him from feeling any undue pain. As this is a surgical procedure the patient must provide his consent.

The patient is placed in an upright position and will require an overbed table to lean on in order to expand the thoracic cavity and help him to rest during the procedure. The site for the intercostal catheter is chosen according to the chest X-ray and a local anaesthetic is injected. A small incision is made and the catheter and its obturator are inserted through the chest wall and into the pleural cavity. The obturator is then removed and the catheter connected to underwater-seal drainage. The catheter is sutured in place and a dry dressing may or may not be applied to the wound. This is an aseptic procedure.

Preparation of the equipment is mandatory prior to insertion of the catheter. A sterile dressing pack containing the instruments required for insertion of the catheter and all the necessary equipment must be on hand. The underwater-seal drainage apparatus must be assembled in an aseptic manner. This may not be necessary in the case of a prepackaged, assembled and sterile set of equipment.

Nursing care of the patient with an intercostal catheter in situ

The patient is nursed in an upright or semi-upright position to enable good chest drainage and full lung expansion. Strong analgesia such as morphine is usually only required before the tube(s) are inserted (if there is time) and when the tubes are removed. If the patient has significant pain whilst the catheter is in situ, codeine phosphate compounds or paracetamol are usually sufficient to enable him to deep breathe, cough, and move freely around the bed. Chest physiotherapy is of major importance and the patient must cough and deep breathe according to exercises set by the physiotherapist.

Care of the tube(s) and underwater-seal drainage equipment. The tube(s) are attached to underwater-seal drainage to allow the escape of air and/or fluid from the pleural cavity and to prevent their re-entry.

The entire system should be airtight and the bottles, or disposable unit, securely sitting in a cradle or secured to the side of the bed. The glass or plastic rod must be beneath the water seal which is normally sterile normal saline. Air is expelled from the chest with each exhalation and bubbles from the rod under the water seal. The fluid also rises up the rod on inhalation and down on exhalation (swinging), thus indicating that the tubes are patent. The tubes must be pinned to the patient's clothing to prevent drag and there must be adequate length of tubing to allow free movement of the patient in bed. The nurse must observe for kinking and clots in the tubing, and prevent the pooling of drainage in the tubes by assisting its flow into the drainage bottle and milking the tubing as necessary. Cessation of swinging and bubbling, not re-established by milking of the tubing, indicates either a blockage in the tubing or that the lung has successfully re-expanded. This will be confirmed by chest X-ray. At no stage should the bottles be lifted above the patient's chest, but if this is unavoidable the tube(s) should be clamped to prevent back flow of fluid from the drainage system into the chest.

The amount and type of drainage is observed and recorded over each 24 hour period. If negative pressure is to be applied to the drain tube, a two bottle drainage system will be required and the pressure should be checked at regular intervals. When the suction is discontinued, the overflow bottle is removed and a patent airway left in the drainage bottle to allow the free escape of any remaining air from the chest cavity. This will prevent the development of a tension pneumothorax.

Tension pneumothorax

When a pneumothorax occurs, irrespective of whether it is open or closed, the wound in the lung or chest wall may create the effect of a one-way valve which permits the entry of air during inhalation but prevents the escape of this air during exhalation. Over a period of time, a build up of air on the affected side will occur. This pressure will ultimately cause a mediastinal shift, pushing the trachea, heart, and great vessels across to the opposite side of the chest with a resultant loss of cardiac output and effective ventilation, rapidly causing death.

Clinical manifestations

These are identical to those of an uncomplicated pneumothorax and the only clinical signs of a tension pneumothorax are increasing and worsening dyspnoea, increasing cyanosis, and restlessness. In any patient with a pneumothorax the possibility of tension pneumothorax should always be suspected.

Surgical management

Tension pneumothorax is a surgical emergency and management consists of the insertion of a wide bore needle or intercostal catheter into the pleural cavity to allow the release of air with an immediate spontaneous recovery. A wide bore needle is usually the instrument of choice as the insertion of an intercostal catheter is often too time consuming. Valuable life-saving seconds and minutes can be lost in deliberating the institution of such a simple first aid measure. If mediastinal shift has occurred, treatment may require cardiopulmonary rescuscitation.

OTHER RESPIRATORY EMERGENCIES

Pulmonary oedema

Pulmonary oedema, as its name suggests, refers to fluid in the lungs. For consideration of oedema in general refer to Chapter 9; pulmonary oedema and its management is discussed in detail in Chapter 33.

Pulmonary oedema is associated with many conditions such as nephrotic syndrome, shock, severe allergic reactions where the lungs are target organs, and lung infections. However, pulmonary oedema is most often encountered as a principal manifestation of cardiac failure, specifically left ventricular failure.

Pathophysiology

Heart failure results in pulmonary venous congestion and oedema due to the increased back pressure in the pulmonary venous system.

If pulmonary oedema is the result of cardiac failure it may be compounded by sodium retention and hypervolaemia.

Pulmonary oedema is usually an acute condition and in itself is life threatening. The lungs are susceptible to oedema because of the minimal tissue resistence offered by the thin flattened

alveolar cells, the large spaces within the alveoli, and the considerable exposure of capillaries which enhances the formation of oedema. The fluid in the alveolar spaces results in generalized hypoxia, which in itself leads to increased vasopermeability and increased oedema. It may be confined to the basal lobes but can involve all lobes. The lungs are wet and heavy with air, blood, and water, which combine to produce a frothy, sanguineous fluid.

Clinical manifestations

The patient presents with a productive cough accompanied by dyspnoea and tachycardia. In its mild form, the patient produces clear, frothy sputum and exhibits some respiratory difficulty. In its extreme form, the patient has pink, frothy fluid flowing passively up his trachea and into his mouth. The patient is severely orthopnoeic and has marked tachycardia.

Diagnosis

Diagnosis is made on clinical manifestations, relevant past history, and chest X-ray.

Medical and nursing management

The great danger is that the patient will, quite literally, drown in his own fluid. The principles of management are much the same as they would be for somebody who was drowning – 'Get him out of the water; get the water out of his lungs; and ensure that he can breathe properly'.

In pulmonary oedema, fluid is removed from the patient's lungs by upright positioning and oropharyngeal aspiration.

Prevention of further fluid entering the lungs is achieved by the use of some or all of the following measures:

– Diuretic therapy
– Narcotic analgesia
– Rotating venous tourniquets (see Fig. 34.11, page 331).

Ventilation may be improved by:

– Endotracheal intubation and assisted ventilation.
– Oxygen therapy
– Bronchodilator therapy.

Pulmonary embolism and infarction

Pulmonary embolism is one of the most common and lethal forms of embolism. Pulmonary emboli result from thrombosis of the veins in the calf muscles and, to a lesser extent, the other larger veins of the lower legs (see Chapter 32). Other sources include the pelvic veins and right atrium of the heart. An embolus is defined as a mass, either solid or gaseous, that dislodges from its place of formation and is carried by the blood to a site distant from its point of origin. The obvious result is that of either partial or complete occlusion of the vessel, resulting in either partial or complete ischaemia and/or necrosis of tissue distal to the embolus. Dislodgement of large or complete thrombi or smaller fragments of thrombus will result in their passage through the venous system.

Depending on its size, the embolus may either lodge in the right atrium or pass through the large cardiac chambers and lodge in the bifurcation of the pulmonary artery, creating what is termed a 'saddle embolus'. If this occurs, the clinical manifestations are acute, severe, life-threatening, and usually fatal. If the embolus does not lodge in the bifurcation of the pulmonary artery it will pass through to occlude either a major or minor pulmonary vessel, causing clinical manifestations of varying severity. Alternatively, the patient may experience multiple minor emboli which may be totally asymptomatic, or may have the effect of a large embolus in toto.

The embolus will eventually contract, followed by fibrinolytic activity with total lysis of the clot. However, in situations where the embolus is unresolved, and particularly in the case of multiple small emboli, there may occur conditions such as pulmonary hypertension, pulmonary vascular necrosis, and chronic cor pulmonale. In patients with good cardiovascular circulation, blood flow to lung paranchyma can be adequately sustained by the bronchial artery despite obstruction to the pulmonary arterial system. Pulmonary embolism causes infarction in patients where circulation is already inadequate.

Approximately 90–95% of all pulmonary emboli come from thrombosis of the deep veins of the calf muscle. Pulmonary embolism and infarction are frequently complications of other conditions such as cardiac disease, pregnancy, chronic debilitating diseases, and long term immobilization.

Clinical manifestations

These will vary according to the size and site of the embolus. Large emboli that completely occlude blood flow to the lungs (and therefore back to the heart) present an acute and dramatic picture. The patient may appear to be well and then suddenly collapse in a state of cardiac arrest. If the embolus is slightly smaller, it will allow blood flow through the lungs and back to the heart. The clinical picture may mimic that of acute myocardial infarction. The cardiac output will be significantly reduced and therefore the patient may suffer hypotension, tachycardia, chest pain, dyspnoea, profuse sweating, and possibly haemoptysis. In a patient with normal cardiovascular function small emboli may produce transient symptoms and signs as a result of pulmonary haemorrhages. Patients with inadequate bronchial circulation will suffer pulmonary infarctions and may experience jaundice as a result of reabsorption of the haemolysed blood.

Diagnosis

Diagnosis of pulmonary embolism on a clinical basis is not difficult, particularly where the patient already has a confirmed deep vein thrombosis. However, in the event of a silent deep vein thrombosis, pulmonary embolism needs to be differentiated from an acute myocardial infarction. Chest X-ray and pulmonary angiography aid in this differential diagnosis. For less fortunate patients diagnosis may be confirmed at postmortem examination.

Medical and nursing management

Cardiac resuscitation measures are commenced in the event of collapse, but usually without success. Some patients are fortunate enough to be rushed to the operating room for an emergency embolectomy which may or may not be successful. Patients with less severe symptoms are treated with oxygen, bed rest, and intravenous anticoagulants (which may already be prescribed for treatment of a deep vein thrombosis).

The degree of respiratory distress accompanying the condition will depend entirely upon the size of the embolus and the extent of its impaction. Nevertheless, the patient is usually dyspnoeic, extremely anxious and experiencing feelings of suffocation, and is cyanotic. Oxygen therapy is usually given via an intranasal catheter, as oxygen via a face mask will only increase the patient's fear of suffocation. Vital signs will need to be assessed frequently, and the nurse should be prepared for frequent blood gas analysis as a means of assessing patient progress during the treatment phase.

Standard anticoagulant therapy is only capable of preventing the development of further thrombi. As a result, some patients with large, non-fatal pulmonary emboli may be treated aggressively with a fibrinolytic agent that will hasten the breaking up and eventual lysis of the thrombus. The drug used is streptokinase and skilled nursing assessment and management is required to prevent and/or treat the side effects of hypersensitivity and intradermal haemorrhage.

The prevention of pulmonary embolism, and infarction, lies principally in recognition of patients at risk of developing a deep vein thrombosis.

37

Infections of the respiratory system

Jenny Kidd

ACUTE CORYZA – COMMON COLD

Pathophysiology

This is a condition characterized by acute inflammation of the upper respiratory passages. It is of viral origin and is spread rapidly from person to person. The incubation period is short, 24–36 hours, and the onset abrupt. The common cold is one of the most common causes of economic time loss through sick-leave.

Clinical manifestations

The essential feature is rhinitis which produces a mucoid nasal discharge. The patient may be unable to breathe through his nose, the senses of smell and taste may be impaired, and constant nose-blowing gives rise to inflamed ali nasi which may be followed by the onset of herpes simplex on the upper lips or ali nasi themselves. Other symptoms may include general malaise, headache, chilly sensations, and sore and swollen neck glands. The inflammation often spreads to the pharynx, larynx, or trachea causing a pharyngitis, laryngitis, or tracheitis, respectively, and producing a husky voice and a painful trachea. Secondary bacterial infection is common, resulting in the production of purulent sputum, cough, and mild fever.

Medical and nursing management

The treatment is largely symptomatic and consists of bed rest, inhalations, cough depressants containing alcohol and codeine, mucolytics, antipyretics, nasal decongestant drops, and anaesthetic lozenges. Isolation of the patient is desirable due to the highly infectious nature of the condition. A broad spectrum antibiotic may be ordered if a secondary bacterial infection is present. Symptoms usually abate inside one week and recovery is complete.

Complications

Otitis media may occur as a result of an ascending infection into the eustachian tubes. In children and elderly patients there is a possibility of pneumonia. It is important to note that coryza may be the presenting symptom of more serious diseases, such as measles, whooping cough, and meningitis. This should be kept in mind with children, especially those with a history of contact with such diseases.

LARYNGITIS

Clinical manifestations

Laryngitis may occur as an isolated condition. Other causes include excessive inhalation of irritant fumes, including cigarette smoke; allergy; over-use of the voice; and papilloma of the vocal cords. The possibility of neoplasia should be excluded, particularly when symptoms do not appear to be subsiding. The danger of laryngitis in children is that of airway obstruction due to the narrowness of their airways. In severe cases, children are nursed in steam tents and observed constantly for increasing dyspnoea or other obstructive signs. Equipment for a tracheostomy should be readily available in these situations.

TONSILLITIS

The tonsils are composed of lymphatic tissue and are situated on either side of the oropharynx and play an important role in the body's defence against disease.

Tonsillitis (inflammation of the tonsil) may be acute or chronic.

Acute tonsillitis

This is usually due to a bacterial infection, most commonly a streptococcus. It can occur at any age but is more common in children.

Clinical manifestations

Tonsillitis usually begins with a sore throat, painful and difficult swallowing and enlarged, tender cervical lymph nodes. Other symptoms include fever, malaise, muscle pain, and headaches.

On investigation the tonsils are swollen, red, and painful. Exudation may be diffuse over the tonsils and collect in the tonsillar crypts, or the tonsils may be studded with follicles of yellow pus if the infection is due to a streptococcus. Symptoms usually peak at 48 hours and subside within 5–7 days. Recovery is complete.

Management

The management of acute tonsillitis is principally symptomatic and consists of bed rest, and throat gargles of warm saline and aspirin. Analgesics such as aspirin can be used to control pain and fever, and the patient should be kept well hydrated. Broad spectrum antibiotics should be used and a throat swab taken and sensitivity tests done if infection is persistent and recurring. Antibiotic therapy should be continued for 7–10 days.

Complications

Complications due to the streptococcus include pneumonia, osteomyelitis, nephritis and rheumatic fever. Those due to the local infection itself include peritonsula abscess, acute otitis media and chronic tonsillitis.

Chronic tonsillitis is not a common condition and manifests as a persistent sore throat between bouts of acute tonsillitis, with pus expressed from the tonsils at any time. Surgical removal is the treatment of choice.

Peritonsillar abscess – quinsy is a rare condition and is associated with an acute streptococcal or staphylococcal tonsillitis. It is an extremely painful condition causing gross swelling of the soft palate and often uvula displacement. The abscess may rupture spontaneously or may require surgical excision. High doses of antibiotics are also given – penicillin is the antibiotic of choice.

Nursing management of the patient following tonsillectomy

Haemostasis of the tonsillar bed is usually achieved by either diathermy/oblique cautery, and pressure on or ligation of the tonsillar arteries.

It is normal for the tonsillar bed to discharge small amounts of frank blood for the 4–6 hours postoperatively. This then becomes haemoserous. The nurse must ensure that the patient has frequent mouth rinses to keep the oral cavity free of stagnant secretions which may become a focus for secondary infection. Analgesia must be adequate for the first 24 to 48 hours to provide maximum rest and comfort and to reduce swallowing. Antiemetics are also administered to reduce the likelihood of tonsillar bed trauma due to postoperative vomiting. Iced clear fluids will provide local relief and are soothing, and may be commenced as soon as the patient feels well enough to tolerate them. Solids are introduced as the patient desires. Nursing observations are performed to detect the early onset of primary haemorrhage. Excessive swallowing is an early indication of haemorrhage and the patient may vomit or expectorate frank blood and clots. Should the tonsillar bed bleed excessively the patient must be returned to the operating room for ligation and cautery of bleeding points.

Recovery is usually complete within 48 hours and the patient is able to go home.

Secondary haemorrhage may occur as a result of a throat infection and it is not uncommon for the patient to be discharged with a 7-day course of prophylactic antibiotics.

INFLUENZA

Influenza is a highly contagious generalized respiratory disease. It is caused by viruses which are capable of mutation and therefore multiple strains can occur, giving rise to a proportionate number of influenza outbreaks. It is therefore impossible to develop a vaccine for prophylactic use in all types of influenza. The disease typically occurs in epidemics and may also be pandemic. Over the past decades, the world has experienced several massive outbreaks of influenza in which the mortality rates have been very high.

The incubation period varies from hours to days depending on the individual's susceptibility and the virulence of the virus. Both the frail and the elderly are susceptible to a more severe and life threatening form of the disease.

Clinical manifestations

In general it is the systemic symptoms that are severe and debilitating; these include: fever, rigors, joint and muscle pains, general malaise, lethargy, headache, and anorexia. Respiratory involvement need not necessarily be severe. Initially, the cough is dry and unproductive with an accompanying sore throat. The cough may eventually become productive with mucopurulent sputum, as secondary bacterial infection is common.

Prophylaxis

Vaccination against the various strains of influenza is available and is recommended on an annual basis to people at risk, such as the elderly, people in institutions (where influenza can spread rapidly) and people with chronic pulmonary diseases who could not cope with an attack of influenza in an already compromised respiratory state.

Medical and nursing management

Most people can be nursed at home, and treatment is largely symptomatic. Bed rest, antipyretics and analgesics treat the bulk of the symptoms, and the patient must be kept well hydrated. The accompanying chest infection may require cough suppressants at night to enable the patient to rest, and expectorants during the day. Antibiotics are given to treat the secondary bacterial infection. Symptoms usually begin to abate within a 72-hour period leaving the patient weak and exhausted.

If there is no improvement in the patient's condition it may be necessary to admit him to hospital.

ACUTE TRACHEOBRONCHITIS

This condition is characterized by inflammation of the tracheobronchial tree. It is most prevalent in industrial areas due to air pollutants, and occurs also as a result of allergic reactions to pollens. It may complicate an attack of coryza and/or tracheitis.

Pathophysiology

Irritants alone do not cause the disease but rather cause inflammation which stimulates mucus production and weakens normal defence mechanisms. This renders the area susceptible to invasion of microorganisms both viral and bacteriological. The pathogens most commonly involved are streptococci, *Staphylococcus aureus*, *Haemophyllus influenzae*, pneumococci and a variety of viruses including adenoviruses and influenza viruses. The increase in mucus production causes reflex coughing which can further traumatize the trachea and bronchial mucosa. Principally, the lower portion of the trachea and major bronchi are involved.

Clinical manifestations

The significance of clinical manifestations varies with both the aetiology and the age of the patient. The classic symptom is a productive cough with mucopurulent sputum as a result of microbial invasion. Other symptoms such as those seen in coryza and influenza may accompany this condition, particularly when these diseases co-exist. In general, children are more susceptible to acute bronchitis than are adults. This is due to the fact that their tracheobronchial airways are shorter and more narrow.

Acute bronchitis in children can fulminate into a life threatening disease due to the possibility of airway obstruction.

Medical and nursing management

Treatment is symptomatic. The most exhausting symptom is the persistent coughing. During the day mucolytics, steam inhalations, and chest physiotherapy help to loosen the secretions and enable more effective expectoration of sputum. Rest, however, is important for the patient, and cough suppressants at night will enable the patient to gain adequate rest. Broad spectrum antibiotics are commonly ordered to counteract secondary infection. The patient should rest, keep warm, and continue chest physiotherapy until symptoms abate, as exhaustion and retained secretions can predispose to further attacks.

Acute bronchitis is in general terms a mild self-limiting illness, particularly when causative agents can be reduced or controlled. Repeated attacks may however lead to chronic disease with more serious consequences. (See Chronic bronchitis, page 367.)

ATELECTASIS

Pathophysiology

Atelectasis is a condition that refers to incomplete expansion of the lungs, or to the partial or complete obstruction of all or part of a lung resulting in airlessness of that part.

Most often, atelectasis is segmental and may involve patchy, diffuse areas of the lungs, or may be isolated to one or two lobes. Atelectasis can be classified as obstructive or compressive.

The diagnosis of atelectasis should only be made when the alveoli involved are of normal structure and are capable of re-expansion once the underlying cause has been removed.

Obstructive atelectasis

The obstruction may occur anywhere between the trachea and the terminal bronchioles. When obstruction occurs, the air that is trapped in the alveoli distal to the obstruction is absorbed – leaving the lung airless and in a state of collapse. Obstruction may be due to a plug of sputum, inhalation of a foreign body, or bronchial neoplasms. It is important to note that blood flow directed to the obstructed alveoli will continue but remain deoxygenated. This is known as arterio-venous shunting and will subsequently give rise to cyanosis and hypercapnia. Overall, lung volume will be diminished and the mediastinum will be displaced towards the obstructed lung.

Compressive atelectasis

This will result in incomplete expansion of the lung and may be due to compression in the form of a solid tumour mass, pleural effusion, pneumothorax, or an abnormally elevated diaphragm resulting from abdominal distension. The latter would result in basal atelectasis. Conditions such as peritonitis, subdiaphragmatic abscesses, and abdominal carcinomas can cause basal atelectasis. It is also one of the most common postoperative complications, as abdominal distension, particularly in association with a recumbent, bedridden patient, the association of pain, and the difficulty of coughing, will result in an accumulation of secretions and hence atelectasis. Compressive atelectasis will result in a mediastinal shift away from the atelectatic lung.

Clinical manifestations

Clinical manifestations will depend on the cause of the atelectasis and their severity will depend largely on the extent of the condition. If the obstruction is sudden and involves a large proportion of the airway, and subsequently the lung, the patient will experience sudden onset of chest pain, dyspnoea, and cyanosis. Alternatively, smaller areas of obstruction or compression will cause a mild to severe degree of respiratory embarrassment, or may even be asymptomatic.

Investigative procedures

An anteroposterior chest X-ray is taken. If diffuse, the atelectatic areas will appear as whitish, smokey areas; or if highly localized they will appear as a consolidated 'whiteout'.

Medical and nursing management

The extent of the atelectasis will determine the aggressiveness of treatment. Basically it involves prophylaxis, treatment of the atelectasis itself, and treatment of the cause of the atelectasis.

Patients who are to undergo a general anaesthetic should have preoperative chest physiotherapy; this takes the form of teaching the patient deep breathing and coughing.

Postoperatively, one of the goals of the nurse should be to prevent the development of atelectasis. With good nursing care, atelectasis should never form the basis of the patient's debilitating and sometimes life threatening chest infections; this, unfortunately, is not always the case. The nurse must provide adequate pain relief to allow easy coughing and expectoration of sputum. The patient should be sat up as soon as possible after a general anaesthetic and early ambulation should be encouraged. The nurse and/or physiotherapist must assist with and supervise deep breathing exercises and coughing. Postural drainage and frappage (percussion of the chest) are useful to assist the patient to loosen tenacious secretions, whilst the use of a nebulizer may help to liquify the secretions to assist easier removal. Oversedation must be prevented in patients with existing respiratory problems as this leads to exhaustion and reduced lung expansion. Frequent change of position in bedridden and unconscious patients will help to prevent pooling of secretions.

Treatment of other specific causes of atelectasis may involve: removal of a foreign body via bronchoscopy, thoracic aspiration, surgery to remove a compressive lesion, chest physiotherapy, and perhaps even a tracheostomy to allow aspiration of secretions. Antibiotics may be of assistance in the treatment of infected sputum.

Complications

Bronchopneumonia, bronchiectasis, and lung abscess may develop as a result of chest infection with atelectasis. Atelectasis is a reversible condition which, if unrecognized or untreated will cause permanent lung damage.

PNEUMONIA

The general definition given to pneumonia is infection of lung tissue. This, however, is a nonspecific definition due to the fact that pneumonia can be classified into two different types: bacterial and viral.

The classification of pneumonia is made according to the causative organism, the nature of the body's reaction to the disease (for example, suppurative or fibrinous), and the anatomic distribution of the disease (for example, lobular as in bronchopneumonia, lobar as in lobar pneumonia, and interstitial as in viral pneumonia). Anatomically, however, disease patterns can overlap; therefore, it is of primary importance from the clinical aspect to identify the causative agent and extent of the disease.

Bronchopneumonia

The principal characteristic of bronchopneumonia is diffuse patchy areas of consolidated lung tissue.

Aetiology

Common causative organisms are staphylococci, pneumococci, streptococci, and *Haemophyllus influenzae*. Fungi such as aspergillus and candida are often the cause of bronchopneumonia in socalled 'vulnerable' patients with predisposing factors.

Pathophysiology

Bronchopneumonia is a condition that commonly occurs in the very old, the very young, and very ill persons, due to their vulnerability to infection, and is often the end result of a pre-existing illness. In adults diseases such as chronic bronchitis, atelectasis, and upper respiratory tract infections can be antecedents, as can whooping cough and measles in children. It can, however, occur as a primary infection. Significant other predisposing factors to the development of bronchopneumonia include: malnutrition, debility, exposure, long term unconsciousness (which gives rise to the development of hypostatic pneumonia), chronic alcoholism and disseminated carcinoma. Bronchopneumonia is a common finding at postmortem and is often the ultimate cause of death.

Microorganisms gain access to the lungs via the respiratory airways, infecting the bronchi, bronchioles, and ultimately the alveoli. Basically, bronchopneumonia results in the accumulation of large amounts of suppurative exudate in alveolar tissue. It is most often multilobular and bilateral, and due to gravitation of secretions it largely affects the basal lobes of the lung, causing consolidation.

Clinical manifestations

These will depend upon the patient's pre-existing state of health, the virulence of the invading organism(s), and the extent of the total lung involved. In general the common features are: pyrexia; cough with copious, purulent, tenacious sputum; anorexia; exhalatory rales; and varying degrees of tachypnoea and dyspnoea. Air entry to the lower lobes of the lung is poor or nonexistent due to consolidation.

Medical and nursing management

Any underlying cause is treated, and the patient's general state of health is improved with a good diet, adequate fluids, and vitamin supplements. Sputum microscopy, culture and sensitivity is carried out, and treatment is commenced with the appropriate antibiotic. To help prevent broncho-pneumonia developing, patients with any predisposing factor should receive adequate chest physiotherapy and good hydration, and be sat up as soon as possible postoperatively. Early ambulation is encouraged.

Complications

Complications are rare, but may include lung abscess; this most often results if a staphylococcus is the invading organism. A lung abscess can spread to the pleural cavity, causing empyema, and on rare occasions to the pericardium, causing a suppurative pericarditis. Bacteraemia or septicaemia can occur with the resultant formation of metastatic abscesses in other organs or tissues of the body.

Lobar pneumonia

This is an acute bacterial infection involving a large portion of a lobe or one whole lobe of a lung. It commonly occurs in young adults (15–30 years), and more rarely in infancy and later life. Males are affected approximately 3 times more often than females. This form of pneumonia is now rarely seen, due to the effective use of antibiotics.

Aetiology

The pneumococci account for 90–95% of all lobar pneumonias. The remaining percentage is caused by organisms such as staphylococci, *Haemophyllus influenzae*, streptococci and klebsiella; and, due to the problem of antibiotic resistance, gram-negative organisms such as *Proteus vulgaris* can also be responsible.

Pathophysiology

It is thought that the probable route of entry for organisms is via the respiratory tract. The extent of the lobar distribution, however, appears to lie in the virulence of the organism and the vulnerability of the host. There is often an associated predisposing factor such as prolonged exposure, but it can develop in a previously healthy person. It is thought that wide distribution of the lobar form of pneumonia throughout the lung may be due to greater virulence of the organisms, and that the extensive exudation that occurs leads to spread through the pores of Kohn. The spread of the disease is also favoured by the fact that the pneumococcus produces extensive mucoid encapsulation which protects it against phagocytosis, and it is common for one whole lobe to be involved.

The affected lobes or segments undergo the typical pattern of inflammation, beginning with congestion, followed by vascular engorgement, then by exudation of fibrin. In addition, bacteria proliferate in the alveoli. The lobe is heavy and oedematous with a blood stained serous exudate. The bacterial infection invariably extends into the pleural cavity causing pleuritis and/or intrapleural empyema. As the inflammation progresses, the affected lobe becomes dry and granular with a progressive loss of redness. At this stage pleuritis is still significant. As the final stage of the inflammatory reaction occurs there is progressive disintegration of red and white blood cells, resulting in the lung becoming wet and soggy again with a suppurative exudate that is either absorbed or expectorated. Resolution is usually complete.

Clinical manifestations

The onset is very rapid and begins with fever and malaise. The patient has a cough which is either dry and unproductive, or productive with watery mucoid sputum. This is typical of the initial stage of congestion. Symptoms of pleurisy are quick to manifest and may severely compromise ventilation. As the inflammatory response progresses, the sputum becomes productive, purulent and a typical rusty colour due to the presence of blood. During this stage the patient suffers hyperpyrexia and rigors which are presumably the result of episodes of bacteraemia.

Other signs and symptoms may include anorexia, general malaise, lethargy, malar flush, tachycardia, and continued pleuritic chest pain. A continuing high temperature may cause the patient to hallucinate and may be due to an underlying empyema. Shortness of breath, dyspnoea, or even orthopnoea and cyanosis may present if the vital capacity of the lung has been grossly reduced.

The cough is painful, as is ventilation, due to the accompanying pleurisy. As a result ventilation may be shallow with an associated exhalatory grunt. The patient tends to sit favouring the pleuritic side, and attempts to splint the chest wall with his arm in order to reduce the pain. Coarse crepitations are audible as is the pleural rub. Breath sounds in the affected lobe(s) are diminished.

Investigative procedures

A microscopic examination and culture of sputum is required to identify the causative organism. A plain chest X-ray will identify the lobe(s) involved, the extent of consolidation, and evidence of pleural effusion. Blood cultures may be required and these should ideally be taken during a rigor.

Medical and nursing management

The patient's chest pain should be relieved with morphine. The patient will have an intravenous line inserted for hydration and drug administration. Penicillin is the drug of choice, and is given in large doses. Blood gas analysis is not necessary unless the patient is exhibiting signs of respiratory failure.

A large pleural effusion may need to be aspirated if it is affecting the patient's vital capacity. A cough suppressant will be required initially. Morphine will act in this capacity and a linctus containing codeine and alcohol is also an effective cough suppressant. When the cough becomes productive the medication must include a mucolytic.

The patient will require full fever care including drinks of clear iced fluids which are high in carbohydrate content, tepid sponging, frequent change of linen, and the use of a fan may be required to make the patient more comfortable. Antiemetics and antipyretics are important in the symptomatic management of the patient.

In addition to chest physiotherapy, active limb movements must be performed by the patient, as the period of bed rest combined with extreme lethargy can lead to complications. The patient must not be allowed to continue splinting his chest with his arm, as this also leads to complications; therefore, analgesia must be adequate to control the pain, and the patient should be positioned 'arm chair' style with the appropriate number of pillows. When the patient is afebrile, normal activity should gradually resume.

Complications

Complications can be life threatening and diverse:

• Pulmonary organization of the exudate can convert the lungs into solid tissue
• Pleural effusion, empyema, and adhesions of the pleura may occur
• Cardiovascular complications consist of pericarditis, subacute bacterial endocarditis, deep vein thrombosis, and septicaemia
• Neurological complications: meningitis and brain abscess may occur.
• Septic arthritis and frozen shoulder are not uncommon.

Outcome

It is rare today to see the classic complete clinical course of lobar pneumonia as occurred prior to the advent of antibiotics. Then, the patient's temperature rose uncontrollably and rapidly to a dangerous crisis point and then broke suddenly, falling to normal with a simultaneous improvement in the patient's condition. The key to successful treatment has been in the early identification of the organism and appropriate antibiotic administration, to the extent that the crisis may be avoided and patients may be afebrile with few clinical signs in 48–72 hours after initiation of therapy.

Primary atypical pneumonia (PAP) – viral pneumonia

This form of pneumonia results in an interstitial pneumonitis. The pathophysiology differs from that of bacterial pneumonia in that the inflammatory reaction is virtually localized within the septal walls of the alveoli. It is atypical because the alveolae are remarkably free of exudate, which is in contrast with bacterial pneumonia.

Aetiology

It is not known what exacerbates the common cold to result in PAP, but infancy, malnutrition and general debility are known to be contributing factors. In approximately one half of cases no aetiologic agent can be found. The number of viruses known to cause respiratory infection is continually increasing. They are highly contagious, and in general cause a high incidence of upper and lower respiratory tract infections.

Any one of the following viruses may cause respiratory tract infections such as PAP: *Mycoplasma pneumoniae* (Eaton agent) – the largest cause of PAP; influenza types A & B; parainfluenza virus; respiratory syncytial virus (RSV) – the most common cause of PAP in infants; rickettsia; coxsackie and ECHO viruses; and the viruses of rubella and varicella. PAP is itself endemic but may cause epidemics in crowded populations. PAP was responsible for the highly fatal influenza pandemics of 1915 and 1918.

Clinical manifestations

Many cases appear as upper respiratory tract infections, or lower respiratory tract infections commonly termed 'chest colds' or 'the flu'. The symptoms of fever, muscle pains, headaches, and general malaise are common; and a cough, if present, is usually dry and hacking due to the fact that the inflammation is interstitial. The clinical course is usually mild with a low mortality, but can be quite debilitating leaving the patient weak and exhausted for days to weeks.

Outcome

Complete resolution is expected, symptoms abate and the lung parenchyma returns to normal.

DISORDERS OF THE PLEURA

Disorders of the pleura consist of pleurisy, haemothorax, hydrothorax, chylothorax, empyema, and effusions. Pathologic involvement of the pleura is usually secondary to some other underlying disease; however, such secondary pleural disease may indeed be the dominant feature of the overall clinical state of the patient. For example, a patient with carcinoma of the lung may regularly present to hospital for drainage of a pleural effusion, which may cause more respiratory embarrassment than the carcinoma itself. Disorders of the pleura can be divided into three main groups: inflammatory, non-inflammatory and neoplastic.

Inflammatory pleuritis – pleurisy

Common causes of inflammatory pleuritis are pneumonia, (lobar in particular), tuberculosis, lung abscess, bronchiectasis, rheumatic fever and systemic lupus erythematosis. Pleurisy can be classified as wet or dry. Dry pleurisy is extremely painful and is associated with an audible pleural rub. It is not associated with an effusion. Wet pleurisy is associated with development of an effusion due to the often copious serous exudation that accompanies the inflammation. In general, in uncomplicated cases, the effusion consists of a relatively clear, straw coloured fluid; but some, particularly those associated with carcinoma of the lung, can be mildly to heavily blood stained. If the effusion is relatively small it may be re-absorbed with complete resolution. However, these effusions can comprise several litres and can therefore encroach considerably on lung space with accompanying respiratory distress. Pleural effusions can also be a focal site of infection due to both the static nature of the condition, and the potential culture medium for bacterial growth.

Clinical manifestations

The severity of these will depend largely on the size of the effusion. Most are insidious and often asymptomatic. Breathlessness, dyspnoea, and chest pains usually accompany only large effusions.

Infective pleuritis – empyema

This refers to a collection of pus in the pleural cavity. It results most commonly from intrapulmonary suppuration and therefore lung abscess often co-exists. It may also occur as a result of lymph- or blood-carried spread from a separate focus of infection, or may follow injuries such as compound fractured ribs. As a result it may present weeks or months following the patient's discharge from hospital.

Clinical manifestations. Characteristically, the pus is thick, yellow green, and creamy. The inflammatory reaction of the pleura is greater than in other pleural effusions. In addition to the respiratory symptoms and signs outlined above, the patient is toxic and displays a high temperature, rigors, and general malaise.

Non-inflammatory pleuritis

Haemothorax

This refers to blood in the pleural cavity. It is a rare condition and is most often seen as a fatal complication of aortic aneurysm.

Hydrothorax

This is a collection of non-inflammatory serous fluid in the pleural cavity. The most common cause of hydrothorax is cardiac failure, and because of this it is often found together with pulmonary congestion and oedema. The hydrothorax may be unilateral but is often bilateral. The degree of pulmonary oedema and the size of the hydrothorax are not related. Hydrothorax can also be found in other systemic conditions associated with generalized oedema, such as renal failure, nephrotic syndrome and cirrhosis of the liver. Hydrothoracies can, and often do, consist of large amounts of fluid and therefore produce varying degrees of respiratory embarrassment.

Chylothorax

This is an accumulation of chyle in the pleural cavity. Chyle is a milky white fluid containing emulsified fats. A chylothorax is usually confined to the left side of the chest but may be bilateral. The cause is often a malignancy in the thoracic cavity causing obstruction in the major lymphatic ducts; or metastatic involvement in either the right lymphatic or thoracic duct causing obstruction and destruction, and a resultant discharge of chyle into the pleural cavity. The volumes are usually small as compared with inflammatory effusions and hydrothorax.

Diagnosis of disorders of the pleura

All pleural effusions are diagnosed by chest X-ray. Differential diagnosis is by aspiration and analysis of pleural fluid.

Medical and nursing management

Inflammatory effusions and hydrothoracies are dealt with by thoracic aspiration; that is, an aspiration needle is inserted into the pleural cavity and the fluid is aspirated via a syringe.

Preparation of the patient for thoracic aspiration. An explanation is given to the patient as his co-operation throughout the procedure is important. The patient is asked not to sneeze or cough or take a sudden deep breath without indicating that such an occurrence is imminent. The patient is sat in an upright position with his arms resting on an overbed table in order to expand the thoracic cavity. An anxiolytic drug may have been given to help him relax. A local anaesthetic is injected and the aspiration needle is passed between the ribs, through the intercostal muscle, until fluid can be withdrawn.

At this stage an artery forcep is clamped onto the needle, at the point of entry, in order to prevent deeper penetration of the needle. The fluid is then withdrawn, the needle removed, and a small dressing placed over the puncture site. Samples of the fluid may be sent for bacteriological, cytological and biochemical analysis. Following the procedure, the patient's respiratory symptoms should abate, and often the patient is free to return home. Thoracic aspiration may be required by some patients on a regular basis.

Pneumothorax caused by needle puncture of the lung is the main complication of this procedure. Infection is always a possibility where an invasive procedure is performed.

Neoplasia of the pleura

Tumours of the pleura may be primary or secondary. The most common primary tumour of the pleura is classified as a mesothelioma. It has invasive characteristics similar to that of a sarcoma. It is interesting to note that many patients with these tumours have had an association with asbestos, which suggests a causative link. Secondary tumours of the pleura most often result from metastatic spread from carcinoma of the lung and breast, but may arise from any organ in the body.

Metastatic involvement almost always causes a pleural effusion. Cytological examination of the fluid will reveal neoplastic cells and is therefore of significant diagnostic value.

TUBERCULOSIS

Pathophysiology and incidence

Tuberculosis has existed since prehistoric times. In the early 19th century it was responsible for the deaths of one-third of all bodies autopsied in Paris. In Australia the incidence of tuberculosis has decreased from a peak of 5000 cases in 1954 to just over 1000 cases in 1985. Until early this century it was referred to as consumption. Tuberculosis is a notifiable disease.

Tuberculosis is a chronic infectious disease primarily of the lung. It is caused by bacteria from the genus Mycobacterium, and the most usual infecting organism in man is *Mycobacterium tuberculosis*, although the respiratory form of the disease can also be caused by *Mycobacterium avium* and *Mycobacterium bovis*. These bacteria are intracellular parasites that mainly infect macrophages and have a respiratory route of entry. As with most infectious diseases the severity of the illness is a result of the interaction between the virulence and number of the organism, and the resistance of the host.

Since the discontinuance of compulsory annual chest X-rays by the Commonwealth Department of Health, community attitudes to tuberculosis and its incidence have undergone a change. As with the public perceptions of other infectious diseases, such as pertussis and diphtheria, the attitude prevails that tuberculosis no longer exists, or is at least less virulent. However, these diseases still exist in the community and the move away from compulsory vaccination poses a potential danger of further outbreaks. Also, a variety of strains of the mycobacterium, new to Australia, are being isolated and identified in the children of some recent immigrants. Therefore the screening of children for tuberculosis through school health programmes remains a necessary public health measure in the control of this disease.

Lesions are divided into two types: exudative lesions, and productive lesions. An exudate lesion is due to an acute inflammatory process in which the organism is engulfed in fluid which contains polymorphoneuclear leucocytes and monocytes. The lesion may heal or progress to necrosis and the development of a productive lesion (tubercle). The tubercle produces tissue which is called a granuloma, as it resembles a tumour. It consists of a core of large multinuclear cells (giant cells) which are formed by a coalescence of mononuclear leucocytes, surrounded by modified macrophages (epitheloid cells); these are further surrounded by lymphocytes, monocytes, and fibroblasts. The mycobacteria live in the centre of this tubercle, usually within the giant cells.

The tubercle ultimately deteriorates in one of two ways: either it becomes fibrous on the outside and calcifies within; or the centre of the tubercle becomes soft and cheesy – caseation. Within both of these types of tubercle, live bacteria may exist for years. The soft, cheesy tubercles occasionally rupture, leaving their contents into the surrounding tissue, causing a cavity which will eventually heal by fibrosis and calcification. Spread of the organisms throughout the body occurs through direct contact of tissue adjacent to a broken tubercle and through the blood stream or lymphatic system. Such diffuse spread of the organism results in the formation of tiny tubercles throughout any organ of the body and is called miliary tuberculosis because the tubercles are small and firm and resemble millet seeds. Spread of the disease may be to one other organ only, and small numbers of cases of tuberculosis of the pleura, lymph glands, bones and joints, genito-urinary tract, meninges, and peritoneum are reported.

Clinical manifestations

Clinical manifestations of tuberculosis depend upon the target organ of the infection and the resistance of the patient; however, the clinical manifestations of pulmonary tuberculosis vary greatly from no symptoms at all, or mild non-specific symptoms, to the normal range of symptoms such as cough, fatigue, general malaise, weight loss, low grade evening fever and night sweats. Occasionally these are accompanied by pleurisy associated with pleuritic pain. Blood staining of sputum must always be strongly suggestive of pulmonary tuberculosis. In extreme cases the clinical manifestations are rales, retraction of the chest wall, wheezing, deviation of the trachea, haemoptysis, and pulmonary consolidation. Patients with pulmonary tuberculosis may exhibit symptoms caused by secondary involvement of another organ.

Investigative procedures

Skin tests

There are several of these and the most commonly used for community screening is a multiple puncture test (Tine test) using purified protein derivative (PPD). The Mantoux test is more reliable and uses a single intradermal injection of PPD. Both of these tests should be read within 24–72 hours.

A positive Tine test usually requires a Mantoux test for confirmation and a Mantoux test resulting in an area of 10 mm of induration indicates past or present infection; an area of 5 mm of induration in a person recently exposed to tuberculosis should be considered as significant enough to cause him to undergo a course of prophylactic therapy.

Bacteriological studies

Identification of *Mycobacterium tuberculosis* in sputum, pleural effusion fluid, gastric washings, or biopsy of lymph node specimens, ensures a positive diagnosis. Acid-fast stains are made of these specimens (usually after centrifuging) and a search is made for the organism. Acid-fast stains, whether positive or negative, should be confirmed by culture, but the organism is slow and relatively difficult to grow and this procedure will take 4–6 weeks. Gastric washings are taken in the early morning after the patient has fasted for 8–10 hours; this is a particularly effective way of obtaining a specimen from those patients who cannot produce early morning specimens of sputum, or who cannot co-operate.

Chest X-ray

Almost all cases of pulmonary tuberculosis will be seen on X-ray. The usual indications of primary infection are enlargement of hilar lymph nodes and small parenchymal lesions with calcification. Several X-ray views may be necessary to confirm disease.

Pulmonary tuberculosis can be mistaken for other pulmonary diseases, and these must be ruled out in order to make a definitive diagnosis.

General principles of management

The aims of treatment in tuberculosis are to:

1. Isolate 'open' cases (that is, cases in which the sputum culture is positive). Isolation of these patients is for as short a time as possible (usually 2–4 weeks) until there is complete compliance with the drug therapy and the sputum cultures are no longer positive
2. Effectively and safely treat established cases

3. Follow up and treat appropriately those people who have had contact with the disease.

Effective treatment and follow-up of both established cases and contacts is best achieved by the institution of public health programmes at both state and national levels. The major aim of these programmes is to educate the public either to prevent the disease occurring or to minimize its spread in the event of established cases. Public health measures involve: improving living conditions; isolating sputum positive patients for 2–4 weeks; providing early prophylactic drug therapy; searching for contacts; educating patients in personal hygiene, particularly in relation to coughing and spitting; notifying the appropriate health authority when established cases are identified; screening high risk groups; carrying out vaccination programmes; and ensuring that all milk products are effectively pasteurized.

Establishment of a prophylactic programme ensures that all those members of the population who so wish, and those who are at risk, may be rendered partially immune to the disease.

The prophylactic programme is to a great degree dependent on the compliance of the public. It is therefore necessary that an education programme (particularly of the parents of school age children) be carried out, because subject to permission from their parents all school children are Mantoux tested and those with a negative Mantoux test (and therefore no natural immunity) are given BCG (Bacillus Callmete Geurin) vaccinations.

Medical, surgical, and nursing management

Drug therapy

Initially drug therapy should be selected from isoniazid, rifampicin, streptomycin, ethambutol, and pyrazinamide. Until the sensitivities of the bacteria are known, or bacterial conversion is achieved, (and the patient is no longer classified as 'open') the patient should be on a rotating regime of any 3 of the above drugs, followed by a minimum period of 9 months of any 2 of these drugs; the most popular being rifampicin and isoniazid. A rotating regime of drug therapy is used because there is a very real chance of

bacterial resistance to the antibiotics. Every second month one drug is replaced. Drug therapy should be regularly checked and this is best achieved by the patient's regular attendance at a chest clinic. Each patient has a 100% chance of cure if the first-line drugs are administered correctly.

Para-aminosalicylic acid (PAS) was once used as a front-line drug in the treatment of tuberculosis, however its many side effects reduced its effective use. Since the advent of rifamprin and ethambutol, PAS is now only used as a second-line drug and even then only as an alternative to pyrazinamide. Capreomycin and cycloserine are likewise second-line drugs, but due to their extreme toxic effects they are only used as treatment in drug resistant cases.

In non-pulmonary tuberculosis similar drug therapy is used, but is usually continued for 15 months.

Chemoprophylaxis

Chemoprophylaxis is used where the individual is tuberculin positive, but shows no clinical or radiological signs of disease; the drug used is isoniazid over a period of 6–12 months in single daily dosages of 5–10 mg/kg of body weight.

Surgical management

Pulmonary resection may be performed where a positive diagnosis of tuberculosis cannot be made and a malignancy cannot be excluded on radiological findings, or when scar tissue causes bronchial stenosis. Occasionally thoracoplasty is performed to reduce pleural dead space following a large resection.

Nursing management

The patient with tuberculosis requires as much rest as possible, and little if any nursing or paramedical care except reassurance that his symptoms will abate as soon as drug therapy becomes effective and that he will be able to resume his normal life. Even while isolated, the patient is encouraged to maintain his independence. Whilst in hospital, and on return home, all sputum from the patient should be incinerated, and he must cover his mouth when coughing. A linctus may be of value if the patient has an irritating cough.

There are no special dietary requirements in the treatment of tuberculosis; the aim is simply to obtain and maintain the patient's best possible condition and weight.

Complications

The complications of pulmonary tuberculosis are: empyema, pulmonary fibrosis, and pleurisy. Spread of tuberculosis to other body organs causes non-pulmonary tuberculosis of the meninges, the skeleton, the genito-urinary system and the diffuse form, miliary tuberculosis.

The outcome of medical/nursing intervention, according to the Commonwealth Department of Health (1982) is that 'with the anti-tuberculosis drugs available in Australia percent conversion to negative bacteriology and an insignificant relapse rate are achievable targets'.

ANTHRAX – WOOLSORTER'S DISEASE

Aetiology and incidence

Anthrax is an acute infectious disease caused by a gram-positive encapsulated bacillus known as *Bacillus anthracis*. It occurs in sheep, cattle, horses, pigs, and goats and is transmitted to humans by direct or indirect contact with infected animals or their products. The spores are also harboured in soil and remain infective for many years. Approximately 100 000 cases of anthrax occur worldwide annually and most of these are in countries with poor community health regulations. The disease may take one of three forms: cutaneous anthrax, which accounts for 95% of cases; pulmonary (inhalation) anthrax, which accounts for 5% of cases; and gastrointestinal anthrax, which is extremely rare.

The cutaneous form results from direct innoculation through a break in the skin. Agricultural workers handling hides, fur, wool and bones of infected animals are a high risk group. Pulmonary anthrax results from inhalation of spores, causing a diffuse and permeating pneumonia, and rare cases of gastrointestinal anthrax result from the ingestion of under-cooked infected meat.

Diagnosis

Persons presenting with a macular skin lesion with a history of exposure to animals or animal products is suggestive of anthrax. Diagnosis is confirmed by a positive culture of vesicle exudate growing *Bacillus anthracis* and a positive Gram stain of same.

Clinical manifestations

Cutaneous anthrax

The appearance of a lesion consisting of a red macule similar to that of a flea bite occurs after an incubation period of several days. The lesion then rapidly progresses, involving the development of oedema. The macule fills with a haemorrhagic fluid which becomes a thin, bloody, puralent exudate which makes the macule appear like a purple blister. Within a week the vesicles rupture, oozing a serosanguinous fluid followed by the development of a blue-black eschar over the vesicle. These lesions persist for approximately 2 weeks then loosen and fall off, leaving granulation tissue. Satellite vesicles often develop and the surrounding lymph nodes become enlarged and inflamed. The infection may remain localized or the patient may develop a bacteraemia resulting in meningitis or spread to the lungs or other tissues. Cutaneous anthrax may produce relatively mild systematic manifestations, consisting of low grade fever, general malaise, and lymphadenopathy. The mortality rate in untreated anthrax is approximately 20%.

Pulmonary anthrax

The inhalation of spores leads to a diffuse pneumonia resulting in large areas of the lung becoming consolidated. This can also be accompanied by septicaemia and death may follow rapidly. The patient suffers high fevers, respiratory distress, pleural effusions and non-productive cough and often severe prostration. The mortality rate of untreated pulmonary anthrax is higher than that of the cutaneous form.

Medical and nursing management

The antibiotic of choice is penicillin intravenously in large doses, and patients are isolated to prevent spread by airborne or direct contact, even though person to person spread is unlikely.

In cutaneous anthrax the vesicles are covered with sterile dressings. In the pneumonic form the patient's vital signs are closely monitored, oxygen is administered and the nurse must observe closely for signs of respiratory failure (see page 337) and appropriate steps taken to give ventilatory support. The nurse must monitor isolation precautions, including safe disposal of dressings.

Anthrax is a notifiable disease and all cases must be reported to the appropriate health authority.

Prevention measures include: vaccinations; the wearing of gloves; covering of cuts and abrasions; and the wearing of masks by high risk persons.

38

Obstructive disorders of the airways

Jenny Kidd

ASTHMA

Bronchial asthma is a condition characterized by paroxysms of severe dyspnoea, accompanied by wheezing resulting from temporary bronchospasm. The episodes themselves are usually completely reversible.

Aetiology

Asthma is often divided into two types – extrinsic and intrinsic – but may be a combination of the two. Extrinsic asthma is caused by environmental allergens such as pollens, house dust, some foodstuffs, and animal dander, to name a few. Intrinsic asthma is caused by a wide variety of stimuli not related to allergens, such as emotional upset, changes in temperature, upper respiratory tract infection, and perhaps in some cases could be classified as psychosomatic. However, it is still suspected that allergens may play a role in intrinsic asthma.

The largest group of patients who suffer from asthma are those vulnerable to stimuli of both intrinsic and extrinsic origin. Often a history of the asthma sufferer will demonstrate familial allergic tendencies such as eczema, hayfever, or urticaria.

Incidence

It has been estimated that up to 20% of children and 30% of adults in Australia suffer from some degree of asthma. Asthma is a major factor in the cause of death of approximately 200 Victorians each year.

Pathology

Ishizaka and Ishizaka (1967) identified the immunoglobulin IgE, and found this to be present in minute amounts in normal sera, but in increased amounts in persons suffering from extrinsic asthma. IgE-forming cells are found in the mucosa of the respiratory tract, skin, stomach, small intestine, tonsils, adenoids, and rectum. When a person is exposed to an antigen, IgE is produced and becomes attached to lymphocytes and mast cells. This sensitizes the organ which then becomes a target organ. When next exposed to that antigen an immunoglobulin/antigen reaction occurs, causing rupture of the mast cells and the release of both the fast acting vasoactive compound, histamine, and a slower acting vasoactive compound, bradykinin. This results in increased vessel permeability, oedema formation, contraction of smooth muscle (bronchospasm), and an increased mucus production.

The exact pathogenesis of intrinsic asthma has not yet been clearly defined, although various theories exist. The trachea is involved, but principally it is the lumen of the bronchi and bronchioles that is considerably reduced due to bronchospasm and oedema. Mucus plugging can also co-exist, and the alveoli become hyperinflated.

Clinical manifestations

In light of the pathophysiological changes that have occurred in the respiratory passages, it is reasonable to expect the onset of severe ventilatory difficulty. There is associated wheezing on inhalation which worsens on exhalation. In the asthmatic, exhalation is no longer passive; rather, it is an active process in which air is forced out through the narrowed passages, and exhalation is therefore prolonged. The patient suffers hyperinflation of the lungs due to his inability to exhale completely. It is not uncommon for the patient to use his accessory muscles to breathe. The patient may also suffer a dry, irritating cough, or a productive cough with clear mucoid sputum. The patient may be sweating, restless, anxious, dyspnoeic and orthopnoeic; ventilations, although rapid, are laboured. Hypoxia and peripheral cyanosis are a feature, and often coexist with hypercapnia. Tachycardia is common due to anxiety and hypoxia, and may be compounded by the effect of bronchodilators. Exhaustion can occur rapidly, as can respiratory failure, and the patient must be constantly and intelligently observed to enable early detection of these complications.

Diagnosis

Diagnosis is made on both the clinical picture and past history. Skin sensitivities and other exposure to allergens may be of help in isolating the cause(s) of the patient's asthma.

Investigative procedures

A detailed history from the patient of what precipitated the attack is a good baseline from which to begin further investigation. Investigations can be diagnostic but are only practical when performed after the attack has subsided. The two main investigations are: lung function tests such as an FEV1 (forced exhalatory volume in one second) – prolonged FEV1 indicates loss of lung elasticity and perhaps underlying fibrosis; and skin sensitivity tests which can be diagnostic in terms of identifying the causative allergens.

Medical and nursing management

Due to the varying severity of bronchial asthma, management of the attack at home can often be successful. The initial treatment of known asthma sufferers is with a bronchodilator such as salbutamol and/or a corticosteroid such as beclomethasone via a metered dose inhaler. A steamy environment may also be of assistance in reducing bronchospasm.

It is usually only when this treatment fails, or in extremely severe cases, that patients require admission to hospital. Even then, a large percentage of these patients are successfully treated in the emergency department and able to return home. It is therefore only the minority of severe cases which result in hospitalization.

In severe episodes blood gases will be taken to assess the degree of respiratory acidosis and these can subsequently be used as a baseline upon which to assess physiological improvement. A chest X-ray is also taken to assess normal heart size and clarity of lung fields. In the emergency department the patient is given oxygen via an intranasal catheter at 4–6 l/minute. This is often the preferred method of administration due to the claustrophobic effect of a mask. The patient may also be given further doses of a bronchodilator via a small nebulizer. Strict nursing supervision is necessary to ensure that the patient is using the equipment properly and gaining the maximum benefit of the drug. A common cause of failed home treatment with metered dose inhalers is that the patient is not using the inhalation correctly, and therefore not receiving the drug. An IV infusion will provide hydration of the patient and a route for adminstration of drugs.

The drug regime consists of: bronchodilators; sodium bicarbonate to correct respiratory acidosis; antibiotics if there is an underlying or precipitating upper respiratory tract infection; and hydrocortisone, ideally given in a bolus dose. Hydrocortisone acts as an anti-inflammatory drug and also enhances the effectiveness of bronchodilators. Bronchodilators may be given intermittently or by titration.

The patient is observed constantly for signs of clinical improvement, such as improved rate and quality of ventilations, improved colour, a slowing of the pulse back to normal, reduced anxiety, and a more rested emotional and physical state. It should be noted that most bronchodilators are beta-1 as well as beta-2 stimulators, and therefore may cause and/or exacerbate the patient's tachycardia. This can be avoided by slow and careful administration of bronchodilators by the nurse, together with frequent monitoring of the pulse. It may be advisable to use a bronchodilator with an excellent beta-2 effect but a small beta-1 effect, particularly if the patient has severe hypoxia and cardiac strain. Some patients will require a nurse in constant attendance in order to administer drugs and monitor their vital signs and general clinical state. It is of major importance that the nurse understands the significance of blood gas results in order to use this information in assessing the effectiveness of medical treatment. Should the patient's blood gas levels not improve, it is apparent that treatment is not successful and needs reassessment. As exhaustion is a potential problem for the patient he must be observed carefully for signs of respiratory failure (see page 337) and must never be sedated, as this will lead to increasing tiredness, enhance the exhaustion, and worsen the potentially fatal respiratory failure. In the event of respiratory failure, patient exhaustion, or unsuccessful medical treatment, the patient will require intubation and assisted ventilation. Only at this stage is it acceptable to sedate the patient.

Complications

Spontaneous pneumothorax may occur due to rupture of a bleb or bulla. These are small congenitally acquired sac-like formations that are situated on the external surface of the lung. They are prone to rupture under high intrapulmonary pressures such as occur in bronchial asthma. Long-term complications may consist of emphysema, cardiac failure, and pulmonary fibrosis.

Habilitation

Prophylaxis is the major objective and can be achieved by avoiding known allergens and other causative factors. Some patients are required to take prophylactic medication in the form of prednisolone and drugs such as sodium cromoglycate. Other prophylactic measures include chest exercises such as swimming and rope swinging, and effective use of metered dose inhalers. It is the nurse's responsibility to make sure that the patient understands and can use a metered dose inhaler; this can be achieved by practice and supervision with placebo inhalers.

People with asthma must be instructed to contact their physician if a previously adequate prophylactic measure no longer controls their symptoms, as this may signify a dangerous deterioration in their condition. They should also be advised to seek medical aid early in a serious attack, as many deaths are due to late presentation.

CHRONIC OBSTRUCTIVE AIRWAYS DISEASE

Chronic obstructive airways disease (COAD) is a term used to describe disorders that lead to obstructive and/or resistant dysfunction of the lungs. The disease states involved are chronic bronchitis, emphysema, asthma, and bronchiectasis. Chronic bronchitis, the chronic presence of a productive cough, produces obstruction to air flow. Emphysema, the structural dysfunction of the alveoli resulting in lowered gaseous diffusion, produces airway resistance. Asthma, the inflammatory disease characterized by bronchospasm; and bronchiectasis, the profound production of airway secretions, both result in obstruction to airflow. Except in the case of bronchiecstasis, rarely do the diseases present as a single entity – COAD is the multiplicity of the effects of these disorders. Therefore the patient may present clinically with an obstructive disorder, or a disorder of airways resistance, or a combination of the two.

Many patients with clinical evidence of emphysema also suffer varying degrees of airway obstruction similar to those seen in asthma and chronic bronchitis. Therefore emphysema is often equated with, or termed, chronic obstructive airways disease. This is not a clear or concise diagnosis, as many (but not all) patients with emphysema also have chronic bronchitis. A chronic bronchitis sufferer may go on to develop emphysema, and there are those patients with both chronic bronchitis and emphysema who experience little or no airway obstruction. It would therefore seem reasonable to define COAD as a condition referring to emphysema alone or emphysema accompanying chronic bronchitis, and this may be with or without airway obstruction. Emphysema is defined anatomically, whereas chronic bronchitis is defined clinically and the term COAD refers to an overall set of symptoms and signs of any or all of the above.

The significance of understanding the basic difference between emphysema and COAD does not lie in their different medical and nursing management, but rather in the nurse's awareness of the presenting pathophysiology.

COAD is alternatively termed chronic obstructive lung disease, or chronic obstructive pulmonary disease.

PULMONARY EMPHYSEMA

Pulmonary emphysema is a chronic destructive lung disease characterized by gross airway resistance. There is overdistention of the alveoli resulting in loss of elasticity and destruction of the alveolar walls. Fibrous repair destroys the selective permeability of the membrane and therefore reduces the area available for gaseous exchange.

There is resistance to the movement of air because on inspiration the alveoli can distend no further, and on exhalation the alveoli have lost the ability to contract. Therefore, there is an increase in stagnant, dead space air in the lungs.

Types of emphysema

The two major forms of emphysema are centrilobular and panlobular. In centrilobular emphysema there is destruction of the central septum of the lobule of the lung whilst the peripheral alveoli are normal. In panlobular emphysema the destruction occurs uniformly over the entire lobule; that is, the terminal bronchiole, alveolar duct, and alveoli. It is obvious which type of emphysema is likely to have the more remarkable clinical manifestations.

Men are affected with centrilobular form more than women, whereas panlobular emphysema affects both sexes indiscriminately.

Pathophysiology

There is to date no significant evidence to suggest why some patients develop centrilobular as opposed to panlobular emphysema. There are, however, many theories as to the genesis of the two forms of emphysema. One of the oldest hypotheses suggests that chronic bronchitis causes partial obstruction of the airways, particularly of the bronchioles. Irritants such as inhaled pollutants, the most significant being cigarette smoke, cause increased mucous production and thickening and scarring of the bronchioles, resulting in narrowing of the lumen and increased airway resistance. Other noxious airborne substances include coal dust, silicates, and organic residues. The bronchi and bronchioles normally expand and contract on inhalation and exhalation. However, due to the altered narrow lumen and associated loss of elasticity, exhalation becomes a difficult active exercise which tends to further reduce the lumen of the bronchioles, which leads to air trapping and consequently to the characteristic overdistention of the alveoli and the lungs in general. Air trapping and over-distended alveoli squash the septal capillaries, causing ischaemia and destruction of the septal walls. Secondary bacterial infection of retained secretions is common, and the inflammatory response further disturbs blood supply to the bronchial walls and alveoli, leading to their atrophy and eventual collapse.

Another hypothesis suggests that the emphysematous changes that occur in the septal walls are primary, and may lead in fact to chronic bronchitis (Pratt & Kilburn, 1970).

In short, what actually initiates septal destruction is still disputed.

Lastly, genetic factors do play a role in the pathogenesis of emphysema. In a small percentage of patients there is an hereditary deficiency of alpha-antitrypsin, and it would appear that the genetically susceptible individual is more sensitive to environmental pollutants. In spite of the continuing research into the pathophysiology of emphysema the cause or causes remain unknown.

Clinical manifestations

Clinical manifestations become evident when approximately one-third of the total lung paranchyma is diseased, and in general begin to appear from the fourth decade onwards. As with so many other respiratory diseases, dyspnoea is usually the presenting symptom. If the disease is advanced the patient may even have orthopnoea, and the smallest physical activity can cause severe respiratory distress and cyanosis.

Ventilation in the emphysematous patient is not effortless. Exhalation in particular is active, forced, and difficult, and in order to maintain positive pressure in the airways, the patient often breathes out through pursed lips which causes a reflex contraction of the upper abdominal muscles bringing them into play as accessory muscles of ventilation. This prolongs the ventilatory phase and makes exhalation easier. Rapid exhalation is impossible due to the hyperinflation of the lungs and the loss of lung elasticity.

The hyperinflated state of the lungs also raises the intrathoracic pressure and the patient may therefore show signs of a raised jugular venous pressure and general engorgement of the veins of the head and neck. Even small vessels of the lips can be overtly distended.

Other accessory muscles are often required to assist the patient in ventilation. Many patients sit forward to breathe to prevent abdominal pressure on the diaphragm which encroaches on the thoracic cavity. The hyperinflated lungs cause expansion of the ribs with a resultant barrel chest which is usually rigid. The patient has an accompanying chronic productive cough and there may be some associated wheezing. Fatigue, anorexia, and weakness are common complaints, and patients are at risk of developing upper respiratory tract infections. Frequently there is a derangement of ventilation/perfusion ratios, producing chronic hypoxia, hypercapnia, and polycythaemia. Clinically the patient may be peripherally cyanosed, flushed in the face due to hypercapnia (CO_2 being a vasodilator), or may have a purplish hue across the malar area due to polycythaemia.

In acute exacerbations of the disease the patient may develop a respiratory acidosis; but, because the disease is of a chronic and insidious nature, the body's buffer system may be able to maintain the blood pH within normal limits despite abnormal pO_2 and pCO_2 levels.

Respiratory failure is always a possibility. In advanced disease normal activities such as walking short distances, combing hair, laughing and taking a hot shower, may cause life threatening coughing attacks.

All patients with emphysema will present with varying degrees of lung disease and activity tolerance. This is significant when planning appropriate medical and nursing management.

Investigative procedures

The patient's symptoms and clinical findings on examination provide the basis for diagnosis. Pulmonary function tests are performed as these aid in the differentiation between restrictive and obstructive lung disease. Spirometry showing a reduction from normal in FEVI and Forced Vital Capacity (FVC) indicates restrictive lung disease. A pronounced reduction in all parameters of pulmonary function tests highlights the presence of obstructive disease, as the patient takes a longer time to exhale. Blood gas analysis and chest X-ray will further assist in the determination of the stage of the disease and the degree of its effect.

Complications

Complications may include corpulmonale, respiratory acidosis, respiratory failure, and pneumothorax due to a ruptured bulla.

Medical and nursing management

Oxygen will be necessary during an acute exacerbation, and in severe disease will be required on a regular basis just to enable the patients to perform the basic tasks of life. Oxygen is given at controlled percentages to prevent overcoming the patient's so-called 'hypoxic' drive for ventilation.

In cases of emphysema with associated airway obstruction, small doses of a bronchodilator may be administered orally, subcutaneously, intravenously, rectally, or via a nebulizer. Side-effects from these drugs are common and therefore dosage is carefully adjusted according to the patient's tolerance and clinical response.

Treatment of infection. Antibiotics should be administered at the first sign of lung infection. Since many patients with emphysema are prone to lung infection, annual vaccinations against influenza are recommended.

Most patients with emphysema take shallow breaths using the upper part of their chest. This type of breathing is relatively inefficient and the patient can be taught diaphragmatic breathing. This should reduce the rate and increase the efficiency of ventilation by increasing tidal volume. Pursed lips breathing helps the patient to control the rate of ventilation and dyspnoea.

Avoidance of large meals will also prevent unnecessary respiratory distress. During a severe attack, soft foods are necessary, as chewing solid foods is exhausting and occupies potential breathing time. Assistance during meals may also be necessary. It is important to keep the patient well hydrated, to keep sputum moist, and clear fluids are preferable to milk (which increases the viscosity of oral secretions). Tasks such as washing, dressing, shaving, and combing hair may cause severe respiratory stress. Therefore when planning the patient's care, nursing staff should consider the amount and type of assistance the patient requires.

Chest physiotherapy is mandatory. The aggressiveness of the physiotherapy will depend on the extent of the respiratory manifestations. Postural drainage, coughing and deep breathing exercises can be taught to the patient for use at home as well as in hospital. Frappage and chest vibration also play a significant role in loosening tenacious secretions so that they may be easily and effectively coughed up. Many patients with emphysema develop a lazy cough, and secretions are not effectively removed from the respiratory passages.

General physical fitness is important and graded exercise programmes are useful in increasing the patient's exercise tolerance; this in turn has a positive effect on ventilation. This is not always possible in elderly patients with emphysema.

Emotional support and reassurance to both the patient and their relatives is extremely important during acute exacerbations of this crippling respiratory disease.

Patient education

To enable the patient to enjoy a better quality of life he must understand his disease process and the aims of treatment. One of the major medical and nursing objectives is to help the patient accept a compromised lifestyle and to improve his physical condition. If the respiratory condition is severe, the aim is to preserve present pulmonary function and provide effective relief of symptoms. If the disease is mild the aim is to prevent further loss of pulmonary function. In the younger age group removal of causative inhaled pollutants, such as cigarette smoke will aid a return to optimal health.

CHRONIC BRONCHITIS

The widely accepted clinical definition of chronic bronchitis is based on the presence of a persistent, productive cough for at least 3 months over at least two consecutive years. It is most frequent in middle-aged men, but both sexes and all ages can be effected. It is so prevalent that it can be no longer considered as a minor ailment. The condition is exceedingly common amongst cigarette smokers and people who live in industrialized and smog-laiden cities.

Pathophysiology

Chronic irritation caused by inhaled pollutants causes the classical characteristics of hypertrophy and hyperplasia of the mucous glands of the tracheobronchial tree, with resultant excessive mucus production. Normal ciliary action is also impaired. It is thought that the chronic irritation and excessive mucus secretion reduces defence mechanisms and the person becomes more vulnerable to recurrent bacterial and viral secondary infection. This could be due to the fact that the normal ciliated columnar epithelium is replaced by squamous epithelium. However, it is not proven that chronic infection always accompanies chronic bronchitis, or indeed whether the infection precedes or results from the bronchitis. Principally the smaller airways, bronchi, and bronchioles are the most severely affected, and may even be totally obstructed with mucopurulent sputum. The gross changes are similar to those of acute bronchitis; with oedema of mucous membranes, hyperaemia and increased mucus production which is often purulent.

Clinical manifestations

Chronic cough with purulent sputum is the most outstanding, and in fact may be the only presenting symptom for years, and furthermore may not cause the patient any problem. However, the onset of underlying functional impairment is often insidious and consists of increased airway resistance leading to a ventilation/perfusion imbalance with resultant hypoxia, hypercapnia, and dyspnoea.

Medical and nursing management

Management is of the presenting symptoms, which are usually those of acute bronchitis or airway resistance. The patient should be taught to avoid irritants, especially cigarette smoke.

39

Chronic disorders of the lung

Jenny Kidd

BRONCHIECTASIS

Bronchiectasis is a condition characterized by abnormal dilatation of the bronchi and bronchioles resulting from or associated with chronic respiratory infection. It occurs in a higher incidence in young people and is common in childhood. All ages and both sexes can be affected.

Aetiology

The cause of this dilatation is still not certain. Bronchiectasis develops as a result of infective or obstructive respiratory disease such as asthma, tuberculosis, pneumonia, bronchitis, and tumours; and inhaled foreign bodies.

Pathophysiology

As a result of partial or complete obstruction, infection will ensue. This is associated with necrosis which injures the elastic tissue and musculature of the respiratory passages, and weakens the walls of the airways, resulting in their permanent dilatation. If the foreign body or obstruction can be removed prior to the onset of infection, the bronchiectasis may be either prevented or reversed. Atelectasis will occur where total obstruction of the airway, due to significant suppuration, has resulted in alveolar collapse. This exacerbates the problem, as shrinkage of the affected portion of the lung exerts outward traction of the walls of the medium sized bronchi, causing them to become dilated. Areas of bronchiectatic lung are also formed distal to tumours and inhaled foreign bodies. Bronchiectasis in the young often follows whooping cough, and measles where there has been associated respiratory involvement. The bronchial dilatations may be cylindrical, fusiform, or saccular in shape. Although bronchiectasis may involve any part of the lung it usually affects the lower lobes bilaterally, but it is not uncommon for presentation to be unilateral. It rarely affects the middle and upper lobes, and when associated with obstruction due to foreign bodies or tumours, may be very localized. The bronchi and bronchioles may be dilated up to 4 times their normal size. The affected bronchi are filled with copious amounts of suppurative exudate. The sputum may be infected with many different organisms.

Clinical manifestations

The patient suffers a severe chronic cough with expectoration of copious amounts of tenacious yellow-green purulent sputum. The sputum has a foul odour and may be blood stained. The patient also often suffers chronic halitosis, which is extremely difficult to treat. The cough itself is often induced by changes in posture and a coughing paroxysm may occur when a person rises from a sleeping position. If the condition is severe the person may suffer dyspnoea, orthopnoea and even clubbing of the fingers.

Investigative procedures

Diagnosis is made on the clinical picture and a past history of respiratory infection. A bronchogram demonstrates bronchial dilatation, its distribution, and extent. Sputum analysis is performed to exclude conditions such as tuberculosis and to determine sensitivity of antibiotics, should these be required in the event of a superimposed upper respiratory tract infection.

Medical, surgical, and nursing management

This can either be conservative or surgical.

Postural drainage is the most effective conservative measure in keeping the dilated bronchi empty of secretions. It is of great value in reducing the severity of the symptoms of this disease. Since rising from bed can precipitate a coughing paroxysm it is appropriate for the patient to use this time to effectively expectorate sputum that has pooled whilst sleeping. It is recommended that the patient undertake some form of gravitational regimen for at least 20 minutes every morning. The patient lies over the edge of the bed for 20 minutes whilst tilted to one side and a further 20 minutes whilst tilted to the other side. He should cough and expel as much sputum as possible during these postural drainage sessions. Family members can help to loosen secretions by percussing the patient's chest. If the patient suffers severe bronchiectasis he may need to perform some form of postural drainage during the day and again at night in order to keep the bronchial tree as free of sputum as possible. Mostly patients can manage their condition at home and do not require hospitalization. However an upper respiratory tract infection may place the patient in severe respiratory embarrassment and hospitalization may be necessary with oxygen therapy, rigorous chest physiotherapy, good hydration, mouth rinses and gargles, and the administration of antibiotics. Only in severe cases of bronchiectasis may it be necessary for the patient to undergo bronchoscopic aspiration. A light general anaesthetic will be administered for this procedure. Surgical treatment may be indicated if a bronchogram demonstrates sharply localized involvement of segments or lobes of the lung. In such cases a lobectomy or pneumonectomy may indeed be curative.

Complications

Complications consist of: lung abscesses, bronchopleural fistulae, empyema, chronic fibrosis of the lungs which can lead to corpulmonale, and anaemia due to chronic blood loss in sputum.

Prophylaxis

The incidence of bronchiectasis can be reduced by the prevention or effective treatment of tuberculosis, whooping cough, and respiratory infections associated with measles.

Anticipated outcome

In most cases patients with bronchiectasis manage well at home. They and their families are encouraged to take an active and responsible role in their day to day management. The significance of bronchiectasis to the life span is still uncertain. If the disease is acquired in adult life, it appears not to interfere with longevity. However, if the onset occurs in early life it appears that it may reduce the person's lifespan to a degree. Few childhood bronchiectatics live beyond 40 years of age, unless treatment has been consistent and of high quality.

LUNG NEOPLASIA

Bronchogenic carcinoma is the most common primary malignancy of the lung. In industrialized nations it is one of the most common visceral neoplasms, especially in the male population, and in Australia bronchogenic carcinoma is the second major cause of death in males over the age of 45 years. However, the incidence of carcinoma of the lung in females is rising rapidly and there seems to be a correlation between this increased incidence and the rise in the rate of female cigarette smoking since the end of the second World War. Other significant classifications of primary malignancies of the lung are bronchial adenoma, and alveolar cell carcinoma. The lung is more often affected by metastatic growth than by primary neoplasm. Metastatic spread from both sarcomas and carcinomas takes place via the blood or lymphatics, and the result is usually scattered multiple metastatic growths rather than one isolated metastasis of the lung.

Incidence

Whilst the death rate for lung neoplasia is lower in females, it should be noted that the death rate for females has almost doubled in less than twenty years. The disease commonly manifests in the fourth, fifth, and sixth decades of life (but can manifest earlier) and can be viewed perhaps as a consequence of an ageing population as well as of environmental factors. Improved screening and diagnostic tests have resulted in a greater success rate in the treatment of this disease, although total cure and increased longevity is still rare.

Aetiology and pathophysiology

There is strong evidence to suggest that both cigarette smoking and environmental factors are the two most common causes of bronchogenic carcinoma. Genetic predisposition is also of some importance. 90% of bronchogenic carcinomas occur in smokers. Cigarette smoke has been shown to cause loss of ciliated cells, and cellular hyperplasia in the respiratory tract. Most carcinomas of the lung in non-smokers are not of the squamous cell origin seen in smokers.

Bronchogenic carcinomas are divided into basic cell types; squamous cell (most common) adenocarcinoma, undifferentiated carcinoma, and small cell and large cell carcinomas. The tumour mass itself has a cauliflower appearance, and may remain in situ for some years and eventually infiltrate and invade surrounding lung parenchyma. Recent studies have shown that lesions may take many years to grow to a size of 2 cm in diameter. It is not surprising, therefore, that the potential for metastatic spread before diagnosis is high. Areas of the body most susceptible to metastatic spread are the thoracic lymph nodes, adrenal glands, liver, brain, bone, and kidneys.

There have been many studies done on the effects of cigarette smoke on the respiratory tract involving large numbers of the human population in addition to animal testing. In summary it appears that evidence to date strongly suggests that as a cause of lung cancer cigarette smoke far outweighs all other factors. The risk of lung cancer increases with the amount of smoke inhaled and thus with the number of cigarettes smoked each day and the duration of the habit. Pipe and cigar smokers have a reduced incidence of lung cancer compared with cigarette smokers, and a higher incidence compared with non-smokers.

Industrially, fluorocarbons have been shown to be a contributing factor: miners of nickel, radium, cobalt, and coal show 15–30% increased incidence over control populations in the same areas.

Clinical manifestations

As the disease usually manifests between the fourth and sixth decades of life it is viewed as one of the most insidious and quietly aggressive neoplasms in oncology. Symptoms occur late in the disease and patients typically present with a cough of several months' duration, occasionally accompanied by haemoptysis, weight loss, chest pain, dyspnoea and/or breathlessness. A hoarse voice due to involvement of the recurrent laryngeal nerve and persistent pneumonia, anaemia, pleural effusions, and bone pain may be other presenting symptoms.

Investigative procedures and diagnosis

Lung neoplasia can be suspected on clinical evidence alone. Diagnosis is confirmed by chest X-ray, sputum cytology, lung biopsy via bronchoscopy or mediastinoscopy, or thoracic aspiration for cytology. It is not unusual to discover bronchogenic carcinoma on routine chest X-ray, or in the course of investigating a primary neoplasm elsewhere. The presence of lung metastases reduces the chance of total cure of another primary neoplasm, which is one of the reasons why routine preoperative chest X-rays are taken.

Some undifferentiated bronchogenic tumours secrete adrenocorticotrophic hormone, and as such can have additional clinical implications, for example, the patient may exhibit some of the features shown in Cushing's disease.

Medical and nursing management

It must be decided clearly from the time of diagnosis whether treatment is to be merely palliative, or an attempt to cure. This is a critical decision for the patient, medical, and nursing staff. The patient is entitled to a full explanation of the treatment available, the consequences, and the life expectancy which may result from such treatment.

Some 15% of lung neoplasms of primary origin can be successfully treated by lobectomy or pneumonectomy with associated cytotoxic chemotherapy. Conservative management is reserved for patients with invasive spread of tumour and metastatic involvement, and consists mainly of symptomatic treatment, chemotherapy or deep X-ray therapy, and pain control in the terminal stages of the disease. Most patients die within 1 to 5 years of diagnosis, with or without treatment.

LOBECTOMY

Indications for lobectomy include: carcinoma, benign tumour, bronchiectasis, abscess, tuberculosis, and lung trauma. Preoperative nursing care and preparation is the same as for any patient undergoing major surgery. However, the physiotherapist will teach the patient the chest and breathing exercises that will be required in the postoperative phase.

Nursing management

On return to the ward following a lower lobectomy the patient is placed in a semi-upright position, well supported with pillows to allow full expansion of the lungs. An upper lobectomy requires the patient to lie flat for 24 hours postoperatively, to enable full expansion of the remaining lobe(s).

Two drain tubes are inserted intraoperatively, one anterior to the apex, and the other posterior to the base. This is not necessarily demonstrated by the external positioning of the tubes. Both drain tubes are attached to underwater-seal drainage (see page 343) and pleural suction. The drain tubes are removed when the pneumothorax is resolved and when drainage from the intercostal catheters is minimal and serosanguineous, which may take up to 2 weeks. Both tubes are removed simultaneously. The patient can sit out of bed and walk short distances with the drain tubes in situ. Recovery is generally rapid and uneventful.

Complications

1. Pleural effusion, due to blocked or malpositioned drain tubes
2. Empyema and/or wound infection
3. Bronchopleural fistula which may either heal spontaneously or require further surgery
4. Failure of residual lung to fully inflate due to secretions in one or more branches of a bronchus or bronchioles
5. Persistent pneumothorax due to a leak around the drain tube
6. Haemorrhage.

PNEUMONECTOMY

This refers to removal of a whole lung.

Indications for pneumonectomy include: carcinoma, lung trauma and, less commonly, tuberculosis and bronchiectasis. Preoperative nursing care and preparation is the same as for any patient undergoing major surgery. However, the physiotherapist will teach the patient the chest and breathing exercises that will be required in the postoperative phase.

Nursing management

On return to the ward the patient must not be allowed to lie on the operative side for at least 48 hours if the pericardium has been opened. Otherwise the patient should be positioned upright or on the affected side.

There are usually no drain tubes in situ. If a drain tube is in situ it will usually be double clamped and attached to underwater-seal drainage (see page 343). Some surgeons request that the clamps on the drain tube be released briefly every hour. It is of importance for the nurse to, firstly, only release the clamps during quiet ventilation and, secondly, remain with the patient in order to clamp the tube should the patient need to cough. A cough is a full inspiration followed by forced expiration. The drain tube is in the space left by the lung that has been removed and this space is full of air and fluid. If the patient coughs and the drain tube is unclamped, the air in the thoracic cavity is forced out through the drain tube. As this occurs the mediastinum can shift suddenly, causing acute circulatory failure. The tube is unclamped on an intermittent basis to check if the patient is haemorrhaging, although systemic symptoms and signs of haemorrhage will accompany this complication.

The drain tube is usually removed 12–24 hours postoperatively, and patients make a complete recovery.

Complications

1. Mediastinal shift causing kinking of the great vessels resulting in reduced cardiac output.
2. Herniation of the heart through the pericardium following surgical opening, if a radical pneumonectomy has been performed for carcinoma.
3. Shortness of breath both of physiological and psychological origin.

Physiological. This can be due to the following:
● Post anaesthetic atelectasis causing arterovenous shunting and reduced area for gaseous exchange.
● Pain and therefore difficulty in expansion of the remaining lung.
● Reduced function of remaining lung, often due to an associated past history of lung disease of some form.

Psychological. This can be a problem if the patient believes he should be breathless due to the fact that he has lost an entire lung. This can be overcome by a thorough preoperative explanation of what to expect, reinforced by the nurse postoperatively. A calm confident approach by the nurse, in conjunction with intravenous narcotic pain relief should overcome any breathlessness of psychological origin.
4. Infection of remaining lung due to retained secretions (that is, atelectasis leading to pneumonia).
5. Bronchopleural fistula, which may be due to an infection in the bronchial stump.
6. Empyema.
7. Haemorrhage

What happens to the space?

The space fills with haemoserous fluid which becomes organized. The diaphragm moves up to fill the cavity, the mediastinum moves across, and the ribs approximate with the result that within a 2 year period the residual space is filled with fibrous tissue.

SARCOIDOSIS

Sarcoidosis presents as an acute multisystemic, granulomatous disease of unknown aetiology, principally involving the lungs, the hilar lymph nodes, and other areas of the lymphohematopoietic system. It occurs most often in young adults of 20–40 years and occurs more frequently in blacks than in whites. The disease runs an acute course of 2 years' duration and usually resolves. Chronic sarcoidosis is rare and usually results in pulmonary fibrosis.

Suggested causes include a genetic predisposition (there is a higher incidence in families of patients), a hypersensitivity reaction to an agent such as an atypical mycobacteria, or fungi.

Clinical manifestations

In addition to the lungs and lymph nodes lesions can affect the skin, liver, eyes, bone, genitourinary, heart and central nervous system.

The patient usually presents with arthralgia of the smaller joints, such as the wrists, elbows and ankles. This may be accompanied by general malaise, weight-loss, muscle weakness and polyarthralgia. Respiratory symptoms include breathlessness, chest pain and a non-productive cough. Skin lesions present as erythema nodosum and a macropapular nodular rash, and eye involvement as anterior uveitis.

Lymph involvement includes hilar and right paratracheal lymphadenopathy, and splenomagaly.

Cardiac arrhythmias can range from premature beats to complete heart block. Cardiomyopathies are rare.

Patients may also suffer hypercalciuria, hepatitis, cranial or peripheral nerve palsies, convulsions, and pituitary and hypothalamic lesions producing diabetes insipidus. A large number of cases are asymptomatic and often diagnosed incidentally at autopsy.

Investigative procedures

A suggestive history supported by laboratory and radiological findings suggest sarcoidosis.

- Chest X-ray – lymph adenopathy.
- Lung function tests – reduced vital capacity.
- Arterial blood gases – reduced pO_2 tension.
- Negative tubercular skin tests, sputum cultures from mycobacteria and fungi in addition to negative lung and skin biopsies help rule out the possibility of infection.

A positive Kveim Siltzbach skin test supports the diagnosis. The patient is given an intradermal injection of sarcoidal antigen and if the patient has active disease a granuloma develops at the infection site within 6 weeks. Biopsy of the infection site will show granuloma.

Medical and nursing management

Symptomatic sarcoidosis is treated with systemic or topical steroids for a period of 1 to 2 years, however a few patients require life long therapy.

Mild analgesics are given for arthralgia. Nursing management consists of providing a nutritious well balanced diet – low in calcium if the patient has hypercalcaemia. Respiratory function should be monitored closely noting sputum production and difficulty with ventilation. Cardiac arrhythmias will be detected by regularly monitoring the pulse rate and rhythm. Side-effects from steroid therapy must be expected (see page 263) and the patient will need an explanation of the importance of his drug regime over the next 2 years with careful and regular follow-up examinations.

Asymptomatic sarcoidosis requires no treatment.

SECTION D – REFERENCES AND FURTHER READING

Texts

Anderson J R (ed) 1976 Muir's textbook of pathology, 10th edn. Edward Arnold, London
Anthony C P 1984 Structure and function of the body. Mosby, St Louis
Baum G L, Wolinsky E (eds) 1983 Textbook of pulmonary diseases 3rd edn. Little, Brown & Co, Boston
Cahill M (ed) 1984 Respiratory disorders: nurse's clinical library. Springhouse, Pennsylvania
Cameron I R 1983 Respiratory disorders. Edward Arnold, London
Cherniack R M 1983 Respiration in health and disease, 3rd edn. Saunders, Philadelphia
Creager J G 1982 Human anatomy and physiology, Wadsworth, California
Dantzker D R (ed) 1986 Cardiopulmonary critical care. Grune & Stratton, Orlando
Gershwin M E (ed) 1986 Bronchial asthma: principles of diagnosis and treatment 2nd edn. Grune & Stratton, Orlando
Glauser F L (ed) 1983 Signs and symptoms in pulmonary medicine. Lippincott, Philadelphia
Havard M 1986 A nursing guide to drugs, 2nd edn. Churchill Livingstone, Melbourne
Kirby R R, Taylor R W 1986 Respiratory failure. Chicago Year Book
Kryger M H (ed) 1981 Pathophysiology of respiration. Wiley, New York
Luckmann J, Sorensen K C 1980 Medical-surgical nursing: a psychophysiologic approach, 2nd edn. Saunders, Philadelphia
Macleod J 1987 Davidson's principles and practice of medicine, 15th edn. Churchill Livingstone, Edinburgh

McPherson S P 1985 Respiratory therapy equipment, 3rd edn. Mosby, St Louis
Martz K V 1984 Management of the patient – ventilator system: a team approach 2nd edn. Mosby, St Louis
Nelson E J 1983 Critical care respiratory therapy: a laboratory and clinical manual. Little, Brown & Co, Boston
Read A E, Barritt D W, Langton Hewer R 1986 Modern medicine, 3rd edn. Churchill Livingstone, Edinburgh
Robinson S, Russo P (eds) 1983 Providing respiratory care: nursing photobook, 2nd edn. Springhouse, Pennsylvania
Sabiston D C, Spencer F C 1983 Gibbon's surgery of the chest 4th edn. Saunders, Philadelphia
Schonell M 1984 Respiratory medicine, 2nd edn. Churchill Livingstone, Edinburgh
Society of Hospital Pharmacists of Australia 1985 Pharmacology and drug information for nurses, 2nd edn. Saunders, Sydney
Spencer H 1985 Pathology of the lung, 4th edn. Pergamon Press, New York
Storlie F J (ed) 1984 Diseases: nurse's reference library, 2nd edn. Springhouse, Pennsylvania
West J B 1985 Respiratory physiology: the essentials, 3rd edn. Williams & Wilkins, Baltimore

Journals

Carroll P F 1985 Dislodged tracheostomy tube. Nursing 85 15 : 1 : 46
Carroll P F 1985 Tension pneumothorax. Nursing 85 15 : 9 : 41
Carroll P F 1986 Aspirated feeding solution. Nursing 86 16 : 1 : 33

Carroll P F 1986 Caring for ventilator patients. Nursing 86 16 : 2 : 34–39

Carroll P F 1986 Laryngospasm. Nursing 86 16 : 5 : 33

Carroll P F 1986 Artificial airways = real risks. Nursing 86 16 : 8 : 56–59

Carroll P F 1986 The ins and outs of chest drainage systems. Nursing 86 16 : 12 : 26–28

Chisholm S, Jaros T 1986 Duck-bill prosthesis: words of hope for the laryngectomy patient. Nursing 86 16 : 3 : 29–31

D'Agostino J S 1983 You can breathe new life into your COPD patients. Nursing 83 13 : 9 : 26–28

D'Agostino J S 1983 Set your mind at ease on oxygen toxicity. Nursing 83 13 : 7 : 55–56

D'Agostino J S 1984 Teaching tips for living with COPD at home. Nursing 84 14 : 2 : 57

Dalrymple D 1984 Setting up for thoracic drainage. Nursing 84 14 : 6 : 12–14

Dennison R D 1987 Managing the patient with upper airway obstruction. Nursing 87 17 : 10 : 34–41

Dunlop C I, Marchionno P 1988 Help your COPD patient take a better breath – with inhalers. Nursing 83 13 : 5 : 42–43

Eggland E T 1987 Teaching the ABC's of COPD. Nursing 87 17 : 1 : 60–64

Ensuring Intensive Care 1983 Coping with tube problems. Nursing 83 13 : 8 : 20–21

Fuchs P L 1983 Before and after surgery stay right on respiratory care. Nursing 83 13 : 5 : 47–50

Fuchs P L 1983 Using humidifiers and nebulizers. Nursing 83 13 : 6 : 6–11

Fuchs P L 1983 Providing tracheostomy care. Nursing 83 13 : 7 : 19–23

Fuchs P L 1983 Providing endotracheal tube care. Nursing 83 13 : 9 : 6–7

Fuchs P L 1983 ARDA: physiology, signs, and symptoms. Nursing 83 13 : 11 : 52–53

Fuchs P L 1983 Asthma: physiology, signs, and symptoms. Nursing 83 13 : 12 : 36–37

Fuchs P L 1984 Streamlining your suctioning techniques: part 1 nasotracheal suctioning. Nursing 84 14 : 5 : 55–61

Fuchs P L 1984 Streamlining your suctioning techniques: part 2 endotracheal suctioning. Nursing 84 14 : 6 : 46–51

Fuchs P L 1984 Streamlining your suctioning techniques: part 3 tracheostomy suctioning. Nursing 84 14 : 7 : 39–43

Hahn K 1987 Slow-teaching the COPD patient. Nursing 87 17 : 4 : 34–41

Hoyt K S 1983 Chest trauma. Nursing 83 13 : 5 : 34–41

Ishizaka K, Ishizaka T 1967 Identification of IgE antibodies as a carrier of reaginic activity. Journal of Immunology 99 : 1187

Karnes N 1987 Don't let ARDS catch you off guard. Nursing 87 17 : 5 : 34–38

Montanari J, Spearing C 1986 The fine art of measuring tracheal cuff pressure. Nursing 86 16 : 7 : 46–49

Mlynczak B A 1985 Ventilation disorders: a guide you can use with an air of confidence. Nursing 85 15 : 4 : 12–13

Nurse's Clinical Library 1985 Your role in COPD. Nursing 85 15 : 2 : 13–15

Palmer L 1984 Arterial blood gas analysis. Nursing 84 14 : 1 : 24–25

Patry-Lahey R 1985 Helping a laryngectomy patient go home. Nursing 85 15 : 3 : 63–64

Polacek L 1984 Teaming up to send the end-stage COPD patient home. Nursing 84 14 : 11 : 17–21

Rifas E M 1983 Teaching patients to manage acute asthma. Nursing 83 13 : 7 : 11–15

Romanski S O 1986 Interpreting ABGs in four easy steps. Nursing 86 16 : 9 : 58–63

Schluttenhofer N 1984 The special challenge of empyemas. Nursing 84 14 : 12 : 57–60

Schultz S 1983 Oxygen therapy – a long-term view. The Australian Nurses Journal 12 : 9 : 36–37

Sumner S M, Lewandowski V 1983 Guidelines for using artificial breathing devices. Nursing 83 13 : 10 : 54–57

Taylor D L 1984 Respiratory acidosis: physiology, signs, and symptoms. Nursing 84 14 : 10 : 44–45

Taylor D L 1984 Respiratory alkalosis: physiology, signs, and symptoms. Nursing 84 14 : 11 : 44–45

Taylor D L 1985 Assessing breath sounds. Nursing 85 15 : 3 : 60–62

Warren B 1985 Is your patient's job or home killing him? Nursing 85 15 : 3 : 9–11

Weaver T 1985 Chronic ineffective gas exchange: when your patient goes from bad to worse. Nursing 85 15 : 5 : 7

Westra B 1984 "I can't breathe". Nursing 84 14 : 5 : 34–39

White R C 1985 Dislodged chest tube. Nursing 85 15 : 12 : 25

Wimsatt R 1985 Unlocking the mysteries behind the chest wall. Nursing 85 15 : 11 : 58–63

E

The haemopoietic system

40

Introduction to the haemopoietic system

Robyn Anderson

Haemopoiesis (blood formation) occurs in the fetus predominantly in the liver but at the time of birth the bone marrow has become the major source of blood production, and blood is produced in almost all bones. As age progresses haemopoiesis decreases in the shafts of the long bones until only the cancellous ends produce blood, although marrow may reappear in the shafts in time of crisis. After the age of 50 years almost all blood production is confined to flat bones.

Erythropoiesis is a complex process in which blood cells change character several times, starting from large nucleated cells called haemocytoblasts. The stages are:

HAEMOCYTOBLAST
RUBRIBLAST
PRORUBRICYTE
RUBRICYTE
METARUBRICYTE
RETICULOCYTE
ERYTHROCYTE

The haemocytoblast also acts as a precursor to the three major blood cells, erythrocytes, leukocytes and platelets.

Erythrocytes

As the cell passes through the various stages it becomes smaller in size, until it reaches erythrocyte stage at which time it has reached the size of 7 μm in diameter, has lost its nucleus and has attained its classic flattened shape. There are normally 5×10^6 red cells per cubic centimetre of blood, and each erythrocyte contains 200–300 molecules of haemoglobin.

A clear clinical estimation of the rate of blood production can be obtained by measuring the number of reticulocytes in circulating blood. This may be of value in assessing the cause of anaemia and instituting the appropriate treatment. The average life span of an erythrocyte in the blood stream is 105–120 days, after which they fragment in the capillaries and the fragments are removed from circulation by the reticuloendothelial tissue in the liver, spleen and bone marrow.

Leucocytes

There are 5 different types of white cells, which are divided into 2 groups depending upon whether or not they have granular cytoplasm. Table 40.1 shows the normal distribution of these cells.

Neutrophils, eosinophils, basophils and some monocytes and lymphocytes are formed in bone marrow, however most of the lymphocytes and monocytes are produced in lymphatic tissue. The life span of white cells is to a large degree unknown; some granular leucocytes live less than three days whilst some lymphocytes may live as long as 5 years. Lymphocytes are approximately 8 μm in diameter while monocytes are 15–20 μm

Table 40.1 Normal distribution of leucocytes

Leucocytes	Normal % range
Those cells with granular cytoplasm	
Neutrophils	65–75
Eosinophils	2–5
Basophils	0.5–1
Those cells with non-granular cytoplasm	
Lymphocytes	20–25
Monocytes	3–8

on average in diameter. A cubic millimetre of blood contains 5000–9000 leucocytes.

White blood cells are one of the body's most important defences against microorganisms and the changes in percentages of these cells are indicative of a variety of disease states. For this reason white cell differential counting is important. All leucocytes are mobile and can 'squeeze' through the intracellular spaces of the capillary wall by diapedesis and move toward areas of infection or infarction, thereby helping to cause inflammation (see Chapter 9).

Upon reaching tissue level, the neutrophils and monocytes phagocytoze dead tissue and microorganisms, while lymphocytes are predominantly responsible for the formation of antibodies. Eosinophils are weak phagocytes and probably function by detoxifying protein and other substances produced by cellular injury or allergic reaction.

The function of basophils is largely unknown but they may be responsible for the prevention of intravascular coagulation, as heparin can be extracted from their granules.

Thrombocytes

Thrombocytes (platelets) are formed predominently in red bone marrow, however some are formed in the spleen by fragmentation of megakaryocytes. The life span of a platelet is about 10 days. They are 2–4 μm in diameter and are oval or spindle in shape.

CLOTTING

Platelets are largely responsible for haemostasis, that is the stopping of blood flow, and play a large part in blood clotting. They adhere to one another and to the lining of damaged vessels causing the formation of a plug. In the capillaries this occurs within 1–5 seconds of injury. When the injury is extensive the clotting mechanism (or clotting cascade) is activated. This mechanism is as yet not completely understood but it is known that there are at least 13 factors involved in the process. They are:

Factor I	Fibrinogen
Factor II	Prothrombin
Factor III	Thromboplastin/thrombokinase
Factor IV	Calcium
Factor V	Proaccelerin/labile factor
Factor VI	Not named
Factor VII	Serum prothrombin conversion accelerator (SPCA)
Factor VIII	Antihaemophilic globulin (AHG) or Antihaemophilic factor (AHF)
Factor IX	Plasma thromboplastin component (PTC); Christmas factor
Factor X	Stuart factor
Factor XI	Plasma thromboplastin antecedent (PTA)
Factor XII	Hageman factor
Factor XIII	Fibrin stabilizing factor

When the clotting cascade is activated, prothrombin is converted into thrombin, and this takes place only if thromboplastin is released from platelets or damaged tissue, and calcium ions are present. If platelet thromboplastin is released, factors IV, V, VIII, IX, X, XI, and XII must also be present for thromboplastin to be converted to thrombin; this is referred to as the intrinsic system. The extrinsic system utilizes thromboplastin from damaged tissue and requires the presence of factors IV, V, VII and X.

The second major step is the conversion of fibrinogen to insoluble strands of fibrin, and this cannot occur without the presence of thrombin and factors IV and XIII. Fibrin strands form entangled threads which trap blood cells to form a clot.

41

Disorders of the erythrocytes

Robyn Anderson

DECREASED ERYTHROPOIESIS/ANAEMIA

Anaemia is a reduction in the oxygen carrying capacity of the blood and it is usually considered to be present when the haemoglobin concentration is below 13.5 g/dl in adult males and 11.5 g/dl in females. Usually anaemia comprises a low haemoglobin and a reduction in the number of erythrocytes. However, this is not always so, as in long standing iron-deficiency anaemia, for example, the cell count may be normal but the cells are pale and understained by haem.

Clinical manifestations

The clinical features common to all anaemias vary from person to person and depend upon the speed of onset of the anaemia; generally speaking, the faster the onset the more severe the symptoms. They are also dependent upon the severity of the anaemia, the age of the patient and his general physical condition. Some patients, even those with moderately severe anaemia, may remain asymptomatic, whilst others with mild anaemia may have quite marked symptoms. Elderly people tolerate anaemia less well than do the young.

The symptoms of anaemia are weakness, tiredness, headache, palpitations, and shortness of breath, particularly in response to exercise. In elderly patients, or those in whom the development of anaemia has been extremely fast, symptoms of angina pectoris, cardiac failure, intermittent claudication, and confusion may occur; only in extreme cases do visual disturbances from retinal haemorrhage occur.

The signs present in most patients include pallor of mucous membranes, tachycardia and cardiomegally. Any other signs are specific to the individual anaemia.

There is no specific nursing care relevant to a patient with anaemia except to bear in mind the patient's symptoms and to treat them appropriately.

Because the patient is tired and lethargic he should be nursed in bed with short periods of gentle exercise spread over the day. He should be nursed upright to assist ventilation, and oxygen may on occasion be administered. However, since the problem is lack of haemoglobin and not a lack of oxygen the very small amount of extra oxygen that can be carried in the plasma is of little value, as his haemoglobin is already saturated (see oxyhaemoglobin dissociation curve Fig. 9.2, page

Table 41.1 Overview of types of anaemia

Abnormalities of blood production
  Deficiency anaemia
    Iron deficiency
  Megaloblastic anaemias
    B_{12} deficiency
    Folate deficiency
  Aplastic anaemia
  Marrow infiltration by malignant disease
Increased blood destruction – haemolytic anaemia
  Abnormality of erythrocytes
    Hereditary spherocytosis
    Hereditary elliptocytosis
    Sickle cell anaemia
    Thalassaemia
  Abnormalities of plasma
    Haemolytic disease of the newborn
    Severe infection
    Drugs and chemicals
    Mechanical causes
    Liver disease
    Malignancy
    Incompatible blood transfusion
  Autoimmune haemolytic anaemia (AHIA)
Increased blood loss – haemorrhagic anaemia

87). Also, the patient may be distressed by the mask or oxygen catheter to a point which completely overrides any value derived from the extra oxygen.

Table 41.1 shows the categorization of anaemias.

DEFICIENCY ANAEMIAS

Iron deficiency anaemia

A normal diet supplies approximately 14 mg of iron each day and of this only 1–2 mg is absorbed. Iron bonds to substances in the stomach to form chelates whilst some iron is bound to gastric acid and remains soluble.

Iron is absorbed from the proximal 40 cm of the small intestine and the absorption of iron is enhanced by substances such as ascorbic acid, cystine, and hydrochloric acid. Iron absorption is inhibited by phylates and phosphates.

There are no significant mechanisms for the excretion of iron. However, the body has quite elaborate mechanisms for its conservation.

The body contains 3000–4000 mg of iron, and the amount of iron absorbed daily should be exactly equivalent to the amount lost in the shedding of skin, gut, and uterine cells. Absorption of iron is controlled by ferritin. When there is a high marrow demand for iron less ferritin is produced and large quantities of iron are absorbed; conversely when the marrow demand for iron is low, large quantities of ferritin are produced, causing less iron to be absorbed.

There are 4 mg of iron present in plasma, linked to beta-globulin called transferrin. Most plasma iron is derived from the breakdown of erythrocytes and some iron comes from the body stores and from the gut.

The normal serum iron is 100 mg/dl but because its measurement varies greatly between laboratories the normal range for each laboratory should be given.

Iron deficiency anaemia is one of the most common deficiency states encountered clinically and is seen far more commonly in women than in men; this is due primarily to the monthly blood loss of menstruation.

Iron deficiency anaemia usually occurs between the ages of 20–45 years or during periods of active growth. It is quite common in premature infants as they are born before the iron has been laid down which normally occurs during the last weeks of pregnancy.

Aetiology

Iron deficiency anaemia is most commonly caused by increased demands during pregnancy, lactation, and menstruation, and by chronic blood loss from the uterus; and from the gastrointestinal tract, in conditions such as hiatus hernia, chronic gastritis, peptic ulceration, carcinoma of any part of the gut, worm infestation, haemorrhoids, colitis, diverticulitis, and oesophageal varices. It is also seen as a consequence of dietary deprivation of iron, although this is uncommon in Australia due to the high consumption of red meats. Also, 'It has been estimated to take eight years for a normal adult male to develop iron deficiency anaemia solely due to a poor diet or malabsorption causing no iron intake at all.' (Hoffbrand & Pettit, 1984). Lack of dietary iron is most commonly seen in elderly women who live alone and who fail to prepare proper meals for themselves. Premature infants and full term infants from 3 to 6 months of age may exhibit iron deficiency anaemia due to improper laying down of iron or excessive delay in commencing solid foods in the normal baby.

Patients who have had a gastrectomy or repeated attacks of hyperchlorhydria, gastritis, or gastric ulceration may be unable to absorb iron efficiently from the gut.

Clinical manifestations

In addition to the general symptoms of anaemia, the patient's fingernails are prone to brittleness and cracking, particularly on the fingers of the dextrous hand. The process can progress through a stage in which the nails flatten and then become concave and discoloured (koilonychia). Angular stomatitis and atrophic glossitis occur although these may also be present in other disease states. Oesophageal atrophy, causing dysphagia, and gastric atrophy result and these lesions are often premalignant.

Investigative procedures

1. Erythrocyte indices and FBE. This shows a decrease in the number of circulating erythrocytes, the cells are hypochromic and microcytic, the reticulocyte count is low, and the thrombocyte count may be moderately raised where there is continued blood loss.

2. Serum iron and total iron binding capacity (TIBC). Serum iron will be low whilst TIBC rises causing less than 10% saturation of iron.

3. Bone marrow iron. Although this test is not necessarily performed in simple iron deficiency anaemias, it is routinely performed on all bone marrow samples taken for any reason. In iron deficiency anaemia there is complete absence of iron from macrophages and developing erythrocytes; these are small and have a ragged cytoplasm.

4. Serum ferritin. In iron deficiency anaemia the serum ferritin is very low except where the anaemia is associated with a chronic disorder.

5. Free erythrocyte proloporphyrin (FEP). This is increased in the early stages of iron deficiency before anaemia is clinically obvious.

6. Detection of the site of chronic blood loss. Blood can only be lost on a chronic basis from two places without the blood loss being obvious. Firstly, from the uterus/vagina where, due to fear, embarrassment, or ignorance, menorrhagia is not treated promptly. A thorough gynaecological history is therefore mandatory. The nurse should not ask a patient 'Is your menstrual cycle normal?' as the answer is invariably 'Yes'. The nurse should ask 'Would you please describe your menstrual cycle'; to elicit a more specific response.

Secondly, blood can be lost from the gut, and depending on the type of blood found on testing the faeces, further investigations such as barium meal with or without follow through, and barium enema may be performed. Direct gastroscopy, duodenoscopy and/or colonoscopy may also be required.

Blood may also occasionally be lost through the urinary system.

Medical and surgical management

The underlying cause of the anaemia is sought and treated if possible. In extreme cases, blood transfusion or infusion of packed cells may be undertaken although this is rarely necessary unless a chronic, severe iron deficiency is detected in conjunction with another major insult to the body. For example, major road trauma in a patient with a pre-existing iron deficiency anaemia will necessitate not only replacement of blood lost due to the trauma but correction of the anaemia.

There are three ways of administering iron, but orally is by far the safest route. Ferrous sulphate is the cheapest form of oral iron, but it often causes nausea, vomiting and diarrhoea, and is best tolerated in the form of sustained-release tablets and Ferrogradumet is usually prescribed. Clinical trials have shown that the haemoglobin can be raised by 1 g/dl in one week with the twice daily administration of one Ferrogradumet. Oral iron should be given long enough to correct the anaemia and to replenish the iron stores throughout the body.

Parenteral iron is generally unnecessary as the haematological response is no faster to parenteral iron than it is to orally administered iron. The only advantage of using parenteral iron is that the body stores are replenished more quickly.

Intramuscular iron is not popular as it is painful and can permanently stain the skin. For this reason when intramuscular iron is administered the nurse should use a 'Z' technique and the needle used to inject the substance should not be the one through which it was prepared.

Intravenous iron, although widely used, has the potential to cause an anaphylactic response in the patient.

Diet

Where necessary the patient's diet should be adjusted to ensure an adequate supply of iron; green leafy vegetables, and meat are an ideal source.

THE MEGALOBLASTIC ANAEMIAS

Both vitamin B and folic acid are necessary for DNA synthesis and deficiencies of either cause anaemias with morphological changes, predominantly of the erythrocytes, which become megaloblastic. This occurs because the reduced synthesis of DNA allows longer periods of erythrocyte growth, thus causing large cells to be produced. Changes may also be seen in granulocyte precursors and megakaryocytes and in other rapidly dividing tissue such as the cells of the gastrointestinal tract. Many of the megaloblastic cells never mature and are destroyed in the bone marrow, liberating enzymes and causing the serum lactate dehydrogenase (LDH) to become very high, eventually causing significant aplasia with a consequent aplastic anaemia.

Vitamin B₁₂ deficiency anaemia

Vitamin B_{12} is synthesized by animals and by bacteria, and it is taken into the human by eating animal foods and some bacterially contaminated foods. It is found in liver, fish, and dairy products, and in fruit, cereals and vegetables only when they have been bacterially contaminated.

Normal diets contain considerable excesses of vitamin B_{12}, to the order of 7–30 μg/day. The minimum daily requirement is 1–2 μg and the body stores 2–3 mg of vitamin B_{12} – enough for 2–4 years, the limit of absorption is 2–3 μg/day. It combines with a glycoprotein which is excreted from the parietal cells of the stomach (this glycoprotein is called intrinsic factor). Vitamin B_{12} is absorbed from the lower ileum and thence into the portal blood where it attaches itself to a protein called transcobalamin II which carries it to bone marrow and other tissues. Vitamin B_{12} also combines with transcobalamin I but in this form is relatively useless to the body as it does not transfer from this form to the bone marrow.

Vitamin B_{12} deficiency occurs for one of four reasons:

• The diet may supply inadequate amounts of vitamin B_{12}, as is seen predominantly in true vegans.
• There may be a deficiency of intrinsic factor, as in pernicious anaemia, following a total gastrectomy, or on rare occasions congenital deficiencies may be present.
• The terminal ileum from which the vitamin is absorbed may be absent following surgery, or it may be diseased as in Crohn's disease.

• Vitamin B_{12} may be removed from the bowel by intestinal parasites such as fish tapeworms.

Addison's pernicious anaemia is that form of vitamin B_{12} deficiency which results from a deficiency of intrinsic factor from causes other than surgery. It is seen more commonly in females than in males and occurs usually between 45 and 65 years of age. The patients often have grey hair and blue eyes, there is a strong familial tendency and it is associated with other diseases of immunological significance such as ideopathic hypothyroidism, rheumatoid arthritis and diabetes mellitus.

Clinical manifestations

The onset of vitamin B_{12} deficiency anaemia is often insidious and the degree of anaemia may be great before the patient seeks medical assistance. He will present with the clinical manifestations common to all anaemias (see page 381).

For all megaloblastic anaemias, the blood film shows a marked anisocytosis and poikilocytosis. There is a raised level of unconjugated bilirubin in the plasma and iron deposition in the liver, kidneys, bone marrow and spleen; the spleen may be palpable. The mucosa of the stomach and tongue may be fragile and atrophic. If the condition remains untreated or is treated inadequately, degenerative changes may occur in the lateral and posterior tracts of the spinal cord (subacute combined degeneration of the cord) leading ultimately to paralysis and death.

The patient may have glossitis and angular stomatitis. The skin may have a pale yellow tint, there may be infertility in females, and dementia may occur in either sex.

Investigative procedures

A blood film shows megaloblastic changes, anisocytosis and poickilocytosis is present and there may be some fragmentation of erythrocytes. The reticulocyte count is low, leucopenia is present, and commonly hypersegmentation of the neutrophils is seen. The thrombocyte count may vary from normal to extremely low. The bone marrow is megaloblastic, the serum vitamin B_{12} is low. Schilling's test will show that there is a deficiency in the absorption of vitamin B_{12}.

Medical management

Packed cells may be administered only when the Hb level is low enough to threaten the patient's life. It is usual however to administer 200–1000 µg hydroxocobalamin weekly for one month and then monthly for the remainder of the patient's life. 48 hours following the first dose the bone marrow will start to show normal cells and the blood count will rapidly return to normal. Occasionally this return to normal may be so rapid as to deplete iron stores in the body and hence iron is also given (see page 382) and may be ceased when the Hb level is normal.

Complications

Mild peripheral neuropathy and subacute combined degeneration of the spinal cord may ensue as a result of this anaemia. Adequate maintenance therapy should prevent these from occurring.

Habilitation

In most forms of vitamin B_{12} deficiency anaemia the patient's ability to absorb vitamin B_{12} does not improve and therefore a maintenance dose of hydroxocobalamin 200–1000 µg/month is necessary for the remainder of the patient's life. His life expectancy is normal but there is statistical evidence of a significant increase in death from carcinoma of the stomach in patients with pernicious anaemia.

Folic acid deficiency anaemia

Folic acid and its related compounds are often referred to as folates. The body obtains folates from the breakdown of polyglutamates in food with the aid of an enzyme called folate conjunctase. Folate is seen in the plasma as methyl tetrahydrofolate and is changed to tetrahydrofolate (THF) by a chemical pathway which requires the presence of vitamin B_{12}. THF is necessary for DNA production.

Another folate type, formyl THF (folinic acid), will bypass the metabolic blocks created by either the folate antagonist methotrexate or by vitamin B_{12} deficiency. As high doses of folates can cause

nerve cell damage, it is imperative that folic acid is not used to treat vitamin B_{12} deficiencies as, although it may temporarily correct the anaemia, it will hasten neurological damage.

Folic acid is absorbed into the body predominantly from the jejunum. Deficiencies occur because of inadequate food intake or in situations where fresh vegetables and meats are excluded from the diet or when food is significantly overcooked; diseases of the small bowel such as coeliac disease may inhibit absorption. Deficiencies of folate also occur where the body's demand for folate exceeds the supply, for example, during periods of extreme cell proliferation as seen in haemolytic anaemia, leukaemia and other malignancies, and during pregnancy. It is interesting that there is no evidence that the fetus is ever folate deficient despite the condition of the mother and often (especially in countries where famine is present) to her great detriment; however, females deficient in folate may be infertile.

Drugs may also cause folate deficiencies by interfering with the enzyme reduction system. The drugs occasionally responsible for this are methotrexate and pryimethamine. Phenytoin and primidone may also cause folate deficiencies but the mechanism by which this occurs is not understood.

Clinical manifestations

The anaemia is very similar to that caused by deficiency of vitamin B_{12} (see page 383). Glossitis is less common and it is extremely rare for any signs of neurological damage to be present.

Investigative procedures

The investigative procedures used in folate deficiency anaemia are the same as those used in vitamin B_{12} deficiency anaemia (see page 383). The results are indistinguishable except that both the serum and the erythrocyte folate levels are low.

Medical management

Folic acid 5 mg daily is given by mouth and is more than adequate. Preparations considerably stronger than this exist, and although not harmful are useless. Folate supplements are almost always given during pregnancy.

It must be noted that folic acid must never be administered without vitamin B_{12} to patients with B_{12} deficiencies, as it may hasten or indeed precipitate neurological problems (see page 384).

APLASTIC ANAEMIA

Aplastic anaemia occurs when there is a marked reduction of haemopoietic stem cells in the bone marrow. There is no infiltration of malignant tissue and the patient's nutritional status is normal. The majority of cases of aplastic anaemia occur as a result of suppression of the bone marrow from substances such as the alkylating agents (busulphan is the most dangerous), chloramphenicol, the sulphonamides, gold, penicillamine, phenylbutazone, phenytoin, the oral hypoglycaemic agents, and chlorpromazine.

Other chemicals such as glue solvents, toluene, benzene, and DDT are also capable of suppressing bone marrow as is exposure to gamma irradiation. Viral infections (particularly hepatitis) may be responsible for marrow suppression.

Congenital aplastic anaemia may be found, but is extremely rare. It may affect only the erythrocytes as, for example, in Diamond-Blackfan syndrome. This is in contrast to most cases of aplastic anaemia, where not only is erythrocyte production severely reduced but leucocyte and thrombocyte production also ceases.

Clinical manifestations

The patient is pale, listless and lethargic. He is severely anaemic, he may have a variety of minor infections especially a sore throat, tonsilitis, and pharyngitis. Skin infections are common. He will have thrombocytopenia and show bruising, purpura and ecchymosis of the skin and mucous membranes, and possibly haemorrhagic retinopathy. The patient is usually extremely ill.

Investigative procedures

Hb levels and a blood count will show anaemia which will probably be severe, and granulocytes and thrombocytes are severely depleted in number. The erythrocytes are usually normocytic but may on occasions be macrocytic. Bone marrow biopsy is performed to exclude other causes of pancytopenia and studies with Fe^{59} are performed to assess the speed of erythropoiesis. HLA typing is performed on the patient and his siblings in the event that bone marrow transplantation becomes necessary.

Without the correct investigation it is possible to confuse the condition with some types of leukaemia, infiltration of the bone marrow by malignant disease, severe megaloblastic anaemia, hypersplenism, or miliary tuberculosis.

Medical and nursing management

The administration of any drug which is suspected of having caused the condition is ceased immediately. Chelating agents (see page 389) are used where toxicity from gold or heavy metal poisoning is suspected. Management is basically symptomatic and is aimed at sustaining life in the hope that the bone marrow will regenerate and function normally. Management involves preventing and treating infection, treating the anaemia with repeated blood transfusions, and the thrombocytopenia (and therefore the bleeding tendencies) with repeated thrombocyte transfusions. Thrombocyte transfusions are not a viable long term treatment, as the patient will become resistant to the transfusions because of antibody formation.

Corticosteroids may reduce the bleeding tendency. Androgenic steroids may be used and it may be 3 or more months before any change in the patient's condition is observed.

Neutropenia will cause widespread infection and broad spectrum antibiotics should be given to either treat or prevent infection; established infection should be treated aggressively.

Bone marrow transplantation is the only truly curative method of treating the patient, but is successful in only a small percentage of patients.

The patient will be nursed in reverse isolation as, because of agranulocytosis, he is at risk from a variety of bacteria and viruses (see page 393 for the nursing management of the immunosuppressed patient). Extreme care is taken to prevent skin abrasions, as they will not heal well, may bleed profusely, and become infected. On a weekly basis the nurse will be responsible for obtaining bacteriological swabs of all orifices and wounds, specimens of skin, hair, urine, and sputum. Should any culture of these produce a potentially harmful organism, treatment is instituted to effect its eradication at this stage.

The patient will need psychological support and counselling. Financial help may also be necessary and the social worker may be of value in finding assistance for the patient and his significant others.

If bone marrow transplantation is planned, the nursing management is as for the patient undergoing bone marrow transplantation for acute leukaemia (see page 403).

Anticipated outcome

50% of patients recover, with or without bone marrow transplantation, however, 50% die within one year and as many as 90% of severely affected patients die.

HAEMOLYTIC ANAEMIA

Haemolytic anaemia occurs when the erythrocytes are prematurely destroyed (that is, before their normal 100–120 days of life) and the compensatory ability of the bone marrow is greater than normal.

Haemolytic anaemias can be broadly divided into two groups, those where the defect is in the erythrocytes, such as hereditary spherocytosis or elliptocytosis, thalassaemia and sickle cell anaemia, and those where the abnormality is in the plasma such as incompatible blood transfusion, haemolytic disease of the newborn, and infections, particularly malaria. Procedures involving extracorporeal blood lines such as haemodialysis and cardiopulmonary bypass, and following massive blood transfusions (particularly where the blood is given quickly) also cause haemolysis as in these procedures some cells are fragmented by the apparatus. Drugs and a variety of chemicals, and renal and liver disease can also cause haemolysis.

Clinical manifestations

The patient is anaemic, and pale. There may be haemoglobinuria, and ulceration of the legs, and the skin is pruritic, the spleen is enlarged, and there may be skeletal changes due to enlargement of marrow spaces. The patient will be mildly jaundiced and may have gall stones if the anaemia is of long standing, due to excessive production of bilirubin and bile salts.

Investigative procedures

These are aimed at discovering the cause of the haemolysis. A blood film will show abnormalities in the number, size, and shape of erythrocytes. Coomb's test is performed, as is immunofluorescence, to detect autoimmune factors. The serum bilirubin is high in haemolytic anaemia.

Nursing management

The nursing intervention for a patient with any of the haemolytic anaemias is similar, in that they will need the same care as a patient with anaemia (see page 382) but special care will need to be taken of the patient's skin which is often fragile and pruritic. The pruritus is caused by the presence of bilirubin in the skin causing irritation to the nerve endings. Effective management of pruritis is difficult to achieve, as local treatments such as heat or cold (whichever is most effective for the patient), calamine lotion, or the application of alcohol or antipruritic oil, give only transitory relief. Drug therapy for pruritus is usually contraindicated because the antipruritic drugs are detoxified in the liver, and the liver is already overloaded by trying to cope with the amount of erythrocyte breakdown product with which it is being presented. In some patients the wearing of cotton gloves (particularly at night) may be enough to remind them not to scratch. Children may need to have their arms bandaged into soft well-padded splints to prevent scratching. The patient may be distressed by the alteration in his body image made by jaundice, and will need emotional support.

Hereditary spherocytosis

Hereditary spherocytosis is the commonest form of congenital haemolytic anaemia in Caucasians. It is an autosomal dominant condition but with incomplete penetrance and therefore there may be no familial history of the condition. It is probable that there is a defect in the protein of the cell membrane, causing spherocytic cells to be produced and then destroyed at an abnormal rate by the spleen.

Clinical manifestations

The patient has recurrent episodes of anaemia and jaundice due to temporary increases in the rate of haemolysis. He may, however, present with bone marrow depression following infection. Gall stones and intractible leg ulcers may on occasion be the mode of presentation. The spleen is palpable and folate deficiency may also occur.

Investigative procedures

The clinical picture in combination with a full blood examination and a family history will easily confirm diagnosis. Serum bilirubin levels will be raised.

Medical management

Splenectomy should be performed as soon as possible following a confirmed diagnosis as this will reduce the rate of erythrocyte breakdown, although of course it will not alter the underlying spherocytosis.

Following splenectomy the leg ulcers may also improve and complications such as gall stones may be prevented.

Sickle cell anaemia

Sickle cell anaemia is a genetic condition seen often in negroid people and also in people from Middle Eastern and Mediterranean countries. Haemoglobin synthesis in this condition is disturbed at a genetic level and the most common form of haemoglobin seen in these patients is haemoglobin S (HbS). The high incidence of this condition in African peoples is presumably because HbS is usually very resistant to falciparum malaria and over centuries of selective advantage the gene pool has been concentrated with high levels of this malaria resistant gene.

The erythrocytes are sickle shaped due to the formation of pseudo-crystalline substances inside the cell produced by the degradation of HbS. These substances are called tactoids and distort the erythrocyte membrane. Sickle cells increase blood viscosity as they tend to obstruct flow in capillaries. This leads to thrombosis which may in turn be followed by infarction. Because of their unusual shape the cells are readily destroyed by the spleen and jaundice results.

Clinical manifestations

The patient has a chronic anaemia which commences about the fourth month of life and the Hb level rarely rises above 10 mg/dl. A secondary folate deficiency is usually also present and this exacerbates the condition.

The patient may present because of delayed puberty and retarded growth patterns, although he may have periods of excessive bone growth causing skeletal deformity, particularly in the spine. These periods of excessive bone growth are often accompanied by massive erythrocyte destruction, a very fast fall in haemoglobin level, and a rapid enlargement of the spleen and liver. The patient may also have an increased susceptibility to infection, gall stones, cardiomegally, and leg ulcers.

'Infarction crises' occur with episodes of severe pain usually in the bones and spleen. In infants, these infarctions occur in the fingers and toes and may cause permanent deformity due to epiphyseal damage. Mesenteric infarctions may cause extreme abdominal pain, while infarction of the renal papillae can produce painless haematuria. In adults the head of the femur may become necrotic.

These episodes may be spontaneous or precipitated by dehydration, extreme cold, or infection. The pain during these exacerbations is extreme but abates after 24 hours. The patient has fever, increasing jaundice, and malaise.

Investigative procedures

A full blood examination will show the presence of sickle cells and the presence of HbS can be easily demonstrated on a small blood sample. The diagnosis is confirmed by electrophoretic analysis of haemoglobin, and family studies will demonstrate inheritance.

Medical management

There is no cure for this condition and management is directed towards relieving symptoms and reducing the effects.

The patient should avoid extreme temperature changes (especially cold) and dehydration, and infections must be treated quickly and effectively. Folic acid 5 mg orally should be given daily to help prevent deficiency as a result of the massively increased erythropoiesis.

During exacerbation of the pain is caused by tissue infarction; the patient will need narcotic analgesia, and may require blood transfusion if the Hb falls below 6 mg/dl. Minor analgesics may be used for less severe pain. The patient must be kept well hydrated at all times.

Nursing management

During exacerbation these patients are acutely ill, in great pain and are extremely frightened.

The nurse should be aware that he/she will be required to administer narcotic analgesics at least every 4 hours. Pain relief is paramount and any aid such as sheepskins, foam pads, bed cradles, or soft bandages which may relieve pressure on the infarcted area should be employed.

The patient is often severely hypoxic and may be confused, disorientated and dyspnoeic. A semi-upright position and the use of oxygen via a mask may help to reduce both the hypoxia and the dyspnoea.

The patient will need to be helped to understand his condition and to live in a manner which will avoid potential trauma. The social worker may be able to help upgrade social circumstances where necessary.

Anticipated outcome

These patients can lead reasonably normal lives providing their symptoms are properly treated. In the depressed areas of Africa most patients die in infancy or in childhood. In developed countries the patients usually survive into adulthood but rarely reach old age.

The thalassaemias

Thalassaemia is an inherited impairment of haemoglobin synthesis in which either alpha, or more commonly, beta chain synthesis may be affected. In the heterozygous form the patient is only mildly affected and the haemoglobin rarely falls below 10 mg/dl. This is called thalassaemia minor. The homozygous form is named thalassaemia major and is a condition relevant to beta chain synthesis. The homozygous alpha chain synthesis condition may produce a still-born fetus.

Thalassaemia minor

Clinical manifestations. The patient with this condition is rarely ill. He has a mild anaemia and little or no clinical disability and diagnosis is often made only after the patient has been unsuccessfully treated for iron deficiency anaemia, which this condition resembles on blood film.

There is no specific treatment.

Thalassaemia major

This is a severe and debilitating condition in which there is an overwhelming anaemia. It is seen classically in people of Mediterranean origin, Indians, some Northern Europeans, and in some East Asians and usually affects children. As a result of patterns of immigration, Australia's incidence of thalassaemia has risen significantly over the last 40 years.

Clinical manifestations. The patient is severely anaemic, and his erythrocytes are hypochromic and microcytic. Anisocytosis and poikilocytosis are also present. Huge numbers of newly formed erythrocytes are present in the bone marrow and these cells do not mature. Their large numbers cause marrow cavity expansion with resultant skeletal deformity. These are particularly obvious in the skull and face causing overgrowth of both of these areas; the patient's general growth is stunted and his liver and spleen are grossly enlarged. The child is pale, has mild jaundice and brown skin pigmentation caused by the laying down of iron in the skin cells.

Medical and nursing management. The only form of treatment is to administer large and frequent blood transfusions to the order of 1–2 units of blood every 3–4 weeks. This is done in an attempt to suppress the child's own haemopoietic system and thus reduce skeletal abnormalities and hepatosplenomegaly. Transfusional haemosiderosis (the laying down of iron in soft tissue) becomes a problem and the heart is primarily affected; chelating agents such as desferrioxamine will help to slow down this process. Splenectomy may be performed in order to reduce the amount of blood required but the later this can be done the better.

The nurse must be aware that these children spend a great deal of their lives in hospital, they are critically ill and require gentle handling and a great deal of emotional support. If the child is of school age, the nurse should ensure that school work is undertaken. Most large hospitals in Australia with facilities for nursing children are also registered primary schools and maintain a staff of primary teachers.

Blood transfusions must be closely supervised and the child should have a well balanced diet. His parents must understand the significance of chelating agents and must be prepared to ensure that they are administered to the child on his short visits home. A chelating agent is any chemical which changes a toxic heavy metal into a non toxic insoluble substance. These are used in any heavy metal poisoning, but are predominantly used where the body's iron levels are extremely high due to massive erythrocyte breakdown. Chelating agents are usually given to these children through a silastic cannula into the abdominal wall.

Parents may need counselling sessions with members of the clergy and the social worker, as the anticipated outcome of the condition is death, probably before the child reaches his teens.

Autoimmune haemolytic anaemia (AIHA)

AIHA is a condition where erythrocytes are destroyed by autoimmune antibodies. The condition presents in 2 ways depending upon the type of antibody involved. Where IgG antibodies are involved the condition is referred to as warm antibody AIHA whilst cold antibody AIAH involves IgM antibodies.

Aetiology

The condition can be divided into two groups: primary ideopathic AIHA, which can occur at any age; and secondary AIHA, which occurs in response to other conditions, such as lymphoma, Hodgkin's disease, other autoimmune diseases such as SLE, viral infections, and in response to drugs, for example methyldopa.

Warm antibody AIHA

In this condition there is mainly extravascular haemolysis.

Clinical manifestations

Clinical manifestations are the same as for any haemolytic anaemia (see page 386). The onset is acute and the anaemia may be severe.

Investigative procedures

The patient should be thoroughly investigated in an attempt to find a secondary cause for the condition. The blood film shows spherocytosis and diagnosis is confirmed with a Coomb's test. Erythrocyte survival studies will indicate whether or not a splenectomy should be performed.

Medical management

Treatment of the condition is with large doses of steroids to the order of 60–80 mg of prednisolone per day and this is continued until the haemolysis ceases. A splenectomy may be indicated to reduce erythrocyte breakdown, and immunosuppressive drugs such as azathioprine may prove useful.

Blood transfusion should not be performed as it serves only to worsen the haemolysis. Patients with AIHA caused by drugs will almost always recover completely if the drug is withdrawn.

Cold antibody AIHA

In cold antibody AIHA there is agglutination of erythrocytes and intravascular haemolysis. The agglutination is predominantly confined to the small peripheral blood vessels and causes peripheral ischaemia.

Medical management

There is usually no treatment necessary except to avoid cold climate and to wear warm clothing. However, if haemolysis persists, a cytotoxic agent can be used in small dosages. Steroids and splenectomy are rarely useful in this condition.

Other causes of haemolytic anaemia

Malaria

All patients with malaria have haemolytic anaemia, the severity of which is usually related to the severity of the malaria. As the patient recovers from malaria the blood stream is flooded with new, normal red blood cells; this sudden production of cells may produce deficiencies in iron or folate.

Inflammatory and malignant diseases

Both these conditions shorten the life of erythrocytes and therefore speed haemolysis. The mechanism for this is not completely understood.

Transfusion with incompatible blood

Whatever the reason for incompatible transfusion occurring, it may well develop into an iatrogenic disaster. Clinical manifestations of incompatible blood transfusion begin after the infusion of the first few millilitres of blood, and may be mild or severe. Mild reactions consist of skin rashes, slight fever, and tachycardia and in many instances will not require cessation of the transfusion. However,

the transfusion rate may be slowed and the nurse must closely monitor the patient's physical condition for any increase in severity of the reaction.

Severe reactions are usually of rapid onset and the patient will be restless, shivering and nauseated and he may vomit. He may complain of precordial and lumbar pain, his skin will be cold and clammy, and he may become cyanosed. He will have a tachycardia, tachypnoea and his temperature will be elevated to 39–40°. His blood pressure will fall and he will become shocked.

In severe reactions both haemoglobinaemia and haemoglobinuria may be present and the urine output will fall to below 20 ml/hour. This may progress to anuria as acute tubular necrosis occurs. In extreme situations this may lead to renal failure and possibly death. In most instances, following cessation of the transfusion a diuresis will occur within 24–48 hours and the other symptoms resolve.

Investigative procedures. The blood that precipitated the reaction should be re-grouped and cross-matched. The patient's blood is taken for grouping and crossmatching.

Blood and urine specimens are collected and examined for the presence of free haemoglobin.

Medical and nursing management. Obviously prophylaxis is paramount, and most institutions have strict regimes that must be followed to ensure that correct blood is given. These checking regimes are for the benefit and protection of the staff as well as the patient and should be adhered to rigidly.

Should a reaction occur the transfusion should be stopped immediately, the blood saved (in an aseptic manner) and the line kept open with normal saline.

The principles of treatment of a severe reaction involve giving large doses of hydrocortisone intravenously, promoting a diuresis, and treating shock (see page 109) and renal failure (see page 590). Mild reactions are usually self-limiting, and recovery is spontaneous.

Mechanical causes

Anaemia may occur in situations where blood cells may be crushed or fragmented such as during a very fast, large blood transfusion or where extracorporeal blood lines are used, as in haemodialysis or cardiopulmonary bypass. The condition is self-limiting and no treatment is necessary.

HAEMORRHAGIC ANAEMIA

Haemorrhagic anaemia is anaemia due to acute or chronic blood loss.

Acute blood loss

A healthy adult can lose about 500 ml of blood without any ill effect. If more blood is lost the patient's compensatory mechanisms will become active reducing the blood flow to the skin and peripheries and causing the symptoms of shock.

Immediately following a haemorrhage there is no fall in the Hb level, even though the blood volume may be greatly reduced; but if the volume is replaced with fluid other than whole blood, the patient's blood is diluted and the Hb level starts to fall. In order to prevent and to treat this condition, it must be remembered that *when whole blood is lost, whole blood must be replaced* (see Chapter 11).

Chronic blood loss

Chronic blood loss does not cause blood volume depletion as the body's compensatory mechanisms keep the amount of blood stable. Chronic blood loss itself is never responsible for anaemia as such, but for depletion of iron stores and thence iron deficiency anaemia.

Chronic blood loss can only occur in 2 areas without the patient being aware of the loss. Blood can be lost in excessive amounts over long periods via the vagina and may be allowed to continue because of the patient's ignorance of what is normal. Chronic blood loss can also occur from high in the gastrointestinal tract, and, because of partial digestion, it may go unnoticed because it does not appear to be frank bleeding. A full gastrointestinal examination must always be performed whenever chronic blood loss is the suspected cause of iron deficiency anaemia.

INCREASED ERYTHROPOIESIS

Polycythaemia

In polycythaemia there is an increase in the number of erythrocytes. This is often accompanied by an increase in thrombocytes and granulocytes. Polycythaemia may be relative or actual.

Relative or spurious polycythaemia occurs when the plasma/cell ratio is altered in dehydration, burns, and (for unknown reasons) stress. Spurious (stress) polycythaemia occurs usually in middle aged males with high stress levels; it may be accompanied by hypertension and vascular disease. Actual polycythaemia occurs when there is a physiological stimulus such as chronic hypoxia, which causes excess haemopoietin to be produced and there is a resultant increase in erythrocyte mass. It can also occur as a consequence of a pathological increase in haemopoietin, which may occur in response to a tumour of the liver, kidney, bronchus, uterus, or cerebellum (haemangioblastoma) and in the presence of renal cysts.

In both relative and actual polycythaemia, the leucocytes and thrombocytes are usually normal. When erythrocytes proliferate without the stimulus of erythropoietin, primary polycythaemia, or polycythaemia vera, is present.

Clinical manifestations of polycythaemia vera

This condition occurs more commonly in males than in females and is seen predominantly over the age of 40. It may be asymptomatic and is diagnosed incidentally. The patient may present with peripheral vascular disease, loss of concentration, headache, dizziness, syncope, pruritis of the legs, epistaxis, and indigestion. The patient will usually have a red face, suffused conjunctiva, a dark red palate, and dark red-purple hands. On examination of the eye, retinal vein engorgement may be seen; the spleen is palpable in 75% of cases. Peptic ulceration is common in these patients.

Investigative procedures

The diagnosis is made on the clinical history and examination together with the fact that the Hb is greater than 18 g/dl in the male and 16 g/dl in the female. Leucocyte and thrombocyte counts may be raised, and the bone marrow is very active. Neutrophil alkaline phosphatase (NAP) is normal to raised and the urate levels are often high.

Medical management

Venesection is the simplest and most effective therapeutic measure and 500 ml of blood may be removed every second day until the Hb and haematocrit levels are normal. This will cause the patient to become iron deficient, and this deficiency is usually not corrected as the low serum iron will serve to reduce erythropoiesis. Venesection must be performed with extreme care if the thrombocyte level is high as it may induce thrombotic episodes. Radioactive phosphorus (P^{32}) may be used when a positive diagnosis is made; this is an extremely effective form of treatment, the full effects of which will not be seen for 3 months. (See Chapter 13 for the nursing management of the patient undergoing radioactive therapy.) Cytotoxic therapy with busulphan or melphalan may be used.

There is no specific nursing care for these patients as the majority undergo venesection at a local blood bank, or may be hospitalized on a daily basis for venesection. Patients with pruritis, leg ulcers or other accompanying conditions will require nursing care according to the presentation of these conditions.

Anticipated outcome

The average life span after diagnosis in patients undergoing treatment exceeds 10 years and some patients survive for more than 20 years.

The patient may enter a refractory state with a chronic anaemia which progresses to myelofibrosis or acute leukaemia; however this occurs in only a minority of persons with polycythaemia vera.

42

Disorders of the leucocytes and lymph

Jenny Cater   Robyn Anderson

NEUTROPENIA AND AGRANULOCYTOSIS

Neutropenia (leukopenia) is a reduction in the number of leucocytes whilst agranulocytosis is the complete absence of these cells. Therefore, the ability of a patient to produce an inflammatory response will be severely compromised.

Aetiology

Agranulocytosis is often the result of idiosyncrasy or a sensitivity to, or poisoning by, a variety of drugs and chemicals. Amongst these substances are chlorpromazine, chloramphenicol, chlorothiazide, chlorpropamide, phenindione, phenylbutazone, sulphonamides, and the thiouracil derivatives. Insecticides, cytotoxic drugs, and large irradiation doses may also cause the condition, and it may accompany leukaemia and hypersplenism. In some cases there is no discernable cause (ideopathic agranulocytosis).

Investigative procedures

A bone marrow biopsy will show an almost complete lack of granular cells, and in some patients early myelocytes may be seen. There may be indications of an underlying blood disease.

Full blood examination and differential count will show an absence or marked lowering of the number of granulocytes.

Clinical manifestations

The history may show exposure to one of the toxic agents mentioned above. The onset may be gradual or sudden. Often the presenting symptom is a sore throat which may be accompanied by fever and rigors. The patient may be extremely ill. The surface layers of the mouth and throat may ulcerate and there may be obvious patches of necrosis. Death from toxaemia may occur in this early stage. In more chronic cases the neutropenia may appear in 3–4 week periods in regular cycles. The patient presents with malaise, mild fever and sore throat without the necrosis and ulceration.

Medical and nursing management

All substances capable of causing this condition must be used with great care and the patient should be informed of what symptoms and signs to be aware.

The treatment involves removal of the precipitating factor, chemical, or drug, and prevention or treatment of septicaemia.

High dose IV infusions of antibiotics are used to treat and to prevent this condition. The patients mouth may become colonized with *Candida albicans* and should this occur, nystatin solution or lozenges together with parenteral nystatin in large doses will be given.

If the condition resolves quickly the patient should recover without any lasting problems. However, if the bone marrow does not return to normal bone marrow transplantation may be undertaken (see page 403). Although technically this is not particularly difficult and donors are relatively easy to find, the procedure is not enormously effective. Blood transfusion or transfusion of white cells may be effective as an intermediary measure. The patient must be nursed in reverse isolation (see page 399). All orifices must be swabbed and the swabs cultured on at least a weekly basis. Wounds, hair, skin, sputum, and urine specimens should also be regularly cultured and any potentially dangerous organism eradicated.

The patient and his significant others will need to completely understand his condition, and counselling is mandatory.

The patient is ill, looks and feels unwell and may have an ulcerated mouth and lips; his teeth may loosen and he will have significant halitosis. He requires gentle and understanding care and a great deal of attention to oral hygiene.

Anticipated outcome

The patient may return home and can live a normal life if and when his bone marrow is functioning normally and his blood count returns to normal.

INFECTIVE MONONUCLEOSIS (GLANDULAR FEVER)

This is an acute benign infectious disease which is caused by the Epstein-Barr virus. It is seen predominantly in adolescents and young adults of both sexes. It may occur sporadically or in epidemics and is frequently spread by oral contact. The incubation period is 10 days to 4 weeks.

Clinical manifestations

The patient will present with tiredness, malaise, headache, anorexia, and low grade fever. The superficial lymph nodes, particularly of the neck, are enlarged and tender, and petechial haemorrhages may occur at the junction of the soft and hard palate. In 9–10% of patients in whom ampicillin may have been used to treat the sore throat a drug rash will occur, the liver is tender and the spleen may be palpable. Mesenteric adenitis will be indicated by pain in the right iliac fossa.

Investigative procedures

In the early stages the leucocyte count is normal to low, and after the first few days mononucleosis will become obvious. After the first week the Paul-Bunnell reaction becomes positive in more than 80% of cases and will remain positive for weeks. The Monospot test is simple to perform and is used for initial screening.

Medical and nursing management

There is no specific treatment; symptoms are treated as they occur and the patient should rest in bed during the acute phase. Recovery will be complete but the convalescent period may last for months with the patient feeling weak and with an intermittent fever; depression and poor concentration are common during this period.

LEUKAEMIA

Leukaemia is the neoplastic proliferation of haemopoietic or lymphopoietic cells. The cells are of incomplete maturation and their function is compromised. Leukaemia originates in the bone marrow and may infiltrate lymph nodes, liver, spleen, and other tissues.

The leukaemias differ in presentation, age of onset, course of disease, response to treatment, and prognosis. Therefore it is important to identify whether a patient has acute or chronic leukaemia and if the leukaemia is myeloid (granulocytic) or lymphoid in histology.

Aetiology

Environmental and genetic causes have been implicated. However in the majority of cases no definite cause can be identified. Aetiological factors include:

• Ionizing radiation. Following the bombing of Hiroshima and Nagasaki there was a considerable increase in the incidence of acute and chronic myeloid leukaemia. Patients previously irradiated for Hodgkin's disease have an increased risk of developing leukaemia. Also, maternal irradiation during pregnancy increases the likelihood of the child developing leukaemia.
• Chemical and drug exposure. Leukaemia may develop as a second malignancy following treatment using alkylating agents (for example

melphalan) or combination chemotherapy, for example in Hodgkin's disease.
• Genetic factors. When an identical twin has leukaemia there is a considerably increased risk that the other twin will also develop leukaemia.
• Viruses and immunologic deficiencies have been implicated although this is not proven.

Chronic myeloid leukaemia (CML)

CML is the proliferation of the myeloid cells in the bone marrow, and extramedullary sites, liver, and spleen. These cells are mature or partially immature with mild functional impairment. The age of onset varies; CML rarely occurs before the age of 20 and increases in frequency in middle and advanced age. The onset of CML is insidious and is often diagnosed incidentally during routine medical examination.

Clinical manifestations

Symptoms at presentation include malaise, fatigue, heat intolerance, sweating, pallor, and weight loss and are associated with anaemia and increased basal metabolic rate. Abdominal discomfort and early satiety or fullness whilst eating is due to splenic enlargement.

On examination of the patient the physician or nurse will note pallor, warm moist skin, low grade fever, and splenomegaly. Bone tenderness, particularly the sternum, occurs when the marrow's cellularity increases within a short period of time. Lymph nodes are rarely enlarged.

Investigative procedures

A full blood examination will reveal an increased leucocyte count in the range of 100 000–300 000 per mm^3, and anaemia and thrombocytopenia may be present.

Bone marrow biopsy demonstrates a hypercellular marrow with decreased fat; and granulocytes (myeloid cells) are greatly increased in number and resemble those in the circulation, but are less mature.

Biochemical analysis of blood often reveals hyperuricaemia, due to the breakdown of granulocytes.

Clinical course

During the early stages of the disease patients may be asymptomatic or show the above symptoms. This is referred to as the chronic stage of disease and patients may remain in this stage for 3–4 years. However, many patients will undergo acute transformation or 'blastic crisis'. In these patients the disease appears to be under control when they rapidly develop an increased leucocyte count. There is a large number of blastic (immature) cells in the blood and bone marrow. Symptoms of increased fatigue, fever, haemorrhage, weight loss, infection, and hepatosplenomegaly are noted. At this stage CML responds poorly to treatment and death ensues in a matter of months.

Medical management

During the chronic stage of CML, treatment with chemotherapy has not shown an increased life span, although it does improve the quality of life. Therefore the aim of therapy is to control symptoms. The drug of choice is busulfan. It is given orally and the patient managed as an outpatient. Localized radiotherapy to the spleen has been used to reduce splenomegaly. However, as it does not improve survival time, chemotherapy is still thought to be more effective.

Once a patient has entered the acute stage of their disease, response to treatment is very poor. The blood cells in this stage are extremely resistant to aggressive chemotherapy and radiotherapy.

Nursing management

During the chronic stage of CML patients generally have a good quality of life, and rarely require hospitalization. Once the disease has entered the acute or blastic stage a patient requires hospitalization and frequent packed cell transfusion. The nursing management is akin to that of a patient with acute leukaemia (see page 399).

Chronic lymphocytic leukaemia (CLL)

CLL is the most common form of leukaemia seen in Western countries. In this disease there is an increased proliferation and a prolonged survival time of lymphocytes leading to their accumulation in the marrow, blood, liver, spleen, and lymph nodes.

The age of onset is generally older than that seen in CML. 90% of patients with CLL are over 50 years of age, and nearly two-thirds are over 60. CLL occurs more frequently in males.

Ionizing radiation is not a factor in the aetiology of CLL, however there is a strong familial pattern. There have been many cases of multiple family members affected with CLL and this has led to genetic factors being implicated as the cause, although research has not proven this.

The onset is insidious and the patient is often asymptomatic. Diagnosis is often made on routine medical examination or when the patient presents with an unrelated illness. When symptoms are present they include malaise, fatigue, weight loss, enlargement of superficial lymph nodes, and splenomegally.

Physical findings frequently include superficial lymph node enlargement and splenomegally.

Investigative procedures

These include:

• Full blood examination, which may show mild anaemia: anaemia increases when the lymphocyte count increases. Thrombocyte count is often normal or may be slightly decreased. There is a marked increase in the leucocytes, with a predominance of lymphocytes. Positive diagnosis can be made on the FBE.
• Bone marrow biopsy is rarely necessary for a positive diagnosis. Indication for marrow biopsy is when diagnosis is in doubt (usually early in the disease).
• Lymph node biopsy is only performed if the nature of the enlargement is in doubt.

Routine investigations to assess a patient's general health should be performed. These include serum urea and electrolytes, chest X-ray, and ECG.

Medical management

CLL is an indolent disease, and may continue to be asymptomatic for years. Treatment does not result in a cure, and the aim is to palliate symptoms. Patients should be assessed regularly and an FBE performed. When the patient presents with symptoms of anaemia, infection, bleeding, lymph node enlargement causing obstruction, or progressive splenomegally, then treatment should be initiated to control the symptoms and improve the quality of life.

Treatment of choice is chemotherapy. The drugs that have been most valuable include chlorambucil, cyclophosphamide and prednisolone. Medication is often given orally and patients rarely require admission to hospital. However, as the disease progresses the patient may require regular packed cell transfusion for persistent anaemia. Radiotherapy may be useful in reducing the size of lymph nodes or the spleen.

Splenectomy may be helpful in the treatment of CLL if thrombocytopenia and anaemia is not controlled by chemotherapy. An enlarged spleen produces cytopenias due to increased destruction or excessive pooling of thrombocytes and erythrocytes and therefore removal of the spleen may be of benefit.

Nursing management

A patient with CLL is mainly managed as an outpatient, however as the disease progresses and anaemia becomes more marked, he may require frequent packed cell transfusion. At this stage the patient often feels lethargic, tired, and has dyspnoea on mild exertion. The nurse needs to give psychological support and suggest frequent rest periods and a high nutrient diet. Activities should be encouraged and planned around rest periods. When the disease becomes resistant to therapy, the patient will require hospitalization as a result of infection and haemorrhagic episodes. (See nursing care of the patient with acute leukaemia, page 399.)

Anticipated outcome

CLL may continue in the chronic phase for up to 10 years and these patients may lead a relatively normal life. When the disease becomes resistant to treatment prognosis is poor and death results in 2–6 months. A few patients die of causes unrelated to their CLL and this is mainly due to disorders occurring in old age.

Acute myeloid leukaemia (AML)

AML is characterized by the uncontrolled growth of immature, functionally impaired cells. These cells are referred to as blast (or leukaemia) cells and arise in the bone marrow. The presence of blast cells in the bone marrow prevents normal haemopoiesis of erythrocytes, granulocytes, and megakaryocytes, leading to the symptoms of weakness, fatigue, pallor, infection, and haemorrhage.

Classification of AML

There are several histologic classifications of AML which include:

– Acute myeloblastic leukaemia
– Acute myelomonocytic leukaemia
– Acute monocytic leukaemia
– Acute erythroleukaemia
– Acute megakaryocytic leukaemia.

The blast cells responsible for each of these leukaemic forms arise from the same haemopoietic stem cell, and as each leukaemic form is similar in behaviour and response to treatment they shall all be discussed as AML.

AML occurs more frequently in adults (80% of cases), however it is seen in all age groups.

Clinical manifestations

Patients commonly present with symptoms of:

● Fatigue, dyspnoea on exertion, palpatations, or pallor due to anaemia.
● Bruising, petechiae, epistaxis, or gingival bleeding as a result of thrombocytopenia.
● Infection, skin abscess, failure of a minor cut or wound to heal, or systemic infection causing fever and chills due to neutropenia.
● Anorexia and weight loss.
● Abdominal fullness due to splenomegally (occurs in approximately 30–35% of patients).
● Bone tenderness and aching joints due to leukaemic infiltration.

On examination the patient is often pale, has an obvious loss of weight, is febrile and has bruises or petechiae. He may also have symptoms and signs of a chest infection and/or splenomegaly.

Investigative procedure

These include:

● FBE. This reveals anaemia, thrombocytopenia, and neutropenia. Leucocyte count may be normal or slightly increased, however there are immature blast cells present, which may range up to 95% of the total leucocytes.
● Bone marrow biopsy. There is a marked decrease in normal erythropoiesis, granulopoiesis, and megakaryopoiesis, with an overcrowding of immature cells of the myeloid series.
● Serum electrolytes. Hyperuricaemia may be present due to increased cellular turnover.

Routine investigations should include chest X-ray and ECG.

Medical management

The aim of treatment is to induce a remission; that is, there are no blast cells on FBE and less than 5% on bone marrow biopsy, associated with a return to normal haemopoiesis.

Prior to commencing treatment it is important to correct any bleeding abnormalities and infections.

Chemotherapy is the treatment of choice and the drugs that have proven to be most clinically effective include cytosine arabinoside, adriamycin, and 6-thioguanine; numerous other cytotoxic agents have been tried but these are the most effective. Of all patients treated with chemotherapy the majority achieve remission. However, remission induction is also associated with morbidity and mortality due to severe marrow hypoplasia and pancytopenia caused by the disease and cytotoxic drugs. Complications of anaemia, thrombocytopenia and neutropenia inevitably occur. Transfusion with packed cells, thrombocytes and leucocytes is often necessary following initial diagnosis. Intravenous antibiotic therapy is frequently necessary during remission induction, and antibiotics should be commenced whenever the patient's temperature reaches 38°C. Should the patient develop pyrexia then blood cultures, MSU, nose, throat, axilla and groin swabs, stool culture, and swabs of any wounds are obtained in an attempt to locate the source of infection. As well, weekly microbiological and virological swabs and/or specimens are routinely obtained in the management of AML patients in many haematological units.

Once remission is induced the patient commences the next stage of treatment, maintenance chemotherapy. The aim of maintenance chemotherapy is to increase the length of remission. The drugs used are similar to those used to induce remission, however they are given in smaller doses on an outpatient basis. Pancytopenia is rarely a problem during maintenance chemotherapy. Patients are usually reasonably healthy and may continue a normal daily routine, within their physical tolerance. The length of time a patient remains on maintenance chemotherapy varies according to the response of the condition to treatment and the medical regime being instituted.

Bone marrow transplantation is proving to be successful in the treatment and possible cure for patients with AML. Prior to transplantation supralethal doses of total body irradiation and chemotherapy are given to render the patient's bone marrow aplastic, thereby eradicating the leukaemia. The condition of marrow aplasia exposes the patient to the extreme risk of overwhelming infection.

Nursing management

The nursing management of the patient with AML is covered on page 399, and of the patient undergoing bone marrow transplantation on page 405.

Anticipated outcome

Following diagnosis of AML, the patient will require lengthy hospitalization during remission induction treatment. The patient is often nursed in a single room to protect him from infections. However episodes of infection and anaemia are common, due to marrow hypoplasia.

Most patients relapse (that is, display the presence of blast cells in bone marrow and peripheral blood) between 1–2 years following remission induction.

The patient is hospitalized when relapse is diagnosed, and attempts are made to produce a second remission. However second and subsequent remissions are difficult to attain and are short lasting. Death most commonly occurs due to an overwhelming infection, for example septicaemia, and some patients may die from haemorrhage. Prior to the advent of chemotherapy the survival time for patients with AML was extremely short – as little as 8 weeks from diagnosis. With intensive chemotherapy programmes the survival time has been increased to over a year and some patients survive 5 years or longer following treatment. Hope lies in lengthening remission times and achieving cure with bone marrow transplantation.

Acute lymphocytic leukaemia (ALL)

ALL is a malignant proliferation of lymphocyte precursors (lymphoblasts) originating in the bone marrow and perhaps in lymph nodes and the thymus. It effects mainly children, and is the most common neoplasm in children. With excessive lymphoblasts in the marrow there is a decreased production of granulocytes, erythrocytes, and megakaryocytes due to overcrowding. This causes anaemia, thrombocytopenia, and neutropenia.

The peak incidence of ALL is between 2–4 years and a second, smaller, peak is seen in the 60–70 year age group.

Clinical manifestations

The onset is acute with a short history; symptoms are usually present for no more than a few weeks prior to diagnosis. Fatigue, lethargy, fever accompanying recurrent infections, bleeding and bruising, and pallor, are nearly always present. Other symptoms and signs include: generalized lymphadenopathy, bone or joint pain, abdominal fullness (hepatosplenomegally), anorexia, nausea, and vomiting.

Physical findings include: pallor due to anaemia, petechiae and bruising caused by thrombocytopenia, febrile episodes with sweating related to infection, and neutropenia. There may also be superficial lymph node enlargement, and hepatosplenomegaly. Bone pain and tenderness is related to lymphoblastic activity.

Investigative procedures

Investigations carried out to determine the diagnosis include:

- FBE. The total leucocyte count may be normal or slightly elevated, however there is a predominance of blast cells. Granulocyte and thrombocyte counts are low and anaemia is present.
- Bone marrow biopsy. This will reveal a hypercellular marrow with mainly lymphoblasts. Normal haemopoietic cells are decreased.
- Serum urea and electrolytes. These will vary according to the extent of disease and the disturbance to normal systemic function, however they are usually normal.

Other investigations should include: lumbar puncture to assess for CNS involvement, and a routine chest X-ray.

Medical management

Treatment is aimed at inducing a remission. Drugs of most benefit in treating ALL include prednisolone, vincristine, adriamycin, and L-asparaginase. Following treatment with these agents, complete remission is achieved in nearly all children under 10 years of age and most teenagers and adults.

Maintenance chemotherapy is given to lengthen the period of remission because if treatment is ceased at remission then relapse soon follows. By continuing maintenance chemotherapy, long term remission is attained along with the possibility of cure. Maintenance treatment is therefore continued for 2–3 years. Drugs used in maintenance chemotherapy include 6-mercaptopurine and methotrexate orally.

ALL has a high incidence of central nervous system involvement, which commonly presents when the bone marrow is in remission. Therefore to prevent this involvement most haematologists recommend prophylactic cranial irradiation and intrathecal methotraxate once remission is achieved.

Nursing management

Nursing management for the patient with acute leukaemia is covered below.

Anticipated outcome

Treatment of childhood ALL with intensive remission induction chemotherapy, followed by maintenance treatment and prophylactic central nervous system therapy has led to long-term remissions. Survival commonly is 5 years with the majority of patients appearing to be cured of their disease.

Relapses are more noted in males and there is a high incidence of recurrence involving metastizing tumours of the testes; treatment for testicular involvement is irradiation of the testes.

For patients who relapse, remission induction treatment is recommenced and most achieve a second remission. However second remission is inevitably shorter and is associated with a poorer prognosis.

In patients who are 15 years or older ALL is less responsive to treatment leading to survival of only approximately 2 years. A small proportion of adult patients remain in remission for several years and there are few survivors after 5 years.

Nursing management of the leukaemic patient

The leukaemic patient frequently requires intensive highly skilled nursing care. A health team comprising medical and nursing personnel, a dietitian, social worker, and pharmacy staff is essential in co-ordinating the care necessary for a leukaemic patient.

Patients often present with marrow hypoplasia manifested by anaemia resulting in lethargy and fatigue; thrombocytopenia leading to haemorrhagic tendencies; and neutropenia leaving the patient susceptible to infection. All of these problems are further compounded by any active treatment. Complications of treatment frequently encountered include nausea, vomiting, anorexia, stomatitis, mucosal ulceration, alopecia, constipation, diarrhoea, electrolyte imbalances, possible infertility, and renal damage.

The psychological effects of a diagnosis of leukaemia is often devastating for the patient and his significant others. It is difficult for people to face their own mortality and this is compounded by the fear of suffering and what is to be endured as part of the disease and its treatment. Being nursed in protective isolation can reinforce a patient's feeling of loneliness and produce a reactive depression. Other areas of consideration in treatment choice include: whether or not the patient attends school; the effect the diagnosis will have on his relationship with his peers; how he will maintain his studies; and if the patient is the bread-winner in the family, how the family will cope with his lengthy hospitalization and convalescence.

As nursing staff spend more time with patients than do medical staff, dietitians, or social workers, it is not uncommon for a patient with leukaemia to express his fears and feelings to the nursing staff caring for him. The nurse needs to have excellent listening skills, to be understanding and not judgemental, and to appreciate the problems and stresses that the patient is enduring. If necessary the nurse will need to seek a referral for the patient to a chaplain or a social worker.

Building rapport with the patient's family and/or significant others is also important as their co-operation often enhances the degree of patient compliance with treatment; it also involves them in the patient's care. The establishment of a therapeutic relationship with the patient's family and/or significant others also minimizes their stress, and the stress on the care givers, during crisis periods in the patient's treatment. Care must be taken, however, that the patient does not feel that his significant others are 'siding' with hospital staff against him.

The nurse must be prepared to provide care for a patient who will most probably have: thrombocytopenia and therefore have a bleeding tendency; leucopenia with absolute neutropenia and therefore be unable to fight infection; anaemia and therefore have a poor tolerance to exercise and effort; and be experiencing a variety of effects from the treatment of the disorder and their response to the illness.

Nursing management may therefore include:

• Measures to reduce and/or prevent haemorrhage, for example: regularly check skin and mouth for signs of petechiae; perform daily urinalysis for haematuria; test faeces for occult blood; provide a soft toothbrush or cotton buds to clean teeth and gums and thereby reduce the risk of trauma and bleeding; provide an electric razor to shave instead of a blade razor; inform the patient to be careful not to bump or injure himself; apply lanoline to the lips to prevent dryness and cracking that can lead to bleeding; withhold asprin or asprin-containing substances; apply a pressure bandage following any venepuncture; and avoid the needless taking of blood pressure readings.

• Measures to reduce and/or prevent infection. The nurse must realize that the pathogen is commonly one of the patient's own normal flora and all nursing care should aim at minimizing opportunistic infection, for example: reverse barrier nurse the patient in a single room (see page 404); prohibit patient contact with staff and visitors who have infections; record temperature, pulse, and ventilation on a regular basis and report any rise in temperature over 37.5°C; organize nursing care to occur in blocks of time rather than allowing constant contact with the patient; examine the patient's skin daily for reddened or broken areas; inspect the patient's oral cavity daily for signs of fungal infection; provide mouth care strictly as ordered and ensure at least 2–4 hourly mouth rinses with an antifungal agent; ensure that the patient washes daily; and regularly inspect skin folds for moisture as these are likely sites for fungal infection.

• Measures to relieve the effects of anaemia. Nursing measures should ensure that the patient receives adequate sleep and rest, and that he avoids overexertion.

• Measures to minimize effects of treatment:

– Alopecia. Inform the patient that this may occur and reassure him that hair will regrow when the treatment is completed. If necessary refer the patient for the fitting of a wig.

– Nausea and vomiting. Offer small meals, free of fried and fatty foodstuffs, and position the patient comfortably at all times. Administer antiemetics as ordered. Maintain an accurate fluid balance chart; excessive vomiting may lead to dehydration and electrolyte imbalance, thus further compounding the effects of treatment.

– Anorexia. Encourage the patient to eat when he is hungry; this may not necessarily be at established mealtimes; offer smaller meals more frequently and ensure that they are attractively served; offer food that the patient prefers; offer wine or beer prior to meals if this is permitted; ensure that the patient's environment is conducive to eating at meal times, for example, remove offensive articles prior to meals being served.

– Stomatitis and mouth ulcers. During the day the patient should be provided with mouth washes 2-hourly and teeth should be cleaned and gums massaged with a very soft bristled toothbrush. If the patient wears dentures these should be removed and only replaced at meal times or when he has visitors. Regular oral fluids and a soft diet free of acid and spicy foodstuffs should be provided and the patient should be advised to avoid extremely hot or cold foodstuffs and fluids. Lanolin should be applied to the lips to avoid dryness and cracking.

– Diarrhoea. The nurse must maintain an accurate record of fluid balance as excessive, untreated diarrhoea may lead to electrolyte imbalance. Ensure a high fluid intake, and avoid foodstuffs high in fibre, such as raw fruit and vegetables, whole grain cereals, nuts, and citrus fruit juices. Administer antidiarrhoeal drugs as ordered. These measures must be balanced by the need to avoid constipation (see below). The patient's perianal area should be kept clean and swabbed with povidone-iodine twice a day to avoid infection; it may be necessary to apply lanoline to the anal area.

– Constipation. This can be avoided by increasing fibre in the patient's diet in the form of bran added to breakfast cereal or by allowing some fruit and raw vegetables. If necessary, administer an aperient or a faecal wetting agent. The nurse should be observant for the symptoms and signs of a possible bowel obstruction (see page 528).

– Manifestation of alteration to sexual/reproductive function. In women amenorrhoea may result but if menstruation occurs a record is kept of the approximate amount of blood lost. The female patient may be ordered hormonal therapy to prevent menstruation and therefore any risk of excessive bleeding whilst undergoing treatment. The female patient should be advised to avoid pregnancy and the male should be advised to avoid fathering a child, as foetal deformities may result. However, infertility is the usual result

from treatment for both sexes. For males sperm may be deposited in a bank prior to commencement of treatment.

– Renal damage. The nurse must maintain an accurate record of fluid balance and observe and report any symptoms or signs of fluid retention or dehydration. Intravenous therapy should be maintained as ordered.

Caring for the leukaemic or immunosuppressed patient can be demanding both physically and emotionally. There is a challenge for the nurse to coordinate and administer efficient care, as well as to be aware of the possible problems of treatment that may occur and to be able to recognize them early. Nursing leukaemic patients can become very rewarding, especially when rapport is built with the patient and his significant others.

The nursing management of a patient with a Hickman's catheter in situ

The Hickman's catheter is a flexible silicone rubber catheter which is inserted into a large vein to provide long term venous access for the infusion of fluid, blood products, chemotherapy, other medications, and nutrients. It eliminates the need for repeated cannulation and/or venepuncture for blood sampling.

Insertion of the catheter is performed in the operating room and the patient is prepared for surgery as for any general anaesthetic. In addition the anterior chest wall is shaved. The operative procedure involves a subclavicular incision and identification of the subclavian vein. A tunnel is made by separating the skin from the chest wall. The tunnel extends from the initial incision to the level of the base of the mediastinum where a second incision is made. The catheter is pulled through this tunnel until the small roughened cuff on the catheter is positioned at the opening made by the second incision (Fig. 42.1).

The catheter is initially held in position with sutures which are removed 8–10 days postoperatively. As the cuff initiates an inflammatory reaction at its site, fibrosis of the surrounding tissue occurs and it is this which holds the catheter securely in position.

An incision is made in the subclavian vein and the tip of the catheter is passed through this inci-

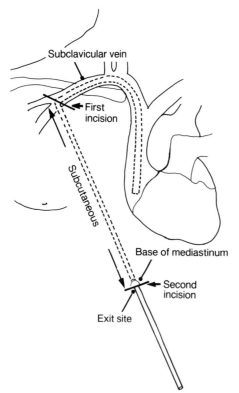

Subclavicular vein

First incision

Subcutaneous

Base of mediastinum

Second incision

Exit site

Fig. 42.1 Hickman catheter in situ.

sion and fed along the vein and into the right atrium. An image intensifier is utilized in ascertaining the correct position of the catheter, and once in position the subclavicular incision is sutured. These sutures may be removed 8–10 days postoperatively, or when healing has occurred.

Postoperatively the nurse must observe the patient for any signs of haemorrhage, or displacement of the catheter. An intravenous infusion will, in most cases, be in progress.

The Hickman's catheter may remain in situ for up to 2 years and it does not require continuous intravenous infusion to remain patent. It may be 'worn' capped, covered by a small dressing which is easily hidden under clothing. The exit site is dressed daily and heparin flushed through the catheter 3 times a week when not in use. Therefore it is important that the patient is taught how to dress and flush the catheter and to be aware of the signs of infection, and a blockage in or damage to the catheter.

The nurse must dress the wound, take blood samples, and flush the catheter. The techniques

utilized vary between health care agencies and local policies and regulations will apply.

When caring for a patient with a Hickman's catheter in situ the nurse must:

● Be proficient in aseptic technique and dressing change procedure.
● Educate the patient in care and self-care of the catheter.
● Be proficient in taking blood samples and setting up intravenous infusions via the catheter.
● Be aware of the symptoms and signs of catheter blockage and be able to observe the patient for signs of onset. Risks of blockages will be minimized if the catheter is flushed with heparin following blood sampling, at the completion of intravenous therapy, and every second day whilst the catheter is not in use. Blockage rarely occurs when infusions are kept running and the catheter is not allowed to empty.
● Be aware of the possibility of infection of the exit site, or infection via the catheter. To prevent infection, the nurse attending the dressing must use an aseptic technique.
● Know that when changing the cap, or commencing/completing intravenous therapy, that the catheter *must* be clamped to prevent either haemorrhage from an unstoppered vein, or air entry due to a negative central venous pressure.

It is the responsibility of the nurse to educate the patient about catheter care and to advise the patient against swimming to minimize the incidence of infection. However, the patient may continue to shower or bath with no restriction. He should be advised to attend to his dressing after showering/bathing. The patient must be warned that he should carry clamps with him at all times and a spare cap, in case damage to the catheter occurs and results in leakage. Should this happen he must apply the clamps between himself and the damaged area of the catheter to prevent further leakage, and attend the hospital immediately to have the catheter repaired.

He must also be taught how to perform a sterile dressing change, and how to flush the catheter. The patient should note any sign of infection, for example redness or exudate from around the catheter exit site. When flushing the catheter with heparinized saline he should be aware of any resistance to the flow of fluid or an inability to flush the catheter. He must report to hospital immediately should he experience any difficulty with catheter management.

BONE MARROW TRANSPLANTATION

Despite the advances which have been made in the treatment of leukaemia, prior to bone marrow transplantation there were few long-term survivors. 95% of patients with acute myeloid leukaemia and 50% of patients with acute lymphocytic leukaemia died due to the complications of their disease. With the advent of bone marrow transplantation there is now hope for a cure but, unfortunately, the procedure is not without its problems.

The availability of a donor, and the intensive workup regime required are problems encountered prior to transplantation. Following the transplantation there are a number of complications which may prove fatal. The most common include immunosuppression, graft versus host disease (GVHD), graft rejection, and resistant leukaemia.

Bone marrow transplantation involves the harvest of marrow by aspiration from the donor, and its intravenous infusion into the patient. This is a hazardous procedure and there are several factors that contribute to its complexity. The pre-transplantation conditioning of the patient involves supralethal doses of chemotherapy and radiotherapy. This is followed by the 'rescue' or transplantation. The aim of the chemoradiotherapeutic regime is to eradicate all leukaemic (blast) cells from the patient, to achieve immunosuppression and myelosuppression, and to minimize GVHD.

There are 4 types of bone marrow transplantation, classified according to the source of transplanted marrow. This may be:

- A related donor, for example a sibling (allogenic transplantation)
- An unrelated donor
- An identical twin to the patient (syngenic transplantation)
- The patient's own marrow (allogenic transplantation).

The allogenic transplantation is the most common and occurs when the donor and patient are human leucocyte antigen (HLA) cross-matched identical. The donor is usually a sibling as there is a 25% chance that 2 siblings will be HLA identical.

The possibility of finding an HLA identical individual who is unrelated is 1 : 10 000. The use of unrelated donors is therefore uncommon.

A syngenetic transplantation occurs when the patient is the identical twin of the donor. The advantage of a syngenetic transplantation is that the patient does not require treatment for GVHD. Unfortunately the chance of leukaemic relapse is higher in this type of transplantation.

As can be appreciated, a suitable donor is often difficult to find and this has led to experimentation with autologus bone marrow transplantation. Whilst in remission, bone marrow is taken from the patient and cryopreserved. Following the harvest of bone marrow the patient receives conventional therapy until relapse occurs. He is then treated with high doses of chemotherapy and radiotherapy followed by rescue with the autologous, cryopreserved remission bone marrow.

Patient selection for bone marrow transplantation

1. *Diagnosis.* Prior to selection for bone marrow transplantation, a definite diagnosis is necessary. Patients with the following conditions are usually the only persons considered:

- AML – during first remission
- ALL – during first remission if prognosis is poor, or after the first relapse. This is because long term remission may be gained by conventional therapy. Also children may be cured with conventional treatment
- CML – whilst the patient is in the chronic stage of his disease
- Aplastic anaemia
- Severe immune deficiency disease.

Research is continuing and perhaps in the future transplantation will be considered for other malignancies.

2. *Histocompatibility.* Compatibility of the donor is assessed on HLA cross-matching. ABO incompatibility does not necessarily preclude the possibility of transplantation.

3. *Remission.* Ideally, transplantation is performed during remission. The rationale being that the

leukaemic cell mass is minimal during remission of the disease state and the potential for total eradication of disease is greater, as the leukaemic cells have less opportunity of becoming resistant to therapy.

During remission the patient's condition is optimal, he is more able to cope with the grafting procedure, and the pre- and post-graft treatment regimens.

4. *Age*. The younger the patient the better he will tolerate the procedure. Overall survival statistics are highest for the under 20 age group. Patients over 30 years have a much lower survival rate. This has led to many centres refusing transplantation to those over 45 years of age.

5. *Assessment and investigatory procedures*. The remaining requirements prior to consideration for bone marrow transplantation are that the patient is in good health, has no cardiac insufficiency, and has no irreversible renal, hepatic or pulmonary disease.

Investigative procedures

Extensive investigatory procedures precede the transplantation and include:

– Full history, including doses of cytotoxic drugs previously given, previous radiotherapy, transfusions of blood products, and any previous infections, plus details of previous relapse.
– Medical and nursing history and physical assessment.
– Haematology: FBE, bone marrow aspiration, blood grouping, ABO cross-match with the donor.
– Biochemistry: urea and electrolytes, uric acid, creatine clearance, 24-hour protein, serum protein and immunoglobulins, liver function tests.
– Cardiology: ECG, ejection fraction.
– Immunology: lymphocyte surface markers on peripheral blood.
– Microbiology: routine nose, throat, and skin cultures.
– Virology: stool culture, MSU, baseline virology titres of cytomegalovirus (CMV), herpes zoster, herpes simplex, measles, hepatitis B.
– Full lung studies, chest X-ray.

The majority of these investigations are performed prior to admission thus decreasing the period of hospitalization.

Isolation

The patient is neutropenic during the period of admission covering transplantation, due to the induction therapy and thus requires isolation to protect him from infection.

Some units nurse the patient in a single room and visitors and staff wash their hands prior to entering the room. Visitors and staff with any infection are not permitted to visit or care for the patient, and he is not permitted to leave the room until his white cell count and neutrophil count have been restored to a level that affords protection against infection.

Other units may nurse the patient in a laminar flow room or bed. The room is cleaned with an antiseptic solution; all articles are sterilized before being taken into the room. Visitors are restricted to one or two per day. The patient is fed a sterile diet and receives antifungal agents to sterilize the gut. Staff and visitors entering the room wear sterile gowns, gloves, hats, boots, and masks, and any contact with the patient is kept to a minimum. Usually there is a phone or intercom system to enable the patient to communicate with people outside the room. In an attempt to reduce the likelihood of introducing infection to the patient, only one nurse per shift is assigned to care for the patient's needs; this has the disadvantage of increasing the patient's social isolation during this stressful period.

Even with stringent rules of total isolation some patients still acquire infection during the neutropenic phase. Therefore it is debatable if such strict isolation is worth the expense and pyschological stress to the patient. The patient in isolation can feel as if he is in solitary confinement; his only 'crime' being that he is a victim of disease. The nurse needs to have excellent communcation skills, and he/she should be able to meet not only physical aspects of patient care, but to also ensure that his psychosocial and spiritual needs are met.

Induction of neutropenia

A Hickman's catheter is inserted into a large, central vein soon after admission (see page 402). Gut sterilization (if it is to be performed) commences on day 1 or 2 after admission and includes antifungal medications and the patient begins a sterile diet.

Chemotherapy

Prior to commencement of chemotherapy an anti-emetic and possibly a sedative is given. Cyclophosphamide is the chemotherapeutic agent given as part of the preparation for bone marrow transplantation. The dose given is 60 mg/kg on 2 consecutive days. Toxic effects of cyclophosphamide are common and the nurse should observe the patient for any signs of nausea and vomiting, fever, fluid retention, stomatitis, haemorrhage, cystitis, potential urate nephropathy, bone marrow suppression, alopecia and hypokalemia.

Where possible, these side effects are prevented; however, if they occur symptomatic treatment is given. The patient will receive 4-hourly flasks of intravenous fluid, to which are added sodium bicarbonate, potassium and posibly a diuretic to prevent haemorrhagic cystitis, hypokalaemia, and fluid retention. Intravenous therapy continues for at least 48 hours.

Antiemetics should be continued as ordered for at least 3 days and an accurate record of fluid balance is essential if output is not adequate to prevent renal complications then diuretics will need to be increased. The pH of all urine is examined. Alkaline urine will reduce the risk of bladder irritation, and thus the pH must be maintained above 7, with the aid of alkalizing drugs.

Total body irradiation

Total body irradiation may be given in one dose lasting approximately 1 hour or it may be 'fractionated' and divided over several days. Fractionation is associated with fewer of the potential complications of total body irradiation, which include: parotitis, alteration of taste, and reduction of saliva; mucositis leading to ulceration; pyrexia and chills for up to 48 hours; somnolence, which may persist for 6–8 weeks post therapy; lassitude; anorexia; nausea, vomiting, and diarrhoea; aspermia or ovarian failure; alopecia; and cataracts, which may occur 2 3 years post total body irradiation.

Harvest of marrow

The harvest of marrow from the donor is performed under a general anaesthetic. Marrow is aspirated from the anterior and/or posterior iliac crests. The procedure is similar to a bone marrow biopsy except that 5–10 ml are aspirated from each of 120–160 different sites. The marrow is collected in heparinized tubes to prevent coagulation, and filters remove bone chips, fat lobules, and clots as the marrow passes into a collection bag similar to an IV flask. Specimens of marrow are assessed for cell counts. The total amount harvested is between 600–1000 ml, and the procedure takes approximately 1–2 hours.

Postoperative nursing management of the donor patient is as for any person undergoing a general anaesthetic (see page 48) and the nurse must observe the patient carefully for any signs of haemorrhage from, and inflammation and/or infection of the donor sites. Narcotic analgesia will be required for at least 24–48 hours to control pain and the donor will need assistance when ambulating.

Transfusion of marrow

The marrow is similar in appearance to packed cells and is infused intravenously via the Hickman's catheter over 1–2 hours. During infusion the patient is observed for any reaction to the marrow – fever, chills, urticaria, and or pulmonary oedema may occur.

Following infusion of the marrow there is a temporary delay in its transit through the liver and spleen, however the donor's marrow will be found correctly located after one week. The marrow begins to 'take' or reproduce 2–3 weeks after infusion. Bone marrow biopsies are then performed regularly to assess whether or not there is adequate functioning of the donated marrow.

Nursing management of the immunosuppressed patient

The patient can be expected to be pancytopenic for a minimum of 3–4 weeks. The lengthy period of pancytopenia increases the possibility of infection and therefore nursing care is geared towards prevention of infection.

Immunosuppression increases the patient's risk of experiencing overwhelming infection and the nurse should aim to minimize patient contact with other persons, and/or infecting agents, until functional marrow produces protection against infection (see also page 393).

The patient's skin must be cleansed with an antiseptic soap once or twice a day. The skin is examined daily for petechiae, abrasions, and examined for integumentary signs of graft versus host disease (see below). An antiseptic solution, for example, povidine-iodine, is applied to the anal area twice a day and after each bowel action as perianal abscess is a common occurrence and when it occurs, the organism cultured is usually one of the patient's commensals.

The patient must receive 2-hourly mouth care during the day and 4-hourly at night. A soft toothbrush is used to prevent trauma to the oral mucosa and is changed every second day. The oral cavity is examined 3 times a day for signs of candidiasis, mucositus, and/or ulceration.

Patients who shave must use an electric razor, as blade razors cause trauma and lacerations to the intact skin surface. The patient's hair is brushed gently with a soft hairbrush.

The risk of haemorrhage and infection can be further reduced by ensuring that the patient does not receive intramuscular or subcutaneous injections, and that all parenteral medications are given via the Hickman's catheter. Blood samples are taken via the Hickman's catheter, thus eliminating the need for venepuncture, Care is taken to avoid injury: sharp instruments, for example safety pins, are not used to secure dressings, and scissors are not used to pare nails.

Blood pressure is not taken routinely, and invasive procedures such as urinary catheterization are discouraged unless absolutely necessary.

All urine, faeces, vomitus, and sputum are tested for blood. Suppositories and enemas are never given.

All persons entering the room must be free of infection and take appropriate hand-washing measures.

If the patient's temperature exceeds 37.5°C routine swabs of body orifices and any lesions, as well as specimens of urine, faeces, and blood are taken for virological and bacteriological examination. Antibiotics are commenced immediately the specimens are collected, and are changed as indicated by the results of sensitivity studies. The importance of early aggressive treatment cannot be

sufficiently stressed, as infection often leads to septicaemia which may be fatal.

The nurse is also responsible for the management of IV infusions for the replacement of depleted blood products, for example, packed cells, granulocytes, and/or platelets. All blood products are irradiated to 15 Gy prior to administration to inactivate lymphocytes which may contribute to graft versus host disease. Observation for transfusion reactions is essential (see page 386).

Accurate fluid balance recording is essential to detect fluid retention or a negative balance. The patient should be weighed daily to assess either weight loss or fluid retention.

The Hickman's catheter must be dressed and the IV line changed daily.

Complications of bone marrow transplantation

Failure of the transplant to take (graft rejection) is fatal. The patient is aplastic from the pretransplantation conditioning and, if the graft fails, the patient will die from an overwhelming infection and/or haemorrhage.

Graft versus host disease (GVHD)

GVHD is caused by the immune reaction of the donor lymphocytes acting against the tissues of the immunosuppressed patient and ranges from mild to severe. It may involve only one organ or it may be widely disseminated and even fatal. The organs involved are the skin, liver, and gastrointestinal tract.

Skin involvement presents as a maculopapular rash and may progress to generalized erythroderma. The skin reaction is most commonly seen on the palms of the hands and soles of the feet, thus distinguishing it from a drug reaction.

Signs of liver involvement are jaundice and abnormally high serum bilirubin levels. Gastrointestinal involvement presents as nausea, vomiting, abdominal pain, and diarrhoea. These may be so severe that fluid and electrolyte imbalances result. Severe cases of GVHD result in sloughing of intestinal mucosa.

Approximately 70% of patients experience some GVHD following bone marrow transplantation.

The discovery and use of cyclosporin A prophylactically has proved to be a breakthrough in the successful prevention and treatment of previously fatal GVHD. Cyclosporin A acts as an immunosuppressive agent by acting on lymph nodes to suppress T-lymphocyte production and therefore prevent rejection of the graft. The side effects include hirsuitism, anorexia, lethargy, hepatotoxicity, viral infections, tremor, and gum hypertrophy. However, side effects are dose dependent and are reversible on cessation of the drug.

Infection

Infection is a frequent cause of death in the bone marrow transplantation patient. For at least 3 months following transplantation the patient, regardless of the leucocyte count, is highly susceptible to infection by any opportunistic organism, for example, bacteria, fungi, viruses, and parasites. The sites most commonly affected are the blood, perianal region, and the lungs. The mucous membranes are highly susceptible to infection with *Candida albicans*. Interstitial pneumonitis affects approximately 60–70% of patients and is fatal in more than 50% of patients. The organism most commonly responsible is the cytomegalovirus.

Resistant leukaemia

Resistant leukaemia is another cause of treatment failure. Patients who receive bone marrow transplantation whilst in relapse have an increased incidence of developing resistant leukaemia. Also, a patient who has been treated with many cytotoxic medications in an attempt to induce remission, may become resistant to treatment.

The frequency of resistant leukaemia is considerably lower in those patients who receive bone marrow transplantation during their first remission.

Anticipated outcome

Leukaemia has long been considered a death sentence by most people. Unfortunately, depending on the age and general health of the patient and the histology of the leukaemia, it still remains a fatal disease for many patients.

Some patients are fortunate in that their disease goes into remission, they have an HLA identical sibling, they are less than 45 years of age, and they are in good general health. These patients qualify for bone marrow transplantation and this offers a hope for a cure. This is an opportunity few people refuse, despite the many side effects and the possibility of fatal complications.

Prior to giving a written consent to the procedure, the patient is given a comprehensive explanation of the transplantation, the need for isolation, the conditioning regime, harvest of marrow, complications which may occur, and the probability of cure. The cure is not without enormous cost to the patient, both physically and emotionally.

HODGKIN'S DISEASE

Hodgkin's disease is a haematological malignancy originating in lymphoid tissue. Prior to 1950 all patients diagnosed with Hodgkin's disease, regardless of staging, died from the condition or its clinical effects. Since the advent of megavoltage radiotherapy and chemotherapy (especially nitrogen mustards) all patients with Hodgkin's disease now have a chance of achieving long term remission or, in some cases, cure.

The site of the disease is initially localized but then spreads in a contiguous fashion, involving lymphoid structures and, ultimately, disseminating to non-lymphoid tissue.

Pathologically, Hodgkin's disease is characterized by the presence of giant bi- or multinucleated cells: Reed-Sternberg cells. The presence of these cells is required for positive diagnosis of Hodgkin's disease of which there are 4 main histological subtypes:

1. Lymphocyte predominance. This occurs in about 5–10% of cases and carries the best prognosis.
2. Nodular sclerosis. This occurs in approximately 50% of patients with Hodgkin's disease and also has a good prognosis.
3. Mixed cellularity. Occurs in approximately 35% of cases and the prognosis is unfavourable.

4. Lymphocyte depleted. This group constitutes 5–10% of cases of Hodgkin's Disease and carries the poorest prognosis.

Histopathological classification is made on the proportion of Reed-Sternberg cells, lymphocytes, and fibrosis found at biopsy.

The aetiology of Hodgkin's disease is unknown. Environmental, infectious, and genetic causes have been examined: there is an increased incidence of Hodgkin's disease among family members; manifestations such as fever, chills, and the predictable spread of the disease has been likened to a viral infection; and there is an increased incidence in some geographic localities. However there is no proof as to the cause of the disease. Hodgkin's disease is more common in males than in females. Age at onset is variable, however it is more prevalent in the 15–34 year age group.

Clinical manifestations

The most common presenting sign is painless superficial lymph node enlargement. Classically, a person will present with a lump below the ear. The cervical lymph nodes are the most commonly involved, followed by axilliary and mediastinal nodes. The patient is often asymptomatic at presentation, especially in the early localized stage of the disease.

With widespread disease the presenting symptoms may include fever, which is low grade; night sweats; weight loss; pruritis; alcohol-induced pain at the site of disease.

The cause of these symptoms is unknown and they are often referred to as 'B' symptoms. Other symptoms may include nerve compression; abdominal pain, due to hepatosplenomegaly or compression by enlarged nodes; and tiredness and lethargy which are usually caused by the anaemia that results from bone marrow involvement and are a very late sign.

Investigative procedures

These include a detailed history, a thorough clinical examination, and a lymph node biopsy. The largest node should be biopsied.

Table 42.1 Modified Ann Arbor staging classification

Stage I	Involvement of a single lymph node region, for example cervical nodes.
Stage II	Involvement of 2 or more lymph node regions on the same side of the diaphragm.
Stage III	Involvement of lymph node regions on both sides of the diaphragm. May have splenic involvement.
Stage IV	Diffuse or disseminated disease involving extralymphatic areas.

Presence of systemic symptoms: each stage is subdivided into either 'A' or 'B' categories. 'A' indicates the absence of systemic symptoms. 'B' classification indicates that systemic symptoms are present and may include unexplained weight loss, fever, night sweats, pruritis, and alcohol induced pain.

Once a positive diagnosis is made it is essential that further investigations are performed to determine the extent, or stage, of the disease, as this will affect the selection of treatment modalities. Table 42.1 lists the staging of the disease based on the extent of lymph node involvement.

The routine investigations that are carried out after diagnosis to determine the extent of the disease include:

• Full blood examination. This is usually normal in early stage disease. However with bone marrow involvement (Stage IV) there may be pancytopenia.
• Serum electrolytes. These are usually normal in early stage disease except for a possible elevated serum copper. The reason for this is unknown. In later stages, biochemical changes will be consistent with the systemic effects of the disease.
• Bone marrow biopsy is performed to determine any bone marrow involvement which indicates Stage IV disease. Biopsy will also confirm the clinical presentation of anaemia, thrombocytopenia and neutropenia.
• Chest X-ray may demonstrate enlarged mediastinal nodes.
• Lymphangiogram will define involved areas, especially retroperitoneal nodes.
• CT thoracic scan. This will confirm the findings of the lymphangiogram and chest X-ray and will give a clearer picture of any enlarged nodes.
• CT abdominal scan will show involvement of any intra-abdominal pelvic and para-aortic nodes. It may also demonstrate liver involvement.

- Urinalysis is routinely performed to ascertain the presence of a urinary tract infection which, if present, must be treated.
- Laparotomy and splenectomy for liver and nodal biopsies respectively. This enables accurate pathological staging of the disease. It is undertaken only in patients with clinical stages I–IIIA disease, as accurate staging is essential in determining the course of treatment, and in locating the areas of disease. All suspicious nodes are biopsied. Splenectomy is performed because a biopsy specimen of the spleen is usually inadequate to determine involvement, as splenic involvement is usually microscopic and profusely scattered.

Once the involved areas have been determined, treatment with radiotherapy can be targetted accurately. Also patients may have more widespread disease than is clinically evident and they may therefore require chemotherapy. Patients with stage IIIB or IV disease do not routinely undergo laparotomy, as the treatment of choice in widespread disease is chemotherapy.

Other reasons for staging Hodgkin's disease are to assess the success of treatment, to aid in prognosis, and to assist in clinical research.

Medical and nursing management

Hodgkin's disease is potentially curable, therefore treatment is aimed at cure or long-term remission. The treatment of choice depends on the stage of the disease and consists of radiotherapy and/or chemotherapy.

In early stage disease, that is stages I–II, the accepted medical treatment is radiotherapy to nodal areas. The areas irradiated are referred to as upper mantle or inverted 'Y' treatment areas (Fig. 42.2A). Nodes irradiated in the upper mantle treatment area are the mediastinal, hilar, cervical, axilliary, supraclavicular, and infraclavicular nodes.

Inverted 'Y' treatment area includes the pelvic, para-aortic, inguinal and femoral nodes, plus the spleen or splenic pedicle (Fig. 42.2B).

For patients in stages II–III it may be decided to treat with total nodal irradiation which incorporates both upper mantle and inverted 'Y' techniques. In women of child-bearing age, the ovaries

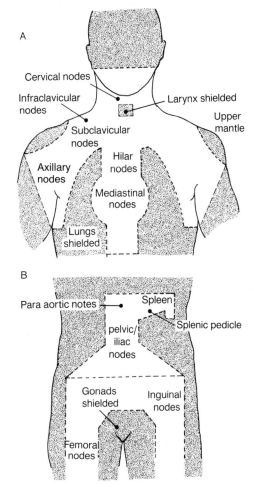

Fig. 42.2 Areas treated with (and shielded from) radiotherapy for Hodgkin's disease. A – Upper mantle. B – Inverted 'Y'.

are moved so that when radiotherapy is given the ovaries may be shielded in an attempt to preserve fertility.

For a detailed discussion on the nursing management of the patient undergoing radiotherapy refer to Chapter 13. The specific side-effects that may be expected include: skin reactions, bone marrow suppression, radiation pneumonitis, dry mouth, oesphagitis, epilation of axilliary hair, tiredness, anorexia, nausea, and diarrhoea.

Patients with stage IIIB or IV disease are treated with chemotherapy with or without radiotherapy. The chemotherapeutic regime that has yielded the best results is MOPP (nitrogen mustard, vincristine, prednisolone and procarbazine). Patients with widespread disease can be treated successfully and expect long term remission or cure with this treatment.

The nursing responsibilities when caring for a patient with Hodgkin's disease are generally the same as those for the care of a patient undergoing abdominal surgery (see page 499), and subsequently for the patient receiving radiotherapy and/or chemotherapy (see page 127). Following recovery from laparotomy most patients complete their treatment as outpatients.

The diet of patients receiving treatment for Hodgkin's disease will need to be modified, especially if the patient is receiving chemotherapy. Procarbazine exhibits monoamine oxidase inhibiting properties, therefore food with a high tyramine content should be avoided. These include matured cheese, yeast, meat extracts, yoghurt, bananas, canned meat and fish, and beer. Patients may become nauseated due to treatment or have difficulty swallowing due to upper mantle radiotherapy.

The nurse must be aware that the psychological needs of patients with Hodgkin's disease must be met. The diagnosis of cancer is traumatic for anyone. It must be remembered that the age of the Hodgkin's disease patient is young compared to many other forms of cancer. Thus problems arise in areas such as schooling, obtaining and maintaining a profession or job, the need to be the same as their peers, feelings of being 'cheated', and having to conform to treatment regimes.

Patients who are to receive treatment need to be advised on contraception. It is important that female patients do not become pregnant whilst undergoing either radiotherapy or chemotherapy, as treatment may cause deformity of the fetus. The pregnancy would need to be terminated or the patient may choose to stop treatment, putting her own life at risk until the baby is born. It is unknown what effects chemotherapy has on sperm and whether deformity of the fetus will result, and male patients are advised not to father children whilst undergoing treatment. Males should be offered the opportunity to bank some sperm prior to commencing treatment, as they will probably be infertile as a result of treatment.

Anticipated outcome

There are several factors that affect a patient's prognosis or response to treatment. These include:

- The stage of disease at presentation. The earlier the diagnosis the less toxic or more effective the treatment.
- Situations where lymphocytes predominate, which carry a better prognosis than those where lymphocytes are depleted.
- The presence of systemic symptoms, or 'B' symptoms, indicate a poor prognosis. The age and general health of the patient. The younger the person and the healthier he is at the time of diagnosis, the better the prognosis and his response to treatment.

LYMPHOMA

Lymphoma (or non-Hodgkin's lymphoma, as it is often known) is a malignant proliferation of cells within the lymphatic system. Unlike Hodgkin's disease, lymphoma spreads in a disorganized manner and may involve extranodal sites early in the disease, for example bone marrow, liver, or spleen. Lymphoma varies greatly in its rapidity of onset and spread.

Pathophysiology

Lymphoma is divided into histologic subtypes based on lymph node biopsy. Because lymphoma varies in its presentation, and the age of the patient also varies at onset, the mode of treatment and the prognosis will depend on the histologic

Table 42.2 Rappaport classification of lymphoma

Nodular
    Lymphocytic, well differentiated (NWDL)
    Lymphocytic, poorly differentiated (NPDL)
    Mixed, lymphocytic and histiocytic (NML)
    Histiocytic (NHL)

Diffuse
    Lymphocytic, well differentiated (DWDL)
    Lymphocytic, poorly differentiated (DPDL)
    Mixed, lymphocytic and histiocytic (DML)
    Histiocytic (DHL)/Large cell (DLCL)
    Undifferentiated (DUL)
    Burkitt's lymphoma (BL)

subtype. Therefore histologic classification is of great importance in lymphoma. The Rappaport classification (Table 42.2) is most commonly used. The histologies are grouped together and graded as low, intermediate, or high. The Ann Arbor staging classification (see page 408) is used to determine the clinical staging of the disease, and facilitates the determination of the treatment modality.

Low grade lymphoma

Patients with low grade lymphoma are generally middle-aged or older; the disease is slow growing or indolent and patients with stage I or II disease are potentially curable. However late stage disease is not amenable to cure. As a patient may continue to be asymptomatic for years, treatment is aimed at reducing the likelihood of symptom development.

Low grade lymphomas include those classified as DWDL, NPDL, and NML.

Intermediate grade lymphoma

Intermediate grade lymphomas include those classified as NHL, DPDL, DML, DHL, or DLCL.

The patient with intermediate grade lymphoma is usually middle-aged or older. The disease follows a more aggressive course; it may not respond well to treatment (particularly Stage III or IV) and often relapses soon after treatment is ceased. Diffuse large cell lymphoma (DLCL) lies between being intermediate grade and high grade malignancy. It occurs more frequently in late adolescence and usually presents as a bulky mass that is often localized; it responds well to initial treatment (either chemotherapy or radiotherapy), however it often relapses within 1–2 years following treatment.

High grade lymphoma

High grade lymphomas are very aggressive and associated with a poor prognosis. DUL usually occurs in adults over 50 years of age, whilst Burkitt's lymphoma occurs primarily in older male children and young male adults. Both DUL and BL may present as an obstructive lesion in the gastrointestinal, urinary, or respiratory tracts. There is widespread lymphatic involvement and most show rapid progression involving the bone marrow and central nervous system. Patients with these forms of lymphoma are treated with aggressive chemotherapy to which they respond well initially. However, early relapse and short survival is characteristic.

Aetiology

The aetiology of lymphoma is unknown although a variety of causes have been examined, including genetic abnormalities, disturbances in immune function, and viruses.

There are significant predisposing factors in the incidence of lymphoma development, and these include;

● Immune deficiencies
● Long-term immunosuppression, for example following renal transplantation to prevent graft rejection
● Treatment with immunosuppressive radiotherapy and chemotherapy for Hodgkin's disease.

Clinical manifestations

In about 70% of cases lymphoma presents with painless lymphadenopathy. The patient often first seeks medical advice regarding a lump in the cervical, axilliary, or inguinal region. Upon investigation these patients are frequently found to have more widespread disease. Other symptoms may include:

● Fever, weight loss, anorexia and/or lethargy
● Sore throat, nasal obstruction or bleeding, or dysphagia, which are symptoms related to nasopharyngeal or tonsillar involvement
● Abdominal distention, gastrointestinal bleeding, abdominal pain, vomiting and weight loss, which are due to gastrointestinal tract infiltration. Abdominal distention may also be due to splenic and/or liver involvement
● Ascites, which may result from liver involvement or indicate extensive peritoneal deposits
● Infection, anaemia resulting in fatigue, lethargy, and dyspnoea. Haemorrhagic tendencies are symptoms of bone marrow involvement

• Dyspnoea, dry cough, and signs of superior vena caval obstruction, which are indicative of involvement of mediastinal nodes

• Pruritis and skin nodules, which are symptoms of skin infiltration

• Pain, if present, may be a result of a variety of causes, for example, skeletal involvement, pressure from enlarged nodes, or pressure from excessive accumulation of body fluids.

Investigative procedures

Investigations carried out are similar to those performed for patients with Hodgkin's disease.

• History and physical examination. This assists in determining the clinical stage of the disease.

• Lymph node biopsy. Confirms a positive diagnosis and identifies histology.

• FBE. The result will depend upon the stage of the disease. With bone marrow involvement, anaemia, thrombocytopenia, and neutropenia are expected.

• Serum electrolytes. These correlate with the clinical extent of the disease.

• Bone marrow biopsy. Confirms the evidence of marrow involvement and identifies the degree of cellular interruption.

• Lymphangiogram. This may demonstrate involved retroperitoneal nodes.

• Chest X-ray and CT thoracic scan. Mediastinal nodes may show evidence of enlargement and therefore disease.

• CT abdominal scan. This is useful in detecting retroperitoneal nodes, mesenteric nodes, and liver involvement.

• Exploratory laparotomy. This procedure has revealed a substantial increase in the incidence of hepatic, mesenteric, and gastric involvement, not previously detected by other investigations. However, laparotomy cannot be justified if it has already been decided to treat with chemotherapy.

Medical and surgical management

Surgery

Laparotomy is performed only as part of the staging process in some patients. During an exploratory laparotomy it is possible to 'debulk'

the lymphoma particularly in DLCL. If the lymphoma is causing obstructive problems it may need to be partially removed in order to relieve the obstruction. The nursing management of these patients is as for any patient undergoing abdominal surgery (see page 499).

The patient may develop spinal cord compression due to tumour pressure or infiltration. When this occurs it is treated by laminectomy to prevent para- or quadriplegia. For nursing management of the patient undergoing spinal surgery see page 724.

Radiotherapy

Most cases of lymphoma are quite sensitive to radiotherapy, therefore patients with early stage disease (Stage I or II) may be considered candidates for curative radiotherapy. Radiotherapy is administered to the primary site and any adjacent lymph nodes. However, lymphoma often spreads early in the disease and an extent of the spread may not be evident when radiotherapy is instigated. Thus the patient can relapse soon after treatment due to the effects of the lymphoma in areas not irradiated.

Radiotherapy is not considered a cure regime for patients with Stage III or IV disease; for these patients radiotherapy may be used only as palliative treatment. Palliative radiotherapy can control local problems, for example ureteric obstruction, spinal cord compression, or superior vena caval obstruction due to tumour compression.

Chemotherapy

The aims of chemotherapy are to control the disease by inducing remission and, in some cases, cure. Patients with low grade lymphomas are often not treated with chemotherapy until such time as the disease becomes symptomatic beyond uncomplicated lymphadenopathy. This is because there is no realistic cure and the disease may continue on a benign clinical course for many years. Therefore treatment is usually aimed at palliating and controlling the symptoms once the disease manifests. Agents used are oral chlorambucil or cyclophosphamide with or without prednisolone; this treatment is relatively non-toxic and tolerated well by the person whose treatment can be managed on an outpatient basis.

Combination chemotherapy is used in the treatment of intermediate grade lymphomas with advanced disease (stage III and IV). There are a number of chemotherapeutic regimes that are effective for these lymphomas. Agents commonly used include adriamycin, cyclophosphamide, prednisolone, and vincristine. Patients usually receive treatment on an outpatient basis, treatment generally being given every 3 or 4 weeks for 6–8 courses.

Aggressive combination chemotherapy is used in the treatment of high grade lymphomas. Chemotherapy should begin as soon as a positive diagnosis is made, because the disease may quickly grow out of control. These forms of lymphoma often respond well initially, leading to complete remission. However remission is very brief, ranging from weeks to a few months, after which the lymphoma becomes resistant to treatment and death soon results.

Nursing management

General nursing principles apply to patients with lymphoma. The psychological impact of diagnosis and treatment needs to be considered. The nurse needs to be attentive to psychological needs and demonstrate good listening skills.

Physical care is as for any patient undergoing surgery (see page 33), chemotherapy (see page 127), and radiotherapy (see page 125).

Anticipated outcome

The course and prognosis of lymphoma varies greatly and depends upon the histology of the disease, the stage of the disease at presentation, the patient's response to treatment, and the general health and age of the patient.

Modern chemotherapy regimes have revolutionized the prognosis for many patients. The median survival time has increased from a few months to greater than 2 years. With improved treatment regimes and a better understanding of the disease survival times may continue to increase, and a cure may eventually be available.

MULTIPLE MYELOMA

Multiple myeloma (or myeloma, as it is more commonly called) is a malignant proliferation of plasma cells in the bone marrow. The cancerous plasma cells are scattered throughout the skeleton, and form tumours. There are also abnormal immunoglobulins in the blood serum.

The disease occurs predominantly in older patients and rarely occurs before the age of 40 years. The aetiology remains unknown.

Pathophysiology

Bone marrow infiltration by plasma cells leads to a reduction in normal haemopoiesis, causing anaemia, thrombocytopenia, and leucopenia.

The ability of the plasma cells to produce functional immunoglobulins is affected. Patients will continue to produce immunoglobulins, but the production will be depleted. Therefore the patient is prone to repeated infections, and it is significant that the same infecting organism is usually responsible.

There is diffuse osteoporosis due to abnormal plasma cells invading the bone marrow; these erode adjacent bone, resulting in osteolysis.

Clinical manifestations

The most frequent symptom of myeloma is bone pain. The pain is often aggravated by movement and may fluctuate for weeks or months. Areas commonly affected are the vertebrae, ribs, clavicles, pelvis, and skull. A sudden onset of severe pain often signifies the collapse of a vertebra, or a spontaneous fracture.

Pallor, weakness, fatigue, palpitations, and dyspnoea are often presenting symptoms, and these are due to the resultant anaemia. Symptoms related to thrombocytopenia may be present and include bruising or excessive bleeding after minor injury. Dyspnoea, a productive cough, and a 'tight chest' may be present and are due to a chest infection or pneumonia; these are also common symptoms at presentation.

Other symptoms for which a patient may seek medical advice include anorexia, nausea and vomiting, polyuria, polydipsia, constipation, and

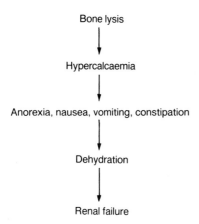

Bone lysis

↓

Hypercalcaemia

↓

Anorexia, nausea, vomiting, constipation

↓

Dehydration

↓

Renal failure

Fig. 42.3 The clinical effects of unchecked osteolysis.

dehydration. Hypercalcaemia, due to bone destruction and the release of calcium into the circulation, triggers an attempt by the body to excrete high levels of urinary calcium. Calcium has a strong osmotic pull and hypovolaemia may ensue due to excessive water loss. Vomiting may also increase the degree of hypovolaemia (Figure 42.3).

Investigative procedures

Investigations that are usually performed initially include:

● History and physical examination. These will reveal the symptoms and signs of the clinical presentation of myeloma and identify the areas of skeletal involvement.
● FBE. There will be a normocytic anaemia, a possible thrombocytopenia and a leucopenia. Erythrocytes show a characteristic 'rouleaux' formation.
● ESR. This will be elevated due to the increase in plasma proteins.
● Blood urea and serum electrolytes. These may reveal hypercalcaemia, an increased urea, and alkaline phosphatase will be normal or slightly elevated.
● Chest X-ray. This will demonstrate the extent of rib involvement in the disease and should be routinely performed to assess the lung fields for the presence of any consolidation or infection.
● Immunoelectrophoresis. This will show a peak in the plasma immunoglobulin affected.

In many instances, the patient may be admitted to hospital but this is usually only so that bone pain can be controlled and more sophisticated investigative procedures can be performed. Such procedures include:

● Bone marrow biopsy. This will reveal the presence of both mature and immature plasma (myeloma) cells in the marrow and confirm the degree of the disease presentation.
● 24-hour urine collection. Bence Jones protein will be positive in nearly 80% of persons with myeloma. Creatine clearance is increased in the presence of proteinuria due to renal damage.
● Skeletal survey. This may reveal multiple, round, 'punched out' osteolytic bone lesions and confirm the extent of skeletal involvement.
● Intravenous pyelogram. This will show the extent of any renal damage present. The patient is never fasted from fluids prior to this procedure as acute renal failure, due to dehydration, may result.

Medical management

The most important aims of treatment of the myeloma patient are to relieve pain, and maintain ambulation. Ambulation is important so that further demineralization and weakening of the bone structure is avoided.

Plasmaphoresis may be carried out to reduce the viscosity of the blood and remove the excessive plasma proteins. However, transfusions of packed cells may be needed to correct any underlying anaemia.

Pathological fractures of the long bones are usually treated surgically with internal fixation. Fractures should never be treated with the application of plaster casts, as immobilization increases the degree of demineralization. Laminectomy and vertebral fusion may be necessary to relieve and/or prevent spinal cord compression.

Radiotherapy is most commonly used to palliate bone pain. However, large osteolytic lesions should also be irradiated in order to reduce the likelihood of pathological fracture.

Chemotherapy is used to decrease the tumour mass and relieve bone pain. The most effective agents in the treatment of myeloma include cyclophosphamide, melphalan, BCNU (carmustine) and prednisolone. Cytotoxic drugs may be given as single agents or used in combination.

There is no cure for myeloma and treatment is therefore aimed at palliating symptoms and giving a better quality of life to the patient. Treatment can induce a remission and therefore prolong life, and median remission duration is 21 months. The average life expectancy, with treatment, is 2–3 years from diagnosis.

Nursing management

The nurse will be responsible for the care of a patient who will have bone pain, but who will be required to maintain ambulation in order to diminish the osteolytic process (Figure 42.4). Additionally, renal function may be impaired and the patient may also be prone to overwhelming infections. Added to this is the potential for nursing problems associated with the treatment regimes of radiotherapy (see page 125) and chemotherapy (see page 127). The nurse must therefore ensure that the patient with myeloma:

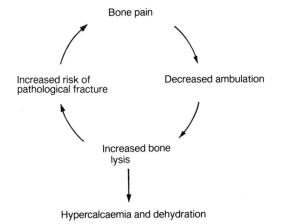

Bone pain

Increased risk of pathological fracture

Decreased ambulation

Increased bone lysis

Hypercalcaemia and dehydration

Fig. 42.4 The osteolytic cycle.

• Drinks 2–3 litres of fluid per day. This will maintain an adequate urinary output, which is required for the excretion of protein and calcium and prevent the onset of renal failure.

• Maintains ambulation. Pain permitting, this will prevent further demineralization and weakening of the bone structure. The patient should never remain on prolonged bed rest.

• Has frequent analgesia in order to maintain continual pain relief. Initially asprin will provide this relief but as the condition progresses stronger analgesia such as codeine phosphate or morphine are often necessary (see also Chapter 12).

Commonly, respiratory pathogens are the infecting organisms in the immune suppressed patient. Therefore constant monitoring of the patient's respiratory function, and early detection of infection is necessary in preventing the overwhelming pneumonia that commonly accompanies myeloma. It is extremely important to note that any physical form of chest physiotherapy is contraindicated, as such therapy may result in skeletal fractures.

Anticipated outcome

During the course of the disease the patient with myeloma may experience complications, for example a pathological fracture, spinal cord compression, hypercalcaemia, repeated infection, bone marrow suppression, or renal failure. The patient is treated with a view to preventing or minimizing complications and palliating any symptoms.

The cause of death is often due to infection, for example, overwhelming pneumonia; haemorrhage from vessels involved in the infective process; or from renal failure.

43

Haemorrhagic disorders

Robyn Anderson

Haemorrhagic disorders can be clearly classified into 3 major groups:

1. Disorders due to defects of the blood vessels

This type of disorder can be caused by a wide range of infections, for example measles, typhoid fever and septicaemia. Chemical agents may also be responsible for damaging vessels, and chemicals such as aspirin, frusemide, indomethacin, phenytoin and snake venom can cause vessel changes. Anaphylactic reactions (Henoch-Schonlein purpura) and conditions such as hepatitis and renal failure may also be responsible.

2. Disorders of the thrombocytes

Conditions where there are reduced thrombocytes include the different types of thrombocytopenia. Thrombocythaemia can also cause haemorrhage as can thrombasthenia.

3. Disorders due to defects in the clotting mechanism

Conditions such as haemophilia, Christmas disease, von Willebrand's disease, and a deficiency of other clotting factors may cause haemorrhage, as can lack of vitamin K, oral anticoagulant therapy and advanced hepatic failure.

The significant haemorrhagic disorders will be discussed but whatever the cause, the basic nursing management remains the same for all these patients.

NURSING CARE FOR A PATIENT WITH A HAEMORRHAGIC CONDITION

Patients with clotting problems bleed easily from vascular areas of the body such as the nose, gums, and kidneys; and gentle thumb pressure on a patient's skin can easily result in bruising. When caring for such patients the nurse must observe for signs of bruising or extended bruising, bleeding from the nose, haematuria, and blood in the faeces. Padding of pressure points such as elbows, heels and sacrum will help to reduce the likelihood of bruising. Patients must be lifted and turned with extreme care to avoid trauma and bruising and if bed rails are required they must be padded.

Constipation should be prevented in patients with haemorrhoids as blood loss from a haemorrhoid can be quite substantial. Intramuscular and subcutaneous injections must also be avoided. The use of soft tooth brushes will prevent gum abrasion and shaving must be with an electric razor. The nurse must also observe for signs of internal haemorrhage (see page 331) which may occur spontaneously or following a fall by the patient. Consequently, the frail patient with a haemorrhagic condition must not ambulate without supervision. If an intravenous line is necessary the site must be securely taped and supported to prevent further trauma and continuous bleeding.

Topical thrombin or an absorbable cellulose pad which acts as an artificial clot can be used to cause haemostasis in such situations where a life-support IV line is required.

THROMBOCYTOPENIA

Thrombocytopenia is present when there is a significant decrease in the number of thrombocytes. It occurs either because thrombocytes are destroyed virtually as soon as they are produced, or because thrombocytes are simply not being produced.

Idiopathic thrombocytopenic purpura

In this condition there is an extreme reduction in the number of thrombocytes, and it is believed that there may be an IgG type antibody causing their destruction. There are 2 forms: the acute form, which is most often seen in young children and is self-limiting; and the chronic form, seen most commonly in females and occurring at any age.

Clinical manifestations

The patient will present with purpura of the skin and mucous membranes, and haematuria and bleeding from the gastrointestinal tract are common. Rarely, the patient may have an intracranial haemorrhage and warning signs of this are headache, dizziness, and confusion (see also page 175). The condition is usually chronic and has a series of exacerbations and remissions.

Investigative procedures

A full blood examination will show marked thrombocytopenia and a normal or possibly increased number of megakaryocytes. In some patients antiplatelet and antimegakaryocyte antibodies can be demonstrated.

Medical management

In young children no treatment is necessary unless there is evidence of intracranial bleeding.

The adult patient is prescribed 60 mg/day of prednisolone; this usually causes the platelet count to rise rapidly to normal levels, and the drug is then slowly withdrawn. Should a relapse occur, higher dosages for a longer period of time should be given. If the platelet level does not rise in 3–4 weeks, splenectomy should be considered. If a splenectomy is performed it should be done under a prednisolone cover and platelet transfusions given only after the splenic artery has been ligated.

Anticipated outcome

Total remission occurs in most cases, although some patients will continue with a low grade bleeding tendency for many years.

THROMBOCYTHAEMIA

In thrombocythaemia there is a raised level of thrombocytes in the blood (in excess of 1000 × 10^9/l which may predispose the patient to either a bleeding or a clotting tendency.

Clinical manifestations

These are the same as for thrombocytopenia with the addition of the symptoms common to vascular insufficiency, for example, petechiae, retinal occlusions, multiple mini cerebrovascular accidents, and problems with peripheral circulation.

Medical management

The condition responds well to radioactive phosphorus P^{32}, and aspirin is given on a daily basis in very small doses as this will help to reduce thrombocyte 'stickiness' and therefore reduce agglutination.

THROMBASTHENIA

In this condition the thrombocytes are normal in number but are unable to function effectively. The hereditary forms are extremely rare and the patients frequently die in infancy or early childhood. The acquired form is more common and may be seen in severe uraemia and following exposure to some drugs, such as aspirin. Thrombasthenia is often a symptom of chronic myeloid leukaemia.

There is no effective therapy but platelet transfusions may be performed, especially to cover surgical procedures.

HAEMOPHILIA

Haemophilia (haemophilia A) is genetically determined and is seen in males at an incidence rate of

1 per 10 000 live births. It is characterized by an abnormal bleeding tendency. The condition is carried on the X chromosome, and in haemophilia the person's ability to produce factor VIII is disturbed and the factor VIII that is made, is abnormal. Females can have haemophilia, but it is extremely rare as it requires the mother to be a carrier and the father to be a haemophiliac. Female carriers may, however, bleed abnormally, especially after surgery.

The important points to remember about genetic inheritance of the disease are that:

• The female children of a haemophiliac (male) who is married to a normal female will be carriers of the condition, and the male children will be unaffected.
• The female children of a female carrier married to a normal male will also be carriers of the condition, and the male children will have a 1 : 2 chance of having the condition.

Clinical manifestations

The patient usually presents because he is bleeding into a joint cavity. This type of bleeding may occur spontaneously, particularly into the large weight bearing joints. The joint will be extremely painful and swollen. Bleeding can also occur into soft tissue, for example muscle, retroperitoneal tissue, from the gastrointestinal tract or from the urinary system. Intracerebral haemorrhage occurs rarely. Haemarthroses can cause severe deformity, leading eventually to osteoarthritis. Bleeding into soft tissue may compress other vital structures, for example, nerves, arteries and the airways.

The patient may have an associated iron deficiency anaemia.

Investigative procedures

Coagulation screening tests will show prolongation of the activated partial thromboplastin time (APTT), and a factor VIII assay will confirm that the factor is missing or extremely low. Occasionally in conditions such as systemic lupus erythematosus, malignancy, and pregnancy, antibodies may be produced that destroy factor VIII. This causes an acquired form of haemophilia.

Medical and nursing management

Any haemorrhage must be stopped. This is done by giving factor VIII intravenously until appropriate levels have been reached. The half-life of factor VIII is 8 hours and therefore at least twice daily administration is necessary. Almost all haemophiliac patients commence their own treatment at home before venturing into hospital. This is done by giving cryoprecipitate intravenously (cryoprecipitate must be of the correct blood group).

From the nurse's point of view, there is little specific treatment except that pain in the affected joint must be relieved. This can be done with prescribed drugs, and local therapy such as ice packs may be useful.

The haemophiliac patient should be encouraged to live as normal a life as possible. The social worker may be able to find employment for the patient, and the occupational therapist can be of assistance in advising modifications to the patient's home or work place to make day to day living safer and easier. The patient should not indulge in contact sports as injury could be disastrous. This is obviously a problem in children who, because they feel perfectly well decide that 'just this once' they will play football or whatever the other children are playing.

The patient and his significant others must understand the condition and be helped to become responsible for the patient's well being.

Because these patients must have repeated doses of blood product, despite the fact that it is all tested, they almost always become hepatitis antigen (Australia factor) positive and may also develop AIDS.

Christmas disease

Christmas disease (haemophilia B) is a sex-linked genetic condition, but in which Factor IX is the missing factor. It is a rarer condition than haemophilia A but is identical in description, treatment and outcome except that Factor IX must be administered to the patient.

Von Willebrand's disease

Von Willebrand's disease is an autosomal dominant conditon and can therefore affect both sexes.

There is defective factor VIII production and therefore defective thrombocyte function.

Clinical manifestations

The patient will display an abnormal bleeding tendency, which may manifest as epistaxes, gastrointestinal bleeding, menorrhagia and extensive bleeding after minor surgery.

The treatment of this condition is exactly the same as for haemophilia and Christmas disease and cryoprecipitate or factor VIII are given.

DEFICIENCY OF FACTORS DEPENDENT ON VITAMIN K

Vitamin K is needed in order for the liver to synthesize prothrombin (factor II) and factors VII, IX and X. Vitamin K deficiencies occur whenever fat metabolism is disturbed, as the fat soluble vitamins are not absorbed. The liver is unable to synthesize prothrombin without vitamin K and also in situations where there is profound hepatocellular dysfunction.

Clinical manifestations

The patient will present with excessive bruising and possibly haemorrhage from the gastrointestinal tract or the genitourinary system. Epistaxes and menorrhagia are common.

Medical management

Administration of phytomenadione (vitamin K_1) will correct the deficiency within 24 hours, and the liver will recommence the production of normal prothrombin within that time. Where greater speed is necessary, for example, in the presence of significant blood loss, a transfusion of fresh, frozen plasma, platelets or whole blood may be performed. It is dangerous to use concentrated factor II, VII, IX and X as such a concentrate can precipitate thrombotic episodes, however in profound hepatocellular disease the use of this material may be essential.

44

Disorders of the spleen

Robyn Anderson

The spleen is a bean shaped, blood filled, fragile organ which lies in the left upper quadrant of the abdomen, and is protected by the lower 4 ribs. It lies adjacent to the stomach and the tail of the pancreas. Approximately 350 l of blood is pumped to the spleen each day. The spleen is full of white and red pulp: 25% of all lymphatic tissue in the body is found in the spleen and makes up the white pulp: the red pulp is a loose honeycomb of reticular tissue containing the splenic sinusoids.

The spleen is a filter for blood cells. Normal cells pass through it without change, but elderly or damaged cells are trapped; these are then broken down and the remnants disposed of basically by phagocytosis. The spleen is also an important part of the immune system, where particulate antigens are filtered off and phagocytosis-promoting peptides are produced, as are some immunoglobulins. It has been suggested that the spleen may have humoral effect on bone marrow, stimulating erythropoiesis and depressing the levels of leucocytes and thrombocytes. (Forrest, 1985). It should be noted that if the spleen is removed other body systems will eventually assume its function.

Under normal circumstances the spleen is not palpable but when it enlarges it extends downwards and can be palpated beneath the costal margin. An enlarged spleen can be seen on soft tissue X-ray and detected by CT scan or ultrasound.

TRAUMA TO THE SPLEEN

The spleen is one of the organs most frequently damaged in abdominal trauma and is particularly susceptible to damage when it is enlarged. There are 3 classic injuries to the spleen: rupture; avulsment from the splenic pedicle; and a tear beneath the splenic capsule. Rupture and avulsion of the spleen cause immediate intraperitoneal bleeding. Delayed rupture occurs in approximately 5% of splenic injury and is due to the enlargement of a subcapsular haematoma; this usually occurs within 2 weeks of the injury but may take months and on rare occasions even years.

Clinical manifestations

The patient presents with pain, tenderness, and guarding in the left upper quadrant of the abdomen and referred pain in the tip of the left shoulder. There are associated signs of shock and in 20% of cases fractures of the lower left ribs are found.

Medical, surgical, and nursing management

Splenectomy is the treatment of choice, except in children. The patient is prepared for surgery, and a nasogastric tube is inserted as the stomach will be handled during the surgery and it must be empty at the time of handling. A thrombocyte count is performed to ensure that it is normal and if necessary a preoperative transfusion of platelets will be given, or be available for infusion during surgery.

The most common surgical approach for a splenectomy is a long vertical or subcostal abdominal incision, but if the spleen is grossly enlarged a thoracoabdominal incision may be necessary.

Postoperatively the patient should recover quickly from the surgery, and drain tubes are not usually left in situ but occasionally a low pressure vacuum apparatus may be used.

There is no specific nursing care following a splenectomy and care is as for any patient following abdominal surgery (see page 499).

Complications of splenectomy

The complications of splenectomy are bleeding from the splenic pedicle, and pancreatitis which may be due to bruising of the tail of the pancreas during surgery. Collapse of the lower lobe of the left lung may occur and therefore there is a need for high quality chest physiotherapy. On rare occasions an abscess may occur in the splenic bed.

Following splenectomy there is often a transient increase in the thrombocyte and leucocyte counts, and therefore an increased risk of venous thrombosis.

Due to the loss of lymphoid tissue there is an increased risk of infection. Most infections occur within 3 years of splenectomy and for this reason some surgeons suggest an antibiotic cover for this period, and this cover is mandatory when the patient is a child. Splenectomy in children should be avoided if at all possible.

HYPERSPLENISM

Hypersplenism is a syndrome consisting of splenomegaly and pancytopenia. The bone marrow is normal and there is no autoimmune disease clinically present.

Primary hypersplenism is due to hypertrophy of the spleen due to the need to destroy abnormal blood cells. Secondary hypersplenism occurs when inappropriate cell destruction is secondary to the splenic enlargement, due to conditions such as:

– Inflammation, caused by malaria, leishmaniasis, sarcoidosis, and rheumatic fever
– Congestive splenomegaly in portal hypertension, caused by bilharziasis and portal vein stenosis
– Infiltration of the spleen by malignant tissue, in myeloproliferative and lymphoproliferative disorders.

Other conditions causing splenic enlargement are the haemolytic anaemias, idiopathic thrombocytopenic purpura, secondary thrombocytopenia, myelofibrosis, and lymphomas. Tumours of the spleen other than those mentioned are rare.

Splenic cysts are rare but fall into 3 groups: congenital dermoid-like cysts, which are often full of creamy material containing hair and teeth; degenerative cysts, as a result of previous infarction or haematoma; and hydatid cysts due to invasion of *Echinococcus granulosus*.

Abscesses of the spleen are rare and are suspected when there is splenomegally accompanied by bacteraemia or septicaemia.

Splenectomy may be undertaken in many of these conditions and the haematologist must make the decision taking into account the degree of trauma which would be caused by removing an enlarged spleen, and weighing the possible beneficial effects against the deleterious effects of such surgery.

SECTION E – REFERENCES AND FURTHER READING

Texts

Anderson J R (ed) 1976 Muir's Textbook of pathology, 10th edn. Edward Arnold, London

Anthony C P 1984 Structure and function of the body. Mosby, St Louis

Beck W S 1983 Haematology, 4th edn. Massachusetts Institute of Technology Press.

Berkow R (ed) 1977 The Merck manual of diagnosis and therapy, 13th edn. Merck, Sharpe & Dohme, New Jersey.

Bulley F, Bartinate L 1983 Multiple myeloma. Unpublished notes.

Bunn H F, Forget B 1986 Hemoglobin: molecular, genetic and clinical aspects. Saunders, Philadelphia

Casciato D A, Lowitz B B 1983 Manual of bedside oncology. Little Brown, Boston

Cater J L Acute leukaemia. Personal notes, unpublished lecture

Cater J L Bone marrow transplantation. Personal notes, unpublished lecture

Cawley J C (ed) 1983 Haematology. Heinemann, London

Chanarin et al 1984 Blood and its diseases, 3rd edn. Churchill Livingstone, Edinburgh

Colman R W et al 1987 Haemostasis and thrombosis: basic principles and clinical practice, 2nd edn. Lippincott, Philadelphia

Creager J G 1982 Human anatomy and physiology. Wadsworth, California

Forrest A P M, Carter D C, MacLeod I B 1985 Principles and Practice of Surgery. Churchill Livingstone, Edinburgh

Gale R P 1979 Bone marrow transplantation in acute leukaemia: current status and future directions. In: R Neth et al (eds) Modern trends in human leukaemia II, Springer-Verlog, Berlin 71–77.

Gruchy G C De 1978 Clinical hematology in medical practice. Blackwell, Oxford

Gunz F W, Henderson E S (eds) 1983 William Dameshek and Frederick Gunz's leukemia, 4th edn. Grune & Stratton, Orlando

Havard M 1986 A nursing guide to drugs, 2nd edn. Churchill Livingstone, Melbourne

Hoffbrand A V, Pettit J E 1984 Essential haematology, 2nd edn. Blackwell Scientific, Oxford

Holland J F, Frei E 1982 Cancer medicine, 2nd edn. Lea & Febiger, Philadelphia

Isbister J P 1986 Clinical haematology. Williams & Wilkins, Sydney

Keller R H, Patrick C W 1987 Miale's laboratory medicine: hematology, 7th edn. Mosby, St Louis

Keopke J A (ed) 1984 Laboratory hematology. Churchill Livingstone, New York

Luckmann J, Sorensen K C 1980 Medical/surgical nursing: a psychophysiologic approach, 2nd edn. Saunders, Philadelphia

Macleod J 1987 Davidson's principles and practice of medicine, 15th edn. Churchill Livingstone, Edinburgh

Miller D R et al (eds) 1984 Blood diseases of infancy and childhood, 5th edn. Mosby, St Louis

Nathan D G, Oski F A (eds) 1981 Hematology of infancy and childhood, 3rd edn. Saunders, Philadelphia

Read A E, Barritt D W, Langton Hewer R 1986 Modern medicine, 3rd edn. Churchill Livingstone, Edinburgh

Rubin P, Bakemeier R F, Krackov S K 1983 Clinical oncology: a multidisciplinary approach, 6th edn. American Cancer Society

Society of Hospital Pharmacists of Australia 1985 Pharmacology and drug information for nurses, 2nd edn. Saunders, Sydney

Storlie F J (ed) 1984 Diseases: nurse's reference library, 2nd edn. Springhouse, Pennsylvania

Thompson R B, Proctor S J 1984 A short textbook of haematology, 6th edn. Pitman, London

Thorup O A 1987 Fundamentals of clinical hematology, 5th edn. Saunders, Philadelphia

Wiernik P H et al (eds) 1985 Neoplastic diseases of the blood. Churchill Livingstone, New York

Williams W, Beutler E, Erslev A, Lichtman M 1983 Haematology, 3rd edn. McGraw-Hill, New York

Wintrobe M M et al 1981 Clinical hematology, 8th edn. Lea & Febiger, Philadelphia

Journals

Beaudoin K 1983 Going the distance with the patient who's a real fighter. Nursing 83 13 : 4 : 6–11

Benson M L, Benson D M 1985 Autotransfusion is here – are you ready? Nursing 85 15 : 3 : 46–49

Bortin N M et al 1982 Factors associated with interstitial pneumonitis after bone marrow transplantation for acute leukaemia. The Lancet February 20: 437–439

Burrell C J, Davis K G 1985 The blood story, Part II: AIDS The Australian Nurses Journal 14 : 7 : 45–47

Davis K G 1985 The blood story, Part I: the phenomenal bank. The Australian Nurses Journal 14 : 7 : 42–44

Davis K G 1985 The blood story, Part III: the storage and administration of blood and blood products. The Australian Nurses Journal 14 : 5 : 40–43

Davis K G 1985 The blood story, Part IV: adverse reactions to blood transfusions. The Australian Nurses Journal. 15 : 6 : 40–43

Gale R P 1981 Bone marrow transplantation in acute leukaemia. Annals of Clinical Research 13: 367–372.

Geary C G, Evans D I K, Scarffe J H 1982 Bone marrow transplantation. British Journal of Hospital Medicine April: 393–399.

Graft A W et al 1981 Fatal dissemination of cytomegalovirus after bone marrow transplantation. Journal of Clinical Pathology 34: 1047–1051

Griffin J P 1986 Be prepared for the bleeding patient. Nursing 86 16 : 6 : 34–40

Hagan S J 1983 Bring help and hope to the patient with Hodgkin's disease. Nursing 83 13 : 8 : 58–63

King L 1981 Blood brothers. Nursing Mirror September 30, 35–37.

Koch P M 1984 Thrombocytopenia: don't let it make a big problem out of nothing. Nursing 84 14 : 10 : 54–57

Lyons F 1985 Malignant melanoma: the sunburnt country's dilemma. The Australian Nurses Journal. 14 : 10 : 48–50

Mauldin B C 1982 Harvest of hope: bone marrow transplant. AORN Journal 36 : 3 : 385–390.

McConnell E A 1986 Leukocyte studies: what the counts can tell you. Nursing 86 16 : 3 : 42–43

McConnell E A 1986 APTT and PT: the tests of time. Nursing 86 16 : 5 : 47

McKinney Wiley F, De Curr-Whalley S 1983 Allogenic bone marrow transplantation for children with acute leukaemia. Oncology Nursing Forum 10 : 3 : 49–53.

Mercado S B 1986 The latest protocols for blood transfusions. Nursing 86 16 : 10 : 34–44

Moeller K I, Swartzendruber E J 1987 Suppressing the risks of bone marrow suppression. Nuring 87 17 : 3 : 52–54

Nurse's Reference Library 1983 Quick guide to common anemias. Nursing 83 13 : 12 : 20–21

Nurse's Reference Library 1984 Cell proliferation disorders. Nursing 84 14 : 1 : 34–41

O'Donoghue 1983 Plasmapheresis using the continuous flow cell separator. The Australian Nurses Journal 13 : 2 : 57–59

Powles R L et al 1985 Cyclosporin A to prevent graft versus host disease. In: Man After Allogenic Bone Marrow Transplantation. The Lancet February 16, 327–329.

Querin J J, Stahl L D 1983 12 Simple, sensible steps for successful blood transfusions. Nursing 83 13 : 11 : 34–43

Rice L, Schottstaedt M, Udden M, Jackson D 1981 Transplantation of bone marrow: graft versus host disease. Heart & Lung 10 : 5 897–900.

Siskind J 1984 Handling hemorrhage wisely. Nursing 84 14 : 1 : 34–41

Stream P, Harrington E, Clark M 1980 Bone marrow transplantation: an option for children with acute leukaemia. Cancer Nursing June: 195–199.

Vogel T C, McSkimming S A 1983 Teaching parents to give indwelling C.V. catheter care. Nursing 83 13 : 1 : 55–56

Westmead Centre 1982 Hickman's catheter: procedure manual. Sydney

F

The liver, biliary system, and pancreas

45

Introduction to the liver, biliary system, and pancreas

Mavis Matthews

Because the liver, biliary system and pancreas are directly involved with the chemical digestion and subsequent absorption of nutrients, their structure and function needs to be understood prior to studying the gastrointestinal tract (Section G) which specifically includes the mechanical and physiological processes of digestion.

THE LIVER

This is the largest organ in the body weighing approximately 1350 g, and is positioned on the undersurface of the diaphragm in the right hypochondriac and epigastric regions. It is divided into 4 lobes which in turn are further subdivided into numerous tiny functioning units called lobules. The inferior surface of the liver contains the porta hepatus (hilum) where all vessels enter and leave. Vessels entering the porta hepatus are: the hepatic artery carrying oxygenated blood indirectly from the abdominal aorta; and the portal vein which carries oxygen and approximately 75% of the liver's blood supply, and is rich in nutrients because it drains the gastrointestinal tract. Vessels leaving the porta hepatus are: the hepatic veins carrying the total blood from the liver to the inferior vena cava; the right and left hepatic ducts carrying bile into the biliary system; and the lymphatic vessels draining the lobules. Hepatic and portal blood flows through every lobule via channels called sinusoids, thus allowing the liver cells to select and deal with the products of digestion and other transported substances (Fig. 45.1).

The liver can be likened to a large chemical factory; it takes in raw products, alters and/or stores them, and then passes the refined

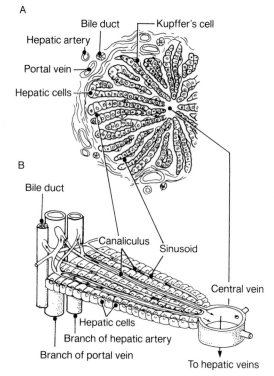

Fig. 45.1 Liver lobule, showing blood and bile flow. **A** – Cross section of lobule. **B** – Lobule.

substances out into the body systems for metabolic needs via the biliary system or the hepatic veins. The liver has numerous functions; among the most important for the nurse to know are:

● The formation and excretion of 600–800 ml of bile daily. The chief constituents of bile are soluble bilirubin, bile salts, cholesterol, bile acids, lecithin, electrolytes and water. Bile is necessary for the breakdown and absorption of fats, fat soluble vitamins, iron, and calcium. It is a natural aperient in that it stimulates peristalsis, it also deodorizes faeces.

- Synthesis of plasma proteins and lipoproteins.
- Regulation of blood glucose concentration by converting glucose to glycogen for storage, then reconverting the glycogen to glucose as the blood glucose level drops. The liver is also able to convert amino acids and lactate into glucose (gluconeogenesis) when glycogen stores are depleted.
- Conversion of metabolically produced ammonia (a potential toxin) to the relatively safe compound urea, which can then be excreted in the urine.
- Desaturation of fats for production of heat and energy. Fatty acids and their metabolic products are used for the synthesis of such complex lipids as lecithin and cholesterol.
- Storing of iron, copper, and vitamins A, B, D and K.
- Detoxification of many hormones, bacteria, drugs, and poisons including alcohol, thus rendering them harmless for excretion.
- Production of heat. This is achieved as the end result of the multitude of cellular activities which occur in the liver.
- Destruction of pathogens from the gut by the Kupffer cells which line the sinusoids.

THE BILIARY SYSTEM

This system comprises the gall bladder and bile ducts. The gall bladder is a pear-shaped sac with a capacity of approximately 50 ml and is attached to the undersurface of the liver. Its function is to concentrate and store bile, and then to eject the bile into the alimentary tract when it is required for the digestion and absorption of fat. The ejection of bile is under hormonal control: cholecystokinin, secreted by the duodenum when fat enters from the stomach, stimulates contraction of the gall bladder muscles and forces bile into the common bile duct. This hormone is also thought to relax the sphincter of Oddi to allow the flow of bile into the duodenum.

Bile travels from the liver to the gall bladder via the right and left hepatic ducts, the hepatic duct, and the cystic duct; in its concentrated form, bile travels from the gall bladder to the

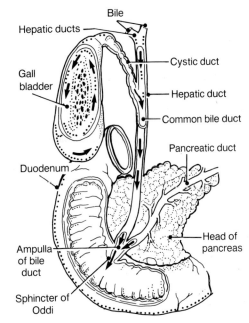

Fig. 45.2 Bile flow from the liver and the gall bladder into the duodenum.

duodenum via the cystic duct and the common bile duct (Fig. 45.2).

THE PANCREAS

This is a glandular organ with combined exocrine and endocrine functions. It is leaf-shaped, approximately 20 cm long, and has three nominal parts: a head, a body and a tail. It lies behind the stomach with its head in the curve of the duodenum, and the tail tapering off towards the spleen. The exocrine secretions pour into the main duct, which runs the internal length of the pancreas. This duct, on leaving the pancreas, joins the common bile duct just as it enters the duodenum. The exocrine secretion is an alkaline substance essential for counteracting acidic gastric juice, and is thus responsible for making the pH of the intestinal juices suitable for enzyme and bile reactions.

Pancreatic juice also contains 3 major enzymes: trypsinogen which, once activated by enterokinase from duodenal cells, aids in the digestion of proteins; amylase which converts any remaining starches to maltose; and lipase, which in the presence of bile, converts fats to fatty acids and glycerol. The presence of food in the stomach stimulates the vagus nerve to excite pancreatic exocrine cells, and the entry of chyme into the duodenum stimulates the secretion of two duodenal hormones – secretin and pancreozymin. Secretin is thought to stimulate the production of pancreatic alkaline substance, and pancreozymin is said to stimulate the production of pancreatic enzymes.

The endocrine functions of the pancreas are discussed in Chapter 28.

Conditions commonly associated with diseases of the liver, biliary system, and pancreas include jaundice, ascites, and haemorrhagic tendencies.

JAUNDICE

In this condition, all body tissue including the sclerae and skin assumes a yellow/green tinge, due to an increased concentration of bilirubin in the blood ($> 35\ \mu$mol/l). Bilirubin is produced by the breakdown of the haemoglobin of erythrocytes in the reticuloendothelial cells of the liver, spleen, and bone marrow. Figure 45.3 illustrates the formation of conjugated and unconjugated bilirubin.

There are numerous causes of jaundice, the majority of which can be grouped according to the origin of the problem.

Haemolytic jaundice

This is caused by excessive haemolysis and can be the result of fragile erythrocytes breaking up prematurely; some agent attacking the erythrocytes in the blood stream, for example an immune response; or an overactive spleen. In haemolytic jaundice too great an amount of erythrocyte breakdown product is presented to the liver. The liver functions at above normal capacity and conjugates more bilirubin than under normal circumstances. This is excreted via the bowel. However, some of the excess unconjugated bilirubin remains in the circulation and is therefore fat soluble. In this unconjugated form it cannot be excreted in urine

and causes jaundice. The faeces may be darker than normal due to increased levels of stercobilinogen, however the urine is normal. The alternative name for this condition is acholuria.

Haemolytic jaundice is not caused by liver disease – the jaundice occurs because the healthy liver has difficulty in dealing with the excessive amounts of insoluble bilirubin that is delivered to it. Treatment is that of the cause, and is discussed under haemolytic anaemia (see page 386).

Hepatocellular jaundice

This most common type of jaundice is due to degenerative or inflammatory processes which either destroy the liver's ability to conjugate bilirubin and/or prevent its drainage into the biliary system. In this instance the liver is diseased and is only able to conjugate a portion of the bilirubin that is presented. The most common causes of hepatocellular jaundice are hepatitis and cirrhosis of the liver. Many toxic substances such as snake

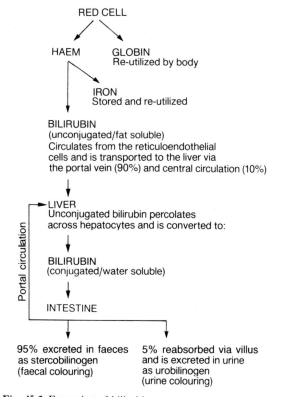

Fig. 45.3 Formation of bilirubin.

venom, carbon tetrachlorides, chloroform, and the sulphonamides may also produce hepatocellular jaundice. Paracetamol in excessive dosages will cause liver damage and subsequent jaundice.

Only a percentage of that portion of the bilirubin which is conjugated is able to drain into the biliary system. The remainder is forced back into the central circulation being unable to reach the ducts because of sclerosis and/or inflammation of the hepatocytes. An examination of the serum of this patient will show raised levels of both conjugated and unconjugated bilirubin. The conjugated bilirubin in the serum can be excreted via the kidney and urine will be darker than normal and slightly frothy. The faeces will be pale and foul-smelling due to the reduced amount of stercobilinogen reaching the intestine.

Obstructive jaundice (cholestasis)

In any situation where there is an obstruction to the flow of bile, whether it be within the ductules of the liver, in the biliary duct system, or at the head of the pancreas, the bilirubin which has all been conjugated (there is no disease of the liver) is forced back into the central circulation. It is water soluble and passes easily through the kidney, however jaundice in this situation can be extreme. The urine contains an extremely high amount of urobilinogen and is very dark and frothy. True steatorrhoea is present and the faeces will be clay coloured due to the absence of stercobilinogen.

It is important to remember that if insoluble bilirubin is reabsorbed the patient will only experience jaundice, but if bile is absorbed the patient will complain of pruritis also. The soluble bilirubin causes the jaundice and the bile salts cause the pruritis.

Extrahepatic causes of obstructive jaundice are: gallstones; tumours which compress or obliterate the biliary ducts, such as carcinoma of the head of the pancreas; stricture of the biliary ducts; and congenital biliary atresia.

As well as jaundice and skin irritation the patient with obstructive jaundice will experience nausea, vomiting, an intolerance for fatty foods; and haemorrhagic tendencies, due to diminished absorption of fat soluble vitamin K.

Medical management of jaundice

Because jaundice is a clinical feature of an underlying disease, it is the causative disease that must be treated if possible. Common specific diseases will be discussed in the following chapters.

Nursing management of jaundice

The yellow discoloration may cause the patient some embarrassment. If so, give him as much privacy as possible and, for the patient in whom recovery is a realistic possibility, reassure him that the colour will decrease as his condition improves.

The skin irritation of obstructive jaundice can be improved by: discouraging the patient from scratching by keeping his nails short; the use of soothing preparations such as calamine or an antipruritic oil; and the administration of an antihistamine if prescribed. Frequent bathing in tepid water without the use of soap is also helpful.

The patient with obstructive jaundice will also be embarrassed by the odour of his bowel actions. If ambulation is restricted he should be allowed to use the commode in the toilet area rather than at the bedside, especially if he is sharing a room. Room deodorizers should be used. The patient should be reassured that the malodorous faeces will return to normal on correction of the condition. The nurse will also be required to observe and record the degree of the patient's jaundice, to test his urine for bilirubin, and to maintain a faeces chart noting colour, consistency, and amount.

In many instances the patient with jaundice has a serious underlying disease, and may even be in a terminal condition; therefore the care of the seriously ill patient must also be considered.

ASCITES

The peritoneum is a thin serous membrane which lines the abdominal cavity and covers the intraperitoneal organs; serous fluid is continuously produced and reabsorbed by the peritoneum. This fluid is contained in the potential space of the peritoneal cavity, and in only just sufficient amount to provide lubrication. Ascites is the marked increase in the volume of either serous fluid or transudate in the peritoneal cavity, due to some serious chronic underlying disease. Ascites is clinically detectable when more than 1 litre has accumulated. It is a serious pathological state with a poor prognosis because the underlying cause is often not treatable.

Pathophysiology

Causes of ascites include:

1. Increased pressure in the portal circulation due to either congestive heart failure, or chronic liver failure.
2. Low serum albumin (hypoalbuminaemia) due to malnutrition, especially from a protein deficient diet; liver cell failure, with a resultant inability to synthesize plasma proteins; or a loss of albumin via the kidneys in some renal diseases
3. Fluid retention due to increased circulating hormones, especially aldosterone and antidiuretic hormone
4. Overproduction of hepatic lymph in chronic liver disease – an inflammatory reaction
5. Overproduction of peritoneal serous fluid in chronic diseases affecting the peritoneum, for example, malignancies or chronic inflammation.

Clinical manifestations

The patient is invariably chronically ill due to the underlying disease; he may be in a terminal state, and will probably exhibit most or all of the following:

1. Dyspnoea, due to the volume of ascitic fluid causing pressure on the diaphragm, and thus restricting normal ventilation.
2. A heavy uncomfortable feeling, and difficulty in moving or repositioning due to extra girth size and debilitation.
3. A tendency to develop pneumonia, deep vein thrombosis, and decubitus ulcers due to associated oedema in sacrum and limbs.
4. Chafing in the groin area due to overlapping skin folds and the weight of excess abdominal fluid.
5. Clothing feeling tight and uncomfortable.
6. Anxiety due to the feeling of unwellness and his possible poor prognosis.

Medical and surgical management

The objectives of treatment are to endeavour to treat the underlying causes, to decrease the production of ascitic fluid, and to decrease the amount of ascitic fluid already formed.

Various techniques are used in order to reduce the amount of ascitic fluid and may include: a low salt diet, a restricted fluid intake, diuretic drug therapy, abdominoparacentesis, and the insertion of a Le Veen shunt (peritoneal-venous shunt).

The Le Veen shunt

This is a relatively new method for managing ascites and enables a continuous re-infusion of ascitic fluid into the venous system, thus preserving valuable proteins and electrolytes. The key to the shunt is a one-way valve which opens at a low pressure stimulus. Once open, the valve allows the peritoneal fluid to flow from the abdominal cavity into a silicon tube; this tube passes under the subcutaneous tissue and empties into the jugular vein (Fig. 45.4).

The patient's own breathing triggers the shunt into action. During inhalation the diaphragm flattens, causing the intraperitoneal fluid pressure to rise, and the intrathoracic superior vena cava

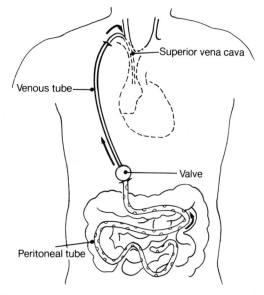

Fig. 45.4 Le Veen shunt in situ. The valve and venous tube are sited subcutaneously.

pressure to fall. The resulting difference in pressure forces the shunt valve to open and fluid to flow into the tubing. On exhalation the valve closes. This one-way valve is so designed that increased venous pressure is prevented. However, in the initial stages following the insertion of the shunt the patient may need a transfusion of packed cells to counteract haemodilution. Restricted fluid intake, low salt diet, and diuretic therapy may also be employed until the initial bulk of ascitic fluid is reduced.

The actual insertion of the shunt is a relatively minor operation performed in the operating room. On return to the ward the patient will have 2 small incisions, one in the abdominal wall and one near the clavicle. Suture removal occurs 5–7 days post-procedure. Increased urinary output, decreasing girth size, and improving general comfort of the patient indicate the success of this procedure; these observations should be recorded in the nursing history.

Abdominoparacentesis

Occasionally it is necessary to withdraw some of the ascitic fluid to relieve severe distension when it is causing difficulty in breathing and/or kidney dysfunction. By use of a trocar and cannula, a catheter is inserted into the peritoneal cavity and allows the fluid to drain slowly into a container. Too rapid removal of ascitic fluid may cause drastic shifts of fluid, minerals, and proteins between the vascular and extravascular compartments with resultant circulatory collapse. The nurse must ensure that the ascitic fluid does not drain off too quickly. An abdominal binder, readjusted hourly, provides a firm support and assists in preventing sudden abdominal organ or fluid shift. Only sufficient fluid is removed to relieve discomfort and this amount will be determined by the physician.

Other complications of paracentesis include perforated bladder, peritonitis due to damage to intestines, and persistent leakage of ascitic fluid at the puncture site. The nurse will ensure that the patient's bladder is empty prior to the procedure being performed and will record observations of vital signs for at least 24 hours post procedure. The dressing to the puncture site must be changed as often as is necessary to prevent soakage onto clothing. The skin around the puncture site must be protected from excoriation by the use of a water repellant preparation.

Nursing management

Nursing care is aimed at preventing or managing the individual patient's identified problems and assisting with the medical management. Nursing responsibilities include:

1. *Oxygenation*. It is important to reduce the pressure of abdominal contents on the diaphragm. This is best achieved by having the patient in a semi-upright position (the fully upright position becomes quickly uncomfortable and is not restful). Hourly deep breathing and coughing exercises are essential and the nurse must teach, supervise and encourage these.

2. *Hygiene*. Because of his debilitated state, the patient must be either sponged or assisted with showering by the nurse; sometimes 2 nurses are needed for this procedure. Particular attention should be given to all pressure areas and chafing in skin folds must be prevented – a light smear of lanoline following each washing of the areas is helpful. Talcum powder in skin folds should be avoided as it becomes moist with sweat and thus serves no useful purpose.

3. *Nutrition*. The nurse must ensure that the patient adheres to a low salt diet. This includes observing that significant others do not bring foodstuffs containing large quantities of salt to the patient. Patients with ascites often need a great deal of persuasion to eat an adequate diet. A fluid balance chart is maintained to monitor the patient's fluid intake, remembering that he will be allowed only restricted amounts of fluid. The fluid balance chart will also be used for monitoring the effectiveness of the diuretic drugs.

4. *Assisting with abdominoparacentesis.*

HAEMORRHAGIC TENDENCIES

The tendency to bleed may have 3 major origins:

1. Lack of bile in the intestine which is necessary for the absorption of vitamin K.

2. Inability of the liver to synthesize prothrombin (coagulation factor II) or coagulation factors V, VI, VII, IX, and X.

3. Portal hypertension. This may result from obstruction of blood flow through a diseased liver, as in cirrhosis, or be due to obstruction of the portal vein. The resulting pressure in the portal circulation often causes portal–systemic communications (collateral circulation) to form at the lower end of the oesophagus, in the stomach, the abdominal wall, and at the anus. These new vessels are usually fragile and readily become varicosed with a tendency to bleed. Oesophago-gastric varices (usually a sign of advanced cirrhosis of the liver) are the most important as bleeding into the gastrointestinal tract from this area can be severe and life threatening.

Medical and surgical management

Vitamin K is administered parenterally until obstruction to bile flow can be relieved. Blood or plasma infusion will replace coagulation factors temporarily until the underlying cause can be determined, and hopefully treated. These patients must be protected from injuries that cause bleeding because once bleeding starts it is very difficult to control.

Diagnosis of ruptured oesophageal varices is made by oesophagoscopy. The aims of management are to:

• Stop the bleeding
• Stop metabolism of blood in the bowel
• Kill the normal flora of the large bowel
• Reduce pressure in the portal vein.

After the site and extent of the rupture has been determined, the gastroenterologist will endeavour to stop and prevent further bleeding by either sclerosing the varicosities or by inserting a compressing balloon (tamponade) of the Sengs-taken-Blakemore type. The oesophageal balloon, once inflated, will exert direct pressure on the bleeding varices (Fig. 45.5).

Stopping metabolism of blood in the gut is achieved by the aspiration of as much blood as possible from the stomach and also by forcing blood that has entered into the duodenum to pass

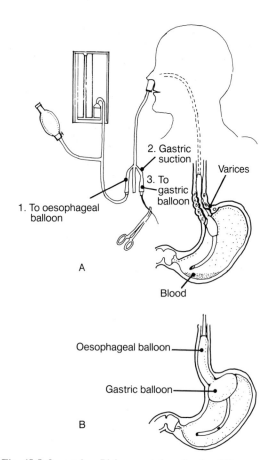

Fig. 45.5 Sengstaken-Blakemore tube, showing (**A**) uninflated tube in position. When (**B**) oesophageal and gastric balloons are inflated, bleeding is stopped and blood is aspirated from the stomach.

through the gastrointestinal tract in as short a time as possible. To accomplish this, a non-metabolizable polysaccharide such as lactulose is given in large quantities to the patient via the nasogastric lumen of the Sengstaken-Blakemore tube. This has dual chemical functions: it irritates the bowel and therefore speeds peristalsis; and it draws fluid into the lumen of the gut because of its high osmotic pressure, therefore increasing the bulk of the gut contents. Lactulose is given until significant diarrhoea is caused and is continued in high dosages until the diarrhoea is free of blood.

During this period it is imperative that the nurse, along with the physician, is aware that the patient's hydration status will alter markedly and IV fluid correction must be instituted and carefully monitored.

Normal flora in the large bowel is responsible for the end metabolism of protein. In a patient with significant liver disease, who has a large amount of blood in the gut, the deamination of protein will cause marked elevation of serum ammonium. To prevent the possibility of acute hepatic coma, the normal flora of the patient's large bowel should be eradicated during this acute phase of illness. The chemical agent used to achieve this must be one that is not metabolized, as the action is needed in the gut, and the load on the liver is already extreme and most drugs are at least partially detoxified by the liver. The substance most commonly used is neomycin.

The administration of the posterior pituitary hormone, pituitrin, is sometimes used as a temporary measure in controlling oesophageal bleeding, as it is thought to lower portal blood pressure. The side-effects of this drug can be quite severe and include myocardial ischaemia, uterine contraction, fluid retention, and intestinal colic. Pituitrin has a vasoconstricting action.

A more permanent method of controlling portal hypertension can be achieved by shunting blood from the portal circulation into the systemic circulation. A variety of techniques have been attempted to achieve a satisfactory portal–systemic venous-shunt. The shunt that is most commonly used is the splenorenal (Warren's) shunt. When a splenorenal shunt is performed the overactive spleen is removed, as portal hypertension often causes splenomegaly and leucopenia. The splenic vein (a vessel of the portal circulation) is anastomosed to the left renal vein (a major vessel of the general circulation). Blood that normally drains into the portal circulation via the splenic vein, from the pancreas and the inferior portion of the stomach, now drains into the left renal vein thus greatly reducing the pressure within the portal circulation (Fig. 45.6). This surgery is more satisfactory if it is performed on younger patients who have some liver function, and before oesophageal varices have become a major problem.

This procedure does not cure the underlying liver disease and the ultimate well-being of the patient will depend on his ability to abstain from alcohol. Alcohol is the chief cause of chronic liver failure which in turn is the chief cause of portal hypertension and bleeding oesophageal varices.

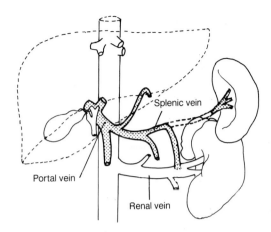

Fig. 45.6 Spleno-renal shunt following splenectomy.

Specific nursing management of the patient with bleeding oesophageal varices

If sclerosis of the varices was performed during oesophagoscopy, the nursing management of the patient post-procedure is similar to that following removal of a tamponade tube.

Care of the patient with a Sengstaken-Blakemore tube

The insertion of a Sengstaken-Blakemore tube is usually only necessary when the patient is in a life-threatening situation. This tube is such that the patient will be unable to swallow secretions and discomfort and apprehension will be key features of his condition. Therefore the nursing management of these patients requires vigilance, technical excellence and skillful communication to provide patient reassurance.

It is essential for the nurse to identify and label each of the three proximal lumina of the tube, which is essentially a nasogastric tube with the addition of two inflatable balloons (see Fig. 45.5). The main lumen leads to the perforated distal end which permits the aspiration of gastric contents. The other two lumina are for inflating the two balloons, which must be checked for any leakages before the tube is inserted. Because the insertion of this tube can be difficult and may cause further trauma, the procedure should be performed by a specialist physician and under fluoroscopic control. The nurse will be responsible for setting up and assisting with this procedure. The larger, elongated balloon exerts direct pressure on the oesophageal varicosities and the more distal, smaller balloon compresses varices in the cardia and also prevents the tube from slipping out of position. The inflation lumina are usually connected to manometers to ensure that the prescribed pressures of 35–45 mmHg are maintained. Too little pressure will not control bleeding, and excessive pressure can cause tissue ulceration. It is essential to empty the stomach of any blood by aspirating via the suction lumen, thus reducing the amount of blood entering the small bowel. Digestion of blood produces nitrogenous wastes that, when absorbed, can contribute to hepatic coma. Accurate measurement and recording of the amount of aspirate is carried out at $\frac{1}{4}$–1 hourly intervals, depending upon the individual patient's needs. The amount of blood should progressively decrease within 1–2 hours after insertion of the tube, and if the blood aspirate continues unabated or increases, the physician must be notified immediately, when he/she may order an ice water stomach lavage in a further attempt at controlling the bleeding.

The oesophageal balloon should be deflated at 1–4 hourly intervals for 5–10 minutes to reduce the risk of tissue damage. During the period of balloon deflation the nurse must aspirate the patient's stomach to ensure that bleeding has not recommenced. If bleeding does recur at this time the balloon must be reinflated immediately and the physician notified.

Whilst a Sengstaken-Blakemore tube is in situ in any patient a nurse should be in constant attendance to observe for any of the common adverse situations which may arise with this procedure, for example, respiratory distress, and difficulty in expectorating saliva that the patient is unable to swallow (because of the inflated tube which obstructs the oesophagus).

Other nursing care includes: constant reassurance to the patient, as he will often have a feeling of suffocation; nasal and mouth care; aspiration of oropharyngeal secretions p.r.n., administration of oxygen; and administration of pethidine or diazepam as ordered. The patient will have complete bed rest whilst the tube is in position and will receive nutrients via an IV infusion or hyperalimentation. At the same time the patient may also require a blood transfusion. Recordings of vital signs and fluid balance are maintained in order to measure the patient's progress. All gastric aspirate and vomitus should be described and faeces should be tested for occult blood where melaena is not evident.

Once bleeding has ceased and prior to removal of the tube, the oesophageal balloon is left deflated for approximately 24 hours and small amounts of clear fluids may be introduced via the tube into the stomach. The tube is removed with extreme caution, usually by the physician, and following this procedure the nurse must observe the patient constantly for signs of recurrence of the bleeding.

When diet is recommended the patient is advised to chew his food well and to avoid such foods as raw fruit, raw vegetables, and nuts, as a large bolus or hard foods may cause further trauma and bleeding at the varicosity site.

The Minnesota four lumen oesophagogastric tamponade tube has the same function as a Sengstaken-Blakemore tube but has a fourth channel that ends proximal to the elongated oesophageal balloon and is perforated at its distal end to allow for the aspiration of oesophageal secretions. This improved tube will probably replace the more common Sengstaken-Blakemore tube.

Splenorenal shunt

If it is necessary for the splenorenal shunt to be performed, nursing care of the patient will be as for any major abdominal surgery. However, the patient will be kept at rest in bed postoperatively for a prolonged length of time, to allow the body systems to adjust to this major reorganization of blood flow. Sometimes these patients are nursed in an intensive care unit in the immediate postoperative phase.

46

Disorders of the liver

Mavis Matthews   Jenny Kidd

HEPATITIS (ACUTE PARENCHYMAL DISEASE OF THE LIVER)

Aetiology

Hepatitis is an inflammatory disease of the liver, which may be of an acute or chronic nature, and is due largely to infective or toxic agents.

The most common infective causes of hepatitis are viruses, namely: hepatitis A (HAV), hepatitis B (HBV), and hepatitis non A/non B (NANB). Cytomegalovirus and Epstein Barr virus have also been known to cause hepatitis.

Nonviral pathogens that may cause hepatitis are *Leptospira icterohaemorrhagia* (Weil's disease), *Toxoplasma gondii* (toxoplasmosis), and *Coxiella burnetti* (Q fever).

Substances that are toxic to the liver cells and can cause hepatitis include an ever increasing list of drugs, alcohol, carbon tetrachlorides, and yellow phosphorus. Some of the drugs that are known to cause hepatitis in susceptible persons include phenothiazines, some of the antitubercular drugs, phenylbutazone, and indomethacin. Tetracycline and paracetamol will cause acute severe liver damage in most people when taken in overdose amounts.

Pathophysiology

Whatever the cause of hepatitis, the liver cells (hepatocytes) and surrounding structures are affected in a similar manner. The whole of the liver is involved, some areas more so than others. There will be patchy areas of necrotic tissue while other areas will show grossly swollen cells. In severe cases there is collapse of the reticulum framework, thus creating an undesirable communication between the portal tracts and the central veins. Cholestasis can be a feature. When the liver is grossly affected with large areas of necrosis, the patient may develop acute or chronic liver failure.

Viral hepatitis

Hepatitis caused by any of hepatitis A (HAV), hepatitis B (HBV) and hepatitis non A/non B (NANB) viruses, is a major health concern throughout the world.

HAV is spread primarily via the faecal–oral route and most outbreaks can be traced to contaminated food. Faecal shedding of the virus is highest during the incubation period, therefore control of the infection is difficult. Sanitary disposal of faeces and thorough handwashing following visits to the toilet are the most effective means of reducing spread.

Many cases of hepatitis A are asymptomatic, but when symptoms do occur the onset is usually sudden and the patient may be incapacitated for several weeks. However, prognosis is good, the mortality rate being less than 0.1%. There is no evidence that chronic liver failure develops or that a carrier state exists. Some measure of protection may be given to high risk persons by using the immunoglobulin γ-Globulin. The development of a HAV vaccine is currently under study.

HBV is spread mainly by direct or indirect contact with infected blood. Contact with secretions, such as saliva, menstrual and vaginal discharges, and semen are alternative modes of spread. People at highest risk include: health workers handling blood or blood products, giving intravenous injections, or performing venepuncture; patients who receive blood, blood products, or injections with contaminated needles or solutions; drug abusers who share needles; people receiving tattoos; and sexual partners of infected people. Male homosexuals appear to be at very high risk. The virus may also spread from a mother to her newborn infant – either during passage through the birth canal or via breast milk.

Hepatitis B is more serious than hepatitis A because although the onset is insidious, the symptoms are often very severe. Later, as symptoms subside, the infection may persist at a subclinical level resulting in chronic liver failure and cirrhosis. The mortality rate may be as high as 10%. A carrier state exists because of the persistent infection, and people may even be carriers of HBV without having had a clinical episode of the disease. A high proportion of infected newborn babies become persistent carriers. The prevalence of carriers in Australia is said to be 0.1%.

The HBV (also known as the Dane particle) has a DNA core and contains several antigens: hepatitis B surface antigen (HB$_s$Ag), hepatitis B core antigen (HB$_c$Ag), and the 'e' antigen (HB$_e$Ag). These antigens together with their immunoglobulins (anti-HB$_s$, anti-HB$_c$, and anti-HB$_e$) which are formed at varying stages of the infection, can be used to identify hepatitis B virus infection and to determine the stage of the disease.

A hepatitis B vaccine is now available for use in Australia.

NANB Hepatitis is diagnosed by excluding HAV and HBV and other identifiable viral infectious agents. It is not known whether one or more viruses are involved, but it is thought that several distinct viruses will eventually be isolated. Viral hepatitis NANB contracted other than through a blood transfusion has been shown to be caused by water borne viruses.

Clinical manifestations

These are the usual symptoms and signs of an acute infectious disease and they vary in intensity. The early symptoms are vague and nonspecific and include mild to moderate fever, headache, and malaise, progressing to anorexia, vomiting, and diarrhoea. The patient often complains of pain in

muscles and joints. This state may or may not be followed by jaundice (the icteric phase). Dark urine and clay coloured faeces may have been noticed prior to the onset of jaundice. There is usually an associated pruritis when jaundice is present. Tenderness in the right upper quadrant is sometimes a feature, and is due to the congested liver. Hepatitis A seems to have a more sudden onset than either hepatitis B or non A/non B, but the inflammatory process is usually much milder. In severe cases, anaemia, haemorrhagic tendencies, leucopenia, and lymphocytosis can occur.

Investigative procedures

1. Viral studies to determine the causative organism and stage of the disease.
2. Serum bilirubin – may be elevated up to 300 μmol/l.
3. Serum enzymes SGPT and SGOT – elevated initially but fall when jaundice appears.
4. Flocculation tests – positive.
5. Prothrombin time – may be prolonged.
6. Full blood examination – may show anaemia, leucopenia, lymphocytosis.
7. Urinalysis – excess urobilinogen in early stages, and bilirubin may be present if there is biliary obstruction.

Medical management

There is no specific treatment for viral hepatitis but because it is an infectious disease a principal objective is to prevent its spread. Another main objective of care is to keep the patient at bed rest during the early active stage of the disease in an attempt to prevent serious liver damage. The patient may or may not be hospitalized.

No specific drugs are used to treat hepatitis. Any drugs which the patient may be taking for other purposes, and which are inactivated or detoxified by the liver, are avoided during the acute illness. Barbiturates and oral contraceptives are included among such drugs.

Diet

These patients often have an aversion to food and in particular to fatty foods. Whilst the patient is at complete bed rest and expending little energy, the nurse is usually able to persuade the patient to take sufficient, high kilojoule/high carbohydrate nutrients in fluid form to avoid having intravenous feedings. As the patient's appetite returns he may eat what he desires except for fatty foods if there has been any evidence of obstructive jaundice. Fat is reintroduced into the diet in the form of butter, eggs, and milk. If these are tolerated lean meats (all meat contains some fat) are added to the diet. As a precautionary measure some physicians advise the patient not to eat fried foods, fatty meat, pastries, or to drink alcohol for 4–6 months following recovery.

Nursing management

For the patient with hepatitis nursing care must always be planned with the patient's specific needs in mind. Patients react differently to their disease state and will therefore present with individual problems to be overcome and individual needs to be met. Not all patients have the same symptomatology nor do they have the same degree of severity of hepatitis. Therefore nursing care is aimed at being individualized and involving the patient and his significant others in the planning, implementation, and evaluation of that care.

The rate of recovery from hepatitis varies considerably between patients. The patient should stay at bed rest until the serum bilirubin and enzymes are within normal levels and until liver tenderness has subsided. Up to 3 weeks in bed is not unusual especially with hepatitis B. Returning to normal activities may take several weeks to months and the patient needs to be supported during this time as he will often feel irritable and depressed because of such slow progress; he may also have guilt feelings about his prolonged stay away from work. See page 427 for nursing management of the patient with jaundice.

Prevention of spread of infection

When hospitalized, the patient with viral hepatitis should be isolated from other patients (see also page 525). Because the organisms may be found in all body secretions of the affected person, particular emphasis is placed on the importance of safe disposal of faeces, urine, and anything contaminated with blood: most hospitals have rigid policies regarding disposal. The wearing of latex gloves, plastic aprons and gowns will assist in protecting all personnel whenever they are caring for the patient. The importance of thorough washing of hands after each contact with the patient or his immediate environment cannot be overemphasized. All linen must be treated as infectious. Some hospitals insist on full isolation nursing for hepatitis patients. Blood, faeces, and urine specimens must be clearly labelled 'hepatitis' or 'highly infectious' to protect the couriers and laboratory workers.

The public, especially school children and foodhandlers, must be taught the importance of thorough handwashing following every visit to the toilet and before handling food. Town councils are responsible for ensuring good sanitation and the complete separation of water supply from sewerage. There must be mandatory screening of all potential blood donors before their blood is used for anything except hepatitis immunization products. The public must also be made aware of the risks of becoming infected when such procedures as tattooing, ear piercing, and self-administration of injections are carried out in nonsterile conditions.

CHRONIC LIVER DISEASE; CHRONIC LIVER FAILURE; CIRRHOSIS OF THE LIVER

The above terms are often used synonymously which is not strictly correct, for it is possible to have chronic liver disease without chronic liver failure, and it is also possible to have chronic liver failure without cirrhosis. However, the most common types of chronic liver disease do lead to cirrhosis; this, therefore, is the condition which will be dealt with in detail.

Aetiology and pathophysiology

For cirrhosis to exist 4 criteria must be met:

1. Evidence of gross liver cell damage
2. Evidence of widespread fibrosis

3. Distorted liver architecture resulting in compression of some blood, lymph, and bile vessels, with congestion of others

4. A characteristic nodular appearance of the liver caused by the fibrosis and distorted liver architecture forcing the regenerating hepatic cells to be clustered into nodules. This nodular regeneration is the 'hallmark' of cirrhosis.

Cirrhosis may be categorized as follows:

Laennec's portal cirrhosis. This occurs when the condition is due to the prolonged, heavy consumption of alcohol. It is also postulated that severe prolonged malnutrition may lead to liver damage and eventually to cirrhosis; but this is debatable because cirrhosis does not occur in kwashiorkor or marasmus.

Post necrotic cirrhosis. This is an uncommon complication of a previous acute viral hepatitis usually of the hepatitis B or non A/non B types.

Biliary cirrhosis. This rare condition, which mainly affects middle-aged women, results from prolonged obstruction to bile flow anywhere between the small interlobular bile ducts and the ampulla of Vater. This obstruction leads to chronic inflammation and destruction of the interlobular bile ducts.

Metabolic cirrhosis. This can be caused by excessive hepatic deposits of iron (haemochromatosis) or bronze diabetes and/or copper (Wilson's disease). Also, some people who are on long term treatment with some drugs that are metabolized in the liver can develop cirrhosis. These include methyldopa and methotrexate.

Ideopathic. In many cases the cause of the cirrhotic state cannot be determined.

Cirrhosis due to alcoholism

This is by far the most common cause of cirrhosis in Australia. It is now believed that alcohol does have a direct toxic effect on liver cells, but why some people are more susceptible than others in developing cirrhosis is not known. About 15–20% of known alcoholics develop cirrhosis. Not all liver cells are affected at the same time, and any of the developing stages (fatty liver, hepatitis, fibrosis, cirrhosis) can be present in the one specimen of liver tissue. During the fatty liver stage, the liver is greatly enlarged due to the liver cells becoming grossly swollen with globules of fat. At this stage the patient has no symptoms, but the enlarged liver may be palpated on routine medical examination and the condition is reversible providing there is complete abstinence from alcohol.

The enzyme nicotinamide adenine dinucliotide (NAD) is necessary for the metabolism of alcohol; it is also necessary for the metabolism of carbohydrate and fat, but because alcohol cannot be stored in the body it is dealt with by the liver to the detriment of normal carbohydrate and fat metabolism. As a result, some of the unmetabolized fat accumulates in the liver. The liver cells are able to adapt to heavy alcohol intake by increasing their activity, thus contributing to alcohol tolerance. However these cells cannot continue to compensate indefinitely and eventually there will be progressive cell failure, death, and necrosis. Ultimately the liver will become shrunken and nodular in appearance. Cirrhosis is an irreversible condition.

Clinical manifestations

Signs of this disease do not appear until almost all of the hepatocytes have been replaced by scar and fibrotic tissue. Because of the numerous functions of the liver the problems for the patient will also be numerous and widespread throughout the body. Table 46.1 shows the major functions of the liver and relates the clinical manifestations of cirrhosis with malfunction. It demonstrates that the symptoms and signs occur either as a result of portal hypertension, or of failing liver cell function.

In chronic liver failure any of the manifestations may appear gradually over a number of years. Rarely do all factors occur together in a single patient. The early signs of digestive malfunction are so vague and nonspecific that the patient is usually not alerted to seek medical aid. Too often the late signs of cirrhosis, for example, jaundice, ascites, and/or bleeding oesophageal varices have developed before the patient is aware of his condition and this, tragically, is often too late for a favourable prognosis.

Table 46.1 Comparison of normal liver function and possible results of malfunction

Normal function of the liver	Possible result of malfunction
1. Receives 20 percent of cardiac output via the portal vein from the lower oesophagus, stomach, spleen, pancreas, small bowel and large bowel.	Any blockage to the blood flow through the liver will result in congestion of blood in the liver which in turn will cause back pressure in the portal vein (Portal hypertension).
	Portal hypertension may cause:
	• Pain in the right hypochondrium due to the engorged liver stretching the liver capsule
	• Formation of collateral circulation between veins of the portal circulation and veins of the systemic circulation especially: – submucosa of oesophagus, fundus of the stomach and the rectum – anterior abdominal wall (caput medusa) – parietal peritoneum
	• Varicosities of the new collaterals – oesophageal varices – haemorrhoids
	• Ascites and oedema
	• Splenomegaly causing rapid destruction of blood cells resulting in – anaemia – leucopenia – thrombocytopenia.
2. Formation of bile. Bile salts are necessary for the breakdown and absorption of fats and fat soluble vitamins A, D and K. Soluble bilirubin is a pigment produced by degradation of haemoglobin. It gives faeces its characteristic colour. Bile has a deodorizing action on faeces.	Engorged or destroyed architecture of the liver reduces either the formation of bile or the outflow of bile. When insufficient bile reaches the gastrointestinal tract there will be: • Maldigestion and reduced absorption of fat and fat soluble vitamins • Malabsorption of vitamin K results in reduced prothrombin formation which leads to bleeding tendencies • Absorption of bile into blood stream causing jaundice, pruritis, dark urine • Pale, malodorous faeces.
3. Stores iron and vitamin B_{12}.	Iron deficiency and pernicious anaemia.
4. Kupffer cells lining the sinusoids trap and destroy bacteria from the gut.	Increased susceptibility to infection.
5. Removes toxic wastes: (a) Drugs	Drug toxicity. Drugs not detoxified may accumulate in the body and reach dangerously toxic levels therefore extreme caution must be used when giving such drugs as digoxin, analgesics and hypnotics.
(b) Hormones • Aldosterone, ADH	Water retention leading to ascites and oedema
• Oestrogen	Excessive oestrogen, especially in the male, can cause gynaecomastia, chest alopecia, altered hair distribution, spider naevi, palmar erythema, testicular atrophy and loss of libido. There will also be menstrual abnormalities in women.
(c) End products of infection.	Natural body responses to infection are decreased. The patient is more acutely ill when infected and may develop toxaemia.
6. Synthesis of plasma proteins: (a) Prothrombin, fibrinogen, factors VII, IX, X	Decreased formation of clotting factors leads to bleeding tendencies.
(b) Albumin.	Decreased formation results in loss of osmotic pressure in vascular compartments and may cause oedema and ascites.
7. Deamination of protein (amino acids).	When there is excessive destruction of protein (damaged liver cells) the enzymes serum glutamic oxalacetic transaminase (SGOT) and serum glutamic pyruvic transaminase (SGPT) are increased. Excessive breakdown of protein also causes increased amounts of the end-product ammonia to be released into the blood stream.
8. Converts ammonia to nontoxic urea for excretion by kidney (NB Bacterial action in the bowel also produces ammonia).	Hepatic encephalopathy. Ammonia is toxic to the brain and can cause confusion, apathy, euphoria, apraxia, stupor, delirium, hallucinations, tremor (liver flap), fetor hepaticus and coma.

Investigative procedures

Some of the more common investigations will include:

1. Blood analysis to determine liver function
   – serum bilirubin and ammonia are both high
   – serum enzymes: SGOT and SGPT are raised
   – plasma proteins: total serum protein and serum albumin are lowered while serum globulin is raised
   – biochemical testing for coagulation factors, which will be reduced
   – prothrombin time: will be extended.
2. Vitamin K test. An injection of vitamin K determines whether hypoprothrombinaemia is due to lack of absorption of vitamin K, or to failure of the liver to synthesize prothrombin.
3. Liver biopsy to determine type and extent of liver damage. (NB. It is mandatory to do a prothrombin time prior to this procedure.)
4. Liver scan will show liver size and is useful for determining functional and nonfunctional areas.
5. Oesophagoscopy to determine if varices are present.

Medical and nursing management

The patient with cirrhosis is usually admitted to hospital in an acutely ill state due to complications of the diseased liver. The main objectives of treatment are to endeavour to control any life threatening situations, for example, bleeding oesophageal varices, severe ascites or oedema; and to then endeavour to treat the underlying cause. For example, the alcoholic must be assisted to realize the importance of abstaining from alcohol for the rest of his life.

The physician will, if at all possible, avoid prescribing any drugs that are inactivated by the liver, such as barbiturates, diazepam, paracetamol, digitalis, opiates, and oral contraceptives. If any of these drugs are used, they will be in reduced dosages to avoid excessive accumulation in the body.

There are no specific drugs for the treatment of cirrhosis. Diuretics may be necessary for the management of ascites but because these are normally detoxified by the liver they may cause an electrolyte imbalance and are therefore usually given in reduced dosages. Chlormethiazole may be prescribed if the patient is in danger of developing delerium tremens. The patient may also require vitamin supplements such as a multivitamin preparation and vitamin K. Electrolyte replacement therapy may be required via intravenous infusion after any needs are assessed by having serum electrolytes evaluated.

Conservation of strength is important, so the patient will remain resting in bed until there is evidence of improvement, such as when tests reveal stabilized liver function. The nurse must assist with the performance of all hygiene needs, and carry out passive exercises until the patient is able to do these for himself. Later, more strenuous activities will be encouraged according to his level of tolerance.

The nurse must observe for developing or resolving ascites and oedema, any signs of bleeding or bruising, and signs of developing hepatic encephalopathy.

Diet

A high kilojoule (10 500–14 700), high protein (100–150 g) diet is ordered in the hope that a reasonable percentage of the nutrients will be absorbed and metabolized. There may need to be restriction of protein if the serum ammonium level is elevated, in which case the amount of protein allowed will be proportional to the serum ammonium level. Fluids and salt may also be restricted in the presence of oedema and/or ascites. The nurse will need to use much ingenuity in persuading the patient to take an adequate oral diet, as these patients are notorious for having no appetite. Frequent small snacks and nourishing fluids may be a better plan than expecting three large meals to be eaten in a day. The nurse should assess the patient's ability to feed himself and be prepared to assist him if necessary. If the patient is acutely ill it is sometimes necessary for hyperalimentation to be instituted so that adequate nutrition can be maintained. In order to monitor the patient's state the amount and type of nutrients and fluids taken must be recorded.

Allied paramedical care and habilitation

The physiotherapist, social worker, and dietician will all be involved in the co-ordinated care of the patient, but perhaps of greatest benefit will be those people who are able to encourage and support him in his endeavours to abstain from drinking alcohol. Such support may be obtained from his family, church, Alcoholics Anonymous, or behaviour modification groups. Once the patient has recovered from the acute episode of the liver complication that necessitated hospitalization, his prognosis and well-being will depend upon ensuring that the remaining functioning liver cells are not compromised. The nurse must ensure that the patient understands that this can only be achieved if he continues with his high protein, high kilojoule, low salt diet, and is prepared to abstain completely from alcohol.

HEPATIC ENCEPHALOPATHY (HEPATIC COMA)

Hepatic encephalopathy results from a rise in the serum levels of neurotoxins, to the point where neurological signs and symptoms occur. These include alterations in personality and intellect, confusion, restlessness, and asterixis ('liver flap' tremor of the hands), and may progress to coma and convulsions. It is a chronic, intermittent condition.

Toxic substances circulate in the body when the diseased liver is unable to carry out its detoxification function; or when portal blood by-passes the liver, for example, with a porto-systemic shunt (see Figure 45.6 page 431) either from pathologically created collateral vessels or surgically created vessels.

Ammonium is the main neurotoxin associated with severe liver disease. Ammonium is produced in the intestine by enzyme and bacterial action on protein derived from diet or from the presence of blood following gastrointestinal bleeding; in the presence of infection; and when there is severe electrolyte imbalance, particularly potassium depletion and metabolic alkalosis.

Factors which precipitate toxic levels of ammonium include:

1. Alcoholic binge in the presence of severe liver disease.
2. Bleeding into the gastrointestinal tract – ruptured oesophageal varices is a common precipitant (see page 430).
3. Excessive protein intake in diet.
4. Abdominoparacentesis causing electrolyte imbalance.
5. Dehydration, hypovolaemia, and diuretic therapy causing electrolyte imbalance.
6. Surgical portocaval shunt.
7. Infections which lead to increased phagocytosis, for example, chest infection.
8. Chronic constipation leading to increased ammonium production.
9. Drugs, for example, narcotics and barbiturates.

Nursing and medical management

Prevention is the most important objective. Individual precipitating factors must be recognized and avoided by both the patient and health workers. Other considerations include: control of haemorrhage; any protein allowed in the diet must be proportional to the blood ammonium level; faeces may be acidified, and constipation avoided, by the use of lactulose; bowel washouts and bowel sterilization may reduce the potential for ammonium production; and diuretics must be used with caution and potassium supplementation given.

Liver by-pass shunts should be avoided unless absolutely necessary to save life; splenorenal circulatory shunts seem to cause fewer cases of encephalopathy than do portocaval shunts because, although portal pressure is reduced, blood from the mesenteries continues to reach the liver. Le Veen shunting of ascitic fluid does not cause electrolyte imbalance to the same extent as does abdominoparacentesis.

LIVER TRAUMA

The most common cause of liver injury is the motor vehicle accident, therefore with their increase there is also an increase in the number of people receiving injuries to the liver. The liver may be pierced, bruised, or lacerated, and the extent of the effect will depend on the amount of haemorrhage, and or damage, to the bile ducts. On admission to hospital the patient must be observed closely $\frac{1}{4}$–$\frac{1}{2}$ hourly for signs of internal haemorrhage and later for biliary peritonitis (see page 447). When there is no evidence of these it is most likely that the injury will resolve by conservative treatment of bed rest and a light, low fat diet.

If, on the other hand, the injury is more severe and haemorrhage or peritonitis is evident the patient will require a laparotomy as soon as possible. Depending on the findings, surgical procedures may include debridement of necrosed tissue, suture repair, ligation of the hepatic artery if haemorrhage is catastrophic, or resection of a lobe of the liver. The surgeon will also carry out a complete exploration of the abdominal contents as there are often associated injuries. In some instances the diaphragm is also involved, causing pulmonary complications such as atelectasis and pleural effusion. When this is suspected the surgeon may insert an intercostal catheter at the time of performing the laparotomy.

Postoperatively the care will be as for the patient following any major abdominal surgery. The gastrointestinal tract will be rested for 2 to 3 days in order to prevent and/or treat ileus and, indirectly, to rest the liver. A nasogastric tube may be in place for aspiration purposes, and also to prevent or detect the onset of ileus. One or more drainage tubes are usually in place to provide adequate drainage of any debris at the operation site. Some surgeons prefer to use a large bore drain, rather than the smaller catheters which are attached to vacuum seal drainage apparatus. Occasionally, a T-tube may be in place if the bile ducts are damaged.

If the patient is in a shocked state due to the extensiveness of the injuries, or due to excessive blood loss, he may have a urethral catheter in place for monitoring urinary volume. He will have an intravenous infusion, preferably via a central venous line, probably a blood transfusion, and possibly an intercostal catheter. When there has been severe associated chest injuries, for example fractured ribs, the patient may be intubated and his ventilation mechanically assisted. It is not unusual for the patient with severe liver injury to be nursed in an intensive care setting for at least the first few postoperative days. When recovery is uncomplicated resumption of oral diet and ambulation should commence between the third and fifth postoperative day.

There is a relatively high mortality rate with severe liver injury, particularly with blunt injuries, and this is mainly due to uncontrollable haemorrhage. Other complications of liver injury include biliary peritonitis, persistent ileus, fever due to necrosis of liver tissue, and subphrenic and sub-hepatic abscesses.

PARASITIC DISEASE OF THE LIVER

Echinococcosis – hydatid disease (see also p. 527)

Aetiology and pathology

Echinococcosis or hydatid disease is caused by the lavae of dog tapeworm. The eggs of the worm are excreted in the faeces of the infected dog. The transmission to man is through the ingestion of eggs from uncooked food, contaminated water and the handling of infected dogs.

Hosts of the tapeworm are man, sheep, pigs, cattle, and other mammals. When the eggs are ingested they hatch in the upper part of the small intestine and enter the bloodstream and lymphatics via the intestinal mucosa. The organisms then lodge in a relatively systematic pattern. In man, over 50% of hydatid cysts are found in the liver with decreasing percentages in the lungs, bones, brain, spleen, and heart. The organisms lodge in the capillaries causing an inflammatory reaction where some are destroyed but others develop into cysts. These cysts can grow up to 25 cm in diameter and are filled with a clear hydatid fluid. The cyst is comprised of 2 layers, the outer having numerous layers similar to tissue paper. The body's reaction to the cyst is one of inflammation and the cysts are surrounded by white cells, giant cells, and fibroblasts.

Cysts that have been present for 6 months begin to develop daughter cysts known as 'brood capsules', which increases the size of the cyst. When cysts form in the bone this results in pressure and atrophy and pathological fractures are not uncommon.

Clinical manifestations

These relate specifically to local pressure and destruction of tissue and occur years after the initial infection. Bleeding can occur due to erosion of blood vessels and pressure of the cysts can cause infarction. Rarely, a cyst ruptures spontaneously, causing leakage of hydatid fluid which may cause an anaphylactic reaction.

Hydatid disease of the liver may incorporate vague symptoms such as abdominal pain, and nausea, and vomiting after ingestion of food. On examination the patient may demonstrate local swelling in the right hypochondrium.

Respiratory symptoms include pyrexia, coughing paroxysms with occasional haemoptysis. The cough may be productive with a typical serous exudate containing threads of tissue.

Osseous cysts cause bone pain and eventual pathological fractures.

Recurrent attacks of urticaria are not an uncommon feature.

Investigative procedures

A history of contact with dogs and recurrent allergic attacks is suggestive of hydatid disease.

Intradermal test – Casoni's reaction. This test involves the injection of antigen prepared from cysts of an infected animal or human. An infected person will respond positively by the appearance of a wheal surrounded by erythema and induration.

Complement fixation test.

X-ray. This will enable the identification, size, location, and number of cysts.

Medical, surgical, and nursing management

Surgery is the ideal treatment, but care must be taken not to rupture the cyst during its removal as this can result in severe anaphylaxis and secondary echinococcosis. It may not be possible to remove multiple or large cysts due to the high mortality associated with massive liver surgery. Mebendazole is an effective alternative therapy.

Lobectomy is the recommended surgery for pulmonary infestation particularly if the lung is badly damaged.

Antihistamines and steroids are of use in controlling allergic reactions.

Nursing care is as for the patient undergoing abdominal surgery (see page 499).

Prevention

In endemic areas dogs should be treated for the disease and should not be fed on uncooked offal.

Personal cleanliness, washing of hands after touching a dog, proper cooking of food, and boiling of drinking water are all important measures in reducing human infection.

Hepatic distomiasis – fluke

Liver flukes are parasites which invade the liver and bile ducts of man. The sheep liver fluke, fasciola hepatica, is the causative organism and is found in all sheep-raising areas of the world. It is also found in goats and cattle, causing 'liver rot'.

The eggs are excreted in faeces of an infected human or animal, and develop in fresh water. From here they are ingested by fresh water snails which become the intermediate host. Excreta from the snails encyst on fresh water vegetation which is eaten by sheep or man and so the cycle continues. Once ingested, the parasite enters body tissues via the intestinal wall. Some lodge in the liver via the portal system and others invade the liver capsule via the peritoneal cavity. Maturation of the flukes occurs in the bile ducts.

Clinical manifestations

Classically there are three phases:

The invasive phase. The patient suffers high fever, general malaise, and weight loss. The liver is swollen and tender with referred pain often occurring in the shoulder. This phase may last weeks.

The latent phase. This occurs once the larvae have settled in the liver and may last for months to years. Patients may be asymptomatic during this time.

The obstructive phase. The flukes are fully mature and obstruct the bile ducts causing epithelial proliferation and eventual portal fibrosis.

Urticaria and oesinophilia are not uncommon features.

The patient is treated conservatively and is rarely if ever hospitalized. Drug therapy has been shown to be effective, however, repeated courses may be required.

TUMOURS OF THE LIVER

Benign tumours of the liver are extremely rare and are removed if they are causing severe pressure symptoms, or are in danger of rupturing and causing severe haemorrhage.

Malignant tumours are usually carcinomas but occasionally may be of the sarcoma group. The carcinomas usually originate in the liver cells (hepatoma) but may be derived from the bile duct cells (cholangioma). The lesions of primary malignant tumours may be singular or numerous, and may affect all or only a section of the liver. Metastases are usually to adjacent organs, the peritoneum, or the lungs. The cause of primary liver cancer is not known but of interest to researchers is the fact that cirrhosis is found in half to two-thirds of patients with this condition.

Secondary carcinoma is said to be about 20 times more common than are primary hepatic lesions. The liver is the most common site of metastatic growths due to the fact that the liver receives large volumes of blood from both the systemic and the portal circulation. Cancer cells can also reach the liver by direct spread from nearby organs such as the stomach and colon, or via the lymphatics.

Clinical manifestations

Unfortunately liver tumours are quite advanced before the patient suffers symptoms severe enough to cause him to seek medical aid. Anorexia, loss of weight, fatigue and abdominal discomfort are the usual initial features, followed by any of the signs of hepatic failure or cirrhosis, for example, abnormal liver function tests, ascites and jaundice. Abdominal pain is a late feature.

Investigative procedures

There are no tests that can be done to elicit liver cancer in its early stages. When the tumour is advanced definite diagnosis may be made by a liver scan showing characteristic filling defects; liver biopsy when the specimen is taken from the tumour; by finding cancer cells in ascitic fluid; and by detecting high concentrations of alphafetoprotein in the blood.

Medical and nursing management

Usually the treatment is palliative and symptomatic and is similar to the care of the cirrhotic patient. For surgery to be considered the tumour must be confined to one lobe and there must be no cirrhosis present; also, liver function tests must not be grossly abnormal. If a hepatic lobectomy is performed, the management is as described in the section dealing with liver trauma (see page 439). Occasionally the patient may be given a course of cytotoxic therapy but results have not proved very successful. Often the nurse is involved with caring for a patient who is dying.

Anticipated outcome

Because most malignant tumours of the liver are well advanced, and causing the grave symptoms of hepatic cell failure before a diagnosis is made, the prognosis is poor. Approximately 90% of these patients die within 1 year of the onset of symptoms.

47

Disorders of the biliary system

Mavis Matthews

Terminology related to biliary disease:

Chole – pertaining to bile
Cyst – bag
Doch – duct
Lith – stone
Cholecystitis – inflammation of the gall bladder
Cholelithiasis – calculi in the gall bladder
Cholecystectomy – removal of the gall bladder
Cholecystostomy – opening and evacuating the gall bladder
Choledochostomy – opening and exploration of the common bile duct, usually to remove calculi
Choledocholithiasis – calculi in the bile ducts
Cholangitis – inflammation of the bile duct(s)
Choledocholithotomy – removal of calculi from the bile ducts
Choledochogram – X-ray of bile ducts
Cholecystography – X-ray of the gall bladder

CHOLECYSTITIS AND CHOLELITHIASIS

Cholecystitis which may be acute or chronic in nature is almost always due to cholelithiasis. Other rare causes of cholecystitis include trauma, ductal occlusion due to previous injury or surgery, or, even more rarely, neoplasm.

Epidemiology

Gallstones are very common in all affluent countries, but the reason why this is so is not known. Until about twenty years ago it seemed that the most likely person to develop cholelithiasis was the fair skinned, obese, middleaged, multiparous woman. However, also for reasons unknown, the incidence is increasing and occurring at a much earlier age, without the sufferer necessarily conforming ro the above description. Cholecystectomy for the treatment of cholelithiasis is one of the most common operations performed in Australia.

Aetiology and pathophysiology

Biochemical analysis has shown that cholesterol is the most usual component of gallstones irrespective of their macroscopic appearance. It appears that whenever there is an imbalance in the ratio of cholesterol to bile acids and lecithin, there is a great chance that cholelithiasis will occur. Gallstones may also contain pigments and salts (especially calcium) and can vary in size (1 mm–50 mm), shape (cuboidal, round, irregular), colour (varying shades of yellow–brown) and number (solitary–numerous).

It is thought that irritation from the stones on the mucous membrane of the gall bladder causes an inflammatory reaction. Later secondary infection may become established and may result in empyema of the gall bladder. *Escherichia coli* and *Streptococcus faecalis* are the most usual offending organisms and the method by which they reach the gall bladder is not clear. If a stone, oedema, or stenosis obstructs the cystic duct a mucocele may develop as the organ distends. Occasionally perforation or gangrene may also occur. Figure 47.1 shows common sites of and conditions caused by gallstones.

Clinical manifestations

Pain. Cholelithiasis can be asymptomatic but may also cause acute or chronic cholecystitis or biliary

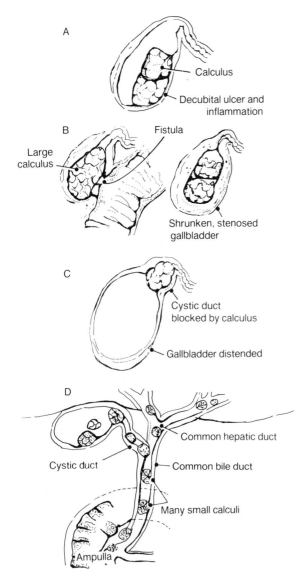

A

— Calculus

— Decubital ulcer and
inflammation

B   Fistula

Large
calculus

Shrunken, stenosed
gallbladder

C

Cystic duct
blocked by calculus

Gallbladder distended

D

Common hepatic duct

Cystic duct

Common bile duct

Many small calculi

Ampulla

Fig. 47.1 A and **B** – Large stones in the gall bladder may
cause ulceration and scarring or fistula formation. **C** – A
stone may obstruct the cystic duct. **D** – Smaller stones may
lodge in the common hepatic or bile ducts.

colic. The pain of acute cholecystitis is so severe
that it may cause extreme restlessness, pallor,
sweating, vomiting, and even severe shock. The
onset of pain is sudden and may last for hours,
localized in the right hypochondrium. Pain may
radiate around the right side of the thorax and
settle between the scapulae. Referred pain in the
right shoulder tip is common; a typical history is
that of pain following the ingestion of a fatty meal.

Tenderness, guarding, and rigidity around the
right costal margin, exacerbated by inspiration
(Murphy's sign), may also be a feature.

'Biliary colic' (a misnomer because there is no
peristaltic action in the biliary ducts) occurs when
a stone or oedema obstructs one of the ducts and
the gall bladder is thought to intermittently
undergo vigorous contractions in an effort to force
its contents past the obstruction. If the stone is
dislodged during this activity the pain may cease
abruptly, however if further stones become
impacted the pain will recur. In chronic cholecystitis the pain is much less severe. The patient may
'put up with it' for years before seeking medical
aid. There is danger of insidious perforation in
these cases.

Nausea and vomiting are common signs.

Fever with rigors is a common response to
inflammation and infection, as is leucocytosis.

Mild jaundice occasionally occurs where there is
ductal obstruction; there may also be an associated
pruritis.

Fat intolerance may occur, and is thought to be
due to the unavailability of bile for digestion of
fat.

Haemorrhagic tendency is a possibility if vitamin
K is not absorbed. This is also due to bile not
reaching the small intestine.

Investigative procedures

If the stones contain more than 10% calcium, a
plain abdominal X-ray will show cholelithiasis.

Oral cholecystogram. A radio opaque substance
is taken orally 10–14 hours prior to the X-ray.
This dye is absorbed into the portal circulation,
secreted by the liver, and concentrated in the gall
bladder. When the X-ray is taken, any stones
present may show up as filling defects.

Intravenous choledochogram/cholecystogram.
Radio opaque dye is injected intravenously when
it is not appropriate for the patient to take the dye
orally. X-rays are then taken.

CT scan can assist in differentiating between
stones and tumours.

Ultrasound may show stones when a cholecystogram has been unsuccessful.

Duodenoscopy followed by endoscopic retrograde cholangiopancreatography (ERCP) is another

method of injecting radio opaque dye prior to X-ray and is also helpful in visualizing the duct system.

Prothrombin estimation may help in determining whether obstruction of bile flow has caused nonabsorption of vitamin K. The degree of jaundice present will be indicated by a serum bilirubin estimation. Serum amylase may be elevated if there is an associated pancreatitis.

Medical, surgical and nursing management

The surgeon has 7 alternatives when deciding on the best method of treatment for a particular patient. They are:

- Do nothing if the patient is asymptomatic.
- Commence the patient on a low fat diet, if symptoms are mild or the patient refuses other treatment.
- Dissolve the stones if they are small and composed chiefly of cholesterol.
- Remove the stones via cholecystostomy.
- Remove the stones via endoscopy and sphincterotomy.
- Cholecystectomy with or without choledochostomy.
- Choledochostomy.

When symptoms are severe, the stones must be removed. Cholecystectomy with choledochostomy is still the preferred method as the stones are then not likely to recur. However, because of inherent dangers of surgical intervention during any acute illness, most surgeons prefer to wait, if feasible, for the acute attack of cholecystitis to subside. The patient may need to be admitted to hospital for medical management of the acute attack, but usually does not come to hospital until elective surgery has been arranged.

Small gallstones with high cholesterol content may be dissolved by the ingestion of chenodeoxycholic acid over a period of 1 to 2 years. The dissolved particles are excreted in the bile. This may be the treatment of choice for patients who either refuse surgery or who are not suitable for surgery. Of course, if the patient suffers from episodes of acute cholecystitis during this prolonged treatment surgical intervention may be necessary. Gallstones can recur following

conservative treatment. Cholecystostomy may be used to evacuate stones when it is not feasible to perform a cholecystectomy, for example when the patient is a poor operative risk, has a short life expectancy, or when the results of severe inflammation have obliterated anatomical landmarks.

Endoscopic techniques have now been developed whereby some stones may be removed following sphincterotomy via endoscopy. This method of treatment also saves the patient from abdominal surgery and many days in hospital. Once again, however, gallstones can recur.

Conservative management of the acute attack of cholecystitis

Principles of management are:

1. Rest in bed with nursing measures to control fever and rigors.
2. Pain relief. Pethidine is the drug of choice because morphine causes spasm of the sphincter of Oddi. However, when morphine is necessary, atropine, phenobarbitone, or hyoscine butylbromide may be given concurrently, as the action of these drugs as muscle relaxants will overcome the increased tone of the sphincter.
3. Relieve vomiting and reduce gastric irritation by keeping the stomach empty.
4. Maintain fluid and electrolyte balance intravenously if the patient is having nasogastric aspirations, otherwise oral fluids may be given.
5. Eliminate or prevent infection with broad spectrum antibiotics as ordered.
6. Pruritus may be relieved by the application of calamine lotion or anti-pruritic oil. In more severe cases an antihistamine may be necessary.
7. Prothrombin time estimation should be carried out and vitamin K given if necessary.
8. Advise patient of possible later surgery.

Surgical management

Cholecystectomy with choledochostomy

Cholecystectomy together with choledochostomy is the treatment of choice for cholelithiasis. Choledochostomy is indicated if there is evidence of stone(s) in the common bile duct, obstructive jaundice, recurrent biliary colic, dilatation or thickening of the wall of the common bile duct, or thickening at the head of the pancreas.

A right subcostal (Kocker's) incision is specific to biliary surgery, but if the patient is obese or if a wider exposure is required then a high, right paramedian incision is preferred. The gall bladder is freed from the undersurface of the liver, leaving a raw area which may need to be oversewn. A drainage tube is usually placed in the area of the gall bladder bed and brought to the skin surface via a stab wound. The drainage tube is usually connected to a low pressure vacuum seal drainage apparatus. The purpose of this drainage tube is to prevent blood or bile from escaping into the peritoneal cavity, and causing peritonitis and/or paralytic ileus.

Following exploration of the common bile duct, most surgeons will leave a T-tube in situ (Fig. 47.2). This tube is anchored in place with a suture at the skin surface and is then connected to a drainage bag. It is vital that this tube not be accidently removed, therefore it must be firmly secured to the patient's thigh or abdomen. The purpose of the tube is to act as a safety valve to allow the drainage of bile while there is oedema and inflammation of the common bile duct, due to surgical intervention. On the first postoperative day as much as 500 ml of bile may flow into the drainage bag, but as the inflammation and oedema subside more bile will flow into the duodenum through the T section of the tube and less out into the drainage bag. T-tubes are made of rubber or

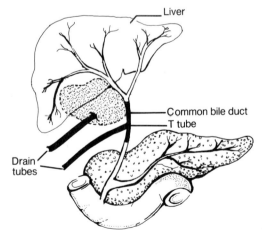

Fig. 47.2 T-tube in place following cholecystectomy.

latex as these materials excite tissue reaction which causes a meshwork of fibrous tissue to form around the tube creating a fistula between the bile duct and the exit site of the T-tube. This is a desirable situation as the track allows for the drainage of any residual bile, after removal of the tube. Most surgeons request that the T-tube remains in place for 8–10 days to ensure that this track has formed. Removal too soon may allow for leakage of bile into the peritoneal cavity resulting in biliary peritonitis. The fistula heals within 2–3 days after removal of the T-tube leaving the common bile duct as the only route for bile flow.

Postoperative nursing management

In addition to the postoperative nursing care that is given to any patient having abdominal surgery, the nurse may be aware of the possibility of problems due to:

– The site of the incision
– The irritant nature of bile on the skin and peritoneum
– Management of the T-tube.

Problems due to the site of the incision

Because of the high abdominal incision, with its close proximity to the intercostal nerve endings, the patient experiences very severe incisional pain and is therefore most reluctant to perform his deep breathing and coughing exercises. This, in turn, makes the patient more susceptible to atelectasis and pneumonia. The patient will require a narcotic analgesic for at least the first 48 hours. The analgesic must be administered regularly, whether the patient is in pain or not to enable him to perform his exercises. The patient can always be reversed sufficiently to enable him to effectively perform these exercises. Initially, the nurse must splint the wound during coughing exercises but as the patient's condition improves he will be able to do this for himself. This must be taught in the preoperative stage.

The patient should be nursed in an upright position in order to assist in the prevention of pulmonary complication. Following the first 24 hours of bed rest with the proper assistance by the nurse, limited ambulation can be achieved, even though the patient may have an intravenous line and drain(s) in situ.

The irritant nature of bile on the skin and peritoneum

Following surgery to the biliary system there is a possibility that bile may leak onto the skin at the T-tube or tissue drain site, causing severe excoriation. If leakage does occur the skin must be protected. 'Stomahesive' compounds, zinc, silicon, or lanolin may be used for this purpose and the patient will require dressings as appropriate. The amount of bile leakage must be estimated, recorded and reported. Bile may also leak into the peritoneal cavity and may cause biliary peritonitis (which will display the same symptoms as does peritonitis of any cause; see page 508) and associated paralytic ileus. Observations for early warning signs of these conditions are an important function of the nurse. Because of the enhanced danger of these patients developing paralytic ileus, the surgeon may take precautionary measures and order the insertion of a nasoenteric tube for drainage purposes. The patient is usually allowed only occasional sips of water (30–50 ml per hour) until bowel sounds are well established. Biliary peritonitis can also occur following removal of the T-tube.

Management of the T-tube

When a T-tube has been inserted into the bile duct, its management is another important function of the nurse and can be considered under the following headings:

- Care of the T-tube
- Indications of bile duct patency
- Removal of the T-tube.

Care of the T-tube. The nurse should explain the purpose of the T-tube and drainage bag to the patient. Tension on the tubing is avoided by fixing the bile drainage bag to the patient's leg. This allows the patient free movement whilst decreasing the chance of the tube being accidentally pulled out.

The tubing must not be allowed to become kinked or compressed, as this will prevent free drainage of the bile, resulting in congestion of bile in the bile duct system. This in turn may lead to further complications, for example biliary stasis which may then lead to liver damage.

The amount of bile drainage must be measured and recorded daily. Between 300–500 ml of bile will drain from the T-tube in the first 24 hours post operatively, but this amount should decrease to nil over a period of 7–10 days. Continued loss of large amounts of bile indicates that the common bile duct is not resuming patency; the most likely causes being continued inflammation and oedema or a missed stone blocking the duct. When there is sudden cessation of bile drainage the nurse should suspect a blocked, kinked, or compressed tube. Too much or too little bile drainage, must be reported. When the bile drainage bag is emptied or changed, aseptic technique must be used.

The colour of faeces and urine must be observed as these are indicators that bile is re-entering the duodenum.

The skin at the drain site must be observed for leakage of bile, inflammation, and excoriation.

Indications of bile duct patency. These include a gradual decrease in bile drainage, the return of faeces and urine to a normal colour, and the gradual fading of jaundice.

The T-tube should be clamped to test the patency of the common bile duct. This is done for increasing lengths of time, 2–3 times a day before meals and released after the meal. Mealtimes are the most likely times for bile to be excreted. There should be no complaints of abdominal pain while the tube is clamped, and there should be no sudden gush of bile when the clamp is released. If there is pain while the tube is clamped, the nurse must release the clamp immediately and observe for sudden bile flow. The incident must be recorded and reported.

Following the clamping regime the surgeon will order an X-ray of the ducts following injection of a radio opaque substance into the T-tube (T-tube choledochogram). If this shows satisfactory filling of the full length of the common bile duct then the T-tube will be removed

Removal of the T-tube. This procedure may cause the patient some considerable pain. Recommended steps to follow are:

1. Give a strong analgesic (for example pethidine) half an hour prior to the procedure.
2. Remove skin suture.
3. Exert a firm, steady pull on the T-tube until it begins to slip out. Do not give a sudden jerk or use any force when attempting to remove the T-tube as the tube could readily snap. Refer to the surgeon if any difficulty is experienced.
4. Once the tube is removed, observe for the amount of bile flow onto the skin.
5. Protect the skin around the drain site with a protective cream, for example silicon, zinc, or lanolin, and cover with a small dressing.
6. Change the dressing as necessary.
7. Observe the patient for early signs of biliary peritonitis for at least 48 hours.

Anticipated outcome and habilitation

When recovery from biliary surgery is uncomplicated most patients are discharged 10–12 days postoperatively. They will be instructed to take the usual precautions following any abdominal surgery. Some patients may find that they tolerate a low fat diet best for a few weeks, after which they should be able to eat a normal diet. The patient should be advised that without a gall bladder, bile will flow continuously into the duodenum. As there is no longer a reservoir of bile, he must avoid eating a large meal with a high fat content.

The prognosis is good and the patient should be able to resume normal activities 4–6 weeks following discharge from hospital.

Complications

Most of the complications of biliary disease and biliary surgery have been described throughout this chapter; they are summarized as follows:

Complications of untreated cholelithiasis:
- Chronic cholecystitis resulting in a fibrotic nonfunctioning gall bladder.
- Haemorrhagic tendencies
- Obstructive jaundice
- Perforation of the gall bladder
- Biliary peritonitis – paralytic ileus
- Empyema of the gall bladder
- Pancreatitis

Complications of biliary surgery:
- Bile leakage
- Biliary peritonitis
- Skin excoriation
- Respiratory complications related to incision site
- Subhepatic abscess
- Pancreatitis
- Post operative obstructive jaundice due to a missed stone or ductal stenosis obstructing the common bile duct
- Iatrogenic disruption of the ducts

48

Disorders of the pancreas

Mavis Matthews

ACUTE PANCREATITIS

Acute pancreatitis is an acute inflammatory condition, with resultant loss of pancreatic function, thought to be caused by the digestion of the gland by its own enzymes, particularly trypsin. Pancreatitis may be mild and transient, or it may be severe and protracted with a mortality rate cited as high as 50%. Some patients have a history of repeated acute attacks which can, on rare occasions, lead to chronic pancreatitis.

The cause of acute pancreatitis is often not known but possible causes are many and varied and include:

- Chronic alcoholism. Pancreatitis is more common in countries such as Australia where there is a high incidence of alcoholism.
- Biliary tract disease
- Infection – bacterial and viral
- Drugs, including certain thiazide diuretics and corticosteroid agents
- Trauma. Crushing or penetrating injuries and more recently as a complication of the procedure ERCP.
- Hyperparathyroidism – pancreatic calculi
- Hyperlipidaemia
- Cancer of the ampulla of Vater
- Chronic pancreatitis

Pathophysiology

Normally proteolytic (trypsin) and lipolytic (lipase) enzymes are activated in the duodenum, but in pancreatitis they are activated in the pancreas. The exact mechanism of this phenomenon is not fully established. Oedema and ischaemia of the gland may in some way be a causative factor; there is also a theory that reflux of bile into the pancreatic duct may in some way trigger the premature enzyme activation. This reflux could be due to spasm of the sphincter of Oddi of which there are many causes including alcoholism or gallstone obstruction. The end result of this abnormal enzyme activity is auto-digestion with varying degrees of oedema, haemorrhage, necrotic tissue, and even abscess or cyst formation. The activated trypsin is believed to cause the activation of other enzymes, for example elastase, which digests the tissue of blood vessels, causing haemorrhage; phospholepase A, which digests parts of all membranes; and kalli-krein, which has an important effect in local damage and system hypotension, causing vasodilation, and increased vascular permeability, and invading leucocytes. Apart from the damage to the pancreas in severe cases, the activated enzymes, particularly trypsin, escape into the peritoneal and retroperitoneal spaces and attack other body tissues, particularly around the aorta, vena cava, and mesenteries. The release of lipases cause fat necrosis in areas adjacent to the pancreas and in the omentum. This results in areas of calcification and may lead to hypocalcaemia and even tetany.

Clinical manifestations

Occasionally, patients may have only mild abdominal symptoms, but usually presentation is in an acutely ill state with pain, shock, and vomiting

Epigastric pain is the most prominent feature and cannot be over-exaggerated. It often is described as 'boring through to the back', causing the patient to be extremely restless.

Shock may be:

1. Neurogenic, due to the close proximity of the pancreas to the coliac plexus of nerves;
2. Hypovolaemic, due to the massive escape of up to 3 litres of plasma from the inflamed pancreas into the peritoneal cavity (see also Chapter 11). The associated vomiting which is almost always a feature will also contribute to hypovolaemic shock.

There is usually marked guarding, abdominal rigidity, and tenderness. Bowel sounds are usually diminished. Paralytic ileus and peritonitis are features of the disease in its most severe form. Other manifestations such as fever and leucocytosis may be present. Obstructive jaundice may occur if pancreatic oedema has been sufficient to compress the common bile duct. Peri-umbilical and/or flank bruising, if present, will be due to haemorrhage into the retroperitoneal spaces.

Diagnosis is suspected from the patient's history and on clinical examination. Peritonitis from any of its many causes, and myocardial infarction must be excluded.

Investigative procedures

Activated amylase escapes into the blood stream in high concentrations. Diagnosis is strongly suggested when the serum amylase is found to be more than 5 times the normal. This test however is valid only if performed within 48 hours of the onset of the illness. Urinary levels of amylase remain elevated for about 10–14 days, therefore the nurse may be asked to collect a 24 hour specimen of urine. Exploratory laparotomy may be performed when diagnosis is doubtful. However this can be dangerous with an acutely ill and shocked patient.

Faecal fat will be estimated, and plain X-rays may show evidence of paralytic ileus in loops of gut adjacent to the pancreas. Ultrasound, pancreatic scan, and ERCP may all be helpful in outlining any structural derangement.

Somogyi units are raised in both serum and urine specimens. Aspiration of peritoneal fluid is performed and will show high amylase levels. Serum calcium is lowered and may produce ECG changes the same as those seen after mycoardial infarction.

Medical and surgical management

The medical management of this disease, for which there is no specific cure, is symptomatic. For relief of pain, pethidine is the drug of choice. Morphine or its derivatives, is used only in extreme circumstances as it causes spasm of the sphincter of Oddi.

Shock is corrected by adequate replacement of fluid, plasma and electrolytes.

The acutely ill patient is rested to decrease body metabolism, and an antibiotic may be used to prevent intercurrent infection, although the practice of using prophylactic antibiotics is controversial.

The underlying cause is sought and, if possible, treated. This may include therapy to overcome an alcohol problem. The activity of the gland is reduced by one or more of the following measures. There is now controversy as to the efficacy of many of them, and those chosen will vary from physician to physician.

- Cessation of all oral feeding
- Continuous gastrointestinal drainage
- Intravenous hyperalimentation
- Vagal inhibition with antivagal drugs, for example atropine or probanthine
- Neutralization of trypsin with aprotinin
- Inhibition of enzyme activity with acetazolamide and glucogon
- Administration of pancreatin, or pancrelipase, an extract of hog pancreas, which is given to maintain reduced stimulation of function once oral diet is recommended
- Monitor and correct electrolytes and deficiencies in fat soluble vitamins.

Only a minority of patients with acute pancreatitis require surgery, however a laparotomy may be the only method of obtaining a definitive diagnosis. During a severe attack of pancreatitis the patient may develop either a pancreatic abscess or a pseudocyst (an accumulation of fluid in the peritoneum adjacent to the pancreas). Either of these conditions may require surgical drainage. If there has been any complication involving the patency of the biliary duct system or the duodenum, corrective surgery will be necessary. Finally, as a life saving measure, and only on extremely rare occasions, partial or complete pancreatectomy may be the only alternative for the patient with acute pancreatitis.

Nursing management

During a severe attack of pancreatitis the patient will require complete bed rest and assistance with all basic needs. The patient will be suffering from shock, therefore the responsibilities of the nurse will be to keep the patient warm, maintain intravenous fluid replacement and monitor the patient's response. This is done by assessment of blood pressure, pulse, urinary output, general colour, and the overall appearance of the patient's clinical state, all of which must be accurately documented (see also Chapter 11). Part of the fluid balance will include the assessment and measurement of gastric aspirate.

Analgesics must be administered with the aim of alleviating pain or reducing it to a tolerable level. Unresolved pain will add to the patient's restlessness and shocked state.

The nurse must observe for signs of hypocalcaemia (see page 246) and also for signs indicating a low blood sugar. Serum blood sugar levels should be monitored regularly so that mild diabetes can be diagnosed and treated appropriately (see also page 252).

When the shock and pain are under control the patient's condition will markedly improve and he may begin to drink clear fluids. Once this is tolerated, commencement of low fat solid foods may begin with the avoidance of caffeine and alcohol.

If the patient is responding to medical management a general improvement should be noticed, with a return to normal of the vital signs.

The patient will be encouraged to attend to his own hygiene and ambulation as his general condition improves.

Other responsibilities of the nurse will include;

• Care of the nasogastric tube, aspiration of the stomach and recording the amount of colour, and viscosity of the aspirate on a fluid balance chart.
• Constant observations for signs of any sudden deterioration of the patient's condition. An observation chart noting skin colour, blood pressure, TPR, degree of pain, and alertness should be maintained hourly during the critical stage of the attack.
• The fluid balance chart will also be utilized to record the parenteral infusion given, urinary output, and number and type of bowel actions.

• Helping the patient who is in extreme pain is difficult but the nurse must attempt to do so by assisting the patient into positions that he feels will give him some relief, by staying with him and by giving analgesics on time as ordered.

Anticipated outcome and complications

Authorities variously quote a 5–50% mortality rate and most deaths are due to shock in the first 5 days. The majority of the survivors recover fully within 19 days but a few develop abscesses or pseudocysts, or continue to have repeated acute attacks at varying intervals. Latest data indicates that rarely does acute pancreatitis lead to chronic pancreatitis, but this point of view is controversial.

Habilitation

If the cause of acute pancreatitis is known and is treated successfully, the patient can be assured that he should not have any further attacks. If alcoholism is suspected as being the major factor, the patient must be informed that recurrence with possible fatal outcome depends entirely on his ability to abstain totally from drinking alcohol. If the patient requires assistance to do this he should be referred to a specialist counsellor therapist.

CHRONIC PANCREATITIS

Aetiology and pathophysiology

Chronic pancreatitis follows a long, slow, insidious course and is characterized by progressive destruction of the organ and replacement by fibrotic tissue and calcification. The ducts become obstructed and the secreting cells slowly cease to function. Usually, the first indication that the pancreas is chronically impaired is when the resultant obstruction and oedema causes an acute attack of pancreatitis, to be followed at irregular intervals by further acute episodes lasting for several days (chronic relapsing pancreatitis). It is not known what the triggering mechanism is that causes the initial chronic inflammatory reaction. Most references suggest that the typical case of chronic pancreatitis is due to alcoholism. Other possible causes are thought to be the same as for acute pancreatitis. With the consumption of alcohol beginning at an alarmingly earlier age and the amount consumed increasing throughout the population, the incidence of this disease is also increasing in this country. The condition is more common in males and alcoholic men as young as 30 years are affected.

Clinical manifestations

Epigastric pain, radiating through to the back, may be present only during acute exacerbations or it may be chronic and persistent. Often, recurrent attacks follow an alcoholic binge, but are not necessarily of equal severity.

Loss of weight is a feature and may be due to anorexia from persistent pain, malabsorption, or malnutrition associated with alcoholism.

Malabsorption, manifesting as steatorrhoea, is a late symptom and is an indicator that 85% of the functioning cells have been destroyed. There will also be a corresponding malabsorption of fat soluble vitamins.

About one-third of patients who have exocrine failure will also develop endocrine dysfunction and will become diabetics.

Mild recurrent jaundice occurs occasionally if fibrosis of the head of the pancreas causes obstruction of the common bile duct.

Investigative procedures

These will be as for acute pancreatitis, except:

- Plain X-ray. This may show areas of calcification.
- Serum amylase is not usually elevated.
- Glucose tolerance test and serum insulin estimation to detect diabetes mellitus.
- Laboratory tests for evidence of malabsorption, for example faecal fat, vitamin A, D and K estimation.
- Duodenoscopy may show obliteration of duodenal folds due to inflammation.
- Pancreatic scan may show poor uptake.

Medical, surgical, and nursing management

Management of chronic pancreatitis is symptomatic. It involves the replacement of pancreatic enzymes, for example, pancrealipase, which will enable the patient to eat an 18 g fat diet and will control steatorrhoea.

Various surgical procedures may be performed, for example, pancreatolithotomy if calculi have formed in the duct, sphincterotomy to relieve pancreatic or bile duct obstruction, and drainage of any abscess cysts, or pseudocysts. Should the patient develop diabetes, the management will be specific to this condition (see page 252).

The persistent pain of chronic pancreatitis in some patients requires prolonged narcotic analgesia. Patients who abstain completely from alcohol and have malabsorption and diabetes mellitus well controlled, can be given a 50–65% expectancy that pain will gradually subside in approximately 5–10 years. Surgery for the control of intense pain is sometimes undertaken but has no proven value. Procedures include pancreatic nerve block, afferent nerve section, sphincterotomy, and partial or even total pancreatectomy. Total pancreatectomy with islet cell auto transplantation into the liver is a new procedure being used in some centres. It is performed in an attempt to preserve endocrine tissue in order to reduce the severity of diabetes that the patient experiences following pancreatectomy.

Anticipated outcome and habilitation

With chronic pancreatitis the gland is permanently and sometimes progressively damaged; therefore at best the condition can only be controlled. Alcoholism, the major cause of the problem, is also the major prevention of its effective treatment. Very few of these patients are able to abstain from drinking alcohol, and unless they do their condition will worsen. For the successful treatment of chronic pancreatitis that must continue for years, the patient will need constant intensive support from appropriate professionals, friends, and family.

Patients who suffer long term pain which genuinely requires the regular administration of analgesics, are so afraid of the pain being unrelieved or worsening that fear of the pain may become more of a problem than the pain itself.

These patients may eventually become psychologically dependent on the analgesic when in fact the pancreatitis may be well controlled. In such situations, psychological counselling, support from persons close to the patient, and gradual withdrawal of the analgesic may overcome the problem. Alternative pain control therapies may be utilized.

CARCINOMA OF THE PANCREAS

Aetiology and pathophysiology

Adenocarcinoma is the most common type of malignant tumour of the pancreas, and is usually located at its head. It is twice as common in males as in females and usually affects the 50–70 year age group. In Australia the incidence appears to be increasing but the reason for this is not known. The lesions often cause pancreatic duct obstruction, resulting in chronic pancreatitis; and biliary duct compression, resulting in obstructive jaundice. The onset is insidious and the malignancy is highly invasive, affecting the nearby organs, especially the liver, spleen, biliary system, and peritoneum. The lungs are a common site for metatasis. Because the tumour is often in an advanced stage before severe symptoms occur, pancreatic cancer is rarely operable and life expectancy is about 8–12 months following diagnosis.

Clinical manifestations

Initially there is vague abdominal discomfort followed by symptoms that mimic acute or chronic pancreatitis; epigastric pain that radiates through to the back being the major complaint. As the condition advances and affects nearby structures, obstructive jaundice, severe weight loss, and ascites are to be expected.

Investigative procedures

These will be numerous and include pancreatic function tests, liver function tests, glucose tolerance test, pancreatic scan, and examination of pancreatic juices for cytotoxic cells. There will also be investigations to determine the existence and extent of metastases in the liver and lungs for example prothrombin time, serum bilirubin and chest X-ray.

Medical, surgical and nursing management

Pancreatic tumours are sensitive to neither radiotherapy nor chemotherapy. Rarely is surgery curative but may bring temporary relief of symptoms and anastamosis of the gall bladder to a loop of small intestine will relieve obstructive jaundice. Biliary drainage into the small intestine can sometimes be achieved by using an endoscopic technique and thus avoiding surgery.

Pancreatoduodenal resection (Whipple's procedure) may be worthwhile if the tumour is small and confined to the head of the pancreas. This involves removal of all but the tail of the pancreas, the duodenum, the antrum of the stomach, and the gall bladder. The remnants are anastomased to the jejunum (Fig. 48.1). The procedure is complicated by leakage, abscesses, and fistulas, and the mortality rate is high. Only 2–5% survive 5 years.

Regardless of the choice of medical or surgical management the nurse will be involved in caring for a seriously ill patient who may be in a terminal state.

Following surgery, and prior to discharge from hospital, the patient and his significant others must receive full instructions regarding his care at home. Such instructions may include: wound care and T-tube drain care; dietary management and dietary supplements, for example pancreatic enzymes; knowledge of complications such as malabsorption, weight loss, diarrhoea, leakage from anastomosis, and abscess formation; and complications of diabetes mellitus if the patient has become insulin dependent as a result of the surgery.

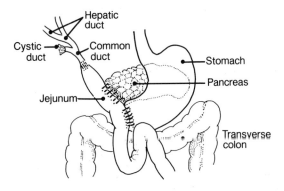

Fig. 48.1 Whipple's procedure.

ZOLLINGER-ELLISON SYNDROME

This syndrome manifests in the outpouring of large amounts of gastric acid, causing intractable peptic ulcerations, and is due to a noninsulin secreting islet cell (delta cell) tumour. This tumour is usually located at the head of the pancreas, but may be found in other endocrine glands outside of the pancreas. It causes hypersecretion of gastrin which, in turn, is responsible for the abnormal excessive production of gastric acid. Treatment is unsatisfactory and may include routine peptic ulcer therapy, total gastrectomy, or even Whipple's procedure. The mortality rate is as high as 80% with the complications of the ulcerations being the usual direct cause of death. (See treatment and complications of peptic ulceration in Chapter 52).

Tumours of the other islet cells have been included in Chapter 28 as they cause hyperinsulism and hyperglycaemia.

SECTION F – REFERENCES AND FURTHER READING

Texts

Anderson J R (ed) 1976 Muir's textbook of pathology, 10th edn. Edward Arnold, London

Anthony C P 1984 Structure and function of the body. Mosby, St Louis

Anthony C P, Thibodeau G 1979 Textbook of anatomy and physiology, 10th edn. Mosby & Co, St Louis

Brunner L S, Suddarth D S 1982 The Lippinoott manual of nursing practice, 3rd edn. Lippincott, Philadelphia

Brunner L S, Suddarth D S 1984 Textbook of medical surgical nursing, 5th edn. Lippincott, Philadelphia

Chaffee E E 1974 Basic physiology and anatomy, 3rd edn. Lippincott, Philadelphia

Chilman A, Thomas M 1987 Understanding nursing care, 3rd edn. Churchill Livingstone, Edinburgh

Cohen L Z, Holmes N, Shirehouse P M, Moclock L C (eds) 1985 Gastrointestinal disorders: nurse's clinical library. Springhouse, Pennsylvania

Creager J G 1982 Human anatomy and physiology. Wadsworth, California

Davenport H W 1978 A digest of digestion, 2nd edn. Year Book Medical Publishers, Chicago

Elmslie R G, Ludbrook J 1976 An introduction to surgery: 100 topics. Heinemann, London

Ganong W F 1977 Review of medical physiology, 8th edn. Lange, Los Altos

Gillespie I E, Thomson T J 1977 Gastroenterology: an integrated course, 2nd edn. Churchill Livingstone, Edinburgh

Given B 1979 Gastroenterology in clinical nursing, 3rd edn. Mosby, St Louis

Guyton A C 1981 Textbook of medical physiology, 6th edn. Saunders, Philadelphia

Havard M 1986 A nursing guide to drugs, 2nd edn. Churchill Livingstone, Melbourne

Luckman J, Sorensen K C 1980 Medical-surgical nursing, 2nd edn. Saunders, Philadelphia

Macleod J 1987 Davidson's principles and practice of medicine, 15th edn. Churchill Livingstone, Edinburgh

Netter F H 1972 The Ciba collection of medical illustrations, 3rd edn. Ciba Pharmaceutical Company, New Jersey

Read A E, Barritt D W, Langton Hewer R 1986 Modern Medicine, 3rd edn. Churchill Livingstone, Edinburgh

Rice H V 1978 Gastrointestinal nursing. Medical Examination Publishing Co, New York

Society of Hospital Pharmacists of Australia 1985 Pharmacology and drug information for nurses. 2nd edn. Saunders, Sydney

Storlie F J (ed) 1984 Diseases: nurse's reference library, 2nd edn. Springhouse, Pennsylvania

Toohey M 1978 Toohey's medicine for nurses, 12th edn. Churchill Livingstone, Edinburgh

Urosevich, P R (ed) 1984 Performing GI procedures: nursing photobook, 2nd edn. Springhouse, Pennsylvania

Watson J E 1979 Medical-surgical nursing and related physiology, 2nd edn. Saunders, Philadelphia

Wilson K J W 1981 Foundations of anatomy and physiology, 5th edn. Churchill Livingstone, Edinburgh

Journals

Altshuler A, Hilden D 1977 The patient with portal hypertension. Nursing Clinics of North America 12 : 317

Ammann R W et al 1979 Pain relief by surgery in chronic pancreatitis? Relationship between pain relief, pancreatic dysfunction, and alcohol withdrawal. Scandanivian Journal of Gastroenterology 14 : 209

Auslander M O et al 1979 Drug therapy of acute pancreatitis. Clinical Gastroenterology 8 : 219

Bossone M C 1977 The liver: a pharmacologic perspective. Nursing Clinics of North America 12 : 291

Boyer C, Oehlberg S 1977 Interpretation and clinical relevance of liver function tests. Nursing Clinics of North America 12 : 275

Buschiazzo L 1985 Ruptured oesophageal varices. Nursing 85 15 : 11 : 33

Daniel E 1977 Chronic problems in rehabilitation of patients with Laenneo's cirrhosis. Nursing Clinics of North America 12 : 345

Dexter D 1982 New hepatitis B vaccine. A hepatitis prevention. American Journal of Nursing 306–307

Khuroo M S 1980 Study of an epidemic of non-A, non-B hepatitis. Possibility of another human hepatitis virus distinct from post-transfusion non-A, non-B type. American Journal of medicine 80 : 818–820

La Sala C 1985 Caring for the patient with a transhepatic biliary decompression catheter. Nursing 85 15 : 2 : 52–55

Lawrence A G, Ghosh B C 1977 Total pancreatectomy for carcinoma of the pancreas. American Journal of Surgery 133 : 244

McElroy D B 1977 Nursing care of patients with viral hepatitis. Nursing Clinics of North America 12 : 305

Nurse's Reference Library 1984 Contrast radiography fact sheet. Nursing 84 14 : 8 : 22–23

Quinless F 1984 Portal hypertension: physiology, signs, and symptoms. Nursing 84 14 : 1 : 52–53

Quinless F 1984 Teaching tips for T-tube care at home. Nursing 84 14 : 5 : 63–64

Smith C E 1986 Assessing the liver. Nursing 85 15 : 7 : 36–37

Tandon B N et al 1984 Associated infection with non-A, non-B virus as a possible cause of liver failure in Indian HBV carriers. The Lancet 8405 : 11 : 750–751

Taylor D L 1983 Gallstones: physiology, signs and symptoms. Nursing 83 13 : 6 : 44–45

Taylor D L 1983 Jaundice: physiology, signs and symptoms. Nursing 83 13 : 8 : 52–54

Wimpsett J 1984 Trace your patient's liver dysfunction. Nursing 84 14 : 8 : 56–67

Zuckerman A J 1982 Viral hepatitis. World Health 19–21

G

The gastrointestinal system

49

Introduction to the gastrointestinal system

Mavis Matthews

OVERVIEW OF ANATOMY AND PHYSIOLOGY

The gastrointestinal system can be likened to a canal (hence alimentary canal) that extends from the mouth to the anus. The lumen of this canal or tract is in direct contact with the external environment. Nutrients taken into the tract serve no useful purpose until they have passed into the mucous membrane of the tract, and thus on into the internal environment of the body. Therefore the first function of the gastrointestinal system is to render nutrients:

• To microscopic size
• To a suitable chemical composition
• Microbiologically safe in order to enable the tract to carry out its other major function of actually absorbing the nutrients.

Any substances that are indigestible or nonabsorbable are discharged via the rectum in the form of faeces. The first sections of the tract, that is, the mouth, oropharynx, oesophagus, stomach, and duodenum, are primarily concerned with receiving and digesting the food; the jejunum and ileum complete the digestive process and are the main absorptive areas. The colon absorbs water and electrolytes and eliminates the residue. Figure 49.1 shows the digestive process.

If there is a defect in the wall of the alimentary tract and contents escape into the internal environment without first having been processed as outlined above, a severe inflammatory reaction will ensue, (for example mediastinitis or peritonitis, see page 508).

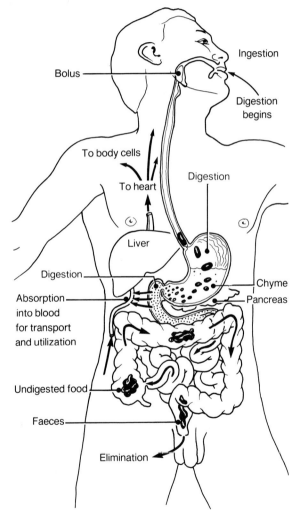

Fig. 49.1 The digestive process.

Digestion

The full length of the digestive tract is surrounded by 2 sets of muscles, circular and longitudinal. (In the stomach there is a third set of oblique muscles.) These muscles are necessary to churn and break up the contents within the tract (mechanical digestion) and to propel the contents along at a definite rate (peristalsis).

Bile, produced by the liver, and enzymes are necessary for bringing about chemical changes to food (chemical digestion). Table 49.1 summarizes the sources, actions, and end products of digestive enzymes. Digestive juices, apart from containing enzymes, also contain mucus, water, electrolytes, and bacteriocidal agents necessary for both mechanical and chemical digestion. Digestive juices are produced in the mucous membrane of the stomach and bowel, and also the pancreas.

Specific hormones produced in the mucosa of the pylorus and intestines stimulate some muscular activity, and control the secreting activity of the stomach, pancreas and liver.

The activities of the gastrointestinal tract are controlled by nerves from the autonomic nervous system and by nerves situated in the submucosa (Meissner's plexus) and between the circular and longitudinal muscles (Auerback's plexus).

Indigestible foods are important because they add bulk causing distension of the canal walls. The distended walls excite nerve endings which stimulate muscular activity, that is, peristalsis and mechanical digestion.

Absorption

In the small intestine the mucous membrane is specifically modified to increase the surface area

Table 49.1 Sources, substrates and products of digestive enzymes. (From: Hubbard J L, Mechan D J 1987 Physiology for health care students. Churchill Livingstone, Edinburgh)

Enzyme	Source	Substrate	Product(s)
Salivary amylase	Salivary glands	Some starches	Maltose
Pepsin	Stomach	Starch	Polypeptides
Trypsin	Pancreas	Proteins, large peptides	Smaller peptides Amino acids
Chymotrypsin	Pancreas	Proteins, large peptides	Smaller peptides Amino acids
Elastase	Pancreas	Elastin	Peptides Amino acid
Carboxypeptidase	Pancreas	Proteins & peptides containing acidic amino acids	Acidic amino acids
Amylase	Pancreas	Starch	Maltose Maltriose Dextrins
Lipase	Pancreas	Triglycerides	Monoglycerides Free fatty acids
Ribonuclease	Pancrease	RNA	Nucleotides
Deoxyribonuclease	Pancreas	DNA	Nucleotides
Membrane peptidases	Intestinal mucosa	Peptides	Amino acids
Cytoplasmic peptidases	Intestinal mucosa	Peptides	Amino acids
Maltase	Intestinal mucosa	Maltose, maltotriose	Glucose
Lactase	Intestinal mucosa	Lactose	Glucose Galactose
Sucrase	Intestinal mucosa	Sucrose	Glucose Fructose
Dextrinase	Intestinal mucosa	Dextrins	Glucose
Nuclease	Intestinal mucosa	Nucleic acids	Pentoses Nitrogenous bases

for absorption (Fig. 49.2). Villi extend into the lumen of the bowel and these villi also have miorovilli extending from them. Under the microscope the microvilli have a brush-like appearance, hence the description 'brush border of the villi'. The presence of villi and their microvilli increase the surface area of the small intestine by several hundred times. Each villus contains an arteriole, venule, and lymph vessel (lacteal). The venules transport absorbed amino acids, glucose, and some fats into the portal circulation for delivery to the liver; the lacteals are the main collecting ducts for transporting digested fats indirectly to the liver via the thoracic duct and the general circulation. Absorption of nutrients into the cell can be by diffusion, filtration, osmosis, or by active transport, depending on the specific nature of the substance being absorbed.

The peritoneum

This is a large expanse of serous membrane that covers most of the organs of the alimentary tract and holds them loosely together (Fig. 49.3). The peritoneum has 2 surfaces; an outer parietal layer which lines the abdominal cavity, and an inner visceral layer which is that part which dips in and around the abdominal organs. The greater omentum is a section of the visceral peritoneum that hangs down, apron-like, in front of the intestines; the mesentery is a fan-shaped extension of the parietal membrane that extends from the lumber region and is attached to the full length of the jejunum and ileum; and the mesocolon is that section of the peritoneum which attaches the colon to the posterior abdominal wall. The

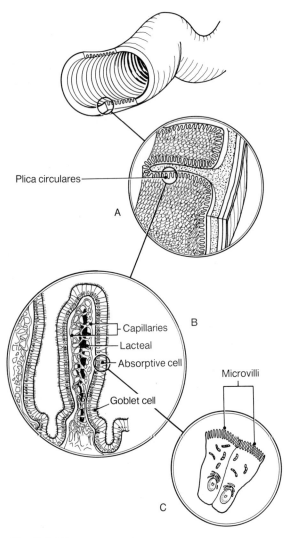

Fig. 49.2 Microstructure of the small intestine. **A** – Villi. **B** – Cross-section of villi. **C** – Microvilli, showing 'brush border'.

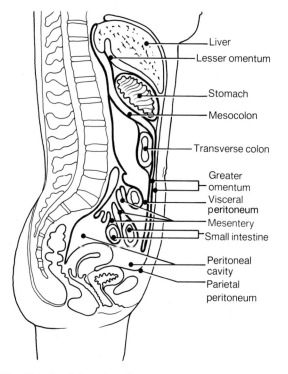

Fig. 49.3 Saggital section of peritoneal cavity.

mesentery allows for free movement of the coils of bowel upon itself, but prevents strangulation. The mesentery also transmits blood vessels, lymphatics, and nerves. Friction between any two peritoneal surfaces is prevented by the secretion of serous fluid.

The peritoneal cavity is normally only a potential space that becomes an actual cavity if fluid accumulates between two peritoneal surfaces. The peritoneum acts as a protection against the spread of infection within the abdominal cavity, due to the presence of lymph nodes and the ability of the greater omentum to surround and isolate an area of inflammation or infection.

COMMON MANIFESTATIONS OF GASTROINTESTINAL DISORDERS

Because the autonomic nervous system plays a major role in the activities of this system, psychological as well as physical stress can be the cause of a wide variety of digestive upsets.

Anorexia, nausea, and vomiting

Anorexia is the loss of appetite, nausea is the unpleasant urge to vomit, and vomiting is the ejection of upper gastrointestinal contents through the mouth. These 3 symptoms often but not always accompany one another. They can be due to any acute or serious physical illness or stress situation.

The vomiting centre, in the medulla of the brain, receives sensory stimuli from many sources. Receptors occur throughout the length of the alimentary canal. There are three other general areas where sensory receptors for vomiting may be found:

1. Throughout the body in such organs as the liver, gall bladder, heart, uterus, kidneys, visceral peritoneum, and semicircular canals
2. Severe pain and other unpleasant sensations of fright, hearing, taste, smell, sight, and thought can trigger the vomiting centre via the cerebral cortex
3. A group of neurones situated at the base of the brain and referred to as the chemoreceptor trigger zone are sensitive to certain chemicals in the blood, and will send impulses to the vomiting centre when stimulated. Such toxic agents include emetic drugs, morphine, digitalis, and toxins of acute infectious diseases.

It was once thought that reverse peristalsis caused the actual act of vomiting, but now it is thought that the following sequence of events occurs:

1. Nerve impulses, from the vomiting centre, travel to the diaphragm, abdominal muscles, and through the vagus nerve
2. The pyloric sphincter relaxes, allowing duodenal contents to fill the stomach. Following a period of nausea there is a sudden, deep inspiration; the glottis, epiglottis, and nasopharynx close and the oesophagus, cardiac sphincter, and stomach relax
3. Whilst this is happening, there is contraction of abdominal muscles and the diaphragm against the dilated stomach, forcing the contents into the oesophagus and out through the mouth.

Sometimes no warning sensation of nausea occurs, or the period of nausea is so short that vomiting occurs before a receptacle can be brought for receiving the vomitus. The nurse must remember this, and not become irritated when a patient vomits suddenly without warning. It is also of importance for the nurse to know that when the unconscious or stuporose patient vomits, the glottis may not close, and these patients are in danger of inhaling the vomitus unless they are placed in a head down, side lying position to facilitate drainage of vomitus from the mouth.

Prolonged vomiting can cause the patient to become seriously ill because:

1. Nutrition is interfered with resulting in fatigue and loss of weight
2. Fluids and electrolytes are lost from the gastrointestinal tract, resulting in fluid/electrolyte imbalance
3. Muscular contractions (occurring during vomiting) can cause exhaustion
4. Postoperatively, vomiting can place a strain on a new suture line. Of particular importance is the hyphaema that can occur following intraocular surgery
5. Vomiting increases intracranial pressure, so must be prevented in the patient who has had a head injury or brain surgery

6. The patient becomes anxious and depressed because of the unpleasantness of the actual vomiting, and through worrying about the underlying cause.

The 4 main principles of management are to:

1. Remove the stimulus if possible
2. Give an antiemetic drug as ordered, for example, metoclopramide
3. Keep the stomach empty, for example, by aspiration via a nasogastric tube
4. Maintain fluid and electrolyte balance by intravenous infusion.

In addition, the nurse must provide the patient with comfort measures such as a clean, quiet, restful environment, and oral hygiene after each vomiting episode. Observations of the amount, frequency, and type of vomitus must be recorded. The nurse should also observe for signs of the effects of prolonged vomiting described above.

Dysphagia, dyspepsia, eructation, and haematemesis are often associated with anorexia, nausea, and vomiting. Dysphagia is difficulty in swallowing and is usually due to problems in the mouth, oropharynx, or oesophagus.

Dyspepsia is indigestion, and occurs when the stomach cannot handle ingested food; the person experiences a feeling of fullness in the stomach and discomfort retrosternally. This discomfort may be severe enough to be described as burning ('heartburn') and is usually due to acid gastric contents regurgitating into the oesophagus. Eructation often accompanies dyspepsia. This is the expulsion of gas from the stomach; to 'belch'. Some foods produce gas in the stomach, but mostly it is derived from swallowed air and it is quite normal to belch following a hearty meal or after drinking aerated drinks. When eructation is associated with dyspepsia there is usually some underlying organic problem, such as peptic ulcer, gastritis, hiatus hernia, or carcinoma of the upper alimentary tract.

Haematemesis is the vomiting of blood. It will be bright red if fresh, and dark brown (resembling used coffee grounds) if old and partially digested. The bleeding site may be the oesophagus, stomach, or the duodenum; haematemesis is always treated as potentially life threatening.

Whereas anorexia, nausea, and vomiting may be related to any illness, dysphagia, dyspepsia with eructation, and haematemesis are more specific to upper gastrointestinal disorders and as such should be fully investigated by the physician.

Pain

Abdominal pain is a common feature in disorders of the gastrointestinal system and in many instances, by knowing its site, intensity, and duration, the pain description can be a useful aid to diagnosis. The nurse should record careful observation of pain characteristics. Because of its usefulness in diagnoses, pain is not usually relieved by analgesia until the full physical examination is completed.

In gastrointestinal diseases pain may be caused by irritation of the mucous membrane, strong contraction of muscular tissues, stretching of a viscus, or inflammation of the peritoneum. Visceral pain is usually deep and diffuse, and described as an ache or burning. It often causes pallor, bradycardia, hypotension, sweating, nausea, and vomiting. In many instances when visceral organs are diseased, irritated, or damaged, the pain may be felt in a superficial area some distance from the affected organ (Fig. 49.4), (see also referred pain, page 115). The nurse needs to be aware of this phenomenon when assessing the patient.

Following abdominal surgery there are 2 distinct types of pain: incisional pain, which is most severe in the first 48 hours postoperatively; and 'wind' pain which occurs 2–4 days postoperatively.

Incisional pain is controlled with analgesia, and gentle and comfortable positioning.

'Wind' pain, which can be very severe, is caused by the inability of gas (normally present in the stomach and bowel) to move along the alimentary tract at its normal pace. This is due to decreased peristalsis which usually occurs following any surgery where the bowel has been handled. As the gas increases it causes bowel distension. Gas pains occur because peristalsis begins to return in the small bowel about 24 to 48 hours before mobility of the colon returns. Therefore, the active small

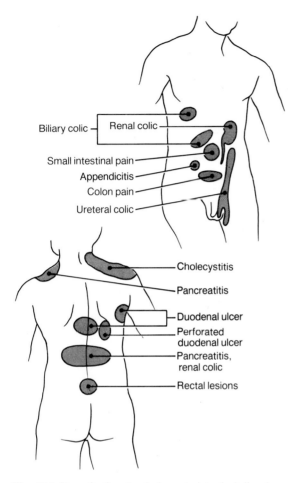

Biliary colic
Renal colic
Small intestinal pain
Appendicitis
Colon pain
Ureteral colic

Cholecystitis
Pancreatitis
Duodenal ulcer
Perforated
duodenal ulcer
Pancreatitis,
renal colic
Rectal lesions

Fig. 49.4 Sites of referred pain in gastrointestinal disorders.

bowel is working against a less active colon and is not able to move the gaseous contents along. Knowledge that the nurse can apply when assisting the patient during this stressful time includes:

- Pain, apprehension, and very hot or iced drinks increase the amount of air swallowed
- Aerated drinks, milk, and high glucose fluids tend to produce gas, and therefore should be avoided
- Until full mobility of the tract is observed, no solid food should be given, and only small sips of water allowed. (See also adynamic ileus, page 532)
- Early, gentle ambulation will help to free pockets of gas caught in loops of small bowel.

Diarrhoea

Diarrhoea is said to be present when there is an excess of faecal water, that is, more than 300 ml/day. The faeces have a fluid consistency and tend to be passed frequently; however, a high frequency of bowel evacuation is not synonymous with diarrhoea. Watery stools are due to excessive bowel mucosal secretions and/or abnormal osmotic forces within the bowel lumen. Less commonly, diarrhoea may be due to decreased transit time of the bowel contents, thus not allowing time for water to be absorbed from the faecal mass. Some of the more common causes of diarrhoea are: reaction to drugs, lactose intolerance, bowel infestation, reaction to foods, malabsorption, diverticular disease, and neoplasia.

Clinical manifestations

Systemic effects. The patient with diarrhoea will lose sodium, potassium, and bicarbonate. If this loss is prolonged, dehydration, acidosis, and hypokalaemia can develop and even cause secondary renal damage. If there is vomiting as well as diarrhoea, complex electrolyte imbalances can occur, and the patient may develop a metabolic alkalosis. Because the body cannot tolerate sustained acid-base or electrolyte imbalances, diarrhoea is a serious condition and must be controlled as soon as possible. Electrolytes and blood gases must be monitored at least daily, and any imbalances must be corrected with intravenous replacement therapy.

The patient who has chronic, severe diarrhoea will have incomplete absorption of nutrients (see malabsorption syndrome, page 504) and will be suffering from fatigue. Local effects. The irritating nature of faecal fluid causes pruritus ani and excoriation of the anal area. The excoriated epithelium can then break down and become ulcerated. Fissures, fitsulae, and perianal abscesses may also develop. When there is associated frequency, the constant pressure on the anorectal mucosa can cause haemorrhoids to develop. These conditions are described in Chapter 54.

Emotional effects. Diarrhoeal stools tend to be malodourous, and when there is frequency there may also be a tendency to some degree of incontinence. The patient who has chronic diarrhoea often experiences feelings of embarrassment and low self-esteem, and because of this often becomes reluctant to socialize.

Investigative procedures

Because of the numerous possible causes of diarrhoea the patient may have to undergo many exhaustive investigations, including rectal and colonic examinations, biopsies, and X-rays. Such investigations usually require bowel preparation, for example, an enema or a bowel washout. The nurse will be required to collect faeces specimens for laboratory testing. The nurse must be aware of the discomforts that many investigatory procedures cause the patient, and should provide adequate explanations and support to minimize these discomforts. For example, a bowel washout can be both embarrassing and exhausting. A faeces chart giving details of the frequency, consistency, colour, and amount of faeces being passed is often required, and must be maintained by the nurse.

Medical and nursing management

The management of patients with severe diarrhoea involves:

– Identifying and treating the underlying cause
– Prescribing antidiarrhoeal drugs
– Replacement therapy of nutrients and electrolytes
– Treating any perianal problems
– Providing nursing care to the fatigued patient
– Providing emotional support.

The management of the common specific conditions where diarrhoea is a feature is described in the relevant sections of this book.

Antidiarrhoeal drugs are useful only for symptomatic treatment, and their mode of action is either to alter intestinal motility or to absorb liquids. Some combination drugs have both actions (see Table 49.2). Antidiarrhoeal drugs must not be given to patients unless they have been prescribed by a physician.

The patient can be assisted to feel less embarrassed if the nurse:

Table 49.2 Common anti-diarrhoeal agents classified by mode of action. (From Havard, 1986.)

Action	Nursing notes
Alteration of intestinal motility	
Codeine phosphate	If dose is $\geq$ 30 mg warn patient of reduced alcohol tolerence and possible dizziness or drowsiness.
Diphenoxylate with atropine	Not for use by children. Possible side-effects include drowsiness, dizziness, depression, nausea, and paralytic ileus, and tachycardia from atropine.
Lopermide	Not for use by nursing mothers. Should be discontinued if no improvement in 48 hours.
Reduction of free water in bowel	
Aluminium hydroxide gel with kaolin Aluminium hydroxide gel with kaolin and pectin Kaolin with pectin	Reduce absorption of many drugs, especially oral iron and the tetracyclines, so give 2 hours apart if possible.

Underlying cause of diarrhoea should always be investigated.

- Does not display embarrassment or disgust
- Does not joke about the situation
- Allows the patient to believe that he/she is anxious to help
- Provides privacy. This may involve allowing the patient to use a bed pan or commode in the toilet area rather than at the bedside
- Keeps the environment clean and fresh smelling
- Is discreet when speaking about the patient's situation and when disposing of faeces or soiled items.

Constipation

Constipation is manifested by the infrequent passing of hardened faeces, and is related to increased transit time along the colon. Constipation cannot be defined in terms of the number of bowel movements in any given period, because the range of bowel movement frequency is from 3 times per day to 2 times per week. It is suggested that the normal segmentation waves of bowel motility become hyperactive and inhibit the

Table 49.3 Causes of chronic constipation

Lack of physiological needs
  Insufficient fibre in the diet
  Insufficient physical activity
  Reduction diets or food lack
  Insufficient fluids
  Constipating foods, e.g. cheese
Psychological causes
  Lack of response to defaecation urges
  Mental stress
Local lesions of the gut
  Obstructing lesions, e.g. carcinoma
  Haemorrhoids and other peri-anal lesions
Defective electrolyte transfer
Aganglionosis, e.g. Hirschsprung's disease
Endocrine dysfunction
  Hypothyroidism
  Hypoparathyroidism
Drugs
  Opiates, anticholinergics, some antacids, antihistamines,
  tranquillizers, prolonged use of mineral oil laxatives

Table 49.4 Conditions associated with chronic constipation. It is suspected that chronic constipation may be a causal factor

Diverticular disease
Large bowel carcinoma
Ulcerative colitis
Irritable bowel syndrome
Haemorrhoids
Peri-anal lesions
Appendicitis
Varicose veins
Gallstones
Hiatus hernia
Ischaemic heart disease
Diabetes mellitus
Obesity
Dental caries

forward movements of peristalsis, thus increasing the transit time. It would appear that the longer the bowel contents remain in the colon, the more faecal water is absorbed, causing the faecal matter to become hardened. It is not clear what actually causes the excessive segmentation activity, but in some way the conditions listed in Table 49.3 are predisposing factors. Table 49.4 lists conditions associated with chronic constipation.

Diet

As successive generations are eating more and more refined and highly processed food, and much less of the foods containing unabsorbable fibres, constipation has become more of a problem.

Research suggests that lack of fibre in the diet is the most common cause of chronic constipation and, more importantly, that this in turn causes many important common diseases. Whether or not lack of fibre in the diet causes constipation, there is no doubt that a high fibre diet helps to correct constipation, unless the bowel is atonic.

Medical and nursing management

Fundamental to the management of constipation is an accurate diagnosis of the underlying cause. Appropriate treatment of the primary cause, for example, may be all that is necessary. Usually patients need to be taught measures to correct faulty bowel habits.

The introduction of high fibre foods, especially bran, into the diet, along with the ingestion of at least 2 litres of fluid per day will correct most chronic cases of constipation. Foods high in fibre include: fruits, nuts, whole grains, raw vegetables, and bran.

Physical exercise, especially brisk walking, should be encouraged, particularly in the elderly and those recovering from surgery.

Specific medications and treatments can be divided into 2 groups: oral medications (laxatives) and rectal medications and treatments.

Oral medications. The laxatives commonly used fall into 4 types: bulk forming, stimulant, faecal softener (lubricant), and osmotic (saline) laxatives (Table 49.5). Bulk forming laxatives, of which natural, unprocessed bran is the best for providing natural fibre, absorb fluid and maintain the faecal mass in a bulky, soft form. They encourage peristalsis and avoid the patient having to strain at defaecation.

Bran is the cheapest and safest method of preventing or treating constipation; however, any bulk forming laxatives should be avoided by persons with intestinal ulcerations, strictures, or obstruction. The other laxatives noted in Table 49.5 are useful for more refractory cases of constipation or when cleaning the bowel prior to bowel investigations or surgery. If these drugs are abused they can become habit forming, cause systemic upsets, or increase the constipation problem by weakening the bowel muscle tone ('lazy bowel').

Table 49.5 Common laxatives classified by mode of action. (From Havard, 1986.)

Action	Nursing notes
Bulk-forming Ispaghula Psyllium Sterculia	Adequate amounts of water must be given with bulk-forming laxatives to avoid danger of obstruction or faecal impaction
Stimulant Bisacodyl	No antacids within $\frac{1}{2}$ hour of taking oral bisacodyl
Castor oil Senna	May colour urine yellow or red
Lubricant Dioctyl sodium sulphosuccinate Liquid paraffin	Avoid liquid paraffin within 2 hours of other medications. Prolonged use may interfere with absorption of fat-soluble vitamins. Possible risk of aspiration pneumonia or anal seepage and irritation
Saline Magnesium sulphate Sodium sulphate Sodium phosphate Sodium citrate with sodium lauryl sulphoacetate	Most oral magnesium salts reduce absorption of oral iron, digoxin, tetracycline, and chlorpromazine. Excessive use may cause dehydration and electrolyte imbalance

All oral laxatives are contraindicated with nausea, vomiting, undiagnosed abdominal pain, or faecal impaction.

Rectal medications and treatments. Suppositories containing stool softeners and/or bowel irritants may be used to relieve constipation, but are more useful for clearing the lower bowel prior to bowel treatments. Suppositories for evacuation purposes usually contain glycerin, bisacodyl, senna, or some chemical compound that releases carbon dioxide after insertion. Carbon dioxide gas increases the pressure within the rectum, thereby providing a stimulus for evacuation. The longer the patient can retain the suppository, the greater the expansion of the rectum, and hence the more likely the complete evacuation of faecal contents.

Evacuant enemas are liquid substances instilled into the rectum and used for the same purpose as suppositories. The enema fluid may be tap water, normal saline, soapy water, oil, or a bowel irritating chemical. The volume of the enema can vary from 5 ml to 2 litres depending on the nature of the fluid. Large volume enemas cause evacuation by adding bulk; oils of lesser volume (100–200 ml) soften and lubricate hardened faeces; and chemical irritants require only a small volume to be effective.

Every year hundreds of thousands of dollars are spent by the 'well' public on proprietary laxatives, which is evidence that these drugs are abused and that chronic constipation is a community problem. The nurse can do much to help overcome this problem by education. Each patient should be questioned carefully about his bowel habits, and if there is any hint that he has a problem with constipation or laxative abuse, he must be commenced on a bowel retraining programme. This programme should include information about high fibre diets and the value of bran; the need for at least 2 litres of fluid a day; the need for habitual exercise; and information about the dangers of laxative abuse. It is not sufficient to commence a person on such a programme while he is in medical or nursing care. The caregiver must ensure that the patient understands the significance of a well balanced diet, and the establishment and maintenance of good bowel habits, so that he will not slip back into faulty bowel habits once he is caring for himself.

GASTROINTESTINAL INTUBATION

An upper gastrointestinal tube is a plastic or silicon rubber tube which is passed into the stomach or upper small bowel for the purposes of aspiration (decompression) and/or feeding (gavage). The tube may be passed via the nose (the most common route), the mouth or through a skin stab wound leading to the oesophagus, stomach (gastrostomy, Fig. 49.5), or upper small bowel (nasoenteric, Fig. 49.7).

Tubes of varying size and construction are used depending on the size of the patient and the purpose of the tube. For an adult the average sized nasogastric tube used for general aspiration or feeding purposes is 100 cm in length, with a 2–3 mm bore. Tubes that are used for washing out stomach contents (lavage) of undigested food have a much wider bore (10–15 mm) and therefore are passed into the stomach via the mouth.

Gastrointestinal tubes are produced by numerous manufacturers who each give their products different names. This can be very confusing for

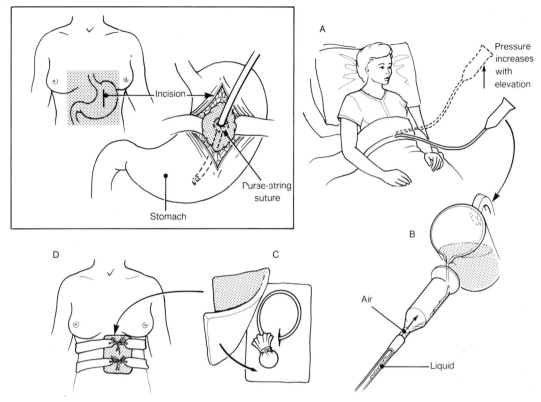

Fig. 49.5 When feeding via gastrostomy (**A**) recepticle must be tilted to allow escape of air (**B**). When not in use, the end of the tube is covered with sterile gauze, and the whole covered by a pad (**C**) and held in place with straps (**D**). The boxed insert shows gastrostomy incision and procedure.

the nurse, therefore it is important to read the description on the package before use.

Aspiration of the stomach (or, more rarely, the upper small intestine) is performed:

● Prior to emergency surgery when there is insufficient time for fasting
● To prevent or treat adynamic (paralytic) ileus
● Following surgery to the upper gastrointestinal tract
  – to rest the operative site
  – to check for haemorrhage
  – to check emptying rate of the stomach
  – to keep the internal sutured area relatively dry
  – to prevent distention and strain on the internal sutured area
● Following poisoning to wash out the stomach
● Prior to feeding via the tube, to check if the distal end of the tube is positioned correctly and to check if the previous feed was tolerated
● To prevent vomiting
● For collection of specimens of gastric and/or duodenal secretions.

Aspirations may be performed intermittently by using a large syringe, or continuously by having the tube connected to a low pressure pump.

Feeding via a gastrointestinal tube

A tube should be used for feeding purposes only when the patient cannot chew or swallow in the normal manner, for example, with the unconscious patient or patients who have disease, trauma, or surgery of the mouth, pharynx, or oesophagus.

A triple lumen combination gastrointestinal decompression and feeding tube has been designed for use immediately postoperatively. A balloon segment is positioned in the stomach just below the cardia and is inflated via the first lumen. The section of the tube which lies in the lower oesophagus and the stomach contains small holes to allow for aspiration of these areas via the second lumen. The third lumen extends to the distal end of the tube which lies in the duodenum and allows for an elemental liquid diet to be instilled at a slow continuous rate. The chief advantage of using this tube is that by providing enteral nutrition immediately postoperatively, positive protein and caloric balance is maintained and wound healing and recovery occur more rapidly.

Patients are usually fed a liquid elemental diet via the gastrointestinal tube. Elemental diets are commercially produced and contain synthetic L-amino acids, sugars, electrolytes, and minerals. They are readily absorbed in the proximal small bowel and cause little stimulation of pancreatic, biliary, or intestinal secretions.

It is the responsibility of each nurse to determine the types of gastrointestinal tubes being used in the particular hospital in which he/she is working. He/she also needs to know the hospital policy regarding physician and nurse responsibility in relation to insertion of tubes, timing of aspirations, and timing and type of feeding required via the tube. Extreme care should be taken when managing the patient who has a gastrointestinal tube in situ.

INSERTION OF A GASTROINTESTINAL TUBE

Requirements

Disposable tray containing:

- 2 containers for aspirate and rinsing water
- 20 ml syringe
- Gastrointestinal tube
- Lubricant
- Adhesive tape

Other requirements include paper towel, paper tissues, emesis bowl, and a glass of water.

Method

A clean procedure. Nasal toilet may be required first.

Conscious co-operative patient. Explain the procedure to the patient and tell him how mouth breathing and swallowing can help in passing the tube. Measure and mark length of tube to be passed. See Fig. 49.6 for nasogastric intubation. For nasoenteric intubation add a further 10 cm.

Lightly lubricate about 10 cm of tube. Have the patient sitting up if possible, with his neck flexed; place paper towel across the patient's chest. Insert

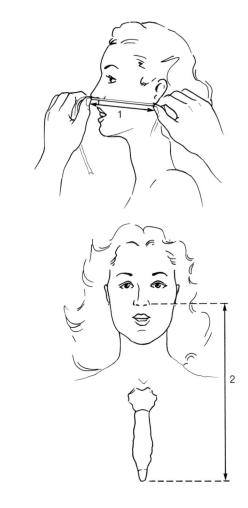

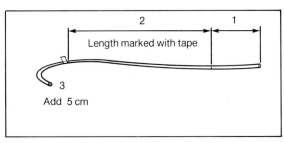

Fig. 49.6 Measurement of length of nasogastric tube.

the tube into a nostril and gently pass into naso-pharynx, aiming backward and downward. When the tube reaches the pharynx, the patient may gag; withdraw the tube a few centimetres and allow him to rest a few moments.

Offer the patient several sips of water, which he may swallow. Then ask him to hold some water in his mouth until told to swallow, advancing the tube as he swallows.

Continue to advance the tube each time he swallows, to the required length. If an obstruction appears to prevent tube from passing, do not use force. Gently rotating the tube may help. If unsuccessful, remove the tube and try the other nostril. If there are signs of distress such as gasping, coughing, cyanosis, or whistling in the tube, remove the tube immediately.

Aspiration is performed with a 20 ml syringe. Do not persist if no aspirate can be obtained: dry suction damages gastrointestinal mucosa. It may be necessary to advance the tube a little further. With a stethoscope over the epigastrium, inject 10 ml of air into the tube. Gurgling sounds indicate air entering the gastrointestinal tract rather than the bronchus.

With tape, secure the tube in a position away from patient's line of vision and avoiding pressure against the nostril.

Unconscious patient. The patient is placed in lateral position, with no head pillow and his neck slightly flexed. Advance the tube between ventilations. The correct location of the tube must be verified by the physician. Medical assistance must be obtained if difficulty is experienced in passing the tube.

Aspiration of the stomach/upper small bowel

When aspirations are to be performed more than once in any 4-hour period, a 'gastric aspiration' tray should be left at the bedside. This tray will be incorporated with the tray for the insertion of the nasogastric tube where applicable.

Requirements

Disposable tray containing:

- 8 containers for rinsing water and aspirate
- 4 small paper towels
- 20 ml syringe in small tray.

Method

Place paper towel under the patient's chin. Connect the syringe and aspirate the stomach contents gently and away from patient's view. Continue until the stomach is empty. If no aspirate is obtained, ensure tube is patent by injecting 10 ml of water.

Rinse the syringe well and return to tray. Record the amount, nature, and colour of aspirate on the fluid balance chart. Dispose of aspirate.

The complete tray is changed every 4 hours, or more frequently if necessary.

Intermittent feeding via a gastrointestinal tube

Prior to every feed aspiration is performed to ensure that the tube has remained in position, and to ascertain how much of the previous feed remains.

If no aspirate is obtained, the tube could be blocked. It may be cleared by injecting 10 ml of water.

If the amount of aspirate is equal to or greater than the previous feed:

- Do not give the feed
- Save the aspirate
- Chart the amount of aspirate
- Notify the nurse-in-charge.

If the aspirate is less than 20 ml it is discarded and not recorded. The normal amount of feed is given.

If the aspirate is more than 20 ml but less than the previous feed:

- It is returned via the tube, as it contains valuable enzymes and other gastric juice components
- The prescribed amount of feed is given, minus the amount of aspirate. The amount of subsequent feeds will be reviewed by the nurse-in-charge of the unit.

Requirements

Add to the aspiration tray:

- 30 ml syringe
- Medicine cup
- Beaker for measured amount of prescribed feed.

Method

Wash and dry hands. At the refrigerator, where feed is stored, the required amount is measured into the beaker. Taking care to do so away from the patient's view, remove the plunger from the syringe, and using the syringe as a funnel, pour in the aspirate (if appropriate), then the feed, allowing it to gravitate to the stomach/intestine.

Follow feed with 10–20 ml of water to rinse the tube. Rinse the syringe well and return it to the tray. Record the feed on fluid balance chart. Discard any feed left after 24 hours. Fresh feeds must be obtained each day.

Continuous feeding via a gastrointestinal tube

Continuous feeding is achieved by connecting the gastrointestinal tube to a drip system similar to an intravenous infusion (Fig. 49.7).

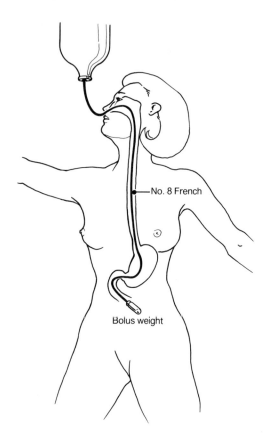

No. 8 French

Bolus weight

Fig. 49.7 Nasoenteric continuous feeding.

The type of commercial feed and giving set is variable; therefore, check the physician's orders before setting up the system. The volume of feed given over a 24-hour period should be ordered by medical staff.

It is not necessary to dilute tube feeds to half strength but this may on occasions be ordered. Once continuous gastrointestinal feeding is commenced there should be no need to aspirate the tube. Change feed giving set every 24–48 hours.

Removal of a gastrointestinal tube

Loosen the adhesive tape and, holding a paper tissue around the tube close to the nostril, gently withdraw the tube through the tissue. Perform nasal toilet if required.

INTRAVENOUS NUTRITION

When for some reason it is not possible for the patient to receive nutrition via the enteral route, either by normal oral feeding or via a gastrointestinal tube, then the parenteral route is used.

Peripheral nutrition. If the patient is in a reasonable state of nutrition and hydration but is to be deprived of an oral diet for a relatively short period (2–7 days) his nutritional needs can be maintained by normal intravenous infusion of dextrose, L-amino acids, and electrolytes. The individual needs of each patient will be assessed by the physician taking account of the patient's electrolyte, fluid, and nitrogen balances.

Central venous nutrition. When the patient is in a malnourished state and/or is in a seriously ill condition, he will require all the components of a normal diet. Because many nutrient solutions are hypertonic and irritant to small veins, a catheter or cannula is inserted into a more robust central vein, usually the subclavicular or internal jugular vein. The risk of thrombosis is also reduced when these solutions are infused into a large, fast-flowing vein. When nutrition is supplied via a central vein the terms hyperalimentation or total parenteral nutrition (TPN) are used interchangeably.

INTESTINAL STOMAS

Definitions

Stoma: an artificial orifice or opening, surgically created between a hollow organ and the skin surface. Its purpose is to replace the function of a nonfunctioning or excised natural orifice.

Ostomy: a suffix denoting a stoma, hence tracheostomy, nephrostomy, colostomy, ileostomy. The prefix denotes the organ or the part of the organ affected.

Colostomy: the formation of a stoma by bringing to and fixing an incised portion of colon to the abdominal wall. Its purpose is to act as an artificial anus, that is, to evacuate the bowel of its contents.

Ileostomy: the formation of a stoma by bringing to and fixing an incised portion of ileum to the abdominal wall. Usually performed when all of the colon has been resected. Its function is to evacuate the small bowel of its contents.

Colostomies are usually named according to their situation in the colon, hence caecostomy, ascending colostomy, transverse colostomy, descending colostomy, and pelvic colostomy. Almost all ileostomies are created in the terminal ileum.

Colostomies are performed when there is some functional colon proximal to the affected area. Permanent ileostomies are performed when there is no colon present or functional. Because some section of the small bowel can be anastomosed to the large bowel, permanent ileostomies are not performed for small bowel disease. However a temporary ileostomy may be created as an emergency measure to relieve small bowel obstruction. See also Figure 49.8.

Temporary stomas

Temporary stomas are created to relieve acute bowel obstruction, to rest an inflamed distal bowel, or to prevent bowel contents escaping into the peritoneal cavity following some cases of bowel perforation. Temporary stomas are usually performed as a surgical emergency. When the underlying problem has been corrected, the stoma is closed and bowel evacuation via the anus is reinstituted. Occasionally a temporary colostomy is refashioned to become a permanent stoma. This may occur if evacuation via the anus cannot be re-established. For example, an emergency temporary colostomy may be performed to allow evacuation of faeces that have suddenly become obstructed due to carcinoma of the pelvic colon. If the surgeon attempts to resect the tumour at a later date, but discovers it to be inoperable, the temporary colostomy would then be converted into a permanent one. Had the tumour been operable an anterior resection would have been carried out; the temporary colostomy would be closed and healthy remaining bowel anastomosed to the rectal stump.

Two methods of creating a temporary stoma may be used: the loop temporary stoma (most

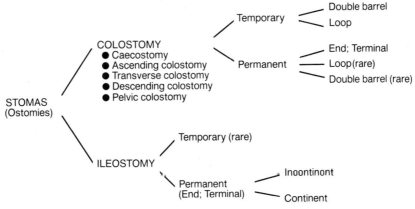

Fig. 49.8 Stoma types.

commonly employed Fig. 49.9) and the double barrel type. In forming the loop stoma a segment of healthy bowel, proximal to the diseased area, is brought to the abdominal surface and an opening is made into the lumen without completely severing the bowel. A plastic retainer is placed on the skin but under the loop, and sutured into place thus preventing the loop from slipping back into the abdominal cavity. With the double barrel type, the segment of bowel that is exposed is completely severed, forming 2 stomas which are each sutured to the skin surface.

Both types of temporary stoma have a proximal and a distal loop. The proximal loop is the functioning section through which bowel contents emerge. The distal loop is nonfunctioning and is adjacent to the diseased segment of bowel. It is important for the nurse to be able to identify which orifice leads to which loop as treatment may be ordered for either loop. Medications may be ordered to be instilled in the distal loop, for example, prednisolone enema when treating an inflamed distal loop; and colostomy washouts (see page 476) may be ordered for either or both loops.

Permanent stomas

A permanent colostomy may be called an end (terminal) colostomy, indicating that the bowel distal to the stoma has been removed, for example, a sigmoid colostomy. If no distal section of the bowel has been resected, the permanent colostomy may appear as a loop or double barrel stoma.

Permanent ileostomies are end stomas, but there are different types: incontinent ileostomy (Fig. 49.10) and continent ileostomy (Fig. 49.11). The incontinent ileostomy is the traditional and more commonly performed ileostomy. The severed end of the ileum is brought directly to the abdominal surface, a lip is formed, and is then sutured to the skin. Small bowel contents are liquid and flow constantly via the stoma into an attached bag. The bag must be worn at all times.

The continent ileostomy (also known as the Koch pouch) is constructed by surgically creating a pouch with a non-leak valve using about 60 cm of terminal ileum that leads to the stoma. This pouch, which is sutured inside the abdominal cavity, allows for the accumulation of faeces. No external ileostomy bag is required. To evacuate

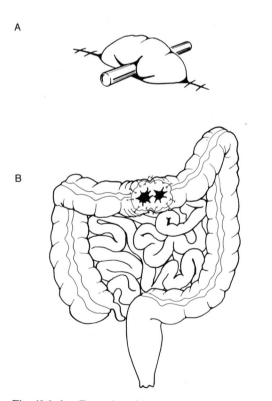

Fig. 49.9 A – Formation of loop colostomy, with section of bowel pulled through incision and held in place by a plastic retainer **B** – Lumen is open, but bowel is not severed.

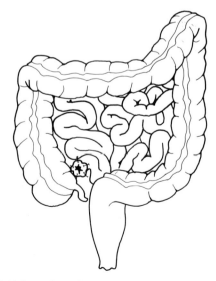

Fig. 49.10 Incontinent ileostomy.

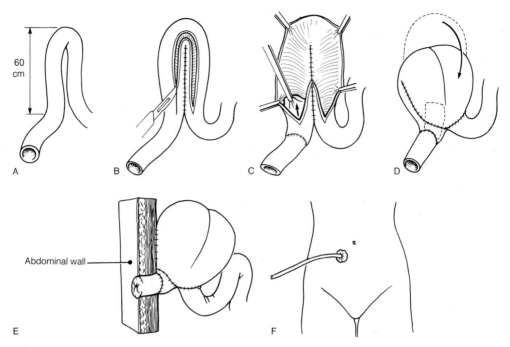

60 cm

A   B   C   D

Abdominal wall

E   F

Fig. 49.11 Formation of continent ileostomy (Koch pouch).

the faecal contents the patient passes a catheter into the pouch via the stoma several times a day. It was hoped that this procedure would have great advantages over the incontinent ileostomy; however, as yet it is not widely employed because the technique, which requires great surgical skill, has not been perfected to guarantee total continency. Also, some patients have difficulty in evacuating the pouch via the catheter.

Nursing management of the patient with a colostomy or an incontinent ileostomy

This is a specialized area and should be managed by a clinical nurse specialist (Stomal Therapist) who has had the necessary education and experience. Unfortunately many hospitals do not employ such specialists, therefore the general nurse practitioner must understand the principles of nursing care for the patient with a bowel stoma.

Nursing management can be considered under the following headings:

- Psychosocial support
- Stoma care and appliances used
- Control of odour, gas, and faecal discharge.

Psychosocial support

The patient who is to have a permanent stoma must have a full explanation of the procedure and its consequences. Each patient will react differently and must be treated individually according to his reactions. Patients may be shocked, angry, depressed, frightened, ashamed, or even revolted, when they realize that they will have little control over their faecal elimination. On the other hand, the patient may be so anxious to have the underlying disease treated or cured that he feels that having a stoma is a small price to pay. Because of these varying reactions it is essential that time is given to allow the patient to search his feelings, ask questions, and to talk about how he thinks he will be able to manage, not only the physical care of the stoma, but more importantly, his social and emotional relationships. Patients may be too timid to ask, but will certainly want to know if they will be able to continue their previous lifestyle, especially in regard to sexual activities, pregnancy, sport, and social outings.

The nurse needs to have the knowledge, as well as a positive attitude, to be able to assure his/her patient that impotency is uncommon because every endeavour is made to preserve the presacral nerves during surgery. Sports not requiring body contact can and should be resumed. Social outings are encouraged. Pregnancy and normal vaginal delivery pose few problems.

How the patient adapts to these concerns will depend to a great extent on how the patient perceives he is being accepted by medical and nursing staff, and by his loved ones. For this reason the nurse who has negative feelings about stomas must call in someone else to give the patient the necessary positive support. Some patients respond well when they meet someone of their own age, sex, and marital status who has adjusted well to having a stoma. It is important that the patient's sexual partner is included in any sex counselling sessions. The patient and his partner must be encouraged to have open, honest discussions about any concerns that either may have. The nurse should be aware of the facilities and literature available in his/her area so that they may be recommended to his/her patient if necessary. Most large towns have an ostomy club or association which serves an important educational and supportive role. The patient needs to be informed of the nearest such facility to allow him the opportunity of joining if he wishes.

Even though a patient has been well prepared emotionally, and appears to have come to terms with the idea of having a stoma in the preoperative phase, it is not unusual for the patient to experience a complete reversal of attitude postoperatively. Once the stoma is a reality, the patient's body image is altered and he will probably go through the stages of grief until he learns to accept, and to feel accepted with, this unnatural body image. Much patience is needed by the medical and nursing team and the patient's family whilst this adjustment is taking place. The patient must not be discharged from hospital without adequate follow up care being arranged.

Stoma care

Because there is no sphincter control at the stomal orifice (except in the as yet uncommon continent ileostomy) bowel contents will flow uncontrolled via the stoma onto the abdominal surface. This is a most unacceptable situation for two main reasons:

- It is aesthetically and socially demoralizing
- The contaminated skin becomes excoreated, ulcerated, and infected.

The nurse's energies will be directed towards minimizing these problems. It would seem a simple matter to attach an appliance (a plastic or rubber bag or pouch) to the stoma to collect the faecal discharge and to change the bag whenever necessary. In the uncomplicated situation this is what is done. Unfortunately the uncomplicated situation is rare, and it is extremely difficult to attach a bag to a stoma so that it is leak-proof and odour proof. Surgeons too are mindful of this problem and choose the site of the stoma very carefully. The site must be clear of natural skin creases, bony prominences, old scars and the new abdominal wound. It must be in such a position that the attached appliance does not shift when the patient moves, walks, or runs. Also, the surgeon ensures that there is a 'lip' on the stoma protruding 1–3 cm from the skin surface in order to fix the appliance snugly around the stoma. Even with a well formed and sited stoma, and a well designed appliance, both the nurse and patient (or significant others) must be skilful in its application.

Another consideration when determining the possibility of leakage is the consistency of the faecal matter. Because water absorption occurs chiefly in the colon, ileostomy discharge is fluid. Caecostomy, ascending, and transverse colostomy discharges are less fluid, and the pelvic colostomy discharge resembles normal firm faeces (unless the patient has diarrhoea). The more fluid the faecal matter, the more likely there is to be a leakage problem and, therefore, associated skin and emotional problems. The nurse might notice that ileostomy stomas protrude further from the skin surface than do colostomies. This is a further attempt to keep the discharging orifice of the stoma away from the skin. Ileostomies discharge continuously, necessitating emptying or changing the bag about every four hours. Pelvic colostomies usually discharge periodically – up to 4 times a day.

Ostomy bags or pouches, which are usually of disposable plastic, may be attached directly to the skin surrounding the stoma. More commonly they are attached to a skin-protecting face-plate, flange, or medicated adhesive gasket which is first fitted around the stoma. Soiled bags can then be lifted from the semipermanent skin protector without disturbing the underlying skin too frequently. In the endeavour to ensure a leak-proof fitting, the nurse must be careful that the opening of the bag or flange is not so small that the stoma becomes strangulated. If this occurs the stoma will become necrosed and the patient may have to return to the OR to have a new stoma created.

Stoma bags can be drainable or nondrainable (Fig. 49.12A & B). Drainable bags are used to save having to constantly change the stoma bag when there is a fluid discharge. A clamp at the bottom of the bag is released when the bag needs to be emptied. Before reclamping the bag it may be cleaned by instilling a little water with detergent and a deodorizing agent into the bag through the opened end. The fluid is gently propelled around the lower part of the bag then allowed to

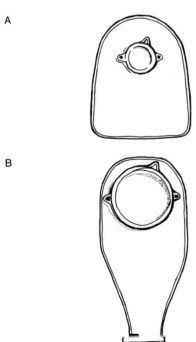

A

B

Fig. 49.12 A – Non-drainable stoma bag. **B** – Drainable stoma bag.

drain. It is important that this cleansing fluid does not come in contact with the stoma site as it could dampen the adhesive causing it to lift and leak. Nondrainable bags are used when faeces are formed or when the patient cannot tolerate the idea of wearing a drainable bag.

If the skin surrounding the stoma does become contaminated and excoriated, there are various products available such as protective powders and adhesive pastes which can be applied to the area prior to fixing the appliance or face plate in place. All stoma appliances and products are packaged with detailed instructions which must be followed carefully.

Control of odour, gas, and faecal discharge

Odours escaping from the stoma or appliance can be controlled to a satisfactory degree by diet, with well-sealed bags, and by the use of deodorizing agents. Foods which cause odours (eggs, fish, onions, cabbage, nuts, and garlic) should be avoided if there is an odour problem. On the other hand, parsley, spinach, and yogurt tend to counteract odours. Intact bags should not allow odours to escape, therefore the first step is to make sure that the bag is attached in a leak-free manner. Drainable bags must be thoroughly cleaned around the drainage opening each time they are drained of faeces. Odour-free bags are available but are more expensive than plain bags. Nondisposable appliances must be washed and dried thoroughly, deodorized, and allowed to air when not in use. If nondisposable equipment is being used, the patient should have 2 or 3 sets to ensure proper cleansing. Deodorizing agents such as charcoal, or commercial products, for example, Nilodor can be placed in the stomal bag. Room deodorizers may also be helpful, but should not be overused as these in themselves can be unpleasant.

Intestinal gas is produced in the bowel during digestion. Some foods such as onions and yeast products, especially beer, are known to produce excessive gas and should be avoided. Swallowed air is also a source of intestinal gas and can be reduced if the patient makes a conscious effort to avoid swallowing air, especially when eating.

Gaseous drinks should also be avoided. The escape of gas via the stoma cannot be avoided entirely and if the stomal bag becomes inflated with the expelled gas the nondrainable bag can be punctured with a needle. After the gas is expelled from the bag the puncture site can be sealed with waterproof adhesive tape. Drainable bags can simply be unclamped. The patient will become embarrassed when gas is expelled from the bag, as the odour is quite offensive. The patient should be warned before the procedure. A light spray of room deodorant is appreciated. When at home, the patient will know to take himself away from other people prior to performing this procedure, but when in hospital he may not have such control.

Control of faecal discharge. Ileostomy patients will have little control over the constant watery discharge in the initial stages. However, the small bowel will eventually compensate for the loss of the colon and its water absorbing function, and will begin absorbing larger quantities of water. The faecal matter will then become less watery and stoma care more manageable. About 4–5 hours following a meal there is usually a large volume evacuation. When possible, this is the best time to change or drain the bag. The lesser volume which flows constantly at other times can easily be contained in the bag hidden under clothing.

Some colostomy patients are able to control the consistency and frequency of the bowel action by careful management of their diet. This control is learned by trial and error, as most people respond differently to similar foods, and therefore no specific diet can be prescribed. If the ostomate can regulate the stoma to act once or twice a day at a specified time, it is not necessary for a collecting bag to be worn at all times. Instead, a disposable, odour-proof stoma cap with an activated charcoal filter for releasing gas is used. Unfortunately, controlling the consistency and frequency of bowel action is not always achievable and most ostomates wear a stoma bag at all times – very often just for peace of mind.

Bowel irrigation

Some patients prefer to control colostomy evacuation by bowel irrigation once a day as an alterna-

tive to natural evacuation. With the irrigation technique a long plastic sleeve is fitted over the stoma and the other open end is situated to allow the washout and faeces to drain into a bowl, bedpan, or the toilet (Fig. 49.13). A soft catheter with a cone attached (to prevent back-flow whilst the irrigating fluid is being instilled) which is also connected to the irrigating system, is inserted no more than 10 cm into the bowel via the stoma. About 1.5 l of tap water at body temperature are allowed to flow in under gravity. The catheter is then removed and the washout flows from the stoma, down the sleeve, and into the receptacle. The washout takes up to an hour to be returned, after which the sleeve is removed, the peristomal area cleaned and dried, and an appliance or stomal cap is replaced. Usually there is no bowel action until the next washout.

The nurse assumes full responsibility for managing a temporary stoma (unless the patient is to be discharged temporarily from hospital) but the patient who has a permanent stoma must, if able, learn self care. Some patients may take days or weeks before they can bring themselves to handle the stoma. These people must be allowed

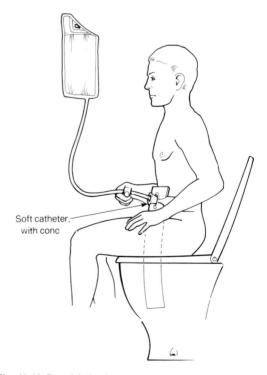

Soft catheter, with cone

Fig. 49.13 Bowel irrigation.

to make this enormous adjustment in the least threatening manner; they must not be rushed into assuming self care lest this puts at risk their acceptance of their altered body image.

Structural complications

Apart from the complications of peri-stomal skin breakdown, altered bowel and dietary habits, and psychological trauma there are 5 main surgical complications of stoma formation that may occur:

● Retraction (inward contraction of the bowel along with its attached skin surfaces)
● Prolapse (projection of the bowel from the skin surface)
● Stenosis (constriction by the surrounding skin which may lead to cyanosis and strangulation).
● Herniation through the divided abdominal muscles
● Bowel obstruction (indicated by increasing diminution of usual bowel evacuations, gas, increasing abdominal distension and pain, loss of appetite, nausea, and vomiting of faecal matter) due to a volvulus, oedema, adhesions, or luminal obstruction with faeces or undigested food.

All these conditions will require further surgical intervention and possibly the re-siting of the stoma. The nurse must be mindful of these possibilities and observe for early signs of such occurrences.

Anticipated outcome.

Numerous people live well adjusted lives even though they have an intestinal stoma. However, this largely depends upon the teaching and support role that both the hospital and the community nurse must play in assisting the patient to become skilled in caring for his stoma and to achieve psychological well being. There must also be continued support from family and loved ones. These people will also need guidance and support and the nurse must ensure that such assistance is available to them.

50

Disorders of the mouth

Mavis Matthews

The general condition of the mouth often reflects the general condition of the rest of the body. Predisposing factors of many of the common disorders of the mouth include: dehydration; severe debilitation; fever; and nutritional or vitamin deficiency. The other common cause of mouth problems is inadequate oral and dental hygiene. Apart from the teeth and gums, the main areas of the mouth which are subject to disease are the salivary glands and the tongue. Dental and periodontal problems do not come under the scope of general medicine and, therefore, will not be dealt with in this book. Although there are numerous conditions of the mouth, only those that the nurse is most likely to deal with are presented here.

STOMATITIS

Stomatitis is generalized inflammation of the mouth and is usually caused by nutritional deficiency or extreme debility. Painful swollen mucosa and excess salivation are the main symptoms. Treatment includes maintaining the patient in a well nourished state, and 2-hourly oral hygiene using mild alkaline solutions. The physician may also order the application of a topical anaesthetic for pain relief and a corticosteriod to reduce inflammation.

MONILIASIS – THRUSH

This fungal infection, caused by *Candida albicans*, is another condition which frequently occurs in the mouth of debilitated persons. It also occurs

following prolonged use of such antibiotics as tetracycline and chloramphenicol because the normal flora of the mouth which usually keep fungi at bay are destroyed by antibiotics. The lesions of thrush develop on the mucous membranes and on the gums. They have a characteristic white, flakey appearance. Antifungal preparations (such as nystatin) given as either a mouth rinse or lozenges, along with oral hygiene, is usually effective treatment.

SALIVARY GLANDS

Saliva, which is chiefly produced in the 3 main salivary glands of the mouth (parotid, submandibular, and sublingual) is transported into the oral cavity via small ducts. Saliva is necessary as a lubricant for mastication and speech, and for aiding in cleansing the mouth. It also contains enzymes which begin the digestive process on some starches. Other enzymes in saliva help to destroy bacteria.

Obstruction to the flow of saliva is a common problem and may be due to either inflammation of any of the glands and/or ducts resulting in a swollen, occluded duct (see sialoadenitis below); or calculi, which sometimes develop in the salivary glands or ducts, particularly the submandibular gland. Sometimes calculi develop because a duct is obstructed.

Mucoceles (mucus-containing cysts) occasionally develop in the gland as a result of ductal obstruction. Mucoceles and calculi are usually treated surgically and with an antibiotic cover.

Sialoadenitis is infection of the salivary glands, the parotid gland being the most often affected (parotitis), and usually occurs in patients who have a severe febrile condition or who have had major surgery. The nurse must be mindful that this condition is preventable, as dehydration and poor oral hygiene during an acute illness, and particularly among the elderly, are the main contributing factors. The staphylococcus organisms are the usual infecting agents. Appropriate parenteral antibiotics and stringent oral hygiene will usually control parotitis, but if an abscess has formed within the gland then surgical drainage may also be required.

THE TONGUE

The tongue often becomes dry, furred and even cracked when the patient is dehydrated or debilitated. It can become inflamed (glossitis) due to local lesions or because of certain nutritional deficiencies, for example, folic acid and vitamin B_{12}. Glossitis may also be a side-effect of alkylating cytotoxic agents. When the underlying cause can be corrected, the tongue returns to normal.

An inflamed, swollen tongue can cause many problems for the patient. He may have difficulty in tasting, chewing, swallowing, speaking, or even breathing. Also, the patient will probably be troubled with pain. The nurse must acknowledge these possibilities when assessing the individual patient who has glossitis. The nursing care plan may include strict 2-hourly mouth cleansing, ice to suck, soft diet, mouth rinses following all food intake, and observations for signs of airway obstruction.

TUMOURS OF THE MOUTH

Aetiology and pathophysiology

Although tumours can occur in any part of the oral cavity and salivary glands, the lower lip, tongue, and the floor of the mouth are the most common sites. Benign tumours are rare and are treated by local excision if troublesome.

Squamous cell carcinoma is the type of cancer that most frequently affects the lip and oral cavity. When the lip is affected, wide excision with plastic surgical repair affords a good prognosis as metas-

tases are uncommon. Occasionally radiotherapy is used for extensive lip cancers.

Carcinoma of the mouth is often preceded by leukoplakia – a white, thickened patch on mucous membranes. The prognosis for carcinoma of the tongue is often poor because the tumour usually grows painlessly on the under surface of the tongue, and may not be noticed until it is well advanced and may even have spread to the floor of the mouth. Also, the tongue is very vascular and has an extensive lymphatic drainage system, so secondary spread is often rapid.

Cancer of the tongue is more common in males and occurs most frequently in the over 55 year old age group. Predisposing factors appear to be poor oral hygiene and chronic irritation, for example, by irregular teeth or ill fitting dentures. Tobacco and alcohol, when taken habitually, are also considered to be important irritants.

Medical, surgical, and nursing management of mouth tumours

Depending on the site, the extent of the tumour, the patient's needs, and the physician's preference, any of the following methods of treatment may be instituted:

- Beam radiotherapy
- Implant radiotherapy
- Excision of the tumour and surrounding tissue, including block dissection of the glands in the neck
- Excision followed by beam radiotherapy
- Radiotherapy (beam or implant) followed by excision.

Because surgery is often very mutilating (see description of Commando procedure below), whenever possible either form of radiotherapy is the first choice of treatment. If the patient is to have implants he will be hospitalized until the temporary implants have been removed or the permanently imbedded isotope's radioactivity has reached a safe level. Only a few hospitals are licenced to treat patients with radioactive isotopes, therefore the patient may have to be hospitalized some distance away from his home. Patients having beam radiotherapy usually attend a department of radiotherapy as outpatients. (See page

125 for care of the patient who is having radiotherapy.)

Commando procedure

The most radical type of surgery that is performed for carcinoma of the tongue, tonsil, and floor of the mouth, is known as the Commando procedure. This procedure can include partial removal of the tongue (hemiglossectomy), mandible (hemimandibulectomy), and removal of the soft tissues comprising the floor of the mouth. Commonly a block dissection of the neck, in which the cervical lymph nodes and surrounding tissues are resected, is also performed (Fig. 50.1). These patients usually have a temporary tracheostomy created to prevent airway obstruction due to gross postoperative swelling. Reconstructive plastic surgery for both functional and cosmetic reasons is also performed, either at the time of the initial surgery or at a later date.

Preoperative nursing management. The patient requires a tremendous amount of emotional support because he will feel devastated when the extent and consequence of the surgery is explained. He will also require a careful explanation of what to expect in the postoperative phase in order to reduce the amount of anxiety he may otherwise experience. Because he will be unable to speak for a few days following surgery the nurse, together with the patient, must develop some communicating signals that can be used postoperatively. Physical preparation includes routine preoperative care plus ensuring that the mouth is as clean as possible. Any dental caries should be treated before the patient is admitted to hospital for the operation.

Postoperative nursing management. The patient will, ideally, be nursed in an intensive care unit until the immediate dangers of asphyxiation, haemorrhage, and shock have passed (24–48 hours). Specific nursing considerations include:

1. Care of the tracheostomy. If present, it is usually only intended as a temporary measure to ensure a clear airway while there is swelling and oedema of the oropharyngeal area. A cuffed tracheostomy tube will prevent inhalation of oropharyngeal secretions, and if used must remain inflated until the danger of secretion inhalation has passed (see page 338 for care of tracheostomy). If no tracheostomy has been created the nurse must ensure that the airway is clear at all times and report immediately any signs of respiratory distress.

2. Mouth care. The patient must be nursed in a sitting position as soon as he is fully conscious, in order to avoid inhalation of any pooled oral secretions or blood, and to aid his ventilation.

Because the patient will have great difficulty in swallowing, gentle oral suctioning will need to be performed quarter-hourly initially, and less frequently as the patient begins to clear his mouth by spitting. An adequate supply of tissues must be kept within his easy reach. The nurse must ensure that the mouth is kept in a clean state at all times. This can be achieved by gentle

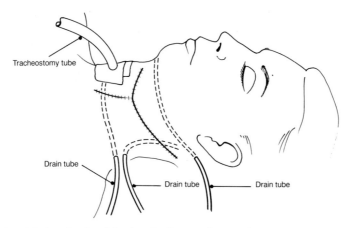

Tracheostomy tube

Drain tube

Drain tube

Drain tube

Fig. 50.1 Possible wound and drain tube sites following the Commando procedure.

suctioning, mouth rinses, and mouth toilets. Usually there are numerous sutures and a grafted area within the oral cavity and these must be inspected for intactness and cleanliness. The lips need to be kept clean and lubricated as they tend to become dry and cracked.

3. Care of the nasogastric tube. The patient usually returns to the ward with a nasogastric tube fixed into position. In the first 36–48 hours post-operatively this should be aspirated at least half-hourly to retrieve any swallowed blood or secretions. Also, apart from checking for haemorrhage, aspirating the stomach may prevent the patient from being nauseated and from vomiting. When the surgeon decides that the patient can have an alimental diet this will be given via the nasogastric tube until the mouth is well healed and the patient is swallowing in a satisfactory manner. The nasogastric tube must be kept clean and patent at all times, as its replacement would be a traumatic and difficult procedure.

4. Maintenance of fluid balance and nutrition. The patient will have intravenous therapy until adequate fluids and diet are taken either by the nasogastric tube or orally. The ease with which the patient resumes oral diet will depend upon the amount of tongue removed, and upon how much the oral phase of swallowing has been affected.

Inhalation is a danger when oral feeding is first attempted, therefore the nurse must make certain that only very small quantities are given with each spoonful. In some instances the patient can manage soft or blenderized foods better than fluids, because the food can be more easily held in the mouth prior to the action of swallowing. Patience and encouragement are essential when the patient is being recommenced on oral diet, and the nurse must ensure that the mouth is thoroughly cleansed following each feeding.

Very occasionally the patient may have to be discharged with either an nasogastric or gastrostomy tube in place, therefore education for self care must be completed prior to discharge. As an adequate diet and fluids are essential for optimum wound healing, the patient must feel confident in managing his intragastric tube.

5. External wound care. This may include care of skin grafts, skin flaps, extensive suture lines, drainage tubes, and a donor site.

The neck is sunken in appearance due to the removal of tissue underlying the skin and will be quite stiff and painful on movement. Gentle neck exercises are commenced after the first 48 hours. Slight nodding and sideways head movements, together with shrugging of the shoulders, progressing to more exaggerated movements are helpful exercises which should be done 3–6 times daily. Arm swinging exercises can also be commenced once the patient is ambulant.

6. Speech and social rehabilitation. The patient will not be able to speak whilst he has a cuffed tracheostomy tube in situ, but can be reassured that this is only a temporary situation. The amount of speech difficulty following removal of the tube is dependent upon the extent of the surgery, particularly the amount of tongue that was resected. With intensive speech therapy, continuing after the patient's discharge, patients can learn to communicate in an understandable manner. The nurse should be aware of the speech pathologist's objectives for the patient and encourage the patient to practise speech exercises.

Socialization must commence well before the patient is discharged from hospital. The nurse can help the patient by explaining that he will feel less embarrassed if he mixes with as many people as possible before discharge. He may be persuaded to move to a 2 or 4 bedded room and to encourage many relatives and friends to visit him. Too often these patients are secluded in a single room during hospitalization and then find great difficulty in coping with resocialization after discharge.

As with all patients who have had treatment for cancer, these patients need to be fully aware of the importance of keeping their appointments for regular progress check-ups.

51

Disorders of the oesophagus

Mavis Matthews

INFLAMMATORY DISORDERS

Acute (corrosive) oesophagitis

This emergency usually arises from the accidental or attempted suicidal swallowing of corrosive substances. The patient will have burns and inflammation of the lips, tongue, mouth, and oesophagus and will be suffering severe pain. Shock is also an expected feature. Diagnosis is made by the history and oesophagoscopy will demonstrate the degree of damage sustained.

Medical, surgical, and nursing management

The corrosive agent must be inactivated immediately if possible, therefore it is essential to know what was ingested. The patient will be given antibiotics and an intravenous infusion. Corticosteroids may also be ordered in an effort to reduce the amount of fibrous tissue that often ensues. When there is resultant gross fibrosis the patient may need repeated dilatations of the oesophagus at varying intervals throughout life. If the oesophagus has been seriously affected, an oesophagectomy may be performed (see page 489). The patient may need to take his nourishment via a gastrostomy tube (see page 467).

Subacute (infective) oesophagitis

The mucosa of the pharynx and oesophagus readily becomes inflamed in cases of mucosal infections arising from lack of effective polymorphonuclear leucocytes. This may occur in such conditions as: toxic granulopaenia (glandular fever) and leukaemia, or when there is an alter-

ation in bacterial normal flora in long-term, broad spectrum antibiotic therapy.

Clinical manifestations

The patient will present with:

- Varying degrees of dysphagia
- Sore throat
- Mild fever
- Retrosternal discomfort.

On examination the physician will find:

- The pharynx to be inflamed
- A white exudate if monilial infection is present
- Generalized debility.

Investigative procedures

A pharyngeal swab culture may demonstrate the responsible organism. Differential white cell count may reveal granulopaenia or leukaemia, and barium swallow X-ray may show a characteristic irregular oesophageal outline.

Medical and nursing management

Those cases that are due to toxic granulopaenia or leukaemia will be helped by constant oral hygiene and gargles, together with an antibiotic.

The cases that are due to long-term, broad spectrum antibiotic therapy will require replacement of the antibiotic with an antifungal preparation.

Chronic (atrophic) oesophagitis

Also named sideropaenic dysphagia, Patterson-Kelly syndrome, or Plummer-Vinson syndrome, this chronic form of oesophagitis usually affects middle-aged women, and is due to chronic iron deficiency anaemia. The group of symptoms that make up this syndrome are chronic oesophagitis, dysphagia, iron-deficiency anaemia, and glossitis. The chronic inflammatory process in the upper oesophagus occasionally leads to ulceration, fibrosis, and finally stenosis and/or the formation of a fold of atrophic epithelial cells (the post-cricoid web), causing partial or complete occlusion. Intermittent dysphagia is due to spasm in the early stages of the condition, but will be due to the web formation or stenosis in the later stages. (Recent research suggests that oesophageal webs can develop in the absence of iron deficiency.)

Investigative procedures

Barium swallow and endoscopy will demonstrate the web and stenosis classically sited at the pharyngo-oesophageal junction.

Medical, surgical, and nursing management

The anaemia is corrected with long-term oral ferrous sulphate therapy. The web may need to be destroyed surgically via an oesophagoscope.

Nursing care is mainly related to care of the patient having an oesophagoscopy (see page 485) and education regarding an iron rich diet, for example, black (blood) pudding, liver (especially if taken raw), eggs, green leafy vegetables and treacle. The nurse must also ensure that the patient understands the need to continue taking the ferrous sulphate for some months following discharge from hospital.

Anticipated outcome

Although this condition does not tend to recur it is a premalignant condition in 10–15% of affected patients.

Recurrent (reflux) oesophagitis

Before considering reflux of gastric contents it is necessary for the nurse to review the mechanisms involved in preventing reflux. These include the lower oesophageal (cardiac) sphincter-like action which normally closes off the oesophagus from the stomach except during swallowing, regurgitation, belching, and vomiting; the mucosal flap valve which is formed by a projection of oesophageal mucosa into the stomach and which lies across the lower end of the oesophagus forming an inert flap valve; the pinchcock action of the crura of the diaphragm; and the effect of the positive intra-abdominal and intragastric pressure on the flaccid intra-abdominal section of the oesophagus (Fig. 51.1).

Reflux of stomach contents into the oesophagus is the most common cause of oesophagitis and may be due to:

- Hiatus hernia
- Gastric hypersecretion
- Associated disorders, such as peptic ulcer or cholecystitis
- Chronic anxiety and nervous strain
- Chronic excessive alcohol intake
- Reduced ability of the lower oesophagus to produce a sphincter-like pressure
- Mechanical factors causing a raised intra-abdominal pressure, such as obesity, tight clothing, pregnancy, or bending.

Inflammation results from the action of the regurgitated gastric juice on the mucosa of the distal oesophagus which, unlike the gastric mucosa, has no natural defence against acid. If this condition is allowed to persist, ulceration and fibrous stricture often ensues.

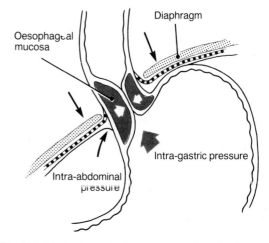

Fig. 51.1 Mechanisms which prevent oesophageal reflux.

Clinical manifestations

Pyrosis (heartburn) is the characteristic symptom. This is the burning sensation felt in the lower retrosternal midline, accompanied by sour eructation. It is classically relieved by alkaline preparations, or on standing and walking if the patient has been lying down.

Disagreeable taste due to reflux of the stomach contents occurs, and it may be described by the patient as sour, metallic, or bitter.

The patient may also complain that he is unable to eat a normal sized meal without reflux occurring. Dysphagia due to oedema, spasm or stenosis may also be a problem.

Investigative procedures

Oesophagoscopy will reveal any inflammation, ulceration, or fibrosis of the lower oesophagus, and barium meal will demonstrate oesophageal reflux.

Medical and nursing management

The rationale for management is to diminish the gastro-oesophageal reflux and to reduce the acidity of the gastric contents.

Frequent, regular doses of a liquid antacid preparation is necessary particularly following meals and prior to bedtime. Most antacid preparations also cause release of gastrin which has the desirable effect of increasing lower oesophageal sphincter-like pressure. Lignocaine may be given to relieve dysphagia. Cimetidine, is occasionally prescribed in an effort to control severe pyrosis and promote healing of any ulcer that may have formed.

Diet. The patient is advised to take small, frequent meals at regular intervals. Solids need to be chewed thoroughly and may need to be washed down with fluids. Spiced and acid foods (for example, tomatoes, citrus fruits) and alcohol should be avoided. Food should not be eaten in at least the 2 hours prior to retiring, and obese patients should be encouraged to follow a reduction diet.

Posture. It is important for the patient to understand that he should maintain a posture that ensures the oesophagus is at a higher level than the stomach. When reaching for things at ground level, bending at the knees should be practised rather than bending at the waist. Lying flat should be avoided. The patient may elect to rest and sleep using extra pillows, or to have the head of his bed elevated by about 15 cm. Sun lounges, which have adjustable back rests, are ideal for these patients when resting.

Oesophageal dilatation. This may be necessary at varying intervals if a stricture develops. Reconstructive surgery may be necessary if the reflux is due to an incompetent lower oesophagus, a peptic ulcer, or an hiatus hernia.

Anticipated outcome

Because the pathology of reflux oesophagitis is nonspecific, the prognosis is determined by the underlying cause. However, most patients learn to live with this condition by following dietary instruction, taking antacids, and being ever-watchful of their posture. These patients also learn to avoid wearing constrictive clothing at waist level.

TRAUMATIC CONDITIONS

Aetiology

Although the oesophagus is well protected against external injury, damage to the oesophagus can occur after a severe epigastric impact, such as a steering-wheel injury, causing rupture of the lower oesophagus.

Internal injuries are more usual and can occur:

- Following impaction of a foreign body (for example, fish or meat bones)
- During attempts to suppress vomiting
- During forceful retching (for example, following alcohol excess causing a linear rupture of the mucous membrane – Mallory-Weiss syndrome
- During endoscopy, particularly in the presence of a stricture or neoplasm.

Clinical manifestations

There may be no immediate signs of oesophageal damage as these can occur up to 48 hours following injury. These may include:

- Mediastinitis, which could lead to fever, shock, toxaemia, and even death
- Restlessness and anxiousness
- Substernal pain
- Dysphagia
- Signs of fluid in, and irritation of, the pleura
- Dyspnoea and cough if the trachea is involved
- Surgical emphysema in the neck region.

Investigative procedures

Oesophagoscopy will usually demonstrate the site and extent of the damage. Chest X-ray may show a widening of the upper mediastinum or any pleural involvement.

Medical and nursing management

The aims of medical and nursing management are to:

1. Provide prompt management of any distressing symptoms and relieve patient anxiety
2. Assess the severity of the injury that has occurred
3. Establish and maintain a patent airway
4. Prevent contamination of the mediastinum.

Specifically, the nurse should allow no food or fluid by mouth as it is important to prevent possible leakage of oesophageal contents into the mediastinum.

Antibiotics are given as ordered, usually intravenously. The patient is prepared for transfer to the operating room as surgical repair will be effected either via the oesophagoscope or by open surgery. Any complicating pleural problem will require its own management (see page 355).

Postoperatively, the nurse will be responsible for: maintaining a patent airway and observing for ventilatory difficulties; management of the IV infusion and observation for circulatory collapse; care of the chest drainage system (if present); and care of the intragastric tube.

DEGENERATIVE CONDITIONS

Achalasia of the cardia

Aetiology and pathophysiology

In this slowly progressive condition, which may occur at any age, there is a disturbance in the motility of the lower two-thirds of the oesophagus. There is an absence of effective peristalsis and failure of the lower oesophagus to relax on the arrival of a bolus of food. The basic defect is thought to be due to degeneration of intramural ganglion cells, resulting in disorganized motor activity. The resulting effect is obstruction of the distal oesophagus, causing it to gradually dilate. The actual cause of this degenerative process is unknown.

Clinical manifestations

- Dysphagia, gradually increasing in severity but there may be a history of periods of remission
- Sudden regurgitation of undigested food, mucus, and swallowed saliva
- Retrosternal pain which is worse following the intake of food
- Gradual weight loss due to inadequate nutrients reaching the stomach
- Inflammation and ulceration of the oesophagus leading to possible haemorrhage
- Respiratory complications occur in a small percentage of patients due to 'spillover' of oesophageal contents into the trachea.

Investigative procedures

Barium swallow will reveal purposeless, nonpropulsive waves and lack of emptying; and the typical X-ray appearance of achalasia. Oesophagoscopy may be performed to visualize the degree of mucosal damage.

Medical, surgical, and nursing management

There is no known way to restore the function of the oesophageal muscle or to correct the disturbance of motility; therefore, treatment is aimed at enlarging the lumen of the lower oesophagus. By the time the diagnosis has been made most patients have already made many adjustments to their eating habits, and further advice on diet is unlikely to be helpful. Dilatation may be achieved by stretching the narrowed area with a mechanical or hydrostatic dilator via an oesophagoscope. If this does not bring satisfactory relief, then an oesophagomyotomy (Heller's operation) is performed. In this procedure the muscle at the lower end of the oesophagus and the cardia is slit to expose, but not to penetrate, the mucosa. A thoracic approach is used therefore postoperative nursing care is as for thoractomy (see page 372).

Anticipated outcome and complications

Good results are reported in 95% of cases following oesophagomyotomy, but the complication of both this and the dilating procedures is reflux oesophagitis. This is due to delayed gastric emptying and loss of integrity of the lower oesophagus during surgery. When this is a problem the nurse must instruct the patient to take the same precautions as described for reflux oesophagitis (see page 483).

Occasionally, further surgery may be necessary. Pyloroplasty (Fig. 51.2) and/or vagotomy may be undertaken to hasten gastric emptying, and to reduce the amount of acidity in the stomach in an attempt to overcome reflux.

Hiatus hernia

There are 2 main varieties of hernias which herniate through the oesophageal hiatus: the sliding hernia, and the much less common para-oesophageal (rolling) hernia (Fig. 51.3). Very rarely a combination of sliding and para-oesophageal hernia may present. In the sliding variety the gastro-oesophageal junction slides up into the thoracic cavity and the mechanism for preventing reflux (see page 483) is lost; gastric juices are then able to come into contact with the oesophageal mucosa giving rise to intense inflammation. With

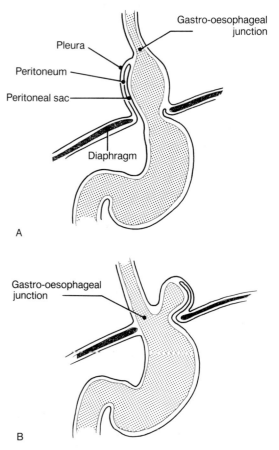

A

B

Fig. 51.3 A – Sliding hernia. **B** – Para-oesophageal (rolling) hernia.

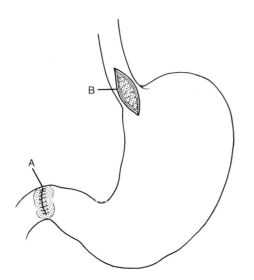

Fig. 51.2 A – Pyloroplasty helps hasten gastric emptying (see Fig. 52.4, page 500 for details of the pyloroplasty procedure) An incision may also be made in the oesophagus to allow the mucosa to bulge (**B**) and relieve oesophageal constriction.

the para-oesophageal hernia the gastro-oesophageal junction remains in the intra-abdominal position, but the fundus of the stomach rises into the thorax alongside the oesophagus. Because the mechanism for retaining the gastric contents is preserved, patients with para-oesophageal hernia usually do not suffer from reflux.

Hiatus hernias occur most frequently in the over 50 year-old age group and are most likely to be due to a gradual weakening of the muscles around the hiatus, due to age. Hiatus hernias can also be due to trauma or can be congenital in origin.

Clinical manifestations

Hiatus hernias are often symptomless. When problems do occur, the sliding hiatus hernia patient will present with the symptoms of gastric reflux (see page 483) which may be extremely severe.

Patients with a large para-oesophageal hernia will have respiratory difficulties, and back pain due to decreased space available for normal lung expansion. Severe pain may also occur when the fundus of the stomach (situated in the thoracic cavity) is distended with food, fluid, or air. The patient often gives a history of this pain being relieved by belching or vomiting. On rare occasions it has been known for the fundus of the stomach to become strangulated at the constriction where the hernia passes through the diaphragm. In this instance the patient presents with severe pain and in a shocked state.

Investigative procedures

Barium swallow X-rays, taken in the erect and Trendelenburg's position, may demonstrate the herniated area. Not all hernias remain fixed in the thorax at all times, therefore absence of evidence of a hernia at the time of X-ray does not rule out the possibility that one is present.

Oesophagoscopy, although not necessary for obtaining a definitive diagnosis, is often performed to determine the extent of incompetence of the lower oesophagus, the presence of gastric reflux, and to obtain biopsy or cytologic specimens.

Medical, surgical, and nursing management

The conservative medical and nursing management of sliding hiatus hernia is as for reflux oesophagitis (see page 483). If these methods fail to give satisfactory relief, then surgical reduction

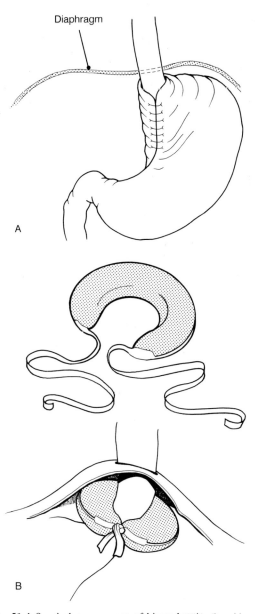

Fig. 51.4 Surgical management of hiatus hernia. **A** – The fundus of the stomach is wrapped around the distal oesophagus. **B** – A silicone collar is tied around the oesophagus, between the stomach and the diaphragm.

of the hernia, together with reduction of the oesophageal hiatus and restoration of gastro-oeso-phageal competence is performed. One of a variety of surgical procedures may be used (Fig. 51.4A & B). An abdominal, thoracic, or combined abdominothoracic surgical approach can be used. The thoracic approach is more satisfactory when dealing with a hernia where shortening of the oesophagus has occurred due to chronic oesophag-itis, ulceration, and fibrosis. Para-oesophageal hernias that cause symptoms should be treated surgically. Reduction of the hernia with repair of the hiatus usually has very good results.

Postoperatively, nursing care is as for the patient having abdominal or thoracic surgery (whichever approach was used). For the first 24 hours only water should be allowed by mouth, and this is gradually increased to a soft, light diet over the next week. The patient is mobilized as quickly as possible to prevent any general complications. The sutures are removed about the tenth day and the patient is usually discharged within 2 weeks from the date of operation.

Oesophageal varices

See Chapter 45.

NEOPLASTIC CONDITIONS

Benign tumours are rare and when they do occur may need to be resected if they cause obstruction.

Malignant tumours

Aetiology and pathophysiology

Oesophageal cancer is particularly serious because of its close proximity to vital structures, and because there is no satisfactory cure. The highest incidence is between the fourth and seventh decades and 3 times as many men as women are affected.

No outstanding predisposing factors have been proven, but there is a slightly increased incidence following chronic irritation due to heavy smoking and inflammation, as in achalasia, stricture, or sideropaenic dysphagia.

Approximatley 25% of tumours occur in the upper third of the oesophagus; 45–50% in the middle; and 25% in the lower third. It is some-times impossible to distinguish between a carci-noma of the gastric cardia extending into the oesophagus, and one originating in the lower oesophagus. These cancers are usually fungating and infiltrating, and 95% of them arise in squa-mous cell epithelium. The remainder are either adenocarcinomas, melanomas, or sarcomas.

Clinical manifestations

Dysphagia is the cardinal symptom and is usually gradual in onset, but may occur as an acute inci-dent particularly when attempting to swallow a solid bolus, especially meat. Substernal discomfort or a sense of fullness may be experienced, and is particularly significant if unrelieved by antacids. In later stages signs of obstruction appear: severe pain; weight loss; anaemia; nocturnal aspiration; and regurgitation. When these late signs appear, the condition is usually inoperable, hence the importance of critical consideration of the early, less obvious clues.

Investigative procedures

X-rays following barium swallow will reveal most tumours but a definitive diagnosis cannot be made on X-ray alone. Oesophagoscopy and biopsy will confirm the diagnosis.

Medical, surgical, and nursing management

The choice of treatment will depend on the site and extent of the disease. In the early stages, before there is evidence of secondary spread, radical surgical resection of the affected area is the treatment of choice. The oesophagus may be rejoined in continuity, or a section of colon or synthetic prosthesis interposed (Fig. 51.5). For tumours of the lower oesophagus, it may be necessary for the surgeon to perform an oeso-phagogastrectomy with anastomosis of the remaining oesophagus and stomach.

Tumours of the upper oesophagus are difficult to resect because of the complicated anatomy in

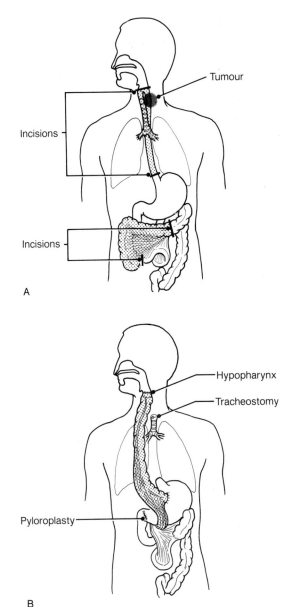

dysphagia (caused by the obstructing tumour) and may be achieved by one or more of the following:

- Deep X-ray therapy
- Palliative resection of the tumour
- Intubation through the tumour area
- Laser therapy. (In some advanced medical centres it is now possible to create a patent oesophagus by using the laser via an oesophagoscope).

Anticipated outcome

Regardless of cell type and site of the tumour, prognosis is poor. Five year survival rates following treatment rarely exceed 10%. The average survival following diagnosis and without treatment is less than 1 year. The tumour often invades adjacent vital organs, which may lead to mediastinitis, tracheo-oesophageal or bronchio-oesophageal fistulas, or fatal haemorrhage due to invasion of one of the major intrathoracic blood vessels. The liver and lungs are the usual sites of distant metastases.

NURSING MANAGEMENT OF THE PATIENT WITH OESOPHAGEAL DISORDERS

The problems common to most oesophageal conditions are dysphagia, aphagia, and discomfort due to reflux or oesophageal obstruction.

Dysphagia, which may be due to obstruction (oedema, stenosis, tumour) or to neurological or psychological conditions, may be of varying degrees of severity. When assessing the patient the nurse must observe for the type of food or fluid the patient is best able to swallow, and under what conditions. For example, the patient may be able to cope with solid food as long as it is chewed thoroughly and washed down with fluid; or the nurse may discover that the patient can swallow food prepared at room temperature, but not when it is very hot or very cold. Other patients may find that they can take adequate nourishment, providing they only swallow a very small mouthful at a time. These patients usually require frequent small meals which are prepared to a soft or thin consistency.

Fig. 51.5 In surgical management of a tumour of the oesophagus, part of the trachea and larynx may be excised (**A**). A section of colon is grafted to the pharynx and stomach, and a pyloroplasty is performed (**B**).

that area, therefore often the treatment of choice is external, high energy irradiation such as radioactive cobalt. All too often, because of the extensiveness of the disease at the time of diagnosis, palliative treatment is all that can be offered to the patient. The main aim of this is to relieve

When the oesophagus is partly occluded, food that is retained in the oesophagus may more easily be moved into the stomach if the patient maintains an upright position and is encouraged to relax following meals. Therefore patients should not undertake activities such as attending to hygiene needs, or physiotherapy for at least 1–2 hours after meals. When the patient is having frequent small meals his day must be planned to allow for these relaxation periods.

Aphagia, the condition where the patient is unable to swallow anything, presents more problems for the patient and the nurse. The patient will need to be nourished via a nasogastric tube, a gastrostomy tube, or be given total parenteral nutrition (see page 470). Saliva and oropharyngeal secretions must be constantly spat out, therefore a disposable container which is renewed frequently, must be with the patient at all times; tissues are inadequate. Mouth hygiene is most important. Lanolin or a similar preparation should be applied to the lips, as constant wiping of them causes irritation and cracking. Some aphagic patients benefit by being allowed to chew and spit out food. Being able to taste food helps them psychologically and also stimulates the secretion of digestive juices, so this is particularly helpful prior to tube feedings.

Discomfort is usually due either to reflux or to distension of the oesophagus by retained food. Antacids given 2–3 hourly will relieve the symptoms of reflux. When the discomfort is due to retained food in the oesophagus, withhold further feedings until the discomfort has eased. If after 2–3 hours there has been no relief, the oesophagus may need to be aspirated via a large-bore tube or an oesophagoscope. Also, the manner in which nutrition is provided may need to be reviewed.

A fluid balance chart and twice-weekly weight recordings will reflect the patient's nutritional and hydration state. Recording the time, amount, and type of any vomiting or regurgitation is essential information that the physician must have; as is the type, duration, and location of pain. The nurse must also assess the patient's psychological reaction to his disease and treatment.

Postoperative nursing management

The main objective is to rest the oesophagus until healing of the oesophageal suture line has taken place. To achieve this aim, no food or fluid will be given orally for about 1 week, and longer in some instances. All necessary precautions will be taken to prevent vomiting. A nasogastric tube is usually inserted during the operation. The purpose of the tube is to allow continuous aspiration of the stomach in order to detect any haemorrhage, and to keep the stomach empty of gastric and oesophageal secretions (see page 466).

Until the patient is able to resume an adequate oral diet, he is usually given total parenteral nutrition (TPN). If the patient was having gastrostomy feedings prior to surgery, these may be recommenced about the second or third postoperative day until oral eating habits are re-established. Following surgery to the oesophagus most patients find taking fluid or food orally to be most uncomfortable. They should start with small sips of water until they learn how much they can swallow at a time. They must also be taught to take small mouthfuls, chew thoroughly, to eat slowly, and to rest after meals.

Specific observations relate to the real danger of the patient developing postoperative complications. For example, the nurse must monitor the patient constantly for signs of shock and fever for at least the first postoperative week. This is to detect mediastinitis and aspiration pneumonia which indicate leakage at the anastomosis.

See page 372 for care of the patient having thoracic surgery and page 338 for management of the patient with a tracheostomy. Also, the nurse may be required to provide emotional care of the patient with inoperable carcinoma.

52

Disorders of the stomach and duodenum

Mavis Matthews

The 3 most common conditions to affect the stomach and duodenum are gastritis, peptic ulceration, and carcinoma. Pyloric stenosis may be associated with these.

GASTRITIS

This condition may be classified as acute, chronic superficial, or atrophic.

Acute gastritis

Acute gastritis is inflammation of the superficial epithelium of the stomach. It may be diffuse or patchy in distribution, and is usually an isolated attack running a brief course.

The common causes of acute gastritis are: thermal (very hot fluids or food); chemical (for example, alcohol, spicy foods, and drugs such as aspirin, digitalis, some antibiotics, and cytotoxic agents); and bacterial (for example, staphylococcal food poisoning). Disease states which may cause gastritis include uraemia, shock, and prolonged emotional tension.

Clinical manifestations

The patient will present with epigastric pain of varying degrees of severity, and nausea and vomiting are common. Haematemesis may occur, and if there has been gastric bleeding there may be melaena.

If the gastritis is due to food poisoning, colic and diarrhoea occur 2–4 hours following intake of the affected food. If the attack is very severe the patient may become dehydrated and shocked.

Investigative procedures

Gastroscopy with biopsy is indicated for recurrent attacks of acute gastritis, or when the acute episode does not spontaneously resolve within 24–36 hours.

Medical and nursing management

Medical and nursing management is largely symptomatic. Oral fluids and food are withheld whilst vomiting is a problem, and re-instituted gradually according to the patient's tolerance. Parenteral fluids may be required if the gastritis lasts longer than 12–18 hours, or if there is evidence of dehydration and electrolyte imbalance.

Drugs that may be prescribed include an anti-emetic to relieve nausea and vomiting, and an anticholinergic to decrease gastric secretions and to relax smooth muscle. Cimetidine is usually given to reduce gastric acid secretion when there is haemorrhage associated with the gastritis. If the acute gastritis produces illness serious enough to require the patient to be hospitalized, then he will need complete bed rest.

Chronic superficial gastritis

Chronic inflammation of the superficial gastric mucosa is not generally believed to be a natural sequela of acute gastritis. It often develops in association with other chronic conditions such as alcoholism, gastric ulcer, thyroid disease, diabetes mellitus, and iron deficiency anaemia. Some authorities believe it may be a premalignant condition. The inflammatory cells invade the superficial mucosa, but the gastric glands are not affected and continue to function.

491

Clinical manifestations

The majority of patients are asymptomatic. However, when symptoms do occur they are similar to those of gastric ulcer or carcinoma. These include dull epigastric pain, anorexia, and weight loss.

Investigative procedures

Gastric contents are analysed to detect any alterations of normal constituents. Cytologic studies may be carried out on gastric contents to differentiate chronic gastritis from gastric carcinoma, however, biopsy is generally more diagnostic. The patient is investigated for any associated condition which may be the cause.

Medical and nursing management

Rarely is the patient acutely ill, therefore he is usually managed as an outpatient. There is no specific treatment for chronic superficial gastritis. Antacids may help the patient who presents with epigastric discomfort. He may need to be educated regarding alcohol intake and altered eating habits. The patient with chronic gastritis benefits by eating small, frequent, bland meals. Chewing food thoroughly also reduces the digestive work of the stomach. Any detected associated condition is treated.

Atrophic gastritis (gastric atrophy)

This condition tends to occur in the elderly, and its incidence increases with age. In atrophic gastritis there is a gradual loss of parietal cells and gastric glands, together with infiltration of the mucosa by plasma cells and lymphocytes. When atrophy is complete the stomach no longer produces acid, pepsin, and finally, the intrinsic factor. This causes the development of pernicious anaemia.

The cause of this phenomenon is not understood. It is often said to be due to the ageing process, and a gradual failure of the immunological mechanism. Researchers are not agreed as to whether atrophic gastritis is a progression of superficial chronic gastritis. There is some evidence that chronic gastritis precedes or may even predispose to gastric carcinoma.

Medical and nursing managment

Medical and nursing management is symptomatic; no treatment is known for stimulating regeneration of gastric mucosa. The patient is advised that known gastric irritants for example, alcohol, irritating foods, and drugs such as aspirin and some antibiotics should be avoided. If the patient develops pernicious anaemia he will require life-long treatment with monthly intramuscular injections of cyanocobalamin. (See pernicious anaemia, page 383).

PEPTIC ULCER

A peptic ulcer (Fig. 52.1) is a circumscribed ulcer extending into the muscularis of any part of the alimentary tract which is exposed to acid-pepsin contained in gastric juice. Common sites are lower oesophagus, stomach, and duodenum. Peptic ulcers may also develop at a gastrojejunal anastomosis, in a Meckel's diverticulum, and in people who have Zollinger-Ellison syndrome. When a peptic ulcer is located in a specific organ it is usually named accordingly. Thus, oesophageal ulcers, gastric ulcers, and duodenal ulcers are all peptic ulcers.

Peptic ulcers may be acute or chronic. Acute ulcers are often multiple and are usually located in the fundus of the stomach (Fig. 52.2). These ulcers are thought to be stress related, superficial, and self-limiting. However, occasionally they penetrate a blood vessel causing haemorrhage of varying degrees of severity.

Chronic ulcers, which are more common than acute ulcers, are likely to be found at the sites shown in Figure 52.2. These ulcers usually occur as a single lesion with margins that are thickened, hyperaemic, and oedematous. Chronic ulcers tend to recur frequently, causing extensive scarring. They sometimes penetrate deep into the muscularis causing haemorrhage and/or perforation.

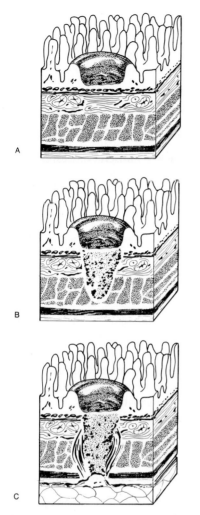

Fig. 52.1 Acute peptic ulcer. **A** – A cavity forms in the mucosa. **B** – The ulcer penetrates the muscle. **C** – Perforating peptic ulcer.

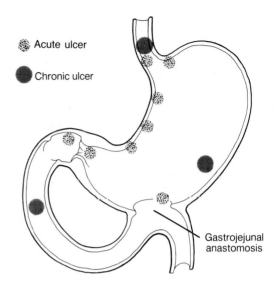

Fig. 52.2 Sites where peptic ulcers and inflammation commonly occur.

Incidence

About 10% of adults living in westernized societies develop peptic ulcers; they are more common in males. Duodenal ulcers are believed to be up to 10 times more common than gastric ulcers, and occur more often in the 20–45 year age group; gastric ulcers occur more often in the 40–65 year age group. Duodenal ulcers occur more frequently in people who have blood group O; gastric ulcers occur more frequently in people with blood group A. Duodenal ulcers develop more often in people who are prone to stress and who smoke heavily.

Siblings of ulcer patients are 2–3 times more likely to develop peptic ulcers.

Aetiology

The cause of peptic ulcers is not fully understood and many of the theories and concepts suggested below have not been substantiated to all researchers' satisfaction. However it is agreed that gastric secretions are capable of breaking down any living tissue, and that peptic ulcers do not occur where there is complete achlorhydria.

Duodenal ulceration tends to be associated with hypersecretion of acid and pepsin. The duodenal mucosa is not ordinarily digested by gastric secretions because these secretions are diluted, neutralized, and buffered by alkaline secretions present in the duodenum. However, when there is excessive gastric acid secretion it may not be neutralized in the duodenum and autodigestion may occur. Increased gastrin secretion which influences acid–pepsin secretion may be a factor in peptic ulceration. Other causes of hypersecretion of acid–pepsin include:

• Increased vagal stimulation; hence any increased physical or mental stress can initiate the formation of a peptic ulcer. Patients with burns or head injuries commonly develop stress ulcers

- Increased number of parietal and pepsin producing cells. There is usually evidence of these with duodenal ulcers
- People with duodenal ulcers usually have rapid gastric emptying.

Gastric ulceration is associated with normal or hyposecretion of acid and pepsin. These ulcers are thought to be due to some defect in the normally protective nature of the stomach mucosa. The defective area is then susceptible to the action of acid and pepsin.

Oesophageal mucosa, not having the same protective nature as gastric mucosa, may become ulcerated if the acid gastric secretions constantly reflux into the oesophagus.

It has been demonstrated that certain drugs and agents irritate the gastric mucosa and may possibly cause a peptic ulcer to form. Some may cause excessive acid–pepsin secretions while others produce localized mucosal damage. The most common of these include: aspirin, corticosteriods, indomethacin, phenylbutazone, cytotoxic agents, reserpine, vasopressors, caffiene, alcohol, bile salts, and nicotine.

Some researchers believe it to be significant that many patients with chronic gastritis and peptic ulceration have had campylobacter-like gram-negative bacteria isolated in their gastric secretions. That these bacteria are sensitive to a wide range of broad spectrum antibiotics, including clindamycin and erythromycin, may be an important factor in the aetiology and treatment of peptic ulcers.

Clinical manifestations

Peptic ulceration has often been described as a disease of symptoms with pain predominating. Peptic ulcer pain is:

- Chronic and periodic – the frequency is highly variable
- Usually localized to the epigastric region. The patient can often point to the spot with one finger
- Invariably described by the patient as gnawing, aching, boring, or burning. The intensity is highly variable
- Initiated by irritants peculiar to the individual, (for example, alcohol, spices, onions), or acid foods (for example tomatoes and citrus fruits)

- Worse when the stomach is empty, especially at night
- Relieved by antacids or bland food
- Pyrosic when there is reflux of gastric juices into the oesophagus

Eructation, the belching of sour tasting gases due to excessive air swallowing, occurs.

Vomiting is not usually a feature unless there has been dietary indiscretion, especially excessive alcohol intake. It may occur when the pain is extremely severe. If there is duodenal obstruction, as often occurs with chronic peptic ulcers, projectile vomiting may be a feature.

Rupture of a blood vessel at the ulcer site may cause haematemesis.

Investigative procedures

The patient's complete history, including eating, smoking, drinking habits, and emotional status, is taken.

Barium meal X-rays are taken, and gastroscopy and duodenoscopy are performed. The endoscopy is the most informative test.

Faeces are checked for occult blood, and an FBE including haemoglobin level, is performed.

Complications of untreated peptic ulcer

Haemorrhage. This may manifest as a massive, sudden haematemesis with or without melaena, with no previous warning or symptoms. This constitutes an emergency situation with a 10% mortality rate. Mild chronic bleeding is usually only detected when faeces are examined for occult blood, and when haemoglobin is measured.

Perforation. It is important to be aware that perforation can occur in the absence of haemorrhage. When the ulcer perforates through the wall of the stomach or duodenum (5% of cases) the acid contents may flow into the peritoneal cavity causing peritonitis, or into pancreatic tissue causing acute pancreatitis. The acidity of these secretions causes excrutiating pain, and reflex, boardlike rigidity of the abdominal wall. All perforations require urgent surgical intervention in order to save the patient's life.

Obstruction. When chronic peptic ulcers repeatedly heal and break down, the resultant scar tissue sometimes causes a permanent narrowing of the pyloric sphincter, called pyloric stenosis. This requires surgical repair, and discussion of the condition and its management can be found on page 497.

Occasionally temporary obstruction to the flow of chyme may be due to muscle spasm or oedema.

Conservative medical and nursing management

The majority of people with peptic ulcers manage their own treatment (sometimes for years) by relying on taking antacids, milk, and a bland diet whenever their symptoms are causing discomfort. When these measures are no longer effective the patient then consults his physician who usually initiates:

- The promotion of rest
- The relief of pain
- The modification of dietary, smoking, and drinking habits
- The reduction of excessive hydrochloric acid and pepsin secretion

Antacid preparations and dietary control will bring pain relief but have little, if any, effect on the healing of a peptic ulcer.

The promotion of rest

It is thought that taking adequate rest away from stressful situations will benefit the ulcer patient. These people should make a conscious effort to incorporate relaxing activities into their daily lifestyle. Actual bed rest will only be necessary to overcome physical exhaustion due to severe pain during an acute episode.

The relief of pain

Most common analgesics contain aspirin and are contraindicated for ulcer patients. Pain is thought to be due to the action of the hydrochloric acid on the ulcer, therefore neutralizing the acid with antacids and/or bland food usually controls the pain.

Antacids are used to raise the pH of gastric contents and therefore reduce the effect of acid on the gastric mucosa. The most potent antacids

(sodium bicarbonate, magnesium oxide and hydroxide, and calcium carbonate) all have disadvantages.

- Sodium bicarbonate relieves pain rapidly but is absorbed and causes metabolic alkalosis, which is serious in patients with renal insufficiency
- Magnesium oxide and hydroxide acts quickly but causes diarrhoea, (as do all magnesium salts)
- Calcium carbonate is absorbed, but does not significantly alter pH unless taken with large quantities of milk. However, with excessive milk ingestion hypercalcaemic (milk-alkali) syndrome may occur. Milk-alkali syndrome manifests as headache, weakness, anorexia, nausea, vomiting, abdominal pain, constipation, thirst, and polyuria, with temporary, or occasionally permanent, renal damage. All calcium salts constipate.

There are alternative antacids of the magnesium and aluminium groups that relieve peptic ulcer pain but which are not readily absorbed through the gut. These compounds therefore do not significantly affect acid–base balance. The most common forms of these compounds are magnesium trisilicate and aluminium hydroxide, which is believed to inactivate pepsin but causes constipation.

Antacids also come in many forms as 'over the counter' preparations.

Liquids and powders are generally more effective than tablets. Tablets are best sucked, not chewed. When pain is severe these preparations can be taken hourly or 2-hourly, with or between meals.

Modification of habits

The modification of dietary and drinking habits, and the cessation of smoking is all that is required to control the activity of a peptic ulcer in most people. However, indiscretion in any of these habits can lead to relapse. The most beneficial facet of dietary control is to ensure that the patient eats something (not necessarily a large meal) at least every 2 hours, and to have milk and perhaps a biscuit at the bedside in case he awakens during the night. The milk should be kept cold or hot in an insulated container. Ulcer patients know which foods aggravate their condition and soon learn to avoid them. Usually, acid (for example, citrus fruit, tomatoes) and spiced (for example curry, pepper) foods are not tolerated. Some patients have benefitted from drinking a litre of milk per day; however, excessive milk intake is not advised as it is thought that calcium stimulates gastric acid secretion.

Reduction of secretions

Rest, the use of antacids to relieve pain, alterations to diet, a reduction of alcohol ingestion, and the cessation of smoking, will reduce the production of gastric secretions and relieve ulcer symptoms in the majority of patients.

Aggressive medical and nursing management

Should conservative measures prove to be no longer effective, the patient will require more aggressive medical intervention, usually in the form of drug therapy initially. Surgical intervention may prove necessary for the chronic ulcer patient and a discussion of this follows on page 499.

Generally speaking, drug therapy consists of using a variety of chemotherapeutic agents which will in some way reduce the ulcerative irritation of the mucosa, and possibly promote ulcer healing.

Anticholinergic drugs

These act by opposing the action of acetylcholine at post-ganglionic parasympathetic (cholinergic) nerve endings. Because of the effect at the vagus nerve endings, these drugs are also called antivagal drugs. Atropine and atropine-related drugs block the effect of acetylcholine, particularly on smooth muscle and glands. In the stomach this reduces the amount of acid secreted and delays gastric emptying.

Side-effects are those of atropine: dry mouth, blurred vision, difficulty with micturition, tachycardia, constipation, and mental confusion.

These drugs are never used in patients with glaucoma, pyloric obstruction, or symptoms of urinary obstruction.

Anticholinergic drugs are usually given before meals with an additional dose at night.

Histamine (H₂) receptor antagonists

These relatively new drugs have greatly simplified the management of peptic ulcer and also greatly reduced the need for surgery. Histamine (H_2) found in the parietal cells of the stomach and the intestines, regulates various secretory activities. Cimetidine and ranitidine are histamine (H_2) receptor antagonists and, therefore, inhibit gastric acid secretion. These drugs have proved to be more effective than the anticholinergics but may have to be taken continuously for 1–3 years, as cessation of treatment often results in relapse.

Intravenous cimetidine has proved to be very effective in controlling haemorrhage from ulcer sites. When used intravenously, hypotension may be a side-effect; therefore, the nurse must observe the patient's vital signs while the treatment is in progress.

Since the symptoms of gastric carcinoma mimic those of peptic ulcer, a gastroscopy and biopsy should precede the administration of either of these drugs because they effectively mask neoplastic symptoms. Otherwise, there are no known contraindications for the use of cimetidine and ranitidine. Side-effects such as diarrhoea, dizziness, bradycardia, gynaecomastia, altered mental state, and decreased sperm count are usually only mild and more likely to occur in those patients who are on high dosages for life. Oral cimeditine or ranitidine should be taken with meals as they are absorbed rapidly in the stomach.

Inhibiting gastric reflux

Gaviscon, a proprietary antacid marketed in the form of chewable granules or a mixture, is active only in the stomach and is not absorbed. The granules are chewed thoroughly, a little at a time, and followed by sips of water. An alginic acid gel forms on the gastric contents, inhibiting reflux. Side-effects are unknown, but the granules contain sugar and this should be taken into account when treating diabetic patients.

Multifocal action (sucralfate)

While conventional anti-ulcer therapy focuses on reducing gastric acid by neutralization or by inhibition of secretion, sucralfate is a new anti-ulcer drug which protects the mucosa, inhibits the action of pepsin, and has an acid-buffering capacity. Sucralfate binds to the ulcer crater, thus providing a barrier to erosive factors. It appears to be more effective with duodenal ulcers than with gastric ulcers. The incidence of side-effects to this drug is less than 4%, and when they do occur, they are mild and transient. Side-effects include constipation, nausea and dizziness.

Antibiotic therapy

There has been some interest in prescribing antibiotics such as clindamycin and erythromycin to those ulcer patients who have campylobacter-like bacteria in stomach secretions. There is as yet no conclusive evidence that this is curative therapy for peptic ulcer patients.

PYLORIC STENOSIS IN ADULTS (See also page 495)

Obstruction due to stenosis occurs around the pyloric region and may extend from the antrum of the stomach into the proximal third of the duodenum. The stenosis is due to scarring and fibrosis associated with chronic inflammation and ulceration, and causes gastric dilatation, gastritis, and gastric stasis.

Clinical manifestations

The patient has a constant feeling of epigastric fullness which is more pronounced towards the end of the day and which is relieved by vomiting. Nausea and anorexia are present. Large volumes of retained food and gastric secretions may be vomited, and the vomitus contains no evidence of any bile.

The patient will be constipated and show weight loss and other signs of malnutrition, including coated tongue, thirst, debilitation, increased haematocrit, and electrolyte imbalance

Investigative procedures

Barium meal will demonstrate a dilated stomach, motor inactivity, and delayed emptying of the barium.

Gastroscopy enables the physician to view the extent of the obstruction, and blood tests will indicate the degree of electrolyte imbalance and haemoconcentration, and may also show an elevated blood urea/nitrogen level (BUN).

Medical and surgical management

Decompression of the stomach by intermittent aspiration of stomach contents via a nasogastric tube, allows the stomach to regain its contractability and tone. Nutrients and fluids and electrolytes will be restored via intravenous infusion or hyperalimentation.

Surgical intervention will be required to relieve the obstruction and to treat the ulcer. Common surgical procedures include pyloroplasty or partial gastrectomy with gastroenterostomy. Vagotomy may also be performed.

ZOLLINGER-ELLISON SYNDROME

This rare syndrome is characterized by a triad of features:

1. A nonspecific non-insulin producing islet cell tumour of the pancreas, which produces a hormonal substance that has a gastrin-like action but is said to be 30 times more potent than gastrin. The tumour is malignant in over 60% and multiple in about 25% of cases
2. The gastrin-like hormone causes a huge increase in gastric secretions
3. Severe multiple peptic ulcerations that may appear at unusual sites such as the jejunum and oesophagus, and which tend to recur in spite of normal peptic ulcer treatment.

Removal of the tumour frequently abolishes the hypersecretion of gastric juices with subsequent healing of the ulcer(s). Unfortunately, when the tumour is of an advanced malignant nature, or is too diffuse, satisfactory resection of the tumour cannot be achieved. Other methods used to attempt to reduce the acid secretion include using large doses of cimetidine, or resorting to the formidable procedure of total gastrectomy (see page 499). The outlook for the patient with this syndrome is usually grim, because whatever treatment he has he will still suffer one or more of the following outcomes:

- Severe debility due to the peptic ulcerations
- The problems associated with total gastrectomy
- The fatal consequences of having an inoperable malignant tumour.

The nursing care of these patients will be primarily aimed at relieving the symptoms along with great emphasis on meeting the emotional needs of both the patient and his family.

GASTRIC CARCINOMA

Carcinoma of the stomach is quite common throughout the world, whereas primary carcinoma of the duodenum is rare. Gastric carcinoma is more common in males, affecting chiefly the 55–70 year age group.

Aetiology and pathophysiology

Some of the predisposing causes of gastric cancer that have been suggested by researchers include:

- Diets high in carbohydrate, but low in fat and fresh fruit and vegetables; food preservatives have also been implicated as possible carcinogens
- Genetic factors: gastric carcinoma has an increased incidence in the close relatives of these patients; a majority of patients with gastric cancer have blood group A
- Chronic atrophic gastritis
- Long-standing pernicious anaemia
- Chronic gastric ulceration, polyps or surgery
- Heavy cigarette smoking.

Cancer of the stomach is an adenocarcinoma and may be polypoid, ulcerating or diffuse infiltrating (linitis plastica). Gastric carcinoma occurs mainly along the lesser curvature with a preponderance in the pyloric region and gastro-oesophageal junction. Metastasis is by direct extension to nearby structures, especially to the liver. There is also spread by lymphatic channels to regional nodes; one characteristic site is in the supraclavicular fossa (Verchow's node). Dissemination by the blood stream can involve the lungs, brain, bone, and even the skin.

Clinical manifestations

Patients will usually present to their physician with a history of persistent nonspecific symptoms of long standing. These may include:

- Vague gastric symptoms similar to those of peptic ulcer
- Anorexia, which is consistent with but nonspecific to gastric carcinoma
- Symptoms caused by secondary deposits in other sites, for example, hepatomegaly, ascites
- Late local symptoms, such as vomiting, causing weight loss and general malaise
- Epigastric pain which may be present but which is usually not a prominent feature.

Investigative procedures

Barium meal X-rays will reveal the majority of lesions, showing the ulcerative types as filling defects, the polypoid types extending into the stomach cavity, and the infiltrating lesions as displaying decreased motility of the affected areas of the gastric wall.

Gastroscopy will reveal the majority of tumours in the pyloric antrum and body of the stomach, but those in the cardia are extremely difficult to see. Biopsy taken at the time of gastroscopy usually confirms the diagnosis; but on occasions, where there is accompanying extensive inflammation, it can be difficult to differentiate between carcinoma and peptic ulcer.

Exfoliative cytology and gastric function tests are sometimes performed, but are of limited value and have in the main been superseded by gastroscopy and biopsy.

Medical and surgical management

There is as yet no effective medical therapy for gastric cancer. Radiotherapy is occasionally used in palliative care. Surgery, following early diagnosis, gives only about a 40% 5-year survival rate. When metastasis has occurred, surgery is not indicated unless for the purpose of overcoming obstruction or haemorrhage.

The most common surgical procedures used are partial gastrectomy (Billroth II, see page 501) and total gastrectomy. In total gastrectomy (Fig 52.3) the oesophagus can be anastomosed:

1. Directly to the duodenum (Fig. 52.3B)
2. To the side of a loop of jejunum (Fig. 52.3C)
3. To the side of a loop of jejunum with a further side-to-side anastomosis of the afferent and efferent limbs of the jejunal loop. This latter procedure provides a greater capacity for food intake (Fig. 52.3D).

Other variations of total gastrectomy such as the Roux-en-Y anastomosis are falling from favour because of their high rate of complications.

When total gastrectomy is performed for carcinoma, the omentum, spleen, and regional lymph nodes may also need to be removed. Also, in order to anastomose the oesophagus to the jejunum, the surgeon will have to enter the thoracic cavity. It is usual, therefore, for these patients to have underwater seal chest drainage as well as 1 or 2 abdominal drains.

Complications following total gastric resection

Total gastrectomy is a radical procedure usually reserved for those patients in whom there is some hope of cure. A major organ has been removed and potential complications include:

Pulmonary complications due to pleural involvement during surgery. It is essential that the nurse ensures that the patient deep breathes, coughs, and has hourly positional changes. Ideally a physiotherapist should be in attendance for at least the first 72 hours postoperatively. Management of the underwater-seal drainage is another responsibility of the nurse (see page 343).

Dumping syndrome due to the absence of the stomach, and (more importantly) the lack of pyloric sphincter control of flow of ingested nutrients into the gut (see page 502).

Malnutrition due to poor digestion and hence poor absorption of nutrients. This results in weight loss and general debilitation.

Absence of intrinsic factor and gastric secretions, resulting in pernicious and iron deficiency anaemias if vitamin B_{12}, iron compounds, and folic acid are not replaced for the rest of the patient's life.

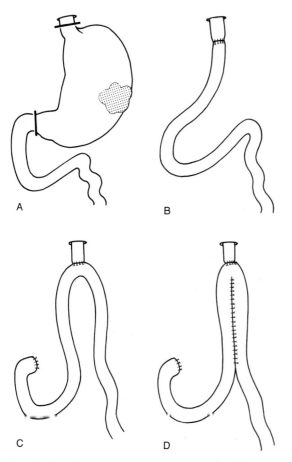

Fig. 52.3 Total gastrectomy. **A** – Resection. **B–D**. Methods of anastomosis of oesophageal stump.

UPPER GASTROINTESTINAL TRACT SURGERY

Surgery for upper gastrointestinal tract disorders is considered in the following situations:

1. To control haemorrhage when conservative methods fail. If haemorrhage is acute and life threatening, surgery is performed as an emergency and the bleeding site is oversewn, cauterized, or excised. With chronic persistent bleeding, surgery will be elective and may involve partial gastrectomy, vagotomy with pyloroplasty, or gastroenterostomy

2. To repair a perforation. This is always performed as a surgical emergency, because of the life threatening danger of peritonitis

3. To relieve pyloric stenosis due to fibrosis from recurring ulceration around the pyloric region
4. To relieve intractable pain
5. If malignancy is suspected
6. To cure or remove an ulcer when conservative methods fail to keep the patient in a reasonable state of good health.

It is not enough to simply excise peptic ulcers, because there is a high tendency for them to recur; therefore, the aim of surgical intervention is the same as for medical management, that is, to alter the local environment in order to reduce the amount of acid produced by the stomach. Surgically this can be achieved by interrupting the vagus nerve (vagotomy), and/or resecting the gastrin and acid producing area of the stomach (antrectomy or partial gastrectomy). Because no one operation can give total success, a variety of procedures have been devised.

Vagotomy with pyloroplasty or gastroenterostomy

Vagotomy eliminates or reduces the neural stimulus to gastric secretion of acid, and reduces gastric tone and motility. With reduced tone and motility there may be undesirable delayed emptying of the stomach, therefore a drainage operation such as pyloroplasty (Fig. 52.4) or gastroenterostomy (Fig. 52.5) is usually performed at the same time.

Vagotomies may be trunkal, selective, or highly selective (Fig. 52.6). The highly selective vagotomy is the most sophisticated and recent procedure, but requires the skill of a specialist surgeon. It involves dividing only those fibres which supply the gastric body and fundus, and does not usually require an associated drainage procedure.

Partial gastrectomy

Billroth I. This procedure entails removing one to two-thirds of the distal stomach and anastomosing the proximal end of the duodenum to the stomach remnant. This operation is often reserved for gastric ulcers. Not only is the ulcer removed but also the gastrin secreting antrum,

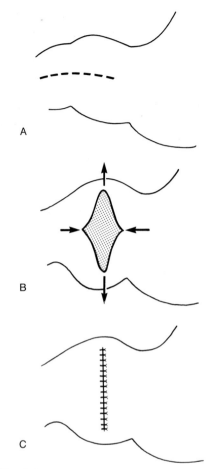

Fig. 52.4 Pyloroplasty. Longitudinal incision in the pylorus (**A**) is stretched (**B**) and sutured (**C**).

along with some of the acid and pepsin secreting cell mass.

Billroth II, also called Polya (see Fig. 52.7). The difference between this operation, performed for duodenal ulcers, and Billroth I is in the manner in which continuity of the alimentary tract is achieved. The proximal stump of the duodenum is oversewn and a loop of jejunum is incised and anastomosed to the stomach remnant. Usually the actual ulcer is not removed; the duodenum must be preserved to allow entry of the pancreatic and bile ducts. Note: There is an afferent and efferent loop of bowel adjoining the stomach remnant

Total gastrectomy

See page 498.

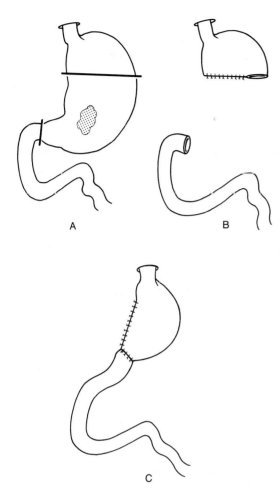

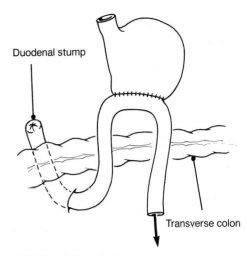

Fig. 52.7 Billroth II method of partial gastrectomy.

Fig. 52.5 Billroth I gastrectomy.

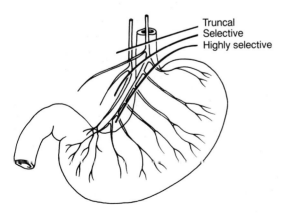

Fig. 52.6 Sites of vagotomies.

Other procedures

Some surgeons modify the above basic procedures. For example, vagotomy may be done without a drainage procedure, or a vagotomy with antrectomy may be the operation of choice. Very rarely, if ever, is a total gastrectomy performed for peptic ulceration.

Complications of gastric surgery

Immediate complications

All surgery carries with it the possibility of resultant complications such as shock, haemorrhage, and respiratory difficulties; in addition to these potentially life-threatening problems, intraabdominal procedures bring the threat of adynamic (paralytic) ileus. (This condition and its nursing management are described on page 532). Other complications include:

• Excessive aspirate via the nasogastric tube. This is thought to be due to irritation of the mucosa during surgery, and if its significance is not recognized, severe electrolyte imbalance will ensue.
• Bile aspirated. This could mean that either the nasogastric tube has slipped into the duodenum or that there is reflux of bile into the stomach.
• Leakage from anastomosis or rupture of the duodenal stump. These can give rise to peritonitis,

pelvic or diaphragmatic abscess, or fistula formation.

• Pancreatitis. This may be caused by handling of the pancreas during surgery, or by temporary obstruction of the duct due to oedema and inflammation of the sphincter of Oddi.

Intermediate complications

• Afferent loop syndrome (following Billroth II procedure or gastroenterostomy procedures). This occurs when there is an obstruction to the flow of bile and pancreatic secretions proximal to the gastroenterostomy anastomosis. The cause is usually local oedema at the anastomosed site, or kinking of the loop. The symptoms of pain, shock, and vomiting of bile usually appear in the first postoperative week, particularly when the patient commences oral diet. The condition usually resolves as oedema subsides, but if it does not further surgery may be necessary to overcome the obstruction.

• Efferent loop (postprandial dumping) syndrome. This is the result of the rapid passage or 'dumping' of food from the stomach into the jejunum. Dumping occurs when there is no pyloric sphincter control of the rate of emptying of the stomach, for example, following gastroenterostomy and more rarely following gastroduodenoscopy. This condition often becomes evident when the patient returns to solid food, that is, 5–7 days postoperatively. If the reintroduction of the amount of food has been well controlled whilst the patient is in hospital, dumping may not be a problem until he returns home and forgets to follow the instructions regarding his diet for at least 3 months following discharge. These are:

1. Take small bulk meals
2. Eat frequent meals (2–3 hourly)
3. Observe a high protein, low carbohydrate diet
4. Take fluid between, not with, meals
5. Lie flat for 30 minutes after main meal.

Dumping syndrome causes sudden abdominal discomfort, and palpitations, nausea, sweating, giddiness and fainting. Steatorrhea and diarrhoea may also occur. These manifestations are more common following high carbohydrate meals or the taking of fluids with meals. They are thought to be due to a sudden shift of extracellular fluid into the jejunum to aid digestion, and to the sudden demand for insulin. Signs due to the sudden fluid shift occur 15–30 minutes after meals, and those due to insulin reaction typically occur 2–3 hours after meals.

Occasionally the patient may require a sedative or an anticholinergic drug to delay stomach emptying. If he is nauseated, metoclopramide must not be prescribed as it hastens emptying of the stomach.

Late complications

Complications which may occur 3–12 months following surgery are:

• Anaemia. As hydrochloric acid is essential for the absorption of iron, patients who have undergone gastric surgery may develop iron deficiency. Removal of the part of the stomach which secretes the intrinsic factor will result in pernicious anaemia due to vitamin B_{12} deficiency. Pernicious anaemia may also be due to chronic gastritis which is sometimes a sequela of gastric surgery.

• Folic acid and calcium deficiency. Because acid is required for the absorption of these elements this can be a rare complication.

• Malabsorption syndrome can occur due to persistent dumping.

• Stomal or anastomotic ulcer. No surgery can guarantee 100% cure from peptic ulceration, and ulcers tend to recur at sites of anastomosis causing the original symptoms and the same risk of complications, for example, haemorrhage, perforation.

Nursing management of patients undergoing gastroduodenal surgery

All gastroduodenal surgery is a traumatic experience for the patient. He will have been experiencing some degree of discomfort and dysfunction for quite a period of time, and the prospect of surgery and its sequelae will only add to his anxiety. The principles of nursing care are to:

• Manage pain
• Ensure adequate nutrition
• Promote healing

- Prevent infection
- Prevent postoperative complications.

The nurse, therefore, must prepare to meet the needs of a person:

– Who will usually have an extensive abdominal wound and associated drainage tubes, both of which may result in extreme discomfort and/or pain, and considerable threat to body image
– Whose normal means of nutrition is by-passed and whose parenteral nutrition must be managed carefully. The nurse may also need to prepare the patient for long-term changes in food habits and elimination patterns
– Whose surgery may carry with it the potential for gastric secretions to interrupt the normal healing of mucosa.
– Whose intestine has been exposed and handled, and hence will not function normally for a period of time.
– Who will, therefore, usually return to the ward with a nasogastric tube in situ. This nasogastric tube will have the twofold purpose of removing gastric secretions from the wound site, and relieving potential intestinal obstruction until the bowel resumes normal function
– Who will need close observation of vital signs and of the amount and nature of nasogastric aspirate. The nurse must detect early signs of the potentially life-threatening postoperative complications of haemorrhage and leakage of an anastomosis.

It is important for the nurse to determine how much of the stomach was resected, or its function reduced, in order to appreciate the capability of the altered anatomy. Close cooperation with the surgical and health team is essential for the successful management of these patients.

The general nursing management of the patient who has a nasogastric tube in situ is described in Chapter 49. In gastroduodenal surgery nasogastric intubation is used mainly for aspiration in order to determine any bleeding, stasis of secretions, or regurgitation into the stomach of bile. The

amount of secretions being aspirated should gradually decrease over a 2–4 day postoperative period. A careful record of the amount and type of aspirate must be maintained and evidence of bleeding or increasing amounts of secretion must be reported to the surgeon without delay. However, a decrease in the amount of aspirate (either gradual or sudden) accompanied by abdominal distension and pain must be viewed with suspicion. These symptoms and signs may herald leakage of the anastomosis and should be recorded carefully and reported immediately.

Oral fluids and diet are introduced when aspirations are minimal and when there is evidence of peristalsis. Oral intake can be commenced usually between the second and fourth post-operative day, under the surgeon's orders. In the interim the patient will be nourished intravenously either by a peripheral or central vein.

Accumulation of intestinal gases causing severe 'wind' pain is a common feature following gastric and bowel surgery and should not be discounted by the nurse as it can cause severe distress (see page 462).

SURGERY FOR CONTROL OF MORBID OBESITY

When all else fails in an attempt to assist grossly obese persons to lose weight, surgical intervention may be performed either to reduce the capacity of the stomach or to reduce the absorptive area of the small bowel by carrying out a bypass operation. Neither approach to this problem has proved very successful as there is a significant morbidity and mortality rate. Most patients do lose weight initially but many regain it when the body learns to adapt to its altered anatomy. With the ileal bypass operation some patients develop severe malnutrition due to insufficient absorption of nutrients (see malabsorption syndrome, page 504). Currently, surgery for obesity is not favoured by most surgeons.

53

Disorders of the small and large intestine

Mavis Matthews

The numerous diseases of the small and large intestine can be grouped into 4 main categories:

1. Malabsorption syndrome
2. Inflammatory bowel disease
3. Intestinal obstruction
4. Neoplasm of the intestine.

It is necessary for the nurse to realize that there can be overlap between the groups. For example, inflammatory bowel disease can cause intestinal obstruction, malabsorption syndrome, or be the forerunner to a neoplasm or anorectal lesion. On the other hand, neoplasm can be the cause of inflammation in the intestine, intestinal obstruction, or an anorectal lesion.

Generally, malabsorption syndrome and chronic inflammatory bowel conditions cause debilitating diarrhoea, and are usually treated conservatively. If there is danger of perforation or severe stricture, then surgical intervention is required. Intestinal obstruction almost always requires surgical release of the underlying cause. A neoplasm is resected whenever possible.

MALABSORPTION SYNDROME

Many of the diseases which cause malabsorption have already been discussed. Here, the syndrome together with the more common intestinal disorders that are directly associated with malabsorption are discussed.

Aetiology and classification

The fundamental basis of this syndrome is faulty absorption of one or more essential nutrients. It occurs as a result of a large variety of diseases (Table 53.1). Faulty absorption is commonly due to either faulty digestion, where nutrients are not changed into an absorbable nature, or because nutrients which have been digested are not being transported across the brush border of the villi. The unqualified term 'malabsorption' usually refers to fat malabsorption, because the absorption of fat is often impaired early in many of the diseases listed in Table 53.1.

Table 53.1 Common causes of malabsorption

Faulty digestion
  Defects in the fat-splitting phase of digestion
    Chronic pancreatitis
    Carcinoma of the pancreas
    Fibroplastic disease of the pancreas
    Pancreatic resection
  Defects due to lack of bile salts (fats and/or bile salts remain insoluble and cannot be absorbed)
    Biliary obstruction
    Chronic liver disease
    Abnormal bacterial proliferation in the small bowel
    Extensive disease or resection of the ileum
  Decreased intestinal transit time (insufficient time for complete digestion to occur)
    Chronic inflammatory bowel diseases
    Hyperthyroidism
    Extensive gastric or bowel resection
Faulty absorption
  Reduced absorptive surface
    Atrophy of the villi as in coeliac disease, tropical sprue, Crohn's disease, and Whipple's disease
    Small bowel resection or bypass (NB this may be purposely done to induce malabsorption as one method to treat morbid obesity)
    Gastrocolic or jejunocolic fistula
    Damage of intestinal mucosa by radiation or drugs (e.g. cytotoxic agents)
  Reduced intestinal mucosal enzyme activity
    Lactose intolerance due to lack of enzyme lactase in epithelial cells

Coeliac disease (gluten-induced enteropathy; nontropical sprue)

Coeliac disease is a metabolic defect due to abnormal sensitivity to gluten protein (gliadin) which is found in wheat, rye, oats, and barley. Contact with gluten results in jejunal mucosal inflammation and severe villous atrophy, giving the mucosa a flattened appearance.

The disease can occur at any age, even as young as 3 months when the baby is first introduced to any of the above cereals. The reason that some adults develop a sensitivity to gluten is unknown. The outcome of villous atrophy is general malabsorption, but particularly of fat and fat soluble vitamins. The condition is reversible when gluten is excluded from the diet; however, this is not easy when one considers all the food products that contain the offending cereal. In addition to breads and cakes, less obvious gluten-containing foods include sausage, pasta, synthetic cream, battered or crumbed foods, flavoured potato crisps, some milk flavouring, most tinned foods, and barley water. Life-long adherence to a gluten-free diet is absolutely necessary.

Tropical sprue

This cause of malabsorption is similar to that of coeliac disease. Jejunal biopsy shows a similar villous atrophy pattern, but the condition does not respond to a gluten-free diet. The cause is unknown. It is especially prevalent in tropical or subtropical regions and although there is no specific cure, patients do improve with Vitamin B_{12}, folic acid, and broad spectrum antibiotic therapy. This suggests an infective origin, although no specific bacterium or virus has been demonstrated. Tropical sprue is seen in Australia, either in those Australians who have visited tropical countries, or in immigrants from tropical countries.

Whipple's disease

This is a rare but important cause of malabsorption. The disease can affect most parts of the body, therefore the patient has signs and symptoms other than those associated with malabsorption. These include arthralgia, lymphadenopathy, skin pigmentation, pleural effusion, and fever. The small bowel mucosa, lymph glands, and other tissues are infiltrated with large numbers of macrophages which stain with periodic acid Schiff (PAS). Diagnosis is determined by small bowel biopsy which reveals the characteristic PAS staining of macrophages, and abnormally shaped villi. Aetiology is unknown, but it is thought to be related to bacterial infection even though no organisms have been identified. The disease responds to prolonged (1–2 years) antibiotic therapy. Penicillin and streptomycin are usually the drugs of choice. Relapses occur if only a short course of therapy is given.

Lactase deficiency

Malabsorption of lactose due to lactase deficiency is fairly common, especially among Asian immigrants who begin consuming milk and milk products in Australia when previously this was not part of their diet. The bowel symptoms which follow milk ingestion are the result of fermentation of the non-absorbed lactose and production of excessive gas and irritating metabolic products. The patient will complain of distension, borborygmi, and diarrhoea. The treatment is to avoid milk and milk products.

Clinical manifestations

The patient who is admitted to hospital with malabsorption may be in a state of starvation and therefore acutely ill. He will display some or all of the following features.

Steatorrhoea, which is the excretion in faeces of more than 7 g of fat daily and accepted as evidence of malabsorption. The stools are characteristically pale, bulky, offensive, and difficult to flush down the toilet. In less severe cases the stools may appear normal and are greasy only after a fatty meal.

Wasting, due to failure of absorption of essential body building nutrients. Weight loss may not be evidenced by weighing because the patient may have ascites and/or oedema.

Abdominal distension, borborygmi, flatulence, and abdominal discomfort, due to increased bulk of intestinal contents and gas production.

Symptoms and signs of specific deficiencies are commonly seen:

- Fatigue due to anaemia and/or hypokalaemia
- Oedema due to hypoproteinaemia and/or anaemia
- Tetany due to hypocalcaemia
- Haemorrhage (in the form of ecchymosis) due to failure of absorption of vitamin K
- Koilonychia due to iron deficiency
- Glossitis and stomatitis due to folic acid and vitamin B deficiencies
- Osteoporosis, osteomalacia, and bone pain due to hypocalcaemia and vitamin D deficiency
- Infections due to globulin deficiency
- Pigmentation of skin and mucous membranes due to hypoadrenalism
- Hypotension, hypothermia, and inhibition of growth due to depression of endocrine activity
- Mental changes occur, particularly in gluten enteropathy. Patient irritability and the difficulty in management of these patients are both often strikingly improved after treatment.

Investigative procedures

The term malabsorption syndrome is not a diagnosis and should be replaced by the name of the specific disease, or the name of the substance(s) not being absorbed, for example, coeliac disease, Whipple's disease, or lactase deficiency. To reach this diagnosis the patient may have to undergo numerous tests which are designed to confirm that malabsorption is occurring, assess the extent of any deficiencies, and determine the primary cause of the malabsorption.

These aims are not entirely dissociated from each other; for example, low serum levels of iron may indicate deficiency but may also, in the absence of obvious blood loss, suggest malabsorption. In the same way, a follow-through X-ray may show a malabsorption pattern and may also demonstrate the primary cause, for example, jejunal diverticulosis.

Faecal fat estimation. The measurement of faecal fat is the most reliable single test for establishing malabsorption. The normal average daily fat excretion on a diet containing at least 75 g of fat is less than 5 g measured over a 3 or 5 day period.

Figures above this level indicate that further investigations are necessary. It is absolutely essential that all faeces are saved during the prescribed collection period. If a specimen is lost the collection period must be recommenced.

D-Xylose absorption test. Less than 20% urinary excretion of a 25 g oral dose of d-xylose within 5 hours suggests a mucosal defect. This is because this substance does not require any digestion prior to being absorbed.

Glucose and lactose tolerance tests. These may also be used to determine carbohydrate absorption.

Haematological studies. If serum albumin levels are low in the absence of hepatic or renal disorders, they may indicate protein malabsorption. Specific absorption tests for other elements are often done, for example, Schilling test to determine whether vitamin B_{12} is being absorbed, and/or serum levels of folate, iron and calcium. Full blood examination is performed to determine the type and degree of anaemia.

Radiography. A barium meal and follow-through is usually performed, as it may demonstrate the primary cause as well as showing a 'malabsorption pattern'. A plain X-ray of the skeleton may show bony changes due to deficiency of protein, calcium, and vitamin D.

Small intestine biopsies are taken via a per-oral endoscope. The biopsy material and aspirate is examined histologically and chemically for evidence of structural and enzymatic disorders. These techniques are of particular value in mucosal disorders such as gluten enteropathy. A normal biopsy will mean that further tests, such as liver and pancreatic function tests or the culture of intestinal aspirates for bacteria, should be performed.

Breath tests. Bacterial overgrowth may also be determined by measuring exhaled $^{14}CO_2$ after the ingestion of a meal containing ^{14}C glycocholic acid. ^{14}C-triglycerides are sometimes used as a breath test for fat absorption.

Medical and nursing management

The principles of treatment are:

- To treat or remove the primary cause, for example a gluten-free diet in coeliac disease, pancreatic extract by mouth in chronic pancreatic disease or antibiotic therapy in diverticulosis.

- Where specific treatment is not possible, such as following extensive resections of stomach or intestine, to try to overcome the malabsorption by increasing the intake of essential nutrients and kilojoules
- To replace the specific deficiencies detected. Intravenous therapy is often necessary to achieve this
- To reduce the symptoms associated with steatorrhoea

Drugs prescribed for the patient with malabsorption will be dictated by the underlying cause and any known deficiencies, for example:

- Antibiotics for diverticulitis, or Whipple's disease
- Corticosteroids for chronic inflammatory conditions
- Intravenous electrolytes for dehydration and electrolyte imbalance
- Vitamins, minerals, and iron as necessary
- Pancreatic supplements for pancreatic insufficiency.

Diet

If admitted to hospital in an acutely ill state with obvious wastage, dehydration, and diarrhoea, the patient will require total parenteral nutrition, via a central venous line (see page 470).

If or when an oral diet is tolerated the patient is usually prescribed a high protein, low fat, high kilojoule diet with added nutritional supplements. The physician must also be mindful of the underlying cause of the malabsorption and should prescribe a specific diet where applicable, for example, a gluten-free diet for the patient with coeliac disease.

The nurse who is caring for the patient where the underlying cause is unknown or is not treatable, will have his/her resourcefulness taxed to the limit in his/her efforts to ensure adequate nutrition. The patient usually has no appetite and it is difficult to persuade him to eat. The nurse will be helped in this task if he/she has a thorough understanding of the rationale behind each prescribed dietary regime. It may be necessary for a fluid balance chart and a food intake chart to be maintained.

Total parenteral nutrition may need to be continued for prolonged lengths of time. When this occurs the patient may, in suitable situations, be discharged with a Hickman indwelling catheter in place to allow him the opportunity of being at home. The patient and/or a significant other is taught to administer the parenteral fluids (see page 401).

Specific nursing management

The nurse needs to use a problem-solving approach when caring for these patients because of the multiplicity of causes and the varying degrees of severity of the syndrome. The 3 main areas to be assessed are:

1. Problems associated with diarrhoea and steatorrhoea (incontinence, embarrassment, excoriation of the perianal area and fatigue)
2. Problems associated with ensuring that the patient receives adequate nourishment
3. Psychological status. Depression, grief and anger may be a response to the loss of normal good health.

The nurse may also be required to provide full general nursing to the very ill person who is at complete rest in bed. Of particular importance is diligent mouth and pressure area care, as well as deep breathing exercises.

Allied paramedical care and habilitation

The patient's specific needs will be assessed and referrals written if required. Almost always the dietitian is involved and, because of the chronicity of the problem, the social worker is also of great assistance in dealing with any work or social problems.

Where the underlying cause of malabsorption is not known or not treatable, the patient's general condition usually deteriorates over a long period of time. The nurse may be caring for a dying person.

The patient's family and/or significant others will be caring for the patient between the numerous hospital admissions. The nurse should remember to inquire after their welfare whenever he/she is speaking with them, and be prepared to give appropriate advice and support when necessary.

INFLAMMATORY BOWEL DISEASE

The common inflammatory bowel diseases are:

- Peritonitis
- Diverticulitis
- Regional ileitis
- Ulcerative colitis
- Appendicitis
- Intestinal infections and infestation.

Peritonitis

Peritonitis is inflammatory involvement of the peritoneum due to either bacterial or nonbacterial irritation.

Aetiology and pathophysiology

Peritonitis may be caused by:

- Perforation of the hollow abdominal organs (the stomach, duodenum, appendix, intestines, gall bladder, or urinary bladder) due to injury or disease
- Extension of inflammation from the abdominal organs including the viscera in females, and transmigration of bacteria through the intestinal wall in these conditions and in intestinal obstruction
- Infection via the blood stream, for example, septicaemia
- Excessive handling of the bowel during surgery
- Exposure of abdominal contents to the environment during surgery
- Penetrating wounds of the abdominal wall, for example gunshot, stab, and surgical wounds.

Classically, the inflammatory process takes the following course:

1. The inflamed area becomes reddened and oedematous
2. There is exudation of serous, seropurulent, or purulent fluid into the peritoneal cavity
3. Lymphatic exudate adheres to coils of intestine, viscera and/or omentum

4. Hypovolaemia, electrolyte imbalance, dehydration, and shock develop due to loss of fluid, electrolytes, and proteins into the peritoneal cavity
5. Intestinal peristalsis is depressed due to the inhibiting effect of the toxic peritoneal exudate; peritonitis can cause adynamic (paralytic) ileus.

Clinically this inflammatory process presents as:

- General, acute diffuse peritonitis
- Localized acute peritonitis, such as local or intraperitoneal abscess
- Chronic peritonitis.

Clinical manifestations

Symptoms depend on the location and the extent of the inflammation, which is determined by the underlying cause of the peritonitis.

The patient usually presents with:

- Acute abdominal pain and tenderness due to the inflammatory process
- Abdominal rigidity due to muscle contraction which attempts to guard the underlying affected area.
- Vomiting due to irritation of vomiting receptors in the abdominal viscera.
- Fever due to inflammatory process
- Inability to lie flat or stand erect due to abdominal pain. Extended legs causes relayed pull on abdominal muscles
- Dehydration due to vomiting and fever
- Dry mouth, cracked lips, furred tongue, and halitosis due to dehydration
- Hypovolaemic shock due to infection and electrolyte imbalance
- Lethargy and anxiousness due to pain and shock
- Adynamic ileus due to inflamed peritoneum irritating the bowel.

Investigative procedures

A full physical examination and abdominal palpation, is performed, together with a rectal and vaginal examination to palpate pelvic organs for tender spots, for example, appendix, fallopian tubes, ovaries.

Supine and erect abdominal X-rays are taken.

Blood examination will reveal that the white cell count and erythrocyte sedimentation rate are increased.

Midstream urine analysis and basic urinalysis are performed to rule out renal causes of fever and pain.

Medical, surgical, and nursing management

The principles of treatment are:

- To combat infection
- To restore intestinal motility
- To supply lost fluids and electrolytes
- To prepare the patient for emergency surgery.

Nursing management on admission to hospital. Acute peritonitis is a life-threatening emergency which requires prompt surgical attention. The nurse must therefore prepare the patient for surgery whilst concurrently instituting appropriate resuscitative measures.

If the patient is in a collapsed state, oxygen will be required via a mask or intranasal catheter to promote ventilatory function. Artificial ventilation may even be necessary.

The patient is allowed nil orally. An accurate record of intake and output including parenteral fluids, vomitus, and any flatus or faeces must be made. The passage of flatus or faeces should be reported to the physician immediately.

A nasogastric tube is inserted and connected to either free drainage or low pressure suction to decompress the stomach. This is manually aspirated at frequent intervals and the amount, colour, and presence or absence of blood is recorded.

A central venous catheter may be inserted and central venous pressure (CVP) monitoring may be used to check for circulatory overload or severe shock.

An IV infusion to replace fluids and electrolytes will be commenced and maintained. Potassium is added to the infusion, as a deficit may cause a paralytic ileus long after the peritonitis has resolved.

The central venous line is also necessary for the administration of massive doses of broad spectrum antibiotics. Combined therapy is used in adequate doses, based on bacterial sensitivity tests if possible.

If anaemia is severe, the nurse will be responsible for managing a blood transfusion through a side arm of the central venous line.

The patient's conscious state (which can deteriorate rapidly), temperature, pulse, ventilation, and blood pressure are recorded at least half-hourly. There must be constant appraisal of the patient's general condition.

Once the diagnosis is confirmed and there is no risk of masking symptoms a narcotic, for example morphine, will be prescribed for pain relief. This narcotic may also serve as the patient's premedication.

The patient is nursed in a position of comfort and least restriction. Obviously, ambulation is not advisable.

Aims of surgery. These are to remove the cause (for example, an inflamed appendix is removed, or a perforated ulcer is repaired); and to evacuate the peritoneal cavity of fluid, blood, pus, and any detritus; to administer a peritoneal lavage; and to apply topical antibiotics. Any diseased bowel is resected and the healthy ends are anastomosed. Any adhesions are freed.

Postoperative nursing management. Ironically, surgery presents a further assault to an already at-risk patient. The nurse must therefore anticipate the needs of a severely ill person which will include:

- Position. The patient lies flat for 2–3 hours, and is then nursed in a position of comfort. He may prefer to be nursed sitting up, as it makes breathing and coughing easier and reduces the risk of postoperative atelectasis and infection. Leg exercises will be necessary to prevent deep vein thrombosis and subsequent pulmonary emboli.
- Hydration and nutrition. Gastric aspiration and drainage, and parenteral nutrition are continued until peristalsis commences. The patient is returned gradually to oral food and fluids until he is able to tolerate a diet or a modified diet as ordered by the physician. An accurate record of intake and output must be maintained.
- Personal hygiene. The patient should be sponged in bed for the first 2–3 days as he is usually exhausted. Stringent care to all pressure

areas is essential. Mouth and lip care to prevent drying and cracking of the lips may be necessary, particularly if dehydration was marked. Meticulous nasal care is necessary whilst the nasogastric tube is in situ. If a urinary catheter has been inserted, perineal or penile toilets will add greatly to the patient's comfort.

• Elimination. An accurate record of output must be maintained. Bowel stimulants are withheld until there is evidence of return of peristalsis. Once bowel sounds return a bowel action may occur naturally or after a rectal suppository.

• Medication. Pain relief will be provided by analgesics, which should be administered frequently enough to ensure patient comfort. Control of the underlying infection will continue with the administration of antibiotics (intravenously or orally) as ordered.

• Wound care. Care is as for the patient undergoing general abdominal surgery. Drain tubes are either shortened or removed after 48 hours. An accurate record is made of the type of drainage. Sutures are removed 7–10 days postoperatively. Care of the patient's central venous line dressing will be undertaken by the nurse or physician in accordance with the hospital's infection control policy. Such policies should also dictate the frequency with which the line is changed.

• Psychological care. The patient has been through an horrendous experience and will be extremely apprehensive. He will need constant care, reassurance, and explanations. His significant others may also be in need of similar support.

When the nurse observes a decrease in temperature and pulse rate, decreasing distension and rigidity of the abdomen, the return of peristaltic sounds, and flatus or bowel actions, he/she may be encouraged that the acute episode of peritonitis is subsiding.

Complications

The patient with peritonitis may develop any of the following complications. A problem-solving approach to nursing care involves the anticipation of these potential complications and is hence directed towards minimizing their development and observing for early signs of their appearance.

• Hypoventilation, atelectasis, pneumonia
• Adynamic ileus
• Septic shock
• Mechanical intestinal obstruction
• Wound healing complications: infection, disruption, evisceration, and hernia formation
• Intraperitoneal or wound abscesses, for example, subphrenic, subhepatic, pelvic, or the abdominal wound itself
• Thrombosis
• Adhesions.

Diverticulitis

A diverticulum is a blind pouch or saccular dilatation protruding from a tube or main cavity. It may be congenital or acquired. Alimentary tract diverticula are herniations of mucosa through the muscular wall of the tract. Diverticulosis is the condition of having multiple diverticula, and diverticulitis is an inflammation of diverticula.

Congenital intestinal diverticula occur in the duodenum and in the ileum (Meckel's diverticulum) while acquired intestinal diverticula appear throughout the small and large intestines.

Duodenal diverticulum

This is usually a single congenital deformity and is symptomless, although it lies in the head of the pancreas, it may cause inflammation of that organ (pancreatitis). Very rarely it needs to be removed surgically.

Meckel's diverticulum

This diverticulum is a common congenital abnormality occurring in about 2–3% of the population. It is usually 5–8 cm in length and is situated 1 metre above the ileocaecal valve in the ileum. The vitella–intestinal duct of fetal development persists, resulting in a blind-ended pouch leading from the ileum which may remain connected to the umbilicus by means of a fibrous cord. It is usually symptomless, however occasionally Meckel's diverticulum is lined with gastric-type mucosa, so peptic ulceration may develop. Possible but rare problems include ulceration leading to perforation and peritonitis and obstruction due to a loop of bowel becoming caught up in the fibrous band.

Treatment is necessary only if the above occur, and consists of surgical removal.

Small intestine diverticula

These are rare, but multiple in number when they do occur. They are usually symptomless but are potentially liable to become chronically infected, causing stricture and obstruction or malabsorption. Diagnosis is made on barium meal with follow through. The patient who presents with symptoms of malabsorption is treated with long-term antibiotics. If intestinal obstruction or perforation of a diverticulum occurs, the patient will require bowel resection of the affected part followed by end-to-end anastomosis.

If a large section of small intestine needs to be resected this, in itself, could cause malabsorption.

Colonic diverticula

This extremely common condition occurs more frequently in women, and in 30–40% of people over 50 years of age in Westernized countries. (It is believed to be directly related to long-term dietary habits.) However Shearman and Finlayson (1982) suggest that in Australia as many as 25% of males and 40% of females over the age of 20 years may have colonic diverticular disease.

Aetiology and pathology

People in Westernized societies commonly eat highly refined cereal products which do not give enough bulk in the diet, which results in chronic constipation. Chronic constipation is said (although not proven) to be a contributing factor in the development of colonic diverticula, as there is increased intraluminal pressure when there is low bulk content in the bowel. Conversely, it is noted that populations who consistently eat a high bulk diet do not develop colonic diverticula.

Long-term chronic constipation with the prolonged use of cathartics is thought to cause colonic muscle dysfunction and abnormal peristalsis, which causes the increased intraluminal pressure. This in turn forces the mucosa through the weakened section of the bowel wall, for example, penetration of the muscularis by blood

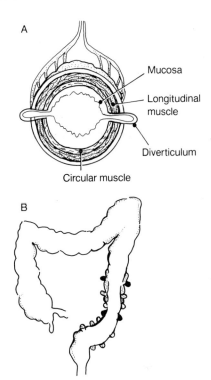

Fig. 53.1 Intestinal diverticula. **A** – Cross section. **B** – Parallel herniations.

vessels (Fig. 53.1A). Hence herniations occur in 2 rows (Fig. 53.1B) and are mainly confined to the descending and pelvic colon.

Clinical manifestations

Most cases of diverticular disease are symptomless and are discovered incidentally; 75% of the cases that do have symptoms complain only of mild, vague abdominal discomfort, and irregular bowel habits with no consistent pattern. At times there may be diarrhoea; at other times the patient may be troubled with constipation. The patient is usually not concerned enough to seek medical attention.

The remaining 25% of patients suffer acute abdominal attacks which may be constant or intermittent, and are usually due to the diverticula becoming blocked with faeces, leading to inflammation and infection. The manifestations may include:

- Anorexia, nausea, and vomiting
- Severe diarrhoea or obstinate constipation

- Severe lower abdominal pain
- A palpable mass in the left iliac fossa
- Malaise with fever
- Bleeding per rectum.

Complications

Diverticulitis is important because the complications of inflammation (Fig. 53.2) readily occur and can become life threatening.

Investigative procedures

Barium enema shows a characteristic picture and is diagnostic. Sigmoidoscopy or colonscopy is often performed, but chiefly to exclude carcinoma of the lower bowel as it is not uncommon for these 2 conditions to coexist.

Full blood examination and ESR are usually performed and will reveal an increase in the leucocyte count and the ESR.

Medical management

Chronic, mild diverticular disease. The underlying principle of treatment is to alter the motility pattern of the colon, which is achieved by educating the patient to eat high fibre foods and to drink at least 3 l of fluid per day. The physician may prescribe an anticholinergic drug for its antispasmodic action, and a bulk forming laxative.

Acute diverticulitis. The objectives of treatment are to:

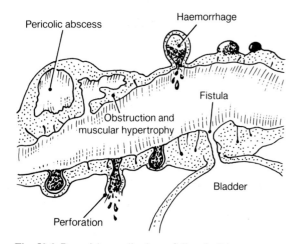

Fig. 53.2 Potential complications of diverticulitis.

- Control infection
- Control pain if the pain is severe
- Rest the bowel
- Maintain fluid, electrolyte, and nutritional requirements.

The medical management of diverticulitis is thus largely symptomatic. However, treatment options become more challenging and complex because of the wide variety of complications that may arise from this disease.

Broad spectrum antibiotics such as tetracycline, amoxycillin, and metronidazole are usually given orally or intravenously to control the infection.

Analgesics and antispasmodics are ordered to control painful spasms. It is sometimes even necessary to give the patient pethidine. Morphine is not used as this has been shown to induce the hypersegmentation and increased colonic pressure that is a feature of diverticulosis.

Bulk laxatives, for example, psyllium (Metamucil) and bran, may be ordered to prevent or treat constipation.

Dietary modification is regarded as the first line of treatment in diverticular disease. However, during an acute exacerbation the patient is usually ordered nil by mouth, and must therefore receive adequate nourishment via the intravenous route.

When oral diet is resumed, most authorities recommend that the patient be introduced to a high-fibre, non-irritating diet, which he must adhere to for the rest of the his life.

Very occasionally a low residue diet may be ordered if there is evidence of marked inflammation and stenosis.

Surgical management

Surgery is contemplated only when diverticulitis becomes complicated. Surgery may involve:

- A temporary transverse colostomy either to relieve obstruction or to rest a persistent acutely inflamed area
- Resection of the affected area, with end to end anastomosis
- Draining of any abscess
- Repair of any fistula
- On very rare occasions the patient may need a left hemicolectomy with or without a permanent

colostomy depending on whether an anastomosis can be achieved.

Nursing management

The aim is that patients with diverticular disease should produce soft formed, bulky stools. This can be achieved with a high fibre diet, the addition of 1 tablespoon of bran 3 times a day, and the drinking of 3 l of fluid a day. It is the nurse's responsibility to ensure that the patient understands the reasons for this dietary regime.

Observation of the patient during an acute episode is important because of the very real danger of complications occurring, sometimes with very little warning. The nurse must observe for signs of fever, haemorrhage per rectum, increased left-sided abdominal pain, signs of shock, and type of bowel action.

Expected outcome and habilitation

Once diverticula form they do not resolve, therefore the patient must learn to live with the condition and alter dietary habits. Most patients do this very successfully. About 15–20% of patients require some type of surgery. The morbidity and mortality tend to increase with age. The overall mortality of patients who have been admitted to hospital for treatment is 3–5%.

Regional enteritis/regional ileitis, and ulcerative colitis

A review of the literature reveals that medical, nursing, and dietary authorities are unable to agree on the definition, incidence, and differential diagnosis of regional enteritis, regional ileitis, and ulcerative colitis.

Generally, regional enteritis is classified as regional ileitis, or Crohn's disease; but, because of the marked similarity of this disease to ulcerative colitis, most authors consider the diseases together.

It should be noted, however, that while Crohn's disease can occur anywhere along the intestinal tract, it appears to manifest most commonly within the ileocaecal region. For ease of student learning, the diseases are considered separately in this text with reference to their similarities where appropriate.

Regional ileitis (Crohn's disease)

Regional ileitis, commonly called Crohn's disease, is a non-specific, granulomatous, usually focal, inflammatory condition of the intestine. It is thought to be due to an abnormal immune response in the gut wall. The disease is most frequently encountered in young adults and it appears to be a race-related disorder (occurring in Caucasians mostly). Males and females are equally affected. The incidence appears to be increasing and it is a relatively common disorder. This is a chronic, remitting disease which undermines health and disrupts the life of its victims.

Aetiology and pathophysiology

The cause of this condition is unknown. Despite the efforts of numerous researchers no specific bacterial agent has been isolated, nor have specific food allergens been demonstrated. Autoimmunity is a possible but unproven factor. Any part of the gut may be involved but the terminal ileum is the most common site. The colon may be involved in continuity with the ileum, and sometimes only the colon is affected (Fig. 53.3). Crohn's disease has often been described as having 4 identifiable morphological characteristics:

1. Granulomas. These are composed of collections of lymphocytes, and epitheloid and giant cells. These granulomas may be found in bowel tissue and nearby lymph nodes
2. Skip lesions. The lesions tend to occur in isolated segments along the length of the intestine.
3. The string sign. Due to stenosis of the affected area, only a thin line of barium is seen on X-ray but there is normal filling of the unaffected intestine.
4. Cobblestone appearance of the mucosa. This is due to deep mucosal ulceration and oedema.

Although it is the mucosa and submucosa that is predominantly affected, there is often also inflammation and hypertrophy of the muscle layers, inflamed serosa, and lymphatic obstruction. The peritoneal reaction often results in

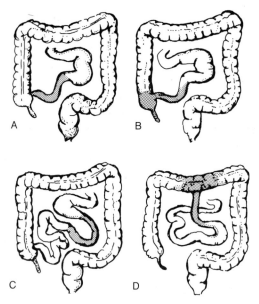

Fig. 53.3 Common sites of regional ileitis. **A** – Terminal ileum. **B** – Terminal ilium and caecum. **C** – Upper ileum. **D** – At ileocolostomy.

adhesions between loops of bowel which may then become obstructed.

Local complications

- Fistula formation, especially in the perianal area and at the site of previous surgery.
- Abscess formation
- Perineal problems – fissure, sinus, and stricture.
- Haemorrhage, perforation, peritonitis.
- Bowel obstruction due to adhesions or stenosis.

Clinical manifestations

Often the young adult is seen with a history of intermittent colic, diarrhoea and weight loss. Sometimes, however, the patient is not seen until the condition is more advanced and he presents with signs of one or more of the above complications.

Pain varies from mild colic to extreme pain with associated vomiting due to obstruction. The site of the pain also varies according to the site of the lesion(s). When the disease is confined to the terminal ileum the clinical presentation is similar to that of acute appendicitis.

Diarrhoea is intermittent initially, but may be severe; a manifestation of steatorrhoea and malabsorption may be due to destruction of the site for bile salt absorption in the ileum. There may be haematochezia (blood with the stool). Weight loss due to malnutrition is a consequence of reduced dietary intake, increased nutritional requirements (of the chronic inflammation process), and malabsorption.

Anaemia may be present and could be due to chronic blood loss, or due to interference with folic acid or vitamin B_{12} absorption.

Fever is often present and of a low grade nature due to the chronic inflammatory process.

Palpable mass may be felt due to adherent loops of bowel which could even be entwined about an abscess.

Extraintestinal manifestations. Shearman & Finlayson (1982) note that 'a wide variety of systemic manifestations have been described in ulcerative colitis, and it is becoming apparent that most also occur in Crohn's disease of the colon. Many, such as those in the eyes, joints and skin, may be due to immune reactions. Occasionally the "complication" or associated disease manifests itself before the bowel disease . . . Thus, inflammatory bowel disease may already exist in an early form in patients who first present with symptoms of the complication.'

These authors cite the following systemic manifestations:

- Skin lesions, especially erythema nodosum, pyoderma gangrenosum
- Joint complications, particularly arthritis and ankylosing spondylitis
- Eye lesions – conjunctivitis, iritis, and episcleritis
- Aphthous oral ulceration
- Finger clubbing
- Thrombosis and embolism
- Hepatobiliary disease.

Investigative procedures

Barium meal with follow through and a barium enema may demonstrate the skip lesions and string sign in the small and/or large intestine.

Sigmoidoscopy and/or colonoscopy are invaluable for direct visualization of the mucosa, and for taking a biopsy. The biopsy can prove diagnostic if granulomas are detected.

Full blood examination will be carried out to establish whether there is any leucocytosis or anaemia.

Serum electrolyte, urea, creatinine and protein measurements are made and the Schilling test is performed to check for vitamin B_{12} absorption.

The patient will have a thorough physical examination, especially checking for known associated extraintestinal features.

Medical, surgical, and nursing management

There is no cure for Crohn's disease, therefore the management for each case will be symptomatic and specific to the individual, and based on careful assessment. Most patients can be managed without being hospitalized (except, perhaps, for investigatory purposes). There will be remissions and relapses probably for the rest of the patient's life.

Management will be aimed at controlling the symptoms and manifestations of the disease; providing surgical relief or correction of any local complication; and offering psychological support to the patient and his significant others.

There is no specific drug therapy for this disorder. Oral steroids, the immunosuppressive agent azathioprine, and sulphasalazine are often tried during an acute attack, but it is disputed whether any of these drugs have any real benefit in the long term

Antibiotic therapy is used if there is evidence of an overgrowth of intestinal bacteria or abscess formation.

Codeine phosphate is often used to treat diarrhoea.

Anticholinergic preparations are sometimes prescribed, but they may predispose to bowel obstruction.

Supplements, for example, iron, folic acid, viatmin B_{12} and potassium, may be required.

The patient's diet should be as nutritious as possible when there is persistent diarrhoea and evidence of malabsorption. Indigestible residue (raw fruit and vegetables, wholegrain cereals, and nuts) may precipitate episodes of intestinal colic and/or obstruction, and should be avoided during and shortly after an episode. Weight loss is reported in 65% of patients, therefore a high kilojoule, high protein, low fat diet is the aim. High kilojoule supplements such as egg flips between meals may be necessary.

During an acute episode which requires hospitalization, the patient may be ordered nil by mouth and may receive total parenteral nutrition until it is assured that there is no bowel obstruction. If the patient is unable to tolerate a normal oral diet, an elemental diet may prove satisfactory in supplying adequate kilojoules and nutrients.

In general the diet will be determined by the individual's problems and deficiencies. A minority of patients demonstrate lactose intolerance and when this occurs milk and milk products are omitted from the diet.

Surgical management. Surgery should be considered only as a last resort as it is known that fistula often develop at the site of surgery; also, surgery will not cure the condition. There are occasions, however, when the surgeon has no alternative but to operate – particularly if there is evidence of bowel obstruction (which does not resolve by conservative methods), perforated bowel, fistula or abscess formation. If extensive resection is necessary there is the added danger that the patient may develop malabsorption.

Specific nursing management. Physical care will be symptomatic. There may be minimal requirements or the patient may be so acutely ill that he will need constant nursing care and observations.

Because there are often associated perianal problems (haemorrhoids, fissure, fistula, extreme excoreation) it is absolutely necessary to ensure that this area is washed and gently pat-dried after every bowel action. A soothing ointment or cream should always be used as a preventative measure. The need for perianal care cannot be stressed too greatly. Perianal problems such as intolerable pruritis and pain, particularly on or following defaecation, are often the patient's main concern. Observations will be similar to those for acute colonic diverticulitis.

Psychological support is one of the patient's greatest needs. These patients will have to live with this debilitating and acutely embarrassing condition for the rest of their lives. Their management provides a challenge for the health team.

There may be:

- Chronic pain and discomfort
- The embarrassment of chronic diarrhoea
- Frequent hospitalization
- Loss of work and income opportunities
- Irritability leading to poor interpersonal relationships
- Self-imposed social isolation and reduced social opportunities.

The nurse who is aware of these possibilities will take the time to allow the patient to talk about such concerns. He should also be encouraged to acknowledge to family and friends that he has Crohn's disease, rather than trying to cope alone, as is often the case. In most instances a social worker will be required to assist the patient's adjustment.

The patient will need advice regarding diet, adequate rest, perianal care, and the need to socialize.

Habilitation and anticipated outcome

This is a disease of remissions and exacerbations over many years and of varying degrees of severity. It is almost impossible to predict the course or outcome of the disease for an individual. Crohn's disease becomes more serious with time but with careful, consistent medical management and family support these patients can live a long, useful life. The overall mortality is quoted at 5–10%.

Ulcerative colitis

As the name implies, this is inflammation of the colon with ulceration. The mucosa and submucosa are affected primarily, but muscle layers of the bowel may be involved when there is secondary bacterial invasion. Ulcerative colitis can occur at any age but onset is usually in the 20–40 year age group and both sexes are equally affected. There appears to be a familial tendency.

Like Crohn's disease it appears to be a racial disorder, occurring most commonly in Caucasians; it is, however, more common than Crohn's disease. There are many similarities between ulcerative colitis and Crohn's disease and sometimes it is difficult to distinguish the two.

Aetiology and pathology

The cause is unknown. Infection, allergy, psychosomosis, and autoimmunity have all been implicated, but none has been proven to be the cause. An immune basis is the most favoured theory because, like in Crohn's disease, there are other systemic disturbances (iritis, arthritis, ankylosing spondylitis, erythema nodosum). The characteristic features are:

- Symptom-free periods between acute episodes
- Diffuse mucosal inflammation which begins in the rectal area and spreads proximally
- Usually only the rectum, sigmoid colon, and descending colon are affected. Occasionally the whole colon is involved. Very occasionally there may be extension of the disease into the terminal ileum
- Histologically there is mucosal destruction, and infiltration of plasma cells, lymphocytes, polymorphs, and eosinophils
- Tiny abscesses form in the epithelial crypts
- Extensive shallow ulcers, which tend to bleed, develop when there is loss of surface epithelium.

The continuous healing process causes thickening and hypertrophy of the underlying muscle, and pseudopolyps form. Eventually the hypertrophy causes the affected colon to become slightly dilated and rigid. On X-ray the rigid colon shows up as the classical 'hosepipe' sign.

When the muscularis is involved muscle tone may be lost and the lifethreatening condition toxic dilatation of the colon (toxic megacolon) may ensue. This development is a surgical emergency as there is a real danger of sudden, massive, perforation.

When the disease is in remission, the mucous membrane continues to be abnormal and easily traumatized.

Clinical manifestations

Ulcerative colitis may present in a mild, moderate, or severe form; therefore, symptoms will vary.

Bowel symptoms. When one considers the state of the mucous membrane, it is easy to realize that the patient will be passing slough, blood, mucus, and debris per rectum. These products of inflammation and ulceration may or may not be mixed with faecal matter. The patient may complain of:

- Diarrhoea or constipation
- Passing blood per rectum
- Frequent passage of small amounts of mucus and blood
- Urgency leading to faecal incontinence
- Perianal excoriation
- Abdominal soreness and colic

Systemic symptoms may include; general debility; weight loss; dehydration and electrolyte deficiencies; fever; shock; and anaemia.

There may be symptoms of the associated conditions, or there may be signs of local complications such as:

- Severe haemorrhage. This is readily recognized as it passes per rectum; emergency surgery may be required to control the bleeding
- Bowel perforation. This is detected by observing for signs of acute peritonitis (see page 508).
- Anal fissures. These cause extreme pain on defaecation and are seen on visual examination.
- Toxic megacolon. This is suspected when there is abdominal distension along with cessation of previously troublesome diarrhoea.

There is a greater risk of malignant change when the whole colon is involved. The percentage incidence approximates the duration of the disease in years; that is, a 20 year case will have a 20% risk of developing cancer. See page 534 for signs of colonic cancer.

Psychological disturbances. Colitic patients are said to be difficult to manage and are often described as fastidious, self-centred, demanding, ungrateful, and having a peculiar resistance to encouragement. There is argument as to whether this personality type has a predisposition to developing ulcerative colitis, or whether this chronic, debilitating, embarrassing disease causes personality changes. It is interesting to note that those patients who have been cured by having a total colectomy no longer display the psychological problems described above.

Investigative procedures

Sigmoidoscopy and/or colonoscopy with biopsy is performed. Barium enema X-ray may show: lack of haustration; lack of mucosal definition; ulcers and pseudopolyps; a dilated colon; the 'hosepipe' sign.

A plain abdominal X-ray may reveal faecal stasis proximal to distal disease, and dilatation of the colon.

Haematological examination may show anaemia, leucocytosis or an elevated ESR.

Serum chemistry may show electrolyte disturbances and evidence of protein loss.

Medical and nursing management

The only cure for this condition is total proctocolectomy. Since it results in a permanent, incontinent ileostomy it is an unacceptable method of treatment to both physician and patient, and will be used only as a last resort.

Conservative management follows much the same rationale as for Crohn's disease, that is, the treatment and nursing care will be symptomatic.

Corticosteriods intravenously, orally, or rectally, are given during exacerbation and withdrawn gradually after the acute episode has subsided.

Sulphasalazine is ordered during exacerbations and a reduced dosage is prescribed indefinitely to maintain remissions for as long as possible.

Broad spectrum antibiotics such as gentamicin or cefoxitin are ordered intravenously only if there is evidence of bacteraemia during an acute severe relapse.

If diarrhoea is troublesome with mild distal disease, antidiarrhoeal drugs such as codeine phosphate or loperamide may be ordered. However, antidiarrhoeal drugs should never be given to patients with total colitis during an acute attack, as they may precipitate toxic megacolon. Sodium cromoglycate (anti-allergy) and azathioprine (immune suppressant) have been used as maintenance therapy, but there appears to be no evidence that either of these drugs are as effective as sulphasalazine.

For those patients where constipation or straining to pass faeces is a problem, bulk forming laxatives such as psyllium should be prescribed.

Diet. These patients were once ordered low residue diets, but this is now not thought to be desirable. During an acute episode the bowel is usually rested, but when food is allowed, the aim is to provide a high kilojoule, high protein intake to compensate for the continual losses from the bowel. As in Crohn's disease, a minority of patients benefit from the introduction of a milk-free diet. It is thought that some patients develop a secondary hypolactasia.

Surgical management. Surgery must be considered:

- Where there are life threatening complications such as toxic megacolon, severe haemorrhage, or perforation
- When acute episodes fail to respond to conservative management
- When there is chronic ill health from colitis and the patient is unable to lead a reasonable life
- In long-term cases of total colitis where malignant changes are suspected.

In the emergency situation a colectomy with ileostomy may be performed. The rectal area is removed when the patient is better able to withstand a longer period of anaesthesia.

Elective surgery, performed during remission, may consist of proctocolectomy with ileostomy, or, if the rectum is not grossly involved, colectomy with ileorectal or ileo–anal anastomosis. When the anorectal area is preserved, the risk of rectal cancer remains but a stoma is avoided and there is reduced incidence of sexual dysfunction.

Nursing care of these patients is as for any general surgery; however, the resultant stoma presents a range of patient problems that require empathic and skilled nursing intervention. Chapter 49 discusses stoma care in detail.

Habilitation and anticipated outcome

Persons with ulcerative colitis should always be managed by a specialist health team that employs a joint medical–surgical approach. The majority of patients are treated on an outpatient basis and usually require hospitalization only during an acute exacerbation of extensive disease. Patients must be instructed that it is imperative that they have regular, frequent follow up, even when they are in long remission. Prognosis is almost impossible to determine, but mortality figures are reduced when the patient and physician work closely together to sustain remissions. Patients whose condition remains localized to the rectal area have a good prognosis; but when the whole colon is affected, mortality may be as high as 40%.

Emotional support for both the patient and his significant others is essential, because these people will have all the emotional and social problems that have been described for the patient with Crohn's disease (see page 513).

Appendicitis

Inflammation of the appendix is a potentially dangerous condition because, if untreated, perforation and life threatening peritonitis is the most likely outcome.

Aetiology and pathology

Appendicitis can occur at any age, but the peak age of onset is 15–20 years, with 12–15% of the population being affected. The direct cause appears to be obstruction of the lumen of the appendix, but the precipitating factors which cause the lumen to become obstructed are not known. It is a disease of modern Western society; therefore, there is speculation that the Western diet of refined foods and insufficient fresh fruit and vegetables is a contributing factor. This diet tends to cause increased transit time of the movement of bowel contents, allowing for faecaliths to obstruct the lumen of the appendix. The lumen may also become obstructed if there is hyperplasia of the mucosa due to infection of possibly viral origin.

When the appendix is blocked it becomes an ideal environment for commensal bacteria to multiply and trigger an inflammatory response. Inflammation may lead to a compromised blood supply, gangrene, and perforation or abscess formation (Fig. 53.4). If a low grade infection is the cause of the inflamed appendix and the lumen is not completely obstructed, the clinical manifestations are not as dramatic as with the obstructed

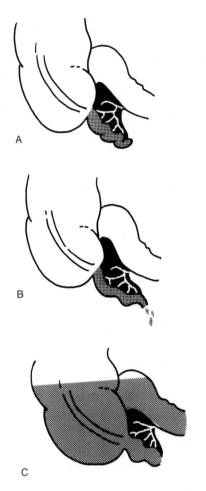

Fig. 53.4 Appendix becomes twisted or obstructed and inflammation results (**A**). If not relieved (usually by appendectomy) either perforation (**B**) or abscess formation (**C**) results.

case. This condition (catarrhal appendicitis) may resolve, may become chronic, or the infection may cause enlargement of the lymphoid follicles of the submucosa leading to acute obstructive appendicitis.

Clinical manifestations

Pain usually begins in the umbilical area but within a few hours moves to the right iliac fossa. Occasionally the appendix is not situated in the normal anatomical position and the diagnosis of appendicitis may be missed because the pain site may be uncharacteristic. If, for example, the appendix is situated in the retrocaecal area, pain will be referred to the umbilicus. The pain is usually of acute onset and is severe, intermittent, and colicky in nature.

Anorexia, nausea and vomiting may be a feature, and the patient may experience fever and general malaise. A moist, furred tongue, halitosis, and a mild tachycardia may be present.

Investigative procedures

Abdominal palpation reveals tenderness with muscle guarding or rigidity in the right iliac fossa. There is usually rebound tenderness. Rectal digital examination reveals tenderness on the right side. Full blood examination may reveal a moderate leucocytosis. These investigations, along with a carefully taken patient history, will lead to a diagnosis which is usually straightforward. However, the physician must be mindful of other conditions with similar features: ovarian cyst; salpingitis; Crohn's disease; infective dysentry; enteritis; biliary, renal or ureteric colic; acute intestinal obstruction; and peritonitis from other than appendix origin.

Medical, surgical, and nursing management

The principles of medical and nursing care are to:

- Remove the site of inflammation
- Relieve pain
- Promote healing
- Prevent complications, including further infection.

Acute appendicitis is almost always treated as a surgical emergency, because of its inherent life threatening dangers. The patient is prepared for the operating room as quickly as possible; usually the nurse has 2–4 hours warning of the surgeon's intent in which to carry out preoperative preparations. Bowel preparation is not performed as it may aggravate the condition. In an acute emergency, premedication may need to be given in the operating room; OR staff must be advised if the premedication is not given in the ward or emergency department.

If the patient has had a meal within 4 hours of expected surgery, or if the patient is vomiting, a nasogastric tube may be passed and aspirations performed prior to surgery. If there appear to be signs of peritonitis (see page 508), or the patient is showing signs of hypovolaemic shock (see Chapter 11), intravenous therapy must be instituted prior to surgery.

The appendix is usually removed via the McBurney's or the right lower paramedian incision.

Postoperatively, routine care for the patient who has had abdominal surgery is carried out. The wound is obvious as a short (10–15 cm) suture line, usually without drainage and covered with a light dressing. Skin sutures, if used, are removed in 6–10 days, often after the patient has been discharged if he makes a good recovery. Alternatively, a continuous subcutaneous skin suture is used, which does not require removal and results in scarless wound closure.

If there is associated peritonitis, the patient's recovery time will be longer and the nurse may be involved with nasogastric tube care, intravenous therapy care, and wound drainage care.

Prior to discharge it is essential to ascertain that there is no wound or pelvic infection, that the patient is eating well, and is having normal bowel actions.

Complications of surgery include the general complications of any surgical procedure – haemorrhage, shock, wound infection, and pneumonia. Additionally, the patient may suffer:

- Difficulty with micturition
- Adynamic ileus
- Secondary pelvic abscess
- Secondary peritonitis
- Faecal fistula.

Intestinal infections and infestation

Intestinal disease due to food poisoning, specific microorganisms, and helminths are categorized in Figure 53.5. This figure is far from complete and some authorities argue the difference between food poisoning, food infection, and intestinal infection; for example, the dysenteries are sometimes included with the food infections. Only those conditions important for the Australian nurse to know are described in the text.

In general, most intestinal infections and infestations are due to poor hygiene, improper food handling, or inadequate food processing and storage. Inadequate fly and vermin control can also be a direct cause of infection via food or the faecal–oral route.

Treatment of affected persons will depend on the seriousness of the attack and is directed towards the symptoms which are invariably nausea, vomiting, abdominal pain and/or colic, and diarrhoea. In some instances there are specific drugs which may be prescribed (Table 53.2).

Apart from cholera and typhoid, which are rare in Australia, most of the conditions described in this section run a mild course and patients do not require hospitalization. However, all of them are potentially serious and some may manifest extra-intestinal symptoms if the offending organism penetrates the intestinal mucosa and escapes into the blood stream.

Food poisoning with microbial toxins

Staphylococcal food poisoning is extremely common. The *Staphylococcus aureus* is harboured in the nose and throat of healthy people, as well as in boils and localized infections. This probably accounts for the frequency of this type of food poisoning. Whilst growing in the contaminated food (cream and custard are excellent culture mediums), the staphylococci release a toxin which, when ingested with the food, causes a severe reaction in the gastrointestinal tract. This enterotoxin is very heat resistant, and therefore is not necessarily destroyed (even though the staphylococci are) when food is cooked or reheated.

The incubation period is 2–6 hours. It is not unusual for affected persons to become violently ill whilst still at a dinner party.

There is a sudden onset of severe abdominal pain, vomiting, and diarrhoea which can last up to 24 hours, and leave the person feeling very debilitated for several days.

Diagnosis is usually made by the characteristic history, and the fact that usually many people who ate the same food are affected at the same time.

Affected persons are encouraged to replace lost fluids and electrolytes as soon as the vomiting settles. Very occasionally there may need to be admission to hospital for intravenous fluid and electrolyte replacement.

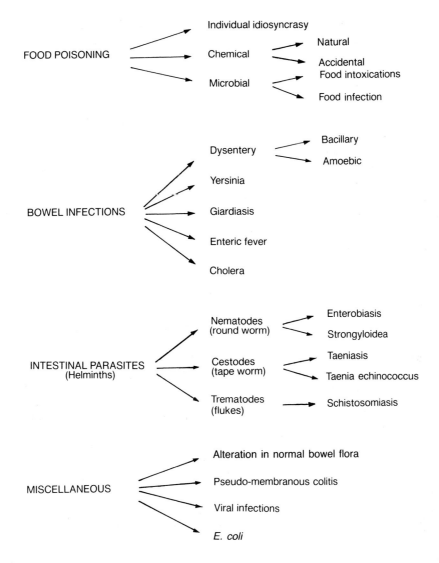

Fig. 53.5 Classification of causes of intestinal infection and infestation.

Staphylococcal food poisoning may be prevented if exemplary hygiene standards are observed when handling food. Food should be refrigerated when not being used.

Clostridium perfringens food poisoning occurs occasionally. It manifests in a manner similar to staphylococcal food poisoning, with the main difference being the incubation period, which is 6–12 hours. Treatment is as for staphylococcal food poisoning.

Botulism is another rare food poisoning, and is caused by eating food containing the toxins of *Clostridium botulinum*. *Clostridium botulinum* will thrive and produce toxins only in anaerobic conditions, therefore preserved non-acid foods (meat, meat products, and vegetables) are possible sources. Modern canning methods have almost eliminated any danger of buying contaminated, commercially produced products; but home preserved vegetables could be suspect.

Table 53.2 Common bowel diseases due to food poisoning, microorganisms, and helminths

Disease	Infecting agent	Manifestation	Therapy
Allergic food poisoning	Individual idiosyncracy	Individual allergic response	Avoid offending allergen (e.g. shell fish, eggs, strawberries, food colouring)
Chemical food poisoning	Some naturally poisonous foods	Onset of GI disturbance after ingesting foods	Avoid offending foods (e.g. mushrooms toadstools) Treat symptoms and signs according to severity
	Poisons accidentally added	Onset of GI disturbance after ingesting food	Avoid offending foods (e.g. plant sprays, food preservatives) Treat symptoms and signs according to severity Poison may need to be neutralized
Microbial food poisoning	Enterotoxins–*S. aureus* (very common)	Incubation 2–6 hr Rapid onset severe GI disturbance	Fluid and electrolyte replacement Anti-emetics
	– *C. perfringens* (rare)	Incubation 6–12 hr Rapid onset severe GI disturbance	Fluid and electrolyte replacement Anti-emetics
	– *C. botulinum* (very rare)	Incubation 12–36 hr Mild GI disturbance → overwhelming CNS collapse → death	Ventilatory resuscitation. Fluid and electrolyte replacement
	Microorganisms – *S. typhimurium* (very common)	Incubation 12–48 hr Sudden onset GI disturbance	Fluid and electrolyte replacement Anti-emetics, anti-diarrhoeals Specific antibiotic if bacteraemia present
	– *Campylobacter jejuni* and *C. coli*	Incubation 12–48 hr Sudden onset GI disturbance	Fluid and electrolyte replacement Anti-emetics, anti-diarrhoeals Specific antibiotic if bacteraemia present
Dysentery Bacillary	*Shigella sonnei* (common) – *S. flexneri* (uncommon) – *S. dysenteri* (uncommon)	Incubation 2–7 days Acute diarrhoea with blood, mucus, and pus in stools	Stringent hygiene to break faecal–oral route Antibiotics if warranted
Amoebic	*Entamoeba histolytica*	Incubation days – months Acute diarrhoea with blood, mucus, and pus in stools. May last for weeks	Stringent hygiene to break faecal – oral route Anti-infective agents, followed by anti-diarrhoeals
Yersinia	*Y. enterocolitica*	Mild-acute lower GI disturbance, lasting 1–4 weeks	Stringent hygiene If severe, tetracycline or co-trimoxazole
Giardiasis	*Giardia intestinalis*	Generalized GI irritation, diarrhoea and possible malabsorption. Symptoms may last months–years Infection is generally commensal, silent and most common in children	Stringent hygiene to break faecal–oral route Metronidazole and tinidazole are specific
Enteric fevers Typhoid	*Salmonella typhi*	Incubation 1–3 weeks	Highly contagious

Table 53.2 (*contd*)

Disease	Infecting agent	Manifestation	Therapy
Paratyphoid	*S. paratyphi* A, B, & C	General malaise, pyrexia, with constipation a feature Not endemic to Australia, but seen following travel to tropical developing countries. Common vector is contaminated water.	Requires strict isolation nursing. Chloramphenicol and co-trimoxazole are specific Active immunization available
Cholera	*Vibrio cholerae*	Incubation 36 hr Rapid onset severe vomiting and profuse watery diarrhoea – dramatic decline – death (high mortality) Not endemic to Australia, but seen following travel to tropical developing countries. Common vector is contaminated water	Highly contagious. Requires strict isolation nursing Tetracycline and furazolidone are specific Active immunization mandatory in travel to endemic countries
Nematodes (round worms) Enterobiasis	*Enterobilus vermicularis* threadworm (very common), pinworm seatworm	Nocturnal pruritis ani Familial infestation	Hygiene measure to break faecal–oral route; familial hygiene measures to prevent transmission Pyrantel embonate and mebendazole are specific. Family treated collectively
Trichuriasis	*Trichuris trichiura* (whipworm)	Heavy infestation produces chronic blood-streaked diarrhoea and tenesmus. Weight loss in children	Hygiene measures to break soil-human route Thiabendazole and mebendazole are usually effective
Strongyloidiasis	*Strongyloides stercoralis*	Dermatitis and cough precede inflammatory bowel response Malabsorption in severe cases	Hygiene measures to break soil-human route Thiabendazole and mebendazole are specific
Ascariasis	*Ascaris lumbricoides* (roundworm)	Widespread and frequently symptomless in tropical countries. Children commonly affected. Mild GI disturbance produces visible evidence of infestation	Hygiene measures to break faecal-soil-oral route Pyrantel embonate and mebendazole are specific
Ancylostomiasis	*Ankylostoma duodenale Necator americanus* (hookworms)	Widespread and frequently symptomless in tropical countries Mild GI disturbance produces visible evidence of infestation Iron deficiency anaemia a feature of heavy infestation	Hygiene measures to break faecal-soil-oral route. (Footwear recommended in contaminated areas) Thiabendazole, pyrantel embonate, and mebendazole are specific

Table 53.2 (*contd*)

Disease	Infecting agent	Manifestation	Therapy
Cestodes (tapeworms) Taeniasis	*Taenia solium* (porcine) *Taenia saginata* (bovine) (common)	Usually symptomless; possible mild GI discomfort and weight loss. Tapeworm segments passed in stools	Avoid undercooked pork and beef Niclosamide is specific for *T. saginata* but not recommended for *T. solium* because it promotes autoinfection
Echinococcosis (hydatid disease)	*Echinococcus granulosus*	Cyst development in liver (usually) and lungs (less commonly) Usually asymptomatic unless excessive growth causes pressure or rupture occurs, causing growth of secondary cysts	Hygiene measures to break canine faecal-human oral route Avoid water and uncooked vegetables in areas contaminated with canine faeces Avoid feeding offal to dogs Mebendazole may be useful
Trematodes Schistosomiasis (blood fluke)	*Schistosoma haematobium* and other species of Schistosomatoidea	Asymptomatic, unless heavy infestation Haematuria Recurrent bouts of loose stools with occasional passage of blood and mucus	In developing countries a major water-borne public health problem Disease not endemic to Australia, no disease-specific agent generally available

Gastrointestinal symptoms of botulism are usually mild, but the extremely potent toxins attack the central nervous system causing generalized muscular weakness and paralysis, leading to death in 70–80% of cases.

Diagnosis is made on clinical observations and demonstration of toxins in the suspect food and/or from the alimentary tract.

Treatment is symptomatic, such as replacing lost fluids and electrolytes, and providing ventilatory resuscitation. Those patients who do survive tend to do so because of their own natural resources, rather than because of medical intervention. Polyvalent antitoxin is of little value once symptoms have developed, but it may have prophylactic value for those who have consumed the affected food but who have not yet developed symptoms. Preventive measures include fastidious cleanliness when preparing food for preservation, and using high temperatures to kill any spores.

Food infections

Salmonellosis. Salmonella typhimurium is the most common species of the Salmonella group to cause food infection. The organism always reaches

the human in food, especially in processed meats, chickens, and reheated foods. The eggs of infected ducks may also be vectors.

The incubation period is 12–48 hours. Manifestations are: sudden onset vomiting, abdominal cramps, and watery diarrhoea, which are short-lived and self-limiting. It can be serious in the very elderly or ill person, causing dehydration. Bacteraemic shock and renal failure have been known to occur on rare occasions. Diagnosis is made when the organism is found in the patient's faeces or on blood culture. Suspected food should also be investigated when determining the source.

Treatment is mainly symptomatic and includes bed rest, replacement of fluids and electrolytes, and the administration of an antiemetic and an antidiarrhoeal. If there is bacteraemia an intravenous infusion will be required for the administration of an antibiotic such as neomycin or tetracycline.

The organisms may be conveyed to food by human carriers, or by flies from infected faeces. Therefore, fly control and high standards of cleanliness wherever food is processed or handled is essential. Cooking food at high temperatures ensures the destruction of the organism. Avoid reheating food at low temperatures, or keeping food hot in warming ovens. Keep unused food refrigerated or frozen. Frozen food, especially chickens, must be thoroughly thawed before cooking, otherwise sufficient heat may not penetrate to destroy any hibernating organisms.

Public health measures to prevent outbreaks of salmonellosis include the education of food handlers regarding food infection hazards and hygiene habits; and meat and poultry inspection of abattoirs, shops, restaurants, and food processing factories.

All diagnosed cases are notifiable to the Public Health Department whose responsibility it is to identify the source of the infection. Persons admitted to hospital should be isolated until cultures of faeces are free from Salmonella for 3 successive days, or until discharge. Some affected people continue to excrete the organisms for many months. This can become a real problem. Carriers must not be employed as food handlers. Nurses must adhere to the principles of isolation nursing, being particularly careful when disposing of faeces.

Campylobacter enteritis. The causative organism is *Campylobacter jejuni* or *coli*. These organisms are also a cause of food infection, and sources of infection include hens, dogs, and milk. The manifestations, treatment, and prevention are as for salmonellosis, except that if an antibiotic is required erythromycin is usually the drug of choice.

The dysenteries

This term is used when the infective organism causes damage to the bowel mucosa, manifesting in diarrhoea that contains blood, mucus, and pus. Bacillary dysentry is usually caused by some Shigella organism, and amoebic dysentry is usually caused by the ingestion of the cysts of the protozoon *Entamoeba histolytica*.

Shigella sonnei is the most common organism responsible for shigelliosis. The incubation period is 2–7 days. Mode of spread is usually the faecal–oral route, and if the condition warrants antibiotic treatment ampicillin or co-trimoxazole are usually prescribed. Co-trimoxazole is also prescribed for chronic carriers.

The incubation period for amoebic dysentery can be from days to months, and the patient may be acutely ill for a number of weeks. The amoeba may travel to the liver via the portal vein and produce an inflammatory response; the resultant hepatic abscess may need to be aspirated.

Metronidazole is used for acute invasive amoebic dysentry, but is not effective against the cysts. A course of metronidazole is followed by a course of diloxanide which usually destroys the cysts. Chloroquine may be prescribed to treat liver abscess.

Very occasionally, patients with either type of dysentery may develop a post-dysenteric irritable colon. Although the faeces culture is negative, these unfortunate few may have intermittent diarrhoea for years. They may need treatment with high fibre diet, antidiarrhoeal drugs, and anticholinergic drugs.

Intestinal parasites (helminths)

Enterobiasis (thread worm, pin worm, seat worm). These small worms (Fig. 53.6A) are extremely common in children and family groups. They live in the colon and lay their eggs in the perianal area at night, causing irritation, perianal lesions (due to scratching), and loss of sleep. Self-infestation is usual. The whole family needs to be treated with pyrantel or mebendazole for 7 days. Gloves worn at night will control scratching and reinfection.

Trichuris trichiura (whip worm). These worms (Fig. 53.6B) which are about 5 cm in length, reside in the caecum, and their eggs are discharged in the host faeces. Reinfection is via the faecal–soil–oral route. Whip worm cause problems because their nourishment is derived by embedding into the mucosa, causing oedema, ulceration, and anaemia if infestation is heavy. There may be right iliac fossa pain, and diarrhoea with blood from the ulcerated areas. Diagnosis is made by isolating the whip worm ova from the faeces. Mebendazole for 3 days is usually satisfactory treatment, but the course may need to be repeated. Thiabendazole is also used.

Ancylostomiasis (hook worm). The *ancylostoma duodenale* (Fig. 53.6C) is common in Australia and lives in human duodenum and jejunum, attached

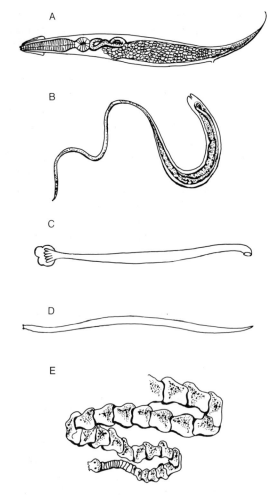

Fig. 53.6 Helminths (not to scale). **A** – Enterobiasis. **B** – Trichuris trichuria. **C** – Ancylostoma duodenale. **D** – Ascariasis. **E** – Taeniasis.

to the mucosa. It is about 10 mm long and is nourished by sucking its host's blood, causing anaemia, malabsorption, and sometimes epigastric pain. The eggs are passed in the host's faeces. The egg develops into a filariform larva which can live in damp soil for months. The larva enters the skin of its host and makes a complicated journey via blood stream, lungs, trachea, and finally into the alimentary tract where it grows to maturity.

The affected person may display irritation at the site of penetration, and respiratory symptoms (cough, wheeze, pyrexia) due to larval migration. There are several effective drugs available for the treatment of hook worm, including thiabendazole,

pyrantel and mebendazole. Anaemia and nutritional deficiencies may need to be corrected.

Ascariasis (round worm). These large worms (Fig. 53.6D) grow up to 30 cm in length and reside in the small intestine, passing their eggs with the host's faeces. Swallowed embryonated eggs hatch in the small intestine, and the larva penetrates into the portal circulation then returns to the small intestine via the liver, inferior vena cava, heart, lungs, trachea, oesophagus, and stomach. Symptoms may be due to irritation during migration, especially in the liver (hepatomegaly) and lungs (pneumonitis and pulmonary eosinophilia – Loffler's syndrome). Allergy to the larva may also occur, manifesting as urticaria. Problems caused by the adult worm may be bowel obstruction (due to the size and number of worms); they may obstruct the common bile duct and pancreatic duct causing obstructive jaundice and/or pancreatitis. The worms may also cause malnutrition by competing with the host for nutrients. Mebendazole and pyrantel are used to treat ascariasis.

Taeniasis (tape worm). Tape worms (Fig. 53.6E) are long (up to several metres) and segmented. The anterior end is called the scolex and contains suckers for attaching to the host. The segments (proglottides) progressively develop from the scolex, ribbon-like, and are shed from the distal end. The shed proglottides contain ova, pass from the host in the faeces, and can stay viable for several weeks until ingested by an intermediate host. The larvae from the ova, called cysticerci, penetrate the intermediate host's tissues. Human disease is acquired when undercooked flesh of the intermediate host is eaten. There are many different types of tape worm, but the ones that commonly grow in humans are *Taenia saginata* (beef tape worm) and *Taenia solium* (pork tape worm). The intermediate host for solium is usually the pig, but may also be human, sheep, canine or feline. Autoinfection is possible with solium, but is most improbable with saginata. Adult tape worms usually do not cause serious illness. There may be loss of weight and diarrhoea, but of chief concern to the victim is the psychological distress of observing worm segments, and perianal irritation by the active proglottides. Diagnosis is made by identifying the ova or proglottides in the faeces. In the larval stage of solium there may be demonstration of larvae in a biopsy specimen taken from a subcutaneous swelling, or X-rays may show calcified areas in muscle or brain tissue.

The incubation period – from time of ingesting affected meat to the elimination of a proglottide – is about 2 months. Tape worms can live in the intestine for up to 20 years. When man is the intermediate host the cysticerci develop in the muscles, and sometimes brain, causing muscle pain, weakness, and epilepsy. The only drug recommended for treating tape worm infestations as well as cysticercosis is niclosamide as it is both effective and non-toxic to the host. Only a single dose is required.

Echinococcosis (hydatid cysts). Echinococcus granulosus is a tiny tape worm (5 mm in length) which causes hydatid disease in man. Man and herbivorous animals are the intermediate hosts, but dogs and other carnivores are the hosts for the adult worm. Ingested ova from the worm hatch in the duodenum and the embryos escape into mesenteric capillaries. From there they lodge in various organs, particularly the liver (65–70%) and lungs (10–15%). There, many embryos are killed by eosinophils, but those which survive produce one or more hydatid cysts. The cysts may be destroyed by the body's defence mechanisms, or they may grow to quite a large size over a period of many years. Some cysts have been known to contain many litres of fluid as well as numerous new scolices. Scolices are transferred to the tape worm host, particularly the dog, when carcasses containing cysts are eaten. They adhere to the intestine of the dog and develop into mature tape worms. The eggs of the tape worm are passed in the dog's faeces. Contamination can be on vegetation, or on human hands after fondling a dog. (See also page 440.)

Symptoms may be due to pressure of a large cyst; a ruptured cyst may cause anaphylactic shock (because the cyst fluid contains a protein foreign to man), or released daughter cysts may obstruct the biliary tree causing obstructive jaundice. Rupture of a cyst into the pleura causes pleural effusion, and rupture into the peritoneum causes peritonitis. Diagnosis is suggested when an X-ray shows a calcified mass in liver or lungs.

Eosinophilia is present in about 25% of cases, and the indirect haemagglutination test confirms the suspicion. Ultrasound and scanning will localize the cyst.

Until recently, surgery to remove the cysts if they were causing problems or were in danger of rupture, was the only treatment. Drug therapy is now proving effective, and mebendazole is prescribed for at least a 3 week period. Allergic symptoms are treated with antihistamines and corticosteroids. Prophylaxis can be achieved by regular deworming of dogs, ensuring that dogs do not eat contaminated uncooked meats, careful washing of possibly contaminated vegetables, and washing of hands following the fondling of dogs.

INTESTINAL OBSTRUCTION

Intestinal obstruction is any situation which results in interruption to the normal flow of contents along the intestinal tract. This is a potentially dangerous situation requiring urgent medical management.

Intestinal obstructions may be complete or incomplete, acute or chronic. They may also be classified as simple where there is no interference with blood supply; or strangulated or incarcerated where blood supply is interrupted and there is danger of necrosis and perforation. Closed loop obstruction occurs with strangulated hernia and volvulus.

Approximately 80% of intestinal obstructions occur in the small intestine, and tend to be acute in nature. Because of its larger diameter, large intestine obstructions usually have a more insidious onset. Partial obstruction occurs initially, but without treatment the obstruction may become complete thus creating an acute situation.

Aetiology

The causes of intestinal obstruction are numerous. The majority are mechanical obstructions which may arise from extrinsic, intrinsic, or luminal problems. Adynamic ileus also causes small bowel obstruction but is neurogenic in origin. Common conditions causing intestinal obstruction are discussed on page 530.

Pathophysiology of acute intestinal obstruction

Regardless of the cause of acute intestinal obstruction the pathophysiological sequence of events follows a similar pattern. The section of intestine immediately above the area of obstruction becomes distended with gas and fluid. The gas is from swallowed air and bacterial action on stagnating bowel contents. The fluid that accumulates is due to the nonreabsorption of fluid that is constantly being secreted into the intestine lumen, plus oedema fluid. When one considers that approximately 8 litres of fluid is secreted into the alimentary tract each day, it can be appreciated that distension can be very rapid if it is not reabsorbed.

Fluid shift from the circulatory system into the intestine lumen, together with fluid losses from vomiting or aspiration and from the skin, will cause the patient to become dehydrated and shocked. In mechanical obstruction there is an initial increase in peristalsis in an attempt to force intestinal contents past the blockage. This activity, together with the distension, causes a build up of pressure which is exerted on the intestine wall. Compression of both venous and arterial blood vessels results, as well as increase of permeability. Gangrene then sets in; bacteria readily escape from the intestinal lumen into the peritoneal cavity, resulting in peritonitis and endotoxic shock.

During this course of events, the intestine becomes progressively fatigued until eventually all peristalsis ceases. Continued strangulation results in necrosis, perforation, and peritonitis. Peritonitis can cause adynamic ileus in adjacent loops of bowel.

Clinical manifestations of acute mechanical obstruction

The five cardinal features of complete intestinal obstruction are:

- Pain
- Vomiting
- Distension
- Shock
- Constipation.

These can be variable depending on the level and length of bowel involved.

Pain is due to distension and excessive peristalsis; it is severe, intermittent colic. Severe constant pain is a sign of strangulation. Decreasing pain and increasing manifestations of shock are signs of atonic bowel or perforation. Pain is sometimes relieved temporarily after vomiting. Borborygmi often accompanies the severe pain.

Vomiting is due to reverse peristalsis and is the body's attempt to relieve the distension. It is an early feature, and is copious when the obstruction is in the proximal small intestine. It is also often projectile in nature. In distal small intestine and colonic obstruction, vomiting is not so dramatic and may even be absent. When vomiting does not completely empty the build up of pooled luminal secretions, gases, and solids, distension continues to increase. In colonic obstruction vomiting occurs only when there is an incompetent ileocaecal valve and distension has progressed into the ileum.

Distension may be palpated, or may even be visible at the abdominal surface of the site of the obstruction. Distension can produce pressure on the bladder, causing urinary frequency; or it may produce pressure under the diaphragm, causing ventilatory problems.

Shock is due to dehydration, electrolyte imbalance, and endotoxins. Chloride, sodium, and potassium are the chief electrolytes affected, and when there is serious imbalance renal failure may result. Metabolic acidosis may develop, depending on the amount of bile and pancreatic juice being vomited.

Constipation. Initially there may be some passage of faeces that had accumulated below the level of obstruction, but once obstruction is complete no further faeces will be formed and constipation becomes absolute. Likewise no flatus will be passed. In colonic obstruction there may be passage of some faecally stained mucus. Bowel sounds will be heard to be quite vigorous whilst there is peristalsis, but are absent when the bowel becomes atonic.

Investigative procedures and diagnosis

Diagnosis is usually made on physical examination when the above features are evident.

Plain abdominal X-rays often show the presence of fluid levels and gas shadows in the affected segment of the intestine. Gastrografin enema X-rays will illustrate colonic obstruction. Gastrografin is safer than barium as it is less likely to augment the obstruction.

Full blood examination, and serum electrolytes will probably demonstrate increased haematocrit and haemoglobin levels, indicating dehydration; increased non-protein nitrogen and BUN levels; and decreased sodium, chloride, and potassium levels.

Medical and surgical management

The principles of medical and nursing management are to:

- Re-establish intestine patency
- Restore fluid and electrolyte balance
- Provide symptomatic relief.

Re-establishment of intestine patency

Acute mechanical intestine obstruction must be relieved immediately by surgical intervention. This may involve resection with end-to-end anastomosis, or the formation of a temporary ileostomy or colostomy (see page 471) for immediate relief of the obstruction. Elective surgery is performed at a later date to deal with the cause of the obstruction. Sometimes, as in intestine obstruction due to extensive ulcerative colitis (see page 516) or carcinoma of the rectum (see page 533), the patient may be left with a permanent stoma.

In sub-acute obstruction, the patient may be managed conservatively (see page 533) until his general condition is such that he will be a better surgical risk.

Restoration of fluid and electrolyte balance

The patient will not be able to take anything orally until the obstruction is relieved; therefore intravenous therapy (preferably via a central vein) must be instituted to correct dehydration, electrolyte, and acid–base imbalance. These measures must be commenced prior to surgery, otherwise the patient's desperate physical state will not be able to tolerate the further trauma of general anaesthesia and surgical intervention.

Serum electrolytes and haematocrit levels will be monitored until normal levels are attained.

Symptomatic relief

Relief of symptoms such as pain, vomiting, and distension is described on page 462.

Nursing management

During the acute phase the nurse must appreciate the seriousness of intestinal obstruction and recognize that the nursing role will include:

- Ensuring that the patient is kept at complete bed rest
- Frequent observation of vital signs and general appearance
- Observing for any changes in the pain characteristics, for example: intermittent changing to constant; changes in severity or location; increase in severity following movement; pain relief following a vomiting episode or gastrointestinal tube aspiration
- Preparation for and assistance with intestinal decompression and intravenous therapy. Aspiration of the gastrointestinal tube as ordered. Maintainance of the intravenous infusion
- Monitoring the amount of vomitus and/or aspirate
- Monitoring the urinary output
- Preparing the patient for emergency surgery
- Demanding the presence of medical staff if the patient's condition appears to be worsening
- Giving the necessary emotional support and explanations to both patient and significant others.

Prognosis and habilitation

Prognosis is good when the patient is diagnosed early and appropriate treatment is commenced without delay. When death occurs it is usually due to electrolyte imbalance, shock, peritonitis, toxaemia, or renal failure. The elderly patient succumbs rapidly.

When the principles of management have been achieved, the patient usually makes a rapid recovery and is discharged from hospital within 10–14 days of treatment.

Common conditions causing intestinal obstruction

Peritoneal adhesions. These are bands of fibrous tissue which commonly develop following inflammation of the peritoneum, or abdominal surgery. These bands adhere loops of bowel together and can produce a constricting effect on the intestinal lumen, causing mechanical extrinsic obstruction. Obstruction is relieved by freeing the adhesions via laparotomy. Occasionally, bowel resection with end-to-end anastomosis is required if the adhesions have compromised blood supply, or if they are tightly enmeshed.

Intussusception. This can be described as a telescoping of one section of bowel into the adjoining distal section. It is common in young children, but can occur in adults. It appears to be due to excessive peristaltic contractions. The enfolding bowel causes obstruction, and requires surgical reduction or resection.

Volvulus. Occasionally a loop of bowel twists upon itself when the bowel rotates on the axis of its mesentery, causing a volvulus. The usual site is the sigmoid colon, although occasionally adhesions can be the cause of a small intestine volvulus. The bowel becomes strangulated where the twist occurs, causing acute bowel obstruction constituting a surgical emergency.

Carcinoma of the colon. This is the most common cause of large intestine obstruction (see page 527).

Strictures. Strictures of the small (and occasionally the large) intestine can cause intestinal obstruction. Chronic inflammatory bowel diseases, for example, Crohn's disease (see page 513), ulcerative colitis (see page 516), and diverticulitis (see page 510) are the usual cause of stenosis of the intestine, due to the recurrent inflammatory processes which lead to fibrosis and hence stenosis. To relieve the obstruction, the affected area is resected.

Indigestible ingestants, gall stones, and constipated faeces are all examples of possible causes of mechanical luminal obstruction. When obstruction is complete, surgical intervention will be required. Ingestants and gall stones may be retrieved via an incision into the lumen of the bowel. Faeces can usually be evacuated per rectum with the patient under general anaesthesia.

HERNIA

A hernia is the protrusion of any part of the internal organs through the structures enclosing them. Hernias are caused by muscle weakness which may be congenital or acquired. Hernias may be acquired through injury or strain, for example, persistent coughing, heavy lifting, straining at stool, or straining to micturate when the bladder is obstructed, or following surgery. They may also be acquired through loss of muscle tone in multiparity, illness, obesity, or old age.

Hernias are either reducible or irreducible. A reducible hernia occurs when the contents of the sac can be returned to the abdominal cavity by manipulation. The sac, however, remains protruding through the muscular defect. When the hernia is irreducible, the contents cannot be returned to the abdominal cavity either because of adhesions, or narrowing of the neck of the hernial sac. Irreducible hernia may also be referred to as incarcerated.

The danger of hernia is that the intestine or its blood supply may become obstructed. If the hernia is strangulated, the arterial blood supply is

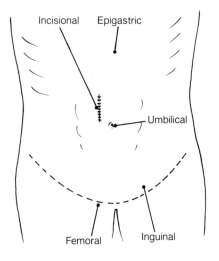

Fig. 53.7 Common sites of abdominal hernia

occluded, predisposing to gangrene and perforation of the bowel.

Abdominal hernia is the protrusion of a viscus or portion of a viscus, usually contained in a sac of peritoneum, through a weakness in the abdominal muscle. The common sites of abdominal hernia are shown in Figure 53.7.

Inguinal hernia

The inguinal canal is an oblique structure about 3.5 cm in length in the lower abdominal muscles. Its upper end is called the internal ring and the lower end the external ring. The inguinal canal transmits nerves, blood vessels, and the spermatic cord in males, and the round ligament in females.

Indirect inguinal hernia is called congenital inguinal hernia. The hernial sac passes through the internal ring of the inguinal canal alongside the spermatic cord or round ligament, and may enter the scrotum or labia (Fig. 53.8).

Because of the narrowness of the canal, strangulation is common, leading to intestinal obstruction or infarction, and pressure on blood vessels and nerves supplying the testes which may cause sterility.

Indirect inguinal hernia is most common in males, and the incidence is highest in childhood or young adulthood.

Direct inguinal hernia is also called acquired inguinal hernia. The sac of the hernia does not pass down the inguinal canal, but emerges in the external ring area through an area of weakness in the abdominal wall. The incidence is highest in the elderly patient. It is not as likely to strangulate and cause intestinal obstruction as is the indirect inguinal hernia.

Femoral hernia

The femoral canal is a funnel-shaped tube in the femoral sheath which passes between the inguinal canal and the innominate bone. The femoral canal has 3 channels containing the femoral artery, the femoral vein, and lymph nodes and fat.

The opening or femoral ring is wider in women than in men. The sac of the hernia passes through the femoral ring and down the canal to protrude beneath the skin just above or slightly below the crease of the groin.

Femoral hernia is most common in females and the hernia can become incarcerated and strangulated. Part of the urinary bladder is sometimes drawn into the sac causing dysuria, frequency, and haematuria.

Umbilical hernia

Hernias of the umbilicus may be congenital, acquired, epigastric, or ventral.

Congenital. Some occur as a result of exomphalos and require surgery at birth because the viscera protrudes through the umbilicus with the cord. Unless the viscera is replaced and the defect repaired, necrosis occurs along with normal umbilical cord necrosis. This type of hernia is rare. More commonly a small hernia develops through a failure of closure of the fascia at the umbilicus. This usually closes spontaneously by the age of 3 years and may be treated by strapping. It does not commonly become irreducible or strangulated, and surgical repair is not usual before the age of 3 years. Females are affected more often than males.

Acquired (paraumbilical). The sac protrudes through a weakness in the muscle near the umbilicus. This type is more common in elderly, obese females who have had multiple pregnancies. This type of hernia is prone to incarceration and strangulation, and is therefore usually corrected surgically.

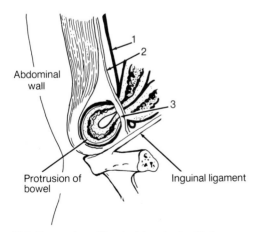

Fig. 53.8 Progression of inguinal hernia. 1 – Peritoneum relaxes. 2 – Weakness in transversalis fascia. 3 – Internal inguinal ring relaxes.

Epigastric. In this rare hernia, the sac protrudes through a weakness in the linea alba between the ziphoid process and the umbilicus. It often contains the falciform ligament of the liver. Most are irreducible and require surgical correction.

Ventral (incisional). The sac of the hernia protrudes through a weakness in the abdominal muscles at the site of a previous incision. This type of hernia is more common if there is post-operative infection of the wound, postoperative distension, obesity, or malnutrition. The hernia may be corrected surgically or by the use of a corset.

Medical, surgical, and nursing management of abdominal hernia

Abdominal hernias are treated by either conservative management or surgical repair. The aim of conservative management is to attempt to reduce the hernia and maintain its reduction by a truss or corset, usually until the patient is fit for surgery. In the case of umbilical hernia, reduction is maintained until it is apparent that the defect will not close spontaneously.

Surgical repair is required immediately if the hernia is strangulated and/or causing obstruction. It is advised if the hernia is irreducible. The types of surgical procedures are:

• Herniotomy. The hernial sac is exposed, opened, and the contents are returned to the abdominal cavity. The hernial sac is excised.
• Herniorrhaphy. Herniotomy is performed and the defect is repaired and strengthened with nylon, braided silk, nylon tricot, or steel wire.
• Hernioplasty. The procedure is as for herniorrhaphy, but the defect is repaired and strengthened with fascia from the thigh.

Postoperatively, the nursing management of the patient who has undergone hernia repair is as for any patient who has undergone abdominal surgery.

Following surgery, the patient should be instructed to flex the hip on the affected side during coughing exercises or other strain, to minimize tension on suture lines.

Given the intrinsic nature of a hernia, patients should be advised and encouraged to avoid situations which may predispose to hernia recurrence. For example, obese patients are urged to lose weight; correct lifting techniques should always be taught; respiratory disorders should be treated, and cigarette smokers should be urged to desist to minimize the effects of coughing.

ADYNAMIC ILEUS

Adynamic ileus (also known as paralytic ileus or functional bowel obstruction) is decreased mobility of a section of the small intestine (usually the ileum). It is thought to be due to either irritation of the sympathetic nervous system, causing hyper-activity, or irritation of the parasympathetic nervous system, causing inhibition of its function.

Adynamic ileus is a potentially serious condition which can, in extreme cases, lead to irreversible fluid and electrolyte imbalance.

Aetiology

Adynamic ileus can occur in the following conditions:

• After extensive surgery. This is the most common cause, especially if the intestine or nerve supply to the intestine has been irritated, for example, in surgery to the intestine, kidney, uterus, or lumbar spine
• Following prolonged anaesthesia
• After hollow viscus perforation
• Peritonitis
• During any prolonged serious illness
• Hypokalaemia.

Pathophysiology

The pathology involved in adynamic ileus is as for any acute intestinal obstruction (see page 527).

Clinical manifestations

Diagnosis is usually made on clinical examination. More often than not the patient is in the early postoperative phase, or suffering from a serious illness. The patient looks and is ill, showing signs of shock with pale, cold, clammy skin. Abdominal discomfort is present but there is no severe pain unless there is an associated peritonitis. Abdominal distension is evident and the patient reports a bloated feeling below the umbilical level. Bowel sounds are diminished or absent, there is no passage of flatus or faeces.

Vomiting (and especially the vomiting of faecal fluid) is a late feature, but should not occur if nursing assessment has been effective and the stomach is being aspirated. There will be large volumes of gastric aspirate.

There may be evidence of dehydration and electrolyte imbalance.

Medical and nursing management

Preventive

Adynamic ileus is not as prevalent as it once was, mainly due to the fact that definite steps are taken in its prevention. The nurse must always recognize the probability of this condition occurring with any seriously ill person, especially any patient who has undergone major abdominal surgery, and must be alert for any of the above warning signs. The following measures should be implemented routinely in the management of these patients:

• Nil orally until bowel sounds are present following any prolonged surgery and particularly following stomach or intestinal surgery.
• Aspirate the stomach via an intragastric tube at 0.5–1 hourly intervals following surgery until bowel sounds recur. To avoid a build up of gastric secretions between manual aspirations, the intragastric tube should either be allowed to drain freely into a drainage bag, or be connected to low pressure suction. It is normal for there to be no bowel sounds (indicating no activity) following any surgery that has interfered with nerve supply to the intestine. Bowel sounds are the first indicators that bowel activity is recommencing and should occur within 18–36 hours of surgery.
• Maintain hydration and electrolyte balance via the intravenous route until an adequate diet is reestablished.
• Once bowel sounds have returned the patient may be, very gradually, reintroduced to oral fluids and food over a period of 3–4 days.

Active management

Should preventive measures fail, or the patient present with an adynamic ileus, prompt nursing assessment and intervention can limit the extent of the pathological process. In addition to preventive measures (nil orally, gastric aspirations and drainage, and intravenous therapy) the following actions may be implemented:

• Rest. The patient must have absolute bed rest and may require sedation with a narcotic analgesic.
• A drug to stimulate the parasympathetic nervous system and hence encourage peristalsis may be ordered. These drugs (for example bethanecol or neostigmine) can be dangerous when given in the presence of an already compromised bowel, therefore the patient must be observed very closely for signs of increasing shock for at least 2 hours following administration of the drug.
• In some instances the physician may order the passage of a flatus tube or a small water enema in order to stimulate bowel activity. These measures are rarely effective.

Should active management, which may be carried out for several days, fail to produce a return of peristalsis the patient will be in a life threatening situation. Resection of the affected segment of the intestine is a last resort. This is rarely necessary as the majority of cases resolve with conservative treatment.

NEOPLASMS OF THE SMALL AND LARGE INTESTINE

Small intestine neoplasms, both benign and malignant, are rare. When they do occur they are usually not detected until they cause signs of obstruction. Treatment is by surgical resection with end-to-end anastomosis. Radiotherapy and chemotherapy do not appear to have any significant effect on the progress of these malignant tumours. As with all neoplastic conditions prognosis depends on whether metastasis had occurred prior to treatment.

Colonic neoplasms

Benign neoplasms

These are usually referred to as polyps, and can be single or numerous in number. Histologically there are many types of polyps some of which are thought to be precancerous particularly polyposis coli (see below). Polyps producing symptoms can be removed (if not too numerous) with a snare or diathermy via an endoscope (Fig 53.9). Polyps can cause intussusception or intestinal obstruction, or they may bleed.

Polyposis coli is an uncommon but important condition. It is inherited as a Mendelian dominant condition and affects many members of a family. Carcinoma of the colon almost always develops some years after the appearance of these polyps, and for this reason colectomy is performed before there is evidence of malignancy. The patient usually has a permanent ileostomy but some surgeons anastomose the ileum to the rectum. When this is done the patient must have annual examinations to ensure that no polyps have developed in the remaining rectum. If further polyps do develop, they are usually removed via a sigmoidoscope.

Malignant neoplasms

Malignant neoplasms of the colon are almost always adenocarcinomas. They are extremely common with the majority (over 50%) occurring in the pelvic and rectal area. Carcinoma of the colon represents the second major cause of death from cancer in Australian adults. Traditionally, Australians have consumed a diet high in red meat, animal fats, and refined cereals; these factors may be implicated in the high incidence of colonic tumours.

Aetiology and pathophysiology

The cause of colorectal carcinoma is unknown and is still subject to debate and research, but some predisposing conditions are thought to include:

● Diet. Persons taking a high-fat and animal protein, low residue diet consistently appear to be at a much higher risk of developing colonic cancer. It is thought that when there is increased transit time of bowel contents, as with chronic constipation, carcinogens have increased exposure time with bowel tissue. This is the theorized relationship between low fibre diet and carcinoma of the colon. Gram-negative bacteria are able to alter bile salts to substances known to be carcinogenic in animals.
● Age. Colonic cancer is more prevalent in the over 60 years age group, except for those cases that are associated with polyposis coli or ulcerative colitis.
● Familial tendency. Cancer of the colon occurs 3–5 times more often amongst first degree relations of patients with the disease than in the general population (Shearman & Finlayson, 1982).
● Polyposis coli.
● Extensive chronic ulcerative colitis of many years' standing.

The tumour may extend around the circumference of the bowel causing a 'ring' stricture or it may extend into the lumen of the bowel. In either case progressive obstruction will occur if the tumour remains untreated. The tumour may spread by direct infiltration of nearby organs, to nearby lymph nodes, or to the liver via the portal circulation.

Clinical manifestations

Colorectal cancers tend to bleed readily, therefore in some patients with left-sided tumours, and

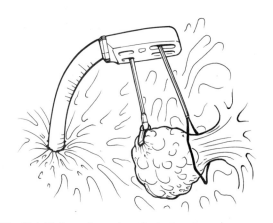

Fig. 53.9 Endoscopic snaring of colonic polyp.

especially those with rectal tumours, there will be obvious fresh blood with the faeces. If, however, the tumour is in the ascending or transverse colon, the blood loss may not be so obvious. Anaemia may be a feature in patients with right-sided tumours due to a chronic blood loss.

The growing tumour will cause partial intestinal obstruction which manifests early in left-sided tumours, because of the formed nature of the faeces. Signs of intestinal obstruction are late signs in right-sided tumours, because the lumen is wider and because of the more fluid nature of the bowel contents. In all cases the tumour is quite large before it obstructs the lumen, and unfortunately total obstruction is an extremely late sign in right-sided colonic cancer.

Not all patients experience a change in bowel function; however, unexplained constipation or diarrhoea may be the clinical feature that prompts the patient to seek medical advice.

But, for the elderly person who, due to diet, probably already suffers from chronic constipation and haemorrhoids, any early warning signs such as altered bowel habits and blood with the faeces would most likely be missed. Other late signs include anorexia, progressive weakness, abdominal pain, and weight loss.

Investigative procedures and diagnosis

The patient's clinical, dietary, and family history will point to the need for a thorough physical examination. Early rectal cancers can be felt on digital examination.

Sigmoidoscopy and/or colonoscopy with biopsy of any suspect areas have a high diagnostic accuracy.

Barium enema may show a filling defect or a stricture.

Testing faeces for blood and checking haemoglobin levels, may prove bleeding and anaemia but are nonspecific.

Tests for cancer-embryonic antigen (CEA) are performed. CEA is a protein found in the mucosa of fetal colon and in colonic tumours. CEA is sometimes also demonstrated in the blood of patients with colonic tumours. When the tumour is removed the CEA blood level falls, but rises again if there is recurrence of the growth. Serial estimations of CEA levels should be carried out when the patient is checked for recurrence.

Surgical management

Surgical resection of the tumour and sufficient adjacent structures in an endeavour to remove all cancerous cells is the treatment of choice (see Fig 53.10).

Nearby lymph glands are also resected in an attempt to control secondary spread. Anaemia will be corrected by blood transfusion. If there is acute intestinal obstruction this may need to be dealt with prior to the removal of the tumour. This may mean that the patient has an emergency temporary colostomy to divert the obstructed intestine contents then, at a later date, the tumour is resected. Depending on the site of the tumour the temporary colostomy may be closed or it may need to be fashioned into a permanent stoma (see page 472).

If the tumour is too advanced for curative surgery, palliative surgery to by-pass the obstructing tumour may be required. This usually involves creating a colostomy or an ileostomy without resection.

Nursing management

Postoperatively, nursing management will involve all the care appropriate to any patient who has undergone abdominal surgery (see page 499). Additionally, nursing care of the patient undergoing surgery for malignant disease must be incorporated (see Chapter 13), and nursing care of the patient with a stoma (see page 473) may be required.

The operations performed for colorectal carcinoma are named according to the segment of the bowel removed and each procedure will produce its own particular nursing requirements. In order to minimize the risks of faecal contamination of the abdominal cavity, most surgeons will insert 2 drain tubes during wound closure. A round bore or a corrugated drain via an anterior stab wound will drain the operative site, whilst a thin, low pressure vacuum suction drain will be inserted to drain the bed of the resected area.

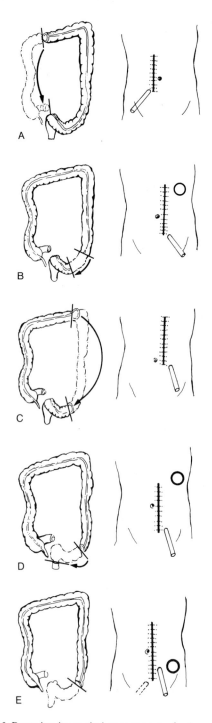

Right hemicolectomy. (Fig. 53.10A) The tumour is resected along with adjacent portions of caecum, and ascending and transverse colon; the terminal ileum is then anastomosed to the transverse colon. In almost all cases of right hemicolectomy, the patient does not require a temporary colostomy and postoperatively nursing care of the patient will involve the wound management of a right para-median incision along with the drain tube(s). Ultimately bowel function should return to normal with formed, soft stools.

Sigmoid colectomy. (Fig. 53.10B) The tumour is resected along with adjacent portions of intestine; an end-to-end anastomosis of the descending and pelvic segments of colon is performed either immediately or following a temporary colostomy formation. It is not unusual for the patient to require a temporary colostomy to allow time for the proximal colon to recover from the effects of the obstruction. A left paramedian wound with drain tube(s) will require nursing management postoperatively, as will a temporary stoma if this has been fashioned. Bowel function following recovery should result in normal, formed stools.

Left hemicolectomy. (Fig. 53.10C) The tumour plus the length of descending colon is removed and an end-to-end anastomosis of transverse to sigmoid colon is performed. A temporary colos-tomy may be required and a left paramedian incision with drain tubes results. Bowel function will result in softer, more fluid stools that can be controlled by the patient taking a faecal bulking agent.

Anterior resection of rectum. (Fig. 53.10D) The rectum and pelvic colon is removed and an end-to-end anastomosis of the sigmoid colon to the anal canal is performed. Nowadays, in almost all cases of anterior resection, stapling is the preferred method of anastomosis as this has enjoyed a high success rate of wound apposition. Often, a tempo-rary, transverse colon, loop colostomy is fash-ioned; this is closed after healing at the site of the anastomosis has taken place, anywhere from 3 weeks to 3 months.

Postoperatively, the patient will have a left paramedian incision, abdominal drain tubes, maybe a loop colostomy, and an anal pack which may or may not incorporate a drain tube. Ulti-

Fig. 53.10 Resection in surgical management of colorectal carcinoma, showing postoperative wound, drain tube and stoma sites. **A** – Right hemicolectomy. **B** – Sigmoid colectomy. **C** – Left hemicolectomy. **D** – Anterior resection of rectum. **E** – Abdominal-perineal resection of rectum.

mately, bowel function should be normal but care must be taken to ensure that stools remain soft so as to avoid stress on the anastomosis site.

Abdomino-perineal resection of rectum. (Fig. 53.10E) With the increasing success of anterior resection using the stapling method, the requirement for this procedure as a method of treatment for rectal carcinoma is decreasing. Most patients see this as a physically mutilating operation as the pelvic colon, rectum, and anal canal are resected along with an extensive pelvic clearance of lymph nodes. There is no alternative to the resulting terminal sigmoid colostomy and an oversewing of the anus. The procedure requires a long anaesthetic with 2 surgical teams for the abdominal and perineal approaches.

Postoperatively, the patient will have a left paramedian incision, abdominal drain tubes, a permanent sigmoid colostomy, and a perineal incision with a drain tube under low pressure suction. Care must be taken to ensure patient comfort, as positioning in the immediate postoperative period will be extremely difficult. Bowel function should ultimately result in soft, formed stools discharging via the terminal colostomy. Flatus can be of particular distress to patients and gas absorbents should be encouraged, for example charcoal tablets.

Anticipated outcome

Most references quote a 50% 5–7 year cure rate when it is believed that all the tumour was removed at operation by radical excision, and when there is no evidence of metastases.

Although chemotherapy and radiotherapy have little effect in the treatment of colorectal cancers, these methods are sometimes used to palliate pelvic spread.

Research continues in an attempt to develop new drugs or immunotherapy which will be suitable for use in managing these tumours.

54

Common disorders of the anorectal area

Mavis Matthews

The majority of conditions related to the perianal region are associated with either chronic constipation or diarrhoea and Figure 54.1 illustrates the relevant anatomy of the region. Excessive straining and bearing down in an endeavour to pass a constipated stool, will eventually weaken the muscles of the pelvic floor, cause congestion of the anal veins and mucosa, and will also cause the mucosa or skin of the anal area to split. The person who has a problem with diarrhoea (for example, ulcerative colitis, Crohn's disease) will experience excoriation of the perianal area. Constant cleansing of this area with toilet paper after each bowel action, together with the irritating nature of watery faeces, will produce microscopic lesions; these in turn become inflamed, grow larger and deeper, and may become infected leading to abscess formation and perianal fistulae.

The skin of the lower margins of the anus is highly sensitive to pain, therefore diseases in this area are acutely painful, especially at the time of

defaecation when the affected skin is being stretched. Many people augment their problems by avoiding defaecation because it is so painful. Thus constipation with its sequelae can develop requiring hospitalization.

SPECIFIC DISORDERS

Pruritus ani

Itchiness around the anal area is extremely distressing as well as embarrassing. Some people say they 'nearly go mad' with the discomfort. The primary cause is thought to be due to some faecal elements entering the skin via microscopic lesions and setting up an irritation. Scratching the irritated area will cause further lesions. Often no underlying cause can be determined but when there is this must be treated if possible. Careful washing and drying of the perianal area after each bowel action (rather than using toilet paper) is essential. Absorbent cotton briefs should be worn at all times to absorb moisture and scratching must be avoided. Betamethasone diminishes the itch and hydroxyquinolone reduces the risk of superimposed Candida infections. When pruritus ani is a chronic problem which resists treatment a condition known as lichenification or chronic neurodermatitis may develop. This is due to constant scratching and causes the skin to become thickened and pigmented with patchy excoriation.

Descending perineum syndrome

Pelvic floor muscles become lax and anal sphincter efficiency is lost when there is a long history of constipation and straining to pass hard faeces.

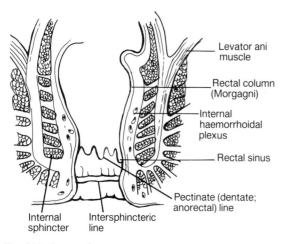

Fig. 54.1 Anorectal anatomy.

Levator ani muscle

Rectal column (Morgagni)

Internal haemorrhoidal plexus

Rectal sinus

Pectinate (dentate; anorectal) line

Internal sphincter

Intersphincteric line

This results in a bulging perineum and faecal incontinence. Attempts at surgical repair are rarely satisfactory. Constipation must be corrected.

Rectal prolapse

This is a circumferential descent of the rectum through the anus and is associated with descending perineum syndrome. A partial rectal prolapse occurs when only the rectal mucosa is affected, and a complete prolapse describes the collapse of the whole rectal wall. Partial prolapse tends to occur in the young, whereas complete prolapse usually occurs only in the elderly.

Rectal prolapse may be reducible manually or it may be irreducible and require surgical repair. The untreated irreducible prolapsed mucosa readily becomes ulcerated and infected. Like many anorectal conditions chronic constipation is the chief cause, but fistula repair, obstetrical tears, or a lax external anal sphincter can predispose to rectal prolapse. The patient complains of a prolapsing rectum on coughing, straining, and defaecating. Faecal incontinence may also be present. Partial prolapses may be treated by correcting constipation and injecting the mucosa with phenol, or by excising the mucosa in such a manner as to preserve anal sphincter control. There is no single satisfactory procedure for treating a complete rectal prolapse, therefore various surgical techniques are employed in an endeavour to fix the rectum in place, repair the pelvic floor, and to preserve or repair the anal sphincter mechanism. An abdominal approach is commonly used, and nursing care is directed towards the postoperative management of the patient having abdominal (see page 499) and/or bowel (see page 529) surgery. Patient education is directed towards preventing constipation (for example, increased dietary fibre, adequate fluid intake, and regular exercise), and it is a nursing responsibility to ensure that the patient (or significant others) understands and is able to implement these self-care measures prior to discharge.

Anal fissure

A fissure is a crack or cleft and when it occurs at the anal verge it usually manifests as an acute or chronic ulcer. It is usually located posteriorly; it is very painful, and may bleed. Forceful passage of constipated faeces is the usual precipitating cause. Chronic anal ulceration is also caused by Crohn's disease, syphilis, leukaemia, and anal carcinoma. If the internal sphincter is exposed at the base of a deep fissure, painful sphincter spasm is marked. Chronic fissures affecting the sphincter muscles cause fibrosis and stenosis. Infection, leading to an abscess and fistula formation, can occur.

Correction of the underlying constipation is essential when treating anal fissures. With acute fissures the use of stool softeners, along with the application of a local anaesthetic ointment will help to relieve pain and usually promote healing. Chronic fissures, where the sphincter muscles are involved, may respond to anal dilatation performed under general anaesthetic; however, many of them require wide surgical excision with healing by granulation.

Abscess

Abscesses commonly form in the anal mucosal, peri-anal, or ischiorectal regions and less commonly in other sites (Fig. 54.2). Infection may commence in fissures, anal tears, or in the ducts of the anal glands at the base of the columns of Morgagni. The bowel commensal, *Escherichia coli*, is the usual offending organism when it escapes from the bowel lumen into underlying soft tissues. Like any abscess these are extremely painful and may cause fever and general ill health. The abscess needs to be opened and drained. Surgery may be via the skin surface or through the anal canal mucosa. The opened wound heals by granulation which may take some weeks. A systemic broad spectrum antibiotic is sometimes prescribed.

Anal fistula

A fistula is an abnormal track, lined with granulation tissue, between two epithelial surfaces. The track of an anal fistula commonly communicates between the anus and skin surface and is almost always the result of underlying suppuration. A fistula may have 2 or more branches with external openings (Fig. 54.3). The patient complains of a

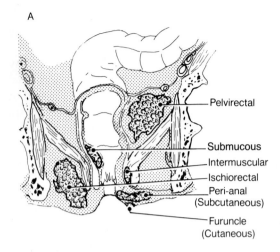

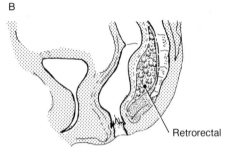

Fig. 54.2 Sites of anal abscesses. **A** – Coronal view. **B** – Median view.

Tracks are cored out when there is danger of dividing the anorectal ring which may cause incontinence of faeces. Healing may be by granulation, primary closure, or there may need to be split-skin grafting of the area. Broad spectrum antibiotics are usually prescribed.

Anal sinus

A sinus is a track leading from an epithelial surface to an inner cavity. An anal sinus usually leads from the anal canal to an abscess cavity in the soft tissues of the perianal region. These sinuses have the same cause and treatment as anal fistulae.

Pilonidal sinus

This is a sinus which contains loose hair. The most common site for such a sinus is in the cleft of the buttock just above the coccyx (Fig. 54.4). Oily skinned, thick haired males are the most commonly affected and there is a familial tendency to the condition. The hair creates the sinus by curling and penetrating the skin, setting up a chronic irritation. Secondary infection is common

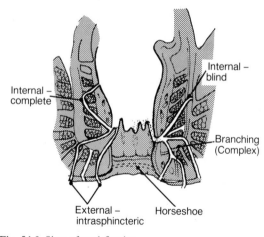

Fig. 54.3 Sites of anal fistulae.

painless discharge, itchiness, and embarrassment. There will be a history of previous perianal infection or abscess.

Treatment consists of laying open or coring out the track(s) and removing the granulated lining.

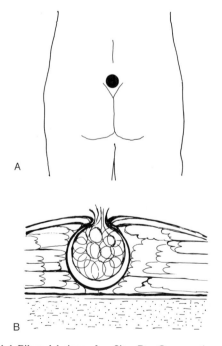

Fig. 54.4 Pilonodal sinus. **A** – Site. **B** – Cross-section.

and may lead to a pilonidal abscess which causes the patient to seek medical attention because of the throbbing pain experienced at the base of the spine.

The infected sinus may respond to antibiotic therapy and hot baths 2–3 times a day. An abscess will need to be surgically drained. After all infection is cleared the sinus should be eradicated by elective surgery. A large surface wound is created, which extends almost to the sacrum. This ensures that all affected areas are exposed and avoids recurrence. The wound is usually left open to heal by granulation over a period of weeks.

Haemorrhoids

Internal haemorrhoids are congestion of the internal haemorrhoidal venous plexus in the anal submucosa, and which project into the anal canal (Fig. 54.5A). They may be classified as first,

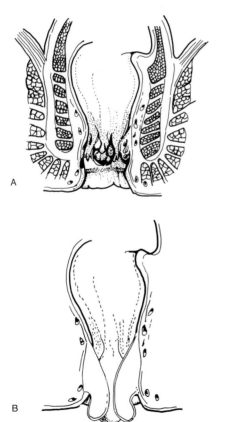

Fig. 54.5 Haemorrhoids. **A** – Internal. **B** – Prolapsing internal.

second, third, and fourth degree to indicate the severity of the prolapse. Irritation of the anal mucosa by chronic constipation or diarrhoea is thought to be the chief cause; but pelvic congestion, due to such conditions as pregnancy and portal hypertension, is also implicated. Bleeding, which can be profuse, is usually the first sign and accompanies defaecation. A large prolapsing internal haemorrhoid may be felt outside the anus (Fig. 54.5B), and if it becomes strangulated by the anal sphincter there will be gross oedema and extreme pain. The haemorrhoid may also become thrombosed. If bleeding is chronic or profuse the patient may develop iron deficiency anaemia. Pruritus ani is caused by the irritating mucus which is secreted by the engorged anal mucosa. Proctoscopy is essential for the diagnosis of internal haemorrhoids.

Medical and surgical management

Conservative measures. Patient education is directed towards:

- Avoiding constipation by taking a high-fibre diet, at least 2 litres of fluid daily, and by taking a bulk forming aperient if necessary.
- Inserting haemorrhoidal suppositories or cream as prescribed. These preparations usually contain local anaesthetic, anti-inflammatory, antiseptic, and antipruritic properties.
- Keeping the anal area clean and dry at all times. It is better to wash the anal area after each bowel action rather than to use toilet paper. Absorbent briefs should be worn.
- Taking hot sitz baths 2–3 times daily.
- If necessary and if possible, manually replacing a prolapsed haemorrhoid inside the anal canal.

The above measures are all that are necessary for the majority of patients, but if these fail to give reasonable relief the physician has a choice of other more definitive treatments, usually undertaken in their room in an outpatient department or clinic.

Injection. The submucous tissue of the haemorrhoid is injected with a sclerosant, such as phenol or carbolic acid in almond oil, with the intention of inducing fibrosis and obliterating the blood vessels. The haemorrhoid then shrinks. The injection is painless and 2 or 3 repeats at 2-weekly intervals may be necessary.

Rubber band ligation (Fig. 54.6). This method of removing the haemorrhoid is widely used. With the aid of a proctoscope and a rubber band applicator, the rubber band is placed around the base of the haemorrhoid. Over a period of 2–4 weeks the haemorrhoid sloughs away.

Incision and evacuation of the haematoma may be required if the area is acutely thrombosed.

Anal dilatation and internal sphincterotomy. The young patient who has developed haemorrhoids because of tight anal sphincters will often gain relief by having the anal area forcefully dilated or from a sphincterotomy. These are extremely painful procedures, therefore they are performed in a hospital, usually under spinal or general anaesthesia.

Haemorrhoidectomy is usually reserved for permanently prolapsed haemorrhoids that are causing distress and which do not respond to, or are unsuitable for, any of the above procedures. Hospitalization is necessary. The nurse needs to be especially aware that these patients will probably have a long history of pain and discomfort, and will be very embarrassed. There are several surgical techniques employed. The main objective is to remove the haemorrhoid(s), while at the same time preserving the integrity of the anal sphincters so that the complications of either anal stenosis or incontinence do not occur.

External haemorrhoids

Some authorities do not consider these to be true haemorrhoids but rather describe them as external anal haematomas that form at the outer anal margin and are covered by skin (see Fig. 54.7A & B). They are almost always due to straining to pass a constipated stool.

These lesions may resolve without interference, or with the application of haemorrhoidal cream. The haematoma may need to be incised and evacuated if it is causing great distress. Anal skin tags (Fig. 54.7C) are often the result of resolved

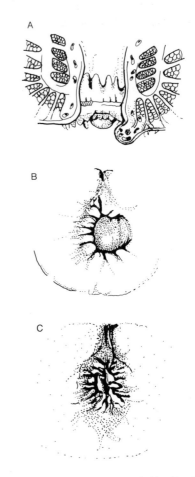

Fig. 54.7 **A** & **B** – External haemorrhoids. **C** – Anal skin tags.

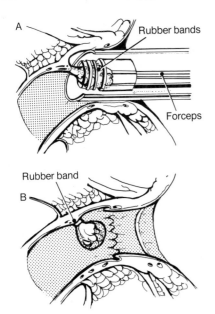

Fig. 54.6 Rubber band ligation of haemorrhoid.

haematomas. Haematomas can become complicated. There may be pressure necrosis of the overlying skin, the development of a fissure, or abscess formation. External anal haematomas are very common and very painful and, like internal haemorrhoids, the great majority are preventable with the avoidance of constipation.

Haemorrhoidal creams containing local anaesthetic must not be used over lengthy periods of time because many people develop allergic perianal excoriation, thus augmenting their problems.

NURSING MANAGEMENT OF THE PATIENT UNDERGOING PERIANAL SURGERY

Preoperatively

Ensure that the patient has privacy during treatments and discussions to reduce his level of embarrassment and anxiety.

Explain all pre- and postoperative procedures carefully, and give assurance that every endeavour will be made to minimize pain. Remember that the patient has been experiencing great pain, especially at time of defaecation or rectal examinations.

Bowel preparation is aimed at ensuring the rectum is clear of faeces prior to and immediately following surgery. This can be achieved by a low residue diet the day before surgery and by fasting 6–8 hours prior to surgery. An evacuant enema or suppository may be ordered, but this will depend on the state of the anorectal area. The patient may not be able to tolerate any invasion of the area. If a bowel washout, enema, or suppository is ordered, it may be helpful to apply an anaesthetic cream to the anal area prior to the procedure.

Observations will include noting: any anal discharges such as blood, pus, or slough; the nature of any faeces passed; and a description of any pain experienced.

Postoperatively

The patient may return to the ward with a rectal pack and/or drain in place; there may be an external raw area that is to heal by granulation, or there may be a visible perianal suture line. The nurse must determine if there are any packs, drains, or sutures to be managed and removed at a later date. Raw edges are usually covered with some type of paraffin-impregnated gauze, for example tulle gras, so that new granulating tissue is not disturbed each time the dressing needs to be renewed. On the other hand, some surgeons prefer plain gauze to be applied as they say it is a better haemostat in the immediate postoperative phase. If plain gauze is used it must be soaked away from the wound at each dressing change or bath time.

Cleanliness of the area is essential. This means that each time the female patient voids or has her bowels opened and when the male patient has his bowels opened, the wound must be cleansed and, if applicable, a new dressing applied. A sitz bath following every bowel action is highly recommended. Some hospital wards have bidets in the toilet areas and these are also helpful for cleansing the perianal area.

Because of the high vascularity of the perianal area, observation for haemorrhage in the first 24 hours postoperative is essential, especially following surgery to the anal canal or rectum, as in internal haemorrhoidectomy. Ice packs may control any haemorrhage, but if it persists the surgeon must be notified and the patient may even need to be prepared for a return to the OR in order to control the bleeding.

Patients usually dread the thought of having an anal pack removed, or of having the first bowel action following perianal surgery, as these can be very painful procedures.

The following is a suggested regime to ensure minimal distress during removal of an anal pack and/or with the first postoperative bowel action.

• Diet should be high-fibre, low-irritant with at least 2 litres of fluid per day, as soon as the patient resumes full diet.
• An aperient should be administered on the second or third postoperative evening
• On the following day:
1. Analgesia as prescribed, for example pethidine, is administered 30 minutes prior to the planned time for removal of the pack.

2. The patient should sit in a sitz bath for at least 20 minutes to ensure that the pack becomes saturated. He may be able to remove the pack whilst in the bath.

3. Alternatively the patient returns to bed and the nurse carefully removes the pack.

4. If the patient is able, he should be encouraged to have a bowel action while the analgesia is still effective.

5. Following bowel action the patient should have a bidet douche or another sitz bath.

6. The area is then dressed and a T-binder is fitted or disposable pants are worn to hold the dressing in place.

It is essential that patients who have had perianal surgery do not become constipated, as the passing of hard faeces will cause pain and trauma to the operative site.

Following each bowel action the patient should have a sitz bath. The perianal area is inspected for signs of healing or problems; and any prescribed treatment is performed, for example, dressing, application of ointment, instillation of suppository, or anal dilatation.

Prior to discharge the patient must understand the need for preventing constipation and for keeping the perianal area clean at all times.

SECTION G – REFERENCES AND FURTHER READING

Texts

Alexander E L 1983 Alexander's care of the patient in surgery, 7th edn. Mosby, St Louis

Anderson J R (ed) 1976 Muir's textbook of pathology, 10th edn. Edward Arnold, London

Anthony C P 1984 Structure and function of the body. Mosby, St Louis

Anthony C P, Thibodeau G 1979 Textbook of anatomy and physiology, 10th edn. Mosby, St Louis

Barbezat G O Rational treatment of diverticular disease. In: Medical Monograph Series 1, ADIS Press, Sydney

Bardhan K D 1977 Perspectives in duodenal ulcer. Smith Kline and French Laboratories Ltd, Hertfordshire

Bateson M C, Bouchier I A D 1981 Clinical investigation of gastrointestinal function, 2nd edn. Blackwell, London

Bonaparte B (ed) 1981 Gastrointestinal care: a guide for patient education. Appleton-Century-Crofts, New York

Bouchier I A D 1982 Gastroenterology, 3rd edn. Bailliere Tindall, London

Brunner L S, Suddarth D S 1982 The Lippincott manual of nursing practice, 3rd edn. Lippincott, Philadelphia

Brunner L S, Suddarth D S 1984 Textbook of medical surgical nursing, 5th edn. Lippincott, Philadelphia

Burton G R W 1983 Microbiology for the health sciences, 2nd edn. Lippincott, Philadelphia

Charters A D 1983 Human parasitology. Imperial Printing Co, Perth, Western Australia

Chilman A, Thomas M 1981 Understanding nursing care, 2nd edn. Churchill Livingstone, Edinburgh

Cohen L Z, Holmes N. Shinehouse P M, Moclock L C (eds) 1985 Gastrointestinal disorders: nurse's clinical library. Springhouse, Pennsylvania

Creager J G 1982 Human anatomy and physiology. Wadsworth, California

Davenport H W 1978 A digest of digestion. Year Book Medical Publishers, Chicago

Elmslie R G, Ludbrook J 1971 An introduction to surgery: 100 topics. Heineman, London

Feutz S A 19 Ostomy at a glance. United Division of Howmedica, Florida

Gillespie I E, Thomson T J 1977 Gastroenterology: an integrated course, 2nd edn. Churchill Livingstone, Edinburgh

Gius J A 1972 Fundamentals of surgery. Year Book Medical Publishers, Chicago

Given B A, Simmens S J 1984 Gastroenterology in clinical nursing, 4th edn. Mosby, St Louis

Guyton A C 1982 Textbook of medical physiology, 6th edn. Saunders, Philadelphia

Hardy K J, Hughes E S R, Cuthbertson A M 1981 Stoma and fistula management: a practical guide. E R Squibb, Melbourne

Hare R, Cooke E M 1984 Bacteriology and immunity for nurses, 6th edn. Churchill Livingstone, Edinburgh.

Havard M 1986 A nursing guide to drugs, 2nd edn. Churchill Livingstone, Melbourne

Hood G H, Dincher J R 1980 Total patient care – foundations and practice. Mosby, St Louis

Hughes E S R, Kyte E M, Cuthbertson A M 1971. All about an ileostomy, 3rd edn. Angus and Robertson, Sydney

Humphrey C (ed) 1982 Surgical nursing. McGraw Hill Book Co, Sydney

Langman L T S 1982 A concise textbook of gastroenterology, 2nd edn. Churchill Livingstone, Edinburgh

Luckmann J, Sorensen K C 1980 Medical/surgical nursing: a psychophysiologic approach, 2nd edn. Saunders, Philadelphia

Macleod J 1987 Davidson's principles and practice of medicine, 15th edn. Churchill Livingstone, Edinburgh

Nash D F E 1980 The principles and practice of surgery for nurses and allied professions, 7th edn. Edward Arnold, London

Netter F H 1972 The Ciba collection of medical illustrations, 3rd edn. 3:II. Ciba Pharmaceutical Company, New Jersey

Passmore R, Eastwood M A 1986 Davidson's human nutrition and dietetics. Churchill Livingstone, Edinburgh

Price S A, Wilson L McC 1982 Pathophysiology – clinical concepts of disease processes, 2nd edn. McGraw Hill, New York

Read A E, Barritt D W, Langton Hewer R 1986 Modern medicine, 3rd edn. Churchill Livingstone, Edinburgh

Shaper K N et al 1975 Medical surgical nursing. Mosby, St Louis

Shearman D J C, Finlayson N D C 1982 Diseases of the gastrointestinal tract and liver. Churchill Livingstone, Edinburgh. p. 816

Sleisenger M H, Brandborg L L 1977 Malabsorption. Saunders, Philadelphia

Society of Hospital Pharmacists of Australia 1985 Pharmacology and drug information for nurses, 2nd edn. Saunders, Sydney

Solomon E P, Davis P W 1983 Human anatomy and physiology. Holt-Saunders, Tokyo

Spence A P, Mason E B 1983 Human anatomy and physiology, 2nd edn. Benjamin/Cumming, Menlo Park, California

Steichen F M, Ravitch M M 1984 Stapling in surgery. Year Book Medical Publishers, Chicago

Storlie F J (ed) 1984 Diseases: nurse's reference library, 2nd edn. Springhouse, Pennsylvania

Sykes M (ed) 1981 Aspects of gastroenterology for nurses. Pitman, London

Tortora G J 1984 Principles of anatomy and physiology, 4th edn. Harper & Row, New York

Urosevich P R (ed) 1984 Performing GI procedures: nursing photobook, 2nd edn. Springhouse, Pennsylvania

Vukovich V C, Grubb R D 1977 Care of the ostomy patient, 2nd edn. Mosby, St Louis

Walker F C (ed) 1976 Modern stoma care. Churchill Livingstone, Edinburgh

Watson J E 1979 Medical-surgical nursing and related physiology, 2nd edn. Saunders, Philadelphia

Journals

Barisonek K, Newman E, Logio T 1984 "My stomach hurts". Nursing 84 14 : 11 : 34–41

Bisacre M (ed) 1983 In: Preston (ed) Insight. Illustrated encyclopaedia of science and the future. Marshall Cavendish, London Pt 1

Brozenec S 1985 Caring for the postoperative patient with an abdominal drain. Nursing 85 15 : 4 : 54–57

Doering K J, LaMountain P 1984 Flowcharts to facilitate caring for ostomy patients: part 1 preop assessment. Nursing 84 14 : 9 : 47–49

Doering K J, LaMountain P 1984 Flowcharts to facilitate caring for ostomy patients: part 2 immediate postop care. Nursing 84 14 : 10 : 47–49

Doering K J, LaMountain P 1984 Flowcharts to facilitate caring for ostomy patients: part 3 recuperative care. Nursing 84 14 : 11 : 54–57

Doering K J, LaMountain P 1984 Flowcharts to facilitate caring for ostomy patients: part 4 discharge outcome assessment. Nursing 84 14 : 12 : 47–49

Ellard J (ed) 1982 Identifying peri-anal problems. Modern Medicine Australia 25 : 3

Feeley J, Wormsley K G 1983 H2 receptor antagonists – cimetidine and ranitidine. In: British Medical Journal 286. February 1983 pp. 695–697

Fleming M 1987 Stomal therapy: an unusual case study. The Australian Nurses Journal 16 : 9 : 39–44

Garnett W R 1982 Sucralfate – alternative therapy for peptic ulcer disease. In: Clinical Pharmacy Vol 1, July–August, 307–314

Gramse C A 1983 Diverticular disease. Nursing 83 13 : 6 : 56–57

Gross L, Bailey Z 1979 Enterostomal therapy: developing institutional and community programmes. Nursing Resources Inc, Massachusetts.

Hartwig M S 1983 Sticking to a gluten-free diet. In: American Journal of Nursing, September, p. 1308

Loustau A, Lee K A 1985 Dealing with the dangers of dysphagia. Nursing 85 15 : 2 : 47–50

Marshall B J, Warren J R 1984 Unidentified curved bacilli in the stomach of patient with gastritis and peptic ulceration. In: Lancet June 16 p. 1311–5

McConnell E A 1987 Meeting the challenge of intestinal obstruction. Nursing 87 17 : 7 : 34–41

Montanari J 1986 Wound dehiscence. Nursing 86 16 : 2 : 33

Nuefeldt J 1987 Helping the IBD patient cope with the unpredictable. Nursing 87 17 : 8 : 47–49

Patras A Z, Paice J A, Lanigan K 1984 Managing GI bleeding: it takes a two-tract mind. Nursing 84 14 : 7 : 26–33

Preston D M 1982 Identifying perianal problems. In: Modern Medicine. 25 : 3 pages 27–30

Ryan S A 1983 Trichinosis. Nursing 83 13 : 10 : 13

Smith C E 1985 Detecting acute abdominal distension: what to look for, what to do. Nursing 85 15 : 9 : 34–39

Sweet K 1983 Hiatal hernia: what to guard against most in postop patients. Nursing 83 13 : 12 : 39–45

Thomson N A 1983 Abdominal trauma. Nursing 83 13 : 7 : 26–33

Tribulski J 1983 Supporting the patient with Crohn's disease. Nursing 83 13 : 11 : 46–51

Wind S, Felice P 1983 Providing ileostomy care. Nursing 83 13 : 11 : 9–10

Wojtklewicz B 1983 Plague. Nursing 83 13 : 8 : 24–25

H

The urinary system

55

Introduction to the urinary system

A. P. Barnett

The normal urinary system comprises 2 kidneys, 2 ureters, a urinary bladder, and a urethra (Fig 55.1). It is the primary function of this system to help maintain homeostasis by eliminating wastes from the body in the form of urine, though the kidneys especially are responsible for a number of other important functions which will be discussed later. This chapter reviews the basic anatomy and physiology of the urinary system and introduces some of the methods used to assess its structure and function.

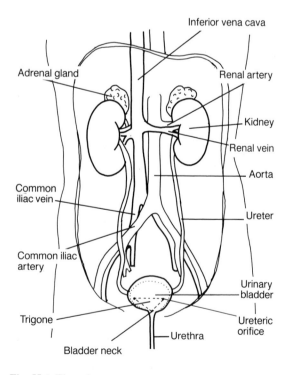

Fig. 55.1 The urinary system.

THE KIDNEYS

The kidneys are retroperitoneal, located on either side of the vertebral column between the twelfth thoracic and third lumbar vertebrae. Both kidneys move downward (1–2 cm) with contraction of the diaphragm during inspiration. This fact is utilised by the renal physician performing a renal biopsy; when the biopsy needle is inserted into the kidney substance it will 'swing' (that is, describe an arc) with ventilation, thereby providing some confirmation of the location of the tip of the needle.

The kidneys are comparatively small, bean shaped organs; the adult kidney is approximately 11 cm in length, 5 cm wide, 2.5 cm thick and normally weighs 120–170 g. The hilus is a notable depression or slit within the medial border and this is the aperture through which various vessels enter and leave the kidney. The kidney presents a smooth outer surface due to the presence of a thin capsule consisting of fibrous tissue which adheres to the parenchyma. Outside this fibrous covering or true capsule, is a layer of adipose tissue known as the perirenal fat. This layer of fat extends some way through the hilus into the renal sinus, and surrounds the renal vessels and the expanded upper end of the ureter. The perirenal fat is enclosed within the renal fascia, a fibrous sheath which assists in maintaining the kidneys' position. Outside the renal fascia is another layer of adipose tissue, the pararenal fat (Fig. 55.2).

A coronal section through the kidney (Fig 55.3) reveals that it may be divided into 3 general regions; the cortex, the medulla, and the renal pelvis. The cortex contains the Bowman's capsules, glomeruli and convoluted tubules of the functional unit of the kidney – the nephron. The

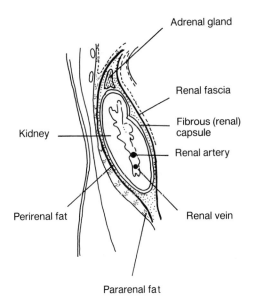

Fig. 55.2 Saggital view of the kidney.

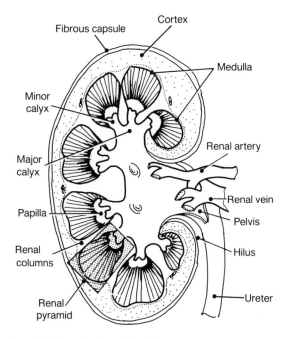

Fig. 55.3 Coronal view of the kidney.

drains urine from the 2 or 3 major calyces found in each kidney.

Nerves and lymphatics. The renal nerves follow and are distributed along the smooth muscle of the renal blood vessels. Predominantly sympathetic efferent fibres, stimulation can cause intense vaso-constriction thus diverting blood flow from the kidney to other organs in time of need. The afferent fibres from the renal pelvis and upper ureter play a role in pain of renal origin. The many lymphatic vessels within the kidney drain into the thoracic duct.

Vasculature. Blood is supplied to the kidney by the renal artery (though there is usually only one renal artery per kidney, multiple renal arteries are not uncommon). The afferent arterioles arise from the smallest divisions of the renal artery – the interlobular arteries (Fig 55.4).

The afferent arteriole travels a short distance then breaks up into a network of glomerular capillaries (these capillaries are collectively referred to as the glomerulus) which reform as the efferent

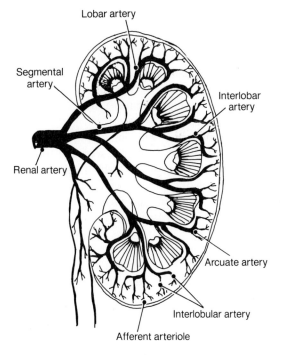

Fig. 55.4 Blood supply to the kidney. The renal substance may be divided into lobes and lobules. The lobes receive blood from the interlobar arteries and the smaller lobules from the interlobular arteries which are derived from the interlobar arteries.

medulla consists of up to 20 cone shaped struc tures, the renal pyramids, which contain the loops of Henle and collecting ducts of the nephron, and the blood vessels which accompany these struc-tures. The renal pelvis is continuous with and arteriole. The efferent arterioles which arise from the majority of glomeruli break up into a network of capillaries which surround the renal tubules. These capillaries are the peritubular capillaries and form the peritubular capillary network. However, the glomeruli situated deep within the cortex (the juxta-medullary glomeruli) give rise to efferent arterioles that break up into long straight capillaries (the vasa recta) as well as a peritubular network. The vasa recta form the major blood vessels of the medulla. Initially they course down the renal pyramids toward the papilla then return back towards the cortex parallelling the loops of Henle and the collecting ducts. Some of the vasa recta arise from 'aglomerular' arterioles situated close to the medulla.

The peritubular capillaries eventually drain into the interlobular veins, and the vasa recta into the interlobular or arcuate veins – these being smaller divisions of the renal vein.

The nephron

The nephron is the microscopic functional unit of the kidney (see Fig 55.5). There are over one million nephrons in each kidney. Though the majority of nephrons arise in the cortex, approximately 15% originate from areas near the junction of the cortex with the medulla. These juxta-medullary nephrons produce a hypertonic urine when necessary.

Anatomically and functionally, the nephron may be divided into 2 distinct sections: the renal (or Malpighian) corpuscle which is primarily concerned with the process of filtration; and the renal tubules which modify the glomerular filtrate through the processes of reabsorption and secretion.

The renal corpuscle comprises the glomerular capillaries and the Bowman's capsule. The glomerular capillaries are held together and arranged around a stalk of specialized connective tissue cells called mesangial cells. Surrounding the glomerulus is Bowman's capsule, a structure consisting of 2 single cell layers of epithelium. The inner or visceral layer is made up of specialized epithelial cells (podocytes) which project pedicles or foot processes onto the basement membrane of the glomerular capillaries. The foot processes of

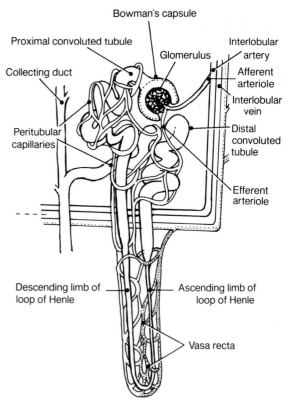

Fig. 55.5 The nephron.

neighbouring podocytes interdigitate, and the small gaps or slit pores between such structures allow small particles to pass quite easily from the glomerular capillaries to the space between the visceral and parietal layers of Bowman's capsule. The space between these structures (the urinary space) witnesses the first step in the formation of urine (Fig 55.6). The glomerular membrane is many times more permeable than most capillaries yet under normal circumstances remains selectively permeable, allowing only smaller particles to pass through easily.

The renal tubules, though microscopic, average approximately 50 mm in length. Continuous with the parietal layer of the Bowman's capsule is the proximal convoluted tubule. Following this is a looped section of the tubule known as the loop of Henle which comprises a descending limb and an ascending limb. Generally, the loops of Henle of the cortical nephrons are shorter than those of the juxta-medullary nephrons which may extend deep into the medulla.

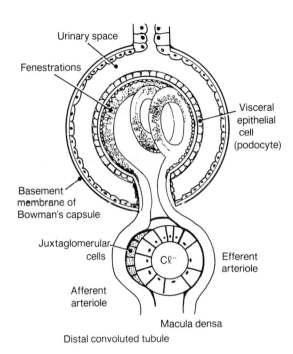

Fig. 55.6 The glomerular and juxta-glomerular apparatus.

As the loop of Henle returns towards its glomerulus, the tubule again becomes convoluted and is called the distal convoluted tubule. Early on in its course, the distal convoluted tubule comes into close proximity with the afferent and efferent arteriole of its glomerulus. In this region some of the tubular cells are columnar and appear more dense than others. These specialized cells are collectively referred to as the macula densa and in some way monitor the concentration of chloride ions in this section of the tubule. The smooth muscle cells of the afferent and efferent arteriole in this region contain granules of the enzyme renin and are called juxta-glomerular cells because of their close proximity to the glomerulus. Together with some extra-glomerular mesangial (or lacis) cells, the macula densa and juxta-glomerular cells constitute the juxta glomerular apparatus, an anatomical area of the nephron which is closely related to the physiology of autoregulation of glomerular filtration rate and blood pressure control (see Fig 55.6)

The distal convoluted tubules of many nephrons are drained by a collecting duct. The collecting ducts pass straight through the cortex and medulla, joining together and eventually forming

the ducts of Bellini which convey urine to the tips of the renal pyramids and thus to the minor calyces and other excretory passageways.

Physiology

The kidneys have major excretory and regulatory functions. By the formation of urine, the kidneys are able to excrete many of the waste products produced by the body and by adjusting the volume and composition of urine, regulate blood pressure and the volume, electrolyte composition and pH of body fluids. The kidneys also produce the erythropoietin (haemopoietin), some prostaglandins, and play a role in the activation of vitamin D.

Formation of urine, excretion of wastes, and conservation of essential substances

The formation of urine has traditionally been described in 3 steps: glomerular filtration, tubular reabsorption, and tubular secretion.

Glomerular filtration refers to the movement of substances (both waste products and substances useful to the body) from the glomerular capillaries to the urinary space of the Bowman's capsule due to a pressure gradient.

The volume of fluid filtered per minute is referred to as the glomerular filtration rate: in the adult it is approximately 120 ml/min in males and a little less in females, though this rate tends to decline with age. The formation of glomerular filtrate depends upon a number of variables:

1. The permeability of the glomerular membrane. The ease with which a substance is able to pass through this membrane is related to its molecular weight. It should be noted however that in certain kidney diseases, the permeability of the glomerular membrane increases, therefore larger sized substances (for example, proteins and blood cells) may be filtered and appear in the urine in significant amounts.
2. The size of the glomerular capillary bed. The surface area has been estimated to be a little less than one square metre for each kidney.
3. The hydrostatic and colloid osmotic pressures within the glomerular capillaries. This is estimated

to be in the region of 60 mmHg and 32 mmHg respectively.

4. The hydrostatic and colloid osmotic pressures within the urinary space of the Bowman's capsule. The hydrostatic pressure has been estimated at 18 mmHg whilst the intracapsular colloid osmotic pressure is negligible due to the lack of plasma proteins in the filtrate. The net filtration pressure can be calculated to be 10 mmHg.

It should be recognized that the major force for glomerular filtration is derived from the hydrostatic pressure of the blood within the glomerular capillaries. Glomerular filtration can be maintained at a rate sufficient to allow for the removal or clearance of waste products from the blood despite quite wide fluctuations in arterial pressure, due to autoregulation. However, if mean arterial pressure should fall below 40–50 mmHg (as in the case of severe haemorrhage or shock) the glomerular filtration rate may fall to zero despite autoregulatory mechanisms, and wastes will be retained by the body.

Tubular reabsorption and secretion follow glomerular filtration in the formation of urine. Both processes occur simultaneously along most parts of the renal tubule and involve either the active transport of substances (for example, the reabsorption of glucose or secretion of hydrogen ions) or the passive movement of substances down a concentration, electrical, or osmotic gradient (for example, the reabsorption of urea, chloride ions, and water).

Under normal circumstances, approximately 99% of the water in the glomerular filtrate is reabsorbed passively along the length of the tubule, a process facilitated by the low hydrostatic pressure within the peritubular capillaries, the active transport of sodium chloride out of the filtrate, and the hypertonicity of the medulla. Approximately 70% of the water is reabsorbed along with the active transport of sodium in the proximal convoluted tubule, 10% in the loop of Henle (primarily by the thin descending limb) and the remainder (19–20%) in the distal convoluted tubule and collecting ducts.

The proximal convoluted tubule actively reabsorbs a large percentage of the electrolytes filtered as well as other substances essential for cellular processes (for example, glucose, amino acids). Because of their large size, the small amounts of protein that are filtered are reabsorbed by pinocytosis. Examples of substances secreted by the proximal convoluted tubule include hydrogen ions, ammonia and some creatinine. The glomerular filtrate eventually leaves this section of the tubule much reduced in volume yet isotonic. As the filtrate passes down the loop of Henle it becomes hypertonic due to the diffusion of sodium chloride into and water out of the filtrate. Upon entering the ascending limb of the loop of Henle, chloride ions are actively (and sodium ions passively) reabsorbed out of the thick portion which, because of its relative impermeability to water, ensures that the filtrate entering the distal convoluted tubule is hypotonic. Within the distal convoluted tubules and collecting ducts, the composition and volume of the filtrate is modified further such that urine leaving the collecting ducts may be hypotonic, isotonic, or hypertonic depending on the fluid and electrolyte needs of the body and the functional integrity of the tubules.

For some substances, the renal tubule's ability to actively reabsorb from or secrete into the filtrate is limited; these substances are said to exhibit a 'transport maximum'. A good example of a substance with a reabsorptive transport maximum is glucose; should the plasma glucose concentration rise too high (for example, with poorly controlled diabetes mellitus), the amount filtered at the glomerulus may exceed the proximal convoluted tubule's ability to reabsorb, thus glycosuria becomes evident. The plasma level at which glucose appears in the urine is referred to as the renal threshold for glucose.

As the filtrate passes along the tubule, it is modified to such an extent that what is excreted represents substances that are either waste products of, or substances no longer required by, the body.

Substances required by the body are effectively reabsorbed and thus conserved, while others may be secreted by the tubular cells or permitted to pass along the length of the tubule as wastes to be excreted. A schematic summary of some of the glomerular and tubular processes involved in the formation of urine appears in Figure 55.7. Table 55.1 shows the typical composition of urine.

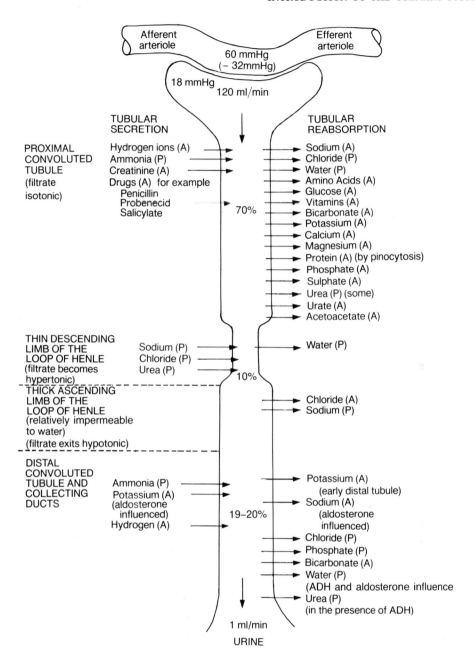

Fig. 55.7 Processes involved in the formation of urine. A = active; P = passive.

Formation of a dilute or a concentrated urine, antidiuretic hormone, and the counter-current mechanism

Whether a person excretes a dilute or a concentrated urine depends to a large extent on the amount of antidiuretic hormone (ADH) circulating in the blood and its effect on the distal convoluted tubules and collecting ducts.

ADH is synthesized in the hypothalamus and stored in the posterior pituitary gland from where its release is stimulated by either an increase in

Table 55.1 Typical composition of urine (in grams excreted per 24 hours)

Urea	30 g
Sodium chloride	15 g
Sulphate	2.5 g
Phosphate	2.5 g
Potassium	3.3 g
Creatinine	1.6 g
Ammonia	0.3 g
Hippuric acid	0.3 g
Uric acid	0.3 g
Calcium	0.3 g
Others	3 g

blood osmolality or volume depletion (for example, due to water loss or large salt intake) sensed by special osmoreceptors located within the hypothalamus.

When released, ADH effectively increases the permeability of the distal convoluted tubules and collecting ducts to water (and to some extent urea), causing these substances to be passively reabsorbed from the filtrate. The primary effects of ADH are therefore to increase circulating blood volume and to reduce blood osmolality by decreasing the volume of urine excreted. Once blood volume and blood osmolality have been restored to normal, ADH secretion is reduced. Conversely, if blood volume should be increased and/or blood osmolality decreased (for example, after drinking a large amount of water), ADH secretion will be inhibited, less water will be reabsorbed from the filtrate and the volume of urine output increased.In the presence of ADH, water is reabsorbed from the filtrate thereby raising the concentration of the remaining solutes and increasing urine osmolality. A reciprocal arrangement is evident in the absence of or with reduced ADH secretion, when the urine volume is increased while the osmolality of the excreted fluid is low. Severe damage to or destruction of the structures involved in the synthesis or storage of ADH will produce diabetes insipidus, a condition characterized by polyuria and polydipsia (see page 237).

A clinical indicator of the concentration of solutes in a specimen of urine is its specific gravity (SG). Under normal circumstances, a direct correlation exists between urine SG and osmolality.

In the formation of a concentrated urine, water moves passively from the tubular lumen of the collecting ducts into the medullary interstitium due to an osmotic gradient. This gradient is initially established by the active transport of chloride ions out of the thick ascending limb of the loop of Henle, positively charged sodium ions passively follow this movement of chloride ions in response to the electrical gradient established by the transport of negatively charged ions across the tubular cell membrane. Because this section of the tubule is relatively impermeable to water, the removal of salts from the filtrate without any loss of water eventually renders the tubular fluid hypotonic.

Once delivered to the medullary interstitium, sodium chloride is free to diffuse into the descending limb of the loop of Henle while water moves out of this limb due to the concentration gradient established. In this way the osmolality of the tubular fluid increases as it passes down towards the papilla. As this process continues, sodium chloride becomes deposited deep within the interstitium of the medulla thereby increasing its osmolality such that the concentration of solutes at the tip of the renal pyramids reaches 1200 mOsmol/l compared to 300 mOsmol/l at the cortico-medullary junction.

The high solute concentration in this area is enhanced by the diffusion of urea out of the collecting ducts into the interstitium in the presence of ADH, and maintained by the flow of blood through the vasa recta which act as counter current exchangers. The vasa recta are freely permeable to both solutes and water, and within their descending limbs water moves out of and solutes (sodium chloride and urea) into the blood in response to concentration gradients. Conversely, as blood flows away from the medulla in the ascending limbs of the vasa recta, solutes move out of and water into them, again along concentration gradients. As well as maintaining the concentration gradient established by the loops of Henle, the vasa recta also remove the excess water and solutes which are added to the medullary interstitium by the loops of Henle and the collecting ducts.

This counter-current mechanism, which ultimately allows for the concentration of urine, entails primarily the long loops of Henle of the juxta-medullary nephrons (Fig 55.8).

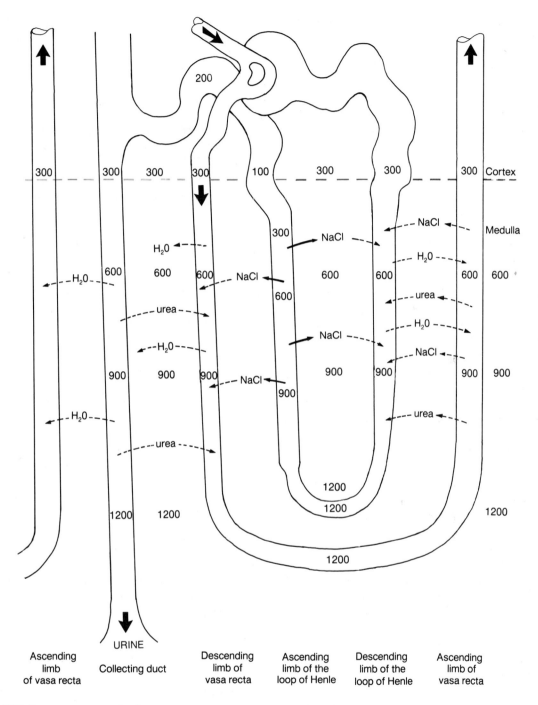

Fig. 55.8 Counter-current mechanism.

Renal regulation of electrolytes, blood pressure and pH

Aldosterone, the principal mineralocorticoid secreted by the adrenal glands, is a major determinant of sodium and potassium concentrations in the extracellular fluids. The adrenal cortex is stimulated to release aldosterone by one or more of:

1. Raised extracellular potassium levels
2. Circulating angiotensin II
3. Decreased extracellular sodium level
4. Adrenocorticotrophic hormone (ACTH).

When released, aldosterone acts primarily on the distal convoluted tubules and collecting ducts causing an increase in the active reabsorption of sodium from the filtrate. With the movement of sodium out of the filtrate an osmotic gradient is established, thus water is also reabsorbed. Accompanying the reabsorption of sodium is the secretion of potassium (and to a lesser extent hydrogen ions) into the filtrate, thus the net effect of aldosterone secretion is to increase extracellular fluid volume, to decrease sodium excretion and increase potassium (and hydrogen ion) urinary losses, thereby reducing the stimuli eliciting its secretion.

In hyperaldosteronism (for example, due to an aldosterone secreting tumour), this negative feedback mechanism is not effective and the condition is commonly characterized by hypertension (due to salt and water retention), hypokalaemia (due to excess potassium urinary loss) and an alkalosis (due to an excessive urinary loss of hydrogen ions). The opposite occurs in hypoaldosteronism (as in Addison's disease) where there is the development of hyperkalaemia, acidosis and a potential problem of shock due to circulatory volume depletion.

Under the influence of parathyroid hormone, the kidneys are able to contribute to the regulation of calcium and phosphate balance. Should plasma calcium levels fall too low, parathyroid hormone is released and acts directly on the renal tubules to increase calcium reabsorption and increase phosphate excretion. Parathyroid hormone also causes the kidneys to increase the rate of vitamin D conversion, thereby enhancing calcium absorp-tion from the intestine and further increasing plasma calcium levels.

The kidneys play a vital role in the regulation of blood pressure by synthesizing and secreting renin in times of need. The juxta-glomerular cells are stimulated to release renin when there is:

1. A decrease in the arterial pressure in the afferent arteriole (for example, due to haemor-rhage, diarrhoea, renal artery stenosis), this decrease in pressure being sensed by the juxta-glomerular cells which act as baroreceptors
2. Decreased chloride ion delivery to the macula densa cells of the distal convoluted tubule due to a reduced glomerular filtration rate
3. Increased sympathetic activity.

When released into the circulation, renin acts on angiotensinogen to form angiotensin I, and this protein is then converted by a converting enzyme in the lungs to angiotensin II. Angiotensin II has a number of major effects which contribute to elevating blood pressure, including measures aimed at increasing circulating blood volume and increasing peripheral vascular resistance. Specifi-cally, angiotensin II stimulates:

1. The release of aldosterone
2. Constriction of arterioles
3. The thirst mechanism
4. ADH secretion.

When afferent arteriolar pressure and glomer-ular filtration rate are restored to normal, renin release is decreased. This important renal mech-anism for regulating blood pressure is referred to as the renin–angiotensin system.

Together with the lungs and the buffer systems in the blood, the kidneys regulate acid–base balance. They are responsible more for the long-term rather than short-term regulation of blood pH, and thus respond more slowly to acid–base changes than the other systems. Because the body's metabolic processes generally result in the formation of an acid excess, which when buffered leads to a depletion of bases, the kidneys are usually required to excrete hydrogen ions and conserve bases, primarily bicarbonate. The processes by which the kidneys accomplish this, and thus regulate pH, are outlined in Chapter 9. Figure 55.9 summarizes the 3 major processes

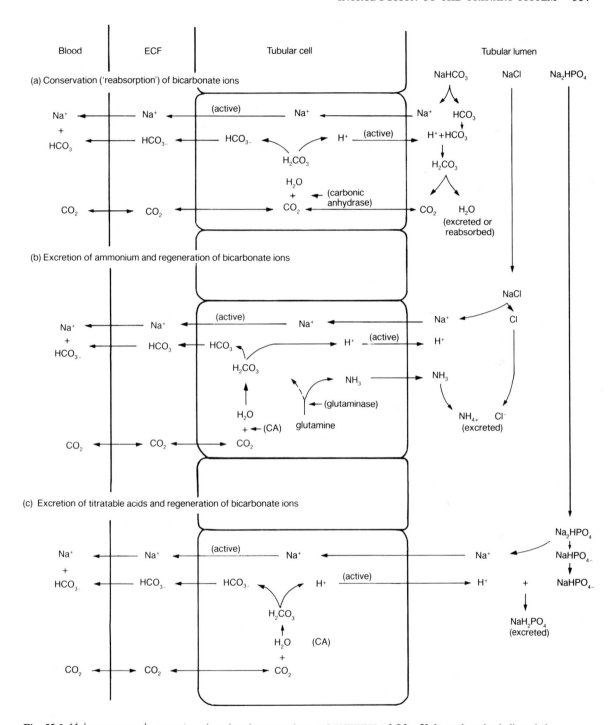

Fig. 55.9 Major processes in excretion of acid and regeneration and regulation of CO_2. Unless otherwise indicated the movement of all substances is passive. The movement of CO_2 from the blood compartment to the tubular cell is favoured when blood CO_2 is elevated.

involved in the excretion of acid and conservation and regulation of bicarbonate by the kidney.

The kidneys as endocrine organs

Though the kidneys are regarded primarily as organs of excretion and regulation, they do have some important endocrine functions. Firstly, they perform the final step in the formation of active vitamin D_3 (calcitriol) from its inactive form. This process is largely under the control of parathyroid hormone since the conversion requires its presence. Secondly, the kidneys are a source of erythropoietin (or a factor which leads to its production), the major stimulus for its release being hypoxia of the renal tissue. Lastly, the kidneys, like many other organs and tissues in the body, synthesize prostaglandins. The prostaglandins have wide ranging effects though in the kidney are thought to increase renal blood flow and have a diuretic effect with an accompanying loss of sodium.

THE URETERS

The ureters are the tubes connecting each kidney to the urinary bladder. They are approximately 25–30 cm long in the adult and pass through both the abdominal and pelvic cavities. The ureter is continuous with the renal pelvis and descends along the posterior abdominal wall retroperitoneally until it crosses the pelvic brim at the bifurcation of the common iliac artery. The ureters enter the bladder at its posterior-lateral base and course through the bladder wall for approximately 2 cm at an oblique angle.

The junction between the ureter and the bladder is referred to as the vesico-ureteric junction and the junction between the renal pelvis and the ureter the pelvo-ureteric junction. At both these points, and in the region where the ureter crosses the pelvic brim, the ureter appears to be more constricted than elsewhere; thus these areas are possible sites for the lodgement of renal calculi. An important feature of the vesico-ureteric junction is that the ureter's oblique entry into the bladder allows its lumen to become constricted when the bladder contracts during micturition,

thereby preventing reflux of urine from the bladder up to the kidneys. The actual ureteric orifices present as slit-like openings on cystoscopy due both to their mode of entry and the fold of mucous membrane which guards the entrances.

The ureters are innervated by both sympathetic and parasympathetic nerve fibres as well as by afferent sensory fibres, the latter being responsible for transmitting the severe pain associated with renal colic. Blood is supplied to the ureters by branches of the renal, testicular or ovarian, and vesical arteries; venous blood is drained into corresponding veins.

Quite narrow in diameter (approximately 0.5 cm), the ureters are composed of an outer layer of fibrous tissue (with some elastic fibres to accommodate distension), a middle layer of smooth muscle, and an inner layer of mucous membrane arranged in longitudinal folds called rugae. This arrangement also allows for distension.

The function of the ureters is to convey urine formed by the kidneys to the urinary bladder by peristalsis. These contractions are initiated as urine accumulates in the renal pelvis thus increasing the pressure within that area. This pressure stimulates waves of muscular contraction which occur at a rate of approximately 2–6/min and are strong enough to overcome quite significant intravesical pressures.

THE URINARY BLADDER AND URETHRA

The urinary bladder is basically a muscular sac which sits below the peritoneum and behind the symphysis pubis in the pelvic cavity. In the female, the uterus is superior to the bladder, an anatomical feature which accounts for at least some of the urinary frequency associated with both pregnancy and the onset of each menstrual cycle, and the vagina is its immediate posterior relation. In the male, the rectum is the major structure lying behind the bladder.

Like the ureters, the bladder is composed of 3 major layers: an outer fibrous coat; a middle layer composed of 3 smooth muscle layers collectively known as the detrusor muscle; and an inner layer of mucous membrane which is arranged in rugae to accommodate increases in vesical urine volume.

(The capacity of the bladder does vary though it usually cannot hold much more than 600–700 ml without discomfort). At the base of the bladder, the mucosa does not form rugae and is firmly attached to the underlying muscle. This triangular shaped area is referred to as the trigone, the 3 points of the triangle being the 2 ureteric orifices and the urethral orifice. The point where the urethra joins the urinary bladder is the bladder neck; around this area the muscle fibres of the bladder form what could be functionally regarded as an internal sphincter, the relaxation or contraction of which is under the control of the autonomic nervous system. The bladder receives its blood supply from the vesical arteries and is endowed with a rich network of lymphatics. The function of the bladder is to store urine until its expulsion from the body via the urethra.

There are a number of significant anatomical differences between the male and the female urethra. The relatively straight female urethra is approximately 3–4 cm long in the adult, much shorter than that of the adult male's which is approximately 15–20 cm in length. The male urethra runs an 'S' shaped course from the bladder neck to the urethral meatus, the proximal 2.5 cm being surrounded by the prostate gland. The female urethra has only an excretory function whilst the male's serves both excretory and ejaculatory functions. As the urethra in the male exits the prostate gland it passes through the urogenital diaphragm, the muscles around this area serving as an external urethral sphincter which is under voluntary control. The corresponding structure in the female is located near the external urethral orifice. In both sexes, the wall of the urethra consists of an inner mucous membrane containing a number of urethral glands and a muscle layer.

Micturition

Micturition involves the coordination of the autonomic and voluntary nervous systems. When filling, the bladder is predominantly under sympathetic control which allows for relaxation of the detrusor muscle and constriction of the internal sphincter. The external sphincter will remain closed due to a learned response until the time and place are appropriate for voiding.

As the bladder fills to around 200–400 ml, stretch receptors located within the bladder wall are stimulated to produce the micturition reflex. Impulses are sent to the conscious portion of the brain which, if the time and place are appropriate, will inhibit the impulses to the external sphincter causing relaxation and (in the absence of obstruction) voiding will commence. The act of voiding can be delayed and the micturition reflex inhibited for a period of time; however as the intravesical pressure increases due to increased urine volume, the micturition reflex will become stronger and stronger and the need to void more urgent. Conversely, even with relatively small amounts of urine in the bladder, the stretch receptors can be stimulated and the micturition reflex initiated by simply holding one's breath and contracting the abdominal muscles (Valsalva manoeuvre), thereby pushing the abdominal contents down onto the bladder, for example, when obtaining a urine specimen.

ASSESSMENT OF THE URINARY SYSTEM

Many of the functions of the urinary system are integrated with and help to maintain other body systems. It is, therefore, necessary that an adequate assessment of this system draws upon data from other systems and that the patient is viewed as a whole. The following assessment procedures represent a brief guide to the assessment of the urinary system.

History

The nurse should obtain a full and accurate history from the patient. In doing this the nurse should be especially sensitive to the cultural and social constraints commonly experienced by some patients, when asked to divulge information or discuss problems associated with the urinary system. Specifically, subjective data from the patient should include reports of any pain or discomfort associated with the kidneys (for example, loin ache or pain), the ureters (for example, 'renal' colic), the urinary bladder (for example, suprapubic pain or a feeling of fullness), or any pain associated with voiding (dysuria).

Changes in voiding patterns of the patient may also provide clues to pathology; questions to elicit information in this regard would include:

– How often does the patient normally void?
– Does the patient have to visit the toilet more often than usual during the day (frequency) or have to get up at night (nocturia)?
– Is there any difficulty in maintaining continence (for example, dribbling, enuresis)?
– Is there any difficulty in starting or maintaining a urine flow?
– Has there been an unusual discharge from the urethra?

Concomitant with possible changes in voiding patterns, the patient should also be questioned about drinking habits (volume and type of fluid), and past history of urinary problems. Subjective data relating to the functioning of other biological and psychosocial systems which may be affecting the patient's health status should be elicited.

Objective data the nurse should obtain during the initial assessment of the patient with urinary problems include observations of body temperature, pulse, blood pressure, and ventilations; the weight of the patient; his hydration status (for example, skin turgour, presence of sacral, orbital, or ankle oedema, jugular vein distension); neurological observations (if neurological dysfunction is suspected); and an assessment of the patient's general physical condition.

Specifically, the skin area around the loin may be observed for the swelling or bruising which may occur following renal trauma, and the physician may, if possible, palpate the kidneys to ascertain their size and shape. If the patient is unable to void, a distended bladder may be palpated as a firm mass above the symphysis pubis. In the case of the patient with a lower urinary tract infection, the urethral meatus will appear red and inflamed and a discharge may be observed.

Analysis of urine

A large number of tests may be performed to assess urinary function and to detect disorders or diseases of the urinary system. One of the most obvious samples required for some form of analysis is urine and the commonest of all the tests performed on urine within hospitals is basic urinalysis. Because the first morning specimen is the most concentrated it is preferred for urinalysis. Urine may also be required for:

• Microscopy to detect the presence of leucocytes, erythrocytes, microorganisms, casts, crystals, or neoplastic cells
• The culture of bacteria present in the urine
• Tests to ascertain the sensitivity of bacteria present to antimicrobials.

Urine may be obtained from the patient in a number of different ways for example, mid-stream specimen of urine (MSU), catheterization of the bladder or ureters, supra-pubic aspiration (SPA), or by drainage of the renal pelvis via a nephrostomy tube or ileal conduit. In all cases it is important that a recognized procedure be adhered to when collecting the specimen.

The other major method of urine specimen collection is a 24-hour collection, a procedure in which all the urine voided by a patient in a 24-hour period is saved. Such collections are useful for quantifying the renal excretion of substances such as electrolytes, proteins, hormones or their metabolites, and creatinine.

Glomerular filtration rate

It is often valuable when managing renal patients to obtain an estimate of their glomerular filtration rate as this is a good overall indication of the kidney's ability to remove (or clear) waste products from the blood.

The value obtained for creatinine clearance is, under most circumstances, a good estimation of glomerular filtration rate because creatinine is freely filtered at the glomerulus and is not reabsorbed by the tubule though a little is secreted.

Concentration and pH of urine

The kidneys' ability to dilute or concentrate urine may be tested by administering a fluid load to the patient which should result in the excretion of a dilute urine; conversely, by imposing a period of water deprivation, the patient should excrete a highly concentrated urine. The kidneys are usually able to excrete urine over a relatively wide pH range, and may be tested by administering an acid load to a patient (for example, ammonium chloride). The urine subsequently voided by a patient undergoing this test should be quite strongly acidic. In cases of distal renal tubular acidosis this will not occur, as in this condition the kidneys are unable to excrete acid.

Blood tests

The measurement of certain constituents of the blood plays a key role in both the assessment of renal function and in monitoring the progress and treatment of patients with renal disease. Two of the more important of these constituents are blood urea and serum creatinine, both of which are used as indicators of glomerular filtration. Urea represents the end product of protein metabolism, thus blood levels can fluctuate quite considerably depending on dietary intake of protein and the rate of endogenous protein catabolism. Blood urea levels, though elevated when there is a reduction in glomerular filtration rate may also be increased in cases of a high dietary intake of protein, severe trauma, or infection, though the increase will be disproportionately high in relation to serum creatinine levels.

Creatinine, on the other hand, is primarily the product of skeletal muscle metabolism and its levels are therefore not influenced by dietary intake. Serial measurements of both urea and creatinine provide one of the simplest and most effective estimates of renal function, though it should be recognized that these levels may not rise above the upper limits of normal until glomerular filtration rate is reduced by up to 50%.

Other blood tests used in the assessment of a patient's renal function include measurements of sodium, chloride, potassium, calcium, phosphate, uric acid, bicarbonate, pH, alkaline phosphatase, total protein, albumin, complement, and immunoglobulins, as well as various haematological studies.

Radiological examination

There are a number of radiological tests and procedures utilized in the assessment of both the

Table 55.2 Radiological examinations of the urinary system

Plain film (of kidneys, ureters and bladder)
Renal ultrasound
Intravenous pyelogram (IVP)
Computerized tomography (CT scan)
Radionuclide studies
Renal arteriogram
Retrograde pyelogram
Retrograde cystogram
Micturating cystourethrogram (MCU)
Retrograde urethrogram
Cystometrogram
Antegrade pyelogram
Percutaneous nephrostomy

structure and function of the urinary system. A list of the more common radiological procedures appears in Table 55.2.

Cystoscopy

A cystoscopy is a relatively common urological procedure involving the insertion of a cystoscope into the urethra in order to visualize the urethra and the inside of the urinary bladder. Within hospitals it is usually performed under a general anaesthetic, but it may be performed under a local anaesthetic providing that the patient is compliant and suitably sedated.

A cystoscopy can be performed for diagnostic or therapeutic reasons. Therapeutically, it may be used in the treatment of bladder neoplasia and the removal of calculi. Diagnostically, it is usually part of a series of tests associated with the investigation of haematuria, recurrent urinary tract infections, or urinary incontinence. Cystoscopy may also be used diagnostically in the assessment of the function of each individual kidney (via ureteric catheterization) obtaining biopsy samples of the bladder wall, and prior to retrograde pyelography. Urinary tract infection usually contraindicates cystoscopy.

If a retrograde pyelogram is to be performed following the cystoscopy, a bowel preparation of some form may be necessary to enhance imaging. In some centres, antibiotics or urinary antiseptics may be ordered for the patient prior to and following cystoscopy to reduce the likelihood of infection.

Renal biopsy

A biopsy of the kidney allows a histological diagnosis of a renal lesion, which will guide the treatment of the disease and aid in determining prognosis. A small cylindrical section of the renal cortex is removed for examination. The material is examined using light microscopy, electron microscopy and immunofluorescent staining techniques. Should the biopsy needle penetrate the renal medulla with its larger blood vessels, the risk of haemorrhage is increased; thus the depth to which the biopsy needle is inserted is critical and needs to be gauged accurately.

A renal biopsy may be performed using a skin puncture technique or an 'open' method in which an incision is made and the lower pole of the kidney exposed. The former method is by far the more common of the two, even though it may carry a greater risk of haemorrhage.

Prior to the biopsy, blood samples should be obtained for coagulation studies to group and cross-match 2 units of blood should haemorrhage occur following the procedure and the patient require a blood transfusion.

The procedure may be performed in the radiology department, operating room, or in the ward treatment room. For safety it is commonly carried out in conjunction with ultrasonography and may be performed in association with a CT scan or following an IVP. Confirmation of the needle position is made radiologically and also by observing the needle for a respiratory 'swing'. Following the biopsy firm pressure is applied to the site for 5–20 minutes to prevent bleeding and a pressure dressing applied. Bedrest is usually recommended for 24 hours and should be continued for a longer period should macroscopic haematuria persist.

A high fluid intake should be encouraged to flush out any blood from the kidney and the urinary tract. All urine should be observed and tested for blood; if there is macroscopic haematuria, 3 consecutive samples of urine should be saved for comparison and the renal physician notified.

The major complication following renal biopsy is haemorrhage and may be recognized by the development of any of the following:

1. Deterioration of vital signs consistent with the development of hypovolaemic shock
2. Macroscopic haematuria
3. Pain, haematoma formation at the biopsy site, or bleeding from the puncture site.

On discharge, the patient should be advised not to lift heavy weights or engage in strenuous exercise for 2–4 weeks, and to seek medical attention immediately should blood be noticed in his urine, or if swelling or pain occur around the biopsy site. Under most circumstances, renal biopsy is a safe and not too uncomfortable procedure for most patients.

56

Urinary tract infection

A. P. Barnett

The urinary tract, except for the lower part of the urethra, is usually free from microorganisms and, unless infected, the urine found within the urinary tract is sterile. A urinary tract infection (UTI) therefore refers to the presence of microbes in any part of the urinary tract and is diagnosed primarily upon finding microorganisms in significant numbers in the urine. The number of bacterial colonies in a specimen of urine is quantified and expressed as colony-forming-units (cfu, or microorganisms) per millilitre. The term 'significant bacteriuria' is used to refer to the presence of more than 100 000 cfu/ml of urine and indicates that there is a high probability that an infection is present, provided that the urine specimen was correctly collected, stored, transported and examined. The presence of bacteria in quantities less than 100 000 cfu/ml does not however rule out the possibility of an infection, and any growth of bacteria from urine obtained by suprapubic aspiration or ureteric catheterization should rate a high index of suspicion.

UTI may be conveniently divided into 2 major groups: upper urinary tract infections (pyelonephritis, pyelitis); and lower urinary tract infections (cystitis and urethritis). Because bacterial infection of the renal pelvis (pyelitis) is rarely documented as a discrete entity and because there is little evidence to support the theory that viruses are the aetiological agents of upper UTI, the only upper urinary tract infection that will be presented for discussion in this chapter will be acute pyelonephritis (a bacterial infection of the pelvis and parenchyma of the kidney). Lower UTI, though commonly caused by bacteria and diagnosed by the presence of a significant bacteriuria, may be 'abacterial'. In these latter cases, the cause of the cystitis or urethritis may be microbes of nonbacterial origin or some irritant (for example perfume sprays, or bath salts). The term 'nonspecific urethritis' (characterized by the symptoms of dysuria and frequency) refers to urethritis of nongonococcal origin which may or may not be caused by a bacterial infection, though the most common cause of this condition is the bacterium *Chlamydia trachomatis*.

INCIDENCE

UTI are prevalent in both community and hospital populations. The incidence of UTI is much higher in females than in males, though the difference decreases with age. Males and females are affected in roughly equal numbers over the 65–70 year old age group (Cameron, 1981; Tiller, 1981). This 'equality' between sexes probably reflects the development of prostatic hypertrophy in later life and the frequency with which males in this age group undergo urethral instrumentation and catheterization.

It has been reported that from 1–12% of all general practitioner consultations are for patients with symptoms of UTI (Forland, 1977; Cameron, 1981; Brooks, 1982), and that 25–35% of women between the ages of 20 and 40 years have had at least one episode of cystitis (Sheahan, 1982). The incidence also appears to be higher in sexually active women who have had children (a phenomenon which may in part be due to the damage done to the pelvic ligaments during childbirth). Other authors have predicted that 10–20% of all females will have a UTI at some time during their life (McConnell & Zimmerman, 1983); for one author, this figure increases to 50% for married women (Uldall, 1977). An even more pessimistic (though probably realistic) view of the prevalence of UTI in women has prompted one urologist to state: 'It is probably true to say that no woman has gone through life without a urinary tract infection at some time or the other' (Hatfield, 1982). On a more optimistic note however, it may be said that lower UTI are more common than the more serious upper UTI.

What has become increasingly clear is that significant numbers of people have had to deal with the problems and disruptions to lifestyle that are frequently associated with UTI, especially recurrent lower UTI. Despite this fact, it would appear that there has been a dearth of information with regard to this type of UTI and it is only in the more contemporary health care literature that the nature and extent of this problem has been recognised and addressed.

One important area in which nurses play a vital role in preventing these infections is in the hospitalized patient. UTI constitute approximately 40% of all nosocomial infections, most of these being related to catheterization or instrumentation of the urinary tract (Meers & Stronge, 1980). On average, 1–2% of these patients develop gram-negative septicaemia (which has a mortality rate of 20–50%), so it must be recognized that such procedures are not without risk. It is therefore imperative that nurses respond to the problem of UTI by adopting effective management and preventive techniques, and utilizing these skills both in the traditional hospital setting and the community.

AETIOLOGY AND PATHOPHYSIOLOGY

A UTI occurs when microorganisms of sufficient virulence gain entry to the tissues of the urinary tract through a defect or deficit in the host's normal defences. An account of the pathophysiology of UTI must therefore consider the types of microorganisms which commonly invade the urinary tract, the portal by which they enter, the normal anatomical and physiological defences which must be overcome, and factors which may lead to defects in these defences.

Microbial causes of UTI

The most common microbiological cause of UTI are the gram-negative bowel flora, the most notable being *Escherichia coli* which is responsible for 50–90% of all UTI. Table 56.1 lists some of the more common causative organisms in roughly descending order of frequency, though it should be recognized that the prevalence of any one type of microorganism will vary from setting to setting and possibly on the age group under study. Also listed are some of the nonmicrobial agents implicated in causing urethritis.

Portals of entry

The most common portal of entry is probably via the ascending route. By gaining access to the external urethral meatus it is possible for microbes to infect the urethra and gain access to the bladder. In males, it is also possible for the prostate gland to become infected; unless adequately treated this infection may serve as a residual source of pathogens leading to recurrent UTI. Should sufficient numbers of microbes gain access to renal tissue by this (or any other) route, acute pyelonephritis will result due to the renal medulla's relative susceptibility to infection. Factors associated with the medulla's higher susceptibility to infection when compared to the renal cortex or other tissues include:

Table 56.1 Urinary tract infections

Causative organisms
Escherichia coli
Klebsiella species
Proteus species
Pseudomonas aeruginosa
Aerobacter aerogenes
Streptococcus faecalis
Staphylococcus aureus
Staphylococcus epidermidis
Candida albicans
Chlamydia trachomatis★
Herpes virus★
Agents implicated in causing urethritis of nonmicrobial origin
Perfumed soaps
Feminine hygiene sprays
Bubble-bath lotions
Spermicidal jellies
Rubber contraceptive devices

★ Associated primarily with urethritis

1. The low blood flow rate in that area (thus the delivery of blood borne defences is reduced)
2. The hypertonicity of the medulla (which tends to inhibit complement activity and phagocytosis).

Though it is apparent that microbes may move in a direction counter to that of normal urine flow, urinary stasis (due to obstruction to the urinary tract) and vesico-ureteric reflux are major contributing factors to the migration of microbes from the bladder to the renal pelvis, and therefore acute pyelonephritis results. Microorganisms may also gain entry via the blood. The kidneys, because of their large blood supply may receive microbes seeded from some other loci of infection. The third postulated pathway is via the lymphatics, though it is unclear how significant a role this particular route plays in the pathogenesis of UTI.

Innate defences

The urinary system has its own local defences which aid in the prevention of infection and, should a lower UTI be present, assist in preventing its spread to the kidneys. Urine itself has antimicrobial properties; changes in urinary pH render it a suboptimal medium for sustained microbial growth. Similarly, the bladder wall is able to produce an antibacterial substance referred to as 'antiseptic paint', and the urethral glands secrete immunoglobulins and other substances which inhibit the growth and multiplication of microorganisms. The flow of urine provides a major defence for the urinary tract, though the efficacy of the mechanism obviously depends on fluid intake, a person's ability to void, and voiding habits. The oblique passage of the distal part of the ureters through the bladder wall normally causes them to become compressed during voiding, thus preventing what may be infected urine passing up to the renal pelvis. In the male, a secretion from the prostate gland, prostatic antibacterial substance, has been identified and demonstrated to be effective against gram-negative bowel flora. In the female, the relative acidity of the vagina during childbearing years helps prevent vaginal colonization by pathogens which would in turn predispose to UTI.

Contributing factors

Despite these defences, pathogens do gain entry and infect the urinary tract. The sex incidence of such infections suggests that there are other important anatomical and physiological factors which should be considered. The first major anatomical difference between the male and female urinary tract which helps explain the sex incidence is the length and course of the urethra: the female urethra, being much shorter and straighter than the male, may provide an easier access for microorganisms to the bladder. The second significant anatomical difference is that in the female, the urethral meatus is in close proximity to the anus, a factor which increases the ease with which transperineal contamination of the urethra with bowel flora may occur. Both of these anatomical features in part underlie the reason why, for some women, attacks of cystitis occur more frequently following, or are associated with, sexual intercourse. It is possible that during coitus there is some trauma to and contamination of the anterior urethra, and that microbes may be massaged from the urethral meatus up the urethra to the bladder by the action of the penis on the anterior vaginal wall. As well as anatomical and mechanical considerations, the presence of prostatic antibacterial substance reduces the likelihood of this occurring in the male.

Pregnant women are a significant 'at risk' group for UTI, though it is unlikely that any single factor can account for this. The enlarging uterus may compress the ureters, preventing complete emptying of the bladder, and the high circulating levels of the smooth muscle relaxant progesterone may allow for dilation of the ureters and predispose to urinary stasis and the development of hydroureter and hydronephrosis. Thus a lower UTI may progress to the more threatening and distressing acute pyelonephritis. For this reason it is usually recommended that pregnant women should be routinely screened for bacteriuria and, if present, the infection should be promptly and effectively eradicated be it symptomatic or asymptomatic.

Table 56.2 lists some selected factors which predispose patients to UTI. The first group of conditions listed are those which predispose to

Table 56.2 Urinary tract infections: predisposing factors

1. Factors which lead to urinary stasis
   Low fluid intake
   General anaesthesia
   Congenital structural anomalies (e.g. horseshoe kidney, duplex ureters, vesical or urethral diverticulum, urethral valves)
   Renal calculi
   Renal papillary necrosis (e.g. as occurs with chronic analgesic abuse)
   Tumours (within the urinary tract or external tumours causing compression to structures of the urinary tract)
   Retroperitoneal fibrosis
   Pregnancy
   Neurogenic bladder (e.g. cerebrovascular accident, spinal injury, paraplegia, quadraplegia, multiple sclerosis, spina bifida)
   Vesical diverticulum associated with urethral obstruction
   Prostatic hypertrophy
   Urethral strictures

2. Vesico-ureteric reflux

3. Conditions which predispose to urethral contamination
   Catheterization and instrumentation
   Coitus
   Faecal incontinence
   Poor perineal hygiene
   Vaginal colonization by pathogens
   Pruritis vulvae

4. Other factors
   Presence of generalized sepsis
   Impaired cellular or humoral defences
   Impaired renal function
   Diabetes mellitus

urinary stasis. Urinary stasis presents a problem in that the small numbers of microorganisms which gain entry to the urinary tract may be provided with the time and conditions in which to multiply and cause an infection, instead of being removed mechanically by peristalsis or the flushing action of voiding.

Congenital abnormalities of the urinary tract may not necessarily predispose to infection, as it is the degree to which the anomaly causes urinary stasis that is of primary concern. For example, a horseshoe kidney (in which the lower poles of the left and right kidneys are fused) may be a benign condition unless it causes the ureters to become kinked when they pass over the fused lower poles of the kidney, thereby causing urinary stasis.

The precipitation of salts out of solution to form calculi, which may become lodged within the renal pelvis, may also cause the stasis of urine; though conversely it should also be remembered that the development of infection within the renal pelvis,

and the subsequent sloughing of necrotic tissue together with bacteria, may provide a nidus for the formation of calculi.

A variety of bladder conditions resulting in problems of micturition and urinary incontinence are conveniently described under the title of 'neurogenic bladder'. Patients with this condition commonly have a higher than normal volume of residual urine due to an inability to empty their bladder completely, unless catheterized or appropriately trained, and it is possible that bacterial populations may thrive within the bladder.

Urethral obstruction, unless relieved, will cause distention of the bladder resulting in a reduction of blood supply to the bladder wall, as well as causing urinary stasis. If prolonged, this will lead to thickening of the bladder wall due to high intravesical pressures and the formation of diverticula from the herniation of the mucous lining through defects in the muscular wall. These diverticula then become filled with residual urine and may serve as foci for infection. Treatment for this condition involves restoring patency to urinary drainage and excising the diverticulum.

Vesico-ureteric reflux is an important abnormality whereby urine from the bladder passes in a retrograde fashion along the ureters to the kidneys during micturition. Should this urine contain microorganisms, renal tissue will become infected and acute pyelonephritis will result. Normally, expulsion of urine from the bladder causes the distal part of the ureters to become compressed. This fails to occur in the case of vesico-ureteric reflux and urine passes up the ureters during micturition, then flows back down the ureters to the bladder following voiding (Fig. 56.1). This results in incomplete emptying of the bladder, a large residual urine and urinary stasis. The problem in patients with this condition is therefore twofold: there is urinary stasis (which predisposes to bacterial growth); and retrograde urine flow (which predisposes to the spread of infection to the kidneys).

Vesico-ureteric reflux is relatively more common in children than in adults (suggesting that the problem resolves itself with age); thus the role of corrective surgery (reimplantation of the ureters into the bladder) as opposed to a more conservative management approach is not clear. In order

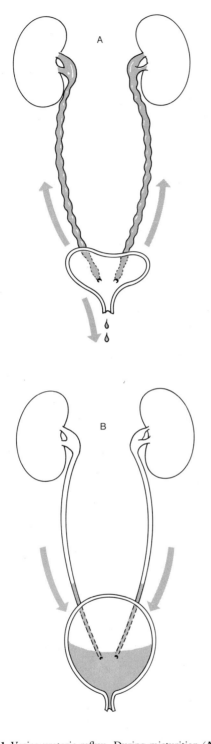

Fig. 56.1 Vesico-ureteric reflux. During micturition (**A**) there is a retrograde flow of urine. After micturition (**B**) urine flows back from ureters into bladder, resulting in a large volume of residual urine.

to prevent renal scarring, however, it is important that measures are taken to prevent UTI in these patients; and, should an infection develop, it should be actively treated.

There are a number of conditions which may lead directly to urethral contamination; in the hospital setting the most obvious of these is catheterization or instrumentation of the urinary tract. Whenever these procedures are performed, it is vital that an aseptic technique is employed to prevent infection. Contamination of the urethra with bowel flora through faecal incontinence is probably a more noticeable factor in the very young or the very old, thus soiled nappies or bed linen should be changed regularly and the perineal area of these patients should be thoroughly cleansed with soap and water.

Poor personal hygiene has been implicated in the pathophysiology of UTI; in females, failure to regularly change underwear or sanitary napkins, and wiping from the anus towards the urethra following bowel actions, have been suggested as possible factors. It would appear that there is no evidence to suggest that tampons are more hygienic than sanitary napkins with regard to the development of UTI during menstruation, and it is probable that regular changes and washing are more important in preventing such infections.

Table 56.2 also lists some other factors which may predispose to UTI. It should be remembered that, whilst patients with impaired renal function or diabetes mellitus may be more prone to UTI, and are frequently 'investigated', the diagnosis of UTI should not preclude consideration of other important clinical causative variables.

CLINICAL MANIFESTATIONS

The clinical manifestations of an acute urinary tract infection generally provide some indication of the site and extent of the infection. An upper UTI usually produces more severe and general manifestations than does a lower UTI, though an acute attack of cystitis may also produce the severe and distressing symptoms more commonly associated with acute pyelonephritis. To complicate matters further, a UTI may also be asymptomatic, these patients being found to have significant bacteriuria only on routine screening.

In the case of urethritis, the symptoms are relatively mild. Dysuria, frequency, and scalding on micturition may be present; a clear, milky-white or purulent discharge from the urethra is common and the meatus may appear inflamed. The male patient with urethritis may also complain of urethral pain when the penis is moved. More severe or general symptoms should suggest that the infection may have extended up the urinary (or urogenital) tract.

The patient with cystitis may present with a variety of symptoms ranging from those associated with urethritis (though a urethral discharge is less common) to more systemic manifestations. Dysuria and frequency are commonly accompanied by urgency, strangury, hesitancy, dribbling (which may develop into enuresis in children or incontinence in the elderly) and nocturia, as well as complaints of suprapubic or lower back pain. The nurse should be empathic in his/her approach to the patient, as the constant desire to urinate, the pain, and the frequent trips to the toilet (especially at night) often results in the person feeling irritable, frustrated, and helpless. If prolonged, cystitis may lead to anorexia and weight loss; recurrent attacks of cystitis have also been cited as a major disruption to interpersonal relationships.

Acute pyelonephritis may evoke many of the problems associated with cystitis. The patient with this condition is usually very sick and is frequently hospitalized. Pyrexia with accompanying chills and rigors is usually a dominant feature until appropriate antibiotic therapy is instigated. There is loin pain on the affected side and the patient will feel listless, anorexic, and often nauseous. Headaches and joint pain may be reported and the patient may become septicaemic.

Observation of the urine of the patient with an acute UTI reveals bacteriuria, pyuria, and there may be some haematuria; the urine is commonly cloudy and foul smelling. When tested for pH, the urine may be alkaline due to the presence of urea splitting bacteria, and some protein could be present if there is additional renal involvement.

Figure 56.2 shows some of the major problems associated with UTI. The listing does not represent a rigid order, as an episode of cystitis may also produce those symptoms and signs listed for acute pyelonephritis. The listing does however draw attention to the notion that as an infection ascends the urinary tract, it is usually accompanied by more severe symptomatology. It should also be recognized that an upper UTI often causes those problems listed alongside cystitis and urethritis in Figure 56.2.

INVESTIGATIVE PROCEDURES

Should a UTI be suspected a ward urinalysis (to observe for odour, transparency, and to detect the presence of blood, protein, and nitrite), an MSU, and, in cases of a urethral discharge, a urethral swab must be performed. The latter 2 procedures allow for the specimen to be microscopied and cultured for pathogens and to ascertain the sensitivity of any microbes present to specific antibiotics. The collection of the urine specimen should be complemented by obtaining a full history from the patient which may elucidate the aetiology of the condition and guide the selection of appropriate interventions. If an MSU cannot be obtained from the patient, in some circumstances a catheter may be introduced aseptically for this purpose or a suprapubic aspirate obtained.

A number of methods have been utilized to help identify the site of infection and if a sterile specimen of urine is obtained from a suprapubic catheter in a patient from whom a continiminated urethral specimen was colected, it would indicate an infection of the urethra rather than of the bladder or kidney. A suprapubic specimen also reduces considerably the amount of contamination which may occur in the collection of an MSU, thus it is of greater diagnostic significance.

Other tests to determine the exact location of the infection are available, but are less likely to be performed because of their prohibitive cost. More practically, sophisticated investigations are rarely performed because, whatever its location, an infection exists and the patient exhibiting symptoms requires treatment for it. The treatment for any UTI is basically similar.

Other investigative procedures that may be performed include a plain abdominal X-ray, an

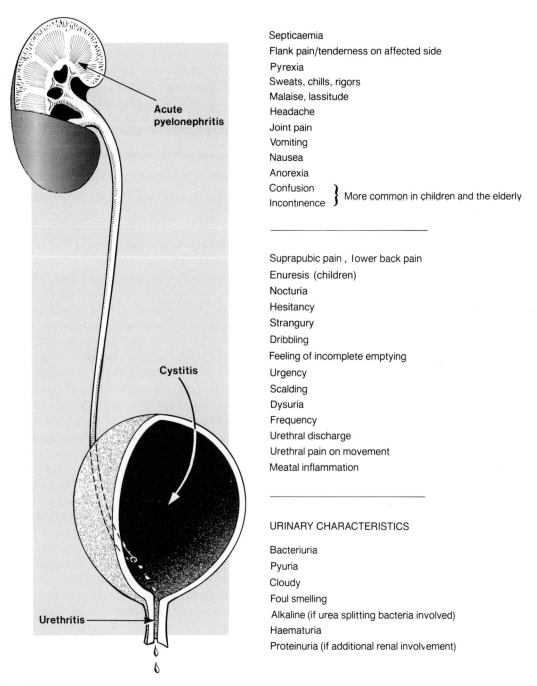

Septicaemia
Flank pain/tenderness on affected side
Pyrexia
Sweats, chills, rigors
Malaise, lassitude
Headache
Joint pain
Vomiting
Nausea
Anorexia
Confusion
Incontinence } More common in children and the elderly

Suprapubic pain , lower back pain
Enuresis (children)
Nocturia
Hesitancy
Strangury
Dribbling
Feeling of incomplete emptying
Urgency
Scalding
Dysuria
Frequency
Urethral discharge
Urethral pain on movement
Meatal inflammation

URINARY CHARACTERISTICS

Bacteriuria
Pyuria
Cloudy
Foul smelling
Alkaline (if urea splitting bacteria involved)
Haematuria
Proteinuria (if additional renal involvement)

Fig. 56.2 Major problems associated with UTI.

IVP, and following the acute infective episode, a micturating cystourethrogram. These investigations are performed primarily to detect structural defects or changes in the urinary tract, and to detect vesico-ureteric reflux. If the patient is hyperpyrexic, blood cultures should also be taken in order to exclude septicaemia, the major complication associated with acute pyelonephritis.

To fully investigate all patients who present with a UTI would be both unwarranted and costly, although it is essential to obtain a MSU and/or urethral swab. The major group of patients for whom more extensive investigation of UTI is warranted include: infants, males below the age of 50–60, women with recurrent UTI, and any patient with acute pyelonephritis.

CHRONIC PYELONEPHRITIS

Chronic pyelonephritis as a specific disease entity has been something of an enigma. On an IVP, the kidneys of patients with this disease are usually small and scarred; there is an irregular renal outline, a reduction in cortical thickness, and the calyces are deformed. The patient may or may not have a history of previous UTI, and on examination there may be no evidence of a current infection. It is probable that chronic pyelonephritis is a disease which originates in childhood with a combination of severe vesico-ureteric reflux and infection producing renal scarring (for example, reflux nephropathy).

Patients with this disease may therefore present with an acute UTI or as the renal damage progresses, may present with hypertension, nocturia, and polyuria. An examination of the urine reveals a sterile pyuria. The management of these patients is aimed at treating any underlying infection (if present), and conserving renal function. In some patients, renal function continues to deteriorate, thus ultimately dialysis and/or renal transplantation is necessary to preserve life.

TUBERCULOSIS OF THE URINARY TRACT

Infection of the urinary tract by *Mycobacterium tuberculosis* is not common. The organism spreads via the blood from the primary site of infection (for example, the lung) to the urinary tract where it may produce the symptoms of a UTI. Suspicion is aroused because of the resistance of the infection to conventional therapy. The disease may also be associated with recurrent epididymitis, orchitis, or prostatitis; the most common urinary abnormalities found are pyuria and haematuria.

Tuberculosis of the urinary tract is diagnosed by identifying the causative organism in the urine; this usually requires serial specimens of urine to be collected from the patient. The tuberculin skin test in most cases of the disease is positive. Treatment of this condition includes antitubercular drugs being administered to the patient over an extended period of time (see page 357).

MEDICAL AND NURSING MANAGEMENT OF UTI

The treatment of a patient with a UTI is largely determined by the site of infection and the severity of the symptoms. Most cases of urethritis can be managed and reviewed on an outpatient basis or from a clinic, whilst patients with acute pyelonephritis are usually hospitalized. Generally, in uncomplicated cases, the major symptoms of a UTI (frequency, pain, and pain on micturition) can be relieved within hours of initiating appropriate therapy. In some cases of urethritis and cystitis the symptoms may undergo spontaneous remission. Not all cases of significant bacteriuria may require treatment; it is thought that, in the absence of any significant urinary tract abnormality, the treatment of asymptomatic bacteriuria in nonpregnant women is probably unwarranted.

Prior to the treatment of the patient with a UTI, an MSU must be taken and swabbing of the urethral meatus performed.

Bacterial urethritis is probably the easiest of all UTI to manage, if it is not complicated by an infected prostate gland. The patient is advised to refrain from sexual intercourse for a 1–2 week period to avoid spreading the infection to a sexual partner.

For the patient with UTI, antimicrobial therapy may be started immediately following collection of the urine specimen (and blood culture specimen if the patient's temperature is elevated and acute pyelonephritis is suspected) and reviewed accordingly when sensitivity patterns are available.

Table 56.3 lists some of the more common antibiotics and urinary antiseptics currently used to treat UTI. Patients with cystitis may be prescribed a course of antibiotics or urinary antiseptics, though single-dose or 'one-shot' therapy has been found to be equally effective and offers the advantage of better patient compliance. With this method of treatment, patients are required to take just one dose of the prescribed drug (for example, amoxycillin 3 g, or co-trimoxazole 2–5 g) rather than a full course.

In many cases of UTI 7–10 day high dose courses, with an initial loading dose of the specific antibiotic may be used in preference to any other regimes.

Follow-up cultures of urine are carried out 2 weeks, 6 weeks, and then 3-monthly for 1 year following commencement of antibiotic therapy to evaluate effectiveness.

In patients with acute pyelonephritis it is common to insert an IV line to administer the antibiotic and thereby achieve therapeutic levels of the drug more rapidly. For these patients, a 5–10 or 7–14 day course of antibiotics is usually prescribed; the IV or IM form is replaced by the oral form of administration as the infection becomes controlled.

When administering antibacterials to patients with UTI, it is often necessary to adjust the pH of the urine to achieve maximum effectiveness or to prevent the unwanted side-effects of the drug. Generally, the urine should be made alkaline when using sulphonamides or the aminoglycosides, and

acidic when using methenamine compounds. Alkalizing of the urine may assist in relieving pain on micturition.

Caution should also be employed when administering drugs to patients with renal impairment, in order to prevent toxicity or further deterioration in renal function. For this reason, serum levels of the antibiotic may be taken so that the dosage can be adjusted accordingly. The effectiveness of the antibacterial agent is determined by obtaining an MSU from the patient at regular intervals for microscopy, culture, and sensitivity testing. If the drug is effective, the bacteriuria will diminish and the symptoms will abate.

Diet

Patients with UTI are encouraged to maintain a fluid intake of at least 2–3 litres per day in order to assist in the mechanical removal of bacteria and debris from the urinary system, and to reduce the risk of dehydration if there is an excessive loss of fluid due to vomiting or sweating. Further, there is a technique described as 'oral' bladder washout in which the patient drinks 1.5 l of fluid over a 20 minute period; this produces a massive flushing effect of the urinary system. This is usually performed only once and is most effective when commencing antibiotics.

A fluid balance chart should be maintained in the patient with acute pyelonephritis to assist in maintaining input and monitoring output. Such patients often do not feel able to drink copious amounts of fluids and may be nauseated, therefore a large percentage of their fluid and electrolyte intake, at least in the short-term, may be by the IV route. A nutritious diet should be encouraged if tolerated by the patient and, if required, the administration of an antiemetic half an hour before meals may aid in relieving the nausea or vomiting and may help to improve dietary intake.

Specific nursing management

The nurse will be responsible for managing a patient who, depending upon the severity of the UTI, may be: pyrexic; in pain; anorexic; nauseated and/or vomiting; and experiencing the distressing symptoms of dysuria and frequency. The patient will be required to have a large fluid

Table 56.3 UTI drugs classified by mode of action

Antibacterial agents
  Antibiotics
    Sulphonamides
    Co-trimoxazole
    Ampicillin or Amoxycillin
    Penicillin
    Aminoglycosides
    Tetracyclines
    Nalidixic acid
  Urinary antiseptics
    Nitrofurantoin
    Hexamine mandelate
    Hexamine hippurate
Urinary alkalizers (used in conjunction with sulphonamides and aminoglycosides)
    Sodium citro-tartrate
Urinary acidifiers (used in conjunction with methenamine compounds)
    Ammonium chloride
    Ascorbic acid
Urinary analgesics
    Phenazopyridine

intake along with high doses of antibiotics. In nearly all cases of urethritis and cystitis the person is managed at home.

Pyrexia should be managed by the implementation of appropriate fever care. Should the patient feel tired and lethargic, bed rest should be encouraged as this will also reduce metabolic demands.

A narcotic analgesic may be needed to relieve the loin pain associated with acute pyelonephritis; milder oral analgesics may be used if effective, though it should be noted that patients with cystitis may also have severe pain requiring a strong form of analgesia. Heat may be applied as an adjuvant to relieving pain in the patient with cystitis. Administration of the urinary analgesic phenazopyridine may relieve dysuria to some degree, and patients receiving this drug should be warned that it stains the urine red or orange for the duration of the treatment.

The urinary symptoms, dysuria and frequency, are usually the most distressing for the patient. If hospitalized, the patient should have ready access to toilet facilities or a clean bedpan or urinal. A call bell should be within reach should assistance be required and, at night, staff should ensure that the night lights are switched on – especially if the patient is ambulant and is able to visit the toilet. The patient will require reassurance that these urinary symptoms will abate in 2–3 days, if not sooner, after instigation of antibacterial therapy.

Some authorities recommend the use of urinary alkalizers to relieve dysuria, though whether a urinary alkalizer or acidifier is used should be primarily determined by the choice of antibacterial administered to the patient. There is an inherent danger in recommending the widespread use of a urinary alkalizer. A patient who has an attack of cystitis at home may gain symptomatic relief by taking a glass of sodium bicarbonate solution at regular intervals, and may not seek medical advice, believing that with the disappearance of symptoms the infection has been cured. This may in fact be far from the truth, and there is a danger that the infection may worsen; thus it must be stressed that medical attention should be sought if the symptoms or signs of a UTI arise.

The patient on oral antibiotics should be advised to empty his bladder just before sleep so that the concentration of antibiotic that rests in the bladder overnight is at its maximum. The patient

with pyelonephritis will require monitoring of vital signs in order to gain some indication of his response to treatment and to monitor for the development of complications. The short-term complications of acute pyelonephritis include: septicaemia (and thus the potential problem of septic shock); dehydration; and (rarely) acute renal failure. To assess for the development of acute renal failure, regular blood tests for urea and creatinine may be performed, and the volume of urine output is closely monitored. A longer-term problem is that of 'chronic pyelonephritis' and progression to end-stage chronic renal failure (see page 595).

The patient should also be assessed for pain and discomfort, and the effectiveness (and possible side effects) of all drugs given. A urinalysis is usually performed daily to provide a rough indication of the patient's progress.

Recovery is generally the rule following an episode of either cystitis or acute pyelonephritis, and there is usually no permanent impairment of renal function; however, recurrence of UTI following an attack of acute pyelonephritis is common. It is therefore important to investigate such patients in order to identify and correct (if possible) any underlying abnormality or factor that may be predisposing him to infection, and to maintain close patient follow up after discharge.

Discharge advice for the patient hospitalized with an acute UTI should include:

1. Ensure that the full course of the prescribed antibacterial is taken, even though the symptoms may have abated. This will ensure that all pathogens are eradicated and may reduce the likelihood of antibiotic-resistant organisms developing.
2. Seek prompt medical attention should any of the symptoms or signs of a UTI reappear.
3. Maintain a high fluid intake (2–3 l/day) to promote urinary lavage.
4. Maintain regular contacts with the physician in order that follow up MSU specimens may be taken for analysis to monitor for possible recurrence of the infection.

For a significant group of women, UTI consistently recurs, despite the fact that no underlying structural or functional abnormality can be found. If such attacks are symptomatic (characterized by frequency, dysuria, and urgency), these patients may tend to limit their fluid intake in an attempt to relieve the need to void frequently. There will be disruptions to their work and social life, and long meetings, theatre visits, car trips, shopping expeditions, and sexual intercourse will be

Table 56.4 Selected preventive measures for female patients with a history of recurrent urinary tract infection

Drug therapy

If any of the signs and symptoms of a UTI or vaginitis appear, seek prompt medical treatment

Be sure to take the full course of antimicrobials if prescribed

If other measures fail, take a prescribed urinary antibiotic or antiseptic at night after voiding. (Taken at night, the agent will remain in the urine for a longer period than if taken during the day.)

Voiding and drinking habits

Drink copious amounts of fluids each day (at least 2–3 litres) to promote flushing of bacteria from the urinary tract

Do not ignore the urge to pass urine and try and void every 2–3 hours

If urinary reflux has been identified or is suspected of being present, use a 'double-void' technique when visiting the toilet. Wait for 1/2 to 1 minute after first voiding, then try again. This will reduce the amount of residual urine left in the bladder

Personal hygiene

Wash hands before and after going to the toilet

Wash the perineal area at least daily, and dry well

Maintain good menstrual hygiene

Wipe from front to back following bowel actions

Wear cotton rather than nylon underwear to minimize moisture around the perineum, and change underwear regularly

Avoid wearing tight jeans or pantyhose, as they may irritate the urethral meatus and encourage dampness

If pantyhose are to be worn, wear those with a cotton gusset

Showers are preferred to baths because there is less risk of bacteria gaining access to the urethra via the dirty water

Avoid the use of possible urethral irritants, such as bubble baths, perfumed soaps, or vaginal spray

Sexual intercourse

If coitus is a major precipitating factor to urinary tract infections, then consideration should be given to the following measures:

• Drink 1–2 glasses of water following sexual intercourse and void immediately. This will flush any bacteria which may have gained access to the urethra or bladder from the urinary tract during intercourse.

• Take a prescribed urinary antiseptic prior to intercourse. Encourage adequate foreplay and/or use a non-irritant lubricant to minimize trauma.

curtailed or avoided due to the unfortunate symptomatology of their infection. The nursing challenge when managing such patients is therefore primarily in the arena of preventive health care and in supporting them should attacks occur. Table 56.4 lists some of the measures which these patients may take to try to prevent the recurrence of their UTI. The list is extensive, therefore the nurse should obtain a full history from the patient in order to identify those measures which are appropriate and most easily introduced to the individual's lifestyle.

Management of catheter associated UTI

As noted previously, catheter associated UTI represent a significant proportion of all nosocomial infections. Although it is likely that any patient

Table 56.5 Nursing management of patients with indwelling urinary catheters

– Use the smallest sized catheter possible (to help reduce urethral trauma during insertion and tissue necrosis when in place)
– Use a catheter with the smallest possible balloon (to help reduce urinary stasis)
– Adhere to aseptic techniques when inserting the catheter and connecting the drainage system
– Use a sterile, closed drainage system
– Secure the catheter to the patient's leg with tape to prevent movement and urethral traction
– Wash hands before and after contact with a patient's catheter or drainage system
– Maintain the drainage bag and tubing below the level of the patient's bladder to allow urine to drain by gravity
– Perform soap and water catheter/perineal toilets bd and prn
– Check regularly that the connections are tight and that the catheter or drainage tube is not kinked
– Do not disconnect the catheter and drainage tube unnecessarily
– Avoid clamping the catheter or drain line for extended periods
– Unless contraindicated, encourage a copious fluid intake
– Do not let the drainage bag fill completely, empty prn
– When emptying urinary drainage bags:
    i) use a clean receptacle for each patient, do not empty more than one drainage bag into the same (unemptied) container
    ii) wash hands before and after the procedure and also between patients
    iii) clean the drainage bag outlet with a disinfectant before and after emptying the drainage bag
Obtain catheter specimens of urine required for microbiology from the rubber specimen port on the drainage line using a small gauge needle and syringe. *Do not* collect microbiology specimens directly from the drainage bag outlet or by disconnecting the catheter and drainage line.

with a long term indwelling urinary catheter will at some time have bacteriuria, every effort should be made to minimize the risk of any patient with an indwelling urinary catheter from acquiring an infection. If a bacteriuria develops it may become symptomatic causing unnecessary distress to the patient, or may spread causing septicaemia.

One of the most important measures that can be taken to guard against infection is handwashing before and after contact with these patients or their catheters and drainage systems. If an infection does occur, it is useful to separate or isolate the patient from other patients with urinary catheters. This will increase the likelihood of staff washing their hands before and after contact with patients, and reduce the risk of the same drainage receptacle being used to empty more than one drainage bag without it being adequately cleaned or sterilized between patients.

Symptomatic UTI in catheterized patients is treated with a course of the appropriate antimicrobial. It is less likely that catheterized patients who are asymptomatic will be treated, because of the high rate of recurrence unless the catheter is removed. Management aims should therefore be: catheterize patients only when absolutely necessary; remove the catheter as soon as possible (or utilize some other form of urinary drainage device); and practice techniques aimed at preventing infection. Table 56.5 identifies nursing guidelines which should be observed when caring for patients with indwelling urinary catheters.

57

Trauma to the urinary system

A. P. Barnett

The major single cause of trauma to the urinary tract is motor vehicle accidents. As the number and severity of such accidents increases, health care centres should expect to be confronted by more patients with this type of traumatic injury. It is not unusual for motor vehicle accident victims to present with multiple injuries, thus nursing and medical care is often directed to managing the 'multiple trauma' patient. In these cases, trauma to the urinary tract is commonly accompanied by fractures (for example, pelvis, ribs, vertebral column, and limbs), lacerations, and various internal injuries. For this reason, urinary tract trauma may go unsuspected for some time, not being noticed until the patient fails to respond fully to interventions aimed at his more obvious injuries.

It is important that as complete a history as possible be obtained from the trauma victim or an accompanying witness on arrival to the health care facility. A knowledge of the nature of the insult will often guide the clinician to the most probable area(s) of damage thereby saving time and enhancing recovery by assuring that the most appropriate interventions are taken.

As noted in Chapter 55, the structures of the urinary tract are relatively well protected. The kidneys with their surrounding layers of fat and fascia are also afforded protection posteriorly by a number of muscles and posteriosuperiorly by the ribs. Anterior to the kidneys are the abdominal organs. The ureters course along the posterior abdominal wall for some distance thus are protected by the muscles of the back and then, as they pass over the pelvic brim, they are protected by the pelvic girdle. The urinary bladder, unless full, sits safely within the pelvic cavity and is surrounded by bony structures; though the urethra in the male, because of its length and fixation, is comparatively unprotected and thus more vulnerable to trauma than that of the female.

Despite these anatomical defences, traumatic injuries to the urinary tract do occur and though not usually life-threatening by themselves, can present a number of short- and long-term problems for the patient and for the health care team. This chapter will discuss the management of patients with trauma to the kidneys, ureters, urinary bladder, and urethra.

Incidence

Injuries to the kidney account for the largest percentage of traumatic injuries to the urinary tract. Most renal injuries are seen in males. Renal injury occurs most often in the 20–30 year old age group.

Although 80% of renal injuries are minor, associated injuries may occur in up to 80% of all renal trauma cases and in 20–30% of cases there is serious injury to other parts of the body (Campbell 1983, McConnell 1983, Mendez 1977).

Damage to the ureter is rare and practically all urethral injuries occur in males (McConnell, 1983). The incidence of injuries to the bladder, urethra, or both, associated with pelvic fractures has been reported to be 13.5% (Palmer et al, 1983) and approximately 10% of male patients with pelvic fractures have some form of traumatic disruption of the prostateomembranous portion of the urethra (Webster et al, 1983).

RENAL TRAUMA

Renal injuries may be conveniently subdivided into two major groups depending on their cause (Fig. 57.1). The first group of injuries are those caused by penetrating trauma (open injuries). Examples of penetrating injuries include gunshot and stab wounds where a foreign object has entered through the skin and caused direct damage to the kidney or its blood vessels. The second group of injuries are those caused by blunt or nonpenetrating trauma (closed injuries) and are responsible for 60–70% of all renal trauma (Mendez, 1977). In these cases, the cause may be either:

1. Direct, where the kidney is crushed between an external force and some internal structure, for example back muscles, vertebrae, or ribs. These latter structures under some circumstances may be fractured and penetrate the kidney.
2. Indirect, where the kidney is torn from its pedicle due to a severe deceleration effect, for example, as seen in motor vehicle accidents.

Renal trauma may also be classified according to the type of injury sustained by the kidney (Fig. 57.2). The mildest of these is a contusion. With contusion injuries, bleeding occurs within the renal parenchyma but the haemorrhage is usually contained by the renal capsule and blood does not escape to the perirenal areas. The renal capsule may therefore help to limit the spread of blood and contribute to haemostasis. The kidney

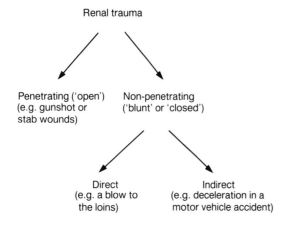

Fig. 57.1 Causes of renal trauma.

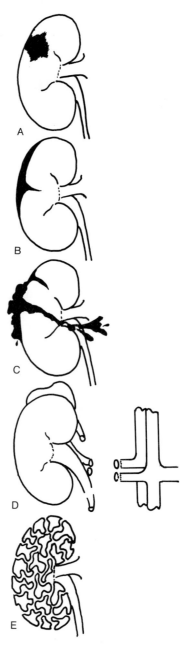

Fig. 57.2 Types of injury sustained by the kidney. **A** – Contusion. **B** – Laceration. **C** – Laceration with extravasation of blood and urine. **D** – Division of renal pedicle. **E** – Pulpefaction of kidney.

may also be lacerated. Lacerations to the kidney may either be minor, for example, with the development of a perirenal haematoma; or major, where there is damage to the parenchyma and pelvis of the kidney and extravasation of urine and blood. The most serious of renal injuries are those involving injury to the major blood vessels as may occur with a stab wound or division of the renal pedicle due to rapid deceleration, and a 'shattered' or pulpefacted kidney where the kidney is fractured into many segments. For these types of injuries, major surgery is usually indicated and if the damage is irreparable a nephrectomy is performed.

Clinical manifestations

The clinical manifestations are varied and depend on the nature and extent of the injury. The most common sign is that of either macro or microscopic haematuria, macroscopic haematuria being present in approximately 80% of all renal trauma patients. The absence of haematuria does not however rule out the possibility of renal trauma, since the renal pedicle may be divided or the ureter disrupted; thus blood may not be conveyed to the bladder. Another common manifestation of renal trauma is that of pain in either the loin or abdomen; the pain may be described as severe, aching, dragging, dull, or colicky (possibly due to the passage of blood clots down the ureter) and may be associated with nausea.

In some cases there may be noticeable abdominal distention or an increase in girth measurements if these are performed serially. Excluding possible damage to the abdominal viscera with resulting fluid leak, the probable cause for this is extravasation from the injured kidney: blood and/or urine collects in the retroperitoneal space causing the abdominal contents to be pushed anteriorly. Another consequence of this extravasation is that it may restrict lung expansion by compressing the diaphragm.

Approximately one-third of all patients with renal trauma present with accompanying shock.

Patients may, however, be asymptomatic or the manifestations of renal damage may be overridden by other more obvious or severe injuries.

Investigative procedures

Urinalysis is the easiest and most valuable investigative procedure and the nurse should observe and test for the presence of blood.

Radiological investigations include intravenous pyelogram to assess the extent of the injury and to confirm (in the case of trauma to only one kidney) the presence and function of the other; it is usually preceded by a plain abdominal film. Other radiological investigations include renal arteriogram, CT scan, and a retrograde pyelogram.

Blood may be obtained for haemoglobin and haematocrit estimations and sent to be grouped and cross-matched should a blood transfusion be required.

Medical, surgical, and nursing management

The management of patients with renal trauma is in part guided by the extent of their injuries, though the broad aims of any intervention are to control haemorrhage, preserve as much renal substance and thus renal function as possible, relieve symptoms, promote healing, and aid recovery.

For most cases of renal trauma, a conservative approach is taken because most patients have contusions or minor lacerations of the kidney, problems which usually resolve without the need for surgical intervention. Total bed rest is mandatory until vital signs are stable and haematuria resolves (or at least becomes microscopic). The patient should be observed for the early signs of reactionary haemorrhage. By resting in bed, the patient will minimize further trauma to the kidney and promote haemostasis. This may take several days, thus nursing care should be aimed at preventing the complications associated with immobility. Once the patient's condition has improved, ambulation should proceed in gradual stages, the patient being warned to avoid straining or lifting as this may precipitate a reactionary haemorrhage.

The patient should be assessed regularly for the type and severity of pain, and a suitable analgesic administered if necessary. For some patients a sedative may also be required to promote rest.

The loin area is observed at least TDS for swelling and bruising, and daily girth measurements may be taken if continued intra-abdominal or retroperitoneal extravasation is suspected. All urine voided by the patient is collected and observed or tested for blood. If the haematuria is macroscopic, it is common to save three consecutive samples in clear specimen containers to compare the colour between specimens, and thereby gain an indication of whether the bleeding is decreasing or increasing. Blood specimens are taken from the patient at regular intervals to assess haematocrit and haemoglobin levels, and if a deterioration in renal function is suspected, blood levels of urea, creatinine and various electrolytes will be ascertained. The patient should be observed for the development of shock and infection.

Unless contraindicated and if tolerated, patients are encouraged to have a liberal fluid intake with the aim that this might help maintain renal function and prevent clotting and urinary tract infection.

Immediate or delayed surgical intervention is usually reserved for severe renal damage and is used only for approximately 10–20% of patients. The aim of surgery is to arrest haemorrhage and to salvage as much renal tissue as possible. The type of surgery will range from a simple exploration and drainage and/or suturing of tears, through to a partial or total nephrectomy. Removal of the kidney is usually reserved for critical injuries involving the renal pedicle or in cases of the kidney being shattered.

Indications for surgery in cases of renal trauma include: penetrating injuries to the kidney; continuing, uncontrollable blood loss; severe injuries resulting in extravasation of urine; injury to the renal pedicle; and evidence suggesting the development of a perinephric abscess.

The prognosis for patients with uncomplicated renal trauma is usually good, providing haemorrhage is controlled.

Complications

Complications which may occur as a result of renal trauma include: haemorrhage, shock, infection, and acute renal failure (rare). Longer term complications include hypertension (probably as a result of renal ischaemia and stimulation of the reninangiotensin system) and persistant haematuria.

Specific discharge advice should be directed toward warning the patient to avoid heavy lifting or straining for several weeks. Patients should be advised to seek prompt medical attention should they notice what may be blood in their urine.

TRAUMA TO THE URETER

Trauma to the ureter is a rare occurrence. Trauma may be caused by external violence though the most frequent cause is iatrogenic. Iatrogenic damage may be suspected postoperatively by any of the following clinical manifestations: pyrexia, loin pain or discomfort, abdominal pain or discomfort, leakage of urine through the vagina or surgical wound, or the signs and symptoms suggestive of peritonitis or a paralytic ileus.

Ureteric trauma is usually confirmed radiologically by performing an IVP and/or a retrograde pyelogram. For lower ureteric injuries, the ureter may be reimplanted into the bladder in such a way as to prevent the possible reflux of urine. Other types of injuries may call for a reanastomosis of the severed ends of the ureter, implantation of the end of the injured ureter into the patent ureter, or for some patients, a form of ureterostomy.

At some centres, a percutaneous nephrostomy may be performed to drain urine from the kidney on the affected side to reduce extravasation and to promote healing. At the time of ureteric repair, a ureteric stent (which acts like a splint) may also be inserted in order to maintain the ureter in a straight course, thereby preventing kinking and maintaining patency of the ureter. The device may be left in place for days to weeks. A urethral catheter is usually inserted to facilitate drainage and to prevent the build up of high intravesical pressures which may endanger the internal sutures. Specific postoperative nursing care for these patients is therefore aimed at observing and maintaining the patency of all drainage systems, and observing the patient for symptoms and signs of possible urine extravasation and infection.

TRAUMA TO THE BLADDER

Injuries to the bladder may be caused by penetrating trauma but the majority are a result of blunt trauma such as a blow or a crush injury.

Because of the bladder's protected position, trauma is frequently accompanied by damage to pelvic structures and other pelvic organs.

Blunt trauma to the bladder may cause a contusion, though if the trauma is severe it may produce a tear in the bladder wall with subsequent extravasation of urine into either the intraperitoneal or extraperitoneal space. Fractures to the pubic bone may result in rupture of the bladder as may a blow to the lower abdomen in the presence of a full bladder.

Clinical manifestations

Clinical manifestations of a bladder rupture usually include: haematuria, lower abdominal or suprapubic pain, suprapubic or abdominal swelling (due to haemorrhage and extravasation of urine), and problems in voiding (for example, an inability to void, or voiding only small amounts). The clinical picture is usually complicated by other pelvic or general injuries though the presence of a ruptured bladder can usually be confirmed radiologically by performing a cystogram or an IVP. A plain X-ray of the pelvis is also carried out to identify possible pelvic fractures.

Medical, surgical, and nursing management

The management of small ruptures usually only requires the provision of adequate urinary drainage, as most will heal spontaneously. Larger ruptures require surgical intervention aimed at an exploration and repair of the lacerations, with subsequent drainage of all extravasated fluid via a urethral or suprapubic catheter. Nursing management is therefore similar to that of a patient with ureteric trauma, and is aimed at maintaining patency of the drainage systems, providing the patient with symptomatic relief, and taking measures to prevent infection until the laceration heals.

TRAUMA TO THE URETHRA

Injury to the urethra occurs primarily in males and may result from: blunt trauma, for example, a fall astride an object, or in association with pelvic injuries; penetrating wounds; insertion of foreign objects; iatrogenic events, for example, trauma caused during catheterization or instrumentation of the urinary tract; or rupture which may occur when forcibly voiding against an obstructive urethral stricture. The trauma usually results in a urethral laceration allowing blood and urine to extravasate to surrounding areas; the laceration may be complete or incomplete. Severe trauma, with a complete laceration of the prostatomembranous urethra may dislodge the bladder and prostate from their attachments to the pelvic floor causing them to become mobile. This condition is generally considered an indication for immediate reparative surgery.

Clinical manifestations

The clinical manifestations of urethral trauma include: blood at the urethral meatus or bleeding from the urethra; difficulty or inability in voiding; perineal or lower abdominal pain; nausea; swelling of the perineum and/or genitals; and later, bruising around the perineum. The physician will, where possible, perform a rectal examination to identify the prostate, a plain X-ray will be taken of the pelvis to assess other possible damage, and a retrograde urethrogram will be performed to determine the extent of the urethral injury. Blind urethral catheterization is generally not encouraged for these patients because of the risks of converting a partial laceration into a complete laceration and introducing infection.

Medical, surgical, and nursing management

The management of urethral injuries remains somewhat controversial. Partial lacerations of the prostatomembranous urethra may be managed by inserting a suprapubic bladder catheter and performing serial urethrograms to monitor the healing process, a voiding trial being performed prior to removal of the catheter. Complete lacerations of the prostatomembranous urethra may be managed by either immediate surgical repair and realignment of the urethra over a stenting urethral catheter, or by suprapubic cystostomy followed by delayed elective urethroplasty. This latter operation may be performed some months after the injury. Injuries to the urethra below the level of the urogenital diaphragm may be treated by inserting a urethral catheter to act as a stent, or by suprapubic bladder drainage to allow the injury to heal.

There are many variations on any of the above management themes, therefore the nurse must be familiar with the specific treatment plan drawn up for any particular patient. Common among a number of patients who have sustained urethral injuries are the unfortunate complications that arise from this type of trauma. Urethral strictures occur in many patients, which may necessitate either repeated urethral dilations or a urethroplasty. Impotence has been reported to occur in up to 50% of patients, and urinary incontinence in up to 44% of patients in some studies (Webster et al, 1983). Current research is directed towards identifying optimal ways in which to manage particular injuries in an attempt to minimize such distressing complications. In the management of these patients, nurses must be cognizant of such complications so that optimal short- and long-term care plans can be drawn up. The goal is to prepare patients for, and to deal with, such problems using the most effective methods available.

58

Disorders of the kidney

A. P. Barnett

GLOMERULONEPHRITIS

Glomerulonephritis is an inflammation of the glomeruli of both kidneys. Glomerulonephritis may manifest itself clinically in several different ways and may also be associated with a number of systemic diseases (for example, systemic lupus erythematosus, SLE, see page 786), Goodpasture's syndrome, Henoch-Schonlein purpura, scleroderma, diabetes mellitus (see page 252) and amyloidosis. On renal biopsy, the glomeruli of patients with glomerulonephritis may also show distinctly different histological lesions, thus glomerulonephritis is a generic term for a variety of clinicopathological entities.

The prevalence of glomerulonephritis in the population is largely unknown, though it has been estimated that some 2–5% of people would, on screening, show some protein and/or blood in their urine which in the majority would indicate some underlying glomerular lesion (Kincaid-Smith, 1980; Kincaid-Smith & Dowling, 1983). This probably occurs most commonly in children who, some 2 weeks following a minor throat infection, spend approximately 7–10 days feeling generally unwell. This malaise is accompanied by obvious dependent oedema towards the evening, however this goes unnoticed by most parents. If the urine were to be tested at this stage it would show a small amount of protein and a few erythrocytes and leucocytes. It is, however, unlikely that the urine will be tested; the child recovers spontaneously. Even in children who have required admission to hospital for the treatment of glomerulonephritis, electron microscopy shows that there is no residual damage to the glomerular membrane within a period of 2 years. 85% of these patients admitted to hospital have no further renal problems for life.

Approximately 15% of all patients admitted to hospital for treatment of glomerulonephritis experience some complication. This is usually a period of classic nephrotic syndrome (see page 586), however a small percentage progress over a period of 5–20 years to end-stage renal failure (see page 595). Glomerulonephritis is the commonest cause of end-stage renal failure in a number of countries and is therefore responsible for a large percentage of patients entering dialysis and renal transplantation programmes (Kincaid-Smith & Dowling, 1983; Australian Kidney Foundation, 1984; Border & Glassock, 1984). It is therefore crucial for both humanitarian and economic reasons that research is ultimately directed toward the prevention and the effective treatment of this disease.

Aetiology and pathophysiology

As noted in Chapter 55, the first step in the formation of urine is the movement of plasma components across a filtration membrane consisting of the glomerular capillary endothelium, glomerular basement membrane and the visceral epithelium. The volume and composition of the filtrate formed is dependent on the integrity of the membrane and the net pressure difference between the fluids on either side of it. Because of the relatively high pressure and rate of blood flow through the kidneys, the renal corpuscle is vulnerable to injury from a number of blood-borne elements (for example, antigens or immune complexes). When trapped within the glomerular membrane they are capable of initiating an inflammatory response. This inflammatory reaction may involve any one, and at times a number, of the components of the renal corpuscle. Swelling and proliferation of particular cells, and various structural changes lead to alterations in the permeability of the glomerular membrane. Leakage of protein and some erythrocytes and leucocytes into the glomerular filtrate occurs. If the inflammatory process persists, the functional components of the renal corpuscle may become obliterated and replaced by scar tissue, with an accompanying reduction in renal function.

It is now evident that immunological mechanisms play a key role in the development of most forms of glomerulonephritis, though in many cases of this disease the particular antigen has not been identified. The antigen most commonly involved in the aetiology of glomerulonephritis is beta-haemolytic streptococcus. To a much lesser extent *Treponema pallidum*, *Plasmodium malariae*, a number of viruses, and various endogenous substances, for example, DNA have been identified.

In glomerulonephritis, immunoglobulin as a result of an immune response can be directed against:

1. A particular part of the glomerulus (for example, immunoglobulin is formed against the glomerular basement membrane in Goodpasture's syndrome)
2. An exogenous antigen which has become attached to the glomerulus
3. Antigens present in the circulation which form immune complexes.

In all three cases, accumulated immune complexes may become larger and induce changes within the glomeruli by activating various other immunoinflammatory processes. The degree of injury produced is related to the quantity of antigen and immunoglobulin reacting in the glomerulus (Border & Glassock, 1984). Other elements such as the enzyme 'complement', neutrophils and monocytes, and the activation of the clotting mechanism may be involved in producing morphological changes within the glomerulus.

In glomerulonephritis, the overall picture at the level of the glomerulus is therefore commonly one of inflammation, congestion, and increased glomerular permeability.

Classification of glomerulonephritis

Following a renal biopsy of a patient with glomerulonephritis, immune complexes, components of the complement system, and other material may be detected and located within the glomerulus microscopically. The major histological categories of glomerulonephritis (which are based on the possible changes to the glomerulus) are listed in Table 58.1 together with a glossary of terms. It should be noted that a patient with glomerulonephritis may show different findings on serial renal biopsies as a consequence of the disease process or its treatment.

Whatever the classification the ultimate problem in glomerulonephritis is that the basement membrane thickens, thereby interfering with filtration. Occasional splits occur in the membrane causing a minor nonselectivity of the filter.

Table 58.1 Classification of glomerulonephritis. (Adapted with permission from Thomson N M, Atkins R C, Ryan G B 1987 Classification, pathology and clinical features of glomerulonephritis. In: Whitworth J A, Lawrence J R Textbook of renal disease. Churchill Livingstone, Melbourne.)

Minimal or no glomerular lesion on light microscopy
Minimal change disease

Diffuse glomerular lesions
Non-proliferative
    Membranous nephropathy
Proliferative
    Diffuse endocapillary proliferation (with or without exudation). (Post-streptococcal GN)
    Diffuse mesangial proliferative GN (with or without mesangial IgA)
    Diffuse proliferative GN with crescents (e.g. Goodpasture's syndrome)
    Membranoproliferative GN (e.g. SLE)

Focal glomerular lesions
Non-proliferative
    Focal glomerulosclerosis (focal and segmental glomerular hyalinosis and sclerosis)
Proliferative
    Focal and segmental GN

Glossary of terms
Proliferative – proliferation of endogenous (endothelial, epithelial, mesangial) glomerular cells
Exudative – infiltration of the glomerulus by polymorphonuclear leucocytes, macrophages, or lymphocytes
Diffuse – involving all glomeruli
Global – involving the whole glomerular tuft
Focal – involving some glomeruli only
Segmental – involving only a segment of the glomerular tuft

Clinical manifestations

Inflammation of the glomeruli inevitably results in changes to the integrity of the glomerular filtration membranes. Therefore substances which under normal circumstances are not filtered by the glomerulus are often afforded passage into the glomerular filtrate and may eventually be detected in some form in the urine. The major abnormal urinary constituents that may be detected on urinalysis (or in some cases observed by the patient) are protein and blood.

Proteinuria is present to some degree in all forms of glomerulonephritis, thus methods used for its detection are useful in screening large numbers of people for the possible presence of this disease. The urinary protein loss may be small and go largely unnoticed, or alternatively the proteinuria may be large (>5 g/day) and lead to nephrotic syndrome. Thus a patient may present with generalized oedema.

Haematuria is also evident in many types of glomerulonephritis (for example, focal and segmental proliferative glomerulonephritis) and may be either microscopic or macroscopic. In some cases, periods of microscopic haematuria are interspersed with episodes of macroscopic haematuria; this may be accompanied by hypertension which is primarily caused by the secretion of renin in response to the change in pressure differential from juxtaglomerular apparatus to glomerulus.

Less commonly, patients may also present with an acute nephritic syndrome, acute renal failure, which may in turn progress to end-stage renal failure. The clinical manifestations may be predominantly those of chronic renal failure. Table 58.2 lists the major ways in which glomerulonephritis may present. It should be stressed however, that proteinuria will be present in all forms of glomerulonephritis.

Table 58.2 Clinical manifestations of glomerulonephritis

Proteinuria
Haematuria – microscopic
           – macroscopic
Nephrotic syndrome
Acute nephritic syndrome
Chronic renal failure
Acute renal failure

Investigative procedures

A urinalysis should be performed looking for the presence of protein and blood cells. An MSU is also obtained to quantify the number of cells present and is cultured if a UTI is suspected. Microscopic examination will often reveal a number of 'casts'. These are cylindrical accumulations of cellular debris from a variety of different cells, which have taken on the shape of the tubules – they have been 'cast'. A 24-hour urine collection may be required to ascertain the amount of protein excreted each day, and a creatinine clearance may be performed to gain an estimation of the glomerular filtration rate.

A number of blood tests are commonly performed and include: urea and creatinine levels to help assess renal function; serum albumin, which may be low if there is heavy proteinuria; serum cholesterol and triglycerides, which are commonly elevated in the nephrotic syndrome. Serum complement (for example, C3 and C4), an immune complex assay, and a clotting profile may be performed to provide some indication of the immunoinflammatory process. Other blood tests may also be conducted to check for underlying disease, for example, SLE.

In many centres, a renal biopsy will also be performed as this procedure remains a mainstay in the diagnosis of glomerulonephritis.

Medical and nursing management

Treatment measures for patients with glomerulonephritis are commonly directed at both the immunological/inflammatory mechanisms involved, and the subsequent tendency for fibrin deposition and coagulation to occur within the glomerular capillaries. To this end, immunosuppressants (for example, prednisolone, azathioprine, and the broad spectrum antineoplastic agent cyclophosphamide), anticoagulants (for example, heparin or warfarin) and antiplatelet agents (for example, dipyridamole, sulphinpyrazone, or aspirin) may be used either singly or in combination against various forms of glomerulonephritis. The combination of dipyridamole, warfarin and cyclophosphamide has been used to treat patients with diffuse membranous glomerulonephritis and diffuse mesangiocapillary glomerulonephritis.

Minimal change glomerulonephritis has probably been the most responsive to drug therapy. Patients with this lesion usually respond to a course of prednisolone; and for those patients who show little response to steroids, cyclophosphamide is used. The rationale for the use of these drugs lies in their ability to dampen down the inflammatory process, minimize cellular proliferation and prevent coagulation. A major nursing implication arising from their use is correct administration, careful observation of patients' responses to therapy and the possible adverse effects such drugs may have. Immunosuppressants will increase a patient's susceptibility to infection. Effectiveness of treatment is monitored by daily estimation of urinary protein and blood. These will both diminish as the patient responds to treatment.

Plasmapheresis (plasma exchange) is performed on rare occasions and has been found to be an effective adjunct to the drug treatment of several types of glomerulonephritis, for example, glomerular lesions associated with SLE, multiple myeloma, and Goodpasture's syndrome. In this procedure plasma is separated from the cellular components of blood by either centrifugal force or filtration. The gradual removal of plasma from a patient with glomerulonephritis in exchange for a replacement fluid of some kind (for example, stable plasma protein solution – SPPS) reduces the amount of immunoglobulin, immune complexes, complement, and clotting factors in the circulation. By removing these (and probably other) mediators of glomerular injury over a period of time (for example, by performing a number of 2–4 litre plasma exchanges over a period of weeks), a number of types of glomerulonephritis may be treated. Following plasmapheresis, the nurse should observe the patient for signs of volume depletion and for longer-term complications such as infection, and anaemia.

Many patients are reviewed regularly on an outpatient basis. The nurse is usually only required to manage such patients when they are admitted for various investigative procedures, or if they develop more acute or serious manifestations. If, over a period of time, the patient's renal function deteriorates, treatment is aimed at controlling blood pressure, maintaining fluid and electrolyte balance, and minimizing blood urea levels. These particular aspects of management are discussed in this chapter under 'Chronic renal failure' (page 595).

Anticipated outcome

In the majority of cases of people with glomerulonephritis there is no widely recommended treatment, thus management is generally directed toward supportive care until the lesion resolves.

IgA nephropathy

IgA nephropathy (Berger's disease, IgA glomerulonephritis) is probably the most common disease of adults with a primary glomerular lesion. A diagnosis of IgA nephropathy is made when, in the absence of a clinically apparent systemic disease, deposits of IgA are found within the mesangium of a renal biopsy specimen (Clarkson et al, 1982). As well as the presence of IgA on immunofluorescence, the glomerular lesions of patients with this disease may be described as diffuse mesangial proliferative glomerulonephritis, focal and segmental proliferative glomerulonephritis, or sometimes focal and segmental hyalinosis and sclerosis (Clarkson et al, 1982; Kincaid-Smith, 1980).

The disease is most common among young men and is characterised by recurrent episodes of macroscopic haematuria which usually follow within 24 hours of a sore throat, a urinary tract infection, a gastrointestinal disturbance (Clarkson et al, 1982), or vigorous exercise (Border & Glassock, 1984). Despite this observation, the exact immunopathogenesis of IgA nephropathy is unknown. Loin pain and more generalized symptoms such as fever, malaise, fatigue, and myalgia may accompany the episodes of macroscopic haematuria; whilst mild proteinuria and microscopic haematuria usually persist between such episodes.

To date, there is no widely recommended treatment for patients with this disease; management is generally conservative and if hypertension is present some form of antihypertensive therapy will be necessary. Patients with this disease may present with the nephrotic syndrome and though bouts of macroscopic haematuria are not usually associated with a raised serum creatinine or urea level, it is possible for patients to present in acute renal failure. The outlook for IgA nephropathy is generally favourable but some patients progress slowly to chronic renal failure.

Acute post-streptococcal glomerulonephritis

Also termed Bright's disease or acute nephritis, acute post-streptococcal glomerulonephritis is a disease which affects males more often than females and is more common in children than adults. Though relatively uncommon in adults, the disease is generally more severe in this age group and the prognosis is less favourable than in children of whom approximately 95% recover fully. In the adult group, only 60–80% make a full recovery; the remainder develop persistent proteinuria and/or haematuria and hypertension, over a period of years. For a small group of patients, glomerular damage continues and renal function gradually deteriorates to such an extent that end-stage chronic renal failure is the result.

Classically, this form of glomerulonephritis follows an infection with beta-haemolytic streptococcus, the most common site being the throat, although other microorganisms may be responsible. The interval between the infection and the onset of this form of glomerulonephritis is on average 10–14 days, thus it is distinguishable from IgA glomerulonephritis. The streptococci do not infect the kidneys; rather it is believed that the glomeruli undergo an allergic and inflammatory reaction in response to antigens and immune complexes become trapped in the glomerular capillaries. Histologically, the glomerular changes are those of diffuse endocapillary proliferative glomerulonephritis. The glomeruli are congested and the reduced blood flow through the glomerular capillaries commonly results in a reduction in the glomerular filtration rate, and leakage of some protein and erythrocytes through the damaged glomerular membrane.

Clinical manifestations

The clinical manifestations of a patient with post-streptococcal glomerulonephritis who presents with an acute nephritic syndrome are predominantly those associated with fluid overload and impaired renal function. Typically, there is oliguria and a raised blood urea level, haematuria, hypertension and oedema. The patient may feel tired and lethargic, and complain of an ache in the loins; the hypertension may cause a headache and there may be a feeling of nausea with subsequent vomiting. The patient may be dyspnoeic or orthopnoeic if there is a degree of pulmonary oedema present.

The disease may be mild, especially in children, though adults usually require hospitalization. Some patients may present in nephrotic syndrome.

Investigative procedures

A full medical history is obtained, renal function is assessed and in some centres, a renal biopsy will be performed.

Blood tests which may be performed include: antistreptolysin-O titre (ASOT) (usually raised); antideoxyribonuclease-B titre (antiDNase-B) (usually raised); serum complement level (C3) (usually low); erythrocyte sedimentation rate (ESR) (usually elevated); serum albumin levels (may be low if there is heavy proteinuria); and haemoglobin (may be low).

Swabs may be taken from an infective lesion for microbiological analysis (for example throat swabs).

MSU will show erythrocytes and casts, and a 24-hour collection of urine is taken to quantify the amount of proteinuria. Urinalysis for blood and protein is performed.

Radiological investigations include plain film of the kidneys, ureters, and urinary bladder, and chest X-ray to assess lung fields and heart size.

Medical and nursing management

The general management aims when caring for a patient with post-streptococcal glomerulonephritis are to treat any underlying infection (if present) with an appropriate ordered antibiotic; to relieve the patient's symptoms; and to prevent the possible complications which may arise from salt and water retention and reduced renal function.

Bed rest is encouraged for the patient until a diuresis begins; this usually occurs several days following the initial onset of symptoms. Rest may be further encouraged by grouping nursing and allied activities.

During the acute phase, if the patient is dyspnoeic, a more upright position in bed should be utilized. Once the patient's oedema decreases, ambulation and other physical activities may be gradually increased as tolerated by the patient.

To minimize and prevent the effects of fluid overload, the patient's total fluid intake should be restricted to no more than 1500 ml per day, and diuretics may be ordered to promote urinary excretion. A fluid balance chart should be maintained to assist in monitoring fluid intake and output, and a mild negative balance should be achieved daily until oedema has resolved.

Diet. In the short-term, dietary protein may be restricted and sodium restriction is indicated if oedema is severe and hypertension present. If serum potassium is raised, dietary potassium must be reduced. Whilst dietary restrictions may be necessary, it is also important that the patient receive an adequate carbohydrate intake in order to meet metabolic demands and to prevent muscle wasting. Dietary manipulations of this order usually require the expertise of a dietician and to ensure the effectiveness of such restrictions, the patient and his significant others should understand the reasons for the restrictions.

Any foods brought in for the patient should be checked by the nurse to ensure they comply with salt and protein restrictions.

Specific nursing management. Assessment is a critical part of the nursing management. Vital signs should be taken regularly and changes and abnormalities reported promptly. As an indicator of fluid status, patients should be weighed daily and the extent of any oedema should be noted at least once per shift. Because uraemia, severe hypertension, and hyperkalaemia may produce sensorial changes, the patient's behaviour may also be monitored for signs of confusion, disorientation, anxiety, restlessness, or drowsiness.

During the oedematous period the patient's skin will require particular care. Mouth care should be performed regularly and to help alleviate the sensation of thirst, ice chips and boiled sweets may be provided. Deep breathing and coughing exercises are encouraged to aid ventilation and

help reduce the risk of the patient developing a chest infection; when the patient is confined to bed, active limb exercises should also be encouraged to prevent deep vein thrombosis, and to promote venous and lymph drainage.

Prior to discharge, the importance of completing the course of any drug therapy prescribed should be stressed. An appointment must be made for follow up visits to an outpatient clinic or medical centre in order that the patient's blood pressure and renal function be monitored. The patient should also be advised to seek medical attention should any urinary abnormality be noticed (for example, haematuria, reduced urine output); if the oedema recurs; or if there is any evidence of an infection, as it is probable that the prompt and effective treatment of infections may reduce the prevelance of this type of glomerulonephritis.

Complications which may occur whilst the patient is oliguric include acute heart failure, hyperkalaemia, uraemia, a hypertensive crisis or infection. Table 58.3 lists some methods for recognizing these complications and suggests methods by which each may be prevented.

NEPHROTIC SYNDROME

Pathophysiology

The nephrotic syndrome is not a specific disease; rather, it is a clinical picture brought about by the excessive loss of protein in the urine. It is characterized by 4 major features: proteinuria, hypoalbuminaemia, oedema, and hyperlipidaemia. It may be differentiated from the acute nephritic syndrome by its much greater degree of proteinuria, and the general absence of hypertension. The diseases which present with nephrotic syndrome include: glomerulonephritis, diabetes mellitus, SLE, and amyloidosis. Nephrotic syndrome may also be precipitated by allergic reactions to drugs (for example, penicillamine) or poisons (for example, bee stings). It is sometimes secondary to an infection such as malaria, tuberculosis, syphilis or hepatitis B.

In adults, the degree of proteinuria (primarily albuminuria) required to produce the nephrotic syndrome is commonly greater than 5 g/24 hours, though a protein excretion rate of 20–30 g/24

Table 58.3 Complications of postinfectious glomerulonephritis

Potential problem	Assessment	Prevention
Acute heart failure (strain on the heart due to retention of water and sodium)	Breathlessness Cyanosis Rapid, irregular pulse Pulmonary congestion Oedema	Restrict Na^+ and water intake Maintain accurate Fluid Balance Chart Weigh patient daily
Hyperkalaemia (retention of K^+ due to impaired renal excretion)	Cardiac arrhythmias Blood K^+ levels ECG changes Usually asymptomatic, may have vague signs or symptoms, e.g. – nausea, vomiting – flaccid paralysis – muscular cramps – anxiety; restlessness – muscle weakness	Restrict dietary potassium
Uraemia (retention of urea and the waste products of protein metabolism due to renal excretion)	Anorexia, nausea, or vomiting Uraemic breath (smells faintly of urine) Deep sighing ventilation Haemorrhagic tendencies – skin (bruising) – gums – nose Drowsiness Confusion	Restrict protein in diet
Hypertensive encephalopathy (hypertensive crisis; associated with severe hypertension and cerebral oedema)	Headache (severe) Blurred vision Nausea or vomiting Confusion Convulsions Cerebrovascular accident	Restrict fluid intake Antihypertensive therapy
Infection	Pyrexia Cough Dysuria Sweating	Personal hygiene Restrict contacts with infected patients Regular screening of secretions for microscopy/culture/sensitivity

hours has been reported. With the loss of albumin in the urine, there is also a loss of complement and immunoglobulin. If albuminuria is prolonged and severe, this reduces the body's internal defences and renders the patient more susceptible to infection. The liver is unable to synthesize proteins at a rate equivalent to their excretion rate, and this results in hypoalbuminaemia. Concomitant with lowered blood albumin levels is a decrease in plasma protein osmotic pressure, and the osmotic gradient thus established causes fluid to pass from the intravascular compartment into the interstitium, producing the oedema characteristic of the nephrotic syndrome. With the loss of intravascular fluid volume, compensatory mechanisms are activated in an attempt to restore circulating blood volume. These mechanisms include: stimulation of the renin–angiotensin–aldosterone system which causes an increase in the reabsorption of sodium and water from the renal tubules; and stimulation of the posterior pituitary gland to release ADH to cause an increase in water reabsorption from the distal convoluted tubules and collecting ducts of the nephron. Both mechanisms therefore reduce the volume of urine output which further exacerbates the problem of oedema. Due to the central dehydration the patient is thirsty. However, any fluid taken by the patient moves immediately into the interstitium and the thirst is therefore insatiable.

A phenomenon associated with the hypoalbuminaemia is hyperlipidaemia. For some reason not fully understood, the liver increases its synthesis of cholesterol and triglycerides, as well as increasing its production of proteins; thus blood levels of these substances will be elevated and may in the long-term predispose the nephrotic patient to atheroma formation. The major points of the pathophysiological processes involved in the nephrotic syndrome are outlined in Figure 58.1.

Clinical manifestations

The most obvious clinical feature of a nephrotic patient is oedema. Upon rising, the patient's face is puffy, especially around the eyes, and as the day progresses, the feet and ankles become swollen and pitting is evident. In addition, there may be scrotal and sacral oedema, ascites, and a pleural effusion. There is a noticeable weight gain due to the retention of fluid and the patient will be thirsty and may feel weak and tired. The skin may appear pale due to the oedema and mild anaemia and, if the condition has progressed for some time, there may be evidence of muscle wasting. An inspection of the nails may reveal transverse white bands attributable to chronic hypoalbuminaemia. The majority of patients are hypertensive.

Investigative procedures

Blood tests performed may be: serum albumin and total protein (usually low); serum cholesterol and triglycerides (elevated); sodium (may be elevated); and potassium (may be low due to hyperaldosteronism or diuretic therapy). The nephrotic syndrome may be associated with an increased coagulability due to the loss of antithrombin III in the urine, so coagulation studies may be carried out.

Full blood examination may demonstrate an anaemia.

Urinalysis will indicate protein, possibly blood, and a raised specific gravity. MSU may reveal red blood cell casts, fatty casts and oval fat bodies. 24-hour urine collection shows decreased sodium and increased potassium excretion, large protein excretion.

Renal biopsy may be performed.

Medical and nursing management

The aims of treatment for a patient with the nephrotic syndrome are to treat or remove the underlying cause and to relieve the symptoms. The hypoalbuminaemia is managed by increasing the patient's dietary intake of protein, often to an amount greater than 1.5 g/kg body weight/day. If renal impairment is present, the need to increase dietary protein will have to be balanced against blood urea levels. Sodium and fluid restrictions may be necessary in severe cases to help control the oedema; the amount of restriction will depend on the degree of oedema and the patient's response to drug therapy. It is also necessary to ensure that the patient receives an adequate carbohydrate intake in order to prevent endogenous tissue breakdown. In some cases, it is necessary to administer salt-poor concentrated albumin in order to raise blood albumin levels in the short term (24–48 hours) and thereby promote a diuresis by increasing circulating blood volume and renal blood flow.

Immunosuppressants are effective in some patients with the nephrotic syndrome (if, for example, the cause is minimal change glomerulonephritis) and diuretics may be used to help increase urine output and reduce oedema once the intravascular osmotic pressure has been corrected. Any patient treated with a short-acting diuretic should be ordered a potassium supplement. The extensive use of diuretic therapy may also produce hypovolaemia which will further reduce renal blood flow and may precipitate the development of acute renal failure. It is therefore important to monitor the patient carefully for signs of hypotension following a response to the diuretic.

Patients with nephrotic syndrome must be nursed in bed, although some may be allowed to walk to the toilet. The nurse should ensure that when a patient is out of bed, he remains mobile, as sitting in a chair will produce gross and painful oedema of the legs. If there is noticeable oedema of the feet and ankles when the patient is ambulant, support stockings may be used.

The nurse should care for the patient's skin, changing his position regularly to prevent skin breakdown. Gentle handling will also reduce skin trauma. Lotions may be applied to the skin to soothe and protect it, and heparinoid preparations

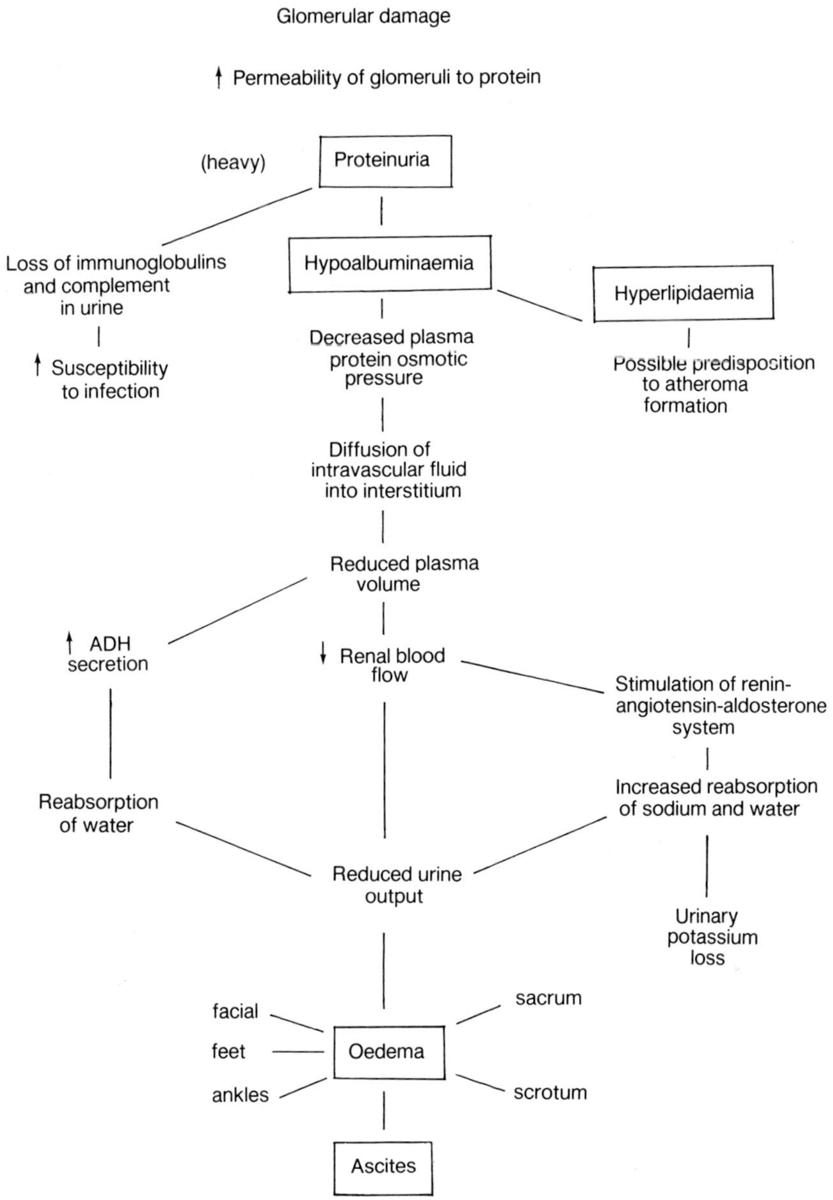

Glomerular damage

↑ Permeability of glomeruli to protein

Fig. 58.1 Pathological processes in the nephrotic syndrome.

may be used to reduce any bruising which may be present. Aids to spread pressure, such as a sheepskin should be utilized.

Observations of the patient which should be performed include: daily weighing (at approximately the same time each day), monitoring of fluid intake and output, daily assessment of the extent and degree of oedema, and regular vital signs.

The gross oedema can prove quite distressing to the patient and his significant others. The nurse should explain the rationale for all interventions and provide support throughout the duration of the disorder.

Physiotherapy in the form of active limb exercises should be undertaken, especially if there is an increased tendency to blood clotting and the patient is resting in bed.

Complications

Complications which should be observed for and guarded against in patients with the nephrotic syndrome include: infection, thrombosis, and protein depletion; and more rarely, hypovolaemic shock and uraemia. The prognosis for patients is determined by the type and presence of any underlying disease and, in cases of a primary glomerular lesion, the morphological type of glomerulonephritis.

ACUTE RENAL FAILURE

Acute renal failure is a medical emergency. Patients with this condition require specialist nursing care and are often maintained on either peritoneal dialysis or haemodialysis (see page 601) until renal function returns. The term 'renal failure' describes a rapid decline in renal function usually in response to prolonged hypotension which, as it progresses, is accompanied by an accumulation of waste products in the blood. Though acute renal failure is usually characterized by a reduction in urine output, it may be associated with polyuria (that is, non-oliguric or high output renal failure) and the inherent problem of fluid depletion. Because oliguria is more commonly observed in patients with this condition, extended discussion will be confined to this type of acute renal failure.

Aetiology and pathophysiology

The causes of acute renal failure are numerous (Fig. 58.2), but have traditionally been grouped under 3 major headings:

1. Pre-renal causes
2. Renal causes
3. Post-renal causes.

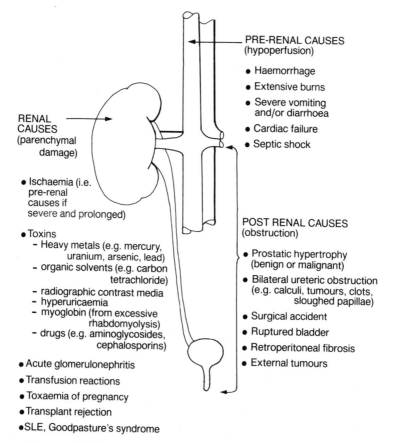

Fig. 58.2 Categorization of causes of ARF, and examples of specific causes.

Pre-renal causes

Pre-renal causes are by far the most common. A pre-renal cause of acute renal failure is any condition which precipitates prolonged hypotension and/or causes the release of free haemoglobin or myoglobin. Examples of pre-renal causes include: severe haemorrhage, burns, gastrointestinal losses (for example, severe diarrhoea and vomiting), cardiac failure, septic shock, and crush injuries. A reduced renal blood flow results in a reduction in glomerular filtration rate, a fall in the volume of urine output, and ultimately a retention of nitrogenous and other wastes. If an adequate renal blood flow is promptly restored renal tissue will not be damaged and renal function will be preserved. If, however, renal perfusion is not improved, renal ischaemia will result and the tubular epithelium will become damaged.

Acute-on-chronic renal failure is an acute deterioration of renal function on a pre-existing state of chronic renal impairment which has been previously undiagnosed. This commonly occurs as a result of dehydration or infection and in such conditions the cause may be considered to be prerenal. The aim of management in such cases is to restore circulating blood volume, thereby increasing renal perfusion and preventing a further exacerbation of already compromised renal function.

An episode of acute renal failure in these patients is a fortunate occurrence as it enables the diagnosis and therefore the management of a chronic underlying illness.

Renal causes

The renal causes of acute renal failure refer to those conditions in which there is direct damage to the renal parenchyma. This may result from: toxins, heavy metals, and some drugs; damage to the glomeruli and microvasculature, for example, glomerulonephritis; or from ischaemic changes as a result of prerenal causes. Damage to renal tissue from prolonged ischaemia or toxicity frequently results in oedema, obstruction, and necrosis of the renal tubular cells: acute tubular necrosis. If acute tubular necrosis is present, management is directed to preserving life and maintaining homeostasis until renal function returns.

Post-renal causes

The post-renal cause of acute renal failure is obstruction to the normal passage of urine along the urinary tract. Causes of post-renal acute renal failure include benign or malignant hypertrophy of the prostate, blockage of both ureters due to calculi or sloughed papillae, tumours external to the urinary tract causing compression of the urinary pathways, and urethral strictures.

Whatever the cause of the renal failure the pathophysiological changes are similar. These are blocking of the glomerulus, due predominantly to stasis of blood flow; and tubular necrosis.

Initially, urine is formed despite the obstruction. As the collecting systems fill with urine pressure is transmitted back to the glomeruli, preventing glomerular filtration. Thus the glomerular filtration rate is reduced and waste products are retained. If the condition is not treated at this stage, the renal parenchyma will become 'waterlogged' resulting in increased difficulty in management. The aims of management are to relieve the obstruction and to maintain fluid and electrolyte balance during the post-obstructive diuresis. In some cases the diuresis may be so great that intravenous fluid and electrolyte replacement therapy may be warranted.

Clinical manifestations

All patients who are shocked are obvious candidates for renal failure. Too often these hypovolaemic patients are said to be in renal failure when all they need is better fluid management. Acute renal failure does not exist until there is evidence of acute tubular necrosis.

The clinical features of acute renal failure are: oliguria, which may be extreme; a rise in urea, creatinine, sodium and potassium levels, leading to azotaemia and eventually uraemia; and a fall in pH producing a metabolic acidosis with a compensatory respiratory alkalosis as the patient increases his rate and depth of ventilation in an attempt to 'blow off' excess carbon dioxide.

Post-renal or obstructive renal failure is usually characterized by anuria. If the obstruction is prostatic or urethral, the bladder will be palpable and the patient may complain of suprapubic discomfort and pain. Urinary dribbling may be evident if there is retention with overflow, and the characteristic signs of fluid overload may be present if fluid intake is not restricted. If the obstruction is located within the upper urinary tract, renal colic may be experienced; and as urine collects within the ureters and renal pelvis, an ache in the loins may be described by the patient. It should be noted that an obstruction to the flow of urine from only one kidney will not produce anuria or acute renal failure providing the other kidney is functional and its drainage system patent; thus in terms of developing acute renal failure, patients with a unilateral kidney are more at risk.

The majority of patients misdiagnosed with renal failure are not in fact in failure but are in desperate need of fluid. A few patients who truly are in renal failure are overhydrated, (due to non-recognition of deteriorating renal function or over-enthusiastic resuscitative measures), oliguric and azotaemic. The characteristics of fluid overload more commonly associated with this condition include oedema, dyspnoea, raised CVP, and weight gain. Changes in mental state (for example, confusion) may be evident. The patient will feel lethargic, may have gastrointestinal disturbances, and haemorrhagic tendencies. This latter manifestation may be related to a defect in platelet function associated with raised urea levels or disseminated intravascular coagulation (DIC, see page 107). The urine of patients with acute renal failure varies in consistency from urine with normal constituents and concentration to a few millilitres of almost black fluid with a treacle-like consistency (this is almost pure haemoglobin or myoglobin).

Investigative procedures

Essential to the effective treatment of acute renal failure is an identification of its particular cause, thus efforts are made to delineate whether there is hypoperfusion, obstruction, or parenchymal damage. Blood tests include urea, creatinine, uric acid and phosphate and potassium levels, all of which are elevated in acute renal failure. Haemoglobin and haematocrit may be checked, and if glomerulonephritis is suspected, tests are performed to identify the particular type of glomerulonephritis causing the renal failure and for the presence of any underlying disease. An assessment of acid–base balance indicates a metabolic acidosis. Bicarbonate levels are depressed, and pH decreased.

Where possible, urine is collected, observed, and tested for specific gravity. Urine osmolality and sodium levels may also be estimated.

An electrocardiograph is performed if cardiac failure is suspected as being either the cause of acute renal failure or a result of fluid overload. An ECG may also be used as an adjunct to monitoring serum potassium levels as hyperkalaemia produces characteristic changes to the ECG pattern.

A number of radiological investigations are commonly performed and include a plain X-ray of the chest (to observe heart size and lung fields) and of the kidneys, ureters and bladder (to observe for obstruction). Ultrasound studies may be performed if obstruction is present and further studies such as an intravenous or retrograde pyelogram may better define the nature and location of the obstruction. Renal angiography may also be performed, especially if renal artery occlusion is suspected.

A renal biopsy is usually undertaken only if glomerulonephritis is suspected, or if the patient remains oliguric for 2 or more weeks.

Medical, surgical, and nursing management

Once the cause of renal failure has been ascertained, appropriate therapies may be instigated. If an obstruction is present, it must be removed. The patient with obstructive acute renal failure may therefore be required to undergo cystoscopic examination and surgery (for example, transurethral resection of the prostate gland, see page 647), or more extensive surgery to remove the obstruction and promote urinary drainage.

In cases where the patient's renal failure has been precipitated by hypovolaemia, rehydration plays an important therapeutic role. Treatment of acute renal failure precipitated by hypovolaemia is divided into two clear stages.

Stage 1 involves stressing the kidneys in order to attempt to force them to function. A reasonable regime for this treatment would be:

1. Administer an aliquot (a predetermined quantity of fluid) of 500 ml of 5% dextrose intravenously as fast as possible, bearing in mind the patient's age, weight, and physical condition.

2. 20–30 mg of frusemide intravenously is administered concurrently. If the patient has produced urine, he is not in renal failure and a suitable regime of fluid management is arranged accordingly.

If no urine is produced, diuretics may be repeated several times. However, osmotic diuretics (for example, mannitol) are given only once, if the patient has not produced any urine. If an osmotic diuretic is not excreted, it can cause cardiac failure by pulling fluid into the vascular system due to an increased osmotic attraction, thus causing a fluid overload. Therefore, it is important for the nurse to observe carefully the patient's cardiac status during this period.

If there is no response to this treatment, that is, there is still no urine produced, then a state of acute renal failure exists.

Stage 2 of treatment is then instigated. This involves fluid restriction to 400 ml plus a volume equal to the previous 24-hour urine output. Most of this fluid should be given orally to keep the buccal and oesophageal mucosa in good condition and allay the patient's thirst. A micro pump will enable an intravenous line to be maintained with minimal fluid input.

In order to monitor urine output accurately, and to exclude a lower urinary tract obstruction, a urinary catheter is inserted initially. In the absence of any other major indication, catheterization of patients with established acute renal failure is probably urwarranted in view of the fact that such patients are prone to developing infections and the prolonged use of a urinary catheter invariably leads to a UTI.

Once established, acute renal failure from whatever cause usually follows a classical course extending over a period of weeks. Traditionally, the clinical course of acute renal failure may be divided into 3 major phases (Table 58.4). The first phase is the oliguric phase, characterized by a period of low urine output. This phase lasts on average for 10–14 days, though may extend on rare occasions for a month or more.

Following the oliguric phase is the diuretic phase which marks the end of renal failure and the beginning of recovery. The normal constituents of urine are present, but the kidneys are still unable to conserve fluids or electrolytes. The patient's urine output may be as high as 10–15 l/24 hours.

Table 58.4 Clinical course of acute tubular necrosis

A. Pre-renal azotaemia (renal function will be preserved if underlying problem is corrected promptly)

B. 1. Oliguric phase (lasts 10–14 days on average)
   Major problems – fluid overload
   – hyperkalaemia
   – infection
   – uraemia
   – hyperphosphataemia
   – metabolic acidosis

   2. Diuretic phase (lasts 2–10 days on average)
   Major problems – hypervolaemia
   – hyponatraemia
   – hypokalaemia
   – infection

   3. Recovery phase (may last for months)
   Major problems – failure of kidneys to regain normal function
   – end-stage chronic renal failure

This phase, on average, persists for approximately 2–10 days until daily urine volume returns to normal and blood levels of urea, creatinine and other retained waste products gradually fall. This is termed the recovery or convalescent phase.

The 4 major principles to be observed when caring for a patient with acute renal failure are to:

1. Monitor and control hydration and serum electrolytes
2. Regulate dietary intake in order to maintain or improve nutritional status
3. Prevent infection and other complications
4. Ensure patient safety, and provide psychological and social support for the patient.

These principles may be applied and extended through the 3 phases of acute renal failure.

Management during the oliguric phase

During the oliguric phase, in order to prevent the complications of fluid overload, daily fluid intake should be restricted to 400 ml plus an amount equivalent to the previous day's urinary output. If there are other fluid losses, equivalent amounts should also be replaced. The patient's intake and output should be recorded accurately, and the patient observed regularly for signs and symptoms of fluid overload and weighed daily in order that any progressive fluid retention may be monitored and controlled. If an intravenous line is inserted, a microinfusion pump must be used to minimize the risk of infusing too much fluid.

To assist in the control of electrolyte levels, blood samples should be taken daily for estimations of creatinine, urea, potassium, and other electrolytes. Blood urea levels may be stabilized or reduced by restricting the patient's dietary intake of protein. A restriction of between 20–40 g/day is common practice; the amount of restriction depends upon blood urea levels and the presence and severity of uraemic symptoms. If the patient is hypercatabolic, it may be unwise to restrict protein intake severely, and in some cases protein intake may be supplemented parenterally. If a protein restriction is necessary, it is important to provide the patient with protein foods of a high biological value in order to provide the body with those amino acids it cannot synthesize. To ensure the energy requirements of the patient are met, and to prevent endogenous protein breakdown, it is also important that an adequate kilojoule intake (8000 kJ) is maintained.

Hyperkalaemia, with its cardiotoxic effects, may produce ventricular fibrillation and cardiac arrest; thus every effort should be made to maintain blood potassium levels within the normal range. Longer-term control of blood potassium levels is achieved by dietary restrictions of potassium (for example, 60 mmol/day) and the administration of an ion exchange resin (for example, Resonium A) on a regular basis either orally or as a retention enema. The immediate treatment of hyperkalaemia, however, may include: haemodialysis; 50 ml of 50% glucose and 5–10 units regular insulin IV; or calcium gluconate or sodium bicarbonate. The last choice is not commonly used because sodium and water are also administered; factors which may potentiate the problem of fluid overload. If a cardiac monitor is connected to the patient, the nurse should observe for ECG changes associated with a rise in blood potassium level. Hyperkalaemia may be exacerbated by the administration of old blood or potassium-containing medications; thus if transfusions are necessary, fresh blood should be available for the patient and medications containing high levels of potassium should, where possible, be excluded from the treatment regime.

Some dietary restrictions on sodium intake may be required during the oliguric phase of acute renal failure. The restriction will be primarily determined by the degree of oedema, heart failure, or hypertension present. A biochemical finding of hypernatraemia may be due to fluid loss or to the excessive use of sodium-containing medications or intravenous infusions. Hyponatraemia is commonly due to fluid overload and may be corrected by appropriate fluid restrictions or dialysis (see page 601). Hyperphosphataemia is controlled by the administration of an oral phosphate-binding agent (for example, aluminium hydroxide) with all meals. These agents bind with dietary phosphates allowing them to pass through the gastroinestinal tract to be eliminated in the faeces. The hypocalcaemia which may be present and the metabolic acidosis rarely requires specific treatment.

The dietary manipulations commonly needed by patients in acute renal failure require the expertise of a dietitian in order that the diet is appropriate to the specific needs of the individual and that necessary adjustments can be made on a regular basis. For a number of patients an oral diet is not possible, thus their nutritional needs must be met parenterally. Alternatively, if the patient can tolerate an oral intake, regular haemodialysis or continuous peritoneal dialysis may obviate the need for the more severe dietary restrictions, providing the patient's condition is stable.

The uraemic patient is susceptible to infection because of the impaired functioning of the immune system. Most common are lung and urinary tract infections. Because sepsis is associated with a higher acute renal failure mortality rate, measures should be taken to minimize the risk of the patient developing an infection. Where possible, patient contact with infected persons should be prohibited; urinary catheters should be removed unless absolutely necessary; and wound, IV insertion sites, tracheostomy, or any other sites where there is a break in the skin should be dressed and regularly observed for any signs of infection. An elevation in the patient's temperature should be reported promptly; swabs and/or samples should be obtained from potential sites of infection; and the infection treated rigorously with an appropriate antimicrobial. Chest physiotherapy, early mobilization, and skin and mouth care should also be included as routine nursing interventions.

Gastrointentinal related upsets are common and are usually associated with rising blood urea levels. Thus, if blood urea can be controlled by dialysis and/or protein restrictions, such uraemic manifestations may be minimized. Gastrointestinal bleeding may occur; cimetidine may be prescribed and the faeces tested for occult blood.

Care should be exercised when administering drugs which are excreted renally; if the dosage of such drugs is not adjusted accordingly, toxic effects may occur. This is especially true when an aminoglycoside is being used to treat an infection. Serum levels of the drug should be monitored and the dosage regulated accordingly.

Careful explanations should be given to the patient regarding all procedures and interventions. The reasons for dietary restrictions should be outlined and the patient's significant others should be involved in developing an individualized care plan to meet his needs. Dialysis can be a frightening and traumatic experience. Its function should be explained clearly and simply in order to allay unnecessary fear and anxiety (see also page 601). The physician should discuss prognosis with the patient and his significant others and the nurse should develop a trusting relationship in order to promote a positive health attitude and patient compliance to treatment schedules.

Acute renal failure is usually reversible. Most patients, providing complications are recognized early enough and dealt with promptly, will regain normal renal function. During the oliguric phase, the major complications are those associated with fluid overload, hyperkalaemia, uraemia, and infection.

Diuretic and recovery phase

A marked diuresis is usually the beginning of recovery, however, a number of problems associated with the oliguric phase may continue through to the diuretic phase.

If the diuresis is massive, the problems of hypovolaemia, hyponatraemia, and hypokalaemia arise. The patient should be assessed on a regular basis and blood will still be taken daily for biochemical analysis until urine output returns to normal. During this phase it is important that fluid and electrolytes are replaced. Any dietary restrictions on sodium and potassium are usually removed. However, because blood urea levels may remain high for some days following the diuresis, protein intake will still need to be restricted. All

nursing measures should be taken to prevent infection as the patient's immune status is still suppressed.

Gradually, the volume of urine output returns to normal. The patient's biochemistry is stabilized and other associated problems are resolved. Dietary and fluid restrictions are removed and the patient is encouraged to maintain a high fluid intake, for example, 3 l/day. This will promote a continuing diuresis. Return of full renal function may take up to 12 months, and for some patients there will always be a degree of renal impairment. Regular follow-up visits at an out-patient clinic are encouraged in order to monitor renal function and recovery. As a general rule, work and social activity may be recommended as tolerated by the patient.

Anticipated outcome

Most cases of acute renal failure are reversible and a near normal return of glomerular filtration rate is common after some months. A small percentage of treated patients fail to recover and require maintenance dialysis or renal transplantation.

CHRONIC RENAL FAILURE

Chronic renal failure is a chronic, progressive, totally destructive disease of the nephrons which if not interrupted and treated effectively leads ultimately to death. This process may take from 5–30 years. Although the damaged nephrons cannot be regenerated the importance of early diagnosis is that further destruction of nephrons may be prevented and the disease progress halted. At that stage dietary modification may allow the patient to have a normal life span and a relatively normal lifestyle. Chronic renal failure develops insidiously because the kidneys have a great deal of functional reserve, thus a large number of nephrons have been destroyed before the patient develops any distinct clinical manifestations.

Chronic renal failure may develop as a secondary outcome of another primary disease (see page 596); or, conversely, the inexorable progress of nephrotic destruction may exacerbate the presentation and management of other diseases (such as cardiac failure or hypertension).

In Australia, there are approximately 600 new patients admitted to dialysis and renal transplantation programmes each year. Unfortunately, this figure is increasing and represents only that proportion of patients who have reached end-stage chronic renal failure; therefore, the incidence of patients who develop, and are treated for, chronic renal failure within the community is probably much larger. Although not clearly defined there are 3 stages in chronic renal failure. In the early or first stage the patient is usually physically well with no clinical manifestations except polyuria, polydipsia and nocturia. The second stage occurs when the patient's renal function is no longer good enough to maintain homeostasis without the patient having to adjust his diet and fluid intake. In this stage the patient's urine volume is normal to low.

The third stage, end-stage renal failure, exists when the patient's renal function can no longer maintain homeostasis despite severe alteration to his diet and fluid intake. In this stage the patient will eventually become uraemic and acidotic.

Aetiology

Gradual destruction of the functional nephron mass may be brought about by a number of causes. The major worldwide single cause is chronic glomerulonephritis. The other major causes of chronic renal failure in Australia are: analgesic nephropathy, brought about by the long-term abuse of analgesics; polycystic kidney disease, an autosomal dominant disorder in which renal tissue becomes obliterated by cysts; reflux nephropathy, also referred to as chronic pyelonephritis or interstitial nephritis; diabetic nephropathy and hypertensive nephropathy, (although it is often difficult to determine whether the hypertension preceded or followed the development of chronic renal failure).

In most patients chronic renal failure develops over a number of years. However, a very small number of patients 'slide' from acute renal failure into chronic renal failure over a period of days or weeks. In the initial stages, although there is a diminution in renal reserve, the kidneys are still able to excrete wastes. Urea and other products of metabolism do not accumulate and the patient

therefore is largely asymptomatic. When the glomerular filtration rate is reduced to less than 20–25% of normal, blood urea and creatinine levels may begin to rise slightly and the patient may be intolerant to a large fluid load. For example, slight dyspnoea and a transient oedema of the ankles may be noticed following the ingestion of excessive amounts of fluids. The patient may also complain of nocturia and thirst, and various non-specific symptoms such as frequently feeling tired or an occasional headache. A risk during this stage of chronic renal impairment is that the patient may develop acute-on-chronic renal failure due to dehydration, therefore the maintenance of an adequate fluid intake should be encouraged at all times.

As the glomerular filtration rate is further reduced (for example, to less than 10% of normal), the patient becomes uraemic. Urea rises to toxic levels, as do other waste products in the blood which in turn affects all body systems. Progression of the condition eventually leads to end-stage chronic renal failure, a state in which dialysis or transplantation is required in order to maintain life.

Clinical manifestations and underlying pathophysiology

The clinical manifestations of the disease develop insidiously. As a result of this, the condition is ignored or goes unnoticed by the patient and his physician. Those symptoms of which the patient does become aware, such as polydipsia, nocturia and polyuria, are rationalized away by statements such as 'Of course I pass a lot of urine – I drink a lot'. However, the polydipsia is secondary to the polyuria and the patient drinks a lot because he must do so to maintain a normal state of hydration. It is often not until renal function has dramatically deteriorated and the more serious systemic effects of the disease such as drowsiness, poor concentration, twitching, muscle cramping, headaches and general malaise are noticed by the patient, that advice is sought from a renal physician.

Urinary manifestations associated with the disease include initially either a normal urine output or polyuria, though as the disease process progresses and more and more nephrons are obliterated, urine output falls and the patient may become oliguric. The increase in urine volume during the early stages may be due to a urea-induced osmotic diuresis and/or hypertrophy of the remaining nephrons in response to decreased functional renal mass. Consequent to these changes is an impaired ability to conserve fluid and concentrate urine; thus the patient may complain of thirst and nocturia and, when tested, the urine will have a low, often fixed, specific gravity (for example, 1.005–1.010). This specific gravity of urine rarely varies, as despite the cause the ultimate problems remain twofold: the filter is partially blocked; and due probably to the reduced amount of time which the filtrate spends in the tubule, concentration of the filtrate is inefficient and hence the resultant urine is always dilute.

With a number of chronic renal diseases, the kidneys become scarred and reduced in size; a major exception to this is the patient with polycystic kidney disease where the kidneys may increase in both size and weight several fold.

As the kidneys fail to regulate the composition of body fluids and to excrete circulating wastes, a metabolic acidosis develops (thus the patient may exhibit Kussmaul breathing) and an accumulation of substances such as urea, creatinine, uric acid, potassium, and phosphate occurs. In some patients carbohydrate intolerance may be noticed; there may be a tendency to develop hyperglycaemia, probably due to an insensitivity of peripheral tissues to insulin. When urine output is high, some patients may lose excessive amounts of sodium in the urine. However, in the later stages of chronic renal failure and in end-stage chronic renal failure, sodium retention is a more common problem, contributing to fluid retention, hypertension, oedema, and heart failure.

Hypertension may be suspected initially because of complaints of headaches, palpitations, and occasionally nausea. The elevation in blood pressure may precede the development of chronic renal failure or may be the result of sodium and water retention associated with a deterioration in renal function, increased renin release, or possibly a reduction in prostaglandin release from the renal medulla. Regardless of aetiology, hypertension,

and its accompanying salt and water retention may precipitate left ventricular hypertrophy and failure, congestive cardiac failure, retinal changes, and, if severe, hypertension may lead to encephalopathy. Oedema occurs as a result of heart failure and the loss of plasma proteins. Pericarditis is occasionally seen in patients with end-stage chronic renal failure in whom blood urea levels are very high; thus it is sometimes referred to a 'uraemic pericarditis'. This condition may be asymptomatic or may be accompanied by chest pain and a low grade fever; a pericardial friction rub may be noticed on auscultation.

The uraemic patient has a tendency to develop respiratory problems such as pulmonary oedema, uraemic pneumonitis, and pleurisy. The patient may thus be dyspnoeic, and orthopnoeic, may have a ·cough and may complain of chest pain.

Haemopoiesis is suppressed in patients with chronic renal failure due to a reduction in the amount of haemopoietin which is produced and as a result there is a reduction in the number of erythrocytes with a consequent anaemia. Other factors also predispose to anaemia such as increased haemolysis of red blood cells due to the uraemic enironment; a bleeding tendency (thus there may be gastrointestinal blood losses); and possible nutritional deficiencies, for example, of folic acid and iron, due to poor dietary intake. Mouth and gastrointestinal ulcerations commonly develop with time as the blood urea level rises, and the patient may therefore complain of bleeding gums or malaena. Loss of blood from the gastrointestinal tract is exacerbated by a qualitative defect in platelet function which is also due to the suppressed haemopoiesis, and the patient may also notice a haemorrhagic tendency. With the progression of uraemia, the patient becomes more susceptible to infection due to impaired immune responses, and a reduced number of leucocytes. An infection in a uraemic patient could further damage renal function and worsen the uraemia, and should thus be treated promptly.

Gastrointestinal manifestations associated with raised blood urea levels include nausea, vomiting, anorexia and weight loss, diarrhoea (or alternatively, constipation). Raised blood urea levels also manifest in hiccoughs and these may be so severe, continuous, and unresponsive to treatment as to eventually cause death from exhaustion. The patient may complain of a foul taste in his mouth and, in some cases, the patient's breath may smell ammoniacal (uraemic fetor).

The neurological problems of chronic renal failure are due to the accumulation of uraemic toxins, and fluid and electrolyte imbalances. The more important of these are insomnia, and a motor and sensory peripheral neuropathy which causes various degrees of parasthesia of the extremities, gait changes, foot drop, and in some patients the 'restless leg syndrome' – a condition characterized by choreic movements of both legs. An important consideration when managing uraemic patients is that they may have decreased concentration, reduced attention span, and some memory impairment; thus patient education programmes should be modified accordingly.

As renal function deteriorates, the musculo-skeletal problems of chronic renal failure become more serious. The inability of the kidneys to excrete required amounts of phosphate ion, and the reduction in the amount of active vitamin D synthesised by the kidneys, tend to result in elevated blood phosphate and depressed calcium levels. The reduction in blood calcium stimulates parathormone release which, by causing an increase in osteoclastic activity, liberates more calcium from the bones and thereby attempts to restore blood calcium levels to normal. This bone demineralization can result in osteoporosis, and as the serum calcium rises calcium is lost through the kidneys leading to the production of calcium calculi in the urinary tract. Bone pain and pathological fractures may result as a consequence of the osteoporosis. The deposition of calcium, phosphate and/or uric acid within the tissues may produce arthritic pain and swelling of the joints and gout may occur. Elevated blood potassium levels may produce generalized muscle weakness and cardiac arrhythmias. The loss of calcium and sodium in the urine during the early stages of chronic renal failure may precipitate muscle cramps.

The child with chronic renal failure will have retarded bone growth due to the lack of calcium despite normal circulating levels of growth hormone.

As urea and other waste products accumulate, various dermatological features become apparent. The anaemia may produce a pallor though the overall complexion is usually one of a muddy-brown colour due to retained pigments. Pruritus may be a problem and is thought to be, in part, related to the deposition of calcium and phosphate within the skin.

If left untreated, patients with chronic renal failure will eventually manifest many of the features outlined in Table 58.5, become comatose and die. However, effective management of patients with this disease may minimize a large proportion of the systemic effects of uraemia for some time.

Table 58.5 Systemic manifestations of endstage chronic renal failure. (Adapted from Read A E et al 1984 Modern Medicine 3rd edn. Churchill Livingstone, Edinburgh. p 276)

General
  Tiredness
  Irritability

Ocular
  Retinopathy
  Band keratopathy
  'Red eye'

Dermatological
  Pigmentation
  Pruritus
  Dry skin
  Purpura

Musculoskeletal
  Bone disease
  Weakness
  Myopathy
  Muscle cramp
  Restless legs

Endocrine
  Secondary hyperparathyroidism

Neurological
  Headache
  Parasthesia
  Convulsions
  Coma

Gastrointestinal
  Nausea
  Vomiting
  Anorexia
  Diarrhoea
  GIT haemorrhage
  Hiccough

Haematological
  Anaemia
  Susceptibility to infection
  Haemorrhagic tendency

Table 58.5 (*contd*)

Respiratory
  Dyspnoea and orthopnoea
  Pulmonary oedema

Cardiovascular
  Oedema
  Hypertension
  Pericarditis
  Ischaemic heart disease

Reproductive
  Impotence
  Subfertility
  Menstrual disturbances

Urinary
  Nocturia
  Enuresis
  Polyuria–Oliguria

Metabolic
  Elevated urea
  Elevated creatinine
  Hyperuricaemia
  Hyperkalaemia
  Hyperphosphataemia
  Metabolic acidosis

Investigative procedures

A thorough history should be obtained from the patient and should specifically include questions aimed at identifying any long term analgesic abuse. A physical examination may reveal any of the clinical manifestations outlined above and blood tests should be performed to assess renal function, electrolyte and acid–base balance, and serum albumin levels. Blood may also be obtained for levels of parathormone and alkaline phosphatase which are elevated in renal osteodystrophy. A full blood examination is undertaken for estimations of erythrocyte and leucocyte cell counts, haematrocrit, and haemoglobin. A clotting profile may also be performed.

Urine is obtained for microscopic examination of the sediment, and tested for protein and blood. A 24 hour urine collection is made to calculate creatinine clearance time and to assess urinary sodium, potassium, and protein losses. If a urinary tract infection is suspected, a midstream specimen is obtained for culture. Nerve conduction studies, a bone biopsy, a renal biopsy (if the kidneys are not too small) and a number of radiological investigations (for example, skeletal survey,

chest X-ray, pyelography, or arteriography), may also be undertaken to investigate the kidneys and the possible extent of bone disease.

Medical and nursing management

There are two major schools of thought regarding the more active treatment of patients with chronic renal failure. Some physicians favour the early introduction of either haemodialysis or peritoneal dialysis. Others prefer to delay dialysis for as long as possible by minimizing the systemic effects of uraemia through dietary controls and drug administration. Obviously, the treatment path ultimately selected for the patient should be aimed at meeting the individual's particular needs and requirements as much as possible. Patient compliance and understanding are essential to the effectiveness of any form of treatment.

The patient must have his fluid intake and output balanced, all fluid taken in (including that in food) and all fluid excreted (including that fluid lost in faeces, respiration and through the skin) must be estimated and recorded. It is reasonable throughout this entire disease process to use the same fluid replacement parameters, that is to ensure the patient takes in a volume of fluid equivalent to the previous day's fluid loss plus 400 ml. Whether the patient is oliguric or polyuric this regime will cater for his fluid needs.

The patient's fluid intake and output must be accurately charted and balanced on a daily basis by altering intake or by increasing output with the use of diuretics. The patient should be weighed daily as a further guide to fluid balance.

If the patient has a fluid overload, pulmonary oedema with a subsequent chest infection is likely and chest physiotherapy is therefore an essential part of treatment. If the patient does contract a lung infection, treatment should be commenced promptly with a high dose short-term antibiotic.

Some patients may require sodium chloride supplements if there is excessive loss of sodium in the urine. As urea and electrolyte imbalances occur, blood should be tested regularly to monitor the effects of treatment and to detect any further deterioration in renal function. A rising blood urea level associated with gastrointestinal upsets is an indication for restricting the amount of protein in the diet. Protein restrictions in the order of 0.3–1.0 g/kg body weight/day are not unusual though the patient's dietary intake should consist of high biological value proteins (for example, milk, eggs, fish, meat and poultry) and a carbohydrate intake of around 8000 kJ should also be maintained to prevent muscle wasting. Advice should be sought from a dietitian regarding the patient's diet and an educational programme initiated for the patient and his significant others in order that the restrictions can be applied in the home. Dietary restrictions should, where possible, be imposed gradually and only when necessary, as very low protein diets (for example 20 g/day) are largely uninteresting and unpalatable.

A reduction in glomerular filtration rate usually causes a retention of potassium ions which may lead to fatal arrhythmias. For this reason dietary potassium restrictions may be necessary in the later stages of chronic renal failure and the patient may also be required to take Resonium A orally. Vitamin supplements (for example, B group vitamins) are commonly prescribed for patients with chronic renal failure as deficiencies may occur.

Hypertension is treated aggressively.

The chronic (usually normochronic, normocytic) anaemia is difficult to manage; most patients adapt to a lowered erythrocyte count, however some may require an infusion of packed cells every few months. When transfusing blood to these patients, care should be taken to infuse it slowly, as their inability to excrete a fluid load rapidly heightens the risk of pulmonary oedema. Before blood is transfused to any patient with chronic renal failure it must be considered that repeated blood transfusions can complicate the patient's tissue classification. Repeated blood transfusions may make it ultimately impossible for a reasonable tissue match to be found and it will therefore be impossible for a renal transplant to be undertaken.

A haemorrhagic tendency in these patients means that extra precautions should be taken to prevent injury (for example, make sure that sharp edges on bed rails are padded if the patient is confused or restless) and when performing venepuncture firm pressure should be applied to the needle site for a little longer than usual. The

increased susceptibility of these patients to infection requires the nurse to be alert for any signs or symptoms of a chest, urinary tract, skin, or any other type of infection, and as a general rule, where possible, these patients should be separated from other infected patients within the ward.

The gastrointestinal-related problems of nausea and vomiting may be relieved by reducing blood urea levels by restricting protein intake or dialysis. The administration of an antiemetic prior to meals, and the imaginative preparation and presentation of foods in accordance with the patient's likes within the imposed dietary restrictions may also help.

Calcium and phospate metabolism is interrelated; if the calcium levels are high, the phosphate levels will be low and vice versa. These patients draw massive quantities of calcium from their bones and 'dump' it into the urine. This process can be slowed down by lowering the phosphate levels and 'deceiving' the body's feedback mechanisms.

Phosphate levels are lowered by administering aluminium hydroxide with meals; this aids in binding dietary phosphate within the gut and allows it to be excreted in the faeces. Dosages of the drug are determined by blood phosphate levels. Depressed blood calcium levels may be further treated by administering calcium carbonate and/or vitamin D analogues. If bones show pathological changes on X-ray and biopsy, care should be taken by the patient and by the nurse when handling the patient, to prevent knocks and falls which may cause fractures. Any bone related pain may be partially controlled by the careful use of analgesia, bearing in mind that some analgesics may worsen the renal failure. If gout is present and blood uric acid levels are high, allopurinol may be prescribed to reduce the formation of uric acid.

Little can be done for the muddy-brown complexion of the uraemic patient. Pruritus is primarily controlled by reducing blood urea levels and through regular skin care. Topical antipruritics and antihistamines are occasionally used.

Cimetidine may be prescribed to help reduce gastric acid secretion and ulcer formation. Frequent mouth washes and regular brushing of teeth may help relieve the foul taste and fetor, and a soft rather than a firm bristled tooth brush should be used to minimize trauma to and subsequent bleeding of the gums. Stools should be tested regularly for occult blood as peptic ulceration occurs in a significant percentage of chronic renal failure patients, and may therefore be a source of blood loss.

Sexual dysfunction related to chronic renal disease is probably best handled by a sex counsellor and an empathic partner. However, the nurse should encourage the patient to talk about any sexual problems he may be experiencing, as sexual behaviour plays a major role in self image and perceptions of interpersonal relationships.

Anticipated outcome

When conservative measures fail to control or minimize the systemic effects of uraemia, then dialysis, transplantation, or death are the only options available. The patient with chronic renal failure should therefore be counselled by dialysis personnel during the course of the disease to allow for some adjustments to occur prior to this therapy being instigated. It is sometimes a useful practice to arrange for discussions to take place between the patient, significant others, and dialysis and transplant patients. Such an exercise is often helpful in allaying the many fears patients have once they realize dialysis is inevitable. Naturally enough, when faced with the prospect of a chronic disease, many patients will undergo periods of depression and some will entertain notions of suicide. It is important, therefore, for the nurse to support the patient and family throughout the illness, to encourage the verbalization of feelings, and to be alert to those indicators which will suggest the need for further specialized supportive intervention.

DIALYSIS

Within Australia, approximately 4000 patients are receiving either some form of dialysis or have functioning renal transplants. At present, haemodialysis is the most common method of treating patients with end-stage chronic renal failure in Australia. With recent advances in peritoneal dialysis techniques, it is likely that this method will become more favoured in the future. A little over 50% of all patients being dialysed are managed at home, thus the concept of 'self-care' is an important philosophy upon which the treatment of a patient is based.

Peritoneal dialysis

Peritoneal dialysis is a process whereby sterile fluid (dialysate) is introduced into the peritoneal cavity in order that fluid, electrolytes, and wastes can diffuse from the blood vessels of the peritoneum into the dialysate. Following a suitable period of time in which the substances in the dialysate and blood equilibrate across the peritoneal membrane, the effluent dialysate is drained out of the peritoneal cavity by gravity and discarded. If this procedure is repeated a number of times, the metabolic disturbances brought about by uraemia may be controlled. Peritoneal dialysis may be employed to treat patients with either acute or chronic renal failure and may also be indicated in cases of poisoning, fluid overload, electrolyte imbalances, and rarely in the treatment of peritonitis (for example, by the addition of antibiotics to dialysate fluid). Peritoneal dialysis is generally contraindicated for patients who have had recent abdominal surgery, who have intra-abdominal adhesions, or who are hypercatabolic.

The dialysate is introduced to the peritoneal cavity by means of a catheter inserted into the anterior abdominal wall. For short-term dialysis a rigid catheter is inserted under local anaesthetic and sutured in place so that it can be easily withdrawn once dialysis is no longer required. Long-term dialysis requires the implantation of a silastic rubber (Tenckhoff) catheter into the abdomen, usually under a general anaesthetic.

The method of dialysis is determined by the patient's condition. If the patient is in acute renal failure, and peritoneal dialysis is the method of choice, continuous cycles are generally maintained until the problem resolves, that is, urea and electrolytes are controlled, or the patient begins an effective diuresis. A 'cycle' in these cases refers to the time required for the dialysate to infuse into the peritoneal cavity, for equilibration to occur, and for the effluent dialysate to drain out again.

This usually takes approximately an hour, thus 24 cycles are usually possible each day.

If peritoneal dialysis is considered the treatment of choice for a patient in end-stage chronic renal failure, the general aim is to train the patient to manage the dialysis largely independently, with due regard to his safety. Such patients may therefore enter a continuous ambulatory peritoneal dialysis (CAPD) training course, or may be selected for some form of intermittent dialysis programme.

CAPD offers the advantages of flexibility, promotes independence and self-care, and prevents the wider fluctuations of urea and electrolyte levels within the blood which are associated more with other forms of dialysis. CAPD requires the patient to carry out 4–6 exchanges (cycles) per day for 5–7 days each week. The equilibration time (that is, the time in which the dialysate remains in the peritoneal cavity) varies from 3–8 hours and, during such times, the patient is free to carry out any reasonable task desired (for example, work or recreation). The patient is responsible for infusing, draining, and aseptically changing the dialysate bags periodically. Figure 58.3 depicts the practical principle of CAPD.

Intermittent peritoneal dialysis, for practical purposes, usually requires the aid of some form of automation. When using this form of dialysis, the patient is required to dialyse for 40–48 hours per week which may involve one extended session of dialysis per week, or the time on dialysis may be divided through a seven day period (for example, 2 sessions per week of 24 hour duration, or 4–6 nightly dialyses each week). If dialysis is performed during the night, the last exchange may be left in the peritoneal cavity during the day and drained prior to commencing automated dialysis at night; this form of peritoneal dialysis is referred to as continuous cycling peritoneal dialysis (CCPD).

Intermittent peritoneal dialysis and cycling peritoneal dialysis have 2 advantages over continuous ambulatory peritoneal dialysis:

- They use machines, and the patient is thus relatively free of the responsibility of changing flasks
- The patient has some time during the day without a fluid load in the peritoneum.

Sterile, commercially available peritoneal dialysate is commonly packaged in 1 or 2 litre plastic packs which contain water, dextrose, sodium, chloride, calcium, magnesium, and lactate. Variation in the concentration of dextrose allows for more or less fluid to be removed from the patient during each exchange. Hypertonic solutions (for example, dextrose 2.5% and dextrose 4.25% dialysate) will remove fluid from the patient, therefore

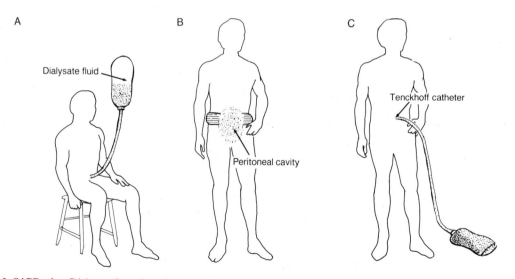

Fig. 58.3 CAPD. **A** – Dialysate flows from bag into peritoneal cavity through Tenckhoff catheter. **B** – Bag is rolled and carried around waist or in pocket. Dialysis takes place. **C** – Effluent flows into bag.

the volume of effluent dialysate will be greater than the amount of dialysate infused. A dextrose concentration of 1.5% will remove little (if any) fluid from the patient, and a hypotonic dialysate (for example, dextrose 0.5%) will allow fluid to be retained by the patient. If required, other electrolytes (for example, potassium) or drugs (for example, heparin or antibiotics) may be added to the dialysate manually, using aseptic technique.

The management of patients on peritoneal dialysis includes regulating the composition of the dialysate to achieve fluid and electrolyte balance, and observing the patient regularly for signs of fluid imbalance, infection, and other complications associated with this procedure. These include: infection, primarily of the peritoneum and the lungs, pain, protein loss, fluid excess or deficit, mechanical problems (for example, poor inflow or outflow), and hyperglycaemia. Leakage around the catheter exit site, electrolyte imbalance (especially hypokalaemia if potassium is not added to dialysate packs), atelectasis, and loss of water soluble vitamins may also occur. The presentation and nursing management of the more common complications associated with peritoneal dialysis are described in Table 58.6).

Table 58.6 Common complications of peritoneal dialysis

Potential problem	Presentation	Nursing management
Poor flow	No drip rate Extended inflow and/or outflow time Positive dialysate balance	Check line for kinks Check roller clamp is on Check catheter under dressing is not kinked Observe line for fibrin threads Change position of patient (e.g. sit up, stand out of bed, roll to side) if possible Using aseptic technique, aspirate and wash out catheter, change lines Add heparin as ordered to dialysate bags if fibrin present
Peritonitis	Abdominal pain Pyrexia Diarrhoea/nausea/vomiting Cloudy effluent Poor inflow and outflow Fibrin threads in effluent Distended abdomen	Obtain effluent sample for microscopy/culture/sensitivity Administer antibiotics as ordered via dialysate Add heparin as ordered to dialysate to prevent blockage of catheter Continuous In/Out cycles until effluent is clear
Fluid overload	Oedema Dyspnoea Orthopnea Hypertension Weight gain	Obtain blood and dialysate for electrolytes assessment Monitor vital signs Weigh patient Restrict fluids Use hypertonic dialysate solutions (e.g. 2.5% or 4.25% dextrose)
Protein loss via dialysate	Postural hypotension Oedema may be present	Often associated with peritonitis, therefore treat if present Check protein intake is adequate Monitor both lying and standing blood pressure
Fluid deficit	Weakness May have a postural hypertension Tachycardia Weight loss	Obtain blood and dialysate for electrolytes assessment Monitor vital signs Weigh patient Increase fluid intake Identify and treat underlying problems (e.g. diarrhoea) If problem due to excess fluid removal via dialysis, use 0.5% or 1.5% dextrose dialysate DO NOT USE HYPERTONIC SOLUTIONS

Haemodialysis

Like peritoneal dialysis, haemodialysis may be used for patients in acute or chronic renal failure. The process involves gaining access to the patient's circulation so that blood may be removed from the patient and directed along a semipermeable membrane. Fluid and wastes diffuse across the membrane to a dialysate which is then discarded. Having passed through the machine, the blood is returned to the patient, creating a continuous circuit. Figure 58.4 illustrates a typical unit.

Patients with acute renal failure are dialysed when necessary to maintain fluid and electrolyte balance. During the oliguric phase this may involve a 4 hour session of dialysis every day or every second day. Patients in end-stage chronic renal failure need maintenance dialysis therapy to sustain life. Most commonly, this involves three 4–6 hour sessions of dialysis each week. Dialysis takes place either in hospital or, when a training programme has been successfully completed, the patient may dialyse himself at a dialysis 'satellite' centre within the community or may be dialysed at home.

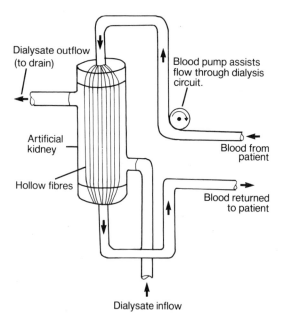

Fig. 58.4 Haemodialysis. Blood is removed from and returned to the patient in a continuous cycle. In the machine, blood is passed through fine, hollow fibres which are bathed in a flow of dialysate. Wastes diffuse from the blood into the dialysate.

Nursing management

Haemodialysis, like many aspects of peritoneal dialysis, requires the specialist attention of specialized personnel. Nursing students should however be familiar with the major potential complications which may follow a dialysis session, and should have a practical knowledge of the most commonly used means of vascular access so that on return to the ward the patient can receive appropriate care.

The most common complications which the nurse may encounter in a patient after dialysis has been completed include; hypotension (due to excess salt and fluid removal during dialysis); headaches, nausea and vomiting; fatigue and weakness (these symptoms usually subside in a few hours); infection (for example, an infection of the arterio-venous shunt or fistula, and septicaemia); muscle cramps and haemorrhage, or thrombosis of the arterio-venous shunt or fistula. If any of these complications are present or suspected, they should be reported immediately and appropriate action taken.

Access to the patient's circulation for haemodialysis may be afforded by the insertion of a central venous catheter(s), or an arterio-venous shunt, or by the creation of an arterio-venous fistula. The former methods are most commonly used to dialyse a patient with acute renal failure because they can be used immediately following insertion. An arterio-venous fistula (or some form of graft material) often requires some weeks before oedema subsides and the fistula is ready for use. The non-dominant arm is the preferred site for an arterio-venous shunt or fistula, though a leg may be used on occasions.

The arterio-venous shunt comprises 2 lengths of silicone rubber tubing joined at one end by a Teflon connector. The other ends of the tubing are inserted into an artery and a suitable vein, thus arterial blood flows through the rubber tubing which is brought out on top of the skin and then straight back into a vein (Fig. 58.5). By disconnecting the silicone tubing, access to an arterial supply is gained for haemodialysis and the dialysed blood can also be returned to the circulation via the venous end of the shunt. Unfortunately, a major complication associated with both arterio-venous shunts and arterio-venous fistulae

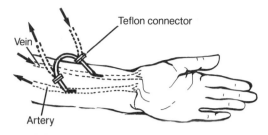

Fig. 58.5 Arterio-venous shunt.

is thrombosis, and because these access devices are the patient's 'life-line', measures should be taken to prevent thrombosis and regular patency checks should be made of the access device to monitor viability.

The patency of an arterio-venous shunt can be ascertained by the following assessment procedures:

1. Observe the colour of the shunt tubing. It should be a uniform, bright red colour. If clotted, the shunt may be dark in colour, and a separation of the serum and cells will be noticed.
2. Auscultate the tubing with a stethoscope. A bruit will be heard if the shunt is patent.
3. The shunt should be warm to touch. It may feel cool if clotting has occurred.
4. Gently squeeze the exposed tubing between thumb and forefinger to feel the pulsating flow of blood through the shunt. If clotted, no pulse will be felt.
5. Kink the exposed tubing sufficiently to occlude the flow of blood and observe the clear white silicone tubing. Upon release of the tubing, blood should immediately recommence flowing. *NOTE: Do not occlude the tubing for any more than 2 seconds as a sustained occlusion of the tubing may lead to thrombosis.*

The arterio-venous fistula (Fig. 58.6) is an artificially created anastomosis between an artery and a vein such that arterial blood is directed through a superficial vein causing it to dilate and thicken. When an arterio-venous fistula is used for haemodialysis, a cannula is inserted into a distended vein from which blood flows to the dialyser. A second cannula is also inserted higher in the same vein to provide a means for returning blood to the patient. The patency of an anterio-venous fistula may be checked by the following procedures:

1. Feel the anastomosis site for the presence of a strong pulse. If no pulse can be felt, the fistula may have thrombosed
2. Auscultate the arterio-venous fistula with a stethoscope. A definite, loud bruit should be heard if the fistula is patent
3. Observe the skin above the anastomosis site. It may pulsate slightly as blood is directed through the anastomosed vein. Also observe for distention of the superficial veins.

General measures to be taken to minimize the risk of thrombosis of the above types of angioaccess include:

1. Do not measure blood pressures on the limb involved in angioaccess
2. Do not allow IV infusions or venepunctures in this limb
3. Do not apply tight clothing, or an identification bracelet or wrist-watch to this limb
4. If an arterio-venous shunt is inserted, ensure that the tubing is free from kinks.

RENAL TRANSPLANTATION

Renal transplantation is widely regarded as the treatment of choice for most patients with end-stage chronic renal failure. However, because the demand for donor kidneys far outweighs current supply, many patients are required to undergo months or years of dialysis before a suitable kidney becomes available. Since 1977, there have been over 300 renal transplant operations per year in Australia. The donor kidney is usually obtained from patients who die in hospital, having been diagnosed clinically as being 'brain dead'. A small proportion are obtained from living donors.

Statistically, grafts transplanted from a living donor have a much better rate of survival than

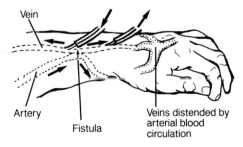

Fig. 58.6 Arterio-venous fistula.

those obtained from cadavers. The one year primary graft survival rate was 86% from living donors and 59% for cadaveric allografts; five year primary graft survival rates were 66% and 40% respectively in the period 1978–1983. One and five year patient survival rates are somewhat higher, being 96% and 89% for living donor transplants and 89% (one year) and 73% (five years) for cadaveric transplant patients.

Donor–recipient compatibility plays an important part in the success of transplanted kidneys. Tests are performed to determine whether donor and recipient have compatible blood groups (ABO match) and similar tissue antigens. Tissue typing utilizes the antigens present on the walls of leucocytes and is referred to as Human Leukocyte Antigen (HLA) matching. When as close a match as possible is made between the prospective recipient and the donor, the kidney and a section of its ureter, artery and vein is transplanted into the recipient's iliac fossa. The renal artery is usually anastomosed to the internal iliac artery and the renal vein to a nearby vein (for example, iliac vein). The transplanted ureter is tunnelled into and attached to the bladder wall in such a fashion as to prevent reflux.

Postoperative medical and nursing management

Post operatively, the patient is nursed in protective isolation for some time because the heavy immunosuppression required to minimize rejection also renders him susceptible to many types of infection. The patient's state of hydration, his vital signs, and his fluid balance should be monitored carefully throughout the postoperative period. Urine output is measured and recorded hourly, urinary drainage being provided by a Foley's catheter inserted during or prior to the transplant operation; a continuous bladder irrigation may also be commenced. The wound should be observed regularly, as for any postoperative site (see Chapter 6). Patency of the angioaccess must be maintained since dialysis may still be required should the transplanted kidney not work immediately, or if it is rejected at a later date. Blood and urine tests are performed regularly to assess the function of the new kidney.

The greatest threats to the transplant patient are infection and rejection of the grafted kidney. The latter may occur within 24 hours of the operation or later on in the habilitative period. For this reason, medications are required to be administered to control and suppress the patient's immune system; agents commonly used include: prednisolone, azothioprine, cyclosporin A, and in some centres antilymphocyte globulin (ALG) may also be used. The signs and symptoms of rejection and other major complications associated with renal transplantation are listed in Table 58.7.

Table 58.7 Complications of renal transplantation

Rejection
    Manifestations:
        Pyrexia
        Pain or tenderness over the graft site
        Swollen graft
        Weight gain, oedema, hypertension
        Decreased urine output, proteinuria, decreased urinary
            sodium
        Elevated blood urea and creatinine levels

    Possible management options:
        Increased immunosuppressive therapy
        Antilymphocyte globulin (ALG)
        Heparin therapy
        Plasmapheresis
        Graft nephrectomy

Infection
    Common sites:
        Respiratory tract
        Urinary tract
        Wound
        Skin
        Blood

    Microorganisms commonly implicated:
        Streptococcus
        Staphylococcus
        Pseudomonas
        Candida
        Herpes virus
        Cytomegalovirus
        Pneumocystic carynii

Obstruction to urine outflow

Haemorrhage

Arterial stenosis

Complications associated with immunosuppressive therapy
    Psychosis
    Bone marrow depression
    Acne
    Cushingoid appearance
    Malignancy
    Hyperglycaemia
    Increased appetite (weight gain)
    Peptic ulceration
    Aseptic necrosis of bones (e.g. hip)

During the postoperative period the patient may undergo episodes of depression. This is often due to misplaced guilt about acquiring a kidney as a result of another person's death. Depression can also be caused by fear of tissue rejection, especially if the graft takes some time to function. The nurse should be aware of these psychological changes which may occur and provide support when necessary. Professional counselling may at times be required.

Physical changes due to steriod therapy (for example, acne, cushingoid facial appearance) may be distressing initially, but they resolve and disappear as drug dosages are gradually reduced postoperatively. Fortunately, most dialysis patients have had close contact with transplant patients and are thus well informed about the procedure and its consequences.

Statistics quoted in the above discussion of dialysis and transplantation are from the Seventh Report of The Australia and New Zealand combined Dialysis and Transplant Registry, 1984.

RENAL CALCULI (UROLITHIASIS)

The presence of calculi in the urinary tract is relatively common. The prevalence of renal calculi in Western society has been estimated at 0.02–2%, the variation being attributable to the population sample studied, its geographical location, and possibly its socioeconomic and occupational characteristics. Males are more commonly affected than females, but this sex incidence is reversed in cases of 'infection stones' (struvite or staghorn calculi) due to the higher incidence of urinary tract infections in women. Renal calculi are relatively rare in Negroes and in children, suggesting that both genetic and environmental factors play a role in the aetiology of the disease. Unfortunately, recurrence of renal calculi following removal or passage from the urinary tract is high (around 60%), thus measures aimed at the prevention of stone formation play a major role in therapy.

Calculi are usually formed within the kidney, but may migrate to the ureters, the urinary bladder, or the urethra. Should they become impacted along the urinary conduit (for example,

renal calyces to urethra), they may cause obstruction to the flow of urine and produce a hydroureter and/or hydronephrosis. A large percentage of patients admitted to hospital with a diagnosis of renal calculi have so called 'noisy' stones, that is, the movement of the stone along the urinary tract or its obstruction to the flow of urine is sufficient to produce severe symptoms. Some stones on the other hand may be regarded as 'quiet', that is they do not produce symptoms and may be found only in the course of investigating the patient for some other complaint.

Aetiology and pathophysiology

A number of factors are implicated in the formation of renal calculi. These include a positive family history of the condition and dietary habits of the patient. High calcium and oxalate diets, and high protein diets are associated with stone formation. Recurrent or persistent urinary tract infections also play a role in the development of particular types of stones. Other factors implicated include prolonged immobilization which tends to increase bone demineralization; dehydration, by causing the formation of a solute-laden, highly concentrated urine; and the stagnation of urine from any cause, for example, low fluid intake, bladder dysfunction, or obstruction to the flow of urine. An excess in the concentration of normal or abnormal urinary constituents may predispose to the precipitation of salt-forming crystals and eventually stone formation. The deposition of crystals is also dependent on the temperature and pH of the urine, and the presence of some substances which can act as a nidus for the development of the stone (for example, mucoproteins, mucopolysaccharides, bacteria, cellular debris, or foreign body).

The 4 major types of calculi are described in Table 58.8. By far the most common are those containing calcium, either in combination with oxalate or phosphate, or as a mixture of both calcium oxalate and calcium phosphate.

In approximately 80% of patients with calcium stones the cause is idiopathic. For the remainder of patients with calcium stones, an underlying cause such as hyperparathyroidism, excessive vitamin D ingestion, bone malignancy, prolonged

Table 58.8 Major types of renal calculi and some measures which may be taken to prevent their formation

Major types	Comment	Prevention
Calcium-containing Calcium oxalite Calcium phosphate	Most common type of calculi	Low calcium, low oxalate diet. Acidify urine, low calcium diet, thiazide diuretic
Struvite	Infection calculi, Staghorn calculi	Acidify urine, treat any underlying infection
Uric acid	Form only in an acid urine	Alkalize urine, limit intake of purine-rich foods, allopurinol
Cystine	Form only in an acid urine	Alkalize urine, penicillamine

immobilization, or, rarely, milk-alkali syndrome may be found.

The second major type of renal calculi are those which occur in the presence of an upper urinary tract infection with urea-splitting microorganisms such as *Proteus mirabilis* or *Staphylococcus aureus*. These are termed infection or struvite stones and are composed largely of magnesium, ammonium, and phosphate. Characteristically, these stones remain 'silent' for some time and grow extensively within the renal pelvis, and the major and minor calyces. Because of their large size and peculiar shape, they are often referred to as staghorn calculi because the conformation of the stone, in line with the collecting system of the kidney, resembles the horns of a male deer.

Uric acid stones form the third major type of renal calculi. They may be produced as a result of idiopathic gout, or secondary to any factor in which excessive quantities of uric acid are released as a result of cellular destruction, for example, malignancy, polycythaemia, cytotoxic therapy, or irradiation. Under certain circumstances, the use of a uricosuric agent may also precipitate the formation of uric acid stones. Because uric acid is the end product of purine metabolism, the incidence of uric acid calculi is relatively high in Western countries due to the large amount of dietary protein ingested.

A less common cause of renal calculi is cystinuria. Cystine is an insoluble dibasic amino acid which may, if excreted in excessive amounts, produce cystine stones. These stones occur in patients with an inherited defect of tubular reabsorption of cystine. Both uric acid and cystine stones are formed only in acidic urine.

Clinical manifestations

If symptomatic, the manifestations of renal calculi are often severe and frightening for the patient, though the type and location of the pain does vary somewhat depending on the location of the calculus. Calculi may become lodged within the calcyes and pelvis of the kidney, at the pelvo-ureteric junction, the pelvic brim, the vesico-ureteric junction, the bladder, or the penis. The pain of an upper urinary tract calculus is usually on one side, though bilateral renal calculi do occur and may produce bilateral flank pain.

Typically, the pain of 'renal' colic begins abruptly and increases in intensity over 10–30 minutes until it becomes so excrutiating that the patient is often doubled over in agony. The attack may last for hours, and characteristically the pain comes in waves interspersed by pain-free periods in which the patient is very apprehensive, anxious, and restless not knowing when the next attack will come. The pain may be of such severity that it is accompanied by the feeling of nausea, sweating, chills, fever, and the patient's skin may be pale and clammy. This type of pain is usually associated with the lodgement or passage of the calculus in the pelvo-ureteric junction or down the ureter. The pain is initially identified in the region of the loin, and radiates laterally around the abdomen to the iliac fossa. As the calculus moves down the ureter, the pain may be referred to the suprapubic region, the groin, scrotum, testis, or labia. A bladder calculus may produce suprapubic pain, dysuria, frequency, strangury (which may also indicate the presence of a urinary tract infection), and perineal discomfort.

Passage of the calculus through the urethra may cause urethral pain, especially at the external urethral meatus. Calculi lodged within the calyces or renal pelvis may not produce severe pain and are usually manifested only by a dull ache in the loin and costovertebral tenderness, probably as a result of the obstruction to urine flow and the developoment of hydronephrosis or pyelonephritis.

Investigative procedures

The patient's history, especially regarding urinary tract problems such as calculi or infection, normal dietary habits, fluid intake, and any medications the patient may be taking (including self-prescribed vitamin supplements and over-the-counter proprietary preparations) is taken. Radiological investigations will include a plain X-ray of the kidneys, ureters and bladder (most calculi are radio-opaque, though uric acid stones are radioluscent); an intravenous pyelogram; and a CT scan of the urinary system to demonstrate the presence of all calculi.

Blood will be obtained for renal function tests as well as for estimations of serum calcium, phosphate, uric acid, alkaline phosphatase and parathyroid hormone levels. Some haematological tests may also be performed (for example, Hb, FBE, erythrocyte sedimentation rate.

If the patient passes a calculus in the urine, it should be sent for analysis to ascertain its chemical composition. Such information will be useful for determining appropriate treatment and assists in planning the prevention of further calculi. Urine will be collected to estimate the 24-hour excretion rate of calcium, oxalate, urate, and cystine. Specimens may also be obtained for microbiological analysis, acid-fast bacilli, and cytological studies. At the ward or outpatients level, the urine should also be tested for blood, protein, glucose, and pH.

Medical, surgical, and nursing management

The aims of management of patients with renal calculi are to treat any underlying cause; to provide measures which assist in the passage (or removal) of the calculus; to prevent the complications associated with treatments, and to minimize the risk of recurrence. The methods of treatment for patients can be divided into two major groups. Conservative management is used for the majority of patients as approximately 90% of renal calculi are small enough to eventually be passed naturally. Surgical intervention is also necessary when conservative measures are ineffective or inappropriate. These measures are summarized in Figure 58.7.

Conservative management

The conservative management approach is utilized for those patients in whom the calculi are small (generally less than 5 mm) and will be passed in urine provided a high fluid intake is maintained. Pethidine is the analgesic of choice to control the bouts of pain as it relaxes smooth muscle. In general, morphine is contraindicated, as it causes spasm of smooth muscle and would therefore increase the pain. If morphine must be given, an antispasmodic such as atropine or hyascine butylbromide is also given. Antiemetics may also be needed if the patient is nauseated, and if vomiting occurs fluid intake may need to be supplemented intravenously.

The application of local heat to the loin, and hot baths may also help to ease the pain. A high fluid intake (for example, 3–4 l/24 hours) should be encouraged for all patients with renal calculi. It may also be necessary to wake the patient during the night to maintain the flushing action of urine over a 24-hour period.

The frequency of observations should be determined by the condition of the patient and special note should be made of the location, type, and duration of pain. All urine voided should be collected and strained, and if calculi are passed they should be sent for analysis and their passage reported. A urinalysis should be performed daily. X-rays are taken on a regular basis, usually every second day, to monitor the progress of the calculus through the urinary tract.

Once the calculus has been analysed, specific therapy for the patient can be instigated. A finding of calcium oxalate calculi may necessitate the patient to adhere to a low calcium, low oxalate diet. Dietary intake of oxalate may be curtailed by avoiding foods such as rhubarb, parsley, beetroot, strawberries, tomatoes, spinach, cola drinks, and tea. Through dietary control and also

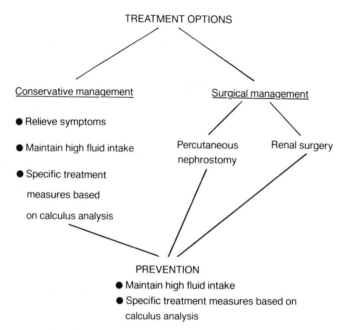

MANAGEMENT AIMS

1. Treat the underlying cause

2. Provide measures which assist in the passage (or removal) of the calculus

3. Prevent complications arising from treatment

4. Minimize risk of recurrence

TREATMENT OPTIONS

Conservative management

● Relieve symptoms

● Maintain high fluid intake

● Specific treatment

measures based

on calculus analysis

Surgical management

Percutaneous
nephrostomy

Renal surgery

PREVENTION
● Maintain high fluid intake
● Specific treatment measures based on
calculus analysis

Fig. 58.7 Schema of management of renal calculi.

by maintaining a high fluid intake, the recurrence of calculi may be minimized.

Calcium phosphate calculi are soluble in an acid urine, thus acidifying agents such as viatmin C or ammonium chloride may be ordered for patients with these calculi. With any form of calcium calculus, dietary restrictions of calcium-containing foods may also be needed. In some cases a thiazide diuretic may be used to reduce the renal excretion of calcium.

The formation of uric acid stones occurs only in the presence of a low urinary pH, and thus may be prevented by administering a urinary alkalizer such as sodium bicarbonate or a citrate solution. For some patients, the administration of allopurinol is effective, however some may need to limit their intake of purine rich foods, including meat, spinach, tea, coffee, and chocolate. In all cases where modifications to the diet are required, the patient and significant others should receive counselling from a dietician.

Patients with infection or struvite calculi pose special management problems. Any underlying infection should be treated with the appropriate antibiotic and the urine acidified to minimize recurrence of calculi. This often requires long-term drug therapy and regular follow up. Short-term management may involve the surgical removal of the calculi or the infusion of a Renacidin (R) solution via a nephrostomy tube or ureteric catheter in an affort to dissolve the calculus.

In cases of cystine stones penicillamine is used for some patients as it increases the solubility of cystine, thus allowing its excretion.

Surgical management

Surgery is indicated for those patients in whom a conservative approach has failed. Specific indications for some form of surgical intervention include: an obstruction of the urinary tract leading to hydroureter and/or hydronephrosis; the presence of calculi that are too large to be passed in the urine; recurrent infection; deterioration in renal function; and when a patient has frequent attacks of pain which are only poorly controlled by analgesia.

One of the least traumatic surgical interventions currently practised is that of the removal of renal calculi via a percutaneous nephrostomy tube. In this procedure, the patient is given premedication and, under radiological control, the tube is inserted through the loin into the pelvis of the kidney following infiltration of the area with local anaesthetic. Once inserted, the tube forms an alternative conduit for the drainage of urine and should be managed on the same principles as an ileal conduit (see page 620).

On the following day, the track made by the nephrostomy tube is gradually dilated until it is of sufficient size to afford the ready passage of a nephroscope. The patient is anaesthetized and a nephroscope is passed into the renal pelvis via the tract created by the nephrostomy tube. This enables visualization of calculi within the calyces or pelvis of the kidney. The urologist then has a choice of treatment: calculi may be removed using a basket extractor or forceps; or they may be disintegrated by means of an ultrasonic probe (Sonotrode), the tip of which is applied to the calculus under direct vision. The resulting fragments may then be aspirated, or manually removed, or they may pass down the ureter in the urine. Following the procedure, the nephrostomy tube is replaced and X-rays are taken to confirm that all calculi have been removed, prior to the patient being returned to the ward. There, in 1–2 days time, the nephrostomy tube is removed and if no extravasation of urine occurs, the patient is discharged.

The advantages of this procedure over conventional renal surgery are that only a small incision is required, and the time of hospitalization is reduced, as is convalescence. Problems which may be associated with the procedure are haemorrhage, extravasation of urine around the nephrostomy tube, and dislodgement of the catheter. The success achieved with this method suggests that it will be used with increasing frequency.

For a minority of patients, some form of open surgery is necessary in order to remove the calculus from the kidney or upper urinary tract. The more common types of operations performed are:

• Pyelolithotomy – removal of calculi through an incision made in the pelvis of the kidney
• Nephrolithotomy – removal of calculi through an incision of the renal parenchyma
• Partial nephrectomy – removal of a part of the renal substance
• Nephrectomy – removal of a kidney.

Complications

The major complications associated with renal calculi are: infection, hydroureter and hydronephrosis, chronic renal failure, and, in some cases, acute renal failure due principally to obstruction. Recurrence of renal calculi is common. Prior to discharge the nurse should ensure that the patient and significant others have a good understanding of the condition, any dietary modifcations needed or medications required, and of the importance of maintaining a high fluid intake. If a urinary acidifier or alkalinizer is prescribed it is useful to teach the patient how to test urine for pH.

RENAL SURGERY

Surgery to the kidney may be necessary for a number of reasons but the general nursing management of patients receiving such surgery subscribes to the same basic principles. For simplicity, the management of a patient undergoing a nephrectomy is outlined.

Nephrectomy is a relatively uncommon surgical procedure, being indicated in cases of malignancy, severe trauma or infection of the kidney, where a kidney is donated for transplantation, or when the kidneys are destroyed by calculi.

The usual operative approach is that of a loin incision, though, in some cases, a transabdominal approach may be utilized (Fig. 58.8).

Specific preoperative prepation should include an assessment of the other kidney's function, usually ascertained by performing an IVP and renal function tests, and a nipple-to-pubic shave. Routine postoperative care should be provided (see Chapter 6), and special note taken of the amount and type of drainage from the wound. Chest physiotherapy should also be carried out regularly to prevent pulmonary infection and collapse. It is also important to monitor urine output as a guide to the function of the remaining kidney.

Postoperative complications include haemorrhage, infection, and atelectasis which is compounded by the patient's reluctance to fully expand his lungs due to the close proximity of the operative site to the diaphragm. Less commonly, a pneumo- or haemothorax may occur if the pleura is cut when the loin approach is used. Peritonitis or an ileus may follow a transabdominal approach.

Patients undergoing renal surgery should be cautioned not to lift heavy weights for 2–4 weeks following the operation, and to maintain a copious fluid intake. Discharge advice should also require the patient to report any unusual pain or swelling of the loin or blood in the urine.

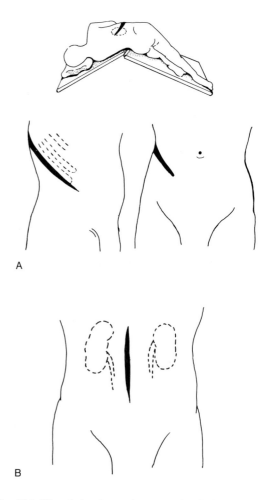

Fig. 58.8 Wound sites in renal surgery. **A** – Loin approach. **B** – Transabdominal approach.

59

Disorders of the ureter, bladder and urethra

A. P. Barnett

CALCULI

Ureteric calculi

Calculi which become lodged within the ureter are of renal origin. They may move from the calyces and renal pelvis down the ureter to cause either a complete or partial obstruction to urine flow resulting in a hydroureter or hydronephrosis. The passage of the calculus may be either 'noisy' (that is, producing severe pain) or 'quiet' (that is, largely asymptomatic), and a dull loin ache may be the only predominant symptom. Approximately 75–90% of ureteric calculi will eventually pass if the patient is given adequate pain relief and a copious fluid intake. Whether surgical intervention is required for the removal of the calculus is largely dependant upon its size. The majority of calculi can probably pass spontaneously if less than 7 mm in diameter.

The indications for the surgical removal of calculi within the ureter are:

- Obstruction (resulting in compromised function of the affected kidney)
- Infection (for example, pyelonephritis)
- Severe pain
- The size of the calculus.

Prior to surgery the patient should have an X-ray to check the location of the calculus and enable the surgeon to make an appropriate decision regarding the operative site. It is not unusual for a calculus to become dislodged along the ureter from one day to the next, especially if a good diuresis is maintained.

The aims of surgical intervention are to relieve the obstruction, prevent postoperative complications and to introduce long-term measures aimed at preventing further calculus formation. A number of surgical approaches may be used to extract a calculus, larger than 7 mm in diameter, from the ureter or calyceal system and these techniques are either invasive or noninvasive.

Percutaneous ultrasonic lithotripsy

This recent advance in surgical technique has markedly reduced the need for open ureterolithotomy and involves the removal of the calculus via a nephroscope using an ultrasonic lithotrite inserted via the skin and onto the portion of the urinary tract in which the calculus has lodged.

The advantages of percutaneous ultrasonic lithotripsy include: the elimination of the need for open surgery; fewer postoperative complications; a reduced hospital inpatient time (4–7 days as compared to 7–12 days for ureterolithotomy); a more rapid recovery to full physical ability (most patients can return to normal working conditions within 1 week of surgery as opposed to a convalescence of approximately 7–8 weeks with uterolithotomy).

Under fluoroscopic and radio-opaque dye control, the surgeon inserts the nephroscope either into the ureter or into the calyceal system via the body of the kidney and positions the nephroscope so that the calculus is within reach or can be suctioned into position. Initially an attempt is made to remove the calculus through suctioning or by seizing and crumbling the calculus using the caliper tongs of the nephroscope.

Should the calculus be too large or be resistant to such force, disintegration is attempted using ultrasound through a hollow probe, passed via the nephroscope. These high frequency sound waves normally result in disintegration of the calculus, forming granular particles of 1–2 mm in diameter. These particles are then removed either by a combination of irrigation and suction via the nephroscope, or by flushing from the urinary system with a postoperative diuresis. The nephrostomy and lithotripsy are normally performed in the one operation although the procedures can be staged over 1 or more days.

The procedure is normally performed under general anaesthesia but can be performed under a high spinal anaesthetic should the patient be considered a high risk for general anaesthesia. The nephrostomy incision is usually 1–2 cm long, and following removal of the calculus a nephrostomy catheter is usually inserted and sutured in place. This catheter is connected to a drainage bag and prevents urine build up in the unlikely event of a piece of calculus obstructing distal ureteral flow. The catheter also ensures drainage of all irrigation fluid from the kidney and reduces the likelihood of postoperative renal oedema.

Postoperative management. The patient will also have a urethral catheter in situ (and may also have a ureteral catheter) and the nurse will be responsible for regular and accurate monitoring of the patient's renal function. All urine passed should be strained through fine gauze and a record made of any calculus fragments passed.

The nephrostomy site dressing must be regularly checked for any copious drainage and/or bleeding. The patient should be advised that a mild degree of haemoserous drainage is to be expected around the nephrostomy catheter for at least the first 3 days postoperatively. Care must be taken when changing the nephrostomy site dressing so as to prevent excessive traction on the catheter and trauma to the incision. The nephrostomy catheter is usually removed on the third or fourth postoperative day and a pressure dressing applied to the wound. Only in the event of postoperative ureteral oedema would the patient be discharged with a nephrostomy catheter in situ.

The urethral and/or ureteral catheter is removed prior to discharge of the patient, usually on the third or fourth postoperative day and many patients are discharged soon after. He should be advised to maintain a high fluid intake in order to effect adequate flushing of the urinary tract and removal of calculi granules. The patient should be advised to change the nephrostomy dressing regularly in order to minimize the colonization of microorganisms. Wound healing should be effected within 7 days.

Although the patient's total pain experience is less with percutaneous ultrasonic lithotripsy than with open ureterolithotomy, immediate pain experienced in the first postoperative 24 hours is greater. This is largely due to both the passage of calculus granules and to the effects of ureteric inflammation and/or ureteric oedema. Pethidine is the pain control drug of choice because of its properties of smooth muscle relaxation and therefore its effectiveness in controlling ureteral colic.

Complications. The complications of percutaneous ultrasonic lithotripsy include: retroperitoneal haemorrhage from the body of the kidney; haemorrhage from the nephrostomy site (although minor bleeding is to be expected for the first 3 days); urinary tract infection either introduced at the time of lithotripsy or subsequently via the urinary drainage apparatus or via the wound; hypersensitivity to the radio-opaque dye used to locate the calculus; retention of irrigation fluid and/or urine; and either a haemothorax or pneumothorax if the nephroscope accidentally penetrates the thorax during insertion.

Extracorporeal shockwave lithotripsy

This totally noninvasive procedure utilizes high frequency shock waves to disintegrate large calculi (over 7 mm in diameter) into granular sand particles for passage in the urine. The shockwaves are administered from the lithotripter whilst the patient is submerged to the clavicular level in a bath of tepid water. The shock waves both enter and exit the body whilst the patient is submerged and the waves are targeted to have maximal effect where the calculus has lodged.

It is necessary for the patient to undergo either a general anaesthetic or a spinal anaesthetic to minimize both movement and pain during the procedure. Following treatment the nurse must ensure care and protection of the patient's limbs until normal sensation and motor function return. It is unusual for the patient to have a urethral catheter in situ post treatment and there is no incision. The patient is normally discharged within 48 hours and care consists largely of ensuring a copious fluid intake and monitoring fluid output for the passage of granules.

Extracorporeal procedures are less commonly performed largely due to the expensive nature of the equipment. Approximately 20% of patients require further treatment with the percutaneous technique and there is an increased risk of respiratory and/or cardiac complications. The ultrasound may cause rupture of alveoli, pleuritis, pleural effusion, or cardiac arrhythmias.

Endoscopic removal

Ureteric calculi may be removed endoscopically following the introduction of a cystoscope into the bladder. The patient is usually given a light general anaesthetic; occasionally, a spinal anaesthetic is used. The endoscopic removal of calculi is usually reserved for relatively small stones located in the lower end of the ureter and commonly involves either:

• The passage of a fine catheter up the ureter, which may enable the urologist to dislodge a partially impacted calculus and thus assist in its spontaneous removal.
• Removal of the calculus using a stone basket extractor, for example the Dormier basket (Fig. 59.1). In this method, the instrument is passed beyond the calculus, the basket is then extended and gently pulled back along the ureter to entrap the calculus and facilitate its removal.

Ureterolithotomy

An open operation for the removal of a ureteric calculus is only required if the stone is so large that it has become firmly lodged within the ureter and lithotripsy is either unavailable or unsuccessful. The site for surgical incision is determined by the location of the calculus on X-ray immediately prior to operation. A calculus within the upper third of the ureter commonly requires a loin approach; if located within the middle third of the ureter a paramedian incision is used; and if in the lower third an oblique incision is made in the region of the iliac fossa (Fig. 59.2). During the

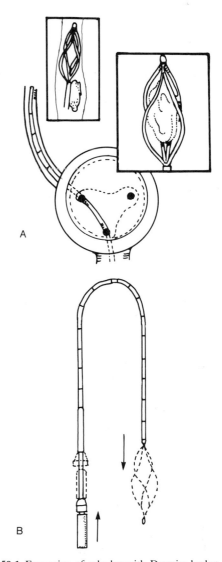

Fig. 59.1 Extraction of calculus with Dormier basket. **A** – Basket is passed up the ureter and traps stone. **B** – Mechanism of Dormier basket.

operation, the surgeon will identify and expose that section of the ureter containing the calculus and place two slings around the ureter, one above and the other below the calculus to prevent accidental dislodgement. The ureter is then incised and the calculus removed (Fig. 59.3) and sent for analysis. Upon completion, care is taken not to close the ureteric incision too tightly to minimize the likelihood of a stricture developing, and a drain tube is inserted to evacuate blood and urine from the operative site.

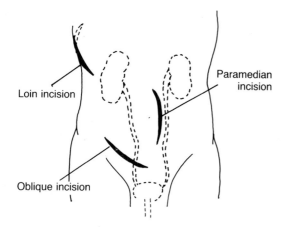

Fig. 59.2 Possible incision sites for ureterolithotomy.

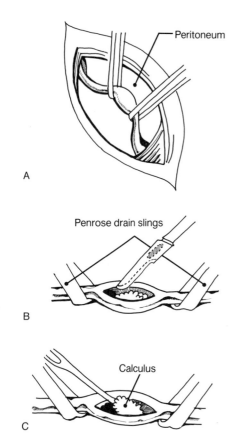

Fig. 59.3 Ureterolithotomy.

Postoperatively, specific care must be taken of the drain tube and, if possible, some form of drainage device should be attached or frequent dressing changes performed and the amount and type of drainage should be noted. The drain tube is left in place until drainage is minimal or ceases; generally, the tube is removed on the second to fifth day postoperatively.

Complications. The major postoperative complications associated with the endoscopic removal of ureteric calculi are a result of damage to the vesico-ureteric junction and include vesico-ureteric reflux and vesico-ureteric stenosis.

Specific complications associated with a ureterolithotomy include:

- Paralytic ileus, due to the extravasation of urine or blood in the retroperitoneal cavity
- Urinary fistula
- Ureteric stenosis, due to fibrosis of the ureter, or the ureter being too tightly sutured
- Damage to pelvic organs or structures.

Vesical calculi

Calculi found in the bladder, like ureteric calculi, usually originate from the kidney. Some, however, may form within the bladder in the presence of:

- Urinary stasis, due to hypertrophy, bladder diverticulum, a neurogenic bladder disorder, or urethral structures
- Infection
- As a result of long-term use of a catheter. The encrustations around the tip of the catheter may become dislodged when the catheter is removed and form a nidus for calculus formation
- As a result of a foreign body being introduced into the bladder.

Patients with bladder calculi may complain of symptoms associated with a urinary tract infection. They may also notice an intermittent stream on urination and an inability to void in certain positions due to the stone occluding the vesico-urethral orifice. If the patient is unable to pass the stone spontaneously, the aims of surgical intervention are the same as those for the removal of ureteric calculi. The 2 major approaches to surgical intervention are summarized below.

Endoscopic litholapaxy

Endoscopic removal of bladder calculi usually involves the passage of a stone-crushing instru-

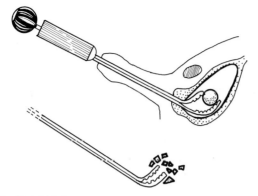

Fig. 59.4 Litholopaxy.

ment (a lithotrite) up the urethra into the bladder. When introduced, the jaws of the lithotrite are manipulated around the calculus which is crushed and the fragments evacuated (Fig. 59.4). Alternatively, ultrasound may also be used on bladder calculi. Postoperatively, the nurse should observe the patient for bladder or urethral trauma and infection (for example, cystitis, pyelonephritis, prostatitis, or septicaemia).

Endoscopic removal of calculi is inappropriate when a calculus is too large and cannot be disintegrated using ultrasound; a bladder tumour is present; the urethra is too narrow to allow the passage of the lithotrite; or a diverticulum is present which requires surgical excision.

Cystolithotomy

A cystolithotomy is the invasive technique used for the removal of large bladder calculi or when other procedures are inappropriate or ineffective.

A transverse suprapubic incision is made and the bladder opened to remove the stone and perform any additional surgery necessary. The surgeon is also likely to insert a self-retaining catheter at the time of operation to facilitate the drainage of blood and urine during the immediate postoperative period. Postoperative care is aimed at maintaining the patency of the catheter and preventing infection.

Urethral calculi

The lodgement of a calculus within the urethra is a rare occurrence, as most are voided spon-

taneously. It most commonly occurs in males and may be due to the presence of urethral diverticulae or strictures. Apart from urethral pain, tenderness, and other related urinary symptoms, the patient may also notice that the stream of urine is split. Surgical procedures for this condition include:

● Direct incision into the urethra and removal of the calculus
● Dislodgement of the calculus back into the bladder by the insertion of a urethral bougie. This procedure is followed by a litholapaxy
● Removal of the calculus with forceps (if the calculus lies within the distal section of the urethra). This procedure may also require a meatotomy to be performed.

The major complication associated with the above procedures is the development of a urethral stricture.

Analysis of the calculus should be undertaken prior to any patient being discharged so that a specific preventive programme can be arranged (see page 609). The patient is also encouraged to seek prompt medical advice should any further problems with urination arise.

NEOPLASIA

The bladder is one of the most common sites for the development of tumours within the urinary tract, secondary only to the prostate.

Ureteric neoplasms

Cancer of the ureters is a rare disease accounting for less than 1% of all genitourinary malignancy. The incidence is higher in males than in females and the most common histological form is that of a transitional cell carcinoma.

Clinical presentation follows much the same pattern as cancer of the bladder. A painless haematuria is the most common finding though some patients may present with flank pain and those symptoms which are associated with obstruction to the flow of urine.

Investigative procedures include urine cytology, pyelography (intravenous, antegrade, and/or retrograde), and in some cases a selective arteriography is also performed.

Management techniques include:

- Partial ureterectomy. If the lesion is localized, the affected section of the ureter is removed and the remaining proximal portion is reimplanted into the unaffected ureter
- Nephroureterectomy. An operation performed for more extensive lesions in which the kidney and ureter on the affected side are removed, as well as a portion of the healthy bladder
- Radiotherapy and chemotherapy may also be used as an adjunct to surgical intervention.

Palliative measures for cancer of the ureter are aimed at relieving pain and the obstruction to urine flow, and include:

- Creation of an ileal loop conduit or some other form of urinary diversion
- Placement of a ureteral stent to support and maintain drainage down the diseased ureter.

Bladder neoplasms

Carcinoma of the bladder is a common form of genitourinary cancer. The incidence is highest in the over 50 age group and males are affected more frequently than females, in a ratio of 3 : 1. Datta (1984) reports that bladder cancer is responsible for some 3% of all cancer deaths; thus early diagnosis, treatment, and follow up are essential to help reduce the mortality associated with the disease.

Aetiology and pathophysiology

Most tumours originating from the bladder are of a transitional cell type, though some do originate from squamous cells, or glandular tissues (adenocarcinoma). Like many other tumours, bladder cancers may be described according to their clinical staging or invasiveness (Table 59.1) and their degree of differentiation or similarity to their normal cell of origin. Thus the most serious of bladder cancers could be described as highly invasive (T4) and the cells poorly differentiated or anaplastic; such a diagnosis would be associated with a poor prognosis. A number of factors have

Table 59.1 TNM staging of bladder tumours

Tis – Tumour in situ
T1 – Tumour invades subepithelial connective tissue
T2 – Tumour invades superficial muscle
T3 – Tumour invades deep muscle or perivesical fat
T4 – Tumour invades one or more of: prostate, uterus, vagina, pelvic wall, abdominal wall.

been associated with cancer of the bladder including cigarette smoking, phenacetin abuse, and various occupations in which workers are exposed to benzidine or beta-naphthylamine (for example, dye, petroleum, and rubber industries).

Clinical manifestations

Approximately 75–80% of patients with bladder cancer present with haematuria. The haematuria is commonly painless and may be either microscopic or macroscopic. At times it is periodic and profuse; in those cases the patient may be prompted to seek medical advice, though unfortunately this manifestation may go unnoticed or even dismissed by the patient as insignificant. In these latter cases, the disease may progress to a more advanced stage which renders medical intervention more difficult and markedly reduces life expectancy.

Other manifestations include: dysuria, frequency, urgency, and hesitancy. In some cases clot retention may occur, which prevents micturition and the patient may therefore present with acute retention. Manifestations associated with invasive tumour growth, especially into other tissues, include: back or flank pain, bone pain, and uraemia (if the vesico-ureteric junction is obstructed or destroyed due to tumour growth). In advanced stages weight loss, anorexia, lethargy, and uraemia may be present. Again, the key to effective management of bladder cancer is the early detection of the tumour growth, appropriate medical intervention, and the implementation of a rigorous follow up programme.

Investigative procedures

Prior to any major investigative procedure being undertaken, a complete physical examination should be performed. A detailed history should be obtained from the patient with specific regard to any abnormalities noticed in relation to urination. Enquiry should also be made of the patient's occupational history and social habits (for example, smoking). Initially, the urine should be observed and tested for the presence of blood, and samples from a whole voided specimen should be obtained for microscopy and cytology, and for microbiological analysis to exclude an infective cause of the haematuria.

Radiological investigations include an IVP, ultrasound studies, chest X-ray, and a bone scan if metastases are suspected. Cystoscopy is commonly performed to allow the bladder to be directly visualized, and a biopsy taken of any abnormal tissue growth. The biopsy specimen is then histologically examined to identify the nature of the tumour so as to guide further treatment measures.

An additional investigative procedure requiring the patient to undergo general anaesthesia is a bimanual examination under anaesthetic (EUA). This procedure requires the surgeon to simultaneously perform a suprapubic abdominal and a rectal (or vaginal) palpation of the bladder to ascertain the presence of a tumour mass, its size, and its mobility.

Medical, surgical, and nursing management

The most common method by which cancer of the bladder is treated is surgery combined in some cases with chemotherapy and/or radiotherapy. Surgical intervention will vary according to the invasiveness of the tumour growth and the severity of the disease.

Transurethral resection of bladder tumour

This operation is usually preferred for the treatment of the more superficial types of lesions in which there has been no invasion of the cancer into the bladder muscle. The urologist introduces a resectoscope via the urethra into the patient's bladder and resects the tumour growth. In some cases, use is also made of a diathermy probe to cauterize the lesion.

Postoperatively, the patient has continuous bladder irrigation in situ to remove blood and tissue from the bladder and to prevent clot retention. The infusion of irrigating fluid (usually sodium chloride 0.9%) via a 3-way self-retaining Foley's catheter should be at a rate sufficient to prevent clot formation and to maintain the outflow at a rose colour. It is therefore important for the nurse to maintain a record of all input and output, to record the colour of the bladder effluent, and to observe for any signs or symptoms of clot retention. These include reduced outflow, poor inflow, bladder distention, bladder fullness, or suprapubic pain. The patient should be encouraged to maintain a high fluid intake as soon as it can be tolerated to promote urine formation and flow, and routine catheter care and pain relief should also be provided.

Unfortunately, the recurrence of superficial bladder lesions is common; thus it is not unusual for the patient to be given topical cytotoxic agents (for example, doxorubicin, ethoglucid, methotrexate, or cis-platinum) instilled into the bladder at regular intervals. This is usually performed on an outpatient basis. The patient is asked not to void for 1–2 hours following the drug instillation, to improve its effectiveness. This therapy is usually continued for 12 weeks.

Regular cystoscopic checks are performed on the patient. A typical protocol following surgery would be for the patient to undergo a cystoscopy 3 months and 6 months following the operation and, if all is 'clear' then cystoscopy is usually warranted only at 12 monthly intervals. Such a protocol needs to be carefully explained to and understood by the patient who should also be instructed to consult his urologist should any signs or symptoms of tumour regrowth be noticed.

Segmental or partial cystectomy

The removal of part of the bladder is usually reserved for a tumour growth localized within the dome of the bladder. The surgeon usually approaches the bladder via a suprapubic incision and resects the tumour growth as well as part of the healthy bladder tissue.

Postoperatively, the patient will have both a suprapubic and a urethral catheter in place, as well as some form of wound drain. The nurse should therefore monitor for the free flow of drainage from all tubes and immediately report any signs of obstruction. A build up of urine or blood within the bladder could raise the intravesical pressure to limits sufficient to cause the bladder to burst and the wound to break down. As a general rule, the catheters are removed when the haematuria and oedema subside (usually 1–3 weeks postoperatively); and following removal, the patient should be observed closely to ensure that he is able to void spontaneously.

Naturally, when a section of the bladder is removed, its capacity to store urine is reduced. The patient should be warned that he will feel the desire to void more frequently following the operation. The capacity of the bladder will gradually increase and the patient in most cases will find that he is able to retain urine for longer periods. During this phase of habilitation, it must be stressed that an adequate fluid intake should be maintained to prevent dehydration and to promote the functioning of normal physiological urinary defences. The initial reaction of the patient to frequency of urination is often to curtail fluid intake.

As with any other form of treatment for cancer of the bladder, regular cystoscopic follow up is essential to monitor progress.

Total cystectomy and creation of a urinary diversion

A total cystectomy is usually reserved for highly invasive bladder tumours. Removal of the bladder is a major operation associated with an operative mortality rate of approximately 10%, and thus is performed in only the most serious of cases. Removal of the patient's bladder disrupts the normal flow of urine down the urinary tract and necessitates the creation of urinary diversion. The healthy ureters are implanted into some other structure to facilitate urinary drainage.

Urinary diversion may take one of several forms. Drainage from the kidneys may be achieved by inserting nephrostomy tubes (usually only a temporary measure), by implanting the ureters into a section of the colon (that is, a ureterosigmoidostomy), or by creating an ileal loop conduit.

The ileal loop conduit is the most favoured method, due in part to the problems of infection and incontinence associated with a ureteric-bowel implantation. Malignancy is not the only indication for an ileal loop conduit. It may also be created in cases where a patient has an untreatable vesicovaginal fistula, a neurogenic bladder disorder (resulting in uncontrollable urinary incontinence), ectopia vesicae, or a greatly contracted bladder (due, for example, to tuberculosis of the bladder).

As with any major surgery, the patient should be counselled with regard to the nature of the operation and its associated risks and complications, and informed consent must be obtained. It is important that the patient is visited by the stomal therapist who will discuss the siting of the urinary diversion, the appliance used to drain the conduit, and its general management. The stomal therapist is commonly the nursing expert in this field and every opportunity should be made for him/her to discuss the operation and its consequences with both the patient and his significant others. Issues should be explored relating to possible changes in body image, sexuality, role perceptions, and social support; both cancer and the type of operative procedure undertaken will mean a radical disruption to the patient's normal lifestyle.

In selecting the site of the stoma, the stomal therapist must consider:

- The manual dexterity of the patient – ideally the stoma must be in a position which allows for easy visualization by the patient and affords ready access for appliance changes and cleaning.
- The position of the patient's waist
- The presence of folds in the skin or any skin conditions.
- The occupation and hobbies of the patient.

All these factors may affect the patient's success in managing the conduit. Stomas are usually sited midway between the patient's anterior-superior ileal crest and umbilicus, the proposed site being carefully selected and marked on the skin preoperatively.

Other preoperative measures include an estimation of the patient's Hb level with blood also being taken for grouping and cross matching. An MSU is obtained so that any underlying urinary tract infection can be identified and treated appropriately. Bowel preparation is also an important procedure prior to surgery; the patient may be ordered a low residue diet some days prior to the operation, aperients are given, and on the operative day a bowel washout may be performed.

In some centres, metronidazole or neomycin may also be administered in an attempt to sterilize the bowel and thus reduce the risk of postoperative infection. Skin preparation requires the patient to be shaved from the nipple line to midthigh and, as with any nursing intervention, a careful explanation must be given to the patient prior to its being performed.

Operative technique. A total radical cystectomy usually requires the surgeon to perform a long paramedian incision and involves the removal of the bladder and regional lymph nodes, a portion of the urethra, the prostate and seminal vesicles, and part of the lower ureters. In the female, the ureter is also usually removed and the operation commonly takes 3–5 hours to perform. As a consequence of such a radical procedure, the male is usually rendered impotent, thus sexual counselling plays an important role in preoperative preparation and discharge planning.

When an ileal loop conduit is constructed, the terminal 10–15 cm of the ileum is isolated along with its mesenteric blood supply, the ureters are anastomosed to it, and the distal end of the conduit is brought through the anterior abdominal wall as a stoma (Fig 59.5). The section of ileum therefore acts not as an artificial bladder, but simply as a conduit through which the urine may drain from the ureters to the external surface of the abdominal wall.

Postoperative management. The patient will have a temporary appliance attached to the stoma to facilitate the drainage of urine. Ureteric stents are inserted into the ureters to maintain patency, and the patient will also have an intravenous infusion, a wound drain(s), and a nasogastric tube. Intensive nursing care during the immediate postoperative period will be required.

Vital signs must be assessed regularly to monitor hydrative status and to monitor for complications such as dehydration, shock, and infection. Special note should be made of the colour, amount, and composition of drainage from the stoma, wound drainage, drainage from the nasogastric tube, and the presence of bowel sounds and flatus. A paralytic ileus is common in

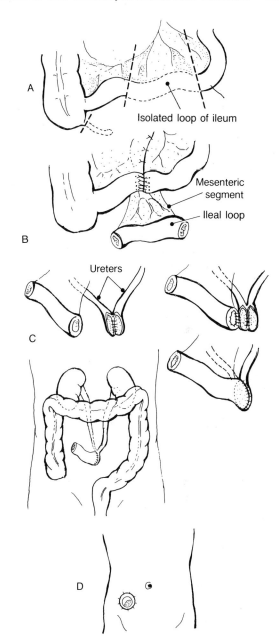

Fig. 59.5 Ileal loop conduit. **A** – Section of ileum is isolated, while retaining the mesenteric segment. Appendicectomy is performed. **B** – Ileum is rejoined. **C** – Ureters are anastomosed together and to end of ileal segment. **D** – Distal end of conduit forms stoma.

most patients due to handling of the bowel during the operation.

The stoma should be observed regularly and, if viable, will appear moist, bright pink in colour, and protrude slightly from the skin. The slight protrusion allows urine to flow directly into the drainage device and prevents skin excoriation. It is not unusual for the initial discharge from the stoma to be bloody and to contain some mucous and debris, and this should clear significantly within 24–48 hours. Should the stoma appear oedematous, dark red, blue, or black, the surgeon should be notified immediately as such changes indicate a poor blood supply to the stoma and consequent necrosis. Such changes will usually require prompt surgical intervention.

The nasogastric tube should be aspirated hourly initially, then allowed to drain freely until drainage ceases. The tube may subsequently be spigotted for 24 hours and then removed. The patient is fasted until bowel sounds return and flatus is passed; thus all nutritional needs must be met parenterally and a close monitor should be kept on fluid and electrolyte balance to ensure that all losses are replaced. With the return of bowel sounds and minimal nasogastric drainage, the patient may commence small sips of clear fluids and if these are tolerated, oral intake gradually increased as his condition improves. As a general rule, a high fluid intake should be maintained at all times.

To prevent the postoperative complications of chest infection and deep vein thrombosis, the nurse should assist and encourage the patient to perform regular deep breathing and coughing exercises and to move his limbs frequently. In most centres, early ambulation of the patient is encouraged in order to improve psychological well-being and to minimize the likelihood of post-operative complications.

As with any postoperative surgical patient, priority should also be given to the relief of pain and nausea, and to the prevention of a wound infection. Wound drain(s) are removed when drainage is minimal usually between the third and fifth postoperative day) and the ureteric stents are removed on the fifth to seventh postoperative day. Following removal of these stents a close observation should be made of urinary output to ensure that the ureters have not become obstructed.

The patient is usually fitted with some form of temporary drainage device which ideally should allow for direct visualization of the stoma and free drainage of urine into some measuring device. If a measuring device is not available, the drainage bag should be emptied regularly to monitor the volume and type of urinary drainage. As the operative site heals, a more permanent type of drainage device is selected and the patient should be taught how to drain, change, and manage it. The patient should also be taught thorough stomal care. Any skin barrier applied around the stoma (for example, Stomahesive, karayagum) should fit snugly in order to prevent skin excoriation from urinary leakage. Should the area around the stoma become blistered or reddened, the skin should be cleaned gently with soap and water, dried, and the inflamed area painted with either mercurochrome or an antacid solution. Creams or ointments are best avoided as they are largely ineffective and may exacerbate the condition.

Advice on stomal care should be sought from a stomal therapist as protocols for the management of urinary stomas vary between institutions and a multiplicity of drainage devices may be used. As a general rule, however, any appliance fitted to the stoma should:

1. Have an adhesive which secures the drainage device to the skin adequately and prevents urinary leakage. If adhesive tapes are used, the patient should first be checked for possible sensitivity to the tape
2. Allow for easy access to drainage and be of a sufficient size to allow 2–4 hours between emptying.
3. Be comfortable to wear and cosmetically acceptable
4. Have a facility which enables it to be connected to some form of drainage at night.
5. Be manageable by the patient.

Fundamental to successful patient habilitation and management of the conduit is the instigation of a thorough educational programme. At all times, the patient should be encouraged to participate in the management of the conduit; nursing intervention should gradually become more advisory as the patient develops an active self-care role and assumes more responsibility. It is also important that any appropriate psychological counselling be provided should the patient be experiencing any problems postoperatively.

Complications. The major complications associated with a total cystectomy and the creation of an ileal loop conduit are:

1. *Early complications*
– Obstruction to urine flow (for example, due to the ostomy site being too small; stricture of the ureteric-ileac anastomosis; kinked ureters)
– Necrosis of the stoma
– Paralytic ileus
– Peritonitis (due to the leakage of urine into the peritoneal cavity)
– Haemorrhage
– Wound infection or breakdown
– Other intestinal obstruction
2. *Late complications*
– Non-acceptance by patient of the stoma (often expressed as non-compliance, depression or withdrawal)
– Stomal stenosis
– Urinary leakage around the appliance (associated with skin problems)
– Herniation
– Recurrent UTI
– Calculi
– Electrolyte disturbances.

After discharge regular outpatient follow up is essential to monitor progress and to ensure that complications are recognized promptly and an appropriate plan of action implemented.

It is also necessary for the patient to be screened regularly for metastases and further treatment with chemotherapy or radiotherapy may be required. Unfortunately, the current outlook for cure of invasive bladder cancer is poor despite such radical surgical interventions; therefore, the procedure of radical cystectomy and urinary diversion is being reassessed and rationalized.

MALFORMATION OF THE URINARY TRACT AND NEUROGENIC BLADDER DISORDERS

A number of malformations may occur in the urinary tract and may involve the kidneys, the ureters, the bladder, or the urethra. Fortunately, many malformations are relatively benign and go unnoticed throughout life. A few may predispose the patient to infection or calculi formation and therefore require investigation and treatment. Some result in the gradual destruction of functioning renal mass and result in uraemia. Only the major malformations will be presented and briefly discussed in this section.

The term 'neurogenic bladder' refers to a condition in which normal nervous system control of micturition is somehow disrupted. The fact that neurogenic bladder disorders have been classified in a number of ways by different authors suggests that some controversy still exists regarding this condition. A detailed and comprehensive classification of the conditions which fall within this heading has been developed by Johnson (1980) and will serve as a foundation for discussion.

Malformations of the urinary tract

Probably the most benign of malformations of the urinary tract are those of:

● Duplex kidney. Two kidneys which arise from a single or duplex ureter on one side
● Renal agenesis. Only 1 kidney is present in the body
● Renal aplasia. One kidney is partially formed or only a part of the ureter is present on one side
● Rotated kidney. The hilum faces anteriorly rather than posteriorly
● Horseshoe kidney. Lower poles of the kidney are fused
● Ectopic kidney. For example, one of the kidneys may be found in the pelvic or thoracic cavities
● Diverticulae in the bladder.

These abnormalities are usually compatible with life and may be discovered only incidentally. If they produce stasis of urine, calculi may form and/or infection result, and the abnormality may require correction.

Ureteric abnormalities may be benign and therefore require no medical intervention unless symptoms associated with obstruction, incontinence, calculi, or infection are present. Duplex ureter on one side may pass unnoticed unless the additional ureter enters the urethra or vagina resulting in an abnormal urinary leakage. In such conditions the ureter may have to be reimplanted or resected.

More serious malformations of the urinary tract include:

• Bilateral renal agenesis. Absence of both kidneys is incompatible with life
• Ectopia vesicae. A condition in which the bladder projects through the abdominal wall and usually requires a cystectomy to be performed and an ileal loop conduit created
• Abnormalities of the urethra in which urine is diverted to some other structure, for example, the vagina in cases of a urethrovaginal fistula or bowel where there is a urethrorectal fistula.

The presence of urethral strictures, diverticulae, valves, and even urethral duplication can usually be successfully corrected by surgical intervention. Providing that infection or recurrence (for example, in the cases of urethral strictures) do not occur, habilitation is usually assured.

Non-malignant conditions which cause eventual destruction of the kidney, and therefore loss of renal function, include:

• Polycystic kidney disease. An autosomal dominant trait in which the kidneys are gradually obliterated by cysts over a period of decades
• Medullary cystic disease. A condition thought to follow an autosomal recessive pattern and characterized by the development of cysts within the renal medulla.

Both these conditions eventually lead to chronic renal failure.

Neurogenic bladder disorders

Should the nerves supplying the bladder and/or sphincters be damaged, problems in the normal pattern of urination will inevitably occur since the act of voiding is the result of the integration of both cortical and autonomic components of the nervous system. A defect in the passage of nerve impulses from and to the bladder and urethral sphincters may therefore produce one or more of the following problems:

• A loss of cortical control over the act of micturition
• A loss of sensation that the bladder is filling

• A loss of reflex emptying of the bladder (due to damage to the nerves or synapses which compose the micturition reflex arc
• Incomplete bladder emptying (resulting in a large volume of residual urine).

Aetiology and pathophysiology

A number of conditions may interrupt the flow of nerve impulses to and from the bladder, the spinal cord, and the brain. The classification of neurogenic bladder disorders presented in Table 59.2 is based upon the ways in which bladder innervation can be disrupted. The micturition reflex arc may be destroyed, or the sensory and/or motor pathways to the cortical regulatory centre may be interrupted, or a combination of both conditions may occur. It is therefore important to identify the exact nature of the defect so that any functional neuronal pathways may be utilized when planning treatment.

Clinical manifestations

The clinical manifestations associated with neurogenic bladder depend upon the degree to which neuronal pathways are disrupted. Manifestations range from stress incontinence and overflow, to frequency, urgency, nocturia, enuresis, and dribbling. Bladder distention may be noticeable, especially in cases where the motor pathways or the micturition reflex arc are destroyed. In some cases, manifestations associated with a urinary tract infection or renal calculi may be present.

Investigative procedures

Assessment of the patient with neurogenic bladder dysfunction should commence with obtaining a detailed history and include a complete physical and neurological examination. Specific regard should be taken of the patient's voiding patterns, his ability to sense bladder distention, and to control and initiate voiding.

Investigative procedures performed include: an MS urine specimen, an IVP, plain X-ray of the vertebral column, uroflometric studies, estimation of residual urine volume, cystometrogram, cystourethrogram, and, in some cases, a cystoscopy.

Table 59.2 Neurogenic bladder disorders: classification. (Modified from Johnson J H 1980 Rehabilitation aspects of neurologic bladder dysfunction. In: Nursing Clinics of North America W. B. Saunders Co. 15:2 (June) pp 293–307.)

Classification	Pathophysiology	Patient problem	Aetiology (examples only)
Uninhibited bladder dysfunction	Lesion destroys pathway for normal inhibition of micturition. Pathway for initiation of micturition intact. Bladder sensation normal. Micturition reflex intact.	Patient unable to voluntarily suppress micturition. Clinical manifestations include: frequency, urgency, nocturia, enuresis.	Cerebral artherosclerosis, CVA, tumours, trauma or infection of the brain, alcohol, Parkinson's disease, delayed toilet training (infants).
Reflex bladder dysfunction	Lesion above S_2–S_4 destroys both sensory and motor micturition pathways of spinal cord. Micturition reflex intact.	Micturition occurs automatically. No cortical control. Micturition may occur following external cutaneous stimulation.	Trauma to spinal cord. Multiple sclerosis, cord compression, infection.
Autonomous bladder dysfunction	Lesion involves both sensory and motor micturition pathways at level of S_2–S_4 Micturition reflex destroyed.	External sphincter relaxed. Dribbling and incontinence common. Large residual urine volume.	Trauma to spinal cord, meningocele, infection, tumours, radical pelvic surgery.
Motor paralytic bladder dysfunction	Motor micturition pathways destroyed. Bladder sensation normal (sensory pathways intact).	Patient able to sense bladder filling, but unable to initiate micturition. Large residual urine volume.	Poliomyelitis, trauma, tumours.
Sensory paralytic bladder dysfunction	Sensory micturition pathways destroyed (motor pathways intact).	Patient unable to sense bladder filling, but is able to initiate voiding.	Diabetes mellitus.

Medical, surgical, and nursing management

The general aims for managing a patient with neurogenic bladder dysfunction are to identify the type of bladder dysfunction present, and to implement a plan of action which ensures that:

• The flow of urine from the bladder is controlled
• The retention of a large residual volume of urine is avoided
• Infection is prevented
• Renal function is preserved.

The patient's progress must be closely monitored and evaluated.

Specific interventions for patients with a neurogenic bladder include:

1. Developing a programme in which the patient is asked to void at specific, regular (for example, 2–4 hourly) intervals. This is useful for patients with uninhibited or sensory paralytic bladder dysfunction.
2. Teaching the patient to stimulate micturition by applying external cutaneous stimuli such as pinching, slapping, or stroking the thigh, pulling his pubic hairs, abdominal massage, or by massaging the perineal area. Stimulation is useful for patients with reflex bladder dysfunction.
3. Teaching the patient to perform simultaneously the Crede manoeuvre (manual application of pressure over the area of the bladder) and the Valsalva manoeuvre, to initiate voiding. This is useful for patients with autonomous or motor paralytic bladder dysfunction.
4. Teaching the patient to perform intermittent self-catheterization. This is useful for patients with motor paralytic bladder dysfunction.

For a number of patients, these interventions may be either inappropriate or ineffective and drugs from the parasympathomimetic group may be prescribed. Alternatively some form of semi-permanent urinary drainage device may be used, for example, urethral catheter, suprapubic catheter, condom drainage, or penile clamps.

Surgical interventions for patients with unresolved problems include a partial resection of urethral sphincters, especially when there is a persistent high residual urine volume; or the creation of an ileal loop conduit. The implantation of electrodes to stimulate contraction of the bladder muscle is a new, largely untrialled technique.

The patient with a neurogenic bladder disorder (from whatever cause) requires intensive support and training from nursing staff. The nature of the disability and the real threats of infection, calculi and, in some cases, an inability to cope with the social effects of the condition, pose a challenge for both the patient and health care team. It is therefore imperative that once a strategy for treatment is developed and implemented, every effort be made to ensure that the patient is well versed and complies with that strategy so that successful habilitation can occur. Referral to an incontinence advisor will be of benefit to the majority of patients.

SECTION H – REFERENCES AND FURTHER READING

Texts

Australian Kidney Foundation 1984 Seventh Report of the Australian and New Zealand Combined Dialysis and Transplant Registry. Queen Elizabeth Hospital, Adelaide

Anderson J R (ed) 1976 Muir's textbook of pathology, 10th edn. Edward Arnold, London

Anderson K H et al 1976 Introduction to medical sciences for clinical practice. Year Book Medical Publisher Unit XI, Chicago

Anthony C P 1984 Structure and function of the body. Mosby, St Louis

Anthony C P, Thibodeau G A 1983 Textbook of anatomy and physiology, 11th edn. Mosby, St Louis, ch 22–24

Asscher A W, Moffat D B (eds) 1983 Nephro-urology. William Heinemann, London

Atkins R C, Thompson N M, Farrell P C (eds) Peritoneal dialysis. Churchill Livingstone, Edinburgh

Black D, Jones N F 1979 Renal disease, 4th edn. Blackwell, Oxford

Blandy J P 1976 Lecture notes on urology. Blackwell, Oxford

Border W A, Glassock R J 1984 Glomerulonephritis. In: Bricker N S, Kirschenbaum M A, The kidney: diagnosis and management. Wiley, New York

Boulton-Jones J M 1982 Diagnosis and management of renal and urinary diseases. Blackwell, Oxford

Breckman B 1981 Stoma care. Billing, Guildford

Brenner B M, Rector F L 1986 The kidney 3rd edn. Saunders, Philadelphia

Brickner N S, Kirschenbaum M A (eds) 1984 The kidney: diagnosis and management. Wiley, New York

Cahill M (ed) 1984 Renal and urologic disorders: nurse's clinical library. Springhouse, Pennsylvania

Cameron F S, Peters D K, Rees A F 1982 New perspectives in glomerulonephritis. In: Jones N F, Peters D K, Recent advances in renal medicine No 2. Churchill Livingstone, London

Cameron S 1981 Kidney disease. Oxford University Press, New York

Catts G R D, Macleod A M 1982 Renal Transplantation. In: Jones N F, Peters D K (eds) Recent advances in renal medicine (No 2). Churchill Livingstone, Melbourne

Clarkson A R, Woodroffe A F, Seymour A E 1982 IgA nephropathy. In: Jones N F, Peters D K, Recent advances in renal medicine No 2. Churchill Livingstone, London

Creager J G 1982 Human anatomy and physiology. Wadsworth, California

Cronin R E 1981 The patient with acute azotaemia. In: Schrier R W (ed) Manual of nephrology diagnosis and therapy. Little, Brown, Boston

Dalton J R 1983 Basic clinical urology. Harper & Row, Philadelphia

De Wardner H E 1985 The kidney 5th edn. Churchill Livingstone, Edinburgh

Earley L E, Gottschalk C W (Eds) 1979 Strauss and Welt's Diseases of the Kidney (3rd edition) Little, Brown & Co, Boston

Fischbach F T 1984 A manual of laboratory diagnostic tests, 2nd edn. Lippincott, Philadelphia

Forland M 1977 Nephrology. Medical Examination Publishing Co, New York

Ganong W F 1977 Review of medical physiology, 8th edn. Lange, Los Altos

Golden A, Maher J F 1977 The kidney (2nd ed). Williams and Wilkins, Baltimore

Gutch C F, Stoner M H 1983 Review of haemodialysis for nurses and dialysis personnel, 4th edn. Mosby, St Louis

Guyton A C 1982 Human physiology and mechanisms of disease, 3rd edn. Saunders, Toronto, part 4

Hamilton W J (ed) 1976 Textbook of human anatomy, 2nd edn. Macmillan, London

Havard M 1986 A nursing guide to drugs, 2nd edn. Churchill Livingstone, Melbourne

Isselbacher K J et al (eds) 1978 Harrison's principles of internal medicine, 9th edn. McGraw Hill, New York

Kagan L W 1979 Renal disease, a manual of patient care. McGraw Hill, New York

Kelalis P P et al (eds) 1985 Clinical pediatric urology 2nd edn. Saunders, Philadelphia

Kincaid-Smith P 1979 Pyelonephritis, chronic interstitial nephritis and obstructive uropathy. In: Hamberger J et al (eds) Nephrology. John Wiley, London

Lerner J 1982 Mosby's manual of urologic nursing. Mosby, St Louis

Luckman J, Sorensen K C 1980 Medical-surgical nursing: a psychophysiologic approach, 2nd edn. Saunders, Philadelphia

McConnell E A, Zimmerman M F 1983 Care of patients with urologic problems. Lippincott, Philadelphia

Macleod J 1987 Davidson's principles and practice of medicine, 15th edn. Churchill Livingstone, Edinburgh

Marsh F 1985 Postgraduate nephrology. Heinemann, London

Miller R B 1981 The patient with chronic azotaemia, with emphasis on chronic renal failure. In: Schrier R W (ed) Manual of nephrology, diagnosis and therapy. Little, Brown, Boston

Newsam J E, Petrie J J B 1975 Urology and renal medicine. Churchill Livingstone, London

Newsam J E 1981 Urology and renal medicine. Churchill Livingstone, Edinburgh

Nissenson A R, Fine R N (eds) 1986 Dialysis therapy. Mosby, St Louis

Older R A, Ladwig S H 1981 Use of radiologic techniques in the patient with renal problems. In: Schrier R W (ed) Manual of nephrology. Little, Brown, Boston

Petersen R O 1986 Urologic pathology. Lippincott, Philadelphia

Rajfer J 1986 Urologic endocrinology. Saunders, Philadelphia

Read A E, Barritt D W, Langton Hewer R 1986 Modern medicine, 3rd edn. Churchill Livingstone, Edinburgh

Reller L B 1981 The patient with urinary tract infection. In: Schrier R W (ed) Manual of Nephrology Diagnosis and Therapy. Little, Brown, Boston

Schrier R W (ed) 1981 Manual of Nephrology Diagnosis and Therapy. Little, Brown, Boston

Schrier R W (ed) 1986 Renal and electrolyte disorders 3rd edn. Little, Brown, Boston

Schrier R W, Gottschalk C W 1987 Strauss and Welt's diseases of the kidney 4th edn. Little, Brown, Boston

Scott R, Deane R F, Callander R 1982 Urology illustrated, 2nd ed. Churchill Livingstone, London

Selkurt E E 1982 Basic physiology for the health sciences, 2nd edn. Little, Brown, Boston

Smith D R 1987 General urology, 12th edn. Appleton & Lange, Connecticut

Society of Hospital Pharmacists of Australia 1985 Pharmacology and drug information for nurses, 2nd edn. Saunders, Sydney

Solomon E P, Davis P W 1983 Human anatomy and physiology. Holt-Saunders, Philadelphia,

Stanton S L (ed) 1984 Clinical gynecologic urology. Mosby, St Louis

Storlie F J (ed) 1984 Diseases: nurse's reference library, 2nd edn. Springhouse, Pennsylvania

Strand F L 1983 Physiology: a regulatory systems approach, 2nd edn. Macmillan, New York

Tortora G J, Anagnostakos N P 1984 Principles of anatomy and physiology, 4th edn. Harper & Row, New York

Uldall R 1977 Renal nursing, 2nd ed. Blackwell, London

Valtin H 1979 Renal dysfunction mechanisms involved in fluid and solute imbalance. Little, Brown, Boston

Walsh P C et al (eds) 1986 Campbell's urology, 5th edn. Saunders, Philadelphia

West R S (ed) 1984 Implementing urologic procedures: nursing photobook, 2nd edn. Springhouse, Pennsylvania

Winter C L, Barker M M 1972 Nursing care of patients with urologic diseases, 3rd edn. Mosby, St Louis

Wood R F M 1983 Renal transplantation a clinical handbook. Bailliere Tindall, London

Whitworth J A, Lawrence J R (eds) 1988 Textbook of renal disease. Churchill Livingstone, Melbourne

Journals

Adu D 1983 Acute renal failure. Medicine International (Australian edn) 1079–1085

Bailey R R 1983 Single dose antibacterial treatment for bacteriuria in pregnancy. Current Therapeutics (Nov) 27–32

Baker L R I 1983 Management of urinary tract obstruction. Medicine International (Australian edn) 1104–1109

Barrett N 1981 Cancer of the bladder: a case history. American Journal of Nursing (Dec) 2192–2195

Betts A 1984 All under control. Nursing Mirror 159:19 (Nov 21) viii–xiii

Bielski M 1980 Preventing infection in the catheterized patient. Nursing Clinics of North America 15 : 4

Binkley L S 1984 Keeping up with peritoneal dialysis. American Journal of Nursing 729–733

Brooks D 1982 Urinary symptoms. International Medicine (Aust edn) 1150–1159

Brown D J 1982 Assessment of osteodystrophy in patients with chronic renal failure. Australian and New Zealand Journal of Medicine (June): 250–254

Bruce P T 1980 Present day status of urinary diversion. Medical Journal of Australia (Nov 1) 477–482

Cain L 1982 The percutaneous nephrostomy tube. American Journal of Nursing (Feb) 296–298

Campbell D 1982 My personal water torture. Nursing Mirror (July 28) 50

Campbell J E 1983 Imaging of the urinary tract. International Medicine (Australian edn) (March): 1054–1061

Chambers J K 1983 Save your diabetic patient from early kidney damage. Nursing 83 13 : 5 : 58–63

Chezem J L 1978 Urinary diversion. Select aspects of nursing management. Nursing Clinics of North America. 11 : 3 : 445–456

Cunha B A 1982 Nosocomial urinary tract infections. Heart and Lung 11 : 6 : 545–55

Datta P K 1984 Carcinoma of the urinary bladder. Nursing Times (April 25) 24–26

Denniston D J, Burns K T 1980 Home peritoneal dialysis. American Journal of Nursing 2022–2026

Dixon S 1984 Renal transplantation. Nursing in Australia 2 : 2 : 22–27

Dugan J S 1984 Winning the battle against incontinence. Nursing 84 14 : 6 : 59

Dunk-Richards G 1981 Prevention and control of cross infection. Australian Nurses Journal 10 : 9 : 44–46

Edwards S 1984 The fashioning of an ileal conduit. Nursing Mirror (May 16) 158 : 20 : 35–37

Engram B W 1983 Do's and dont's of urologic nursing. Nursing 83 13 : 10 : 49

Fennell S E 1975 Percutaneous renal biopsy. American Journal of Nursing 75 : 8 : 1292–1294

Finch M 1978 Management of acute renal failure. Nursing Times (13 April): 631–635

Fox J 1979 Ten day's trauma – and he still wants another motorbike! Nursing Mirror (Jan 18) 25–30

Gogna N K, Nossar V, Walker A C 1983 Epidemic of acute post-streptococcal glomerulonephritis in Aboriginal communities. Medical Journal of Australia (January 22) 64–66.

Gramse C A 1984 Caring for a patient with a urinary diversion stoma. Nursing 84 14 : 7 : 20–22

Gramse C A 1984 Indwelling catheter care: a run-through. Nursing 84 14 : 10 : 26–27

Greenway S M 1982 Renal transplantation in the USA. Nursing Times (15 Dec) 2131–2134

Grey A J 1980 A new lease of life. Nursing Times (Sept 11) 1616–1620

Grimley K 1984 Haemodialysis and the hospitalised dialysis patient. Nursing in Australia 2 : 1 : 51–60

Hadfield J 1981 Griping about renal colic. Nursing Mirror (Jan 22) vi–viii

Hadfield J 1981 Haematuria. Nursing Mirror (Jan 22) viii–xi (supp)

Hahn K 1987 The many signs of renal failure. Nursing 87 17 : 8 : 34–41

Hall B M 1983 Transplantation of kidneys from living related donors in Australia. Medical Journal of Australia 594–595

Hamilton M, Sloman R 1980 Ureteric stone. When do we need to intervene? Australian Family Physician. Vol 9: (May) 360–364

Harvey A 1979 Blunt renal trauma. Nursing Times (Oct 11) 1756–1758

Hatfield J 1981 Urinary tract infections (Clinical Forum) Nursing Mirror (Jan 22) ii–v

Hickman B W 1977 All about sex . . . despite dialysis. American Journal of Nursing 606–607

Hoenich N A 1982 Renal replacement therapy 3–1 haemodialysis equipment. Nursing Times 800–803

Irwin B C 1979 Haemodialysis means vascular access . . . and the right kind of nursing care. Nursing 79 9 : 10 : 49–53

Iveson-Iveson J 1979 Nephrotic syndrome – picture quiz. Nursing Mirror (15 Feb): 5–50

Jackson A S 1980 A conduit for life. Nursing Times. (Sept 4) 1564–1567

Jenner E 1983 Cutting the cost of catheter infections. Nursing Times (July 13) 58–61

Johnson J H 1980 Rehabilitation aspects of neurologic bladder dysfunction. Nursing Clinics of North America. 15 : 2 (June) 293–307

Jones R B 1984 Chlamydia: the most common sexually transmitted pathogen. Medical Aspects of Human Sexuality 18 : 2 : 238–261

Kerr D N 1983 The assessment of renal function. International Medicine (Australian edn) (March): 1049–1053

Kincaid-Smith P 1980 The treatment of glomerulonephritis. Australian and New Zealand Journal of Medicine 10. 340–345

Kincaid-Smith P, Dowling J P 1983 Glomerulonephritis and the nephrotic syndrome. International Medicine (Aust edn) 1070–1075

Knepil J 1983 That figures! Nursing Mirror. (13 April): 44–46

Latimer R G 1980 Comparison of chronic haemodialysis angioaccess procedures. Dialysis and Transplantation 9 : 5 : 499–502

Latos D L 1980 Chronic renal failure: an overview. Dialysis and Transplantation. 9 : 5 : 435–440

Lewis S M 1983 An integrated approach to terminal renal failure. Medicine International (Australian edn): 1089–1094

Leer H A 1982 Acute renal failure. Nursing Times (26 May): 891–896

Mallon D 1986 Renacidin irrigation for struvite stones. Nursing 86 16 : 8 : 26–28

Manley R 1984 Containing the problem. Nursing Mirror 158 : 7 (Feb 15) 37–38

Maguire K 1982 Renal replacement therapy 6–1 renal transplantation – pre and postoperative care. Nursing Times 933–934

Mars D R, Treloar D 1984 Acute tubular necrosis – pathophysiology and treatment. Heart and Lung 13 : 2 : 194–202

Mathew T 1974 Treatment of renal calculi. Current Therapeutics (March) 59–66

Matthews C A 1981 A patient suffering from Goodpasture's syndrome. Nursing Times (September 2). 1543–1546

Mayers A M 1983 Conservative management of chronic renal failure. Medicine International (Australian edn): 1086–1088

McConnell E A 1985 Assessing the bladder. Nursing 85 15 : 11 : 44–46

McGreal M J, Vigneux A M, Young J M 1982 Continuous ambulatory peritoneal dialysis: treatment of choice for some children. Canadian Nurse 21–25

McKenzie S 1981 The role of the dialysis nurse. Australian Nurses Journal 11 : 1 : 50–51+

Meers P D, Stronge J L 1980 Hospitals should do the sick no harm. Urinary tract infection. Nursing Times (Supp) (July 24)

Melman A 1984 Sexual intercourse: a forerunner of female urinary tract infections. Medical Aspects of Human Sexuality 18 : 2 186–192

Mendez R 1977 Renal trauma. Journal of Urology 118 : 5 : 698–703

Metheny N 1982 Renal stones and urinary pH. American Journal of Nursing (Sept) 1372–1375

Noreen J 1980 Tissue typing for renal transplantation. The Lamp 57–60

Norton C 1984 Challenging speciality. Nursing Mirror. 159 : 19 (Nov 21) xiv–xvii

Nunn I N et al 1983 Percutaneous ultrasonic disintegration and removal of renal calculi. Medical Journal of Australia (Nov 26) 543–546

Oestreich S J K 1979 Rational nursing care in chronic renal disease. American Journal of Nursing 1096–1099

Ozanne S 1982 Going home (ileal conduit and bladder tumour) Nursing Mirror. (April 28) pp 56–59

Palmer J K, Benson G S, Corriere J N 1983 Diagnosis and initial management of urological injuries associated with 200 consecutive pelvic fractures. Journal of Urology 130 : 4 : 712–714

Paul M 1982 Renal replacement therapy 1–2 haemodialysis and complications. Nursing Times 704–708

Pavitt L 1982 Renal replacement therapy 2–1 access for haemodialysis. Nursing Times 749–752

Persky L, Hampel N Kedia K 1981 Percutaneous nephrostomy and ureteral injury. Journal of Urology 125 : 3 : 298–300

Perston Y 1981 Ways to help a sensitive problem. Nursing Mirror (Oct 21) 38–42

Potts J 1984 Renal nurse on call. Nursing Times 53–55

Precious A 1978 When nursing vigilance counts. Nursing Mirror (26 Oct) 30–33

Reckling J B 1982 Safeguarding the renal transplant patient. Nursing 82 12 : 2 : 47–49

Reed S B 1982 Giving more than dialysis. Nursing 82 12 : 4 : 58–63

Rigby R J, Butler J L, Petrie J B 1982 Experience with continuous ambulatory peritoneal dialysis. Medical Journal of Australia 331–335

Roberts C 1982 Renal replacement therapy 2–2 home dialysis. Nursing Times 752–753

Rodriguez D J, Hunter V M 1981 Nutritional intervention in the treatment of chronic renal failure. Nursing Clinics of North America 16 : 3 : 573–585

Russ G R, Mathew T H, Caon A 1980 Single day or single dose treatment of urinary tract infection with co-trimoxazole. Australian and New Zealand Journal of Medicine. 10 : 604–607

Sausville P 1980 The nurse's role in haemodialysis. Journal of Nursing Care 12–17

Scott D W, Oberst M T, Bookbinder M I 1984 Stress – coping response to genitourinary carcinoma in men. Nursing Research. 33 : 6 : 325–327

Segasothy M, 1984 Analgesic nephropathy associated with paracetamol. Australian and New Zealand Journal of Medicine 14 : 23–26

Shcahan S L, Scabolt J P 1982 Understanding urinary tract infection in women. The first step to controlling it. Nursing 82 (Nov) 68–71

Shepherd A M, Blannin J P, Feneley R C L 1982 Changing attitudes in the management of urinary incontinence – the need for specialist nursing. British Medical Journal Vol 284 (Feb 27) 645–646

Sieben D M et al 1978 The role of ureteral stenting in the management of surgical injury of the ureter. Journal of Urology 119 : 3 : 330–331

Smith T 1982 A cycler made for one. Nursing Mirror 56–57

Sorrels A J 1979 Continuous ambulatory peritoneal dialysis. American Journal of Nursing 1400–1401

Spencer R C, Fenton P A 1984 Infective complications of peritoneal dialysis. Journal of Hospital Infection 5 233–240

Stark J L 1980 BUN/Creatinine – your keys to kidney function. Nursing 80 10 : 5 : 33–38

Stark J L 1982 Acute poststreptococcal glomerulonephritis. Nursing 82 (May) 31

Stark J L 1982 How to succeed against acute renal failure. Nursing 82 12 : 7 : 26–33

Stark J L 1983 Renal calculi. Nursing 83 13 : 12 : 14–15

Stark J L, Hunt V 1983 Helping your patient with chronic renal failure. Nursing 83 13 : 9 : 56–63

Stevens E 1982 Renal replacement therapy 1–2 introduction and review of dialysis and transplantation today. Nursing Times 700–704

Stewart G 1984 Chronic renal failure. Nursing in Australia 2 : 2 : 16–21

Stewart G 1984 Acute renal failure – caring for people with renal disease. Nursing in Australia 2 : 1 : 34–41

Stewart J H 1978 Analgesic abuse and renal failure in Australia. Kidney International 13: 72–78

Taber S 1982 Renal replacement therapy 6–2 Other aspects of renal transplantation – donor procurement, preservation and alternative rejection therapy. Nursing Times 935–939

Tate D G 1982 Renal replacement therapy 8–1 Tissue typing and its role in transplantation. Nursing Times 1017–1018

Taylor D L 1983 Renal hypertension: physiology, signs, and symptoms. Nursing 83 13 : 10 : 4445

The Royal Melbourne Hospital Pharmacy Department Drugs in current use – Calcitriol. Australian Nurses Journal 9 : 7 : 27–28

Thomas T M, Plymat K R, Blanin J, Meade T W 1980 Prevalence of urinary incontinence. British Medical Journal Vol 281 (Nov 8) 1243–1245

Thompson I M et al 1977 Results of nonoperative management of blunt renal trauma. Journal of Urology 118 : 4 : 522–524

Thompson N M et al 1983 Transplantation of kidneys from living related donors. Medical Journal of Australia (Dec 10/24) 609–612

Thomson N M et al 1983 Continuous ambulatory peritoneal dialysis: an established treatment for endstage renal failure. Australian and New Zealand Journal of Medicine 13 : 489–495

Tiller D J 1981 Urinary tract infections as a disability. Australian Family Physician 10 : 44–47

Tinckler L 1984 The urinary system. Nursing Mirror 158 : 7 : 22–26

Vennegoor M A A A 1982 Dietary management in renal dialysis and transplantation. Nursing Times (19 May): 847–851

Watkins V 1984 Peritoneal dialysis: an alternative. Nursing in Australia 2 : 1 : 44–49

Webster G D, Methes G L, Selli C 1983 Prostatomembranous urethral injuries: a review of the literature and a rational approach to their management. Journal of Urology 130 : 4 : 898–901

Wing A J 1982 Renal replacement therapy. 9–2 hepatitis in European dialysis centres. Nursing Times 1061–1063

Wood A 1982 Continuous ambulatory peritoneal dialysis – an alternative approach to maintenance dialysis therapy. Nursing Times 852–854

Wright E 1983 Double indemnity. Nursing Mirror (April 13) 46–49

Wysocki R 1983 Urinary incontinence and the older adult. Australian Nurses Journal. 12 : 11 (June) 49–50

I

The reproductive system

60

Introduction to the male and female reproductive systems

Helen Farrer

Built into almost every human being is the desire to reproduce. There is a basic biological need to continue the species, and sometimes a more personal desire to ensure that part of one will continue to live on in the next generation. Both the male and the female reproductive systems are designed to achieve this function, and every structure and organ involved has some part to play in this ultimate aim.

This section describes the more common disorders that may arise during adulthood and which the nurse may encounter in her work – both in the hospital setting and in the community. Gynaecology is the specific term used for the study of the female reproductive system; 'genito-urinary' is the corresponding discipline for the study of the male reproductive system.

As most medical conditions of, and/or surgical procedures performed for, reproductive system dysfunction may involve an alteration to the concept of self or body image, a patient may experience a variety of emotional, psychological or physical problems. A multitude of factors influence a person's feelings about sex and reproduction; ethnic and cultural background, upbringing, education, age, life experiences, role in family and society; all go to make up an individual's response. It is the nurse's responsibility to give information and reassurance; consider feelings of shyness and embarrassment; be careful with draping, close screens and doors to minimise body exposure and ensure confidentiality; and to be non-judgemental and professional in approach.

THE MALE REPRODUCTIVE SYSTEM

The reproductive system of the male (Fig 60.1) includes the testes, epididymis, vasa deferentia (seminal ducts), seminal vesicles, prostate and bulbourethral glands, urethra, scrotum, and penis.

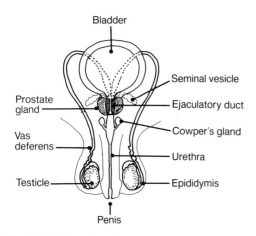

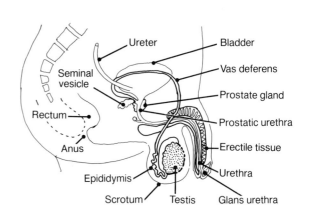

Fig. 60.1 Male genito-urinary system.

Testes

The testes are two small oval structures supported in a sac-like pouch called the scrotum. As the scrotum is outside the body, its temperature is slightly lower than the rest of the body, and this lower temperature is necessary for the production of sperm. The scrotum has a central septum, separating each testis. Within each testis is a mass of convoluted, 'seed-bearing' seminiferous tubules (Fig 60.2), where the spermatozoa originate. Cell division by meiosis occurs and the mature sperm contain only 23 chromosomes.

The seminiferous tubules also secrete the major part of the seminal fluid in which the sperm are transported. The interstitial cells of the testes produce, after puberty, the hormone testosterone, which is responsible for the development of the genitalia and the male secondary sex characteristics.

Epididymis

In each testis the seminiferous tubules unite to form a plexus from which ducts emerge to enter a large convoluted duct; the epididymis. The epididymis, which is attached to the upper part of each testis, is the place of final maturation of the sperm, where they develop their tails and become motile. The sperm are stored in the epididymus until ejaculation occurs.

Vas deferens

From the epididymis of each testicle the semen passes up through the vas deferens, a duct about 45 cm in length, which carries the sperm to the urethra. The vas deferens, and the testicular vessels, nerves, and lymphatics, are enclosed in a fibrous sheath – the spermatic cord.

Prostate gland and seminal vesicles

Surrounding the urethra, as it leaves the urinary bladder, is the prostate gland. Just behind the prostate gland and on the base of the bladder are two seminal vesicle glands. These fluid-producing glands are about 5 cm long. Their ducts join the ductus deferens to form the ejaculatory ducts. The two ejaculatory ducts then empty into the urethra. Just below the prostate gland lie two small glands called Cowper's or bulbo-urethral glands. These add their secretions through the ducts that open into the urethra. The collected secretions from testes, epididymis, seminal vesicles, and prostate and bulbourethral glands are called seminal fluid or semen. The semen passes to the outside of the body through the urethra.

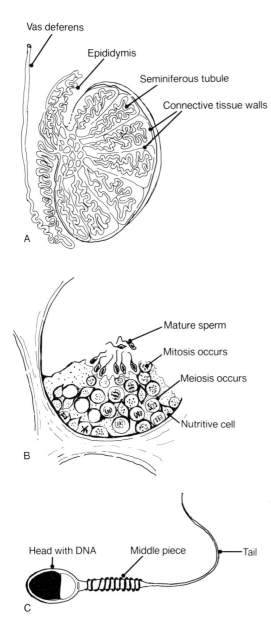

Fig. 60.2 A Structure of testis. B Cross-section of seminiferous tubule. C Mature sperm.

The penis

The penis is a cylindrical organ through which the urethra passes. It consists mainly of highly vascular, sponge-like, erectile tissue, the corpus cavernosum and the corpus spongiosum. When in a relaxed state, the penis is dependent and flaccid. Erection (see page 639) occurs as the capillaries of the erectile tissue become engorged, causing rigidity, and enlargement. The glans penis is the structure at the distal end of the penis containing the urethral meatus. Surrounding the glans is a double fold of skin, the prepuce (foreskin) which is retractable.

THE FEMALE REPRODUCTIVE SYSTEM

The female reproductive system consists of: the internal genital organs (Fig. 60.3) – the ovaries, fallopian tubes, uterus (including the cervix), and the vagina; and the external genital organs of the vulva – mons pubis, clitoris, the labia majora and minora, and the vestibule.

Ovaries

There are two ovaries, lying in the abdominal cavity near the fimbriated ends of the fallopian tubes. The ovaries produce, store, ripen, and release ova, and also produce hormones, the most important ones being oestrogen and progesterone.

Fallopian tubes

Sometimes also called oviducts, the fallopian tubes extend from the cornua (horns) of the upper uterus to the ovaries, and it is within these that fertilization of the ovum by spermatozoa takes place.

The lumen of the fallopian tubes are very narrow. They are lined with ciliated epithelium, which assists in propelling the ovum towards the uterus.

Uterus

The uterus is a thick-walled, hollow, muscular organ, measuring approximately 7.5 × 5.5 × 2.5 cm. It consists of two parts – the corpus and the cervix.

The endometrium consists of two layers of epithelial tissue containing glands and stroma: the surface layer responds to hormonal stimulation, while the basal layer remains constant.

The myometrium consists of three layers of muscle – the outer layer arranged longitudinally, the middle layer arranged obliquely, and the inner layer arranged in a circular pattern. There is also a small amount of fibrous tissue present.

The perimetrium consists of peritoneum, and covers the anterior and posterior surfaces of the body of the uterus. It then extends to the lateral pelvic walls as the broad ligament.

The cervix forms the lower third of the uterus, and half of it projects into the vagina. The hollow part of the cervix is the cervical canal, which opens into the vagina as the external os, and into the uterus as the internal os.

The cervical canal is lined with columnar epithelium, containing large glands which secrete mucus in response to hormonal levels in the blood. That part of the cervix which projects into the vagina is lined with stratified squamous epithe-

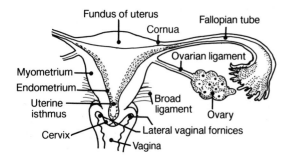
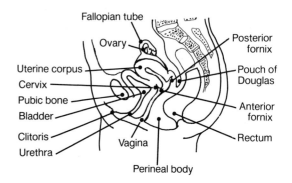

Fig. 60.3 Female internal organs of the reproductive system.

lium, continuous with the lining of the vagina. The point of junction of the two types of epithelium is the external os, and it is here, at the squamocolumnar junction, that abnormal cell changes are prone to occur.

The muscle layer of the cervix is continuous with the uterus, but it contains very much more fibrous tissue.

Vagina

The vagina is a fibromuscular canal extending from the vulva upwards and backwards to the uterus. Its shape is that of a flattened tube, with front and back walls in contact with each other but easily separated. The cervix enters the vagina at a right angle to the sagittal plane, so the posterior wall of the vagina is longer than the anterior wall. A gutter (fornix) surrounds the cervix where it projects into the vagina. The vagina is lined with stratified squamous epithelium. It has no glands, but acidic secretions seep through its wall to provide moisture for comfort and defence against microorganisms. Below the lining is a layer of vascular connective tissue and then two layers of muscle (inner – circular, and outer – longitudinal) which are thin but strong. Loose connective tissue separates the vaginal muscle from the underlying organs – the bladder and urethra anteriorly, and the rectum and Pouch of Douglas posteriorly.

The walls of the vagina are arranged in transverse folds (rugae) which allow for expansion of the canal during intercourse and childbirth.

Vulva (Fig. 60.4)

The mons pubis is a pad of fatty tissue lying over the pubic bone, covered by skin and pubic hair. The fatty pad acts as a buffer during intercourse, and the skin contains apocrine glands which have a distinctive scent believed to be sexually attractive.

The clitoris is the homologue to the penis. It is composed of spongy erectile tissue, has a copious blood supply, and is highly innervated. It responds to sexual stimulation and is one of the major female erogenous zones.

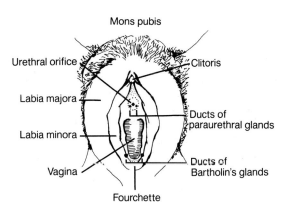

Fig. 60.4 The vulva.

The labia majora extend from the mons pubis to the perineum. They are of the same structure as the mons pubis, with fat, hair on their outer surfaces, and apocrine glands. Their function, together with the labia minora, is to cushion and protect the structures within the vestibule.

The vestibule is the area bounded by the labia minora. Opening on to it are the urethral and vaginal orifices, and the ducts of the Bartholin's glands and the Skene's (para-urethral) glands. The vaginal orifice is surrounded by a fold of thin membrane, the hymen, which does not completely close off the entrance to the vagina. After the first act of intercourse, digital examination, trauma, or insertion of tampons, the hymen is usually torn or stretched open.

Blood supply to the vulva comes from the pudendal arteries, which are branches of the femoral arteries. Venous drainage is by the corresponding veins.

Lymph is drained from the vulva into the inguinal glands, with some drainage to the external iliac glands. Cross drainage occurs from one side of the vulva to the other.

Innervation is from branches of the pudendal nerve and from the perineal nerve.

Pelvic ligaments

The broad ligaments are a raised fold of peritoneum and fibro-muscular tissue extending each side from the uterus to the lateral pelvic walls. They give little support to the uterus, but condense at their base to form the cardinal ligaments, which run from the cervix to the lateral pelvic wall.

The round ligaments run from the anterior surface of each horn of the uterus forward and down, through the inguinal canal, to be inserted into the fat of the labia majora. They help to hold the uterus in its normal anteverted (turned forward) position.

The uterosacral ligament runs backwards from the cervix to the sacrum, dividing for the rectum to pass through it. It pulls the cervix backwards and upwards, and is the major factor in keeping the uterus anteverted.

The pubocervical ligament runs forward from the cervix to the pubic bone, dividing for the vagina and urethra to pass through it.

Pelvic floor

The pelvic floor includes all of the tissues which fill the pelvic outlet and support the organs above.

The levator ani ('lifter of the anus') is sometimes called the pelvic diaphragm or basin, and is the strongest pelvic support. It is a broad sheet extending from the back of the pubic bone to the sacrum and coccyx and from the lateral walls of the pelvis it sweeps inwards and downwards to meet in the centre between the rectum and vagina. The urethra, vagina and rectum all pass through the levator ani, thus weakening it to some extent, but it is normally an adequate support for the pelvic contents.

The superficial perineal muscles lie below the levator ani sheet, arising from the pubis, sacrum and lateral pelvic walls to unite between the vagina and rectum.

The perineal body lies between the lower vagina and the lower rectum and is covered by the perineum (perineal skin). It is a wedge-shaped body of muscle, made up of the inferior surface of the junction of the levator ani and the junction of the superficial perineal muscles.

Blood supply to the internal pelvic organs

Blood to supply the uterus comes from the two large uterine arteries, which are branches of the internal iliac arteries. They run through the base of the broad ligament, then turn to travel upwards along the side of the uterus to the fundus, with coiled branches going off into the uterus. A separate branch turns down to supply the cervix and vagina.

The ovary is supplied from the ovarian arteries, which branch off from the abdominal aorta. A large branch enters each ovary, while the ovarian artery itself continues across to join up with the uterine artery.

Venous drainage is normally beside the corresponding arteries with the exception of the left ovarian vein, which usually drains into the left renal vein.

Lymphatic drainage follows the path of the blood vessels. Lymph channels drain into groups of nodes situated near the major arteries.

Innervation

The uterus is innervated by the autonomic nervous system. The cervix is insensitive to cutting, diathermy and other procedures, but is extremely sensitive to stretch. The ovaries are insensitive to stretch, but are sensitive to pressure (for example, squeezing). The fallopian tubes are sensitive to cutting, touching, crushing and stretching.

THE OVARIAN (MENSTRUAL) CYCLE

Germ cells (ova) are present from birth and are stored and matured in the ovary, contained in ovarian follicles. After puberty, on a regular cyclic basis, one ovarian follicle matures (it is then called a graafian follicle) and ruptures to release its ovum (ovulation). The ovum is picked up by the fimbria of one fallopian tube and transported to the uterus (Figs 60.5 & 6).

If fertilization does not occur within 24 hours of ovulation the ovum dies. The corpus luteum, which has a limited life unless maintained by human chorionic gonadotrophin (HCG), degenerates, causing the levels of oestrogen and progesterone in the bloodstream to fall. As this hormonal support ceases, the surface layer of the endometrium begins to break down and is shed – menstruation.

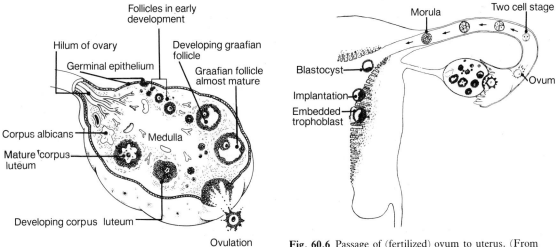

Fig. 60.5 Ovulation. (From Farrer, 1985.)

Fig. 60.6 Passage of (fertilized) ovum to uterus. (From Farrer, 1983.)

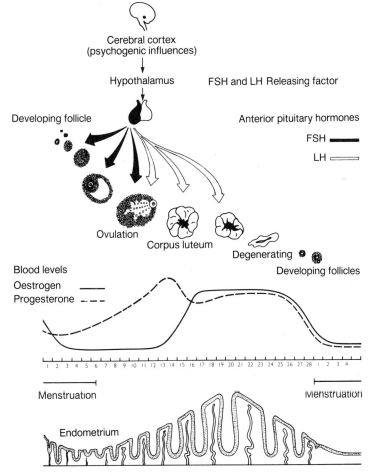

Fig. 60.7 Hormonal control of the menstrual cycle. (From Farrer, 1983).

After menstruation the endometrium proliferates, growing under the influence of oestrogen, produced by the developing ovarian follicle. Following ovulation the endometrium continues its proliferation, but with the additional influence of progesterone. Both oestrogen and progesterone are produced by the corpus luteum, which is the remnant of the ovarian follicle from which the ovum had been released.

Should fertilization of the ovum take place in the tube, cell division and differentiation will commence so that the fertilized ovum is ready to embed in the endometrium by the time it reaches the uterus 5–6 days later.

Finger-like projections grow from the embedded ovum (now called a blastocyst) and invade the endometrial vessels. The outer cells of the blastocyst produce the hormone HCG which, as its levels rise in the mother's bloodstream, acts upon the ovary to maintain the corpus luteum and therefore the production and levels of oestrogen and progesterone. Figure 60.7 shows the hormonal control of the stages of the menstrual cycle.

The menstrual cycle is controlled by oestrogen and progesterone. Their production is governed by the anterior pituitary hormone follicle stimulating hormone (FSH) and luteinising hormone (LH) and these, in turn, are governed by the hypothalamic gonadotrophin-releasing hormone (GNRH) (Table 60.1).

FSH releasing factor and LH releasing factor levels are sensitive to and controlled by the circulating levels of oestrogen and progesterone; a complex biofeedback system. The hypothalamus is also influenced by the cortex of the brain, and cortical influences such as emotion and stresses can affect and interfere with the normal chain of events and so cause a variety of menstrual and fertility problems. Oestrogen and progesterone have widespread affects upon the body, far more than the simple preparation of the endometrium to receive a fertilized ovum. Their effect upon the reproductive system specifically is shown in Table 60.2.

Oestrogen also brings about the body changes at puberty. Together with androgens, it is responsible for the development of secondary sex characteristics. It is also believed to play a part in calcium retention in the bones. Progesterone acts upon all the organs of the reproductive system, but only if they have been influenced by

Table 60.1 The menstrual cycle can be divided into four phases: menstrual phase of 4 days; proliferative phase of 10 days; secretory phase of 11 days; regressive phase of 3 days. (From Farrer, 1983)

Pituitary gland	Ovary	Uterus (endometrium)
Menstrual phase FSH released	Follicles start to ripen	Endometrium is shed, except for basal layer
Proliferative phase FSH continues to be released; level of FSH drops 24 hours before ovulation; LH is released – the LH 'surge'	Follicles continue to ripen, one much more than the others – the graafian follicle; produces oestrogen and some progesterone; graafian follicle grows, distends ovarian capsule, and it ruptures, releasing its ovum – ovulation	Repair and rebuilding of the endometrium
Secretory phase LH continues to be released for a few days then level drops rapidly	Corpus luteum develops from ruptured follicle and produces progesterone and some oestrogen	Endometrium thick and highly vascular. Glands of endometrium become enlarged; secrete and store glycogen, mucus and other substances which can nourish a fertilized ovum
Regressive (or premenstrual phase) Low levels of oestrogen stimulate production of FSH	Corpus luteum degenerates (limited life span); therefore levels of progesterone and oestrogen fall	Endometrial growth and secretion ceases; ischaemia of surface layers; cells die; bleeding below surface; gradual stripping off of whole functional surface – menstruation

Table 60.2 Actions of the ovarian hormones (From Farrer, 1983)

Oestrogen	'Target organ'	Progesterone
Proliferation of endometrium stimulates growth of myometrium	Uterus	Enlargement of stromal cells and glands; mucus and glycogen secretion
Growth of cervical glands; abundant secretion of clear mucus	Cervix	Change of secretion to scant amount of thick mucus
Growth of cells of vaginal epithelium; glycogen appears in cells	Vagina	Maturation of cells of epithelium ceases. Surface cells degenerate and are shed – release of glycogen
Growth and health of vulval tissues	Vulva	
Growth of duct system; enlargement and pigmentation of nipple and areola	Breasts	Growth of the alveoli

oestrogen. With oestrogen it can cause fluid retention in the tissues. It leads to the deposition of body fat in the female shape, and is also thermogenic: it raises the basal body temperature by about 0.5°C.

SEXUAL AND REPRODUCTIVE FUNCTIONING

Sexual response

There are marked similarities in the sexual responses of men and women.

Arousal

Emotional and psychological factors are important in the process of sexual arousal. As well, the senses of sight, smell, touch, and hearing during the period of foreplay act upon the cortex of the brain, giving rise to nerve impulses to the pelvic blood vessels and to the body's erectile tissue.

Psysiological changes

The changes occurring in the body are often divided into four phases.

1. Excitement. Sexual arousal in a woman causes the vaginal blood vessels to become engorged, the vagina and labia minora to swell, and the pelvic floor to relax. Lubricant fluid comes from contraction of the Batholins's glands and also from seepage through the vaginal walls.

In the man, sexual arousal results in engorgement of the vessels of the penis, causing the spaces within the erectile tissue to become filled with blood which is under pressure; the man's penis becomes larger, firmer and erect from the body; and some seminal fluid escapes from the penis. The skin around the scrotum contracts to become thicker and the testes rise higher in the scrotum.

In both sexes the nipples become erect; arm, leg and abdominal muscles become tense, and the heart rate, ventilatory rate and the blood pressure all increase.

2. Plateau. Further stimulation causes the vessels surrounding the lower third of the vagina to become distended with blood and this results in a decrease in the size of the vaginal orifice. The clitoris retracts under its prepuce. During intercourse clitoral stimulation may be achieved by the thrusting movements of the penis, causing traction of the prepuce and thus pressure on the clitoris. The uterus ascends slightly into the pelvis.

In the man, elevation of the testes continues, the diameter of the glans penis increases and seminal fluid continues to escape. Autonomic nerve impulses cause involuntary contraction of the bladder neck, thus preventing urine from escaping from the bladder and retrograde ejaculation of semen into the bladder.

3. Orgasmic phase. During female orgasm, rhythmic muscular contractions begin in the lower third of the vagina and in the uterus. The pelvic floor muscles also contract, and it is during this time that the peak physical feeling of pleasure occurs.

Orgasm in the man is preceded by a sensation 3–4 seconds before ejaculation takes place. The sensation is caused by the expulsion of fluid from the seminal vesicles and prostate gland into the urethra. Contraction of the muscles of the urethra and penis then follow, resulting in ejaculation.

During orgasm in both sexes the ventilatory and heart rates are much increased, the blood pressure rises and most of the muscles of the body become tense.

4. Resolution phase. Resolution is the return of the genitalia to a state of non-arousal. Vascular congestion resolves, resulting in the labia minora, vagina, and penis, returning to their normal size.

The final part of the resolution phase is a general relaxation of the rest of the body's muscles, often resulting in drowsiness and inducing sleep.

Disorders of sexual functioning – female

Inhibited sexual desire

In some women the normal desire for sexual activity is very low or absent (frigidity). There are no arousal feelings even after stimulation, although physiologically there is no abnormality, that is lubrication occurs and orgasm may be achieved, but with little pleasure. Frigidity can cause a variety of emotional disturbances.

The most common cause of inhibited sexual desire is depression, especially when it is accompanied by sleeping and eating disturbances. Stress, certain drugs, hormone imbalance states, and psychological factors can also result in decreased sexual desire.

As the majority of women experiencing frigidity do not have a physiological or pathological basis to their condition, they rarely seek help from their physician or another health professional. Therefore the nurse is likely to only encounter these women in either an informal interpersonal contact or in a community health situation. The nurse must be prepared to recognize the need for referral to the appropriate health professional, for example, sex counsellor.

Dyspareunia

Pain during intercourse may be superficial or deep. Superficial dyspareunia is pain felt at the entrance to the vagina and may be caused by:

* Tenderness of the vulva, urethra or vagina due to infection or allergic reactions
* Haemorrhoids
* Dryness, usually caused by oestrogen deficiency or occasionally by blockage of the Bartholin's ducts
* Tightness of the vaginal orifice, due to a thick or rigid hymen, or following scarring after childbirth or perineal operations.

Deep dyspareunia is pain felt inside the pelvis. It may last for some hours after intercourse. It may be caused by:

* Tenderness in the pelvis due to endometriosis, pelvic infection, or tumours
* Displacements of the uterus (retroversion or prolapse)
* Scar tissue in the upper vagina following operation or radiation
* Psychological factors

Unless the cause is simple and obvious, women suffering from dyspareunia should be encouraged to seek advice from their physician. Local causes are excluded or treated following a gently performed pelvic examination. A general anaesthetic may be necessary if the examination is too painful or if there is vaginismus present.

Lubricants may be recommended for simple dryness. Oestrogen may be given by mouth or locally applied for postmenopausal dryness, or an acid lubrication jelly if oestrogen is unsuitable. Muscle tightness may be relieved by gentle stretching, or by the use of graduated vaginal dilators, or by simple surgery. Local anaesthetic jelly is not recommended as a lubricant for intercourse as it can cause reflex impotence in the male.

Psychological causes are more difficult to treat and the family doctor or gynaecologist will usually refer the couple to a specialist in sexual medicine for treatment and counselling.

Abstinence from intercourse is often recommended during the period of investigation and treatment. If intercourse is attempted before the causative problems have been solved, dyspareunia will most likely return and may be even worse than before.

Psychological factors which may cause dyspareunia include: mental attitude to sex, previous bad experiences, lack of privacy, relationship or financial worries, tiredness, fear of pregnancy or labour, and lack of education or explanation following gynaecological operations or childbirth.

Vaginismus

Vaginismus is a condition of spasm of the muscles of the pelvic floor causing the vagina to close tightly, making intercourse impossible. Sometimes the adductor muscles of the thigh also go into spasm, and the woman is unable even to separate her knees. The spasms cause sharp shooting pains, similar to the pains of proctalgia – they are very distressing. Vaginismus is due to actual, previously experienced, or feared pain with intercourse; and its treatment requires the intervention of a qualified sex-therapist/counsellor.

Disorders of sexual functioning – male

Impotence

Impotence, which means 'without power' can produce strong and complicated emotions. Few men with this sexual dysfunction are able to discuss their impotence easily, or without guilt or confusion – it is a lonely problem.

Impotence is defined as the inability of the male to attain or sustain penile erection satisfactory for normal sexual intercourse. It can be a primary disorder; or a secondary disorder occurring situationally and associated with psychological, pathophysiological and pharmacological causes. It is said to be present if failure occurs in 25% or more of attempts to complete intercourse.

Psychological factors are responsible in 9 out of 10 cases of primary impotence and many cases of secondary impotence. Anxiety, tiredness, depression, fear (especially of failure), problems within the relationship, and work and other stresses may all inhibit the body's responses; from sexual arousal to penile erection.

Other common causes are: general ill-health, diabetes, sedatives, tranquilizers, alcohol, many antihypertensive drugs, and lesions of or interruption to the nerve pathways. The use of local anaesthetic jelly as a lubricant during intercourse can cause reflex impotence.

After physical causes have been excluded or treated, the management of impotence is directed towards psychosexual counselling and education. Ideally, the man's sexual partner is included in this therapy. It is often a slow process and the couple is usually advised to refrain from attempts at intercourse until the counsellor feels that both partners are ready.

Premature ejaculation

Premature ejaculation is the failure to delay orgasm, and thus detumescence, for long enough after vaginal penetration to satisfy the sexual partner.

As in impotence, physical factors are rarely found to cause premature ejaculation. It is fairly common in the adolescent years. Sexual counselling will usually help, by exploring the possible causes and teaching techniques of delaying ejaculation.

Priapism

Priapism is an abnormal condition of prolonged or constant penile erection, usually painful and rarely associated with sexual arousal. Its cause is not fully understood, but it probably involves vascular and neurologic abnormalities wherein pelvic vascular thrombosis inhibits the drainage of venous blood from the corpora cavernosa. This leads to stasis and increasing viscosity of the blood, and inhibition of normal nerve responses, which results in the persistent penile erection. It may also occur in men with acute leukaemia.

Treatment, to be effective, must not be delayed. Cold compresses can be applied as a first-aid measure, but it is important to seek medical attention immediately. Management may include:

● Decompression of the corpora by large-bore needle aspiration, usually performed under general anaesthesia

- Anti-coagulant therapy. This is usually effective only in the early stages of the condition.
- Shunt surgery to re-establish adequate pelvic circulation.

The nurse must anticipate that the patient will be extremely anxious and distressed and that he will require constant support and reassurance. The nurse must also ensure that the patient receives his ordered analgesia as required, until the condition is relieved.

Referral for sexual counselling is necessary in nearly all cases of priapism because the recovery of normal sexual functioning is most difficult unless priapism is treated early, and any underlying condition identified and also treated.

INFERTILITY

A couple is said to be infertile when they have been unable to conceive or maintain a pregnancy until the stage of extra-uterine viability. (20 weeks gestation is the Australian legal age of extra-uterine viability, and modern technology is capable of supporting some neonates at this gestational age). Infertility occurs in 10% of couples, and it can happen to people who have already had children. It is not usually investigated until the couple have been unsuccessful in achieving a pregnancy after a full year of trying.

Causes of infertility

Unless all the structural and physiological factors necessary for pregnancy are present infertility will occur.

Male problems

Sperm quality or quantity may be deficient. The sperm must be alive, motile and present in their hundreds of millions (200–600 million are normally found in a single 2–4 ml ejaculation specimen of seminal fluid) as vaginal acidity can kill large numbers of sperm, as can lubricant agents; also the cervical mucus may be impenetrable to poorly motile sperm.

Absence of sperm can be caused by testicular atrophy (as can occur after mumps orchitis),

undescended testes, irradiation, and cytotoxic drugs. Obstruction of the male genital tract from adhesions following infection (especially gonorrhoea or tuberculosis) or surgery can prevent the passage of sperm. Deficiency in the quality or quantity of sperm may be due to some of these causes even where the condition has affected only one testis. Other factors are chronic infection of the epididymus or prostate; varioceles; prolonged excessive warmth near the testes; heavy alcohol consumption; and cigarette smoking.

Female problems

Female problems with becoming pregnant include anovulation, hormone imbalance, and 'post pill' infertility. Cervical mucus might be absent or diminished following damage to the cervical glands (for example, during cauterisation). Obstruction of the fallopian tubes can occur following gonorrhoea, tuberculosis or other infections can distort the tubes or cause their ends to close. The lining of the uterus can be affected by hormonal disorders, endometriosis, fibroids, foreign bodies, and infection.

Male and female problems

These can include: general ill health, anaemia, overwork, psychological problems, even minor ones which can then be increased by the infertility itself; hypersensitivity to a particular man's sperm by a particular woman's body; failure to coincide intercourse with ovulation.

Investigative procedures

As it is the woman who is not achieving a pregnancy, it is usually she who seeks help first. She will be given a thorough general physical and gynaecological examination and this should exclude obvious causes. Before any further or more detailed tests are performed, the man will be asked to provide a specimen of ejaculate, for assessment of sperm numbers and motility. Alternatively, the woman undergoes examination as soon as possible after intercourse (Huhner's test); this will show, in addition, the sperms' ability to pass through her cervical mucus.

If the sperm tests are satisfactory, the fallopian tubes are examined for patency, either by X-ray (hysterosalpingogram) or by air-pressure (Rubin's test) If the tubes are normal, an assessment of the woman's hormone status, through blood, vaginal smear, or endometrial biopsy examination, would be made, and possibly a laparoscopy performed, to examine the tubes under direct vision.

Any cause discovered is treated if possible. Hormone administration may correct states of imbalance, and microsurgery is being used with increasing success for tubal blockage. Simply learning to recognise the times of fertility within the menstrual cycle has helped many women to achieve pregnancy. Figure 60.8 shows the anatomical and physiological factors necessary for pregnancy to occur.

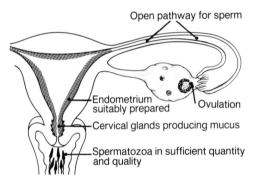

Open pathway for sperm

Endometrium suitably prepared

Ovulation

Cervical glands producing mucus

Spermatozoa in sufficient quantity and quality

Fig. 60.8 Factors necessary for establishment of pregnancy. (From Farrer, 1985.)

Psychological causes are more difficult to manage. Sometimes they require a specialist in sexual medicine or a psychiatrist. More commonly, however, the simple fact that 'something is being done' about the infertility has very positive effects.

In vitro fertilisation (IVF)

In vitro fertilisation has had considerable success in achieving pregnancies for those in whom all other methods of treatment have failed. IVF involves:

1. Removal of mature ova from the ovary, under laparoscopic visualization, just before ovulation. In many cases ovulation is stimulated hormonally.
2. Fertilisation of the ova outside the body (in vitro means 'in glass'), by the addition of a sufficient number of spermatozoa.
3. Preparation of the endometrium by hormone administration so that it is suitably prepared to receive a fertilised ovum.
4. Transferring the fertilised ovum at exactly the right stage of development (the 4–16 cell stage), to the prepared endometrium.

There are many legal and ethical problems surrounding IVF. The issues of surrogate motherhood, the storage of deep frozen embryos, and embryo wastage are just three that are presently being considered, together with the considerable financial cost of the programme.

61

Disorders of the male reproductive system

Chris Game   Helen Farrer

The more common disorders of the male reproductive system are discussed in this chapter.

INFECTIVE AND INFLAMMATORY DISORDERS

A number of the infective and inflammatory disorders affecting the male reproductive system are caused by organisms transmitted sexually. These conditions (syphilis, gonorrhoea, non-specific urethritis, and herpes) are discussed in Chapter 63.

Balanitis and balanoposthitis

Balanitis is inflammation of the glans penis; balanoposthitis is inflammation of the glans penis and the prepuce (in the uncircumcised male). Both conditions involve soreness, irritation and discharge, and result from bacterial infection, phimosis, and/or poor penile hygiene. Balanitis in a circumcised person is extremely rare. Smegma is thought to be a carcinogen, and chronic balanitis is regarded as a pre-malignant condition.

A swab/specimen is taken from the area for culture and sensitivity testing; specific antibiotic therapy is prescribed.

Frequent bathing of the inflamed area with warm normal saline will help to relieve discomfort. Circumcision may be advised in severe or frequently recurring cases.

Epididymo-orchitis

Infection and inflammation of the testis and the epididymus commonly occur simultaneously. The most common cause is ascending infection from prostatitis. It may also occur secondarily to bacterial urinary tract infection, as a complication of sexually transmitted diseases (especially gonorrhoea and non-specific urethritis), and sometimes following prostatectomy. Bilateral epididymo-orchitis, if untreated or allowed to become chronic, may result in blockage of the vasa deferentia and so may cause infertility.

The testes are swollen, tender, and painful; the patient is febrile and may vomit.

Management includes bed rest, high fluid intake, elevation of the scrotum, analgesia, and anti-emetics. Local applications of well-wrapped cold packs for limited periods help to relieve the pain. Antibiotics are prescribed if the infection is bacterial in origin; if viral in origin, it will subside in 7–10 days.

Orchitis without associated epididymitis is most often caused by mumps occurring after puberty. Mumps orchitis may result in atrophy of the testes, and therefore sterility. Males who have not had mumps during childhood should avoid contact with the disease; if they are exposed to it, they should seek medical advice. The early administration of gammaglobulin may reduce the severity of mumps.

Prostatitis

Inflammation of the prostate gland may be acute or chronic; it is usually the result of infection.

Acute prostatitis is usually bacterial in origin. The symptoms are urgency, frequency, and discomfort with micturition; and in severe cases, acute retention, chills, and perineal and low back pain. Sometimes there is also gross haematuria.

The prostate gland is enlarged and tender on palpation.

Acute cystitis soon follows the onset of acute prostatitis, so culture and sensitivity testing of an MSU will determine the appropriate antibiotic therapy. Acute prostatitis is managed by admission to hospital, with bed rest, high fluid intake, antibiotics, and analgesia. If acute retention of urine occurs, the bladder would most likely be drained via a suprapubic rather than a urethral catheter.

Chronic prostatitis is characterized by recurrent low-grade dysuria and frequency, haematuria, fatigue, irritability, backache, and a decrease in libido. On palpation the prostate is found to be enlarged and firm.

Antibiotics are prescribed, but the condition often recurs when treatment ceases. Prostatectomy will relieve bladder neck obstruction.

NEOPLASTIC DISORDERS

Neoplasms, benign and malignant, may arise in any of the structures of the male reproductive system. By regular examination, a number of these growths can be discovered early and treatment begun before they cause complications or, in some cases, become life threatening.

Testicular self-examination

The importance of testicular self-examination cannot be underestimated. Testicular malignancies have a high progression rate, metastasise rapidly, and have a low 5-year survival rate due to most tumours being well advanced when the person seeks medical advice. It is believed that with testicular self-examination techniques, tumours would be found much earlier and therefore medical intervention could occur before metastasis has occurred.

Testicular self-examination should be included in health teaching programs for all males over the age of 15 years. The procedure should be carefully explained and the person given the opportunity to ask questions about any abnormalities that he may encounter. He should be advised that the best time to perform self-examination is immediately after showering or bathing when the body tissues are warm and therefore the scrotum is relaxed making the testes easier to feel.

He should observe the scrotum for any abnormal swelling, colour, or texture and be attentive to feel for any abnormal lumps or swelling in the testes. He should be instructed to hold his scrotum in the palms of his hands and examine each testicle by rolling the testis between his thumb and fingers. Each testicle should feel smooth and approximate the size of a small hen's egg. The epididymis, lying posterior to each testis, should also be palpated and each should feel soft and slightly spongy to touch. The spermatic cords ascending from each epididymus should feel like round firm tubes.

Each man should be encouraged to seek medical advice should he detect any abnormality, no matter how inconsequential it may seem. The majority of lumps or swellings are benign, but early detection of a cancerous lump may be lifesaving.

The penis

Carcinoma of the penis may appear after a long history of irritation from phimosis or chronic balanitis. The lesion, usually on the underside of the glans, begins as a painless wart-like growth which ulcerates and discharges a thin purulent blood-stained fluid. Usually by the time the patient seeks treatment, metastases are found in the femoral lymph nodes.

Following a diagnostic biopsy, treatment is by:

• Irradiation, either surface or by needle implants
• Amputation of part or whole of the penis, and bilateral removal of the pelvic lymph nodes
• Total cystectomy, in advanced cases, or palliative radiation.

The testes

Benign tumours of the testes are very rare. Interstitial cell tumours, fibroids, and lipomas are sometimes found, and these are excised.

Malignant tumours tend to occur most commonly in young men and affect one male in approximately 500 under the age of 50. They are the commonest neoplasms in the 25–34 year age group, and are the leading cause of death in men, from solid tumours, between the ages of 15 and 34 years. Tumours are commonly either: seminomas (45%), which are of gonadal cell origin and arise from the testicular tubules; or teratomas (40%), which are of nongonadal, highly malignant and variously differentiated cell type.

The aetiology of testicular carcinoma is unknown, but there may be an association with hereditary factors, cryptorchidism (undescended testes) or trauma. There is a 10-fold increase in tumour incidence with cryptorchidism regardless of whether or not surgical correction has taken place. As well, malignancy of the remaining testis in the man who has already had a testis removed for cancer is extremely high. No relationship to occupation or social class has been established. The disease spreads early, with metastases in the lungs, liver, and bone.

Clinical manifestations. Testicular carcinoma usually presents as a painless lump in the testis which may be as small as a pea or as large as a tennis ball. The tumour is usually painless at first, but will become painful if haemorrhage into the tumour occurs. Gynaecomastia is a late sign and is due to the production of the hormone chorionic gonadotrophin by the tumour cells.

Medical and surgical management. Diagnosis is by biopsy during surgical exploration, usually after ultrasound scanning. Treatment consists of removal of the testis, radiotherapy, and the administration of cytotoxic drugs.

Seminal vesicles

Neoplasms are rare, apart from fibrosis following chronic infection, and extension of carcinoma of adjacent structures.

The prostate

Benign enlargement of the prostate is a common condition in males over the age of 50 (90% of cases of prostatic enlargement are benign). Because the prostate gland surrounds the urethra at the base of the bladder, its enlargement will interfere with the normal process of voiding. This may ultimately lead to hydronephrosis from back pressure

of urine in the ureters caused by a chronically full bladder.

Clinical manifestations. The patient will experience difficulty in voiding, especially in starting a stream. He may also suffer chronic retention of urine, occasionally with overflow. Occasionally, sudden acute retention of urine associated with acute abdominal distention and discomfort may occur, as may haematuria, due to stretching and rupture of small veins of the bladder neck.

Investigative procedures. Diagnosis is confirmed by rectal examination which demonstrates an enlarged, soft, prostate. Renal function tests are performed. These include: blood urea, which may be elevated if there is associated renal damage; creatinine clearance time, which may be elevated; urinalysis for the presence of protein and blood; and intravenous pyelogram and cystoscopy for identification of anatomical abnormalities.

Medical, surgical, and nursing management. Treatment is by resection of the prostate. Prior to surgery complications such as infection or uraemia are corrected.

An indwelling urinary catheter is used to relieve the obstruction and subsequently to drain the bladder. Care is taken to empty a distended bladder gradually by allowing no more than 500 ml to drain at any one time. A period of 15–30 minutes should elapse before the next 500 ml is allowed to drain. This is done to encourage circulatory compensation into the capillary spaces previously compressed by the very full bladder. Hypovolaemic shock is thus avoided.

Malignant neoplasms of the prostate

These are usually in the form of adenocarcinoma and affect the posterior part of the gland. The tumour grows from the glandular tissue of the prostate, slowly infiltrates the gland, and spreads to the surrounding tissues – the bladder, urethra, and sometimes the rectum. Lymphatic spread occurs with widespread bony metastases, affecting particularly the lumbar vertebrae, the pelvis, and the skull. Carcinoma of the prostate is rare under the age of 50.

Clinical manifestations. At first, the symptoms may resemble those of benign enlargement, thus underlining the importance of regular preventive examination. Rectal examination reveals a firm, irregular, fixed, asymmetrical prostate.

Investigative procedures. Full blood examination commonly reveals anaemia. Serum acid phosphatase levels are markedly elevated. X-rays may show bony metastases. A urethrocytoscopy is performed to assess the degree of prostatic enlargement and any changes in the wall of the bladder. Biopsy is performed by resectoscope, through the perineum, or from the rectum.

Medical and surgical management. Treatment is by radical prostatectomy if the diagnosis was made before the disease has spread to surrounding tissues and if the patient is young. Otherwise a transurethral prostatectomy would be done to relieve the symptoms of obstruction. As the adenocarcinoma is hormone-dependent, the administration of stilboestrol (synthetic oestrogen) will inhibit the growth of the tumour. A bilateral orchidectomy may be performed if the patient is unable to tolerate stilboestrol, with its side effects of fluid retention, nausea, gynaecomastia, and generalized femininization.

PROSTATECTOMY

It is not unusual for the patient with prostatic hypertrophy to ignore the insidious onset of urinary obstruction and not seek medical advice until such time as acute retention, with or without overflow, manifests.

Decisions regarding the need for surgical intervention, the type of procedure, and the method of anaesthesia are based on a variety of factors. These include: the degree of discomfort, inconvenience, and loss of independence in the patient; the degree of renal tract abnormality and dysfunction produced by the obstruction; the degree of haematuria present and hence anaemia; the age of the patient; the presence of recurrent or chronic urinary tract infection; the co-existence of cardiovascular and/or respiratory disease; the amount of residual urine present (over 60 ml is indicative of the need for surgical intervention); and the onset of acute retention.

Men undergoing genitourinary surgery are, on average, elderly, and so general health and condition are carefully assessed and corrected as much as is possible before surgery.

Prostatectomy may be either 'open' or 'closed', that is, the presence or absence of a surgical wound through either the abdomen or perineum.

'Open' methods of prostatectomy are only used if the prostate is quite large (over 50 g).

Transurethral resection of the prostate (TURP)

This common, closed, surgical procedure is usually performed for benign enlargement of the prostate. It involves the paring away of the prostate tissue using a resectoscope, a fine cutting instrument inserted through the lumen of a cystoscope (Fig 61.1). The shavings of prostate fall into

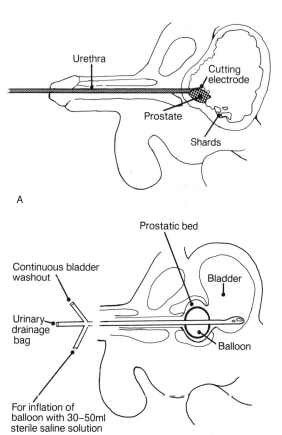

Fig. 61.1 A – Transurethral resection of prostate (TURP). **B** – 3-way catheter in situ following TURP.

the bladder, from which they are flushed by irrigation at intervals during the procedure and any remaining particles evacuated using a special instrument (an ellik) at its completion. As well as removal of the prostate tissue, the operation may include ligation of the vasa deferentia (vasectomy) to prevent ascending infection postoperatively.

TURP is indicated in all cases where the prostate gland is estimated to be below 50 g weight. The procedure can be performed under general or spinal anaesthesia; the use of spinal anaesthesia has considerably reduced the surgical risk in elderly males with cardiovascular or respiratory disorders.

Postoperatively, the patient has a urethral catheter in situ which is usually connected to a continuous bladder washout. The postoperative recovery is usually rapid (5–10 days), but long term urinary incontinence may be a feature.

Retropubic (extravesical) prostatectomy

In this open approach the anterior abdominal incision allows for direct visualization of the prostate and a greater likelihood of complete haemostasis (Fig. 61.2). The bladder is not incised, therefore should covert bladder pathology be present it will not be treated. Osteitis pubis may develop postoperatively but complications are rare. Postoperatively the nurse will be responsible for the care of the patient with a urethral catheter and a low abdominal wound with at least 1 drain tube. Following removal of the abdominal drain

tube there may be some urinary leakage. This usually clears after 24–48 hours, and long term urinary incontinence is rare.

Suprapubic (transvesical) prostatectomy

This surgical approach utilizes a low abdominal incision and an incision into the bladder (Fig. 61.3). Prior to the development of the transurethral technique, this was the preferred surgical approach. Although this procedure allows for a more complete removal of prostatic tissue and extensive examination and treatment of concurrent problems of the lower urinary tract, for example a large bladder calculus, it does have distinct postoperative disadvantages. These include: the likelihood of reactionary haemorrhage is high; extravasation of urine is more likely; severe bladder spasm is common; and a longer postoperative recovery is to be expected. Long term urinary incontinence is rare.

Perineal prostatectomy

In the young male with early malignancy, the perineal approach may be used (Fig. 61.4). This allows for direct visualization of the prostate and facilitates wide resection if early malignancy is confirmed.

However, this approach is rarely used as it produces severe long term problems including: sexual impotence due to the severing of nerves; infection due to contamination of the wound with

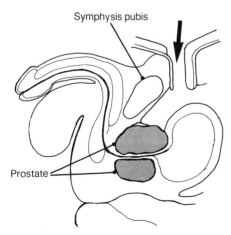

Fig. 61.2 Retropubic prostatectomy.

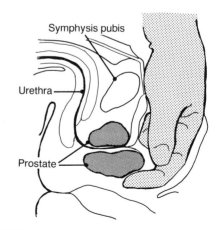

Fig. 61.3 Suprapubic prostatectomy.

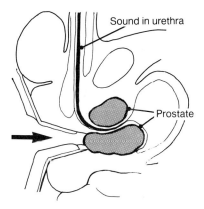

Fig. 61.4 Perineal prostatectomy.

bowel flora; and faecal and urinary incontinence due to interruption of sphincters during surgery.

Postoperatively the patient will have a urethral catheter in situ and at least 1 drain tube with the perineal incision. Healing is fairly rapid and the incidence of reactionary haemorrhage and severe postoperative pain is low.

Nursing management of the patient undergoing prostatectomy

Disorientation and confusion can arise in any elderly person in a strange place. These problems are even greater when associated with the need to void frequently and get up during the night. The nurse needs to be alert to this fact and should provide protection against patient falls.

The nurse should also anticipate, where possible, the patient's needs and thus: provide a urinal at the bedside at all times, especially at night; ensure that a night light is illuminated to assist patient independence; and answer promptly any call for assistance.

Another matter which may disconcert the man who has had urinary problems is his being encouraged to drink copious quantities of fluid. He may well be used to restricting his fluid intake in order to prevent embarrassing or inconvenient situations of having to urinate when away from home or during the night.

Preoperative nursing management

Shaving of the skin is rarely done nowadays. Skin cleansing, using an antibacterial preparation, is

thorough and includes special attention to the pubic and scrotal skin. The evening prior to surgery an enema is given to empty the lower bowel.

The nurse should ensure that the patient has received, from the physician, an explanation of the surgical procedure to be performed, and that the patient understands the nature of the equipment and drainage apparatus that will be used in the postoperative period. It is important to stress to the patient that the nurse will constantly be monitoring his fluid intake and output and that this will also include frequent catheter checks.

Antibiotic therapy (usually a single dose of gentamicin) may be given where catheter drainage is used, to prevent the establishment of infection following surgery.

Fluid intake is encouraged, and an intake-output chart is kept from the time of admission.

Postoperative nursing management

In addition to the routine postanaesthetic and postoperative care the following points are important:

Position. As many genitourinary procedures are performed under spinal epidural anaesthesia, the patient may be nursed in a semirecumbent position for the first 24 hours after surgery, to prevent headache. The spinal anaesthetic will also necessitate observation for the return of sensation and movement of the lower trunk and legs.

Fluid intake. A high fluid intake is important as it ensures the prevention of clot formation by continually washing out the bladder. Intravenous fluid therapy is maintained to ensure a high fluid intake. This is replaced by oral fluids as soon as they are tolerated. Encouragement will be needed to ensure that a high oral fluid intake is maintained.

Following open prostatectomy, the nurse will be responsible for the care of a patient with a low abdominal, or more rarely a perineal, wound and drain tube. After removal of the wound drain it is not uncommon for urinary leakage to occur, but this should cease after 24–48 hours. When a suprapubic catheter is to be removed the nurse should first cut the surface suture(s) holding the catheter in place, and then use gentle but firm traction to remove the catheter. A firm dressing is then applied and reapplied frequently, as urinary leakage is expected for up to 72 hours.

Management of the bladder irrigation system

Continuous bladder irrigation is used in almost all situations following prostatectomy; its major advantage being to prevent the complication of clot retention. A 3-way self-retaining catheter (Fig. 61.1B) is inserted at the completion of the surgical procedure and is attached to the irrigation system. The isotonic irrigation fluid used will depend upon the surgeon's choice: normal saline or 1.5% glycine aminoacetic acid are commonly used; distilled water is an alternative, however water intoxication can occur when hypotonic solutions are used.

Clots may form if the urinary drainage is impeded, and these will then obstruct the catheter. The rate of flow of irrigation fluid should be just enough to maintain a pink to straw/serous colour but not so slow as to allow clots to form.

Urinary irrigation and drainage is frequently observed for: freedom of drainage; amount of return; colour; and the presence of blood clots. A positive return indicates continuing renal function; a negative return may herald the onset of obstruction to flow. A straight rather than tapered connection is used to connect the catheter and tubing.

The entire system should be inspected frequently and 'milked' when necessary to ensure that there are no kinks or that the system is not obstructed. Present day irrigation systems include a compressable 'milking' chamber between the catheter connection and the drainage bag. Care must be taken when 'milking' the system as this may cause pain or discomfort, or even bladder spasm, if done too quickly, too frequently, or with undue force.

Suprapubic catheters may be used as well as urethral catheters, for the introduction of irrigation fluid after 'open' prostatectomy operations.

Removal of the urinary drainage system. Following removal of the catheter, urinary retention or difficulty in voiding may occur. The nurse should therefore record all output and observe for bladder distension, poor urinary stream, pain on voiding, frequency and incontinence. Haematuria is expected, but frank bleeding is abnormal and should be reported immediately. Haematuria should gradually diminish, but a small degree may still be present up to 3 weeks after surgery.

Complications of prostatectomy

Urinary tract infection may arise following prostatectomy. It can be minimized by encouraging a high fluid intake, the use of sterile irrigation fluid and equipment, ensuring that the urethral meatus is kept clear of discharge by frequent penile toilets, and observing aseptic techniques if it is necessary to change urinary drainage tubing and bags. Tubing and bags are not changed routinely.

Clot retention is the major early complication of prostatectomy. Signs of its development are a diminished (or ceased) bladder output. Drainage will become more heavily bloodstained and clots will be present. The patient may complain of lower abdominal pain and distention and an intense desire to void; he may become restless and develop the symptoms and signs of shock.

If these signs appear, continuous irrigation is ceased immediately, and medical assistance is sought. A manual bladder washout, using a Toomey's syringe will be performed, analgesia given and treatment for shock commenced. Only if these measures are unsuccessful is recatheterization attempted in an effort to relieve the clot retention. A whistle-tip catheter is usually used in this instance.

The physician will perform a manual washout until drainage is clear, then the whistle-tip catheter is removed and an indwelling Foley 3-way catheter is reinserted. If these measures are unsuccessful the patient is returned to the operating room for evacuation of the clot through the bladder wall. Emotional support is important at this time, as the patient will be distressed and in pain.

Bladder spasm may occur and is usually due to: irrigation fluid running too fast; the use of irrigation fluid below room temperature; too frequent or too violent 'milking' of the system; bladder distension as a result of clot retention; and, more commonly, a response to irritation from the catheter balloon. Antispasmodic drugs may be prescribed to control bladder spasm, however the most effective treatment is removal of the catheter as soon as possible postoperatively.

Urinary incontinence is to be expected in the postoperative period, but long term incontinence may occur if sphincters have been damaged, for example, in perineal prostatectomy. Urethral stricture is not uncommon and may result from: the instruments used in surgery, for example, the resectoscope; from the presence of the catheter, or from inflammation of the urethra. It is evidenced by a small urinary stream, dysuria, and straining to void, and may develop within 1–2 weeks post surgery. In most instances urethral stricture is treated with the passage of urethral sounds and this procedure may need to be repeated regularly. Rarely, further surgery may be indicated if the stricture is unrelieved.

Sexual impotence may occur transiently in the early postoperative period (up to 2 months) and can be largely prevented by careful and supportive counselling. However, permanent impotence is an expected complication of perineal prostatectomy.

Discharge planning

The patient should be advised that he could expect a degree of urinary incontinence for some time after the catheter is removed. If improvement does not occur within 4 weeks of discharge he should be encouraged to seek medical advice. The reasons for continuing a high fluid intake are stressed: it prevents urinary stasis and therefore infection, and encourages the return of bladder tone and urinary continence.

The patient can be reassured that simple prostatectomy does not cause impotence, but he should be advised to abstain from intercourse until after the follow-up appointment. If his prostatectomy involved ligation of the vasa deferentia he should be reassured that although this means that he is infertile, it does not affect his ability to have normal sexual intercourse.

Strenuous exercise should be avoided at first. The patient should gradually resume his normal daily activity, while setting aside time for extra rest until he is fully recovered. Any more than minimal consumption of alcohol is advised against, to avoid dehydration.

The patient should be told to seek medical assistance if haematuria persists, or if he has any dysuria or lower abdominal pain. He should know when and where to go for his follow-up appointment, and why it is important that this appointment is kept.

TRAUMA

Trauma to the penis and scrotum may occur as a result of penetrating or crushing injuries (for example, ruptured urethra from the cross-bar of a bicycle), or from tearing and separation of the skin (for example, when caught up by clothing into machinery). Hospitalization is required urgently. A search is made for any separated skin, which should be kept cold and reapplied as soon as possible. Skin grafting may be necessary.

The shaft of the erect penis can be fractured (with rupture of one or more corpora cavernosa) by trauma or during intercourse.

Self-mutilation nearly always involves only the penis and the patient presents with severe lacerations or even traumatic amputation. Haemorrhage is usually profuse and the patient deeply shocked. Apart from caring for the patient following extensive plastic surgery, the nurse must be aware of the need for the patient to receive psychiatric referral and follow up, and sexual counselling.

In almost all cases of trauma to the penis, urethral cathererization will be required, and the nurse is responsible for the prevention of catheter induced urinary tract infection. The length of time for catheterization will depend upon the type of trauma, the degree of interruption to normal urethral structure, and the healing process. Nerve injury may also lead to temporary or permanent impotence and the patient requires a large amount of support from the nurse and should be referred for expert sexual counselling.

Other causes of injury, especially to the scrotum, are sexual assault, and sporting injuries – particularly in cricket and football.

Testicular rupture or haemorrhage may result in severe shock, pain, and scrotal swelling. Depending upon the degree of injury, orchidectomy may be performed.

Any trauma to the scrotum invariably results in the development of a haematocele (haematoma) which is usually very painful. A scrotal support should be provided and prescribed analgesia given regularly to ease discomfort. The application of heat is also effective in relieving pain.

Trauma to the male genitourinary tract may result in mild to severe changes in body image and self concept. The nurse must, therefore, provide constant reassurance and support during the recovery phase.

OTHER CONDITIONS

Hydrocele

A hydrocele is a collection of serous fluid in the sac of the membrane (tunica vaginalis) surrounding the testis. It may be preceded by inflammation, or may occur spontaneously. Hydroceles usually occur unilaterally and are painless, but can grow to an embarrassingly large size.

Management may be by aspiration of the serous fluid. Hydrocele can, however, recur and so excision of the tunica vaginalis is preferred as it cures the condition.

Varicocele

Varicocele is a varicose condition of the veins draining the testes, in which there is an abnormal dilatation and tortuosity of the veins of the pampiniform plexus within the scrotum. The condition usually presents between the ages of 15–30 years and approximately 10% of all males have a varicocele. It is interesting to note that over 90% of all varicoceles either become asymptomatic or disappear completely after the commencement of regular sexual intercourse.

In those patients where varicocele is symptomatic and persistent, subfertility is a problem due to decreased number and motility of sperm. The patient will usually seek medical advice due to the persistent scrotal discomfort which is usually described as a dull ache or 'pulling down' feeling in the scrotum.

Examination of the scrotum with the patient in a standing position reveals the dilated and tortuous veins, characteristically feeling like a 'bag of worms'.

In persistent varicocele, scrotal support can relieve the discomfort until treatment by injection of a sclerosing agent, or more rarely, surgical ligation of the veins is undertaken.

Cryptorchidism

The undescended or maldescended testis is a common condition, being seen in approximately 1% of boys after 1 year of age. The condition is usually unilateral and is reported by the parent(s) or found on routine physical examination.

If the testis is retractable, then it is normally found in the scrotum but on stimulation it is pulled into the inguinal canal by an active cremaster muscle. This type of cryptorchidism is usually self correcting and the testis becomes permanently resident in the scrotum at puberty. If the testis is arrested in the line of descent, or is ectopic in presentation, surgical correction (orchidopexy) is required to place the testis in the scrotum.

If orchidopexy is indicated, the surgery is performed prior to puberty to decrease the likelihood of infertility. This is of paramount importance where cryptorchidism is bilateral. If cryptorchidism is left untreated the testis is increasingly susceptible to infertility, trauma, and torsion. Orchidopexy does not reduce the increased likelihood of malignancy in the undescended testis, but does make examination and thus early diagnosis possible.

Testicular torsion

Testicular torsion is an acutely painful condition, where there is twisting of the testis on its spermatic cord and resultant occlusion of the blood supply and lymphatic drainage. It is usually unilateral and presents as an acute inflammatory process within the affected half of the scrotum, accompanied by pain and swelling. It may arise spontaneously or after strenuous exertion. The cause is most likely to be incomplete attachment of the epididymis to the testis.

The pain is usually sudden in onset and accompanied by nausea and vomiting; scrotal oedema and fever then develop. Treatment is required urgently if testicular function is to be saved, and as its presentation is very similar to epididymo-orchitis, all cases of epididymo-orchitis should be considered torsion until proven otherwise. Treatment consists of surgical restoration of the testis to its original position.

Phimosis

Phimosis is a condition in which the prepuce ('foreskin') of the penis is so tight that it cannot be retracted over the glans.

Phimosis is rarely congenital. Before puberty it is commonly due to a poorly performed previous circumcision, or trauma from repeated attempts at retraction of the prepuce. These factors may also give rise to phimosis after puberty, but it is then likely to be due to infection from retained smegma and dirt.

Treatment consists of gentle separation of any adhesions using a probe. In most instances the condition requires recircumcision or, in the case of inflammation, primary circumcision in order to prevent further inflammation and oedema.

In uncircumcised boys health education should be aimed at explanation to the mother that the prepuce does not need to be retracted in order for the glans to be cleaned, and that normal showering or bathing is all that is necessary prior to puberty. Only following puberty is it necessary for the prepuce to be retracted in order to effect good hygiene.

Paraphimosis

Paraphimosis occurs when a tight foreskin has been retracted, becomes oedematous, and is then unable to return to its normal position over the glans. Circulation is impeded and the glans becomes swollen and painful. Careful manual replacement, usually under general anaesthesia, may be possible; and a slit may be made in the dorsal aspect of the prepuce. However, once paraphimosis occurs circumcision is usually advisable to prevent recurrence.

Circumcision

Circumcision is the surgical removal of the prepuce from the penis and is usually performed within 2 weeks of birth. Less frequently it may be performed prior to puberty or, rarely, circumcision may be necessary in the adult male. In Australia approximately 65% of all males are circumcised and only a small percentage of these are performed as part of religious ceremonies.

Although some parents believe that their child should be circumcised for either hygenic or cosmetic reasons, there is no valid medical reason for routine circumcision and strong debate still occurs. There is as yet no statistical support for the theory that circumcision reduces the future risk of the development of penile cancer, or cervical cancer in sexual partners.

Following circumcision the patient must be closely observed and the excision site frequently inspected for reactionary haemorrhage. The original dressing should remain untouched and allowed to fall off, usually within 24 hours. Thereafter a nonadherent dressing of paraffin gauze should be reapplied daily after bathing until healing has occurred, usually within 5–7 days.

If circumcision is performed correctly and all normal pre-, intra-, and postoperative care is provided, complications are unlikely. Most complications, for example phimosis, infection, or penile mutilation, occur as a result of poor surgical technique or operative environment, or inappropriate postcircumcision care.

Hypospadias and epispadias

These are congenital conditions of the male urethra that require surgical correction, preferably before the boy commences schooling.

Hypospadias is the condition when the external urethral meatus is situated on the under surface of the penis, proximal to its normal site. Epispadias occurs when the external urethral meatus is situated on the dorsum of the penis, also proximal to its normal site.

Plastic reconstructive surgery is required, usually in stages, to effect repair and the nursing management is of a highly specialist nature.

62

Disorders of the female reproductive system

Helen Farrer

INFECTIVE AND INFLAMMATORY DISORDERS

The female reproductive system has a natural defence against ascending organisms (Fig. 62.1), with the presence of lactobacilli and the resulting acidity of the vagina being an important part of this defence. There are, however, a number of factors which weaken the natural resistance and allow infection to become established. Those infections which are specifically sexually transmitted are discussed in the following chapter.

Monilia (thrush)

Monilia is caused by the fungus *Candida albicans*, itself often a normal inhabitant of the vagina but usually kept under control by the vaginal lactobacilli.

Monilia causes a thick white cheesy discharge, which is slight but very irritating. The most intense symptom is pruritus vulvae. As well there may be vaginal burning, dyspareunia and dysuria. It can arise:

- During and just after menstruation (the presence of blood in the vagina affects the normal vaginal acidity)
- In pregnancy, when taking oral contraceptives, and in diabetes – all states in which increased glycosuria occurs and in which the fungi thrive
- When taking antibiotics, which kill the lactobacilli.

Monilia is aggravated by wearing tight and/or synthetic underwear and by poor hygiene.

Because monilia can be sexually transmitted, the sexual partner should also be treated and both should abstain from sexual intercourse.

Treatment must be both local and systemic. Antifungal agents are prescribed, to be used locally in the form of creams or pessaries. These should continue to be used, even during menstruation, until the course is completed. Systemic antifungal agents are also given to prevent reinfection from the bowel.

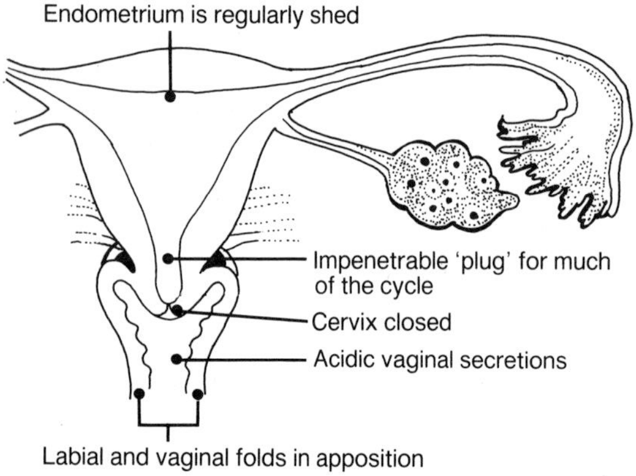

Trichomonal vaginitis

This relatively common infection is caused by the protozoal organism *Trichomonas vaginalis*. It causes a thick, profuse, frothy discharge which may be white or yellow or green in colour. It is foul-smelling and irritating. It is usually spread by sexual intercourse, but may be spread by towels, water, and toilet articles.

Treatment is with oral metronidazole. Vaginal pessaries may also be prescribed as a supplementary treatment. Sexual partners should also be

Fig. 62.1 Defences against ascending infection in the pelvis. (From Farrer, 1983.)

Endometrium is regularly shed

Impenetrable 'plug' for much of the cycle
Cervix closed
Acidic vaginal secretions

Labial and vaginal folds in apposition

treated to prevent reinfection. Extra care with bathing and laundering is advised. Treatment may take up to 6 weeks to clear the trichomonal infection, and for that time sexual intercourse should be avoided.

Pruritus

Pruritus vulvae is an irritative disorder of the vulva. At least 10% of women who seek gynaecological advice do so because of this conditon. Without treatment it can become chronic. Itching leads to scratching, which causes epithelial damage and the damaged area is irritative and itchy – a vicious cycle. Chronic vulval pruritus is associated with chronic epithelial dystrophy, which is a pre-malignant condition.

Causes of pruritus include:

- Irritation from vaginal discharges, especially from monilia and trichomonas
- Urine left on the skin
- Allergies to chemicals in drugs, soaps, vaginal deodorants, and contraceptives
- Tight or synthetic underclothing
- Certain systemic diseases, especially diabetes mellitus, anaemia, liver disorders, and dietary deficiency states
- Poor vulval hygiene
- Carcinoma of the vulva
- Psychological factors.

Psychological factors can be the sole cause of a pruritic condition; many people feel itchy when they see another person scratching. But usually these factors appear in combination with a physical cause.

Pruritus is exacerbated by warmth, anxiety, tiredness, and lack of distraction. It is on retiring to bed that pruritus is at its worst. Scratching most often occurs whilst in bed and commonly continues during sleep. The woman may be quite unaware that she is scratching until such time as a raw area develops and treatment is sought.

Management

Treatment is of little use unless the cause of the condition is removed. All itching that does not respond to good and careful hygiene must be investigated. The simpler causes are eliminated first and a full physical and gynaecological examination is made. After this, tests for diabetes mellitus, blood disorders and allergies may be done. Where carcinoma of the vulva is suspected, a skin biopsy is carried out. When any definite causes are discovered, specific treatment is commenced as soon as possible.

Controlling the urge to scratch may be helped by:

- Local applications of a light dusting of soothing powders such as zinc and starch powder or lotions such as calamine
- Firm pressure over the area
- Taking cool baths, rather than hot showers
- The use of cold applications.
  Other measures include:
- A good diet to aid healing
- Exposing the area to air (but not heat)
- Sometimes antibiotics, to prevent or treat infection
- Use of an anaesthetic cream.

In a small number of women, no cause is found. If the pruritus persists it becomes known as intractable pruritus. In such a case the woman may have no relief until the damaged skin of the area is removed by the operation of simple vulvectomy.

NEOPLASTIC DISORDERS

Ovaries

A number of different types of ovarian neoplasms, both cystic and solid, can arise in the ovaries. They can form at any age and, because the ovaries are insensitive to stretch, can be symptom-free until there is pressure on the surrounding organs, menstrual disturbances arise, or rupture or torsion of a cyst occurs as a surgical emergency. Ovarian cysts can vary enormously in size and can grow to the size of a basketball.

Asymptomatic ovarian neoplasms are often discovered incidentally, at a routine gynaecological examination. As a number of these could be malignant, or of the type that can undergo malignant change, appropriate treatment is usually instituted early.

One benign tumour is the dermoid cyst which is derived from embryonic ectoderm and can contain sebaceous fluid, teeth and hair. Benign tumours are excised, sometimes after diagnostic laparoscopy and aspiration to exclude malignancy. If possible, at least some ovarian tissue is conserved to continue function.

Some ovarian tumours are hormone-producing, causing either excessive oestrogen output or virilizing changes from androgen production.

Ovarian carcinoma is the second most common cancer of the female reproductive system and is the fourth cause of death from all cancers in women. The prognosis is poor, with less than 25% survival at 5 years, regardless of tumour staging (Table 62.1), because the carcinoma spreads rapidly, mainly by seeding directly into the peritoneal cavity. Malignant tumours of the ovary are usually solid rather than cystic.

Surgery involving partial pelvic exenteration, that is total abdominal hysterectomy, bilateral salpingo-oopherectomy, removal of the upper third of the vagina, and pelvic lymphadenectomy (Wertheim's hysterectomy), may be undertaken depending upon the stage of the disease.

Radiotherapy is sometimes used to inhibit tumour growth, and cytotoxic chemotherapy is used to either extend the length of the survival time in early stage disease, or palliate symptoms in advanced metastatic disease. The drugs may be applied locally through a tube into the peritoneal cavity or can be given parenterally or orally.

Uterus

Fibroids

Fibroids consist of fibrous and muscle tissue growing within a 'pseudo-capsule' in the myometrium. They are very common, grow slowly, and vary in size from that of a small marble to that of a large grapefruit. They are oestrogen-dependent and so usually shrink after the menopause. They are benign growths.

The symptoms depend upon the number and size of the fibroids. Large fibroids cause menorrhagia, (and thus anaemia) by interfering with the muscle contractions of the uterus and by increasing the endometrial surface from which bleeding occurs. They can also cause backache and pressure on the bowel or bladder, and are associated with infertility. If pregnancy does occur, they can cause miscarriage, premature labour, obstruction of the birth canal, or undergo degenerative changes.

Table 62.1 TNM and FIGO staging of ovarian carcinoma

TNM categories	FIGO stages		Clinical presentation
TX			Primary tumour cannot be assessed
T0			No evidence of primary tumour
T1	I		Tumour limited to ovaries
T1a		Ia	Tumour limited to one ovary; capsule intact, no tumour on ovarian surface
T1b		Ib	Tumour limited to both ovaries; capsules intact, no tumour on ovarian surface
T1c		Ic	Tumour limited to one or both ovaries with any of the following: capsule ruptured, tumour on ovarian surface, malignant cells in ascites or peritoneal washing
T2	II		Tumour involves one or both ovaries with pelvic extension
T2a		IIa	Extension and/or implants on uterus and/or tube(s)
T2b		IIb	Extension to other pelvic tissues
T2c		IIc	Pelvic extension (2a or 2b) with malignant cells in ascites or peritoneal washing
T3 and/or N1	III		Tumour involves one or both ovaries with microscopically confirmed peritoneal metastasis outside the pelvis and/or regional lymph node metastasis
T3a		IIIa	Microscopic peritoneal metastasis beyond pelvis
T3b		IIIb	Macroscopic peritoneal metastasis beyond pelvis 2 cm or less in greatest dimension
T3c and/or N1		IIIc	Peritoneal metastasis beyond pelvis more than 2 cm in greatest dimension and/or regional lymph node metastasis
M1	IV		Distant metastasis (excludes peritoneal metastasis)

Note: Liver capsule metastasis is T3/stage III, liver parenchymal metastasis M1/stage IV. Pleural effusion must have positive cytology for M1/stage IV.

Management. Iron is given for anaemia, which should be corrected before the woman undergoes surgery. Myomectomy, removal of the fibroids alone, is carried out if the uterus is to be saved for childbearing. Otherwise the best treatment for fibroids causing severe symptoms is hysterectomy.

Polyps

Endometrial polyps are small pre-malignant overgrowths of normal endometrium. They are frequently multiple and may protrude through the cervix.

Polyps can cause menorrhagia, mild cramping pains and irregular or post-menopausal bleeding.

Management. When endometrial polyps are suspected, a dilatation and curettage is always performed. The polyps are removed by the curette or by avulsion – twisting the polyp on its pedicle. As they can undergo malignant changes, all of the curettings obtained are sent for examination to exclude malignancy.

Uterine carcinoma

Carcinoma of the endometrium is the most common of all female reproductive system cancers and is found in the 50–60 years age group rather than in younger women. If diagnosed before it has spread beyond the cervix, treatment will effect a cure in nearly 90% of cases. Table 62.2 describes the staging of endometrial carcinoma.

There is a strong familial tendency in its development and it occurs more commonly in women who are significantly overweight or who have hypertension or diabetes mellitus. A history of uterine polyps, endometrial hyperplasia, or abnormal uterine bleeding are strongly implicated in its development. Oestrogen support therapy for menopausal women has yet to be established as a risk factor in endometrial carcinoma. If it occurs in the premenopausal woman, then anovulatory menstrual cycles or other hormone imbalances are usually a feature.

The first sign is often irregular or unusual bleeding, and any post menopausal woman with that sign must seek medical advice immediately. A clear brown watery discharge, lightly blood-streaked, may appear, and gradually it will

Table 62.2 TNM and FIGO staging of carcinoma corpus uteri

TNM categories	FIGO stages	Clinical presentation
TX		Primary tumour cannot be assessed
T0		No evidence of primary tumour
Tis	0	Carcinoma in situ
T1	1	Tumour confined to corpus
T1a	Ia	Uterine cavity 8 cm or less in length
T1b	Ib	Uterine cavity more than 8 cm in length
T2	II	Tumour invades cervix but does not extend beyond uterus
T3	III	Tumour extends beyond uterus but not outside true pelvis
T4	IVa	Tumour invades mucosa of bladder or rectum and/or extends beyond the true pelvis
		Note: The presence of bullous oedema is not sufficient evidence to classify tumour T4.
M1	IVb	Distant metastasis

become more bloody. Uterine enlargement occurs and pain is rare; when pain does feature it is a late sign. Very occasionally, suspicious endometrial cells are discovered on a routine Papanicolaou smear.

Spread beyond the cervix is fairly rapid and occurs via the fallopian tubes to the ovaries, through the uterus to the peritoneal cavity and the pelvic organs, or via the blood and lymph to distant sites, such as bone and brain.

Management. Regular screening by endometrial aspiration or lavage (a simple outpatient procedure) is important for those in the 'risk' categories. Curettage of the uterus is diagnostic.

In most cases of carcinoma without spread beyond the cervix, treatment is by Wertheim's hysterectomy. Total pelvic exenteration is rarely performed as it involves removal of the bladder, colorectum, and vagina.

Radiotherapy, along with chemotherapy, is usually utilized only when the carcinoma has spread beyond the cervix and, if used either before or after surgery, may inhibit postoperative recurrence and hence increase survival time.

Hormonal therapy with large doses of progesterone is usually utilized only when metastatic disease is manifested.

Choriocarcinoma and hydatidiform mole

Choriocarcinoma is a rare but feared consequence of hydatidiform mole, which is a pregnancy in which abnormal growth of the outer cell mass, the trophoblastic tissue (which would form the placenta), occurs and takes over the entire pregnancy sac, producing enormous quantities of chorionic gonadotrophin.

Choriocarcinoma may also occur following abortion, normal pregnancy, or an extrauterine pregnancy.

Choriocarcinoma metastasizes rapidly through the blood stream to the lungs and liver.

Hydatidiform mole may abort spontaneously or be evacuated immediately upon diagnosis. Careful follow-up is vital as choriocarcinoma may result from the invasion of the uterine wall by remaining hydatidiform tissue or normal placental tissue.

Treatment with methotrexate has brought good results and this was the first disseminated malignancy cured by cytotoxic chemotherapy.

Treatment may also include hysterectomy, and distant metastases may be treated by irradiation; the primary site is not irradiated as choriocarcinoma is radio-resistant.

Cervix

Benign neoplasms of the cervix include polyps, papillomata and Nabothian follicles (blocked cervical glands). They are treated by simple excision, or by cautery or cryosurgery.

Carcinoma of the cervix is the third most common reproductive system malignancy in women. Those most at risk are women:

• Between the ages of 18 and 35 who have had sexual intercourse (especially frequent intercourse)
• Who have had early intercourse
• Who have had multiple sexual partners
• Who have had chronic cervical and vaginal infections, especially genital herpes
• Who have poor personal hygiene.

Cervical cancer is classified as pre-invasive or invasive and Table 62.3 describes the staging of cervical carcinoma. Pre-invasive cancer is curable in nearly 90% of cases if detected and treated early; however, invasive cancer is curable only if treated before stage III is reached. Pre-invasive

Table 62.3 TNM and FIGO staging of carcinoma cervix uteri

TNM				FIGO		
Tis			In situ	0		
T1			Confined to uterus. Diagnosed	I		
	T1a		only by microscopy		Ia	
		T1a1	Minimal stromal invasion			Ia1
		T1a2	Depth ≤ 5 mm, horizontal spread ≤ 7 mm			Ia2
	T1b		Lesions greater than T1a2		Ib	
T2			Beyond uterus but not pelvic wall or lower third vagina	II		
	T2a		No parametrium		IIa	
	T2b		Parametrium		IIb	
T3			Lower third vagina/pelvic wall/hydronephrosis	III		
	T3a		Lower third vagina		IIIa	
	T3b		Pelvic wall/hydronephrosis		IIIb	
T4			Mucosa of bladder/rectum/beyond true pelvis	IVa		
M1			Distant metastasis	IVb		

cancer can only be detected by vaginal examination and the taking of a Pap smear for microscopy. Therefore the importance of annual physical examination, with Pap smear, for all sexually active women over the age of 35 years cannot be overemphasized.

Symptoms appear only after the disease has invaded the cervix. Of significance is abnormal or unusual bleeding, particularly 'contact' bleeding following intercourse or vaginal examination. Pain is a late sign.

Management. If suspicious cells are found, the smear test is repeated, and a punch biopsy or a cone excision of the cervix is performed after colposcopic examination.

Treatment depends upon the extent of the spread. If the malignant change has spread no further than the surface layer of the cervix, then cautery, cryosurgery or cone excision may be sufficient to check the growth. Once spread has entered the cervix, the uterine cavity or the upper vagina, a Wertheim's hysterectomy, preceded by intracavity irradiation, is performed.

If the growth has spread to the lateral pelvic wall, the lower third of the vagina or the neighbouring organs, external irradiation is given, and sometimes Wertheim's hysterectomy is performed.

Endometriosis

Endometriosis is a condition in which endometrial tissue is found in sites other than the lining of the uterus. Figure 62.2 shows the most common of these sites.

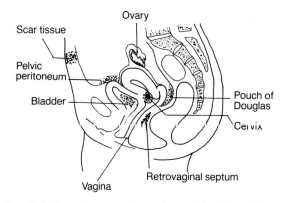

Fig. 62.2 Sites of extra-uterine endometriosis. (From Farrer, 1983.)

Adenomyosis is the growth of endometrial tissue within the muscular wall of the uterus.

Endometriosis is the cause of a number of gynaecological symptoms. It is associated with infertility, menorrhagia, dysmenorrhoea and dyspareunia. Because all endometrium responds to hormonal stimulation, building up and breaking down and bleeding, endometrium situated where there is no escape route will bleed into the surrounding tissue. Much of the fluid content of the blood is absorbed, leaving a dark, tarry residue, thus giving the name 'chocolate cysts' to these collections. Adhesions form and distort the pelvic structures, and the deposits are very tender on examination.

Management. Endometriosis is diagnosed from the history of symptoms, pelvic examination and laparoscopy. It is managed by the administration of progestogens (synthetic progesterone) over several months in an attempt to shrink the growths. Surgical removal of the deposits and division of adhesions may be attempted if the hormonal treatment is unsatisfactory, but the condition is hard to clear without the removal of the ovaries, as part of hystero-salpingectomy.

Vagina

New growths of the vagina are rare. Of importance recently is the condition of adenocarcinoma in a significant number of women whose mothers received large doses of diethyl stilboestrol (DES) to treat threatened abortion from the mid 1940s to the middle to late 1950s. Efforts have been made to trace daughters of these women and they are regularly observed for early signs of malignant change.

The treatment of vaginal carcinoma is by surgery, irradiation, and cytotoxic drugs, but because of the usual lymphatic involvement, few patients with vaginal carcinoma survive longer than 5 years after diagnosis.

Vulva

A number of benign growths arise on the vulva. They include sebaceous, epidermal and inclusion cysts, Bartholin's gland cyst, fibroma and lipoma, warts, and papillomata and urethral caruncles.

Simple cysts are excised. Bartholin's gland cysts are either marsupialized or, if the condition becomes chronic, excised. Vulval warts are treated with podophyllin paint or by cautery or cryosurgery. Papillomata may be cauterized, although sometimes a simple vulvectomy may be advised. All vulval growths are examined carefully because of the possibility of malignancy and early and extensive spread in an area with bilateral cross-drainage of lymph.

Carcinoma of the vulva occurs more commonly in older women than in young. It may be discovered during a routine gynaecological examination or felt as a painless lump. It can arise after many years of skin damage from vulval irritation and scratching.

Management. Skin biopsies are taken from any suspicion lesions on the vulva. If these prove to be malignant the operation of radical vulvectomy is performed. This procedure involves the removal of the whole of the vulval skin and underlying fat and as much of the pelvic lymphatic network as possible. It is a long operation and recovery may be slow, especially in the older patient. Wound breakdown is common.

Radiotherapy is not usually attempted in carcinoma of the vulva as the area responds poorly, but it is used occasionally in those cases where the woman is too old or frail to undergo surgery or where growths have recurred after surgery.

TRAUMA

Trauma to the genital organs is not common. Instances include surface abrasions or rupture in sexual assault, perforation of the uterus during illegal abortion, ectopic pregnancy, and operative injury.

Rape

Rape or attempted rape is a crisis for the victim, and one which the nurse needs to be able to help her meet. If there are no serious associated physical injuries, the acute emotional distress that often arises should be dealt with first, by reassurance, support and sympathy.

There will be a number of major fears in such a situation; those of possible genital injury,

sexually transmitted disease, pregnancy, and the fear of facing the world.

Rarely do any serious genital injuries result from rape of an adult. Surface abrasions will heal rapidly with local treatment. Sexually transmitted disease is a possibility and tests must be conducted to exclude this at the earliest opportunity. If treatment is necessary it will be instituted immediately, before complications arise. Pregnancy fears will continue until either the arrival of the next menstrual period or the negative result of a reliable pregnancy test. The girl or woman should know to report to the doctor if her period is late or scanty.

The emotional aspects of rape are very complex. The victim is usually shocked by the experience and finds the interviewing and physical examination harrowing. If the offender was someone known to her, she may be reluctant to report the offence to the police. Reporting to the police can prevent other people being raped and so is an important and responsible action. If, however, the victim feels unable to do this, she may find help at the Rape Crisis Centre, where counselling, medical and legal advice is offered on a 24-hour a day basis.

Ectopic pregnancy

In this condition, injury is caused to the fallopian tubes, which are the commonest site of ectopic implantation of a fertilized ovum. The tubes have enough elasticity to allow limited growth (up to about six weeks' gestation) and invasion of the wall by the chorionic villi. When the tube can no longer accommodate the growing embryonic sac it may rupture, causing pain, intra-abdominal haemorrhage and shock.

Treatment is surgical, with the affected tube being removed unless the other tube is damaged or absent, in which case an attempt to save it by repair is made.

DISPLACEMENTS

Retroversion of the uterus

Retroversion is backward displacement of the uterus. It is common during the months following childbirth, but usually corrects itself as the pelvic supports regain tone. Fixed retroversion is caused by the uterus being pushed backwards by fibroids or other growths, or pulled backwards by adhesions or endometriosis.

Retroversion may be symptomless, being discovered on routine examination. Sometimes, however, it may be a factor in backache, dysmenorrhoea, dyspareunia, and infertility.

Treatment is not given unless retroversion is causing symptoms. A supporting pessary may be used to hold the uterus forward, and if that relieves the symptoms, the operation of ventrosuspension (shortening the round ligaments) would be considered worthwhile.

Utero-vaginal prolapse

In gynaecology, prolapse refers to the descent of the vaginal walls and the uterus. Prolapse occurs most commonly in parous women and is due to the stretching of the pelvic floor muscles and ligaments and the vaginal walls. It may not appear until old age, when the withdrawal of oestrogen causes a devitalization of the pelvic tissues. Increase in intra-abdominal pressure, as is caused by obesity and chronic coughing, will worsen the condition.

When the pelvic supports fail, the uterus will descend, dragging the vaginal walls down with it. The bladder and rectum, both closely connected by fascial tissue to the vagina, are thus involved: prolapse of the bladder is called cystocele; of the urethra, urethrocele; of the rectum, rectocele (Fig. 62.3).

Clinical manifestations

Prolapse may cause:

● Dragging pains and backache, due to the resistance offered by the pelvic ligaments. In fact, the larger the prolapse, the less the discomfort, as the ligaments have given up the resistance and so there is less tension on them
● A feeling of 'something coming down', or of fullness in the vagina
● Urinary symptoms, especially frequency, stress incontinence and inability to empty the bladder completely, leading to stasis and urinary tract infection. With cystocele, some of the urine in the

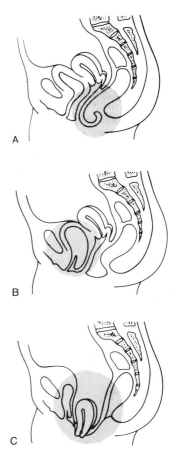

Fig. 62.3 Displacements. **A** – Rectocele. **B** – Cystocele. **C** – Uterine prolapse.

bladder lies below the bladder neck. Unless this is elevated, the urine in that part of the bladder cannot be passed. Many women learn to elevate the bladder neck (via the vagina) instinctively, but may be too shy to mention it to anyone else
● Bowel symptoms may include constipation and inability to empty the rectum completely. As with cystocele, it may be necessary to support the prolapsed wall digitally to empty the bowels properly.

Uterine prolapse is classified into degrees, according to the descent of the uterus:

● First degree. The uterus has descended slightly and there is some elongation of the cervix, but it remains within the vagina
● Second degree. The cervix protrudes from the vulva, is exposed to air, and ulceration may occur

• Third degree (procidentia). The uterus is completely outside the vagina and the vagina is completely inverted

Medical and surgical management

Prolapses are usually treated only if they are causing symptoms.

Supporting pessaries. A vinyl ring is placed at the top of the vagina to extend the fornices and so prevent the uterus from falling down. It is used for women who wish to have another pregnancy, or for those who are too old and frail to undergo surgery.

Surgery. Colporrhaphy is surgery for vaginal repair and may be performed anteriorly to repair a cystocele or posteriorly to repair a rectocele. The aim of surgery is to strengthen the vaginal walls to resist prolapse of adjacent organs, and this is achieved by the use of reinforcing suturing techniques and the excision of any redundant tissue.

Perineorrhaphy is repair of a lax perineum. Manchester repair involves both anterior and posterior colporrhaphy and excision of the elongated vaginal portion of the cervix.

URINARY PROBLEMS

Stress incontinence

Stress incontinence is due to laxity of the bladder supports, particularly weakness of the urethrovesicular junction (the bladder neck), which opens under increased intra-abdominal pressure. It is most common in parous women who are at, or past, the climacteric.

Stress incontinence is a miserable symptom, causing both severe interference with the women's daily life and activity, and vulval discomfort and irritation.

It may be managed by physiotherapy, with special exercises to strengthen the levator ani, or by electrical stimulation of the pelvic floor muscles. Surgical treatment is anterior colporrhaphy or any of the urethral suspension operations, for example, the Marshall-Marchetti procedure, in which a sling is fashioned from perineal tissue to elevate the bladder neck and prevent stress incontinence.

Urgency incontinence

Urgency incontinence is caused by a hypertonic bladder. The woman has warning of the need to void, but the warning is followed almost immediately by strong bladder contractions and the passage of urine.

Treatment is by anti-spasmodic drugs to reduce the force of the bladder contractions.

True incontinence

True incontinence is the continual passage of urine and usually occurs because of a fistulous communication between the bladder or urethra and the vagina or uterus. It can be caused by abnormally prolonged second stage of labour (rare nowadays), invasive malignancy, irradiation, or surgical damage. Treatment is by continuous catheter drainage of the bladder to allow spontaneous healing if possible, or by surgical repair of the fistula.

Chronic urethrotrigonitis ('honeymoon cystitis')

Also called the urethral syndrome, this condition of very acute dysuria is associated with sexual intercourse in that symptoms arise following the act. It affects only some women, and there is no way of knowing who will be susceptible.

The condition is caused by damage to the lining of the short sensitive urethra by the thrusting movements of the penis during intercourse. Bacteria are introduced and may establish chronic infection, which can take years to clear completely.

Symptoms arise about 36 hours after intercourse; because of this delay the association may not be realized at first. It is important that treatment commences early, as intercourse will subsequently hurt and will not be welcomed if it is going to reactivate the symptoms.

A mid-stream specimen of urine will be cultured for antibiotic sensitivity. Often, however, the test is negative, or may show only mild infection, yet the symptoms remain severe. Some relief can be obtained by:

• Increasing the fluid intake to 2.5–3 l/day, to dilute the urine and make it less acid and to physically flush out the urinary system.

● Drinking two glasses of fluid immediately before intercourse

● Voiding immediately before and especially after intercourse, to flush out any organisms before they can ascend further.

These self-help measures will usually treat this condition successfully, as can using a lubricant for intercourse, and, perhaps, altering the position used. Antibiotics are indicated only if the condition persists.

NURSING MANAGEMENT OF PATIENTS UNDERGOING GYNAECOLOGICAL SURGERY

The woman undergoing surgery for gynaecological conditions will do so because of her wish to be relieved of distressing or annoying symptoms, or because of a potentially life threatening condition. In many cases the woman will be concerned at the possible effects of surgery upon her body as a whole, and she may not have found it easy to gain accurate or clear information because of the mystery that surrounds 'female matters'.

Within the Australian community there may still be women who are ignorant about their sexual anatomy and who are strongly influenced by traditional and cultural beliefs. The nurse cannot assume that the patient will be fully aware of the implications of the surgery planned. In some instances the woman may hold totally erroneous beliefs about the surgery and its outcome, for example, believing that pregnancy is still a capability following hysterectomy or conversely that a unilateral salpingo-oopherectomy will render her infertile. The nurse must therefore identify the patient's need for further preoperative explanation by the physician and, where necessary, actively assist her to obtain such information. Health education should also be aimed at ensuring that the patient understands what to expect immediately after the operation, in the way of equipment and procedures, and in the rehabilitation phase.

Many patients undergoing gynaecological surgery experience alteration to their self concept and body image. Empathic nursing, adequate health teaching, and constant support by both the nurse and the patient's significant others will assist most women to a complete physical recovery and emotional readjustment.

Preoperative preparation

Consent for surgery

As well as ensuring that the routine operation and anaesthetic consents have been obtained, a special consent may be necessary if infertility is to be one of the results of the operation.

Investigative procedures

Urinalysis is performed and a mid-stream specimen of urine may be sent for examination to exclude infection. Haemoglobin will be assessed, and blood may be sent for cross-matching of one or more units if bleeding is anticipated during surgery. Vaginal examination is performed as a final check to exclude infection. A sample of any discharge is sent for examination.

Skin preparation

For abdominal operations, the abdominal and pubic areas are shaved. For vaginal procedures, a full (pubic to anus) vulval shave is done, extending to the mid thighs. In most cases no shave is necessary for a D and C (dilatation of the cervix and curettage of the uterus). Preoperatively, skin washing with antiseptic solution is done on skin areas, but not on the vulva. Vaginal cleansing (douching) is now rarely performed in the ward before surgery.

Bowel preparation

A plain water or soap and water enema may be given. For smaller procedures a suppository will be sufficient. Fluid intake is encouraged from the time of admission, and a fluid intake and output chart is commenced.

Postoperative care

In addition to the routine post-anaesthetic and postoperative care the following points are important.

Position and movement

When fully conscious, the patient is helped to a semi-recumbent position and then to a sitting position to prevent chest complications. Movement of the lower limbs is encouraged early, as venous thrombus is a common complication of pelvic operations. The patient is helped out of bed as soon as possible, and early ambulation is supervised.

Observations

Wound and urinary drainage is strictly observed for free drainage and patency of closed drainage systems. The volume of vaginal loss is recorded. If a vaginal pack is in situ, there should be almost no loss from the vagina. Without a vaginal pack, the loss should not fill more than two sanitary pads in one hour.

Bladder fullness is estimated. If there is no urinary catheter, voiding should be observed. Distension of the bladder could cause pressure on newly sutured pelvic structures, as well as causing pelvic pain.

Vaginal packs

These are used to provide pressure to stop bleeding and to prevent adhesions across the vagina. Voiding is difficult when a pack is in situ, and an indwelling urinary catheter is usually left in until the pack is removed, after 24 hours or as instructed. The removal of the pack can be painful, so adequate analgesia must be provided beforehand. Following this, the vaginal loss will increase, and the amount of blood lost should be observed carefully and recorded.

Bladder management

Urinary tract infection and retention of urine are the commonest complications of gynaecological surgery. A high fluid intake is ensured by intravenous therapy until adequate oral intake has been established. Indwelling catheters, either urethral or supra-pubic, are used after major operations and are removed as ordered; urethral catheters usually on the third postoperative day.

After this, residual urine estimations are performed until there is less than 100 ml remaining in the bladder after normal micturition on two consecutive occasions.

Bowel management

Constipation should be avoided as it causes discomfort and can place stress on a new suture line. Mild aperients, suppositories, or a small enema may be commenced on the third night after surgery. Many women fear the first bowel action after surgery, but if the faeces have been softened by suitable agents, the evacuation of the bowel should not be painful.

Vulval care

Vulval washdowns using warm water and perhaps a mild antiseptic are given routinely 4-hourly and after emptying the bladder or bowel, until the patient is able to shower. A clean pad is applied after each washdown. It may be held in place by a T-binder or more commonly by clean personal underwear. Washdowns help to prevent infection and make the area more comfortable.

Perineal care

The area is kept clean by regular perineal toilets. From the fifth day following perineorrhaphy, ray lamps may be used to provide warmth to the area to aid healing. The patient is placed on her side in a comfortable position in order to expose the perineum to the ray lamp. Occasionally, a drying agent is applied to the skin afterwards. Analgesics and aircushions are important for maintaining perineal comfort.

Wound care

Abdominal wound care is the same as for any abdominal operation. Vaginal wounds are not dressed, but observation of the discharge is an important method of assessing the presence of infection. Dissolving sutures are usually used; these fall out about 10 days after surgery, accompanied by a slight, yellow, non-offensive discharge.

Major complications following gynaecological surgery

Thrombosis

Deep vein thrombosis is the major risk in gynaecological surgery. The site of surgery, with its interruption to pelvic venous return, and the fact that lithotomy position may have been used for the surgery, are the specific contributing factors.

Prevention of thrombus formation begins in the preoperative period by eliminating or treating contributory factors; and continues during the operation with special attention to padding and support of the limbs and by electrical calf stimulation. Postoperatively, the supervision of limb physiotherapy, and ambulation are most important, and are very much the responsibility of the nursing staff.

Haemorrhage

Reactionary haemorrhage may occur in the first 12–24 hours and can be severe. Observation of vital signs to recognize internal bleeding must be meticulous. The patient is returned to the operating room for ligation of bleeding vessels.

Secondary vaginal haemorrhage is preceded by warning signs of a minimal but bright loss and a slight elevation of temperature on about the eighth or ninth day postoperatively. Infection causes the suture line to become friable, break down and start to ooze blood. This is soon followed by increasing bleeding which can become severe. Bed rest, antibiotics and vaginal packing are ordered and blood transfusion may be necessary.

Pelvic haematoma

Concealed haemorrhage will drain into the Pouch of Douglas and form a haematoma. The patient will have a high temperature on about the seventh day, lower abdominal pain and a purulent vaginal discharge. Spontaneous discharge through the vagina will eventually occur, but once diagnosed, the haematoma is usually treated by posterior culdotomy, an excision into Pouch of Douglas through the posterior fornix to allow it to drain. Antibiotic therapy is commenced, and special care with vulval hygiene is necessary.

Discharge planning

When the patient and her physician agree that she has recovered from the operation sufficiently to manage at home, plans will be made for her discharge from hospital. Before leaving hospital the patient should know exactly what symptoms to look for and seek help for, when and how to take prescribed medications and treatments, how to look after the wound, when she may return to work, and how much lifting or housework is allowed.

It may be difficult for a woman to observe the necessary requirements for rest, especially if she is used to taking full responsibility for the running of the home. Others in the family may very soon forget that she has recently had surgery, or the house may have become disorganized during her absence, and she may find herself back to full work load very soon. Planning should involve other family members so that they can be prepared to provide assistance at home. Council home help can be arranged to do heavy work or shopping for a few weeks.

If she is sexually active, she should know when it is safe to resume intercourse; most physicians advise women to wait until the postoperative check-up to ensure that full healing has been achieved. The operation may have resulted in her usual form of contraception being now unsuitable, so this should be discussed and appropriate advice given.

A vaginal examination is usually made just before the woman goes home, to ensure that there are no signs of infection and to separate any adhesions that may be starting to form.

63

Sexually transmitted diseases

Helen Farrer

Sexually transmitted diseases have become the most common communicable diseases in the world today. The incidence is rising, despite widespread efforts at education in the methods of prevention. In Western countries the most prevalent sexually transmitted diseases are chlamydia, gonorrhoea and syphilis. These, genital herpes, and a number of other conditions are discussed in this chapter. Acquired immune deficiency syndrome (AIDS) is discussed in Chapter 77.

In all cases, all sexual partners must be traced and treated to prevent reinfection and further spread. The symptoms are unpleasant and/or painful, some conditions have long-term serious effects upon the reproductive potential of the sufferer, and some can cause general body ill-health and even become life threatening.

GONORRHOEA

Gonorrhoea, the second most common and widespread of the notifiable sexually transmitted diseases, is a bacterial infection. It usually enters the body via the genital tract, from where it may spread to other areas of the body. Other portals of entry may be through the eye (causing panopthalmitis) and through the mouth (uveitis).

The organism responsible is the gram-negative *Neisseria gonorrhoeae*. Natural immunity is not acquired after having had the infection. The bacteria first attack those tissues which are not covered by squamous epithelium, especially the urethra.

Clinical manifestations

Male. Symptoms appear 2–10 days after contact. Dysuria, frequency and urgency of micturition occurs, and a purulent discharge is noticed. The urethral meatus may be inflamed. Perianal soreness and a rectal discharge may be present in homosexual men.

Female. 60% of women with gonorrhoea are asymptomatic. When symptoms do occur, they arise within 7–21 days after contact. The condition may settle into a carrier state where the woman is able to infect other people for many weeks. Early symptoms are localized and include dysuria and frequency of micturition, a purulent discharge (which may be slight and so go unnoticed), and vulval soreness, but not pruritus unless a trichomonal infection is also present. Sometimes these symptoms are mild and may be mistaken for a simple bladder irritation.

Occasionally, gonorrhoea is first suspected postnatally, when a newborn baby's eyes are grossly infected from contact with the organism in the birth canal (Opthalmia neonatorum).

Complications

If untreated, the inflammation spreads along the genital tract. In men it passes along the posterior urethra and vas deferens to the epididymis; if bilateral epididymitis occurs, infertility may result. Other structures, such as the Cowper's glands, prostate and seminal vesicles may become infected, sometimes with abscess formation. This may result in initial presentation of a patient in extreme pain.

In women, the inflammation can affect the urethra, and the paraurethral and Bartholin's glands, and spread to the cervix, uterus and fallopian tubes. Thick pus can fill the lumen of the tubes, causing acute salpingitis. This is often referred to as pelvic inflammatory disease and causes acute pain. The fallopian tube may rupture filling the peritoneum with pus. This eventually results in strictures, fibrosis and, finally, infertility. Adhesions cause pain, disturb menstruation and, if they spread to the area of the rectum, cause chronic constipation.

Gonococcal arthritis may also occur; it is more frequent in women than in men. Gonoccocal endocarditis and meningitis, and septicaemia are also possible complications.

Medical management

All patients with dysuria and a history of recent sexual contact should be screened by means of a microscopic examination of a midstream of urine (MSU). If the patient presents with discharge, smears are taken from the urethra (by 'milking' the urethra and Skene's glands), the Bartholin's ducts, endocervix and the rectum, and are sent for examination and culture. Because people who present with gonorrhoea may have syphilis as well, the blood is investigated for the presence of syphilis.

Admission to hospital is not usually necessary unless there are acute or serious complications, for example, salpingitis in women. The medications given to treat gonorrhoea differ at each hospital and clinic. Many still use large single doses of procaine penicillin (3×10^6 units initially, and 1.5×10^6 next day) preceded and followed by oral probenecid to delay the excretion of the penicillin. However, it is recommended by the Veneriological Society of Victoria and the Centre for Disease Control (Atlanta, Georgia) that amoxycillin 3 g orally with 1 g probenecid be used, except where there is a high resistance to the antibiotic, in which case spectinomycin is given IM in a 2 g single dose. Alternatives to penicillin are mainly tetracycline related drugs.

People with gonorrhoea often also have subclinical chlamydia, followed with oral tetracycline or erythromycin.

Because gonorrhoea responds so well to antibiotics and because of their easy availability, a new problem has arisen in the management of sexually-transmitted diseases: self-medication. Self-medi-cation may be sufficient to control the symptoms but not always to eradicate the condition, and rarely are the sexual partners treated.

Advice must be given regarding personal hygiene and abstinence from sexual intercourse to avoid infecting others or being reinfected.

NON-SPECIFIC URETHRITIS – CHLAMYDIA

Chlamydia (in the woman) is caused by the organism *Chlamydia trachomatis*, which is the causal organism of non-specific urethritis in the male. It is now the most common sexually transmitted disease.

Clinical manifestations

Male. In most cases, symptoms of mild dysuria, urethral discomfort, and a mild, sticky discharge arise between 7–28 days after contact. Sometimes the symptoms may be more severe and the discharge profuse and purulent. Proctitis may be present in homosexual men.

Female. There are often no symptoms, or they may be identical with mild gonorrhoea.

Medical management

The infection is suspected when symptoms occur but ordinary cultures are negative. Chlamydia lacks an essential ingredient of cell metabolism, ATP. It is dependent upon living cells for this, so it is truly intracellular and very difficult to grow except by tissue culture. This fact also accounts for its general resistance to common antibiotics. The use of oral doxycycline is at present believed to offer the best chance of controlling the infection.

As chlamydia is highly infectious, abstinence from sexual intercourse is advised until the condition is proven to be cleared. Sexual partners should be traced and treated.

SYPHILIS

Syphilis is caused by the spirochaete, *Treponema pallidum*. It is spread by direct contact, the organisms entering the body by burrowing through cracks and abrasions. Although sexual intercourse is the usual means of transmission, any contact with the organism may, if conditions are suitable, result in its spread. In the first stage of syphilis, the spirochaete is present in all bodily fluids, and can spread to an uninfected person via any broken skin or mucous membrane. Thus lesions may occur on almost any part of the body, but the penis, anus, and perineum in men, and the vulva, cervix and perineum in women are the commonest sites. Occasionally chancres (lesions) are found on the lips, tongue and eye.

Primary syphilis

The incubation period averages about 3 weeks but can range from 10 days up to 3 months. One or more lesions or chancres appear, as painless shallow ulcers about 1 cm in diameter. The sores may not be noticed, especially if on the inner aspect of one of the labia, or on the cervix. The sores usually close and heal after a few weeks, remaining only as skin hardenings. The inguinal lymph nodes enlarge and become hard but are not painful. During this stage, blood tests for syphilis will remain negative, and the patient will be unaware of the infection.

Secondary syphilis

About 2 months later, the spirochaetes invade the bloodstream and a generalized rash may appear. The rash is usually not itchy and is usually copper-coloured, but in some cases may be so mild that it goes unnoticed. Mouth lesions may occur, with a sore throat, glossitis, and small white linear ulcers. Syphilitic alopecia may occur, and its early signs are often the first symptoms of which the patient becomes aware. There is often localized lymphadenitis and the constitutional symptoms of mild fever. The only genital manifestation that arises, and then not always, is the appearance of multiple flat vulval and perineal warts – condylomata lata.

The disease is highly infectious during the primary and secondary stages, that is, when the skin lesions, chancre, rash or warts, are present. These stages can last for up to 2 or more years.

Tertiary syphilis

If the symptoms of secondary syphilis are not treated or pass unnoticed, the disease can remain quiescent and not manifest itself for periods varying from 10–30 years. It is during this period that the millions of spirochaetes in the bloodstream attack various organs and structures in the body, especially the heart, brain, ears, eyes, joints and bones and the major blood vessels, eventually causing soft, nonsuppurative inflammatory changes producing rubbery, grey-white necrotic areas called gumma. Gumma classically invade bone, the liver, and testes, although they can occur anywhere. They respond to long-term antibiotic treatment and eventually shrink to a firm, white scar. The other severe degenerative changes, which may occur are generalized paralysis (often termed tabes dorsalis which is characterized by a classic change in gait) and severe mental disturbances.

Diagnosis

Diagnosis is confirmed by a scraping taken from the chancre in the early weeks. Blood tests are commenced six weeks after possible infection, and if negative are repeated six weeks later. Sexual intercourse must be avoided until a diagnosis has been made and, if necessary, until treatment has been completed. A number of blood tests are performed, including Wassermann reaction (WR) and veneral disease reference laboratory (VDRL), and will usually be positive at 6 weeks. Fluorescent treponemal antibody (FTA) test or treponemal immobilization (TPI) test is often done as an extra check as they are specific for syphilis and are very accurate.

Medical management

Penicillin is still the treatment of choice for early syphilis. Large doses are given, for example IM procaine penicillin combined with benzine penicillin, 1.5×10^6 units daily for ten consecutive days, or LPG (long-acting penicillin G) 1 vial IM weekly for 3 weeks. This will completely cure the condition but will not provide protection against future reinfection. In the later stages of syphilis, the dose may have to be very much higher. Tetracyclines are given in cases of penicillin sensitivity but are less effective. Routine blood tests are continued at intervals over the next 2 years and if a pregnancy occurs during that time, the woman is advised to receive an extra course of penicillin to protect the foetus from congenital syphilis.

HERPES SIMPLEX VIRUS – GENITAL HERPES

There are two types of herpes simplex virus (HSV); type I, which causes common cold sores on the lips; and type II, which causes lesions in the lower genital tract. They can, however, both be found in the opposite sites. Although they are microscopically different, both types produce very similar effects. As with other viruses, HSV are able to remain alive in the body indefinitely after the first infection, travelling along the nerves to a ganglion near the spinal cord where they survive in a dormant state. They may be reactivated at times of physical or emotional stress, or for no obvious reason. Recurrences are generally, although not always, less severe than the initial attack.

Genital herpes infections are becoming a widespread problem. Although not yet a notifiable disease, their incidence is certainly increasing. Herpes genitalia is highly infectious and is spread by direct contact with an active lesion, that is, by sexual intercourse or genital contact. It has an incubation period of 2–7 days, possibly longer, from the time of contact.

Genital herpes occurs more frequently in women who have multiple sex partners and, although the actual cause of cervical cancer is unknown, there appears to be an increased risk of its development in women who have had genital herpes. A factor common to both conditions is the increased frequency of sexual activity.

Recurrences may occur more frequently and are sometimes more severe during pregnancy. Because the herpes virus is comparatively large it does not cross the placental barrier and so the fetus is not affected. But herpes is significant when it is active at the time of delivery, as the baby can be affected as it comes down the birth canal. Newborn infants are particularly susceptible to serious and sometimes fatal infections with either HSV-I or HSV-II.

Obstetricians are careful to exclude active herpes in the 3–6 weeks before delivery in a woman who has a history of genital herpes. If viral cultures taken during this period are negative and if there are no active lesions at the time of labour then vaginal delivery is safe, but if there is any doubt the baby is delivered by Caesarian section.

Clinical manifestations

As with oral herpes, there is a prodrome of tingling and irritation before the lesions appear. Signs and symptoms may include:

- Small red raised spots on the vulva, vagina and cervix in females, and the shaft and glans of the penis, and the prepuce in males
- Blister development, then
- Shallow ulcers which are extremely sore
- Flu-type symptoms: malaise, depression, slight fever
- Intense pain on intercourse
- Rectal pain
- Associated vaginal *Candida albicans* infection
- Cystitis. This can be so severe that natural voiding becomes impossible. Admission to hospital and the insertion of an indwelling (suprapubic) catheter may be the only means of relief, especially in a first attack.

These symptoms may be present for 4–8 days, after which the lesions will heal and the other symptoms subside.

Investigative procedures

Diagnosis is made on history, by examining the lesions, culture of smears, and possibly by blood examination for antibody titre. Syphilis must be excluded.

Medical and nursing management

Herpes, like many viral infections, is 'incurable', but it is usually self-limiting. Much research is being conducted into a cure for the condition and also for a vaccine which may eventually prevent genital herpes.

The most promising specific treatment so far is a non-toxic topical preparation which gives relief from discomfort and promotes more rapid healing. The preparation may also be given parenterally, and this has been shown to shorten the natural history of an acute infection but does not clear the virus from the nerve sheath. The use of interferon for the treatment of herpes is also under investigation.

Symptomatic relief during attacks includes:

• Application of ice applied to the area for 20–30 minutes at the first sign of an attack, which may shorten the attack or make it less severe
• Simple hygienic measures, such as keeping the lesion clean and dry
• Frequent salt or sodium bicarbonate solution baths
• Local skin disinfection, for example, using povidone iodine
• Local anaesthetic ointment
• Avoidance of irritants such as soaps and underclothes.

General measures include:

• Treatment of associated conditions, for example thrush
• Attention to diet
• Rest, and removal of stress if possible
• Abstinence from sexual activity, especially intercourse, during an attack and for a short time after the lesions have healed.

Management in relation to isolation techniques, bathing, and general hygiene procedures, and the disposal of linen and all excreta from the patient, must follow the guidelines issued by each hospital or institution. Where there is a possibility of active herpes, every precaution should be taken, particularly when handling the penis, vulva or perineum; for example, disposable gloves would be worn for perineal shaves or toilets, urethral catheters should not be used.

The patient should be advised that the virus can be spread from one site to another, for example, from the cervix to the vagina, or from the vagina to the vulva; and that it can be passed to the baby during birth. Women with herpes who become pregnant must inform their physician. Oral herpes simplex conditions can be spread (when lesions are active) from the oral mucosa of an infected person to the eyes or genital area during oro-genital sexual activity, and care must be taken by type I herpes sufferers to avoid this.

Persons who have contracted genital herpes need to re-evaluate their whole attitude towards sexual activity and the conduct of their sex lives. To be responsible they must tell prospective sexual partners, because lesions of which the patient may not be aware may be present at almost any time.

Many people feel stigmatized, guilty or self-conscious about this condition, and the nurse should provide appropriate emotional support.

PROCTITIS

Inflammation of the rectal mucosa may result from rectal gonorrhoea, thrush, syphilis or genital warts. In homosexual males, there may be non-specific urethritis in the sexual partner.

The perianal area and rectum are sore and there may be a slight discharge from the anus.

Treatment is of the cause, after culture of rectal smears and blood examination for syphilis.

OTHER SEXUALLY TRANSMITTED CONDITIONS

Chancroid, or soft sore, is caused by a gram-negative bacillus *Haemophilus ducreyi* and is extremely contagious. Within a week of contact with the disease, small papules appear on the external genitalia. They quickly progress to become painful shallow ulcers. Further lesions may develop on the upper thighs and perineum. Inguinal lymph gland involvement usually occurs; abscesses may form and break down to form a single sinus. The diagnosis is usually made on recognition of the ulcer and by seeing its response to sulphonamide drugs. Culture of the discharge from the ulcers is done, but this takes time and most doctors prefer to start treatment immediately. In severe cases, bed rest, with isolation if in hospital, relief of pain, and wash-downs of the affected area are required.

Vulval warts (see page 659), pediculosis pubis (see page 767), and trichomonal (see page 654) and monilial (see page 654) conditions may all be transmitted sexually.

PREVENTION OF SEXUALLY TRANSMITTED DISEASES

Campaigns to educate the community about the symptoms, effects and dangers of these diseases are improving all the time. Where it is suspected that sexual restraint might not be practised, advice is given about the wearing of condoms, washing of the genitalia before and after intercourse, voiding immediately after intercourse and the immediate reporting of any suspicious symptoms.

Routine screening is carried out during pregnancy, at most family planning clinics, and on all blood taken for donation.

Special clinics conduct contact-tracing as well as having diagnosis and treatment facilities. The staff of these clinics are very aware of the reticence of most people to seek and continue treatment and to name contacts, and they are absolutely discreet.

Nursing responsibilities include the prevention of cross-infection to protect other patients and staff. Disposable gloves are worn for all procedures involving the genital region, and all equipment, dressings and linen are disposed of carefully. Often, patients should not know that screening is being carried out for certain diseases; it depends greatly on the circumstances. Care is always taken to ensure that charts and records are not accessible to people who might misinterpret written information.

Nurses will, of course, make sure that their approach to such patients is completely non-judgemental in word, gesture and expression. They must be available and willing to listen to their patients, especially when guilt and worry about the condition and the fear of rejection by family and friends is evident.

SECTION I – REFERENCES AND FURTHER READING

Texts

Anderson J R (ed) 1976 Muir's textbook of pathology, 10th edn. Edward Arnold, London
Anthony C P 1984 Structure and function of the body. Mosby, St Louis
Carey K W (ed) 1984 Attending Ob/Gyn patients: nursing photobook. Springhouse, Pennsylvania
Creager J G 1982 Human anatomy and physiology. Wadsworth, California
Farrer H 1983 Maternity care. Churchill Livingstone, Edinburgh
Farrer H 1985 Gynaecological care, 2nd edn. Churchill Livingstone, Edinburgh
Havard M 1986 A nursing guide to drugs, 2nd edn. Churchill Livingstone, Melbourne
Luckmann J, Sorensen K C 1980 Medical-surgical nursing: a psychophysiologic approach, 2nd edn. Saunders, Philadelphia
Macleod J 1987 Davidson's principles and practice of nursing, 15th edn. Churchill Livingstone, Edinburgh
Read A, Ritt D W, Langton Hewer R 1986 Modern medicine, 3rd edn. Churchill Livingstone, Edinburgh
Society of Hospital Pharmacists of Australia 1985 Pharmacology and drug information for nurses, 2nd edn. Saunders, Sydney
Storlie F J (ed) 1984 Diseases: nurse's reference library, 2nd edn. Springhouse, Pennsylvania

Journals

Bradford D L 1983 Sexually transmitted diseases. The Australian Nurses Journal 13 : 6 : 42–45, 47
Clark N, O'Connell P 1984 Prostatectomy: a guide to answering your patient's unspoken questions. Nursing 84 14 : 4 : 48–51
Helen M 1983 Rape: some facts, myths and reponses. The Australian Nurses Journal 13 : 8 : 42–43
Hurley M, Meyer-Rupple A, Evans E 1983 Emma needed more than standard teaching. Nursing 83 13 : 3 : 63–64
Lutz R 1986 Stopping the spread of sexually transmitted diseases. Nursing 86 16 : 3 : 47–50
West S 1983 Infertility – couples in crisis. The Australian Nurses Journal 13 : 5 : 40–41
Wujcik D 1986 Managing the patient with testicular cancer. Nursing 86 16 : 8 : 42–45

64

Introduction to the breast

Dace Shugg   Peter Braithwaite

The breast plays a key role in nurturing the newborn infant, providing nutrition, and bonding at both physical and emotional levels between mother and child. In many cultures, the breasts are also considered to be symbols of feminine attractiveness and sexuality. For these reasons abnormalities of anatomical size and shape, disordered function, and particularly diseases affecting the breast, are feared by women. The threat to femininity and attractiveness is added to the perceived or actual threat to life from their disease.

ANATOMY

Most women have 2 breasts of approximately the same size, but between women the size is highly variable depending principally on the fat content. The position of the breast is, however, constant, with the base extending from the second to the sixth intercostal space and from the edge of the sternum to the mid-axillary line (Fig. 64.1). The nipple usually projects downwards and outwards but, like the breast contour, may be influenced by posture.

The breast is a subcutaneous structure, deep to skin and superficial fascia, separated from the underlying pectoral muscles by the pectoral fascia which is loose and allows movement of the breast on the chest wall. The breast is supported partly by its shape and also by fibrous bands (Cooper's ligaments) which connect the skin to the pectoral fascia.

The breast is not round, but pear shaped, with the top of the pear extending as an axillary tail into the armpit. There is more glandular tissue in the upper part of the breast than below which may explain why most cancers are in the upper outer quadrant, for this also includes the axillary tail.

The microscopic structure is shown schematically in Figure 64.2 but basically comprises the ductal elements which persist throughout life and the lobular elements which are prominent only during reproductive years. The blood supply to the breast is principally from the internal thoracic, lateral thoracic and intercostal arteries.

The lymphatics in the breast drain to lymph nodes in the axilla, and to the internal mammary, and the infra- and supraclavicular lymph nodes (Fig. 64.3). The nerve supply of the breast is not fully understood but has somatic components via the supraclavicular and intercostal nerves, and

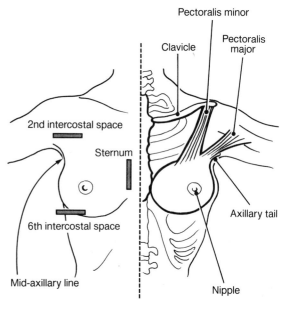

Fig. 64.1 Internal and external position of the breast.

BREAST DEVELOPMENT

The female breast undergoes changes and development at puberty, during menstruation, during pregnancy and lactation, and following menopause. Some hormones which influence breast function are oestrogen, progesterone, prolactin, and oxytocin. The female breasts show the first external signs of sexual development at puberty when they enlarge due to the accumulation of fat within the connective tissue as a response to altered hormone levels.

Under hormonal influence, the breasts of most women exhibit changes during the menstrual cycle. Each month following ovulation, the breasts engorge due to increased vascularity and become 'lumpy', heavy, and tender; most women finding relief with the wearing of a firm-fitting brassiere. At the onset of menstruation the venous engorgement decreases and the breasts return to their pre-ovulation state.

During pregnancy, secretory acini surrounded by contractile myoepithelial cells develop within the breast lobules under the influence of increased progesterone secretion and the lactiferous duct system becomes established due to increased levels of oestrogen; as a result the breasts increase markedly in size. Anterior pituitary secretion of prolactin is also necessary for breast development to occur and its secretion is essential for milk production.

During lactation, milk is secreted by the acini under the influence of prolactin, and the lactiferous ducts collect the milk into 10–20 collecting ducts which open onto the surface of the nipple. Infant suckling at the breast, as well as other stimuli such as smell, touch, voice, cry, and cuddling, stimulates the release of prolactin, thus maintaining lactation. Infant suckling also triggers the release of oxytocin from the posterior pituitary and its release causes myoepithelial contracture resulting in the ejection of milk from the ducts. The cerebral cortex holds an extremely important overriding influence on all of these mechanisms and lactation can be, and is, profoundly affected by attitude, emotion, and personality. However, under normal circumstances lactation can continue for as long as infant suckling persists, regardless of intervening changes in reproductive status. The

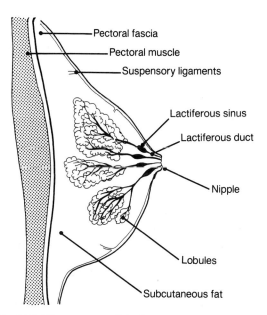

Fig. 64.2 Microstructure of the breast.

- Pectoral fascia
- Pectoral muscle
- Suspensory ligaments
- Lactiferous sinus
- Lactiferous duct
- Nipple
- Lobules
- Subcutaneous fat

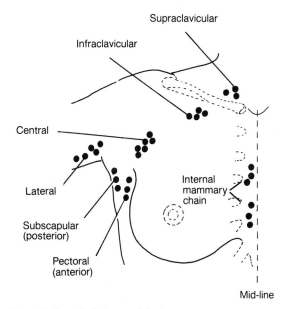

Fig. 64.3 Lymph drainage of the breast.

- Supraclavicular
- Infraclavicular
- Central
- Lateral
- Subscapular (posterior)
- Pectoral (anterior)
- Internal mammary chain
- Mid-line

autonomic supply in the form of parasympathetics with the blood vessels, and sympathetics which produce nipple erection. Pain from the breast may be referred via the supraclavicular nerves to the neck, the intercostal nerves to the chest wall, or the intercostal-brachial nerve to the medial aspect of the arm.

length of breast feeding time for each pregnancy is greatly influenced by personal attitude of the mother, cultural aspects and beliefs, and socioeconomic factors.

Common anatomical abnormalities

Nipple inversion, indrawing, or retraction. This may be congenital or may occur during breast development. It may be present in one or both breasts.

Massive enlargement. This occasionally follows puberty; surgery to reduce the size of the breasts may be indicated.

Extra nipples. These may be tiny or large enough to be considered extra breasts. They usually occur on the torso in line with the normal breasts and are found in both men and women.

Unequal development. A slight discrepancy in size is very common. In some cases one breast may be only a fraction of the size of the other. This can be remedied by plastic surgery.

Gynaecomastia. Hypertrophy of the male breast usually occurs on one side but can be bilateral. This appears most commonly at puberty due to hormonal changes or trauma. In later life it may occur in men with liver disease, endocrine disorders, and as a side effect of some medications such as oestrogens, cimetidine, antihypertensives, diuretics, and sedatives. Gynaecomastia is a functional rather than an anatomical abnormality.

CLINICAL MANIFESTATIONS OF BREAST DISEASE

Any obvious change, particularly if rapid and not during puberty or pregnancy, should be reported to a physician. Changes which may indicate breast disease are listed in Table 64.1.

Table 64.1 Clinical manifestations of breast disease

1. Any lump or lumps in the breast or axilla – painful or painless.
2. Any dimpling of the breast skin or areola.
3. Any skin discolouration over the breast.
4. Any nipple discharge – watery, coloured, or bloodstained.
5. Any inversion of the nipple – indrawing or retraction.
6. Pain, discomfort, or 'sensation' in the breast.
7. Change in shape, contour, or fullness of the breast.
8. Crusting, eczema, or scab formation on the nipple.

BREAST SELF EXAMINATION (BSE)

Over 90% of breast tumours are discovered by women themselves, and many of the smaller tumours are found by women who practise regular and careful breast self examination. Only about one-third of Australian women practise BSE regularly once a month. Twice as many again say that they know how to examine themselves, but fail to carry out this potentially life saving and simple procedure for reasons of embarrassment, lack of confidence, fear of finding a lump, denial of vulnerability, ignorance, and forgetfulness. It is important to remember that 9 out of 10 lumps are not malignant.

Finding breast cancer while it is small means that mastectomy may not be necessary – that the cancer can be treated without the woman losing her breast. This fact should take some of the fear out of finding a breast lump, and encourage more women to perform BSE.

BSE and the role of the nurse

As a predominantly female profession, nursing can play a vital role in increasing the practice of BSE. If nurses themselves practise BSE monthly and are confident and comfortable with it, they are more likely to encourage and teach their patients to do the same.

Studies show that women who are taught BSE through personal instruction by a doctor or nurse:

● Are more competent in the technique (Huguley, 1981)
● Are much more likely to do monthly BSE
● Will find smaller tumours (Foster, 1978)
● Will live longer because they will find cancer while it is smaller (Foster, 1984).

The technique of BSE

Cancer Councils in each State publish detailed brochures on the correct method of BSE; these brochures are often available in physicians' surgeries, in the offices of many other health professionals, and from health agencies. BSE is simple, takes only a few minutes to perform, and provides peace of mind 'at your fingertips'. The technique is best taught in a one-to-one situation but several basic principles apply:

The boundaries of BSE. To make sure that you examine all the breast tissue, feel the area that extends from the collar-bone at the top, to the bra line at the bottom; and from the level of your armpit, to the midline between your breasts (Fig. 64.4).

Timing. All adult women should do BSE once a month just after the monthly period, when a woman's breasts are least vascular and tender. Nonmenstruating women should perform BSE on the first day of each month.

Make time. BSE does not take long but you need to have that time to yourself in private. Choose your time and shut the door.

Inspection. Inspect your breasts in front of a mirror. For this you will have to undress to the waist and have good lighting available. Raise your arms and check that your breasts move symmetrically as you do this; note if any dimples appear anywhere in the breast. Inspect your nipples for any changes.

Lying flat. Lying down comfortably is the simplest and most reliable way to feel your breasts. Getting into position to examine your left breast, first lie on your right side with your knees bent. Then lean back towards the bed so that your shoulders are flat. Put your left arm behind your head. Reverse the position when examining your right breast (Fig. 64.5).

Finger position. Use the flat of your fingers and with a circular pressing motion gently move the skin over underlying tissue. This is called palpation. It sometimes helps to close your eyes and concentrate while you are doing this (Fig. 64.6).

Be systematic. Using the vertical strip pattern as in Figure 64.7, examine your breast in up and down strips similar to the way you would mow a lawn. Start at the armpit and move down towards the bra-line using slow circular movements. Move your fingers across about 2.5 cm and work your way up the next strip towards the collar-bone. Keep moving your fingers in vertical strips. When you reach the nipple, roll back into a position flat on your back. Continue examining in strips until you reach the mid-line between your breasts. Try

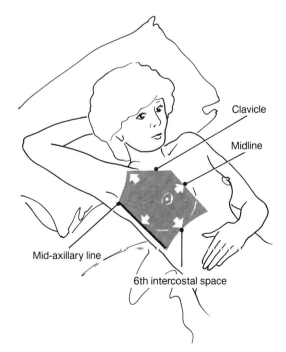

Fig. 64.4 Boundaries of BSE.

Clavicle

Midline

Mid-axillary line

6th intercostal space

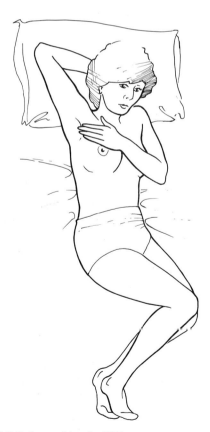

Fig. 64.5 Lying position for BSE.

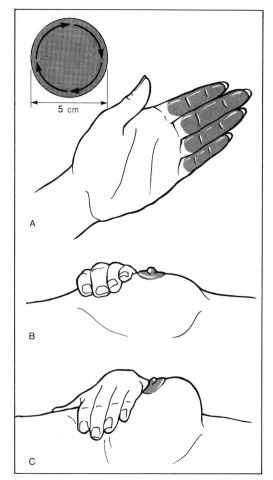

Fig. 64.6 BSE. **A** – Area of fingers used, and pattern of movement. **B** & **C** – At each place tested, both light and firm pressure should be used.

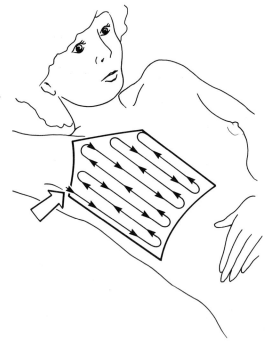

Fig. 64.7 Vertical strip pattern for BSE. Note starting-point (large arrow).

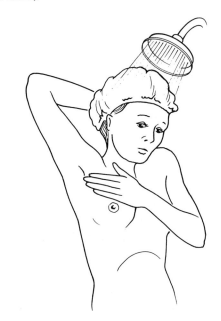

Fig. 64.8 BSE performed in shower.

not to leave too much space between strips. This pattern ensures that you will examine the whole breast thoroughly. Follow the same pattern for the other breast from the armpit to the mid-line.

The nipple. Palpate beneath the nipple and areola and squeeze the nipple gently between your thumb and index finger, to see if there is a discharge.

The axilla. Palpate the axilla carefully to check for any lumps. These may be enlarged lymph nodes.

The shower. Small firm breasts can be adequately examined standing up under the shower, using a soapy hand and elevating the arm on the side being examined (Fig. 64.8). Remember to inspect in front of the mirror as well.

Any worries? If you find anything that worries you, such as a lump, retracted nipple, discharge, soreness, a dimple, or any change, report this to your physician promptly.

65

Benign disorders of the breast

Dace Shugg   Peter Braithwaite

Benign disorders of the breast presenting with the clinical manifestations listed in Chapter 64 are much more common than breast cancer. While not all benign breast disorders require a biopsy, operations for benign disease are 10 times more common than operations for cancer. Most clinical manifestations of breast disease need to be investigated carefully because many of the signs and symptoms for benign disease are the same as those for cancer of the breast.

INVESTIGATIVE PROCEDURES

Breast disease is sometimes diagnosed during a routine physical examination by a physician. More often the patient has drawn the physician's attention to some irregularity she may have discovered herself. The physician will examine both breasts and all gland areas, and take a careful history.

Mammography

A mammogram is a soft tissue X-ray of the breast. Recent developments have provided much safer, 'dedicated' machines which deliver a very low dose of radiation. Indications for mammography are:

• To assess the symptomatic breast. A lump, thickening, retraction, discharge, pain, sensation, or other change may be indication for mammography
• To screen asymptomatic women for early diagnosis of impalpable lesions. The role here is probably best limited to women at a high risk of developing breast cancer (see page 682)

• To assess the opposite breast in breast cancer patients

Even the most expertly interpreted mammograms cannot exclude the possibility of cancer if other clinical signs are present. Suspicious lesions must be biopsied.

Ultrasound

Ultrasound examination uses sound waves to detect tissues of different density and is used in some centres to differentiate solid from cystic lumps. It has the advantages of not using ionising radiation, and efficacy in dense young breasts which may not give a clear mammogram. Its role is much smaller than that of mammography.

Biopsies

No breast lesion can be properly called malignant without pathological confirmation. There are 3 methods of obtaining material for pathologists to determine if a tumour is malignant:

1. Fine needle aspiration cytology. This is a simple procedure often done in an outpatient clinic. No local anaesthetic is used since it only requires the insertion of one needle into the breast. Material obtained is then sent for cytological examination.
2. Trucut biopsy. A special wider bore needle is used for this procedure and it is possible to withdraw solid material inside the cannula. The procedure is carried out under local anaesthetic in a clinic or ward. The core of tissue obtained is examined by a pathologist, who can provide a histological report.

679

3. Excision or incision biopsy. This type of procedure is usually performed under a general anaesthetic. In an excision biopsy, the whole tumour is removed. If only a segment is taken, as in the case of a very large tumour, then it is called an incision biopsy. An incision or excision biopsy may also be performed if the result of a trucut biopsy is negative, or if a lump does not disappear completely after needle aspiration.

Most large hospitals have facilities for a frozen section which means that the patient can have the result of the biopsy within an hour. Sometimes it is necessary to wait for at least 48 hours for the more detailed paraffin section.

BENIGN BREAST DISORDERS

Fibroadenoma

This is a benign condition of lobular tissue which occurs most commonly in women during the early reproductive years (15–30 years). Fibroadenoma usually presents as a firm, mobile, well rounded lump of rubbery consistency. It is sometimes called a 'breast mouse' because it moves so easily within the breast. Surgical management is usually by excision biopsy.

Duct ectasia

This condition occurs when the lactiferous ducts become dilated. Women between 50–70 years are most commonly affected. Possible presenting signs are nipple discharge (yellow, brown or green), localized lump, nipple retraction, skin tethering or dimpling, and an area of inflammation.

Surgical management is by excision of the affected lactiferous duct.

Duct papilloma

In this condition single or multiple papillomas arise from the epithelium and project into the duct. It more commonly occurs in 35–55 year-old women. Presenting signs are bloodstained discharge; and less often a localized lump. Surgical management is by excision.

Cysts

Breast cysts are fluid-filled tumours in the tissue of many women aged 35–50 years; they are not always detectable clinically. They can vary in size from 1 mm to 5 cm in diameter, and frequently more than one is present in the breast.

These cysts present as firm, relatively mobile lump(s) which may be rounded or flat. Surgical management includes needle aspiration which may be curative. If the fluid is bloodstained, excision biopsy is recommended.

Benign mammary dysplasia

This is a fairly common condition principally affecting women in the 24–45 year age group. One or both breasts may be affected and the condition can best be described as abnormal and patchy development and distribution of breast tissue. The 4 pathological components are adenosis, fibrosis, epitheliosis, and cysts. Presenting signs are pain, nipple discharge, distortion of breast outline, and lumps.

Surgical management is by excision biopsy of persistent lesions.

Fat necrosis

This condition may occur at any age and is possibly a response to trauma. It presents as a lump, and surgical management is by excision biopsy.

Acute mastitis and breast abscess

Infection of the breast occurs most often during lactation after the first pregnancy, when a cracked nipple allows entry of microorganisms. Untreated mastitis may develop into a breast abscess. Presenting signs of mastitis are fever, malaise, erythema, heat, tenderness, and pain. Management includes:

– Continuation of feeding from the unaffected breast
– Expression by breast pump from the affected side
– Heat packs followed by ice packs
– Rest

– Antibiotics (as ordered)
– Drainage of the breast abscess if this develops.

Mastalgia (breast pain)

This is a quite common complaint in premenopausal women. It can vary from moderate discomfort premenstrually, to severe pain for most of the month which disrupts all normal physical activity. Management includes reassurance and explanation; breast support with a brassiere, day and night; the application of heat; and mild analgesics. Danazol or bromocriptine may be prescribed for severe pain. Some success has been achieved by the deletion from the diet of all caffeine in the form of tea, coffee, cola or chocolate for a period of 2 months.

NURSING MANAGEMENT

The patient undergoing investigation

Many patients with a breast problem are very anxious about stripping to the waist for examination, and about the possible outcome of the examination or the results of their mammogram. A knowledgeable and compassionate nurse can be of enormous assistance in reassuring and comforting the patient. The need for such reassurance and assistance is most obvious when needle aspiration or needle biopsies are performed under local anaesthetic, but is important in all cases. The nurse plays a vital role in ensuring that the patient has comprehended fully all explanations and advice provided by medical staff.

The patient undergoing general surgery

Each patient will view the prospect of impending breast surgery with her own mixture of apprehension, confidence, and concern. Preoperative nursing assessment will ensure that the patient understands her condition, the procedure to be performed, and its implications. Preoperative nursing management involves preparing the patient physically and emotionally for surgery.

Postoperatively, nursing care specifically involves the management of the wound, a restriction of arm or other movement, and instruction of the patient regarding discharge and follow up. Many hospitals have printed instructions for the patients who have had minor breast surgery.

The patient undergoing plastic surgery

There are 2 types of surgery for benign breast conditions which the nurse is most likely to encounter. These are:

1. Augmentation mammoplasty. This procedure is performed on patients who have inadequate or uneven breast development
2. Reduction mammoplasty. This is usually performed on both breasts for the correction of grossly obese or pendulous breasts. This procedure is also sometimes performed on the opposite breast in conjunction with reconstruction of a breast after mastectomy, to achieve better symmetry

As both these procedures are primarily performed for their cosmetic results, the patient usually approaches surgery confidently and with an air of optimism and excitement regarding the final outcome. Nursing assessment preoperatively still involves ensuring that the patient realistically understands the procedure and its implications. Postoperatively, nursing management is directed towards maintaining the best cosmetic effect: prevention of wound infection is of paramount importance.

66

Malignant disorders of the breast

Dace Shugg   Peter Braithwaite   Chris Game

INTRODUCTION

Incidence

Breast cancer is the most common cancer in Australian women, affecting approximately 1 in 14, or 7% of all women. It is much more common in older women.

It is the first ranking cause of cancer mortality in women, and is the second ranking cause of all deaths in women, behind ischaemic heart disease. In Australia 4500 new cases are diagnosed annually and 1800 women die of the disease every year.

Women in Australia, Europe, and the United States have a much higher incidence of breast cancer than do women in Japan and other Asian countries.

Only 1–2% of all breast cancer cases occur in men, usually at an older age than in women.

Risk factors

Women who exhibit the following characteristics have an increased risk of developing breast cancer:

- Positive family history, especially if more than 1 close relative had breast cancer while premenopausal
- Childless women
- Late first pregnancy – first full term pregnancy after the age of 30 years
- Early menarche and late menopause
- Age – women over 40 years
- High fat and protein intake – obesity is a risk factor.

Women who have a combination of all, or most, of these risk factors need to be especially careful to perform monthly BSE and should have regular breast examinations by their physician.

Tumour types

Mammary carcinoma is not a single entity, but may present as a number of distinctly different histological types. Figure 66.1 illustrates the distribution of tumour types within the infiltrating and the non-infiltrating groups.

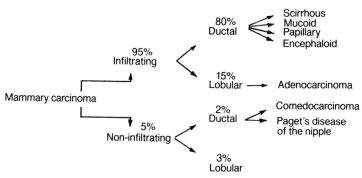

Fig. 66.1 Distribution of tumour types in mammary carcinoma.

Prognostic factors

These include:

• Stage of the tumour. This is determined by the size of the tumour, presence of axillary nodes infiltrated by tumour cells, and presence or otherwise of distant metastases. Patients may be classed as being in stages 1,2,3 or 4; or they may be classified under the TNM system: T = tumour size, N = node status, M = distant metastases.
• Oestrogen and progesterone receptor assays. Tests for these are done by a pathologist on fresh tumour cells before they are frozen or stored. The results determine whether the tumour type will respond to hormone therapy.

Clinical manifestations

Breast cancer most commonly presents as a painless lump. In only about 15% of cases, pain is present in the breast as a symptom. There may be changes in the nipple or axilla. Clinical manifestations which should be reported to the physician are described in Table 64.1, page 676. About 30% of all breast cancer patients present to the physician when they already have distant metastases, that is, with stage IV breast cancer.

Investigative procedures

• Mammogram
• Chest X-ray
• Bone and liver scans – to exclude bone and liver metastases

Aims of medical and surgical management

Medical and surgical management aims at:

• Control of local disease through removal of tumour mass by surgery and/or radiotherapy.
• Control of systemic disease through hormonal or cytotoxic therapy of micro metastases which may be occult; systemic therapy is also used in the treatment of recurrence of disease.
• Palliation – symptom control and management of metastatic disease. Radiotherapy, hormonal or cytotoxic therapy may be used.

Rationale for treatment

Treatment for breast cancer has undergone considerable change in recent years. The change has resulted from the increasing body of evidence which indicates that mammary carcinoma is often a systemic disease even at an apparently early stage. Increasing numbers of cancer therapists now believe that, for patients with small tumours, conservative local therapy and some form of systemic therapy has as good a chance of disease control as does total mastectomy.

SURGICAL MANAGEMENT

Removal, if possible, of the tumour mass is always desirable so that prognostic factors can be assessed and to reduce the 'tumour load' before instigating systemic therapy. Sometimes removal of the tumour mass without systemic therapy is considered adequate treatment.

Surgical approaches

1. Lumpectomy or wide local excision. Only the tumour is removed; this is sometimes called tylectomy
2. Quadrantectomy, segmental mastectomy, or partial mastectomy. The tumour is removed as well as about one-quarter, or a quadrant, of the breast (Fig. 66.2)
3. Lumpectomy and axillary sampling. The tumour is removed with a good margin, and some axillary lymph glands are removed to determine the stage of the cancer
4. Simple (total) mastectomy. The tumour, all breast tissue, overlying skin, and nipple are removed
5. Modified radical or Patey's mastectomy. As in simple mastectomy, all structures are removed; additionally the operation includes the removal of axillary glands, and in some cases the pectoralis minor muscle (Fig. 66.3)
6. Radical mastectomy. All breast tissue, axillary glands and both pectoralis major and minor muscles are removed. This is usually done only if the pectoralis muscle is invaded by the tumour, to achieve local control of the disease (Fig. 66.3)

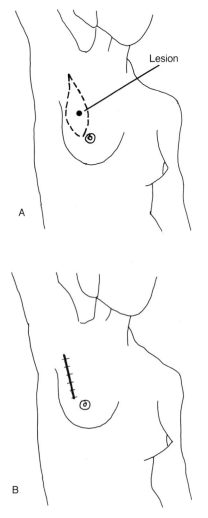

Fig. 66.2 Quadrantectomy. **A** – Area removed. **B** – Resultant scar site.

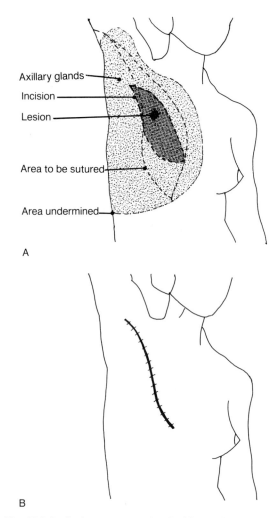

Fig. 66.3 Radical mastectomy. **A** – Incision and area undermined. Note that the area to be sutured is much larger than the incision. **B** – Resultant scar site.

7. Excision biopsy and 'follow through' to mastectomy. If a frozen section reveals malignancy whilst the patient is still anaesthetised and in the operating room, the surgeon may 'follow through' and perform a mastectomy. Permission to do this must be obtained prior to surgery. Some patients still prefer this method to avoid having two anaesthetics, preferring to get it 'over and done with' in one procedure.

Choice of treatment

The health team in consultation with the patient,

will consider all of the following factors when determining the type of surgery to be performed:

– The condition and age of the patient
– The size and site of the tumour
– Presence of distant metastases
– Preference of the patient
– Preference of the surgeon.

Nursing management

The patient awaiting a mastectomy must face and accept a dual assault to her self image: she has cancer, and she is also about to lose a traditional measure of her femininity. These factors will be valued differently by each patient and her ultimate psychological and emotional adaptation will be influenced largely by the nurse. Nurses have a delicate and important role to play in helping the patient (and significant others) to understand the realities of her condition.

Preoperative preparation

The nurse closest to the patient should assess the patient's reaction to this frightening experience, and the degree of understanding that the patient has about her treatment plan. He/she should also try to gauge the amount of family support, or that of significant others, which the patient may be able to mobilize.

Patients having quadrantectomy, lumpectomy, or axillary sampling require similar care.

Allaying fear. It may be useful to call in a Breast Cancer Support Service (BCSS) volunteer to talk to a patient awaiting mastectomy. Such visits can allay much of the fear of surgery and therefore should be encouraged (see page 687).

Information. Nurses need to be thoroughly knowledgeable about all aspects of patient care so that questions can be answered accurately. Ensure that the patient understands the procedure, the method of skin closure, the placement of the suture line and drains, the expected reduction of mobility, the presence of an IV infusion, and the planned postoperative rehabilitation program.

Support. Some patients may live alone or have very little family support for other reasons. In such cases it is most important to make the patient feel she has somebody to talk to who really cares about her.

Skin preparation. Depending upon the surgical procedure to be performed skin preparation usually entails shaving of the axilla, and a shower using a germicidal soap on the day of the surgery. If a skin graft is to be performed (less than 5% of all cases), shaving and preparation of the donor site will also be necessary.

Postoperative management

Recovery phase. If the nurse has the opportunity to get to know the patient, his/her presence in the recovery room will be beneficial. The nurse may be the one who confirms that mastectomy was performed if diagnosis had not been established before surgery, as in the 'follow through' procedure. The nurse should find out before the operation who the patient would like to have present in the first few hours. Many women like to have their husband or closest friend nearby; others wish to cope with the first few hours in privacy.

Immediate care. Regardless of the surgical technique used, the principles of nursing care are to:

1. Manage pain
2. Relieve anxiety and provide support
3. Promote healing
4. Prevent infection
5. Prevent postoperative complications.

The nurse must prepare to meet the needs of a person:

– Who will usually have an extensive chest wall wound and associated drainage tubes, both of which may result in extreme discomfort and/or pain. There are usually at least 2 drainage tubes attached to low pressure suction, one of which is draining the axilla
– Who may have had a skin graft to the chest wall wound which has resulted in an extremely painful donor site. In most instances, the pain of the donor site is greater than the incisional pain of the wound.
– Who may be experiencing grief regarding the perceived loss of her femininity as a result of the alteration to her body image
– Whose surgery may have been so extensive that interruption to blood supply and lymphatic drainage, as well as loss of tissue mass, may interrupt the normal healing processes and predispose to the development of postoperative infection
– Who will need close observation of vital signs, the wound and its drainage, and the donor site. The nurse must detect the early signs of infection, seroma, wound edge necrosis, and lymphoedema in the arm on the affected side.

It is important for the nurse to determine the exact nature of the surgery and how much tissue and muscle was resected. Close cooperation with the surgical and health team is essential for the successful management and rehabilitation of the mastectomy patient.

Pain relief, as ordered, should be sufficient to control pain without depressing the patient's cough reflex (see Chapter 12). Positional changes, including lying on the affected side, and placement of a pillow anteriorly under the affected arm will also help to relieve pain. Coughing and breathing exercises to prevent atelectasis must be encouraged as the patient will be loath to breathe deeply for fear of opening the incision.

Emotional support should be provided, both to the patient and to her significant others. The patient should be encouraged, but not forced, to look at her wound as soon as feasible and an empathic approach by the nurse will assist her to accept her altered body image.

The wound should be inspected anteriorly and posteriorly and any excessive seepage reported. The amount and colour of the drainage via the tubes is recorded; frank bloody drainage should become serous within 12 hours. An occlusive dressing is not normally taken down until the drain tubes are removed, usually after 48 hours.

Any swelling under the wound, accompanied by a fall in tube drainage, may indicate that a seroma is developing; early notification and treatment will prevent wound breakdown. The presence and increase of cyanosis of the wound edges is indicative of necrosis which will result in wound malunion, and healing will be by second intention.

If a skin graft is present, it will be covered by a pressure dressing sutured in place, or the nurse will be responsible for 'rolling' the graft for the first 24 hours (see also care of skin grafts page 780). Wound sutures or clips are removed after 10–14 days. The use of skin grafting ensures that the wound will have viable edges and that there will not be a sizeable defect on the chest wall.

A donor site, if present, will be covered by a fine mesh gauze and a pressure bandage to assist haemostasis. The bandage is commonly removed after 10 days and the mesh gauze is then allowed to remain in place until it detaches by itself, usually after a further 10 days.

Hand and arm exercises. Exercises to prevent contracture and to restore full arm mobility will be instituted with the patient. It is usual to start with hand exercises such as fist clenching, then gentle elbow movements, and gradually progress to hair brushing type exercises. The patient's exercise programme should be monitored closely by the health team. The surgeon, the physiotherapist and the nurse should consult regularly regarding the progress of wound healing in relation to arm mobility exercises. It is desirable that all exercises are done with both arms to preserve symmetry and function and the patient should be encouraged to continue to do exercises after discharge. Patients who are to have postoperative radiotherapy will need to regain full arm mobility before treatment can commence.

Arm care and prevention of lymphoedema. Lymphoedema, or permanent swelling of the arm, is one of the more distressing complications which may sometimes occur following surgical treatment of and/or radiotherapy to the axilla. Gentle exercise and care to avoid any infection in the arm on the operated side are steps which are taken to avoid lymphoedema. Once established, lymphoedema is extremely difficult to reverse, so preventive measures are most important. These are aimed at avoiding infection and swelling due to trauma. For this reason nurses should be aware and the patient advised:

1. Not to permit IV, IM, or SC injections into the affected arm; this includes the IV infusion used in the operating room
2. To obtain treatment for any infection in that arm or hand, even if the infection is very minor
3. Not to have blood taken from or given in that arm
4. That she is vulnerable to secondary oedema for the rest of her life and that trauma may lead to infection and oedema.

Emotional problems after mastectomy. Unanswered questions are frequently a source of anxiety and unproductive worry to patients who may feel diffident about approaching or 'imposing on' their surgeon. Sometimes the surgeon is the only one in a position to explain the facts fully to a patient. The nurse can often help the patient express her questions to the surgeon and also ensure that the patient has at least some opportunity for a private discussion with her surgeon.

Some women feel mutilated and defective after mastectomy, and tend to withdraw from their husbands, fearing rejection. Others may behave with outwardly calm acceptance to avoid upsetting family and nursing staff. In both cases the patient can benefit by skilled counselling from an experienced social worker, chaplain or nurse. Her husband or closest friend should be consulted and included.

Mastectomy rehabilitation

Volunteer visitors from the Breast Cancer Support Service (BCSS) are specially trained women who have had a mastectomy, and who are available to visit patients in hospital. A volunteer can answer non-medical questions, offer practical advice, and provide a boost in morale because she herself is 'living proof' of good recovery. The BCSS also provides a free temporary breast form for use in the immediate post discharge phase.

A visitor from the BCSS will enable your patient to leave hospital better informed and better able to face her new circumstances. Patients should be visited with the surgeon's cooperation, therefore it often falls upon nursing staff to arrange such visits. Telephone numbers for State Co-ordinators are shown below:

ACT	–	(062) 48 0726
NSW	–	(02) 264 8888
VIC	–	(03) 662 3300
QLD	–	(07) 257 1155
SA	–	(08) 267 5222
WA	–	(09) 321 6224
TAS	–	(002) 30 0895
NT	–	(098) 81 3556

Possible complications

Complications are not common: however, wound breakdown; seroma; painful axilla due to trauma to the brachial plexus during axillary clearance; frozen shoulder due to inadequate arm mobility exercises which may be exacerbated by extensive radiotherapy; or lymphoedema may develop. Nursing assessment will determine whether the patient needs advice, education, exercise and/or reassurance. Psychological and emotional maladaptations such as sexual dysfunction, severe depression, and alcohol or tranquillizer dependence require anticipation, referral, and skilled counselling.

Permanent prostheses

The fitting of a permanent breast prosthesis (breast form) a few days after surgery, while the patient is still in hospital, is to be avoided. A good fitting is not possible until all swelling has subsided, and this sometimes takes 6–10 weeks. A temporary breast form can be used until then.

Women with a large remaining breast should particularly be advised that the removed breast needs to be replaced with a properly designed and weighted prosthesis. The volunteer visitor will be able to inform the patient about local guidelines for provision of the first permanent prosthesis.

Breast reconstruction

Rebuilding the breast after mastectomy is possible for the majority of patients; it can be done at the time of mastectomy, or many years later. It is more usual to leave a space of a few months between primary cancer surgery by the general surgeon, and reconstruction of the breast by a plastic surgeon.

Not all patients will choose to have the breast reconstructed. Reasons for not having the procedure include: reluctance to undergo further surgery and anaesthetic, pain, and absence from family. Knowledge that the results will not be as good as the other breast deters some women – also the fact that the nipple construction may necessitate at least one or more additional operations. The opposite breast may need to be reduced to match the newly constructed one.

Despite all the problems and possibilities, many mastectomy patients undergo reconstruction and the vast majority of these patients are happy that they have done so.

MEDICAL MANAGEMENT

Radiotherapy

In the treatment of breast cancer, radiotherapy may be used in the following instances, usually as an outpatient procedure:

● In conjunction with lumpectomy in the treatment of early primary tumours
● In addition to mastectomy for the treatment of lymph node areas

• For the treatment and local control of inoperable advanced local tumours
• For the treatment and palliation of pain due to bone secondaries in advanced disease
• For the irradiation of ovaries to produce artificial menopause (see hormone therapy, page 689).

It is essential for the nurse to be familiar with the procedures carried out in radiotherapy units. Otherwise it is most difficult to reassure, advise and educate the patient having any of the above procedures. There is still a great deal of ignorance, misinformation and fear associated with attending a radiotherapy unit.

Patients having treatment will usually be issued with written instructions regarding special skin care of the area being treated and side effects which need to be reported. These instructions should be available to nursing staff on wards where patients are admitted during treatment. (See also Chapter 13)

Nursing management

Explanation and reassurance. Patients often fail to comprehend explanations which may be offered at the same time as the announcement that radiotherapy will be necessary. The nurse may need to repeat explanations several times and it is important that what is said is applicable to that particular patient.

Radioactivity risk. Patients receiving external beam radiotherapy do not become radioactive. Only patients who have radon chains or radioactive isotopes implanted in the breast become radioactive for the short duration of the implant. They are hospitalized during this time and certain restrictions are placed on visitors.

Side-effects. During the course of radiotherapy, a radiation reaction similar to sunburn may develop in the treated area. Sore throat may develop. The patient will feel tired and require extra rest. Desquamation of skin cells and axillary hair loss temporarily occurs, whereas perspiration will be permanently reduced from treated areas.

The patient needs to be aware of the possible side effects so that, if they occur, she will not imagine that her illness is progressing. She should

be advised that extra rest is necessary, that sore throat can be managed with analgesics, and that she can continue to engage in any activities she normally enjoys, being careful to protect the treated area. Treatment may span 6 weeks, so some disruption to lifestyle has to be expected. Some women continue to work while having radiotherapy.

Chemotherapy

In the treatment of breast cancer, cytotoxic drugs are most commonly used in the following contexts:

• As adjuvant therapy to local management in the treatment of early breast cancer to obliterate any occult micro metastases which might be present. Adjuvant chemotherapy is most often given to premenopausal, stage II patients.
• As therapy for metastatic disease to achieve a remission by arresting the spread of metastases. The aim is to increase life expectancy as well as enhancing the quality of life by producing symptom relief.

Choice of drugs

There are many cytotoxic drugs which are used alone or in combination for the systemic treatment of early, as well as metastatic, breast cancer. Some types of breast cancer do not respond as well as others, and it is sometimes difficult to predict any individual patient's response to this treatment. Commonly used cytotoxic agents include:

Adriamycin
Cyclophosphamide
5-Fluorouracil (5FU)
Methotrexate
Prednisone
Vincristine
Vinblastine

For further information on the use and administration of cytotoxic drugs, refer to Chapter 13.

Side-effects

Cytotoxics act by directly attacking the faster growing cancer cells. Unfortunately some normally functioning cells, such as those of the bone marrow and the epithelium of the gastrointestinal tract, will also be damaged.

Different drugs cause different side-effects, and some patients can tolerate larger doses than others. Mouth ulcers, vomiting, diarrhoea, and hair loss can occur. Bone marrow depression and cardiac toxicity are serious complications of great concern. Most side-effects are known and can be anticipated and, in most cases, controlled. Usually side-effects disappear when treatment is suspended, and the body heals itself. Some disruption to normal lifestyle has to be expected.

The attitude of the nurse

A positive outlook by the nurse towards outcome of therapy with cytotoxic drugs will help the patient to maintain a fighting spirit and cope with all the discomforts of therapy. It also helps to remember that advances are constantly being made in improving the efficacy and reducing the toxicity of cytotoxic drugs.

Hormone therapy

Rationale for treatment

Hormone therapy is most frequently used as a treatment for metastatic breast cancer. Manipulation of the levels of naturally circulating hormones is the aim of hormone therapy. The rationale is that some tumours which are hormone dependent will react to changed levels of circulating hormones and become dormant for periods of months to years.

Surgery to achieve hormone manipulation includes oophorectomy, adrenalectomy, and hypophysectomy.

Non-surgical hormone manipulation can be achieved by: anti-oestrogen therapy with tamoxifen; ovarian irradiation to produce artificial menopause; medical adrenalectomy by the administration of aminoglutethimide; and hormone therapy using oestrogens, progestogens, or androgens.

It should be noted that the use of hormones in treatment will produce a variety of side effects but that these are usually pre-empted by the prescription of specific counter-medications. Patients must understand that it is essential not to discontinue or cut down on any drugs without the physician's knowledge and specific instructions.

ANTICIPATED OUTCOME

Approximately 50% of all patients diagnosed with breast cancer will suffer a recurrence and die of their disease within 5 years despite all treatments. However, 90% of patients with tumours 1 cm or less will be alive and well 20 years after treatment. The value of early detection and treatment cannot be overemphasised.

Individually, the outlook for each person will depend on a number of factors such as tumour type, prognostic factors, early diagnosis, appropriate treatment, the personality of the patient, and the quality of nursing care and support she gets.

Hundreds of women who were treated 5, 10 or 20 years ago for breast cancer are alive and well in the community.

The role of the nurse

There are many ways in which the caring, educated nurse can lighten the patient's load during this difficult time, including:

Practical assistance. Care of the suture line, irradiated area, dressings, exercises, prostheses, and education about self management, side effects, and breast self examination.

Liaison role. Being familiar with methods of referral to voluntary visiting services and urging physicians to involve their patients. Expediting communication between the patient and her physician, and the patient and her family – patients often confide fears to nurses.

Helping the patient cope with recurrence. By understanding the patient's difficulties and giving practical advice on how to cope with each new crisis, the nurse can do much to make the patient feel that she has not been abandoned.

Emotional support. Provide a caring and protected environment for the patient. Warmth, understanding, and encouragement is also needed for the patient's significant others. They all need a person they can talk to who is not afraid to discuss cancer.

A better informed nurse is more likely to have a positive attitude to the outcomes of breast cancer therapy, and a positive attitude is a vital component of successful recovery and rehabilitation.

SECTION J – REFERENCES AND FURTHER READING

Texts

Anderson J R (ed) 1976 Muir's textbook of pathology, 10th edn. Edward Arnold, London

Anthony C P 1984 Structure and function of the body. Mosby, St Louis

Australian Cancer Society, Sydney. Pamphlet: Living with the loss of a breast

Cameron R J 1983 Causes of death Australia 1981. Australian Bureau of Statistics, Canberra

Creager J G 1982 Human anatomy and physiology. Wadsworth, California

Havard M 1986 A nursing guide to drugs, 2nd edn. Churchill Livingstone, Melbourne

Luckmann J, Sorensen K C 1980 Medical/surgical nursing: a psychophysiologic approach, 2nd edn. Saunders, Philadelphia

MacDonald H, Grant P 1982 The art of breast care – a manual for nurse educators. South Australian Health Commission.

Macleod J 1987 Davidson's principles and practice of medicine, 15th edn. Churchill Livingstone, Edinburgh

Pittman R, Sorensen K C 1980 Disorders of the breast. In: Luckmann J, Sorensen K C Medical-surgical nursing: a psychophysiologic approach, 2nd edn. Saunders, Philadelphia, 81 : 1809–1837

Read A E, Barritt D W, Langton Hewer R 1986 Modern medicine, 3rd edn. Churchill Livingstone, Edinburgh

Reynolds P 1979 Living with cancer. Cancer Council of Western Australia

Society of Hospital Pharmacists of Australia 1985. Pharmacology and drug information for nurses, 2nd edn. Saunders, Sydney

Storlie F J (ed) 1984 Diseases: nurse's reference library, 2nd edn. Springhouse, Pennsylvania

Journals

Duncan W, Kerr G R 1976 The curability of breast cancer. British Medical Journal 2 : 6039 : 781–784

Finn K L 1979 Augmentation mammoplasty: the cosmetic surgery with a lift. Nursing 79 9 : 2 : 60–63

Fisher R B et al 1985 Five year result of a randomized clinical trial comparing total mastectomy and segmental mastectomy ± radiation in the treatment of breast cancer. New England Journal of Medicine 312 : 11 : 665–673

Fleagle J M 1980 Helping the patient with breast cancer adjust to teletherapy. Nursing 80 10 : 4 : 60–61

Foster R S, Lange S P, Constanza M C, Worden J K, Haines C R, Yates J W 1978 Breast self examination practices and breast cancer stage. New England Journal of Medicine 299 : 6 : 265–270

Foster R S, Constanza M C 1984 Breast self examination practices and breast cancer survival. Cancer 53 : 4 : 999–1005

Hill D J, Rassaby J, Gray N 1982 Health education about breast cancer using television and doctor involvement. Preventive Medicine 11 : 1 : 43–55

Huguley C M, Brown R L 1981 The value of breast self examination. Cancer 47 : 5 : 989–995

Hutcheson H A 1986 TAIF: new option for breast reconstruction. Nursing 86 16 : 2 : 52–53

Maguire P, Tait A, Brooke M, Thomas C, Sellwood R 1980 The effect of counselling on the psychiatric morbidity associated with mastectomy. British Medical Journal 281 : 6253 : 1454–1456

Mendelson B C 1982 Breast reconstruction. Medical Journal of Australia 1 : 33–35

Rassaby J, Hill D 1983 Patients' perception of breast reconstruction after mastectomy. Medical Journal of Australia 2 : 4 : 173–175

Shugg D, Lee T R, Shepherd J J, Scott A R 1981 Breast self examination, doctors and media. Australian Family Physician 10 : 9 : 691–696

Shugg D 1985 How satisfied are patients with the Mastectomy Rehabilitation Service? An Australian experience. Cancer Forum 9 : 1 : 16–18

Valinoti E 1984 A positive difference. Nursing 84 14 : 5 : 32

Audiovisual

Mastectomy: the patient's experience. 1981 3/4 Umatic Tissue. Australian Cancer Society, Sydney. 3/4 Umatic

BSE 1983 Tasmanian Film Corporation, Hobart. 3/4 Umatic

BSE 1986 Anti-Cancer Council of Victoria, Melbourne. VHS and 3/4 Umatic

SECTION

K

The musculoskeletal system

67

Introduction to the musculoskeletal system

Robyn Anderson

The musculoskeletal system consists of bones, joints, tendons, and ligaments; and the skeletal muscle attached to bones which facilitate their movement.

The bony skeleton supports the remainder of the body, protects delicate organs such as the brain, allows movement, and is the major storage area for minerals such as phosphorus and calcium. It encompasses the majority of the haemopoietic system within the marrow cavity of the long bones.

Bones are divided into 4 groups – long, flat, short, and irregular bones, and examples of each of these respectively are the femur, the bones of the skull, the carpal bones and the vertebrae.

A typical long bone consists of a diaphysis, the main shaft-like portion; the epiphysis which allows bone growth to occur; the articular cartilage, which allows one bone to move on another without too much friction; and the periosteum, which carries the blood supply to the bone (Fig. 67.1). Two types of bone formation exist: compact bone, which is made up of numerous Haversian systems (Fig. 67.2) which make the bone hard and rigid; and cancellous bone, which is a web-like structure filled with bone marrow.

Cartilage is similar to bone in many ways but differs in that the fibres are embedded in a firm gel instead of a calcified cement as is seen in bone. There are no blood vessels in cartilage, which has 2 functions: to protect articulating surfaces, for example, hyaline cartilage, and to give elasticity and therefore protection as in that provided to the intervertebral disks.

There are several different types of joints but the most important type with respect to inflam-

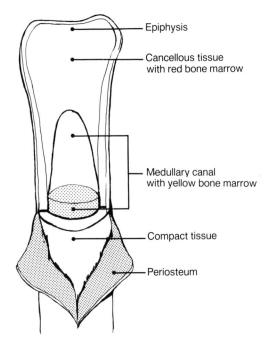

Fig. 67.1 Structure of long bone.

- Epiphysis
- Cancellous tissue with red bone marrow
- Medullary canal with yellow bone marrow
- Compact tissue
- Periosteum

matory or degenerative disease states is the diarthroyic or synovial joint (Fig. 67.3). In this type of joint the articulating bone ends are covered in hyaline cartilage and the joint is lined with synovial membrane and filled with synovial fluid to lubricate its movement.

Ligaments and tendons are made of fibrous tissue which is relatively inelastic. Tendons join muscle to bone to allow bone movement, while ligaments join bone to bone and generally strengthen joints.

Skeletal muscle makes up 40–50% of the body weight of a human being and has 3 major func-

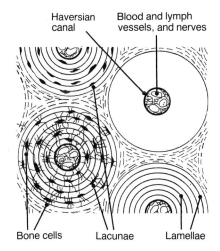

Fig. 67.2 Cross section of long bone microstructure.

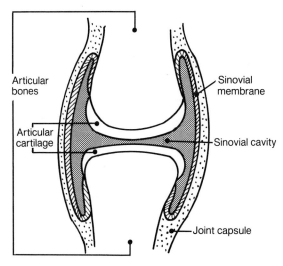

Fig. 67.3 Schema of typical sinovial joint.

tions. Skeletal muscle is responsible for all movement, produces the major part of the body's heat, and is responsible for posture, that is, the continuous partial contraction of skeletal muscle which allows us to maintain any given position.

Skeletal muscle consists of bundles of fibres which generally extend the length of the muscle and they are in turn made up of myofibrils. There are 4 proteins: myosin, actin, tropomyosin and troponin which interact in muscle to cause muscle fibre contraction. The function of skeletal muscle is to contract and therefore allow movement. There are 5 types of contraction: tonic, isotonic, isometric, twitch, and tetanic contraction.

Tonic contraction is a continual, partial contraction of a muscle, i.e. muscle tone, and is seen in all normal people when they are awake. Muscles with less than normal tone are referred to as flaccid, while those with greater than normal tone are called spastic. Isotonic contraction is the normal contraction of skeletal muscle that produces movement. Isometric contraction is the contraction of skeletal muscle that does not result in movement, for example, when maintaining a half-squatting position or pushing against a wall. A twitch contraction is a quick jerking response to a single stimulus whilst tetanic contraction is more maintained than a twitch and is seen as the result of bombardment of the muscle fibres with a series of nerve stimuli. (For discussion of the disorders of muscle caused by neuronal dysfunction see Section A).

The musculoskeletal system is not complete without both parts functioning: bone cannot move alone, and unless muscle is attached to bone it basically has nothing to move.

68

Musculoskeletal trauma

Helga Sabel   Chris Game   Robyn Anderson

Trauma to soft tissue and/or bone is diverse. Soft tissue trauma, as seen in sprains and strains, is often uncomplicated by other injury. However, trauma which is severe enough to cause dislocation of a joint, or fracture of a bone, usually also produces marked soft tissue damage.

SPRAIN

A sprain is an acute, incomplete tearing of the capsule or ligaments within a joint, and of the capillaries within the soft tissue surrounding a joint.

Pathophysiology

A sprain is usually caused by a sudden, twisting force, and is a common sporting injury. When the fibres of a ligament or capsule are torn there is an immediate inflammatory response, with oedema and some capillary bleeding. Later, when healing occurs, dense, fibrous scar tissue is laid down and this is less elastic than the original tissue.

Clinical manifestations

Pain is well localized at first and later becomes more diffuse. It is accompanied by swelling and limitation of joint function. Bruising is a later sign.

Symptoms may not be initially severe or disabling. For example, an athlete may sprain a limb but be able to complete the game. Later, reactive soft tissue swelling and bleeding may be extensive, with the joint being extremely swollen and painful and the person unable to tolerate weight.

Investigative procedures

The diagnosis is usually made on the history of the injury and the clinical features but X-rays with special 'stress' views are performed to exclude complete ligamentous tears, joint instability and fractures.

Medical management

The aim is to reduce pain and restore normal joint function.

1. Ice is applied to constrict the blood vessels and reduce oedema.
2. Elevation aids venous and lymphatic drainage.
3. Compression. A compression bandage provides comfort, support and helps to reduce reactive oedema.
4. Rest. Immobilization is usually not required, other than to protect the joint from repeating the movements that caused the initial injury. If some degree of immobilization is necessary, it is usually only required for a period of 1–3 weeks. Movement must be recommenced early to prevent the development of adhesions.

Analgesia in the form of oral aspirin or paracetamol may be required for pain relief, and nonsteroidal anti-inflammatory drugs may be ordered to reduce inflammation and lessen pain.

Physiotherapy

Heat therapy and active exercises of a sprained joint are carried out to restore full function. A return to normal activity is usually allowed after 6 weeks.

STRAIN

A strain is a similar injury to a sprain, and results from the overuse or stretching of muscles or tendons beyond their normal functional capacity. The terms 'strain' and 'sprain' are often used interchangeably. Strains are very common in sporting activities, and in repetitive manual work.

The treatment principles of rest, ice, compression and elevation (RICE) as a first aid measure, followed by heat and exercise to restore function is the same as for a sprain.

REPETITIVE STRAIN INJURY (RSI)

The RSI syndrome is commonly seen in people required to perform a repetitious physical activity for long periods without adequate rest of the joints involved. It is commonly seen in, for example, typists, computer operators, and people who work on assembly lines. Modern offices have furniture especially designed to reduce the likelihood of this syndrome and to adequately support the limbs and joints being used in the work process. Workers should be encouraged to regularly rest joints used in repetitive work.

Treatment is aimed at reducing the degree of inflammation, resting the limb until such time as the acute symptoms have abated, and then using heat and/or ultrasound and exercise to return the joint and limb to normal function.

DISLOCATION AND SUBLUXATION

Dislocation is the complete displacement of the articulating surfaces of a joint.

Subluxation is the partial displacement of the articulating surfaces.

For a joint to dislocate or sublux, the joint capsule and one or more ligaments must be either torn or stretched. There is often a fracture associated with a dislocation, as the cause is usually a traumatic injury of some force.

Pathophysiology

Tearing of the capsule and ligaments will result in bleeding and an immediate inflammatory response. Joints contain the sensory nerve endings of pain and proprioception, so pain will be severe. The patient will often be aware that the joint is not in its normal position. Muscles controlling the joint will spasm, adding to the pain. The articular cartilage, major blood vessels and nerves may be damaged.

Clinical manifestations

These are the same as for fractures (see page 699), however swelling may not be obvious in deep joints, such as the hip and spine.

Investigative procedures

X-ray is diagnostic. Two views, an AP and lateral, must be taken to clearly identify the dislocation. Some joints may reduce spontaneously and in this situation 'stress' views are taken, and a significantly widened joint space indicates that the ligaments have been torn, and will require treatment.

Medical and surgical management

The aim is to reduce the dislocation as soon as possible to lessen pain and restore joint function.

Closed reduction should be performed as soon as possible following an injury, so that muscle spasm will support the reduced joint rather than prevent relocation. For small joints this may be achieved without anaesthetic. For larger joints, a general anaesthetic is required to relax the muscles and prevent pain.

Open reduction. This is necessary if the joint cannot be reduced by closed reduction, or if there is an associated fracture into the joint. Torn ligaments and the joint capsule are repaired during open reduction. Following reduction, the joint is immobilized for approximately 4–6 weeks. Immobilization may only be required to prevent movement in the direction which caused the initial injury. Early active movement in all other directions may be ordered to prevent adhesions developing in and around the joint and causing contractures. Movement also helps to repair damaged articular cartilage.

Aspiration of the haemarthrosis may be required as the presence of blood in the joint will destroy articular cartilage and cause adhesions.

Nursing management

First aid. With the exception of the elbow, dislocated joints should be placed in as near normal alignment as possible and immobilized. Small finger joints may be immediately reduced by applying a gentle traction force.

A dislocated elbow should be immobilized in the position in which it is found, providing the blood supply to the hand and fingers is adequate. This is because the olecranon process may have been fractured and be mobile within the joint; straightening the joint may lead to damage to blood vessels and nerves. If the blood supply to the hand and fingers is severely compromised, there is no alternative but to straighten the joint whilst applying traction to the forearm.

Shoulder and elbow dislocations are best supported with the arm strapped against the patient's body. Lower limb dislocations will require the two limbs to be strapped together above and below the knee, with the feet brought into alignment.

The neurovascular status of the limb distal to the dislocation is assessed and recorded.

Ice (cold pack) is applied and the limb elevated if possible.

Following definitive treatment, nursing care centres around the patient's need for pain relief, maintenance of neurovascular integrity and restoration of function, and involves:

1. Care and maintenance of the plaster cast or traction
2. Hourly neurovascular observations for 12–24 hours
3. Elevation of the limb to reduce swelling
4. Application of cold packs to reduce pain and swelling
5. Encouragement of active movement and exercises as ordered.

Physiotherapy is essential to maintain joint motion and prevent stiffness and contractures.

Complications

1. Injury to nerves and blood vessels.
2. Avascular necrosis if blood supply to the joint has been affected.
3. Joint stiffness.
4. Joint instability from ligaments healing in a lengthened position.
5. Recurrent dislocation – this is relatively common following dislocation of the shoulder or patella.
6. Osteoarthritis from damage to the articular surface.
7. Infection if the dislocation has been managed by open reduction.

FRACTURE HEALING

Fractured bone, unlike any other tissue that has been injured is capable of healing without a scar. Bone can regenerate and healing of fractures takes place by the laying down of new bone to unite the fracture ends. When the conditions are favourable, healing proceeds through a number of specific stages.

Stages of fracture healing in long (compact) bone

1. Haematoma formation (Fig. 68.1A). A fracture tears blood vessels at the fracture site and bleeding occurs. Both periosteal and nutrient vessels are torn and contribute to the fracture haematoma. In closed fractures, this haematoma is contained by the surrounding soft tissues. The disruption of blood vessels also results in the death, from ischaemia, of cells adjacent to the fracture ends. Consequently there is always a ring of avascular, dead bone at each surface shortly after injury.

2. Cellular proliferation (Fig. 68.1B). During the first week after injury, the haematoma is invaded and replaced by granulation tissue from the ingrowth of new capillaries. Tissue debris and necrotic bone are removed by phagocytosis. Fibroblasts, chondroblasts and the precursors of osteoblasts from the surrounding connective tissue enter the haematoma and form a fibro-cartilaginous bridge between the bone ends. This is usually formed by the third week and is referred to as 'fibrous' union.

3. Callus formation (Fig. 68.1C). Osteoblasts, from the periosteum and endosteum, then begin to lay down osteoid tissue, which is the intercel-

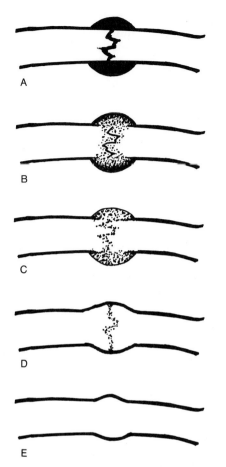

Fig. 68.1 Stages of fracture healing in long bone. **A** – Haematoma formation. **B** – Cellular proliferation. **C** – Callus formation. **D** – Ossification. **E** – Remodelling.

lular matrix of collagen and mucopolysaccaride ground substance. This becomes impregnated with calcium salts, and forms immature bone known as 'primary callus' or 'woven' bone. This callus forms a bridge between the fracture ends, is visible on X-ray, and may be felt as a hard mass. While united, the bone still requires protection, and the fracture line is still seen on X-ray.

4. Consolidation – ossification (Fig. 68.1D). The primary callus is gradually replaced by mature bone, with its typical lamellar structure. At this stage the bone is completely united and no longer requires protection.

5. Remodelling (Fig. 68.1E). In the months that follow consolidation, the bone is gradually strengthened along lines of stress, and surplus bone outside the stress lines is slowly removed by the action of osteoclasts. The medullary cavity is also reformed at the fracture site. This process takes 1–2 years in children and is usually perfect, but in adults the process is slower and the fracture site may be permanently marked by a thickened area.

Factors which influence fracture healing

Type of bone. Cancellous bone heals much more rapidly than compact bone. Because the bone is of a spongy texture and has no medullary cavity, there is a broad area of contact between the fragments and union occurs directly between the bone surfaces. For example, a fracture of the midshaft of the tibia may take 3–4 months to heal while an ankle fracture takes 6–8 weeks.

Bones of the upper limb heal in approximately half the time of those of the lower limb.

Type of fracture. A spiral or oblique fracture heals more rapidly than a transverse fracture, mainly due to the fact that there is a larger fracture haematoma and fracture surface.

Age of person. Children's bones heal in approximately half the adult time. This is because the osteogenic layer of the periosteum is already active being involved in growth. Primary callus may be visible as early as 2 weeks and consolidation in 4–6 weeks in young children. In adults age has little effect on the rate of union: the bones of a person of 65 years will heal at the same rate as those of a person of 25, all other factors being equal.

Blood supply to bone. Inadequate blood supply always delays healing, and may result in nonunion. Avascular necrosis of bone occurs if the blood supply is completely cut off. In the elderly, avascular necrosis of the head of the femur commonly occurs following subcapital fractures of the femur. Other bones which are likely to become avascular following fractures are the scaphoid in the wrist, and the talus in the foot.

Proximity of bone ends. The closer the fractured ends, the more effective the healing. Undisplaced fractures having an intact periosteal sleeve heal twice as rapidly as displaced fractures.

Immobilization. Not all fractures need rigid immobilization, for example, ribs, skull, greenstick. However, rotary and shearing movements between the fracture ends will prevent the normal stages of healing taking place by repeatedly tearing the tiny capillaries.

Diet. To facilitate healing, the diet should be sufficient in protein, calcium, vitamin C and iron.

Infection. Infection of the bone at the fracture site will usually result in delayed or non-union.

FRACTURES

A fracture is a break in a bone. Bones are surrounded by soft tissues, and the forces required to break the bone will result in some degree of soft tissue injury as well. A fracture can vary from an incomplete crack through a bone to a break in which the bone is fragmented and the pieces completely separated.

Causes

1. Violence. A fracture is most commonly caused by excessive violence which may be:
– Direct. The bone breaks at the site of impact (for example, when a car strikes a leg and fractures the tibia).
– Indirect. The bone breaks some distance from the site of impact. A fall on the outstretched hand may fracture the clavicle, or a twisting force applied to the foot may cause a fracture of the tibia and fibula.
2. Repeated continual minor stress which fatigues the bone and causes it to break. These fractures are known as stress or fatigue fractures and are becoming more common as more people become involved in strenuous physical fitness activities, especially jogging. The bones usually affected are the metatarsals, tibia and fibula.
3. Disease of bone. A bone that is already weakened by disease often breaks under a minor force. This is termed pathological fracture and may result from diseases such as osteoporosis, neoplasms of bone, and osteogenesis imperfecta.

Classification

Fractures are classified as closed (simple) or open (compound). Closed fractures are those in which there is no communication between the fracture

and the exterior of the body. Open fractures occur where there is a wound leading down to the site of the fracture. These may be caused by bone ends penetrating the skin or from an object piercing the skin and breaking the bone.

Open fractures carry the serious risk of becoming complicated by infection.

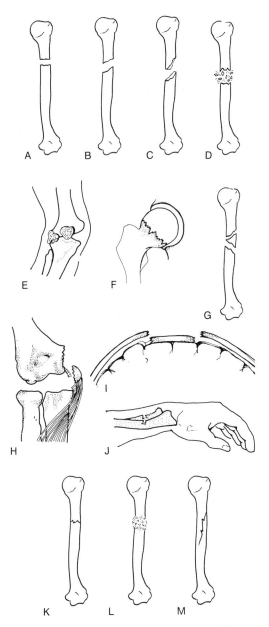

Fig. 68.2 Fracture types. **A** – Transverse. **B** – Oblique. **C** – Spiral. **D** – Comminuted. **E** – Compressed. **F** – Impacted. **G** – Segmental. **H** – Avulsion. **I** – Depressed. **J** – Greenstick. **K** – Stress. **L** – Pathologic. **M** – Longitudinal.

Types of fractures (Fig. 68.2) are:

1. Transverse – a fracture straight across a bone
2. Oblique – a fracture occurring at an angle
3. Spiral – a fracture twisting around a bone
4. Comminuted – a fracture where there are more than two fragments within the fracture site
5. Compressed – the bone is crushed and the fracture comminuted. Occurs in cancellous bone
6. Impacted – a fracture in which the fragments are driven into each other; a feature of this fracture is shortening of the limb
7. Segmental – where the bone is broken into 3 distinct parts with a loose portion of bone between the two fractures
8. Avulsion – a fracture through the bone at the insertion of a ligament or tendon
9. Depressed – a broken bone driven inwards, for example, many skull fractures are depressed.
10. Greenstick – incomplete break in bones of children where the bone is fractured on one side and buckled on the other
11. Stress (fatigue) – a fracture that occurs as a transverse crack in the bone without displacement; most commonly due to repeated pounding stress. Often seen in sports-people.
12. Pathologic – a fracture occurring through a tumour in the bone; most commonly due to metastases
13. Longitudinal – a linear crack in the bone without displacement; most commonly seen in the elderly.

Fractures are also referred to in terms of their location on the bone. They may be proximal, middle or distal fractures; they may occur through the body or neck of the bone; they may be intracapsular (within the joint) or extracapsular (outside the joint).

Fractures can be displaced, undisplaced, angulated, or rotated. As previously mentioned, the forces that cause a fracture always produce some degree of soft tissue injury. A fracture is complicated if it causes damage to major blood vessels, nerves or internal organs.

Clinical manifestations

The clinical features of a fracture will vary, depending on whether the fracture is open or closed, displaced or undisplaced, occurring in a joint, or in the shaft of a long bone. A fracture of the tibia caused by direct violence will have many more observable features than an undisplaced compression fracture of the vertebra caused by indirect violence.

Clinical features of a fracture include local and general manifestations.

Local manifestations

1. Pain may be throbbing, localized and aggravated by movement
2. Loss of normal function results from pain and the instability of the broken bone
3. Deformity, produced by displacement of the bone. This is not always present
4. Swelling results from extravasation of blood from the bone, and soft tissue damage around the fracture site
5. Bruising may not be an immediate sign but is usually apparent after a few days
6. Abnormal movement – may be demonstrated by moving the two ends of the fracture
7. Crepitus – the grating sensation felt when the fragments move upon each other

Tests for crepitus and abnormal movement should *not* be undertaken, as they are extremely painful and can produce further tissue damage.

General manifestations

The broken bone is part of a person. It is important to look for evidence of:

1. Shock from blood loss and pain
2. Haemorrhage. Bleeding from a femoral shaft fracture may be as much as 1–1.5 l, and if the fracture is open may be even greater
3. Associated damage to the brain, spinal cord, viscera, major arteries, or nerves.

Investigative procedures

History – an accurate medical and nursing history, including a description of the possible cause of the fracture is invaluable.

X-ray – at least two views at right angles to each other are essential. A fracture can easily be missed if only one view is taken.

CT scanning may be necessary to identify fractures in complex regions, such as the spine.

Medical, surgical and nursing management

The aim of treatment is to:

- Restore optimum function of the injured part
- Restore as near as possible the normal appearance of the injured part
- Prevent complications of the injury and also of the treatment.

Treatment of fractures falls into the following categories:

1. Emergency management
2. Reduction
3. Immobilization
4. Restoration of function
5. Rehabilitation.

Emergency management

The first aid treatment a person with a fracture receives at the site of the accident is very important, as incorrect handling can cause serious tissue damage; increase pain, haemorrhage and shock; and turn a relatively uncomplicated fracture into a complicated one.

Open fractures must be immediately covered with a dressing to prevent further contamination by bacteria and so lessen the risk of osteomyelitis occurring.

Splinting. The fractured limb should be immobilized prior to the patient being moved. This is best done by a splint which extends from the joints to above and below the fracture. Inflatable air splints, Hare traction splints, and spinal boards are commonly used commercial splints, and are part of the standard equipment of every ambulance. If these are unavailable, any flat board, golf stick, cricket bat, pillow or rolled up newspaper makes a very effective splint. Using the unaffected leg as a splint for a lower limb fracture or the chest wall for an upper limb fracture is also an acceptable way of immobilization prior to transport to hospital. When splinting a fracture, apply gentle traction to the limb below the fracture and bandage the limb firmly to the splint, protecting all bony prominences by padding. Splinting pro-

tects the fracture and prevents further displacement by muscle spasm. No attempt should be made to reduce the fracture.

Elevation. Once the fracture is immobilized the limb should be elevated to aid venous drainage and lessen the swelling.

Observation. The neurovascular status of the limb distal to the fracture must be assessed and regularly observed. Circulation may have been impaired, initially by the fracture or later by the bandage being applied too tightly.

Reduction of the fracture

Reduction is the method by which the displaced bone fragments are brought back into anatomical position. Its aims are to restore bone length, to regain correct alignment, and to provide good apposition of the bone ends.

In reducing a fracture it is much more important to regain correct alignment than to have perfect apposition (Fig. 68.3) and many undisplaced fractures will not need reduction but only protection until union takes place.

Reduction is usually performed under anaesthesia, general or regional, to relieve pain and provide muscle relaxation.

Closed reduction. This is the method of bringing the bones together by manual traction and manipulation. It is the most common method of treatment for the majority of fractures, and the reduction is held by some form of external splint or traction device until healing has occurred.

Closed reduction and internal fixation. After reduction by closed manipulation, some long bone fractures are held by the insertion of an intramedullary rod or nail. This rod is inserted via an incision in the distal or proximal extremity of the bone and directed through the medullary cavity under vision of an image intensifier. The fracture site has not been exposed so this method is

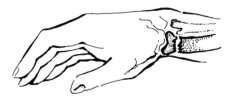

Fig. 68.3 Alignment without apposition in Colles fracture.

referred to as closed nailing. Even though the fracture site has not been exposed there is still the possibility of introducing infection to the bone via the intramedullary rod.

Open reduction. Open reduction is the surgical exposure of the fracture site and the bone ends, which are brought together in apposition and alignment under direct vision.

The reduction is held by internal fixation devices such as metal pins, screws, wires, plates, nails, or rods, until solid bony union has occurred. The metal is usually removed once the fracture has completely healed.

The choice of the internal fixation device depends on the site and type of fracture. For example, a fractured shaft of the femur will have an intramedullary nail inserted, while a fractured neck of the femur will be fixed with a plate and screw.

Internal fixation provides rigidity and enables restoration of normal bone alignment under direct vision. The joints above and below the fracture can be kept fully mobile and early mobilization with weight bearing commenced. The time in hospital is shortened and the patient is able to return to work sooner. Internal fixation may also be associated with external splinting by a plaster cast.

Open reduction converts a closed fracture into an open fracture and so exposes the bone to the risk of infection. It also necessitates the patient having a second anaesthetic later for the removal of the metal. Because of these risk factors, open reduction is undertaken only when there are justifiable indications, for example:

1. Closed reduction may be impossible because of muscle or other soft tissue interposed between the bone ends
2. Precise reduction is essential in certain fractures involving the joint surface, and in fractures involving the growth plate in children
3. Economically and socially it may be unrealistic to keep a patient in hospital for 3–6 months in traction, when open reduction with rigid fixation will have the patient home and back to work in a month
4. Early mobilization is required, especially in the elderly following fractures of the neck of the femur.

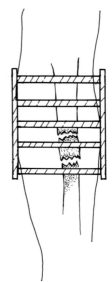

Fig. 68.4 External fixation.

Immobilization

This is the method of holding the fracture in its reduced position until adequate healing has occurred. The aims are to aid healing by preventing displacement, angulation or movement of the bone ends, and to relieve pain. The common methods of immobilization are:

- Plaster of Paris or synthetic casts
- Continuous traction, either fixed or sliding
- Internal fixation.
- External skeletal fixation (Fig. 68.4) may be used when there is severe soft tissue damage associated with open fractures. This device offers rigid immobilization and allows for the wound to be attended to frequently, without disturbing the fracture. Because of the large number of pins inserted into the bone, the complication of pin track infection is a possibility that needs constant observation and care.

Restoration of function

This includes the preservation of function while the fracture is healing.

Treatment is an ongoing process and must begin as soon as the fracture has been reduced. This involves physiotherapy to the immobilized limb and to all other muscles and joints to maintain muscle strength and prevent muscle wasting and joint stiffness. Physiotherapy usually includes:

1. Active isotonic and isometric (or static) exercises to muscles not immobilized.
2. Active isometric exercises to the muscles overlying the fracture. This involves forcefully contracting and relaxing a muscle without moving the joint.
3. Active range of motion exercises to all joints not immobilized. These must be done daily. Passive range of motion exercises are only required if the patient has a nerve palsy or is otherwise unable to participate in his care programme, for example, the patient with head injuries.

Rehabilitation

This is the process of restoring the person to his home, family, community and the workforce with the best possible function. This must be the goal of every member of the health care team and must be borne in mind from the moment of that person's entry into the health care system.

Temporary or permanent splinting may be necessary to assist in the function of the limb, for example, a foot drop splint following injury to the common peroneal nerve.

Occupational therapy may be required if retraining in activities of daily living is necessary.

Vocational and educational retraining may be necessary if function is not restored sufficiently to enable the person to return to his previous position of employment. Home modifications such as rails for bath, shower and toilet, or a ramp and widened doors, may be necessary for the person who requires a wheelchair or walking frame for mobility.

Counselling in marriage, sex and interpersonal relationships may be required for the person who has a permanent physical disability.

The emphasis in rehabilitation must always centre on the function the patient has and not on what he has lost.

Management of open fractures

Compound fractures are those which have communicated with the external invironment. They are caused by violent forces and most commonly involve contact of the bone with road surfaces, gravel and soil. The periosteum will have been torn therefore interruption to the blood supply of the bone occurs. As a consequence there will be an area of necrosis which, although it may be small, will provide an ideal medium for the growth of invading pathogens, particularly anaerobic bacteria. Thus the treatment involves:

Cleansing and debridement of the wound. The patient is transferred to the operating room as soon as practicable following any necessary resuscitative measures. The wound is thoroughly cleaned, tiny bone fragments are removed, the fracture is realigned and where possible the periosteum is drawn together. The wound is then dressed and the limb immobilized. If the wound is extensive and the fracture comminuted this is best achieved by an external fixation device.

Fluid and electrolytes should be replaced as for any patient who has undergone major trauma (see page 109). If blood has been lost then whole blood must be replaced. Plasma expanders may be used in the emergency situation.

Delayed primary closure. In some instances of compound fracture, where there has been a significant soft tissue loss delayed primary closure may be instituted (see page 58).

Antibiotic drugs to combat infection are given intravenously and in very large doses. Therefore the patient will have a central venous line in situ.

Prophylactic therapy in opposition to the invasion of *Clostridium perfringens* and/or tetani must be undertaken if the patient is considered at risk. Therefore anti-gas gangrene serum or tetanus immunoglobulin may be used in previously unprotected persons. Usually, however, tetanus toxoid is given simply as a booster.

Relief of pain. Narcotic analgesia will be required to alleviate pain and reduce shock.

Orthopaedic surgical procedures

Orthopaedic surgical procedures can be divided into the following areas:

- Bone shaft surgery
- Neck of bone surgery
- Epiphiseal surgery
- Joint surgery
- Joint replacement surgery.

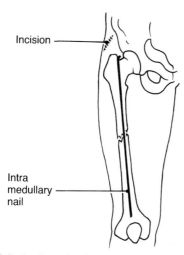

Incision

Intra medullary nail

Fig. 68.5 Reduction using intramedullary nail.

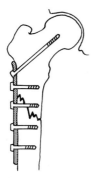

Fig. 68.6 Open reduction using screws and plate.

Bone shaft surgery. The commonest form of bone shaft surgery is the open reduction of fractures. This is done predominantly in one of two ways. Either an intramedullary nail is hammered through the medullary space from a point some centimetres proximal to the fracture, through the fracture site and into the distal medullary space (Fig. 68.5); or a plate is affixed to the proximal and distal pieces of bone, over the fracture site via the use of screws (Fig. 68.6). In some instances of fracture where bone shaft is missing, either through direct trauma or surgical removal of necrotic bone, bone grafting may be necessary to replace the missing tissue. The donor site for this bone is usually the ileum or a rib.

Neck of bone surgery. This usually applies to the neck of the femur but it may apply to the neck of any bone. It is not uncommon for avascular necrosis to occur in the head of the bone affected.

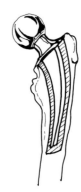

Fig. 68.7 Prosthetic head and neck of femur.

This necessitates the replacement of the head and neck of the bone with a prosthesis (Fig. 68.7). If the blood supply to the bone head is intact then fractures of the neck may be corrected by the use of plates and screws.

Epiphyseal surgery. A fracture of the epiphysis is not uncommon in children and young adults. It is usually immobilized by pinning through the epiphysis. Damage to an epiphysis may result in lack of bone growth and therefore permanent shortening of the limb involved.

Joint surgery. This can be further divided into extracapsular and intracapsular surgery.

Extracapsular surgery predominantly involves tendons and ligaments and is commonly used in the treatment of sporting injuries. Basically, surgery is aimed at either shortening stretched tendons or ligaments, or reimplanting them should they be torn from their point of attachment. Transplantation of a tendon to assume the function of damaged tissue at another location can also be performed.

Intracapsular surgery can be used following articular trauma, to correct joint deformities or to treat arthritis. The types of intracapsular joint surgery commonly performed are:

● Arthroscopy – visualizing the interior of a joint using an arthroscope (Fig. 68.8). This surgery is performed routinely nowadays for the repair of torn menisci or cruciate ligaments of the knee joint.
● Synovectomy – excision of synovial membrane. It is used in the early management of rheumatoid arthritis, especially of the hands.
● Arthroplasty – formation of an artificial joint or the implantation of a new articulating surface.

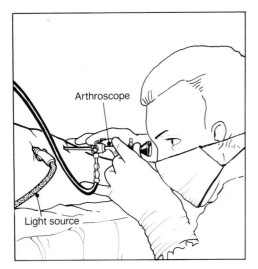

Fig. 68.8 Arthroscopy.

• Arthrodesis – the fixation of a joint by surgery, also known as artificial ankylosis.

Joint replacement surgery. In joint replacement surgery one or both of the articulating surfaces of the involved joint are removed and replaced with an artificial material. The range of materials include metals such as stainless steel, vitallium, titanium, or substances such as silastin, teflon or plastics. Weight bearing joints (hips and knees) are commonly replaced when the patient suffers the severe pain, joint deformity and immobility of either rheumatoid arthritis or osteoarthritis. Less commonly, the shoulder joint, the finer joints of the hand, and the elbow are replaced. The specific nursing management of the patient following joint replacement surgery is covered on page 719.

Specific nursing management of the patient with a fracture

Nursing management of the patient following open reduction is similar to that for the patient following any orthopaedic surgery and may also involve the care of a patient in a plaster cast or traction.

The patient's physical status will vary greatly, depending on the type of injury and the method of treatment. The patient may be quite physically well despite his fracture or joint trauma (as in sporting injuries), or his fracture may accompany other major tissue and/or organ damage. It may also be accompanied by extreme shock which has required vigorous resuscitation (as in multiple trauma following a motor vehicle accident). As well the fracture or joint injury may have occurred in an elderly patient who has co-existing disease of the cardiovascular or respiratory systems.

The principles of nursing care are to:

– Manage pain
– Promote healing
– Prevent infection
– Prevent postoperative complications.

The nurse must be prepared to meet the needs of a person:
• Who has an extensive wound, over a joint or on a limb, and associated drain tubes, both of which may result in extreme discomfort and/or pain. The patient initially requires narcotic analgesics for a period normally ranging from 24–96 hours postoperatively. Minor analgesics may be required for some time; aspirin is the best of the minor analgesics for the relief of pain originating from bone. Additionally, sedatives may be required in the first few nights following surgery, to ensure adequate pain free sleep.
• Whose wound dressing will require frequent observation to detect the early signs of infection and/or wound breakdown. Ideally the wound should be dressed and then not disturbed until sutures are removed. Unnecessarily disturbing a wound dressing results in destruction of granulating tissue and therefore longer healing time and poor cosmetic result, and the possibility of introducing infection. The wound dressing may be reinforced once if exudate is profuse; however, if exudation continues the wound should be inspected and redressed. The patient may have a plaster cast applied to the limb with a window cut over the wound to facilitate easy access for inspection and/or dressing. Low pressure drain tubes are frequently inserted along the operative site through individual stab wounds. These must be kept patent at all times and are usually removed 48–72 hours postoperatively. All precautions must be taken to ensure that the wound is maintained in an aseptic manner, as localized bony necrosis is an ideal culture medium for bacterial growth which may result in osteomyelitis (see page 736).

• Whose fluid balance may have been disturbed by the operative and peri-operative periods. The patient will usually return from surgery with an intravenous line in situ for the administration of fluid for the next 24–72 hours. Blood may also be transfused if large volumes of blood were lost at the accident site or during the operative procedure.

• Who will need assistance to return to optimal physical function as soon as practicable. The patient should be encouraged to perform isometric exercises with the affected limb and active exercises with all other limbs. Weight bearing will be commenced as soon as possible following surgery and this will be determined by: the type of surgery performed; the age and physical condition of the patient; and whether or not traction and/or plaster of paris casts have been used.

PLASTER CASTS

While there are many new forms of external splints available, the plaster of Paris cast still remains the standard method of immobilization for most fractures. It is relatively cheap, easy to apply and remove, and is able to be moulded to limb and body contours. Plaster of Paris is a chalky white powder, derived from the naturally occurring mineral, gypsum (anhydrous calcium sulphate). It is incorporated into gauze bandages of varying widths for ease of application. When the plaster is immersed, it absorbs water and a chemical reaction occurs to form long, slender crystals of hydrated calcium sulphate which interlock with each other through the layers of gauze to form a rigid cast.

During this reaction as the plaster sets, heat is generated and the plaster feels very warm. This 'setting' phase takes from 3–10 minutes, and if movement occurs during this time, the crystal formations will be disrupted and the cast will weaken. Moulding is performed during this stage. A newly set plaster still contains much water which must evaporate before the cast attains its full strength.

Plaster casts take from 24–72 hours to dry completely, depending on the size of the cast. A dry plaster is resonant on percussion.

Circumferential plaster bandages or slabs of the appropriate size are used. Slabs are often used in place of circular plaster bandages when excessive swelling is anticipated (for example, fractured wrist). Slabs are also used to strengthen a plaster at points of stress.

'Stockinette' is used as a lining to protect the skin. Wool padding is required to protect bony prominences from pressure, and is always used under the plaster when swelling is expected following a new fracture or after surgery.

The tepid water used for immersion of the plaster bandage should be changed frequently or the bandages will not take up water evenly, because of the build up of plaster sediment.

Plastic covered pillows and sandbags are used to support the wet cast, and foot or arm supports are used to support the limb.

Adequate explanation should be given to the patient regarding the extent of the plaster, the necessity to hold the limb still during application, and the need to relax the limb completely. Relaxation is important as tense muscles will alter the shape of the limb and result in a plaster that does not fit correctly.

The patient should be warned that the plaster will feel hot while it sets, and that later it will feel cold and heavy while it dries.

The skin should be clean and dry and closely examined for abrasions, bruising, cuts, or pimples. These must be reported and documented and adequate treatment given prior to the application of the cast. This is important, as it will assist in later evaluation should the patient complain of pain or tenderness under the cast.

Rings must be removed as a ring may act as a tourniquet if swelling occurs.

All nail polish should be removed to allow for accurate assessment of vascular sufficiency. Analgesic or narcotic medication may be required to relieve pain and apprehension.

The plaster bandage is immersed in the water and held until bubbling has ceased. Only one roll is immersed at any one time. It is then held at the ends and gently squeezed towards the centre to remove excess water. The operator applies the bandage smoothly in a spiral fashion without tension. Moulding is done with the palms of the hands, and the plaster is constantly smoothed to create one homogeneous mass. On completion, the edges are trimmed and smoothed and the joints proximal and distal to the plaster cast are checked for full range of movement.

Nursing care following application of a plaster cast

Excess plaster should be removed, as the particles may fall inside the cast and cause skin irritation and pressure.

Pillows are used to support the wet cast and to ensure even pressure during the drying period. When lifting a wet cast, care must be taken to ensure even spread of pressure (for example, using the palms of the hands) and the cast must never be lifted directly onto a hard surface. This will cause the cast to be flattened over bony prominences (for example, heel), and cause damage to the underlying skin.

A full leg plaster must be supported its entire length with the heel off the pillow. An arm plaster is fully supported on a pillow or in a wide arm sling.

A patient with a hip spica requires 3 pillows laid crosswise on the bed and 2 lengthwise to support the single leg in the cast. No sharp breaks should occur in the pillow alignment as this could cause the plaster to sag.

Elevation of the limb is required until swelling has resolved and the patient is instructed to elevate his arm or leg during periods of rest.

Instruct the patient not to attempt to move the joints encased in the plaster while the plaster is wet, as this will crack and weaken the cast.

A plaster is best dried by exposure to the air. Rapid drying with the use of heaters or hair dryers may burn the patient or cause the cast to crack. Ideally, a wet plaster should be fully exposed to the air and bed cradles should be used to take the weight of bed linen. However, the patient must be kept warm with special attention paid to the extremities. A plaster cast of a limb takes approximately 48 hours to dry and hip spicas and body jackets up to 72 hours. Absorbent material must be used under a drying cast to prevent sweating, otherwise the plaster will remain soggy. Patients in body jackets and hip spicas must be turned 2–3

hourly to assist in drying. When the cast is completely dry the patient may commence to bear weight.

Observation

Nursing observations of the patient will need to be carried out frequently whilst the plaster is setting and drying, and whilst any soft tissue swelling persists.

Extremities are checked for signs of neurovascular impairment and this is assessed by:

1. *Colour.* The colour of all extremities should be normal and this is best assessed by comparing with the opposite limb, as elderly people may have some degree of peripheral vascular disease and the nurse needs to assess what is normal for that person. To assess capilliary return the nail is compressed and released. The nail should blanch and colour should return to normal within 1–2 seconds. If this reaction is slow, then circulation is impaired and should be reported. Cyanosed and swollen extremities are indicative of impaired venous return, while pale, cold digits are an indication of arterial impairment.

2. *Warmth.* A good blood supply is indicated by warmth. However, this is not a reliable sign while the plaster is wet, as digits may feel cold due to the damp cast. Again, the nurse should compare warmth with the opposite limb.

3. *Movement.* The patient should be able to freely move extremities; swelling of the limb may preclude normal movement. Swelling is caused by: inadequate venous return from a dependent limb, a tight plaster or excessive oedema occurring within the soft tissues surrounding the fracture. If swelling does not decrease in response to elevation and exercise, it may be necessary for the plaster cast to be split.

4. *Sensation.* The feeling in each digit is checked separately. The patient should be able to identify the toe or finger without looking.

Abnormal sensations indicating nerve damage are:
– paraesthesia: pins and needles, tingling
– hyperaesthesia – increased sensation
– hypoaesthesia – decreased sensation
– anaesthesia – no sensation; numb.

Impairment of nerve function within a cast can arise from direct pressure of the cast on a superficial nerve, for example, common peroneal nerve at the fibula head; or ischaemia from a tight cast jeopardizing the circulation.

5. *Pain.* Complaints of pain by a person with a cast should never be ignored. Severe pain is usually an indication of circulatory insufficiency. Accurate assessment needs to be made as to the type, degree and extent of pain and whether elevation, change of position and/or analgesia relieves the pain. If the pain is localized, a window may need to be cut in the plaster to relieve the pressure. The window must be retained and bandaged back in place once the skin has been inspected, otherwise herniation of the soft tissue may occur through the opening, creating further pressure. Generalized, severe pain, together with changes in the neurovascular observations will necessitate splitting of the plaster cast along its full length, including division of the underlying/protective layers down to skin.

Failure to accurately record and report a patient's pain and neurovascular status may result in necrosis of tissue causing a localized pressure sore or, in extreme cases, loss of the limb.

Remember the '6 Ps' for accurate neurovascular assessment:

Pain
Pallor
Paralysis
Paraesthesia
Puffiness
Pulselessness.

Any discharge or bleeding through the plaster should be recorded and reported. Plaster acts like blotting paper, so a small amount of exudate may require assurance that all is well. Discharge at a site not covering a suture line or wound could indicate a pressure sore and it may be necessary to open the plaster either locally or completely to inspect the underlying tissue

Once swelling has subsided, the cast may become loose. This could cause the fracture to displace and may cause skin irritation from friction. A loose plaster will need reapplication.

All joints not enclosed in the cast must be exercised and moved through their full range at least twice daily. Digits distal to the cast must be actively exercised constantly, to prevent joint stiffness and to reduce swelling. Isometric exercises of muscles within the cast are performed to maintain muscle strength and bulk and prevent muscle atrophy.

Complications of plaster casts

1. Areas of necrosis from a rough or tight plaster.
2. Volkmann's ischaemic contracture (see also page 713). This may occur when a group of muscles have been rendered ischaemic due to excessive swelling within the muscle compartment, or a tight plaster.
3. Gangrene from arterial insufficiency.
4. Nerve damage from local pressure of the cast or from ischaemia.
5. Infection of a wound or pressure sore under the cast.
6. Cast syndrome: nausea, vomiting and abdominal distension. This may occur in the patient in a body jacket or hip spica.
7. Joint stiffness from lack of exercise and long period of immobilization.

For the patient who is allowed home with a new cast, the following instructions are given in writing:

1. Elevate the limb as much as possible during the first week.
2. Exercise extremities every hour by flexing them tightly for a few seconds and then relaxing. This helps to reduce the swelling.
3. Exercise all joints not enclosed in the plaster cast.
4. Do not get the plaster wet.
5. Do not poke objects down inside the cast.

Report immediately to your doctor or casualty if you notice:

1. Marked swelling or discoloration.
2. Severe pain or numbness.
3. Inability to move your fingers or toes

Removal of a plaster cast

The procedure should be explained fully to the patient and the equipment demonstrated. The electric saw is noisy and the blade becomes hot as it cuts through the plaster. This may alarm the patient. Reassure the patient that the saw will not cut or burn. Disposable sheeting is needed to protect the patient's clothing from plaster dust.

The skin under the cast often appears dry with yellow scales from dead skin and exudate. It should be washed gently with warm, soapy water, dried thoroughly, and then oiled and the patient informed that with the regular cleansing and oiling it will return to normal. Muscle wasting is noticed and joints when first moved will be painful and stiff. The patient needs to be told that with exercise and normal use the pain and stiffness will disappear and muscle bulk will be restored. Physiotherapy may be necessary.

Swelling will occur after the cast is removed, especially if the limb is allowed to be dependent. An elasticized bandage or stocking may be required initially to support the lower limb and prevent reactive oedema. The period of time that this is worn is reduced each day and it should not be necessary after a week. Full activity should be resumed as early as possible, and the patient informed that once the fracture has healed the bone returns to its original strength.

SYNTHETIC CASTS

These casts are made of fibreglass, polyurethane, or isoprene rubber and have demonstrable advantages and disadvantages over the use of plaster of paris. The advantages include:

– They set quickly and achieve maximum strength within 30 minutes of application, and weight bearing can be allowed almost immediately.
– They are light in weight and less bulky. This is useful in an elderly patient, whose mobility would be restricted by the weight of a plaster of paris cast.
– They are water repellent and immersion does not weaken the cast. However, if swimming or bathing is allowed, it must be ensured that the inner lining and padding of the cast is also synthetic and that the patient has the use of a blow dryer for drying the lining and padding. This must be done thoroughly, otherwise skin irritation and excoriation will occur.

– They do not crumble or crack and do not need to be replaced.
– They can be easily cleaned by wiping with a moist cloth and mild soap.

The disadvantages of synthetic casts include:

– They are very costly and this has restricted their use.
– They are also not as easily moulded as a plaster cast.
– The outer surface of fibreglass casts are rough and may damage the skin of the other limb, snag clothing and scratch furniture. In some cases a cast may consist of plaster of Paris and an outer layer of synthetic material applied to strengthen the cast. This cast must not be immersed in water.

TRACTION

Traction is one of the methods used for immobilizing a fracture. There are, however, many other purposes for which traction is used:

● To immobilize and maintain alignment following a fracture.
● To reduce a fracture
● To prevent or overcome muscle spasm and so reduce deformity and pain, and therefore prevent necrosis of bone ends under extreme pressure
● To rest an inflamed joint
● To correct joint deformity
● Attempt to stretch muscles and ligaments prior to surgery on a joint.

Traction is the method of exerting a pulling force to a part of the body. To be effective there must be an equal and opposite pull – countertraction – otherwise the patient will continually slide in the direction of the traction rendering the procedure ineffectual. Traction is usually continuous, with the pull being maintained without interruption. Intermittent traction may be ordered for the patient who has pelvic traction applied for low back pain syndrome, or halter traction applied for cervical spondylosis.

Manual traction is applied when a fracture is being reduced. Manual traction is also used while skin traction is being re-applied, and when moving a person who has suffered trauma to a bone or the spinal column.

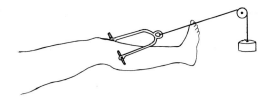

Fig. 68.9 Sliding traction (with skeletal pin).

Skin traction. The traction force is exerted on the skin via extension strapping, and is transferred to the underlying muscles and bone. Adhesive or nonadhesive strapping is used.

Skeletal traction. The traction force is applied directly to bone via metal pins such as Steinmann or Denham pins, Gardner-Wells tongs and halo pins.

After skin or skeletal traction has been applied, it takes the form of either fixed or sliding traction. With fixed traction the pull is exerted between two fixed points. For example, fixed traction in a Thomas splint. The traction cords are tied to the end of the splint beyond the foot. The opposite end of the splint – the ring – rests well up in the groin and fits snugly around the limb. These are the two fixed points. (see Fig. 68.12, page 711).

With sliding traction the traction force is exerted on a part of the body which lies between two mobile points. In sliding traction of the lower limb, the traction force is applied to the leg through adhesive strapping or a skeletal pin, with the cords passing over a pulley attached to freely hanging weights (Fig. 68.9).

The countertraction is the patient's body weight. The foot of the bed must be elevated as the traction will become ineffective if the weights are allowed to rest on the floor.

Skin traction

Adhesive or nonadhesive extension strapping may be used to achieve skin traction. The extension strapping is applied over as large a skin area as possible. This distributes the load and provides for greater patient comfort and traction efficiency (Fig. 68.10). The amount of weight that is used is dependent on what the skin can tolerate. The maximum traction weight that can be safely applied to skin of the lower limb in adults is 4.5 kg for approximately 3–4 weeks. However, this varies considerably according to the size and

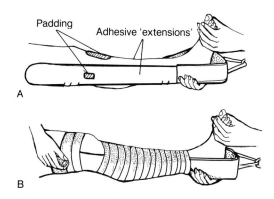

Fig. 68.10 Skin traction. Manual traction is maintained until apparatus is set up. **A** – Padding and extensions in place. **B** – Bandaging. (From Taylor, 1987.)

age of the patient, the condition of the skin and the amount of skin to be covered.

Indications for the use of skin traction

These include:

- Fractures in children. Less weight is needed to maintain alignment and less total time in traction is required. Children's bones heal in approximately half adult time.
- Disorders of the acetabulum and femur in children and adults, for example, inflamed hip joint.
- Hip fractures in adults as a temporary measure to reduce pain and muscle spasm prior to treatment with internal fixation.

Contraindications for the use of skin traction

Adhesive skin traction should not be used in the following situations:

- Abrasions, lacerations or pustules on the skin of the affected limb.
- Patients with peripheral vascular disease.
- Fragile skin, for example, rheumatoid patient on long-term corticosteroid therapy, or the very elderly.
- A patient with any disease of the skin.
- Any patient who has a sensory loss.

Complications of skin traction

- Allergic reaction to the adhesive strapping
- Tearing or blistering of the skin from too much weight

- Total degloving injury
- Pressure sores over bony prominences and from wrinkles or creases in the strapping or bandage
- Nerve palsy from pressure, strapping, or bandages over a superficial nerve
- Circulatory impairment from a constricting bandage.

Nursing management

Specific nursing care of the patient in skin traction is related to preventing the above complications, and involves:

1. Observation of the skin for signs of allergy, itchiness, blistering or pressure necrosis
2. Observation of the neurovascular state of the limb
3. Pain. Any complaint of pain must be assessed, recorded and reported. Local pressure or circulatory impairment may be the cause
4. Daily washing of the limb in traction to ensure that the skin is kept clean and healthy
5. Daily reapplication of the bandage to ensure that the strapping is kept in apposition
6. Regular reapplication of the skin traction apparatus. This is usually performed weekly unless a hypoallergenic strapping is used.

Skeletal traction

Skeletal traction is traction applied directly to bone by using pins, wires or screws through the bone. In cervical traction tongs are applied to the skull (Fig. 68.11).

Indications for the use of skeletal traction are:

- Fractures in adults where large traction forces are required for long periods. Weights of 8–10 kg may be used for as long as 3–4 months
- Where the use of skin traction is unsafe, for example, patients with thin skin.

Skeletal traction may be applied to almost any bone but the most common sites are: proximal end of the tibia for fractures of the femur; calcaneus for tibial fractures; olecranon process for fractures around the elbow; and the skull for cervical spine injuries. The pins are connected to the traction force by hooks or a stirrup.

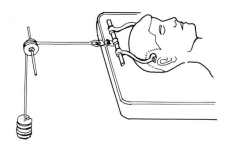

Fig. 68.11 Skeletal traction via cervical tongs.

Complications of skeletal traction

These are potentially serious, and include:

- Infection of the pin track. Pin sites are initially covered with gauze dressings of tincture of benzoin compound or povidone iodine to prevent the entry of microorganisms. Once the wounds are sealed and dry, the dressings may be removed and the sites frequently inspected for signs of infection. Infection is recognised locally by redness, swelling, discharge and local tenderness. Tenderness over the bone between the pin sites may be the first sign of pin track infection. A pin or screw inserted into or through a bone should not, normally, be painful or tender.
- Slipping and rotating of the pin. If the pin rotates or slides back and forth within the bone, the track will be widened, and a serous discharge will develop and so create an ideal medium for the growth of bacteria.
- Tissue necrosis around the pin sites. This may be caused by the skin pressing against the pin or pressure on the skin from hardened gauze dressings. Gauze swabs saturated with tincture of benzoin compound and blood will become rock hard when dry.
- Nerve palsy. The common peroneal nerve which winds around the head of the fibula may be damaged when the pin is inserted into the tibia, or the nerve may be compressed if the leg rests against the bar of a Thomas' splint.

Nursing management

Specific nursing care of the patient with skeletal traction is related to preventing the above complications.

Aseptic technique must be adhered to when dressings are removed or changed. The patient's skin must be kept clean and the exposed pin, hooks or stirrup kept free from dust by wiping daily with alcohol. The pin should be checked for sliding or rotation and any complaints of pain or tenderness must be reported immediately. The neurovascular state of the limb should be assessed regularly.

Thomas' splint

A Thomas' splint (Fig. 68.12) is often used to suspend a lower limb after traction has been applied. Traction may be fixed or sliding, skin or skeletal. The Thomas' splint assists by elevating and immobilizing the limb.

Nursing management

When caring for a patient in a Thomas' splint, the nurse must:

● Check the ring for tightness and pressure. Prevent pressure sores by moving the skin back and forth under the ring. The patient is taught to do this. The ring should be washed and then oiled daily and the groin area kept free of perspiration.
● Check the slings for tightness and unevenness. These may cause pressure. The Achilles tendon is particularly susceptible to pressure sores from a tight sling.
● Check the alignment of the splint. The splint should be straight, abducted, elevated and suspended correctly.

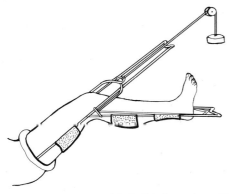

Fig. 68.12 Thomas' splint, with flexible knee piece. (From Taylor, 1987.)

● Check the alignment of the limb, that it is not rotated laterally and resting on the outer bar.
● Supervise exercises. Static quadriceps and active ankle, foot and toe exercises are usually required.

General nursing management of the patient in traction

Once traction has been applied, certain principles must be followed if the treatment is to be effective.

All traction requires a countertraction. If the traction weights are in any way accidentally supported (by the floor, end of bed) effective traction will be lost.

Friction can reduce the effective pull of the traction; therefore, all moving parts must be well lubricated and in good working order.

Traction must always maintain ideal body alignment. The angles are calculated taking into consideration direction of pull (torque and vectors) and muscle bulk of the patient. Nursing activities should be planned so as not to interrupt alignment.

Traction is usually continuous and under no circumstances must it be interrupted. Therefore the nurse must lift the patient smoothly, without jerking the limbs or the traction apparatus, and allow the traction cords to roll smoothly over the pulleys, thus maintaining the correct pull. Conversely, the weight must never be removed, even momentarily, as this may cause the bone ends to slam together, thus undoing days or weeks of work.

Traction must maintain good body alignment. A firm mattress and bed base is required. Mouldable, soft pillows are needed to support the patient's head and shoulders to prevent muscle fatigue. An overhead trapeze is necessary to enable the patient to lift himself.

Traction necessitates that the patient remain in hospital and in bed for a long period of time and care centres around the prevention of the complications of bed rest. The patient is essentially well and can become very bored, frustrated, angry, or depressed by the enforced rest. The nurse must be aware of all the patient's needs and not just those related to the limb in traction and the traction apparatus, and should involve the patient as much as possible in his own care.

Patient education

Noncompliance with treatment is often a result of lack of communication. The patient should be told of his programme during the long and potentially frustrating time in traction. The nurse should also explain the purpose of the traction and how it works, the importance of not interfering with the traction apparatus, and the importance of maintaining the correct position and alignment. The patient should know which positions he may adopt. He must understand the importance of reporting pain, discomfort, itchiness, pressure, numbness or tingling.

The nurse should ensure that the patient understands and adheres to his exercise programme.

Position of the patient

The supine position is required for most tractions. If the patient is allowed to sit up, the nurse must ensure that the line of pull has not altered and that there is still effective countertraction.

Maintenance of the traction apparatus

The nurse should check the cords to see that:

- They are not frayed
- Knots do not impinge on pulleys
- They are correctly positioned over the pulleys.

Weights should:

- Be hanging freely
- Not be knocked or caught against the bed
- Not be lifted up or removed
- Be safe. Knots must be secure and the free end of the knot should be taped to the cord. Weights should not hang over the patient. If a weight has to be positioned over the bed a safety rope is attached from the weight to the overhead bar.

Maintence of skin integrity

The patient must be encouraged to lift himself up with the use of the trapeze 2–3 hourly during the day. This not only prevents pressure sores on the buttocks but also increases the strength of his arm muscles in preparation for crutch walking. Inspect the skin daily and give pressure care 3-hourly to all bony prominences.

The elbow and heel of the unaffected side often become red and sore from continued use. The foot of the leg in traction should be oiled daily to aid the separation of thick skin and prevent the skin from cracking.

Diet

A light diet may be necessary if the patient is nursed in a supine position. A high protein diet with added vitamins C and D aids in bone healing.

Exercises

The complications of chest infection, deep vein thrombosis, pulmonary emboli, joint stiffness, and muscle wasting are prevented by deep breathing and coughing exercises, full range of movement exercises for all uninvolved joints, and muscle strengthening exercises. Exercises of the affected limb must be performed regularly as instructed by the physiotherapist.

Elimination

Urinary. A high fluid intake is necessary to prevent renal calculi and urinary tract infection occurring. Encourage the patient to empty the bladder completely as any residual urine is a focus for infection.

Bowel. Constipation is a common problem of inactivity. Increasing fluids and roughage in the patient's diet will help overcome this problem.

Psychological support

Boredom, frustration, anger and depression are common problems of the patient in traction. Diversional therapy and free access to visitors is important. Involving the patient in his own care and progress is essential. Changing the patient's environment by moving him out onto a balcony, out in the sun for short periods, or just a change of position in the ward, improves his outlook.

COMPLICATIONS OF FRACTURES

Bone complications

Malunion. This occurs when a fracture heals in a position of deformity. Reduction or immobilization of the fracture may not have been adequate, allowing muscle spasm to pull the bone out of alignment. Osteotomy and realignment is usually necessary to correct the deformity.

Delayed union. This occurs when a fracture takes longer to heal than normally expected. It may be caused by: an inadequate blood supply; infection; insufficient splinting, which allowed the bone ends to move; excessive traction which pulls the bone ends apart

Non union. This occurs when the bone ends do not join. On X-ray of this fracture the ends are seen to be widely separated, sclerosed, and rounded. Causes are the same as for delayed union.

Avascular necrosis. If bone is deprived of its blood supply it will die and non union will occur. Certain bones or portions of bone are at particular risk from becoming avascular following a fracture, for example, the head of femur in the elderly, the proximal scaphoid, the lunate and the talus.

Treatment of avascular necrosis and non union is usually surgical and may include bone grafting, electrical stimulation to activate osteoblast activity via a bone growth stimulator, or the removal of the avascular bone and replacement with a prosthesis.

Infection. Open fractures, internal fixation devices, and skeletal pins are all potential sources of infection. Nursing care must be directed to preventing infection in the bone, as any infection in the bone is extremely difficult to eradicate.

Soft tissue complications

Fracture blisters. These sometimes occur when there has been excessive swelling causing superficial layers of skin to be stretched and these are most frequently seen around the elbow or leg.

Nerve injury. Nerves may be damaged by ischaemia, compression, excessive traction, or by complete dissection. Nerves that lie close to bone are at particular risk, for example, radial nerve following fracture of the shaft of humerus, ulnar nerve from fracture of the medial epicondyle of elbow, and common peroneal nerve from fracture of the head of fibula. Nerves have the potential for recovery, but complete dissection may require end to end anastomosis.

Circulatory damage. If a major artery is severed or occluded, the limb distal to the fracture will appear pale, feel cool, and distal pulses will be absent; gangrene will result if treatment is excessively delayed. Treatment includes:

• Splinting to prevent movement
• Cooling to lessen metabolic activity
• Elevation to reduce oedema
• Arteriogram to identify the site of damage and
• Surgery in the form of end to end anastomosis or repair of the artery with a vein graft.

Compartment syndrome occurs when muscles within a closed compartment (in the arm or leg) necrose from insufficient blood supply. Dead muscles will eventually shorten and cause deformity of the joints supplied by that muscle group, (for example, Volkmann's ischaemic contracture is the compartment syndrome of the flexor muscles of the forearm which will result in a claw hand deformity).

Causes of compartment syndrome include arterial damage, and excessive oedema from traumatized muscle or ischaemia. As oedema progresses the pressure inside the compartment increases until the blood supply is completely occluded. The skin overlying the muscle is not affected and peripheral pulses may be present as it is the local blood supply to the muscle group that is initially affected. A rigid plaster cast or tight bandage will aggravate the condition. Permanent joint contracture and deformity will occur if the condition is not recognised and treated early.

Clinical features of compartment syndrome include:

– Severe generalized limb pain

Excruciating pain on passive stretch of the affected muscles (for example, if the forearm flexor muscles are ischaemic, pain will increase if the fingers are moved into extension)
– Swelling
– Paraesthesia
– Paralysis

– Pale or discoloured skin
– The pulse may or may not be present.

Remembering the Ps is a good way of assessing potential compartment syndrome: pain, pallor, puffiness, paraesthesia, paralysis.

Treatment is aimed at relieving the pressure and restoring the circulation. Where a compartment syndrome is suspected the limb is elevated, the physician is notified, and neurovascular observations are undertaken every 15 minutes. If the patient has a plaster cast, it is bi-valved. Tight encircling bandages are removed, distal joints are extended, and the patient is prepared for surgery for a fasciotomy.

A tissue pressure monitoring device may be employed to monitor accurately the pressure within a muscle compartment when it is suspected that this condition may occur. Normally the only pressure within a muscle compartment is that which keeps its blood vessels open, that is 10 mmHg. If tissue pressure rises above this point the blood vessels will close.

Joint stiffness. Immobilized joints will stiffen and there may be a permanent loss of complete range of movement. The elderly patient is more prone to joint stiffening and the use of dynamic splinting may prevent this problem occurring. Joint effusion and haemarthrosis will also result in joint stiffness from adhesions developing within the joint.

Myositis ossificans. This results from calcium being deposited in muscle and most commonly occurs following injuries of the elbow. A haematoma develops in the torn connective tissue of muscle and calcification occurs within the haematoma.

Sudek's atrophy (reflex sympathetic dystrophy). This is a rare, late complication of fracture of the wrist or ankle and is usually only recognized after the plaster has been removed. The hand or foot is swollen, shiny, red and warm. The fingers may have a tapered appearance and movement is restricted and extremely painful. X-ray shows marked localized osteoporosis of bones of the hand or feet. Treatment consists of intensive physiotherapy and the condition may take up to 12 months to resolve.

Osteoarthritis. This is a late complication, which may occur many years after the initial injury, especially where the fracture has been through a joint.

Systemic complications

Fat embolus

Fat embolus occurs when fat droplets circulate in the vascular system and lodge in the microcapillaries of the lungs or the brain, causing a resultant pulmonary oedema and hypoxia. Cerebral emboli cause symptoms similar to those of cerebrovascular accident (see page 174).

While fat emboli occur in almost all patients with multiple, long bone, and pelvic fractures only a small percentage develop symptoms.

Pathophysiology. This is not completely understood but is thought to be a combination of:

• The release of bone marrow fat into the venous circulation
• The mobilization of free fatty acids from adipose tissue subsequent to a catecholamine release. This is seen in major soft tissue injury where bone is not necessarily involved.
• Changes in lipid metabolism resulting in chylomicrons aggregating to form large lipid globules.

These last two effects are thought to be the result of the body's reaction to the stress caused by severe trauma and hypovolaemic shock.

Clinical manifestations. These usually develop 2–3 days after injury but symptoms have been known to occur as early as a few hours to as late as 6 days.

The patient exhibits signs of respiratory distress; the state of consciousness deteriorates and he may become restless, irritable, and disorientated.

He will be pyrexic with an associated tachycardia and multiple petechiae will be seen on the conjunctiva and on the skin of the axilla and chest.

Chest X ray shows multiple opacities with a typical snowstorm appearance.

Blood film shows a sudden fall in haemoglobin; a thrombocytopenia; an elevated serum lipase; free fatty acids will be present in the plasma. Arterial gas analysis will show a low pO_2, a lowered pH, and a raised pCO_2. Sputum and urine will contain frank fat globules.

Medical management. Fat embolism is a self-limiting disease with a high mortality rate which is related directly to the degree of respiratory insufficiency. Treatment is directed to maintaining a satisfactory pulmonary gas exchange through the course of the disease process, and will include:

• Administration of oxygen, and artificial ventilation with a positive pressure ventilator may be required.
• IV diuretics will be ordered to reduce interstitial fluid load on pulmonary oedema, and fluids will be reduced to 1500 ml daily.

Salt and potassium are restricted in the diet and are monitored and corrected IV as necessary.

If the haemoglobin falls below 10 g/100 ml a transfusion of packed cells may be necessary.

IV corticosteroids are administered intravenously.

Nursing management. Any patient admitted with multiple, pelvic and long bone fractures must be closely observed for any signs of fat embolism. It is stressed that petechiae are a late sign.

Once fat embolism has been diagnosed, the patient is best nursed in an intensive care unit where accessibility to artificial ventilation is readily available and the patient can be more closely monitored.

In treating fat embolism it must be understood that death results primarily from pulmonary oedema (see page 330) and therefore treatment is directed towards the prevention of this condition. Early resuscitation of the patient has lessened the morbidity and mortality of this condition.

CRUSH INJURIES

A crush injury occurs when part of the body or limb is caught between two forces and the tissues compressed. A leg pinned to the road by the weight of a motorcycle, or run over by the wheel of a car; an arm caught between rollers; or a foot crushed by the weight of a falling log are some examples of crush injuries.

The extent of tissue damage that occurs is dependent on the cause, the weight, and the length of time under compression.

Crush injuries may result in de-gloving injury or crush syndrome, and often require amputation.

De-gloving injury

In this form of injury the skin is sheared from the underlying fascia, and as a result is deprived of its blood supply. The skin may remain unbroken but swelling and haematoma between the skin and fascia will be extensive, and eventually sloughing of the devitalized skin will occur. Alternatively, as the name suggests, the skin may be totally stripped from the underlying tissue exposing subcutaneous tissue and/or muscle.

Initial treatment consists of elevation, mild compression with a bandage and the application of cold packs. X-rays are taken to identify any undisplaced fractures.

The neurovascular status of the limb distal to the injury is assessed frequently and the degree of swelling and colour of the skin noted. Close observation to determine the extent of injury is important.

Pain will be severe and adequate analgesia will need to be administered frequently.

The limb is supported by a splint even if there is no fracture, in order to rest the tissues and to allow for healing.

An encircling cast is never applied as this will aggravate the condition and embarrass the circulation further, and does not allow for observation of the skin for signs of viability or sloughing.

Later treatment involves removal of devitalized skin and the covering of the defect by a skin graft. Alternatively, the sheared skin is excised and stored in a sterile container in the refrigerator for later grafting. The wound is debrided and dressed with saline soaked dressings until it is ready, as a granulation bed. The stored skin is then laid on as a full thickness skin graft.

Once healing has occurred, vigorous physiotherapy is required to overcome joint stiffness, increase muscle strength and restore function.

Crush syndrome

Crush syndrome occurs when a large bulk of muscle, connective tissue and skin has been compressed, resulting in tissue ischaemia both of the area compressed and of the tissues distal to the compression.

On release of the compressing force there is generalized vasodilation in the areas surrounding the compression point. Ischaemic tissue releases myoglobin and haemoglobin, both nephrotoxins, into the general circulation. This is carried to the kidneys and may block the renal tubules. Renal secretion diminishes and acute renal failure may develop. Death could result.

Clinical manifestations

The patient is in shock, and the crushed area is pulseless and becomes red, swollen and blistered. Sensation and muscle power are lost, and oliguria develops. Underlying bone may be fractured or fragmented.

Medical, surgical, and nursing management

If a limb has been severely crushed for more than 6 hours it should be amputated before the compression force is released, in order to prevent overwhelming nephrotoxicity.

Once compression is released, immediate amputation is of little value as the toxins have already circulated. Treatment must concentrate on preserving the patient's life and restoring normal renal function. Haemo- or peritoneal dialysis may be required should renal failure result and/or to prevent uraemia. Shock must be aggressively treated, and the affected limb(s) are elevated and kept cool.

Nursing management is the same as for the patient following a fracture (see page 700) with emphasis on the management of the patient in shock (see page 105) and/or renal failure (see page 590).

Amputation as a method of medical treatment may be required and the nursing management for the patient undergoing amputation is covered on page 304.

See Chapter 16 for nursing management of the patient with spinal trauma.

69

Degenerative disorders of the musculoskeletal system

Helga Sabel   Chris Game   Robyn Anderson

OSTEOARTHRITIS

Osteoarthritis (less commonly called osteoarthrosis) is a localized degenerative joint disorder and is the most common disease of both axial and peripheral diarthrodial joints. It is characterized by progressive deterioration and loss of articular cartilage, with overgorwth of bone at joint margins resulting in joint deformity.

Pathophysiology

The precise cause of osteoarthritis is unknown. Although biochemical changes in joints occur with age, the ageing process alone does not cause osteoarthritis. Trauma at an early age causing avascular necrosis may influence the early changes, for example, congenital deformity of the hip, Perthes disease, or slipped upper femoral epiphysis. Single or repetitive sports injuries, haemophilia, and inflammatory conditions such as rheumatoid arthritis and septic arthritis, are all known contributing factors.

Osteoarthritis appears to begin in the second decade of life but as degenerative changes take years to manifest, evidence is not seen until middle age and this increases with age. By 55–60 years of age approximately 85% of patients have X-ray evidence of the disease. Men and women appear to be involved equally but only until women reach menopausal age, when they become more severely affected.

Racial differences in prevalence and distribution of affected joints may be related to differences in occupation, lifestyle, and predisposing genetic factors.

Obesity as a cause remains controversial. Apley (1982) states, 'If the load is too great cartilage gives way, but even with normal loads, cartilage gives way if it has been weakened by damage or disease, or if it is unsupported by normal bone.' The pressure of a shoe on a toe joint, for example, may result in the layer of bone and calcified cartilage at the base of the articular cartilage being crushed.

The diet has been discussed by homeopaths as a possible contributing factor but there has been no proven documentation.

Primary osteoarthritis is said to exist when no cause other than wear and tear can be identified. Secondary osteoarthritis develops in a joint previously damaged by, for example, trauma or infection.

Osteoarthritis attacks primarily the weight bearing joints. Early alterations appear in the articular cartilage which becomes soft, irregular and pitted, and undergoes fibrillation. Where pressure is greatest the cartilage becomes thin and gradually wears away.

The bone beneath the stress areas becomes compressed and develops the appearance of shiny ivory (eburnation). Stress fractures occur in the subchondral trabeculae, and cysts develop where pressure is greatest.

New bone is laid down by ostephytes at the joint margins in the nonstress area in an effort to repair the damaged bone. The synovial membrane becomes chronically inflamed, as a result of irritation from minute flakes of damaged cartilage (detritus), and the joint capsule thickens and becomes inelastic (Fig. 69.1). This results in restriction of joint movement.

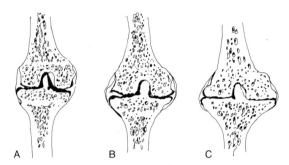

Fig. 69.1 Development of osteoarthritis. **A** – Cartilage begins to wear down. **B** – Lack of cartilage causes bone damage, and compensatory bone growth occurs at joint margins. **C** – Almost complete destruction of cartilage, and significant thickening of joint capsule.

Adult articular cartilage has a limited ability to repair itself, therefore degenerative changes tend to be irreversible and progressive.

Clinical manifestations

As osteoarthritis is not a systemic disease early symptoms are confined to the diseased joint. These changes are characterized by pain, stiffness, and progressive restriction of movement.

Pain is the leading feature, the onset of which is gradual and intermittent. It is aggravated by joint movement and relieved by rest. As the disease progresses pain increases in severity and may occur at rest. Rest pain is thought to result from intra-osseous congestion and wakens the patient at night.

Cartilage has no nerve supply and is insensitive to pain. Pain arising from passive movements is due to the stimulation of pain fibres in other joint capsular structures. Crepitus, a feeling of crackling as the joint is moved, is a significant diagnostic finding.

Joint stiffness is only first noticed after periods of rest. As the disease progresses the stiffness becomes constant and gradually increases.

Swelling is only noticeable in the superficial joints such as the knees and fingers. The joint is swollen due to a mild synovial effusion and is tender when touched but does not feel hot as in rheumatoid arthritis.

Deformity occurs as the joint is destroyed.

Osteoarthritis of the hip may result in a short leg because of a flexion, adduction, and external rotation deformity. The capsular ligaments are stretched resulting in instability and the patient may describe this as a feeling that the joint is 'giving way'. Patients presenting with a limp is not uncommon. Osteoarthritis of the knee may produce a varus or valgus deformity. When osteoarthritis develops in the distal joints of the fingers these are called Heberden's nodes.

Loss of function results more from pain than the deformity and restriction of motion. Fatigue is a feature and results from the need to exert extra physical effort. The opposite limb becomes tired due to compensatory effort and even more so when the patient is overweight, whilst the affected limb develops muscle wasting. Weight bearing certainly aggravates osteoarthritis.

Investigative procedures

Together with clinical examination, X-ray determines the diagnosis and reveals:

- Loss of joint space
- Osteophyte formation
- Sclerosis of subchondral bone.

However, the amount of joint destruction as revealed by X-ray does not necessarily correlate with the severity of the patient's symptoms. A patient may have severe pain in a joint which shows very little destruction while a grossly deformed joint may be relatively painless. However, the lack of pain may be explained by the nerve endings also being destroyed and therefore a pain stimulus is not registered.

Medical, surgical, and nursing management

There is no cure for osteoarthritis and treatment aims to:

- Reduce pain
- Prevent progression of the disease
- Improve function.

Osteoarthritis is most commonly diagnosed by a person's family physician and most likely will be treated conservatively. Obese patients with osteoarthritis in weight bearing joints must be encouraged to lose weight. This will decrease the load on the affected joints and retard the pathological process.

Active joint movement within the limits of pain preserve joint motion. Exercises, grading from isometric to active and resistive, help to restore power to weakened muscles.

Local heat by means of infra-red lamps, wax hand baths, hot packs, and ultra-sound are soothing, help to relieve pain, and lessen stiffness. Heat is often applied prior to exercise. Hydrotherapy by means of a Hubbard tank or heated swimming pool is ideal as the water provides warmth, buoyancy for joint movement, and allows for active exercises against water resistance to increase the strength of muscles.

Removable splints are of value in providing local rest, in relieving pain and preventing deformity. Splints are usually only worn at night and during periods of rest and must be intermittent otherwise sitffness will increase.

A walking stick, especially if combined with a raised shoe, greatly relieves stress on an affected hip. For normal gait the stick should be held in the hand opposite to the affected limb.

When pain, joint stiffness, and restricted movement adversely affect the person's quality of life, then referral for specialist opinion and treatment is usually sought. Surgery to either correct the joint deformity or replace the joint surface(s) and aggressive drug therapy are the treatment methods most commonly used.

Nonsteroidal anti-inflammatory agents are used for their analgesic and anti-inflammatory effect. They do not alter the course of the disease but improve the quality of life by reducing joint pain and swelling, and increasing mobility.

Muscle relaxants. Diazepam may be used to relieve the pain caused by muscle spasm. This is especially useful for patients who have osteoarthritis of the spine.

Intra-articular corticosteroids. Injections of corticosteroids into the affected joint may be used to provide pain relief. This is a temporary measure and frequently repeated may cause further cartilage damage and infection.

Surgical management

Surgery aims to:

• Halt the progression of the disease
• Relieve joint pain
• Improve mobility.

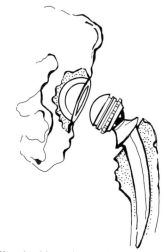

Fig. 69.2 Charnley hip replacement.

Osteotomy. The division and refixing of bone is performed to realign the joint so that the load is distributed through the area of healthy articular cartilage and painless weightbearing is restored.

Arthroplasty. Partial or total replacement involves improving articulating surfaces by changing the alignment of bones, transplanting articular cartilage, patching worn articular cartilage, or replacement of one of the articulating surfaces, for example, Moore's arthroplasty of the hip. Total joint replacement involves replacement of both articulating surfaces, for example, Charnley hip replacement (Fig. 69.2), total knee replacement.

Total joint replacement is the arthroplasty of choice, especially for degeneration of the hip and knee joints.

Arthrodesis. Fusion of the diseased joint provides total pain relief at the expense of motion. Joints proximal or distal to the arthrodesed joint may in time themselves become arthritic because of the increased workload.

Nursing management involves caring for the patient requiring surgery. Total hip and total knee replacement will be discussed as these are common forms of treatment for degenerative joint disease.

TOTAL HIP REPLACEMENT

Total hip replacement is usually performed in the over 60 age group when pain and loss of joint function become severely disabling. The procedure is sometimes used for the younger person if all alternative methods have failed. The patient must realize that an artificial joint does not have the durability of a natural joint and will wear out or loosen in time, and when this occurs further surgery will be required. A total hip prosthesis, if well looked after, should provide the patient with approximately 10–20 years of pain-free use.

In total hip arthroplasty both the acetabulum and femoral head are replaced. The femoral component is usually made of a metal alloy and consists of a spherical head, a neck and a stem which fits into the shaft of the femur. The acetabular component is a cap of high density polyethelene. Both components are fixed rigidly into the bone by plastic cement (methyl-methacrylate).

A ceramic, cementless hip prosthesis is also in use. The ceramic-ceramic articulation produces

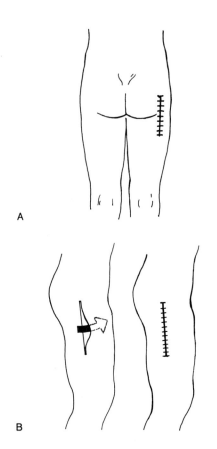

Fig. 69.3 Surgical approaches in hip replacement. **A** – Posterior. **B** – Anteriolateral.

less friction than the metal-polyethylene, and the components are positioned in place without the use of cement.

In performing a total hip replacement the surgeon may approach the hip joint either posteriorly through an incision from the back or anteriorly through an incision from the front or side (Fig. 69.3).

With a posterior approach the joint capsule and soft tissue structures that lie at the back of the hip joint are incised and divided. Postoperatively these structures will be weakest and the new prosthesis may dislocate if the hip is allowed to lie in any position that puts strain on the incision line.

In an anterior or anterolateral approach the joint capsule and soft tissue structures in front of the hip joint are incised and divided and dislocation may occur if the hip is allowed to externally rotate and hyperextend.

It is imperative that the nurse be aware of the type of surgical approach and the surgeon's specific requirements with positioning in order to provide safe patient care.

Preoperative care

The aim is to prepare the patient physically and psychologically for surgery and the nurse will be involved in the education of the patient for the postoperative period.

Assessment. A full nursing history should be commenced and the patient assessed as to his general conditon. Most patients are elderly and may have other medical problems which could affect their progress postoperatively, for example, cardiovascular disease, obesity, rheumatoid arthritis. If the patient has any sign of an infection, surgery will be postponed until the infection has cleared. The presence of infection in a prosthetic joint may require the artificial joint to be removed.

Education. The nurse will need to prepare the patient for his postoperative regime by demonstrating the postoperative position required and the use of the abduction pillow. The patient should practice rolling with this pillow in place and should also practice using a bed pan while maintaining the alignment of his limb and the correct position of his hip. The patient should understand his postoperative physiotherapy requirements regarding chest exercises, muscle strengthening and range of motion exercises, and his ambulation programme.

Physical preparation. As most patients undergoing total hip replacement require whole blood transfusion during the operative period blood will need to be grouped and cross-matched. Skin preparation includes a very careful shave so as not to inflict cuts which provide an entry for bacteria. Some surgeons prefer depilatory creams as these do not abrade the skin. The patient is required to have a shower using an antibacterial agent the night before and the morning of his surgery. Hair must be clean. Large-dose prophylactic antibiotics are usually administered with the patient's premedication.

Postoperative care

The patient has undergone major surgery. The joint capsule has been opened, and a 'foreign body' has been inserted. There is therefore an increased risk of infection occurring in or around the new joint and the prosthesis may also dislocate. Infection in an artificial joint is devastating as it is extremely difficult to gain antibiotic tissue penetration levels in and around a joint. Infection may necessitate removal of the artificial joint with subsequent flailing of the limb.

The specific nursing care is as for any patient undergoing orthopaedic surgery. It is not uncommon for patients following total hip replacement to have the initial wound dressing removed after 48 hours and the suture line sprayed with a plastic skin material.

Prevention of dislocation

Posterior approach

• The patient is positioned supine with the hip extended, abducted, and in neutral or external rotation. An abduction pillow is placed between the patient's legs from knee to ankle; this may or may not be strapped in place.
• The patient's upper body must not be elevated beyond an angle of 30° for the first 3–4 days, therefore a maximum of two pillows is allowed. Elevation to 45° is usually permitted by the end of the first week

• Two nurses are required to turn the patient for any nursing procedures. One nurse controls the affected leg preventing it from internally rotating and adducting while the other nurse assists the patient. The abduction pillow remains in position during the turn
• Only when the patient can maintain hip abduction is he allowed out of bed. This may be as early as day 3 but is usually day 4 or 5. A walking frame is initially used with gradual progression to a walking stick. The patient with a cementless ceramic hip prosthesis is not allowed to fully weight bear for at least 5–6 weeks. Total hospitalization time is around 3 weeks and the patient is discharged when he is ambulating safely and has a good range of movement.

Anteriolateral approach

• The patient is positioned supine with the hip slightly flexed, abducted and internally rotated. A small abduction pillow is placed between the patient's legs; this may or may not be strapped in place
• There are three methods by which the affected leg may be maintained in internal rotation. They are: placement of a small pillow diagonally under the knee with a sandbag on the lateral side; the use of a trochanter roll; or by placing a sandbag on the lateral side of the lower leg
• The patient should be nursed in a semirecumbent position but may sit up for short periods as desired
• When turning the patient for any nursing procedure a pillow is placed between the legs to prevent adduction of the hips
• Only when the patient can maintain hip abduction and his leg in internal rotation is he allowed to walk. Weight bearing is allowed and support with a frame or stick is provided.

Discharge education

Prior to discharge the patient with a total hip replacement requires instructions and education on continuing care. He is advised to:

• Increase his walking distance each day using the walking aid; a walking stick is usually needed for at least six weeks

- Continue daily the exercises taught in hospital
- Sleep on his back with a pillow between his legs
- Lie prone for about a half an hour daily
- Sit on a straight-backed chair and use an elevated toilet seat
- Always dress the affected leg first. Aids such as a stocking/sock dresser may be useful and slip on shoes are preferred
- Showering is preferable to bathing and it may be necessary for the patient to sit using a bath board or seat
- When travelling, the patient should sit in the front seat of a car and low seats of a car should be elevated with a cushion
- Extension aids are useful to reduce the patient's need to bend.

The patient is instructed never to

- Cross his legs
- Bend over
- Sit on low chairs, toilet, bed or bath, or squat.

He is also advised not to participate in active sports, heavy labour, or any activity that places an abnormal load on his prosthetic joint. Swimming is good exercise and is recommended; bowls, golf, dancing, sexual intercourse, and light gardening, may be resumed after 6–12 weeks.

Complications of total hip replacement

Infection of the capsule and surrounding soft tissue. This is treated with bed rest, IV antibiotics, and wound irrigation.

Dislocation. This will require reduction; the limb is then immobilized for 3–6 weeks in traction.

Loosening and/or wearing of the prosthesis. Microscopic flakes of metal and plastic may cause inflammation of the soft tissue and the joint becomes painful. Surgical revision with a new prosthesis is necessary. Loosening and excessive wear of the prosthesis is usually a result of overuse and possibly the abuse of the artificial joint.

Stress fractures through the metal stem. This will require replacement of the prosthesis.

Anticipated outcome

The patient who has had a successful operation has a new lease of life. He is pain free, can sleep at night and is more active than he has been for many years and may be tempted to over-use his new joint. With good care the artificial hip should remain trouble-free up to 20 years.

TOTAL KNEE REPLACEMENT

The outstanding success of total hip replacements has led to the development of artificial knees using the same materials. The diseased articular surfaces are replaced by a stainless steel or vitallium femoral component articulating with a high density polyethylene tibial component. These are fixed firmly in position using bone cement. There are a great many varieties of artificial knee joints available, however, they all aim to simulate the function of the normal knee, retain the collateral ligaments, and remove as little bone as possible.

The aim of knee replacement surgery is to:

- Relieve pain
- Improve or restore normal function.

Preoperative preparation is the same as for total hip replacement (see page 720).

Postoperative care

The knee is immobilized in extension with a bulky compression dressing from mid calf to mid thigh. A bed cradle is required to keep the weight of the bed clothes off the knee, and the foot of the bed is elevated to allow for venous drainage and to reduce effusion in the knee. Ice packs for the first 24 hours may be ordered to reduce pain and swelling.

Isometric and inner range quadriceps exercises are commenced early, graduating to active straight leg raising. Active ankle and foot exercises are performed hourly to prevent deep vein thrombosis and to aid venous return. (In some units a continuous passive mobilizing machine is used to perform increasing flexion and extension of the joint immediately postoperatively.)

The neurovascular status of the extremity is observed and recorded hourly for the first 48 hours. Wound drainage is noted and the low pressure suction kept patent. The drainage apparatus is removed when drainage is minimal.

The compression dressing is usually removed on day 3. A back slab or knee immobilizer is applied during ambulation and at night to prevent the patient flexing the knee. Gentle active knee flexion exercises are commenced and a progressive exercise programme is continued until discharge to increase muscle strength and range of motion. Ambulation is commenced once the patient is able to maintain extension of the leg and is able to straight leg raise. An extension knee support is initially worn and weight bearing is permitted according to pain tolerance. Crutches or a walking stick are usually required for 6–8 weeks.

The patient is discharged home or to a rehabilitation centre in approximately 2 weeks or when he has gained 70°–90° knee flexion and is independent in daily activities. He is given an exercise programme to follow at home and may be required to attend the physiotherapy department on a regular basis for further supervised exercise.

Complications

These are similar to those of a total hip replacement.

Infection is serious and is treated with large doses of IV antibiotics and wound irrigation. If unresolved it may result in the removal of the prosthesis and an arthrodesis being performed.

Joint stiffness and loosening and wearing of the prosthesis may occur.

Anticipated outcome

Following a successful operation the patient should be pain free and have a normal range of joint motion. He should be warned against excessive use of his new knee. Walking, bicycle riding, swimming, and golf are activities in which he may safely indulge.

INTERVERTEBRAL DISC DISRUPTION

Intervertebral disc disruption is the commonest form of lesion requiring surgery on the vertebral column. Cervical spondylosis and herniation of intervertebral discs are the most common forms of disc disruption. Cervical spondylosis is a chronic degeneration of the entire intervertebral discs of the cervical spine and is characterized by the overgrowth of new bone at the periphery of the discs, thereby narrowing the spinal canal and compressing the spinal cord. It is sometimes referred to as osteoarthritis of the spine and occurs more commonly as age increases. As normal movement of the intervertebral discs diminishes, stiffening of the cervical spine occurs.

Herniation of an intervertebral disc can occur at any point in the vertebral column but is most common in the lumbar region. Herniation results when the nucleus pulposus extrudes through the disc's weakened or torn wall (anulus fibrosus). The extruded portion of the disc then impinges on either the spinal cord posteriorly or on spinal nerve roots laterally, giving rise to the common symptoms of lower back pain and sciatica. Herniated discs are most likely to result from severe trauma to, or strain on, the vertebral column; for example, incorrect lifting techniques with the spine in flexion, a fall whilst in a flexed position, or extended periods of poor posture. Herniation may also be related to spondylosis and in this instance minor trauma may be all that is required to effect the rupture of the disc.

Herniation of a disc is a common disorder in industrialized societies and 35% of all cases occur between the ages of 30–40 years; males are more commonly affected than women, in a ratio of 8 : 1. Many occupational health programmes are specifically aimed at reducing the incidence of this disorder by examining and correcting the kinetics of work situations and educating people on appropriate lifting techniques.

Clinical manifestations

The patient will seek medical advice primarily because of the presence of pain. The pain may occur immediately following the injury or may not manifest for some days or weeks after injury. Pain may be felt directly over the affected area or may radiate to points distant from the site of the disc herniation. For example, pain is usually felt in the hands and lower forearms with cervical spondylosis, and the classic symptoms of sciatica exist with lumbar disc lesions. Sciatica presents as pain in the back which is intensified by spinal movement, deep sharp pain in the buttock or thigh which diminishes during rest to a gnawing constant pain. It may radiate down the leg and into the foot and is classically made acutely extreme on sneezing and/or coughing. Normal sensation and movement are generally present but occasionally plantar reflexes are slow, distal sensation may be impaired, and in extreme cases sciatica may be accompanied by foot drop and wasting of leg muscles. With lumbar disc lesions severe muscle spasm at the site of the lesion is not uncommon.

Investigative procedures

- Plain X-ray of the vertebral column may show the results of osteophyte activity which is seen as 'lips' of bone at the edges of the vertebral bodies, narrowing of intervertebral spaces or displacement of vertebrae.
- CT scan and/or myelogram are performed predominantly to exclude tumours. They may demonstrate the compression of the spinal cord and/or nerve roots.
- Rectal and/or vaginal examination may be performed to exclude pelvic pathology as the cause of the pain.
- Physical examination. The straight-leg-raising test is performed to accurately assess the degree of the patient's sciatica and in conjunction with reflex testing determines the degree of spinal nerve root compression. An assessment of the patient's peripheral vascular function will also assist in determining the degree of spinal cord/nerve root compression.

Medical, surgical, and nursing management

In 70% of all cases of patients with intervertebral disc disruption conservative measures of bed rest and analgesia are all that is required. However, these patients may have constant pain for weeks or months and in extreme situations the patient may suffer pain for years. Where pain is constant for months or years the patient's quality of life is severely compromised in that he is seldom pain free and this will ultimately disrupt his work and home environments and make socialization difficult.

Conservative management

The nurse will be responsible for caring for a patient who will be ordered bed rest with minimal ambulatory periods. The patient will be required to lie supine on a firm mattress, on a firm base; one soft pillow will be allowed. The patient's spine may be further immobilized by the use of cervical traction or a variety of lumbar traction methods (refer page 709 for care of the patient in traction). Particularly where traction methods are employed, it may be impossible for the patient to roll in bed or significantly change positions in any way. Nursing activities such as back and skin care and toileting can only be performed by lifting the patient straight up off the bed (so that the patient's spine is kept in alignment during the lift) and a lifting team may be required. When the patient uses a bedpan, his back must be well supported by the use of pillows.

Pain relief must be administered as ordered and asprin is the drug of choice as it also reduces inflammation and oedema at the site of herniation; narcotic analgesics will also be used during the acute phase. Muscle relaxants may also be ordered where pain is accompanied by severe muscle spasm.

Corticosteroids are sometimes ordered during the acute phase to assist in the reduction of inflammation and oedema at the site of the herniation. Heat applied locally may assist in the relief of pain and muscle spasm.

The nurse may also be responsible for assisting the patient with ambulation following the period of bed rest and a cervical or lumbar brace may be required once ambulation is recommenced. A plaster jacket may be utilized to provide total support for the vertebral column whilst ambulating, and the nurse will therefore need to teach the patient regarding the care of the cast (see page 705). However, plaster jackets are more commonly utilized following surgery for spinal fusion.

Physiotherapy referral is necessary to provide a controlled exercise program to prevent further muscle wasting and to strengthen weakened muscles.

Manipulative therapy has been successful in many instances of recurrent disc herniation or chronic lower back pain with or without sciatica, and manipulative follow up may be sought by the patient after his discharge from acute care.

Surgical management

Should conservative methods fail to alleviate pain or improve the patient's quality of life then surgery may be required. In the situation where the herniated disc causes severe neurological or neurovascular impairment, surgery will almost always be considered. Surgery will also be required should vertebral column instability develop secondary to spondylosis; laminectomy and/or spinal fusion are the most common procedures performed.

Laminectomy is the removal of the vertebral laminae to allow access to the herniated disc and subsequent discectomy; lumbar laminectomy is the most common site. If pain is not alleviated by laminectomy, or if segmental instability of the column occurs or is anticipated, spinal fusion may be necessary. Spinal fusion is performed by grafting bone substance (from usually the iliac crest) to the vertebral bodies following discectomy. Once the graft has taken, arthrodesis of the vertebral joints involved results thus immobilizing that section of the spine.

An alternative technique to laminectomy, currently under investigation, is chemonucleolysis. The enzyme chymopapain is injected into the disc (under X-ray control) in an attempt to dissolve the nucleus polposus. Results of this technique remain inconclusive.

Following surgery the patient must lie supine on one small pillow for a period of at least 48 hours. A minimum of 2 nurses are required to move the patient for any nursing procedures that require the patient to roll; log rolling with 1 or 2 pillows between the legs in order to prevent lateral movement in the spine will be necessary.

A drain tube attached to low pressure suction will be in situ for the first 24–48 hours and the nurse must ensure its patency at all times. The drainage must be observed and recorded regularly and the presence of clean drainage may indicate leakage of CSF. The neurovascular status of the patient's lower limbs must be closely observed for the first 48 hours postoperatively and abnormalities recorded and reported, as oedema or haematoma formation may exert undue pressure on nerve roots. Once the drain tube has been removed the nursing management is as for any patient who has undergone conservative treatment.

Anticipated outcome

For the patient with uncomplicated disc rupture, successful conservative management will result in complete recovery over a matter of weeks to months. The patient should be advised to engage in back care techniques, for example maintenance of correct posture, use of correct lifting methods, and exercise to strengthen lumbar muscle groups.

The prognosis for the surgical patient is variable. Some 10% will enjoy a complete recovery; however for the remainder chronic low back pain and related symptoms, and the potential for recurrence of the condition will persist.

70

Inflammatory disorders of the musculoskeletal system

Helga Sabel   Chris Game   Robyn Anderson

RHEUMATOID ARTHRITIS

Rheumatoid arthritis is a chronic, systemic, inflammatory disease of connective tissue. It affects mainly the synovial membrane of joints and surrounding tendons, muscles, ligaments and blood vessels, resulting in eventual joint destruction. Other connective tissue structures in the body may also be involved in the inflammatory process making this a generalized, systemic, polyarticular disease.

Incidence

Rheumatoid arthritis is a relatively common disorder and occurs throughout the world. It is characterized by spontaneous remissions and unpredictable exacerbations. Most patients are able to live a normal life with limited restriction whilst up to 10% of sufferers will be totally disabled from severe articular deformity. It is estimated that 37 per 1000 persons in Australia (3.5%) suffer from a form of arthritis and it is also estimated to be the seventh most frequently reported illness amongst all Australians (McLennan, 1986). Women are affected three times more frequently than men.

The disease may occur at any age but commonly the onset is between the ages of 25–55 years. Juvenile rheumatoid arthritis (Still's disease) occurs less frequently and can manifest itself as early as age 2.

Pathophysiology

Aetiology is unknown, but theories include speculation that the cause of rheumatoid arthritis may be due to a virus or some other microorganism, together with an altered immune response. There is also a possibility that the disease is genetically based. Commonly patients with rheumatoid arthritis exhibit an altered immune response resulting in some of the immunoglobins undergoing changes and themselves acting as antigens (and therefore foreign protein) again stimulating the production of antibodies and producing altered immune complexes. These immune complexes appear particularly in the synovial membrane setting up an acute inflammatory reaction, and are also thought to stimulate the production of anti-immunoglobulins known as rheumatoid factors and antinuclear factors.

Joint pathology

Synovial membrane inflammation. The synovium becomes oedematous and congested. Synovial fluid is produced in excess with an increase of polymorphonuclear leucocytes.

The joints and tendon sheaths show the typical signs of inflammation – swelling, warmth, redness, and tenderness.

Joint destruction and deformity. The onset is insidious and deformity occurs over a long period. Persistent inflammation causes the tissue in the synovium to thicken and proliferate to form a pannus. This pannus creeps over the articular cartilage depriving it of nutrition and causing cartilage necrosis. Proteolytic enzymes produced by the proliferating synovium aid in the destruction of the cartilage. Pannus also erodes the bone at the joint margins and burrows beneath the cartilage to produce local areas of bone destruction (osteolysis). The synovial membrane of the tendon sheaths which provide the tendons with nutrition and lubrication are similarly affected by the rheumatoid inflammatory process and tendons weaken and may rupture. The fibrous capsule and joint ligaments become stretched and weakened leading to joint instability and eventual subluxation or dislocation.

Eventually the inflammatory process subsides and the pannus is replaced by fibrous scar tissue which contracts causing further joint deformity (fibrous ankylosis). If the process continues over many years severe joint damage may lead to bony ankylosis as a result of calcification of the fibrous tissue.

Systemic pathology

Rheumatoid nodules. These are present in approximately 30% of patients with rheumatoid arthritis and consist of small lumps of fibrous tissue which commonly occur at sites of pressure or strain, for example, the elbows, and metacarpophalangeal joints (Fig. 70.1). They may also occur in the connective tissue of the lungs, pleura, sclera, and pericardium. The lumps are firm, mobile and not tender.

Vasculitis. Inflammation occurs in the walls of small blood vessels and may lead to a thrombus causing obstruction. Blood supply to a peripheral nerve may in this way be affected causing a neuropathy which adds to the problems of joint function. Nail fold lesions, skin ulcers and purpuric rashes may also occur as a result of vasculitis.

Muscle wasting. Muscle weakness and wasting is a common problem due to disuse atrophy, to inflammation of the connective tissue in muscle, and to neuropathy. Weakened muscles mean that the joint is even less able to withstand stress.

Pleurisy and pleural effusions, keratoconjunctivitis, scleritis, and pericarditis are other connective tissue problems that may arise as a result of the inflammatory process in those tissues. Anaemia is also a feature due to the constancy of the inflammatory process and the demand for haemopoiesis. However, the dominant feature in rheumatoid arthritis is joint involvement which, if untreated, progresses from synovitis and joint swelling to marked joint destruction and deformity with bony ankylosis occurring in severe cases.

Clinical manifestations

The onset is usually insidious and slowly progressive with:

1. Bilateral and polyarticular inflammation, initially occurring in the small peripheral joints. The joints of the hands and feet and then the wrist are usually the first to be affected. Later the knee, ankle and elbow joints become involved. All synovial joints are susceptible.
2. The joints and tendon sheaths become painful, swollen, shiny, red, and warm.
3. Loss of joint function.
4. Limitation in the range of joint movement.
5. Morning stiffness. Inflamed joints tend to stiffen during periods of rest. These symptoms abate after the person has moved and stretched.
6. Malaise, fatigue, fever, and weight loss are common particularly in the young to middle age

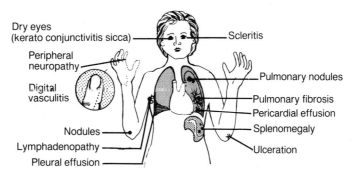

Fig. 70.1 Systemic pathology of rheumatoid arthritis.

group. The patient generally feels unwell and is found to have a low grade anaemia.

7. Muscle weakness and wasting.

8. Subcutaneous modules appear in approximately 30% of patients as the disease progresses.

9. Deformity. This is also a later sign but can develop fairly rapidly from a combination of:

– Muscle spasm. The muscles hold the joint in a position which is least painful – usually flexion

– Muscle atrophy and contraction from disuse and inflammation

– Subluxation from weak ligaments and capsule

– Tendon rupture

– Cartilage destruction.

Most commonly the clinical pattern is one of repeated, acute exacerbations and remissions with the disease eventually 'burning itself out'. The structural damage that has occurred in the joints during the active phase is irreversible. Complete remission with no joint destruction occurs in approximately 10–20% of patients.

Investigative procedures

Haematological tests are made. The erythrocyte sedimentation rate is usually markedly raised when the disease is active and may be persistently raised in patients with long standing disease.

Haemoglobin, serum iron, and serum folate levels are studied because hypochromic and normocytic anaemia is a common feature of rheumatoid arthritis and may also result from an abnormal storage of iron in the reticulo-endothelial system and in synovial tissue. It does not respond to oral iron therapy but improves as remissions occur.

The rheumatoid factor test is positive in about 70% of patients with highly active disease. However, the presence of this factor alone does not establish the diagnosis as approximately 4% of the general population and 40% of patients with other connective tissue diseases have positive tests.

An antinuclear antibodies (ANA) test is positive in 20–35% of patients with rheumatoid arthritis. The test is much more significant in other rheumatoid diseases such as systemic lupus erythematosus (see page 786).

Active phase protein and C-reactive protein titres are raised in active rheumatoid arthritis.

Aspirate of synovial fluid from an actively inflamed joint may show an elevated white cell count and the presence of a polymorphonuclear leucocytosis.

X-ray may only reveal soft tissue swelling with localized osteoporosis in the early phases of the disease. Later there is joint space narrowing, bony erosions, subluxation, and deformity.

The above investigations apart from the late X-ray changes, do not make a diagnosis but rather help in determining the progression and severity of the disease. As stated by Apley (1982) the minimal criterion for establishing a diagnosis of rheumatoid arthritis is bilateral, symmetrical, polyarthritis involving the proximal joints of the hands and feet, present for at least 6 weeks.

Medical, surgical, and nursing management

While there is as yet no cure for rheumatoid arthritis much can be done to alleviate the symptoms and slow the progression of the disease. Not all patients have the same degree of severity or disability; therefore, treatment methods must be individualized and involve the patient, his significant others, and members of the health care team in the implementation of that care. The majority of persons with rheumatoid arthritis are able to lead a normal life despite increasing disablement. A small proportion of sufferers will require hospitalization and aggressive medical, surgical and nursing care.

The aims of treatment are to:

- Halt the inflammatory process
- Alleviate pain and stiffness
- Maintain joint function
- Prevent deformity
- Preserve independence.

Wherever possible the person is managed in the community and methods of treatment include: rest, drug therapy, physiotherapy, psychosocial, and vocational therapy. Only in the event that either surgery or aggressive drug therapy is required is the patient hospitalized.

Rest of the whole body is anti-inflammatory and helps to control fatigue and joint inflammation. Rest of affected joints may be achieved by the use of splints (Fig. 70.2).

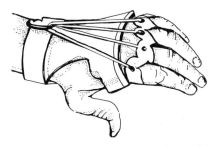

Fig. 70.2 Hand splint for use in rheumatoid arthritis to correct position and rest joints.

Splints support the joints during periods of maximum use, maintain correct alignment during sleep, and lessen pain. When pain is exacerbated by muscle spasm the application of a splint allows the muscles around the joint to relax.

As much as is possible the patient needs to be free from worries about family, work, finance, and about herself and the disease. A multidisciplinary approach is employed and community support systems utilized.

A proper balance between rest and activity is basic to the treatment of rheumatoid arthritis and the amount of rest versus activity is closely correlated to the disease state; rest being required when there is an acute exacerbation, and activity allowed during remissive phases. Activity is necessary to attain and maintain optimum levels of functioning and to keep the patient more stable mentally. Any activity is permissible providing it does not abuse the joints or fatigue the patient. Physiotherapy plays a very important role in the management of the arthritic patient (see page 731).

Drugs are used to halt the inflammatory process and to relieve pain.

Nonsteroidal anti-inflammatory drugs:

1. Salicylates and propionic acid derivatives. These act by prohibiting prostaglandin synthesis and have an analgesic, anti-inflammatory, and antipyretic effect. They are the drugs of first choice in the management of rheumatoid arthritis. These drugs are often used in combination and as the effect on individual persons varies the patient may need a trial before an ideal drug regime is developed. Whichever drug is prescribed it is important that the patient takes the recommended dose at the set times in order to maximize its effect.

Side-effects such as gastric irritation are common but these are reversible and the patient needs to be aware of the potential problems and to be able to recognize early signs of toxicity. These drugs should be ceased prior to surgery because of their effect in the clotting process. They prevent platelet adhesiveness (especially aspirin) and may cause excessive bleeding intraoperatively.

2. Indomethacin. This drug acts by inhibiting prostaglandin synthesis and has an anti-inflammatory and analgesic action. Indomethacin may be taken orally or by suppository. Therapy is commenced with low doses so as to lessen the frequency and severity of side-effects and the dosage is gradually increased as the patient develops tolerance. Side-effects include gastrointestinal disturbances, dizziness, depression and rarely, fluid retention, bone marrow depression, rash and urticaria.

Slow-acting antirheumatic drugs for example, gold and penicillamine are also used. These drugs reduce inflammation and also appear to induce remission. They are tried if there is no significant improvement following the use of nonsteroidal agents. The mode of action of these drugs is unclear and response to treatment is slow; the onset of action is 3–6 months. A low dose is commenced and this is gradually increased until there is significant improvement. The patient then continues on a maintenance regimen. These drugs are much more toxic than nonsteroidal agents and patients need careful and frequent clinical checks and monitoring of blood and urine. Side-effects are many, the most common being pruritis, nonspecific dermatitis, blood dyscrasias (thrombocytopenia, neutropenia, aplastic anaemia) renal problems (proteinuria, nephrotic syndrome), gastrointestinal disturbances (nausea, anorexia, loss of taste, mouth ulcers).

Following injections of gold there may be exacerbations of the rheumatoid arthritis. This is self-limiting and lasts for only 2–3 days.

Antimalarial drugs are an alternate group of drugs if gold or penicillamine fail.

Corticosteroid agents used systemically have a potent anti-inflammatory effect but this diminishes with time, requiring progressively higher doses to produce the same effect. Prolonged use causes serious side-effects such as Cushingoid syndrome, osteoporosis, weight gain, and hypertension. Their use is restricted to patients who have not benefitted from any other therapy. The smallest dose that maintains improvement is used and rarely exceeds 10 mg per day. Short-term use is recommended.

Intra-articular injections of corticosteroids reduce inflammation locally. The effect is immediate and short-lived, however, the dangers are infection and chondronecrosis with repeated injections.

Immunosuppressive-antineoplastic drugs (for example, azathioprine, cyclophosphamide) may be tried in severe, rapidly progressive forms of the disease that remains unresponsive to other medications. These drugs aim to suppress the immune mechanisms responsible for the persistent inflammation. Doses are kept relatively low and given over long periods of time and the patient is monitored carefully for bone marrow depression.

Surgical management

Surgery is aimed at:

- Pain relief
- Improving joint function
- Preventing and correcting deformity.

Synovectomy. Excision of the grossly hypertrophied synovial membrane of joints and tendons often restores function. The synovium will regenerate and it often remains disease free for many years. Synovectomy has been found to be particularly useful in rheumatoid arthritis of the finger joints and knees.

Tendon surgery. Ruptured tendons are repaired and tendons can be transplanted to restore function.

Arthroplasty. Various types of arthroplasty may be performed according to the joint involved.

Replacement arthroplasty. This is widely used in the hip and to a lesser extent in the knee and metacarpophalangeal joints of the hand. The technology is available to replace most peripheral joints but is not necessarily of benefit to the rheumatoid arthritis patient as function of the replaced joint may be less than that of the diseased joint.

Excision arthroplasty. The joint is removed and the gap allowed to fill with granulation tissue. This operation may be used for the metatarsophalangeal joints of the feet. Arthrodesis. This is most suitable for the wrist, subtalar joint in the foot, and the cervical spine.

Excision of nodules. These may be removed if they interfere with joint function.

Surgery is not routinely performed for patients with rheumatoid arthritis, and rarely are cosmetic reasons an indication for it. Grossly deformed hands may look ugly but still enable the patient to be fully employed and independent in activities of daily living.

Specific nursing management

Should the patient require hospitalization or domiciliary nursing services the nurse must be prepared to include physical, emotional, social, and educational factors in such care. Wherever possible, a multidisciplinary approach to care should be given. The nurse must observe for side-effects of medication.

Nursing action must be individualized and will centre around the following needs:

Rest and activity. As stated previously, rest helps to suppress the inflammatory action. The patient will require rest both physically and emotionally and there must be a well planned balance between rest and activity. The patient should have 8–10 hours sleep at night and 1–2 hours during the day but too much rest will result in muscle weakness, decreased range of movement, and osteoporosis.

Posture. Good posture and comfort must be maintained whilst the patient is confined to bed. His back should be well supported to keep the spine straight and limbs positioned in such a way to prevent flexion contractures and foot drop. Pillows should not be placed under the knees and the bed must have a firm base with a firm mattress. A small, soft pillow should be used to support the head and the patient should be encouraged to lie prone, for a couple of hours each day to prevent hip and knee flexion deformities. When lying prone foot drop can be prevented by placing the feet over the end of the mattress.

Joint support and protection. Inflamed joints should be supported when moving the patient. Splints must be comfortable and light. At no time should the splint cause pressure or constriction. If hand splints are required, only one splint is applied at a time so that the patient retains a degree of independence and can attend to personal needs.

Comfort. Clothing and bed clothes should be light and warm. A bed cradle may be required to keep the weight off acutely inflamed knees or feet. Thermal pads to provide localized heat to joints may be used. The patient should be positioned free from draughts and ideally with a pleasant view.

The nurse should anticipate that joint movement will be difficult following prolonged periods of rest. Therefore the patient must be given ample time and, where necessary, assistance to perform tasks, especially in the morning.

Hygiene. Special care is needed when attending to the patient's nails, skin, teeth, and toileting needs. Vasculitis of the digital vessels may have caused nail bed erosion and a podiatry referral may be necessary.

Skin becomes shiny, translucent and papery thin and may tear easily, particularly for those patients on corticosteroids.

Teeth may loosen and gums bleed because of associated periodontal disease (the periodontal ligaments are affected by the disease process) and very careful brushing with a soft brush is required. For those patients with badly affected hands an electric toothbrush is ideal.

A toilet seat raiser and hand rails maybe required to maintain maximum patient independence.

Psychological support. Most patients suffer many episodes of frustration, anger and depression due to the fact that the disease is chronic, is always painful, is generally debilitating, and has no cure. Body image is greatly altered and the simple tasks of life such as doing up buttons, putting on stockings, and unscrewing lids become prohibitive. The nurse can help by being supportive and empathetic; always giving a full explanation of any treatment carried out; encouraging the patient to take an active interest in herself with the use of make-up, attractive, easily managed hairstyles and clothes; planning all care with the patient and allowing the patient to make decisions.

Health education. The patient must recognise the importance of the drug therapy, the side-effects and the need for strict adherence to the regime. Appointments for regular medical check-ups will be required and the patient encouraged to keep them. An adequately balanced 'rest' versus 'exercise' regimen should be maintained and the patient encouraged to use the splints and aids recommended for joint rest and protection and to continue with the exercise programme. The patient may wish to attend the local branch meetings of the Arthritis Foundation. This will provide education and much needed support from others with similar problems.

Diet

There is no specific dietary management for patients with rheumatoid arthritis. During the active phase of the disease when weight loss is a factor a well-balanced diet with added calories in the form of protein is needed. Later, when the disease is quiescent, excessive weight gain may be a problem from inactivity, depression and/or overuse of corticosteroids. Obesity must be avoided as this puts extra strain on weight bearing joints and aggravates the arthritis.

It has been suggested that vitamin C in high doses (10 g daily) is beneficial. While this has not yet been proven it is important that the patient receive sufficient vitamin C in her diet. Rheumatoid arthritis patients tend not to eat well because the effort required to prepare a nutritious meal is very time consuming and exhausting, especially at breakfast when morning stiffness is an added problem.

Allied paramedical care

Physiotherapy is used to.

● Prevent and correct deformity
● Control pain
● Strengthen weakened muscles
● Improve function

Exercises are both isometric to maintain muscle function and strength and isotonic to maintain joint range of movement and prevent joint contractures. Exercises should be gauged according to the patient's pain and fatigue levels and are specific for each joint.

Superficial heat, in the form of hydrotherapy, wax baths, hot bath or shower, or hot packs, has an analgesic effect. Heat also relaxes muscles and relieves joint stiffness and as a result improves exercise performance. Hydrotherapy provides bouyancy as well as heat and so facilitates range of movement exercises.

Deep heat in the form of ultrasound and diathermy is contraindicated in acute rheumatoid arthritis as it may induce enzyme related joint destruction. Superficial heat should not be applied for periods longer than 20–30 minutes and must not be used for patients with sensory loss.

Cold in the form of ice packs or a mixture of alcohol and water may be used as an alternative to heat to relieve pain and reduce swelling. It appears to be most effective when the joints are acutely inflamed and painful.

Splints. Together with the occupational therapist, the physiotherapist provides splints for joints that are deformed and unstable, where muscle power is weak, and where there is persistent pain. Serial plasters may be required to correct a flexion deformity of the knee.

Occupational therapy plays an equally important role in helping the patient to remain as independent as possible. The occupational therapist makes a detailed assessment of the patient's ability to cope with her disability in her home and work environment and is trained to assist with activities of daily living, for example, dressing, bathing, domestic duties. Difficulties in these areas commonly arise from poor grasp and lack of reach. Built-up handles on utensils and long-handled equipment are some of the aids that are employed.

The therapist is able to advise on movements to be avoided and teach ways of performing everyday tasks so that joints are not overly strained and further deformed (for example, picking up a glass).

Splints are used for two purposes: to assist the patient to become independent in an activity that would otherwise be difficult, and to avoid stress and strain on joints thus helping to prevent joint deformity.

Complications

Most problems inherent in treatment stem from the unpleasant side effects of drug therapy, and complications of rheumatoid arthritis are common. These include:

– Infection. The patient has an increased risk of developing infections due to restriction of movement, depression of the immune system by the use of corticosteroids, and the development of abnormal immune complexes.
– Nerve compression. Carpal tunnel syndrome occurs from swollen flexion tendon sheaths of the hand.
– Spinal cord compression in patients with rheumatoid arthritis of the cervical spine.
– Osteoporosis
– Rapid progression of the disease unresponsive to drug therapy leading to total disability.

Rehabilitation

This commences when the patient first presents for treatment and can be said to be achieved when the patient comes to terms with his change of appearance, is coping with his chronic pain, and has adapted his lifestyle to the changing pattern of the disease.

Anticipated outcome

This is variable but most people with rheumatoid arthritis live full, independent lives and have a normal life expectancy.

ANKYLOSING SPONDYLITIS

Ankylosing spondylitis is a chronic inflammatory arthritis, affecting the sacroiliac and spinal joints with occasional involvement of the peripheral joints. It eventually progresses to bony ankylosis of the involved joints.

The condition affects males more commonly than females (in a ratio of 8 : 1) with the age of onset being between 15–30 years. It occurs in approximately 0.4% of the population and is rare among people of African and Asian origin.

Pathophysiology

There is no known cause. However there appears to be a genetic predisposition as it is more common among family members. The HLA-B27 (human leucocyte antigen type B27) gene is present in over 90% of patients with ankylosing spondylitis and in half their immediate relatives, compared with only 7% in the general population.

Ankylosing spondylitis is sometimes associated with genitourinary infections, inflammatory bowel disease, and psoriatic arthritis. The disease is very slowly progressive, taking many years to develop.

The inflammatory process involves the synovial and fibrocartilagenous joints of the vertebrae and sacroiliac joints, and leads to fibrosis and ossification of the joint capsule and surrounding soft tissue, with eventual bony ankylosis of the entire joint.

Ossification across the intervertebral discs results in bony bridges (syndesmophytes) joining the vertebrae; ligaments also calcify. If many vertebrae and ligaments are involved the spine may become absolutely rigid, giving the characteristic appearance of a 'bamboo spine' on X-ray.

Ankylosis of the costovertebral joints may restrict chest expansion.

The disease usually begins at the sacroiliac joint and spreads to the spine. Occasionally inflammation of a large weight bearing joint (hip or knee) precedes the onset of spinal symptoms.

Other associated conditions are recurrent iritis and aortic valve incompetence.

Clinical manifestations

Initially the patient will present for medical advice with some or all of the following:

- Low back pain and stiffness.
- Morning stiffness. The symptoms are most noticeable in the morning and tend to wear off with exercise. Gradually pain and stiffness become more severe lasting most of the day as the disease progresses
- Pain, which may radiate into the buttock and thigh and may mimic sciatica
- Chest pain, which is exacerbated by deep breathing, occurs because of costovertebral joint involvement
- Pain in the heel from associated plantar fascitis or achilles tendonitis
- Unexplained weight loss and general malaise. This may occur in some persons with active disease.

On clinical examination the patient with established disease will be found to have:

- Diminished spinal movement in all directions, particularly in extension. When standing against a wall the heels, buttocks, scapulae and occiput should all touch the wall simultaneously – this is not possible for the patient with ankylosing spondylitis.
- A typical posture, with loss of normal lumbar lordosis (the lumbar spine will be flattened), forward thrust of the neck, slight flexion of the hips and knees, and a flexed spine
- A decreased chest expansion
- Tenderness over the sacroiliac joint.

A monoarticular, peripheral arthritis in the hip, knee, or shoulder with swelling, tenderness and loss of mobility may occur. The patient may also develop colitis.

Early in the disease, spinal movement may be normal with the only symptoms being slight back pain. This makes the disease difficult to diagnose.

Investigative procedures

Typical changes seen on X-ray are narrowing of the joint space, sclerosis and ankylosis of the sacroiliac and spinal joints, squaring of the vertebral bodies, and ossification (bridging) of the intervertebral discs.

Blood tests reveal elevated ESR during the active phase, and presence of HLA-B27 antigen (this is not absolutely diagnostic as only 20% of persons who carry this antigen develop the disease).

Medical, surgical, and nursing management

There is no cure for ankylosing spondylitis but much can be done to prevent the development of severe deformity. Treatment is directed towards:

• Relief of pain
• Reduction of the inflammatory process
• Maintenance of mobility of the affected joints
• Prevention of deformity by maintenance of good posture.

Treatment uses a multidisciplinary approach and involves education, medication, physiotherapy, and surgery. Patient co-operation is essential.

Relief of pain and inflammation

When acute attacks occur, pain is often relieved by rest and analgesic and anti-inflammatory drugs. Complete bed rest should be avoided as it increases stiffness and deformity. Local heat is effective in reducing pain and stiffness.

Maintenance of mobility

Between acute attacks patients must be encouraged to keep active and put their joints through a full range of movement at least twice daily. These are best taught by the physiotherapist. Noncontact sporting activities such as swimming and tennis are encouraged.

Prevention of deformity

To prevent flexion deformity of the spine, patients should:

– Sleep on a firm mattress with a board underneath, and use only one very small pillow
– Lie prone as much as possible
– Sit on hard-backed, upright chairs
– Be encouraged not to sit in one position for too long
– Stand straight at all times. Occupations that require stooping or lifting are unsuitable and will aggravate the condition.

Surgical intervention is restricted to patients who have developed severe deformity. When patients can no longer maintain an erect stance, wedge osteotomy of the vertebral bodies to improve severe flexion deformity of the spine may be performed; internal vertebral braces may occasionally be inserted. Total hip replacement to improve hip joint mobility where ankylosis has occurred may also be performed.

Drug therapy as used in the treatment of rheumatoid arthritis (see page 729) is used to reduce the inflammatory process and control pain.

No specific diet will alter the course of the disease. Patients need to be instructed to eat a well-balanced nutritious diet and to control their weight.

Specific nursing management

Ankylosing spondylitis takes a different course in different people and no two cases are exactly the same. Symptoms are usually intermittent over long periods and eventually settle down. The severity of the disease and of the deformity is variable and hospitalization is usually only necessary if surgery is to be performed. Otherwise, nursing care is as for the patient with rheumatoid arthritis (see page 730) with added emphasis on the need for adequate pulmonary ventilation. Deep breathing and chest expansion exercises must be performed regularly.

The patient and his significant others need to understand: the nature of the disorder; the absolute necessity of following the long-term physical therapy in order to prevent deformity; that the prognosis is good for the well motivated patient; and the importance of taking part in active noncontact sports on a regular basis. This is beneficial psychologically and socially, as well as physically.

Allied paramedical care

Physiotherapy is a most important part of treatment and includes: exercises to restore joint mobility; breathing exercizes to increase chest mobility and vital capacity; strengthening exercises particularly for the extension muscles of the spine; posture correction; back care and general fitness; and relaxation techniques.

Maintenance of physical fitness must be a lifetime commitment for the patient, therefore the physiotherapist prescribes exercises which are pleasurable and can be continued at home or at a Health Training Centre.

Orthopaedic appliances such as spinal supports and collars are not advocated as this decreases spinal mobility and weakens muscles. Splinting devices are only used following treatment of any fracture.

The social worker may be required to advise and assist with change of occupation and lifestyle. Vocational retraining may be necessary. Counselling is needed if the patient has problems adapting to the changes, especially of body image.

Complications

Complications of ankylosing spondylitis include:

– Subluxation or fracture of the cervical spine. This may result from a deceleration injury and commonly occurs at the junction between a mobile and immobile segment. Head supports on car seats are a necessity to prevent this injury from occurring.
– Spinal cord damage from subluxation or fracture of the spine.

Anticipated outcome

The prognosis is good if the patient complies with treatment and most patients live useful, productive lives hardly ever losing a day from work.

71

Infective disorders of the musculoskeletal system

Chris Game

OSTEOMYELITIS

Osteomyelitis is a pyogenic infection of bone most commonly caused by *Staphylococcus aureus*. It occurs more often in children than in adults and results most commonly from a combination of localized trauma and an acute infection appearing somewhere remote from the site of injury. The infection may reach the injured bone directly, as in a compound fracture; at surgery; via the circulation; or via extension from infection in adjacent structures. Acute osteomyelitis is most often blood-borne and commonly affects rapidly growing children. Chronic osteomyelitis, although rare, is more often is present in adults than children, and results from infection of metastatic lesions and is characterized by multiple draining sinus tracts (known as Brodie's ulcers).

Following localized trauma and haematoma development, the infecting organism multiplies rapidly and spreads directly to the bone. Suppuration occurs and the pus collects within the bone. As the condition progresses, pus is forced through the Haversian canals due to increasing intramedullary pressure. A subperiosteal abscess results and, as the abscess increases, the periosteum is stripped from the surface of the bone leading to further bone ischaemia. If this condition is allowed to persist necrosis will result. With necrosis, the periosteum is stimulated to form new bone and the old necrotic bone detaches and moves to the skin surface as sequestrum via the draining sinus tracts. Once this stage is reached, chronic osteomyelitis exists.

Clinical manifestations

The patient with acute osteomyelitis usually presents with sudden pain in the affected bone, and tenderness, heat, swelling and painful, restricted movement over the bone. Generalized symptoms and signs include a sharp rise in temperature, which can be to extreme levels and accompanied by rigors, delerium, tachycardia and nausea. Blood analysis reveals leucocytosis, an elevated ESR and most probably positive blood cultures for the infecting organism. There is very little evidence of bone infection to be seen on X-ray in the early stages of the disease.

In chronic osteomyelitis the onset is insidious and the symptoms may persist intermittently for years.

Medical, surgical, and nursing management

The rationale for treatment is to:

- Control any infection
- Rest the affected limb/part
- Protect the affected bone from further injury
- Provide supportive care.

As it is imperative to arrest the pyogenic process, it is quite common for large dose antibiotic therapy to be commenced intravenously prior to the causative organism being isolated. However, findings from wound swabs and blood cultures, which must be taken before the commencement of antibiotic therapy, may mean that the type of antiobiotic is subsequently altered. As the blood supply to the bone is poor, large dose antibiotic therapy will need to be administered intravenously in an attempt to maximize the effect of the drug on the pyogenic process. Once necrosis occurs the effect of antibiotic therapy is markedly reduced as the blood supply to the affected part has been lost. If the area involved is large, amputation may be the only treatment available for necrosis (see page 304).

Nursing management will therefore include the care of the patient with a central venous line as large dose antibiotics should not be administered via a peripheral line due to the sclerosing nature of the drugs. The patient will usually be confined to bed and, depending upon the site of the osteomyelitis, the affected bone may be further immobilized by way of plaster cast or traction. Nursing care will include the prevention of the complications of bed rest, the care of the patient with a cast or in traction, and encouragement of the patient to continue with isometric and active exercises to prevent muscle wasting.

Immobilization of the limb provides protection against further injury, and stringent hygiene measures along with the use of aseptic technique when changing dressings, will further lessen the risk of infection.

Surgery to adequately drain the affected area may be required to increase the effect of the antibiotic therapy, relieve the build up of pressure, and prevent necrosis developing.

As the recovery period for the patient is lengthy, the nurse will be required to provide long-term supportive care to the patient and his significant others. In particular, as acute osteomyelitis occurs more commonly in children, diversional therapy will be required.

Should the patient fail to respond adequately to treatment, the use of hyperbaric oxygen along with surgery and antibiotics has had some limited success in effecting a cure.

Allied paramedical care

Physiotherapy is mandatory to prevent muscle wasting during the period of immobilization and to effect a return to full range of movement once ambulation is permitted. Occupational therapy may be required with activities of daily living – especially if the patient is elderly or has required

extensive surgery to effect a cure. A referral to the prosthetist will be necessary prior to any amputation surgery being performed.

Anticipated outcome

With the increased use of arthroscopy, adhesive skin drapes, and other measures to reduce wound contamination during joint surgery, the incidence of osteomyelitis due to infection introduced at surgery is diminishing. As well, routine postoperative antibiotic therapy following orthopaedic surgery has led to a lowered incidence of postoperative wound infection. With astute nursing observation and reporting of any incidence of wound infection, the risk of postoperative osteomyelitis will be even further reduced.

The chance of recovery for the patient with osteomyelitis is high and he should be able to return to a normal lifestyle.

SEPTIC ARTHRITIS

Septic arthritis occurs when bacteria invade and infect a joint, causing inflammation of the synovial lining. Should the infecting organism gain entry to the joint cavity then the resulting effusion and suppuration may lead to bone and cartilage destruction with ankylosis and septicaemia occurring in severe cases.

Many bacteria have been isolated as the cause of septic arthritis and both gram-positive and gram-negative cocci are common, along with gram-negative bacilli. In nearly all instances of septic arthritis, the bacteria spread from a primary site of infection in adjacent bone or soft tissue. The primary infection may be due to trauma, especially of articular surfaces as seen in sporting injuries; follow joint surgery; or be introduced during intra-articular injection, for example dexamethasone, following joint injury. However, any concurrent bacterial infection or serious chronic illness may predispose a person to septic arthritis and the elderly and alcoholics are at greatest risk. It is important to note that IV drug users are also at high risk of developing septic arthritis.

Clinical manifestations

The clinical course of septic arthritis is similar to that of osteomyelitis but differs in that it is always confined to joints, especially the large joints of the hip, knee, elbow and shoulder. The onset is rapid and the patient presents with severe pain, inflammation, and swelling of the affected joint. Examination of synovial aspirate will identify the organism and indicate the degree of sepsis present. Joint X-ray will demonstrate the extent of joint damage and blood analysis of ESR and leucocyte count will show the extent of systemic disease.

Medical and nursing management

The medical and nursing management for the patient with septic arthritis follows the same course as for the patient with osteomyelitis (see page 736).

72

Oncological disorders of the musculoskeletal system

Chris Game   Robyn Anderson

Tumours of bone occur as either primary growths or from metastatic spread from carcinomas or more rarely, sarcomas. Metastatic bone tumours are more common than primary growths and once bony metastases have developed the prognosis for recovery is poor.

PRIMARY TUMOURS OF BONE

These may be either benign or malignant; primary malignancy of bone is rare.

Benign tumours occur in the form of osteoma, osteoid osteoma, osteoclastoma, chondroma, fibromas, giant-cell tumours, and cysts. Benign growths are well circumscribed, grow very slowly, remain encapsulated and do not spread to other parts of the body. However, it is not uncommon for a benign tumour to become malignant later in life. Therefore, surgical excision is usually performed as soon as the tumour is diagnosed.

Malignant tumours occur as osteogenic sarcoma, osteoclastoma, chondrosarcoma, fibrosarcoma, Ewing's tumour, reticulum cell sarcoma, angiosarcoma, and multiple myeloma (see page 413). Osteogenic sarcoma is the most commonly occurring primary tumour of bone and manifests in children, adolescents and young adults. When it occurs, it is sited usually in the upper tibia, lower femur or upper end of the humerus. It is a rapidly metastazing tumour and the only accepted treatment is amputation (see page 304). However, less than 10% of patients survive beyond 5 years despite amputation and radiotherapy. Ewing's tumour is a highly malignant tumour occurring in children between the ages of 5–15. The prognosis

is extremely poor with less than 1% 5 year survival despite amputation and radiotherapy.

Metastatic bone tumours most commonly arise from secondary spread from primary tumours of the bronchus, breast and prostate. Renal, ovarian and thyroid tumour have also a high incidence of metastasis to the bone. They are frequently associated with a rise in serum alkaline phosphatase and many are hormone dependent. Therefore, partial or complete remission can occasionally be achieved following hypophysectomy or the administration of the appropriate androgen. Local radiotherapy or cytotoxic chemotherapy may be useful for a time in symptomatic treatment.

Clinical manifestations

Regardless of the type of bone tumour, the symptoms that cause the patient to seek medical advice are similar.

- Swelling, deformity
- Pain, aching
- Warmth over the site of the tumour
- Restriction of movement
- Pathological fractures.

Bone pain with malignant disease is usually severe, persistent and present before metastases can be demonstrated on X-ray.

Investigative procedures

Skeletal X-ray is performed as many tumours show characteristic changes. Biopsy of the suspected tumour area will confirm the presence and types of tumour.

Bone scan will determine the extent of primary disease or secondary spread.

Serum alkaline phosphatase will be raised.

Medical, surgical, and nursing management

The major aim of surgery for a primary malignancy of bone is to remove the tumour as soon as possible, assuming that it has not already metastasized. Therefore, amputation of the limb is performed. Nursing management for the patient following amputation is discussed on page 304. Where the malignancy involves a bone of the proximal skeleton, the bone, or part of the bone, is removed. Follow up radiotherapy and chemotherapy will be adjuvant treatment in these cases and bone scans should be performed at six-monthly intervals for five years.

Specific nursing care of the patient will be as for any person undergoing orthopaedic surgery (see page 720) and/or radiotherapy and chemotherapy (see page 125).

73

Metabolic and nutritional disorders of the musculoskeletal system

Helga Sabel   Chris Game   Robyn Anderson

GOUT

Gout (or gouty arthritis) is an inborn error of metabolism resulting in the deposition of uric acid crystals (monosodium urate monohydrate) within joints and surrounding connective tissue. Occasionally deposition occurs in soft tissue in other areas of the body and accumulation of uric acid crystals in the renal tubules may result in renal calculi (see page 607). Raw uric acid crystals may occasionally be excreted through the skin.

Pathophysiology

Uric acid is the final end-product of normal purine metabolism. In the normal individual there is a constant balance between the production of uric acid by the body and its excretion. Purines are derived from two sources:

1. Exogenous – from high protein foods particularly anchovies, sardines, salmon, organ meats, dried peas and beans
2. Endogenous – synthesized by the body.

Uric acid, a waste product, which must be excreted, is eliminated from the body by urinary excretion (66%) and by biliary and intestinal secretion (33%).

In gout the serum level of uric acid is raised (hyperuricaemia) which results from either overproduction or underexcretion of uric acid or a combination of both. However, many individuals with hyperuricaemia do not necessarily present with clinical symptoms of gout. In one study of 2500 patients (Rohl, 1981), 165 had hyperuricaemia but only 15 had gouty arthritis.

Attacks of gouty arthritis are caused by a sudden deposition of uric acid crystals in synovial membrane. Leucocytes phagocytose the crystals, disintegrate and release lysosomal enzymes which results in acute, severe, local inflammation. Lactic acid is also produced by the active phagocytic leucocytes and this promotes further urate crystallization as urates are less soluble in an acid medium. With more crystallization, more leucocytes are attracted to the area and more lactic acid is produced, resulting in a self-propagating inflammatory reaction.

Early in the disease the crystals are absorbed after each attack, which lasts approximately two weeks, and the joint returns to normal even with no treatment. Attacks are initially infrequent being months or years apart.

Many years later as the disease progresses, nodular deposits (or tophi) develop in one or more sites. Tophi consist of bundles of needles that form from uric acid crystals and commonly occur in the synovial membrane of bursae, especially of the elbow, in tendon sheaths and in the cartilage of the external ear.

When tophi develop the patient is said to have 'chronic tophaceous gout'. Eventually the proteolytic enzymes produced as a result of the chronic inflammatory process destroy the joint cartilage and erode the underlying bone, leading to secondary degenerative joint changes which may be severe.

Gout falls into two main categories:

1. Primary gout (80% of cases). The metabolic defect causing the hyperuricaemia is unknown. There is usually a family history of gout. It is more common in men, usually starting after

puberty and reaching a peak incidence in early middle age. It is rarely seen in women under 45 years of age.

2. Secondary gout. The hyperuricaemia is a direct consequence of the following:

(a) Overproduction of uric acid caused by excessive turnover of cells as in myeloproliferative and lymphoproliferative disorders, chronic haemolytic anaemias, severe exfoliative psoriasis, Gaucher's disease and fructose ingestion or infusion.

(b) Decreased excretion of uric acid by the kidneys as a result of: chronic renal disease; widespread use of diuretics (thiazides and frusemide prevent the re-excretion of uric acid by the proximal tubule); low dose aspirin therapy, which will retain uric acid; and increased levels of organic acids from dehydration, starvation, acute ethanol ingestion, toxaemia of pregnancy and diabetic ketoacidosis.

Statistical data

The full clinical picture of gout is now relatively uncommon due to earlier diagnosis and effective treatment. Mild forms are prevalent (0.3% of total population). Men are most commonly affected with a male : female ratio of 20 : 1. The disease may be present in adolescence but the peak incidence is around age 40. It is rare in females prior to menopause. Gout involves mainly the peripheral joints; it can be monarticular or polyarticular. The most common joint affected is the metatarsophalangeal joint of the big toe. The ankle, knee and small joints of the hands and feet, wrist and elbow follow in decreasing order of frequency.

Clinical manifestations

Acute gout occurs usually only in one joint and the patient presents with a dusky red, hot, swollen and very tender joint, which causes intense, excruciating pain. The patient is unable to move the joint, and may have a slight fever, headache, malaise, and anorexia.

Chronic gout is polyarticular and the patient has loss of function in stiff, swollen, and deformed joints, which are painful. Subcutaneous tophi occur, commonly in the ear and elbow.

Investigative procedures

The patient history may reveal previous episodes of problems with renal calculi.

Serum analysis may show elevated levels of ESR, leucocytes and uric acid. Serum electrolytes, lipids, haematocrit and haemoglobin are also usually performed to determine secondary causes and differential diagnosis.

A 24-hour collection of urine is needed for uric acid determination.

Synovial fluid analysis will determine the presence of uric acid crystals.

Acute gout will reveal only soft tissue swelling and a normal joint on X-ray, but advanced chronic disease will show joint destruction, bony cysts with punched out lesions, and the swelling of tophi containing flecks of calcium. Uric acid crystals are radiolucent but calcification often occurs. X-ray may also show localized osteoporosis. Chest X-ray is also performed for differential diagnosis of other forms of arthritis, for example, SLE or sarcoidosis.

Synovium and tophi biopsy is performed to check for the presence of crystals.

Medical and surgical management

The rationale for treatment is to control the disease to prevent renal calculi and renal destruction, and joint destruction.

Acute attack

Colchicine is specific for acute gout and has no effect on other inflammatory conditions. It is thought to reduce inflammation by suppressing the leucocyte phagocytosis and lactic acid formation. Benefit is usually felt within a few hours and inflammation reduced within 48 hours. Colchicine can be given intravenously if gastrointestinal intolerance is severe.

Nonsteroidal anti-inflammatory drugs are given to reduce the severity of the pain and to reduce the inflammatory process. High doses are required initially until the attack subsides (24–48 hours) and then are continued on a lower dosage for 7–10 days.

Indomethacin is the drug of choice and acts by inhibiting prostoglandin synthesis. Other drugs in this group include naproxen and oxyphenbutazone.

Long-term management

After the acute attack has settled, long-term drug therapy is aimed at reducing the serum/uric acid level and preventing further acute episodes.

Allopurinol is the drug of choice in long-term management. Purine is broken down through a number of steps to uric acid. Allopurinol acts by inhibiting xanthine oxidase, the enzyme responsible for the last two steps in the formation of uric acid. By inhibiting uric acid synthesis it reduces the amount of uric acid in the body and can be safely used for patients with renal disease as it does not depend on functioning kidneys.

Patients must be advised to follow their drug regime strictly as a sudden withdrawal can lead to a rebound attack of gouty arthritis. The drugs are continued indefinitely.

Drugs may be used in combination to enhance the effect and reduce the side effects caused by using single drugs in high doses.

Paracetamol or codeine are the drugs of choice to reduce pain. Aspirin and salicylates are never used with uricosuric agents, as they interfere with the agent's efficiency.

Uricosuric agents are seldom used nowadays because of their gastrointestinal side-effects and also because allopurinol is so effective. However, these agents increase the excretion of uric acid by direct action on the renal tubules. The principal drug in this group is probenacid.

Surgical intervention does not play a significant role in the treatment of gout. Aspiration of fluid followed by intra-articular injection of steroids may be performed in a joint (commonly the knee) where there is excessive swelling with a palpable effusion. Surgical removal of tophi may be required to restore joint function.

Diet

A well-balanced diet should be followed and the patient advised to:

1. Avoid foods that are very high in purines, for example, organ meats, salmon, sardines, anchovies, dried peas and beans. Purine-rich foods produce uric acid and can precipitate or aggravate an attack of gouty arthritis. Cooking does not destroy the purines in these foods.
2. Avoid excessive intake of alcohol. Alcohol promotes formation of lactic acid and ketone bodies.
3. Maintain normal weight – avoid obesity.
4. Avoid 'crash' diets. Diets with few carbohydrates increase the breakdown of normal protein and elevate serum uric acid levels.
5. Increase fluid intake. A minimum of three litres a day is required to prevent uric acid crystallization in the kidneys.

Nursing management

The nursing management of gout is symptomatic and commonsense. It is based on resting the acutely inflamed joints.

For the patient who is admitted with an acute attack of gouty arthritis, nursing care is centred around the following needs:

1. Relief of pain.
(a) The patient is confined to bed until the acute episode subsides
(b) The affected limb is elevated on pillows or with a sling, and protected from the weight of the bedclothes by the use of a bed cradle
(c) Cold packs to the involved joint will help to relieve pain if tolerated by the patient
(d) Provide oral analgesia. Rarely, parenteral analgesia may be necessary until the effect of the drug therapy becomes apparent.
2. Health education.
The patient and/or his significant other must
(a) Understand the disease process
(b) Recognize the importance of drug therapy, the need for strict adherence to the drug regime, and be aware of the possible side effects
(c) Exercise the affected limb gently once inflammation has subsided. Strenuous exercise is to be avoided
(d) Understand the detrimental effects and risks of continued high alcohol consumption
(e) Understand the need to reduce weight and reduce the intake of foods high in purines, and maintain a high fluid intake

(f) Be encouraged to seek medical help if symptoms return or worsen.

For the patient with chronic tophaceous gout the nursing care centres around patient comfort. The many joints affected will need support and protection by the use of pillows, splints and bed cradles. Flexion deformity of the joints must be avoided.

Ruptured tophi exude chalky white crystals of uric acid and will require aseptic wound dressing.

The patient should be encouraged to drink a minimum of 3 l of fluid daily.

Urine pH should be kept alkaline.

Allied paramedical care

Physiotherapy is essential to prevent affected joints becoming stiff and to maintain a full range of movement.

Dietary advice should be arranged for the patient in relation to maintenance of ideal body weight, purine containing foodstuffs and fluid intake.

The occupational therapist may be required to assist the patient in activities of daily living, particularly if the joints on the hand, wrist and elbow are involved.

Complications

Complications of gout are due to uric acid crystallization in the kidneys and renal calculi occur in approximately 10–20% of all patients.

Chronic renal disease and/or degenerative joint disease may result.

Anticipated outcome

Patients with gout should be able to live normal lives without drastic changes to their lifestyle or with little residual damage to their joints, providing the condition is diagnosed early and effective treatment instituted.

OSTEOPOROSIS

Osteoporosis means 'porous bone'. It is the loss of the overall total mass of bone and results in thin, brittle bones which may fracture easily. Both mineral and non-mineralized matrix (osteoid) are diminished but the ratio between the two remains the same as in normal bone.

Pathophysiology and incidence

The cause is an increase in bone breakdown, a decrease in bone production, or a combination of both. The disease develops slowly and is difficult to reverse.

Factors which may contribute to osteoporosis are:

1. Menopause. A drop in the production of oestrogen leads to an increase in bone breakdown (resorption). This is also associated with some degree of calcium malabsorption. Bone loss in women after menopause is approximately 2%/year and continues for at least ten years at which time it may level out (Nordin, 1983).
2. Increasing age. The loss of bone mass is a normal accompaniment of the ageing process and most men and women will develop some degree of osteoporosis after the age of 65. Men begin losing bone after the age of 60 at a rate of 0.5%/year. (Nordin, 1983). In women the bone loss is a combination of both senile and postmenopausal factors and women are therefore at more risk of sustaining fractures. Nordin states that 25% of women over the age of 65 years will have sustained at least one fracture by the time they reach 80, while studies in the United Kingdom suggest that almost half of women over 65 experience at least one osteoporotic fracture (MacIntyre, 1983).
3. Immobilization. Prolonged bed rest, muscular weakness, paralysis, and lack of exercise all result in loss of bone mass. Localized osteoporosis may occur in the bones of a limb that has been immobilized for a long period.
4. Disorders associated with osteoporosis. Thyrotoxicosis, Cushing's disease, acromegaly and diabetes mellitus are all accompanied by osteoporotic changes in bone.
5. Corticosteroid therapy. Prednisolone if given in doses greater than 10 mg/day for long periods reduces calcium absorption, increases calcium excretion from the kidneys and reduces new bone formation.

6. High protein diet. Excessive intake of animal protein causes an increase in calcium loss from the kidneys and results in low serum calcium levels with gradual loss of bone from the skeleton.

7. High sodium intake. Sodium competes with calcium for reabsorption in the renal tubules. The higher the sodium intake the higher the urinary calcium loss.

8. Malignant disease. Carcinoma of the breast, myeloma and leukaemia are all accompanied by osteoporotic changes in bone.

9. Malabsorption of calcium and/or low calcium intake. Decreased serum calcium levels, due either to a low dietary intake or an error of metabolism, triggers the release of parathormone. Calcium is then resorbed from bone to maintain serum calcium levels, thus leading to more porous bone tissue.

10. Hypogonadism, vitamin C deficiency, and decreased production of growth hormone may all contribute to osteoporosis, by decreasing new bone formation.

Clinical manifestations

The person may not display symptoms until such time as a bone breaks. Soft tissue injury is usually minimal. Common sites of fractures that occur as a result of osteoporosis are the neck of the femur, the lower radius and ulna (Colles' fracture), and the vertebral bodies (crush fractures).

The spinal column is most commonly involved in osteoporosis and this leads to a person with a stooped posture, thoracic kyphosis and a loss of lumbar lordosis. Furthermore, loss of height occurs due to increasing fibrosis of intervertebral discs and may be worsened by collapsing of the vertebrae. Commonly, the patient may experience back pain.

Investigative procedures

Thirty per cent of bone mass must be lost before osteoporosis shows on X-ray and collapsing of the vertebrae may be evident.

Bone biopsy from the iliac crest shows a reduction in trabecular bone volume but the trabeculae are normally calcified.

Biochemical studies, including serum calcium levels, fasting urinary calcium, urinary hydroxyproline, and plasma alkaline phosphatase are performed.

Medical and surgical management

With the increase in life expectancy in western society, osteoporosis has become a major health problem costing millions of dollars in hospitalization and institutional care for the elderly, especially those with hip fractures. McIntyre (1983) states that fracture of the neck of femur is the third highest nonpsychiatric factor in bed occupancy in the United Kingdom. Management therefore aims at prevention, the reduction of risk factors, and the treatment of fractures.

Prevention

Research indicates that diet may play a significant role in the prevention of osteoporosis or in lessening the degree of severity. Because bone takes many years to replace itself, any preventive measures to be effective must be initiated during the middle years and continued through life.

The need is for:

• Increased calcium, especially for postmenopausal women
• Increased vitamin C
• Decreased protein. Excessive intake of protein in the form of red meats should be avoided
• Decreased sodium.

Reduction of risk factors

Drug therapy aims at reducing the risk factors. As bone has a turnover period of five to eight years any improvement from treatment will only be noticeable after some years. Drugs, at present, are given only to those in whom risk factors have been identified and who have accelerated bone loss. Drug therapy must be long-term to be effective and is often used in combination as more than one factor is usually involved.

Oestrogen replacement in postmenopausal women lowers urinary calcium loss. Only low doses can be safely given as there is a slight risk of breast and endometrial cancer occurring with long term therapy. Uterine bleeding is an adverse effect which will require the drug to be withdrawn until bleeding stops.

Calcium supplements. Adverse reactions include nausea and constipation. Hypercalcaemia, hypophosphataemia and renal calculi may arise with long term therapy in high doses.

Vitamin D preparations. These are helpful in preventing resorption. Long term therapy may cause nausea, vomiting and constipation, hypercalcaemia, and renal failure.

Androgens. These may be required for the osteoporotic patient with low plasma testosterone.

Treatment of fractures

Fractures occurring in osteoporitic bone heal more slowly than those in normal bone.

Vertebral fractures are usually treated by complete bed rest with hyperextension of the spine at the level of the injury for two to three weeks. The patient is encouraged to continue to sleep with the spine in extension when at home.

Fractures of the neck of the femur are treated by reduction and internal fixation usually with a compression screw and plate. A femoral head replacement (see page 719) may be the method of treatment for subcapital fractures where avascular necrosis of the femoral head is a likely complication.

Fractures of the forearm are reduced and immobilized by a plaster cast for four to six weeks.

In all situations following treatment, patients should be encouraged to be as active as possible and bed rest kept to a minimum.

Nursing management

Patients with osteoporosis are usually only admitted to hospital for investigative procedures, and the treatment of pathological fractures

When a patient is admitted for investigative procedures nursing care centres on the accurate collection of specimens and the accurate recording of data. The patient with osteoporosis is not ill.

For the patient with a fracture nursing care aims at providing for patient comfort, protection of the fractured limb, and early mobilization to prevent the complications of bed rest. See Chapter

68 for the management of the patient with a fractured bone.

Complications

The major complication of osteoporosis is a fracture, with a fracture of the neck of the femur in women being the most common.

Anticipated outcome and habilitation

Most persons with osteoporosis do not know they have the disease and it is identified only when a fracture occurs following a minor trauma such as a fall. Some people have accelerated bone loss and for these back pain and loss of height are symptoms which often go undiagnosed for many years.

In the future, prophylactic drug therapy may be instituted for those with anticipated accelerated osteoporosis, and the number of elderly patients admitted to hospital and institutional care following a fracture of the neck of femur from osteoporosis should thus be reduced.

PAGET'S DISEASE

Paget's disease, or osteitis deformans, is a chronic common disorder of bone which progresses slowly and is characterized by an increase in osteocyte turnover which results in thick, weak, deformed bones.

Pathophysiology

There is an abnormal increase in the number and activity of osteoclasts which causes rapid destruction of bone tissue. In response to the increase in bone resorption there is a compensatory increase in osteoblast activity to repair the process. The new bone that is formed is disorganized and irregular and does not have the normal pattern of mature bone. Blood supply is greatly increased during the active phase of the disease, and the bone radiates warmth and is relatively soft. It is during the active, vascular phase that affected weight bearing bones bend and deform easily. When activity ceases, the bone becomes brittle and breaks easily causing pathological fractures.

The disease progresses very slowly and the extent varies from patient to patient. The disease may be extremely localized or as much as 90% of the skeleton may be involved.

Bones that are most frequently involved in the disease process are the pelvis, the long bones of the lower limb, the skull, the spine, and the humerus.

Many patients with Paget's disease are diagnosed accidentally when X-rayed for an entirely different disorder.

Incidence

It is a disease of middle to old age (it rarely occurs under age 40) and affects men and women equally.

People of Anglo-Saxon origin are more commonly affected and the prevalence in Australasia may be as high as 4% of the population. However, only a small percentage of these are likely to seek medical help as many assume the pain and progressive disability to be the normal process of ageing.

There is no definite known cause but recent research suggests that it may be due to a slow, viral infection of long latency (Rohl, 1981).

Clinical manifestations

Symptoms are variable and any of the following may cause the patient to seek medical help.

Pain in the affected bone(s) varies widely from patient to patient, but is mostly a dull, constant ache which may worsen at night. Severe pain usually indicates a fracture. Limb deformity is most noticeable in weight-bearing bones, and backache, joint stiffness and limitation of movement occur.

Blindness due to pressure of the enlarged skull on the second cranial nerve, and deafness or tinnitus as a result of pressure on the eighth cranial nerve may occur. Headache may be a feature. Nerve compression may lead to paraesthesis.

On clinical examination the following may be present:

1. Bone deformity and thickening. The femur tends to bow laterally and the tibia anteriorly. The skin over the bone feels warm
2. Skull enlargement

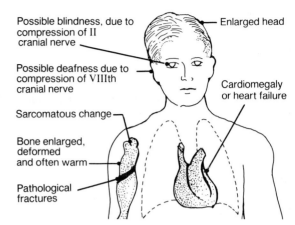

Fig. 73.1 Paget's disease. (Modified from Read AE et al 1984 Modern Medicine 3 Edn. Churchill Livingstone, Edinburgh.)

3. Kyphosis of the thoracic spine
4. In the early stages of the disease the pulse feels full and bounding due to an increased vascularity raising the cardiac output and stroke volume. In the late stage of the disease cardiac failure is evident (Fig. 73.1).

Investigative procedures

Typically, the X-ray will show that the affected bone is thickened and bent with a fuzzy, woven structure. Tiny fissure fractures may be seen on the convex side. Bone scan shows areas of increased vascularity and reveals the extent of the disease.

Serum alkaline phosphatase is raised in active disease and reflects increased osteoblast function.

Urinary hydroxyproline is elevated. Hydroxyproline indicates an increase in the turnover of collagen and reflects osteoclast activity. Serum calcium is usually normal but increases when the patient is immobilized.

Bone biopsy is rarely performed but will confirm diagnosis.

Medical management

The aim of treatment is to relieve pain, suppress the disease process, and prevent the development of complications.

Where possible conservative drug therapy should always precede surgery. Calcitonin is thought to be best as it prevents bone resorption and does not decrease mineralization.

Nonsteroidal anti-inflammatory drugs are effective in relieving mild, intermittent pain and joint stiffness.

Calcitonin acts as a suppressive agent by inhibiting bone resorption. It is also effective in the relief of severe bone pain. It is available from salmon and porcine sources and is administered by subcutaneous injection on a daily or 3 times weekly basis for a minimum period of 8–12 weeks and may continue for up to 12 months. Adverse reactions are common and include nausea, vomiting, diarrhoea, flushing, sneezing, urticaria, and polyuria. These may be minimized by administering the injection at night after giving an oral antiemetic 20 minutes prior to the injection. The patient is taught to give his own injections.

Adverse reactions include gastrointestinal disturbances and these can be minimized by giving the drug after meals.

A combination of calcitonin and diphosphonate drugs may be used.

Cytotoxic agents may be used to inhibit bone growth should all other therapy fail. However, these are rarely used due to their poor tolerance and limited effect.

Patients on suppressive therapy need regular monitoring of their serum alkaline phosphatase, and serum calcium levels, as well as urinary hydroxyproline levels. A fall in these gives an indication of the effectiveness of the therapy.

Surgical management

As Paget's disease is a chronic degenerative disorder, surgical intervention is aimed primarily at improving the quality of life for the patient by correcting deformities that may otherwise cause severe disablement.

Osteotomy may be performed to correct the bowing deformity of the femur or tibia.

Fractures are often treated by open reduction and internal fixation in the form of intramedullary nailing. Any deformity is usually also corrected at the time of surgery.

Total joint replacement of the hip or knee may be necessary in advanced disease where the pain and loss of mobility from secondary osteoarthritis is a major problem.

Spinal decompression is required if bone overgrowth has resulted in stenosis, causing nerve root or cord compression.

Nursing management

Patients with Paget's disease are usually only admitted to hospital for treatment of pathological fractures or corrective surgery.

When planning nursing care the following areas must be considered:

1. Pagetic bone bleeds readily, therefore following surgery blood loss from the wound must be monitored regularly. Haematoma formation can be prevented by ensuring that, if used, the low pressure aspiration device is patent and draining. The limb should be elevated to aid venous return, and vital signs and neurovascular observations are recorded until stable.

2. Immobilization and bed rest increases the rate of bone resorption. Hypercalcaemia with hypercalciuria may develop and predispose to the formation of renal calculi.

Cardiac failure is a possibility in patients with Paget's disease. Therefore the patient's fluid intake should be monitored to ensure an intake high enough to prevent crystallization in the renal tubules and at the same time prevent circulatory overloading.

Fluids high in calcium are restricted and mobilization is commenced as soon as possible with the assistance of crutches or a walking frame, but full weight bearing is usually avoided for several weeks.

3. Pain may initially need to be controlled by narcotic analgesia. Nonsteroidal anti-inflammatory agents and suppressive therapy should continue to be administered.

4. Psychological support may be needed to help the patient come to terms with his chronic disease.

Allied paramedical care

A physiotherapist is involved in helping the patient to regain full mobility, increase his muscle strength, and reduce joint stiffness.

A social worker may be required if the patient is unable to resume normal employment.

Problems associated with treatment

Most problems stem from the unpleasant side effects of drug therapy and the fact that calcitonin has to be administered by injection. Human calcitonin is being developed and when this becomes available it will reduce the allergic type reactions of the salmon and porcine varieties.

Rapid infusion of blood to restore blood loss, which may precipitate cardiac failure.

Complications

1. Osteoarthritis. This occurs most commonly in the hip and knee joints and results from the abnormal stress put through these joints by deformed bones.
2. Deafness and/or blindness from compression of cranial nerves.
3. Nerve root compression or spinal cord compression from spinal stenosis caused by overgrowth of the vertebrae.
4. Cardiac failure.
5. Renal calculi.
6. Osteogenic sarcoma. This is rare but when it occurs it is highly malignant.

Anticipated outcome

The majority of patients with Paget's disease live normal lives without any chemotherapy other than nonsteroidal anti-inflammatory drugs. In many persons the condition is subclinical. For those patients with more progressive disease, treatment with suppressive therapy, corrective surgery and analgesia has improved the quality of their lifestyle and most come to terms with their disease and live useful lives to old age.

OSTEOMALACIA

Osteomalacia occurs as a disorder of phosphorus and calcium metabolism. It produces softening of adult bone and is due to an inadequate dietary intake of vitamin D, or an inability of the body to absorb and/or use vitamin D, and may also result from the underexposure to ultraviolet rays. Ultraviolet rays (sunlight) are necessary for the synthesis of vitamin D, and the commonest cause of osteomalacia is a combination of lack of exposure to sunlight accompanied by a diet low in vitamin D. Consequently it is a condition found in people living in crowded, lower socio-economic areas particularly in the northern part of Europe.

With treatment, bone calcification can be restored and deformities may disappear.

Osteomalacia may result in some persons suffering from malabsorption where the ability to absorb fat soluble vitamins is lost, for example, chronic pancreatitis, biliary obstruction, Crohn's disease, coeliac disease, or following small bowel resection.

Rickets is the term used to describe vitamin D deficiency in infants and children. When the deficiency occurs in this age group, normal bone calcification does not take place and despite treatment, some bone deformities will persist.

Vitamin D-resistant rickets is a poorly named form of rickets which is caused by the inability of the renal tubules to reabsorb phosphate. This is an inherited disorder linked to an X-recessive gene. This form of rickets is also seen in a variety of renal diseases.

Clinical manifestations

Osteomalacia is characterized by generalized bone pain and tenderness, and deformities of the bone. Bending of the long bones due to softening and flattening occurs as a result of a lack of calcium. This is particularly common in the weight bearing bones. Pathological fractures may occur or be demonstrated on X-ray and bone cysts may also be present. Serum calcium and phosphorus levels are reduced.

Medical and nursing management

Following diagnosis of osteomalacia, the cause must be determined and, where possible, corrected. Except in cases of malabsorption, oral supplements of vitamin D preparations, or cod liver oil, plus a diet high in vitamin D and exposure to sunlight will cure the condition, but will not necessarily revert the deformities.

It is important for the nurse to obtain a dietary history, as education of the patient and his significant others will be necessary to prevent the deficiency recurring once the patient returns home.

If long term vitamin D therapy is required the patient should be advised of the side-effects (see page 247) and encouraged to seek advice if headache, nausea, diarrhoea or the symptoms of renal calculi develop.

Prosthetic and orthotic referral may be necessary to assist in the correction of deformities. Splints, calipers or limb supports may be used to straighten deformities as calcium is taken up by the bone.

SECTION K – REFERENCES AND FURTHER READING

Texts

Adams J C 1986 Outline of fractures, 10th edn. Churchill Livingstone

Anderson J R (ed) 1976 Muir's textbook of pathology, 10th edn. Edward Arnold, London

Anthony C P 1984 Structure and function of the body. Mosby, St Louis

Apley A G, Solomon L 1982 System of orthopaedics and fractures. Butterworth Scientific, London

Bogumill G P, Schwamm H A 1984 Orthopaedic pathology: a synopsis with clinical and radiographic correlation. Saunders, Philadelphia

Brashear H R, Raney R B 1986 Handbook of orthopaedic surgery, 10th edn. Mosby, St Louis

Casscells S W (ed) 1984 Arthroscopy: diagnostic and surgical practice. Lea & Febiger, Philadelphia

Corrigan B 1983 Practical orthopaedic medicine. Butterworths, London

Creager J G 1982 Human anatomy and physiology. Wadsworth, California

Crenshaw A H (ed) 1987 Campbell's operative orthopaedics, 7th edn. Mosby, St Louis

Cyriax J 1980 Textbook of orthopaedic medicine. Bailliere-Tindall, London

D'Ambrosia R D (ed) 1986 Musculoskeletal disorders: regional examination and differential diagnosis, 2nd edn. Lippincott, Philadelphia

Duckworth T 1984 Lecture notes on orthopaedics and fractures. Blackwell Scientific, Oxford

Farrell J 1983 Illustrated guide to orthopaedic nursing, 2nd edn. Lippincott, Philadelphia

Fleetcroft J P 1983 The musculoskeletal system: orthopaedics, rheumatology and fractures. Churchill Livingstone, Edinburgh

Havard M 1986 A nursing guide to drugs, 2nd edn. Churchill Livingstone, Melbourne

Laurence D R, Bennett P N 1987 Clinical pharmacology, 6th edn. Churchill Livingstone, Edinburgh 1237

Lawson P K (ed) 1984 Working with orthopedic patients: nursing photobook. Springhouse, Pennsylvania

Lovell W W, Winter R B (eds) 1986 Pediatric orthopaedics, 2nd edn. Lippincott, Philadelphia

Luckmann J, Sorensen K C 1980 Medical-surgical nursing: a psychophysiologic approach, 2nd edn. Saunders, Philadelphia

Macleod J 1987 Davidson's principles and practice of medicine, 15th edn. Churchill Livingstone, Edinburgh

McCrae R 1981 Practical fracture treatment. Churchill Livingstone, Edinburgh

Meyers M H (ed) 1984 The multiply injured patient with complex fractures. Lea & Febiger, Philadelphia

Pauwels F 1986 Biomechanics of the locomotor apparatus: contributions of the functional anatomy of the locomotor apparatus. Springer-Verlag, Berlin

Powell M (ed) 1986 Orthopaedic nursing and rehabilitation, 9th edn. Churchill Livingstone, Edinburgh

Read A E, Barritt D W, Langton Hewer R 1986 Modern medicine, 3rd edn. Churchill Livingstone, Edinburgh

Rockwood C A Jr, Green D P (eds) 1984 Fractures in adults, 2nd edn. Lippincott, Philadelphia

Salter R B 1983 Textbook of disorders and injuries of the musculoskeletal system, 2nd edn. Williams and Wilkins

Schneider F R 1976 Handbook for the orthopaedic assistant. Mosby, St Louis

Sculco T P (ed) 1985 Orthopaedic care of the geriatric patient. Mosby, St Louis

Society of Hospital Pharmacists of Australia 1985 Pharmacology and drug information for nurses, 2nd edn. Saunders, Sydney

Storlie F J (ed) 1984 Diseases: nurse's reference library, 2nd edn. Springhouse, Pennsylvania

Turek S L 1984 Orthopaedics: principles and their application, 4th edn. Lippincott, Philadelphia

Wright V, Dickson R A (eds) 1984 Musculoskeletal disease. Heinemann, London

Journals

Arad D, Ryan M 1986 Low back pain – a survey. The Australian Nurses Journal. 16 : 1 : 44–48

Berkowitz D M 1983 Synovial fluid analysis. Nursing 83 13 : 9 : 11–15

Bayliss C E 1980 Pathophysiology of inflammation in Rheumatoid Arthritis Part 2. Allied Health Professions Section WAARF Issue 2, Dec.

Berzins D 1979 The treatment of Paget's disease. The Australian Nurses Journal Vol 8 : 11, 34, 35

Brooks P M 1981 Propionic acid derivatives. Current Therapeutics, September

Champion S D 1981 The salicylates, Current Therapeutics. September

De Ceulaer K, Buchanan, Watson W 1979 Pathogenosteoarthrosis. Medicine Australia 12

Doyle D 1982 Gout. In: Nursing Mirror, November 11 p. 2

Dunwoody C J, Pais M B 1983 Scoliosis. Nursing 83
13 : 9 : 24–25

Eastmond C J, Wright V 1979 Seronegative arthritis.
Medicine Australia

Evans R R 1974 Osteoporosis, Sandoz Therapeutic Quarterly

Gould P 1980 Management of everyday problems in the
arthritic patient. Patient Management 4 : 5

Hackett C 1983 Limbering up your neurovascular assessment
technique. Nursing 83 13 : 3 : 40–43

Hamilton D, Clements M 1982 The last flush of youth.
Nursing Mirror, January

Health Survey 1977/78. Australian Bureau of Statistics.

Hollingsworth, P N 1982 Why study genetics of rheumatoid
disease? Allied Health Professions Section WAARF Issue
7, July.

Holland C, Jayson M 1979 Rheumatoid arthritis. Medicine
Australia 11 April.

Ibbertson H K (et al) 1979 Paget's disease of bone
assessment and management. Current Therapeutics,
June.

Ingersoll G 1985 Caring for the quadriplegic patient with
ankylosing spondylitis. Nursing 85 15 : 10 : 44–48

Lamphier T A 1980 Current status of diagnosis and
treatment of gouty arthritis. Australian Family Physician.
Vol 9 : 156, 157

Lane P L, Lee M M 1983 Special care for special casts.
Nursing 83 13 : 7 : 50–51

MacIntyre I 1983 Osteoporosis risk factors in the UK.
Osteoporosis Social and Clinical Aspects. First
International Conference, Florence.

Martin T J 1980 Paget's disease. Sandoz Therapeutic
Quarterly No 3: Vol 7.

Merkin D H, Galee M D 1980 Keeping pace with new
problems when your patients exercise. Modern Medicine,
Nov.

Nordin C 1983 Preventing Osteoporosis. Geriatric Medicine,
December.

Nowotny M L 1980 Osteoarthritis. Nursing 80 10 : 9 : 39–41

Nuki G 1979 Gout and hyperuricaemia. Medicine Australia
12, May. 790

Panayi G 1979 The Immunopathology of connective tissue
disease. Medicine Australia 12 May.

Rodts M F 1983 An orthopaedic assessment you can do in
15 minutes. Nursing 83 13 : 5 : 7–15

Rohl P 1981 Metabolic bone disorders: current concepts in
management. Current Therapeutics. September.

Seminar 1981 Antirheumatic drugs. Current Therapeutics,
September

Simpson C F 1983 Adult arthritis. American Journal of
Nursing. February

Soh A 1979 Gout. The Australian Nurses Journal 10 8 : 27,
28

Stevenson R C K 1985 Take no chances with fat embolism.
Nursing 85 15 : 6 : 58–63

Tinsley L 1982 Physical treatment for patients with
ankylosing spondylitis. Allied Health Profession Section.
WAARF No. 6

Tompkins J S, Brown M D 985 Dissolving a lifetime of
lower back pain with chemonucleolysis. Nursing 85
15 : 7 : 47–49

L

The skin and autoimmune disorders

74

Introduction to disorders of the skin

Chris Game

Intact skin and mucous membranes provide the human organism with a primary defence against the invasion of microorganisms, and the absorption or penetration of toxic substances. The skin is the largest organ of the body and is commonly involved in the presentation of many systemic diseases. Primary skin disorders may be due to a variety of causes and it is estimated that there are more than 1000 skin diseases. Although accurate figures are not available, approximately 35% of all persons suffer from a skin disorder that requires treatment, and nearly every Australian will at some time experience a skin disorder.

When obtaining a nursing history and assessing a person for skin lesions, it is imperative that the nurse inspect all areas of the person's body, including nails, nail beds, skin folds, hair lines, and the hairy areas of the body. Many primary lesions are not readily visible and are commonly found in areas normally covered by either hair or clothing. This section will restrict discussion to the nursing management of those skin disorders commonly found in the Australian community, presenting either in children or in adults.

PATHOPHYSIOLOGY OF SKIN DISORDERS

The causes of skin disease are numerous and include those due to: inflammatory reactions; follicular and glandular disorders; bacterial, fungal, or viral infection; parasitic infestation; immunological reaction; and neoplasia.

Lesions may be localized, regional, or general, and less commonly, universal (involving the entire skin, the hair and nails). It is important to note whether lesions occur unilaterally or bilaterally, are symmetrical or asymmetrical, and occur in either a linear or a cluster distribution.

PRIMARY SKIN LESIONS

Primary skin lesions are the visible manifestation of an underlying pathological process; they occur initially as a spontaneous eruption, or as an alteration to skin texture or colour. The majority of primary lesions are benign and, commonly, the person with such a lesion will either not seek medical intervention or will treat himself with the application of a nonprescription ointment or cream. Primary skin lesions can be broadly classified as being macules, vesicles, papules, or cysts.

Macule (Fig. 74.1). A small, flat, circumscribed area accompanied by changes in normal skin colour: for example, freckles, flat moles, rubella, and rubeola. A patch is a macule that is usually > 1 cm in diameter: for example, leucoderma and port-wine stains.

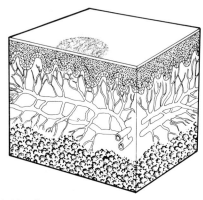

Fig. 74.1 Macule.

Vesicle (Fig. 74.2). A small, elevated, circumscribed, serous, fluid-filled lesion: for example, blister, and varicella.

A bulla is a vesicle that is usually > 1 cm in diameter; for example, blister, pemphigus neonatorum, and pemphigus vulgaris.

A pustule is a vesicle containing purulent fluid; for example, acne, impetigo, and variola.

Papule (Fig. 74.3). A small, solid, elevated, circumscribed, palpable mass accompanied by changes in normal skin colour: for example warts, drug related skin eruptions, and pigmented naevi.

A plaque is formed by a number of coalesced papules; is > 1 cm in diameter; and is flat-topped and rough: for example, psoriasis, and actinic or seborrhoeic keratoses.

A nodule is a round papule that has infiltrated deeper into the dermis and is usually 1–2 cm in diameter: for example, erythema nodosum, and lipomas.

A tumour is a nodular papule that may or may not be clearly demarcated and is usually > 2 cm in diameter; these neoplasms may be benign or malignant.

A weal is a papule characterized by a firm, irregularly shaped area of cutaneous oedema of variable diameter; it is pale pink in colour, transient, and occurs most commonly as a hypersensitivity response to insect bites, and in urticaria.

Cyst (Fig. 74.4). An elevated, circumscribed, palpable lesion which is encapsulated and filled with either liquid or a semisolid substance. The sebaceous cyst is the most common form of this skin lesion.

Telangiectasia (Fig. 74.5). A primary skin lesion caused by the permanent dilatation of groups of superficial capillaries and venules. It occurs commonly in response to prolonged exposure to sun light and in rosacea.

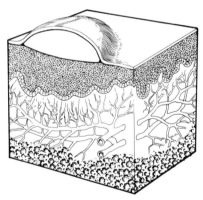

Fig. 74.2 Vesicle.

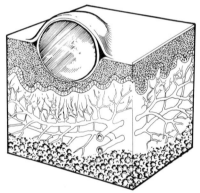

Fig. 74.4 Cyst.

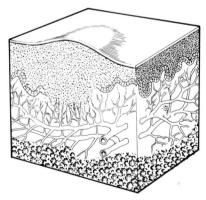

Fig. 74.3 Papule.

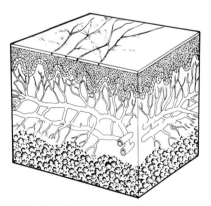

Fig. 74.5 Telangiectasia.

SECONDARY SKIN LESIONS

Should a primary lesion be left untreated, suffer trauma, or fail to respond to treatment, secondary changes can occur. Secondary skin lesions are usually difficult to resolve and may lead to chronic conditions such as psoriasis or dermatitis, or may be permanent in the case of scar or keloid tissue. The following secondary skin lesions are the most common.

Scale (Fig. 74.6). An irregular piled area of loose fragments of keratinized cells in the stratum corneum. The scale is flaky, may be thick or thin, dry or oily, and varies in size according to its cause. Common presentation is in exfoliative dermatitis or as psoriasis.

Crust (Fig. 74.7). Variously sized and coloured dried serum, blood, or purulent exudate from the skin. It is slightly elevated, rough in texture and occurs as a scab on an abrasion or in eczematous dermatitis.

Excoriation (Fig. 74.8). A linear break in the skin with loss of epidermis. The dermis is exposed and becomes inflamed. Excoriation most commonly follows skin abrasion or scratching.

Erosion (Fig. 74.9A). A circumscribed, partial loss of the dermis that produces a moist, glistening depression; it most commonly follows the rupture of a vesicle and is seen in varicella and variola.

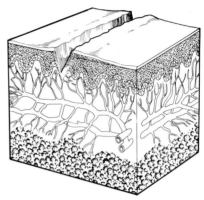

Fig. 74.8 Excoriation.

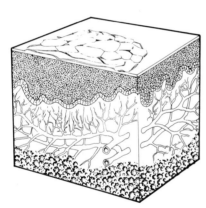

Fig. 74.6 Scale.

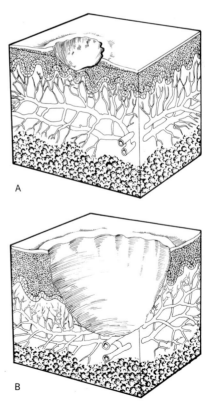

A

B

Fig. 74.9 A – Erosion. **B** – Ulcer.

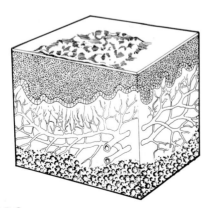

Fig. 74.7 Crust.

Ulcer (Fig. 74.9B). An irregularly sized and shaped concave excavation that penetrates into the dermis. It is usually exudative and commonly occurs as either a decubitus or stasis ulcer.

Fissure (Fig. 74.10). A linear ulcer producing a crack or break extending from the epidermis to the dermis. It is usually small, deep, and inflamed, and most commonly occurs in dermatophytosis.

Lichenification (Fig. 74.11). Areas of thick and roughened epidermis are highlighted by exaggerated skin markings; lichenification is caused by rubbing or irritation and is commonly seen in chronic dermatitis.

Atrophy (Fig. 74.12). Areas of thin skin accompanied by loss of normal skin markings; skin is translucent and paper-thin; commonly seen as a normal process in the elderly or as striae.

Scar (Fig. 74.13). The permanent deposition of fibrous tissue at the site of traumatized dermis; usually irregular in shape and may be either atrophic or hypertrophic; commonly seen in healed wounds or surgical incisions.

Keloid (Fig. 74.14). An irregularly shaped, hypertrophied scar containing excessive collagen, that is elevated and grown beyond the boundaries of the original wound or incision. Some persons are predisposed to developing keloids following injury; keloids are commonly seen in burn scars.

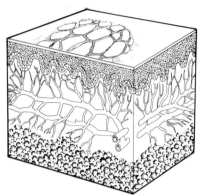

Fig. 74.12 Atrophy.

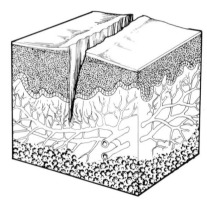

Fig. 74.10 Fissure.

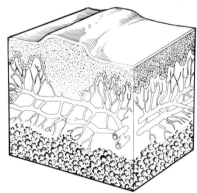

Fig. 74.13 Scar.

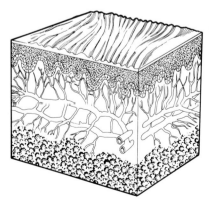

Fig. 74.11 Lichenification.

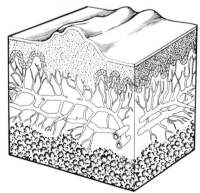

Fig. 74.14 Keloid.

SKIN MANIFESTATIONS OF SYSTEMIC DISEASE

As the skin is the largest organ in the body it is commonly involved in the manifestation of systemic disease and, therefore, the nurse must be prepared to provide intervention for a variety of skin disorders when assigned to care for patients with particular systemic disease.

Systemic disease which manifests with a skin condition include: Crohn's disease (see page 153), ulcerative colitis (see page 516), systemic sclerosis (scleroderma), systemic lupus erythematosus (SLE, see page 786), dermatomyositis, polyarteritis nodosa, pruritus ani (see page 538), pruritus vulvae (see page 655), and systemic malignancy. Skin manifestations include:

Xerosis (dry skin). This occurs most commonly in the elderly and may be accompanied by itching. Xerosis may accompany hypothyroidism, sarcoidosis, and lymphoma. Nursing care includes the topical application of emollient and moisturizing creams.

Pruritus. Itchy skin is probably the most common of all skin manifestations of systemic disease and causes include drug reactions, biliary obstruction, chronic renal failure, anaemia, malabsorption, and parasitic infestations. As antihistamines are poorly tolerated in systemic disease, nursing interventions such as cool, wet compresses, the application of calomine lotion, and encouraging the wearing of light, cool clothing are of tremendous benefit.

Urticaria (see page 768).

Alopecia (see page 772).

Purpura. Bleeding into the skin and mucous membranes may or may not be thrombocytopenic in origin and a drug-induced allergic vasculitis is a common cause. Lesions commonly affect the lower limbs and nursing care includes bed rest and the application of support bandages when the patient is ambulating.

Pyoderma gangrenosum. This is the ulcer commonly seen in rheumatoid arthritis and may also be caused by ulcerative colitis or Crohn's disease. The ulcer has an undermined advancing border with a pustular centre covered by an adherent necrotic crust. Frequent dressings with topical antiseptics are necessary and scrupulous dressing technique by the nurse is required to prevent infection of the lesion.

MEDICAL AND NURSING MANAGEMENT

Unless secondary infection is present the patient with skin disease is managed either in the community or through a dermatological clinic. Once the diagnosis is confirmed, any specific cause is identified and either treated or eradicated. The nursing management for all types of dermatoses aims to:

1. Maintain skin integrity and reduce the physical effects of the skin lesions
2. Prevent the development of secondary bacterial infection of the lesions
3. Ensure maximal patient comfort, relief from the physical effects of pruritus, and a return to normal sleep patterns
4. Restore the patient's self-concept by reducing the factors that give rise to concern with body image.

During the acute stage of any dermatosis, when vesicles and moist exudate are present, wet dressings using normal saline, water, or potassium permanganate are applied and the patient is encouraged to keep the vesicles moist. Any crusted lesions may be gently debrided using an antibacterial soap. Potent steroid creams are also used during the acute stage as topical corticosteroids suppress the inflammatory and/or allergic response, prolong vasoconstriction thus limiting the effect of the pathological reaction, and markedly reduce pruritus. Steroid creams are of great value for the patient who is unable to maintain wet dressings in place, for example, during working hours. As the dermatosis resolves, potent steroids are replaced by weaker preparations so as to reduce unwanted systemic or cutaneous effects. Topical antibacterial and antifungal agents may be prescribed to control or eradicate any secondary infection; and antihistamines may also be prescribed to control pruritus and encourage adequate sleep during the acute phase.

Reassurance and support is required during acute stages as the patient is usually extremely distressed by the sight of the skin lesions, the constant uncontrollable desire to scratch, and by the debilitating effects of disturbed sleeping patterns. Reassurance that treatment can be successful and encouragement to verbalize his feelings regarding his appearance and fear of rejection will assist the patient in maintaining his self-concept and a positive approach to his treatment regime.

As the skin lesions resolve, the wet dressings are replaced with greasy preparations such as oil in water compresses or simple emollient creams. These will usually be sufficient to control pruritus and encourage the skin surface to heal without drying out, becoming scaly, or cracking. Less potent topical steroids are continued as they are a mainstay in controlling the symptoms of the dermatoses.

In chronic dermatoses, keratolytic agents may be used in an attempt to control excessive flaking and scaling of skin surfaces. Coal tar preparations are excellent in controlling pruritus although they are not as cosmetically acceptable as the topical steroids. Oily or greasy compresses are of great value in treating chronic dermatoses; unfortunately patient noncompliance due to the chronicity of the condition has limited their effectiveness.

Health education to improve skin integrity, limit the likelihood of secondary bacterial infection, maintain maximum comfort and rest, and promote body image is the responsibility of the nurse. This will include advice or instruction necessary to:

1. Eliminate or avoid any known precipitating factors such as:
    - heat, high humidity, extreme temperature changes, sweating
    - emotional stressors
    - excessive bathing
    - skin irritants for example, cosmetics, strong soaps, detergents, cleansers
    - woollen clothing, synthetics, tight-fitting clothing, coarse fabrics
    - known, or suspected, primary irritants or allergens.
2. Maintain high standards of skin hygiene. This may include:
    - keeping skin well lubricated
    - wearing loose fitting, light, cotton materials that allow the skin to breathe avoiding extremes of temperature; when bathing, use lukewarm water
    - frequent washing/shampooing of hairy areas if greasy skin is a feature
3. Maintain a well balanced and nourishing diet, including sufficient fluids to maintain hydration and skin turgor.
4. Correctly apply compresses, soaps, and topical medications. Compliance, especially in children, is vital in obtaining long-term results and cure.
5. Recognize the symptoms and signs of any secondary infection and to seek medical advice should they occur.

ANTICIPATED OUTCOME

In most dermatoses the condition can be controlled effectively by eradicating or avoiding precipitating causes, maintaining stringent skin hygiene, and using topical steroid creams. Patient compliance with topical measures is essential in the acute stages to ensure long-term control or cure. Chronic dermatoses can usually also be controlled by these measures and thus enable the patient to maintain his self-esteem. Cure will depend largely upon the type of skin lesion, the degree of pathological change in the skin surface, the type of skin structure, the treatment modality instituted, and the degree of patient compliance with the therapy regimen.

75

Common skin disorders

Chris Game

INFLAMMATORY SKIN DISORDERS

Dermatitis; eczematous dermatitis

The terms 'dermatitis' and 'eczema' are now used synonymously (eczematous dermatitis) to describe a superficial inflammatory response of the skin that is characterized by vesiculation, pruritus, erythema, epidermal oedema, exudate, scaling, and crusting. In the presence of chronic dermatitis the skin becomes thickened and lichenified. In all forms the epidermis breaks down as oedema accumulates from dilated dermal capillaries. Vesicles form and may burst onto the skin surface; thickening of the cells takes place; crusting and scaling occurs and linear fissures may appear.

Many different factors can cause dermatitis and in some instances a variety of causes can be found simultaneously. Generally the causes of dermatitis are either endogenous or exogenous. Medical intervention varies little between the types of presentation; and nursing management, though individualized for each patient, follows principles common to all types of dermatitis.

Eczematous dermatitis may present in a variety of forms. The most common are: atopic dermatitis, seborrhoeic dermatitis, pompholyx dermatitis, primary contact dermatitis, and allergic contact dermatitis.

Atopic dermatitis

Also known as infantile eczema, this is an endogenous, familial condition and is associated with other atopic diseases, for example, intrinsic asthma, hay fever, allergic rhinitis, or urticaria ('hives').

The condition usually manifests during infancy, and clears to re-appear in late childhood and again during late adolescence or early adulthood. The basic cause is an immunological defect in that the person has high serum levels of IgE, responds exaggeratedly to environmental irritants, and has a susceptibility to bacterial and viral infections.

The person has ichthyosis and xeroderma (dry and scaly skin), especially in skin flexures, and a lowered threshold to pruritus. This leads to excessive skin scratching which results in further epidermal breakdown.

Extremes of environmental temperature and humidity are poorly tolerated and high humidity increases vasodilation and the inflammatory response. Food allergies may trigger or exacerbate the disorder, for example, cow's milk in infancy. Psychological factors are not thought to play a role in causation. Secondary bacterial infection is always a risk and commonly occurs.

Seborrhoeic dermatitis

This is a chronic, recurring, erythematous, endogenous eczema that characteristically affects areas in which sebaceous glands are concentrated. The scalp, eyebrows, nasolabial folds, chest, back, and body folds (for example, axillae and groins) are most affected. In infants 'nappy' areas may be involved and the condition tends to affect males with seborrhoea more than any other group.

The lesions may be mild or severe and vary from dry, greasy scales to excoriated, erythematous crusts. In the scalp the lesions are adherent, thick, yellow scales. The disorder is worse during the winter months when thick clothing is worn, and secondary bacterial infection is extremely common.

Psychological factors have been shown to influence the degree of presentation of this dermatitis.

Pompholyx dermatitis

A common condition in which the eczema affects the palms of the hands and the soles of the feet and is usually endogenous in causation, but may also be exogenous. There is usually marked hyperkeratosis which prevents the vesicles from bursting so that they form large, fluid-filled blisters (pompholyx); painful fissures are also present. The condition is exacerbated by excessive perspiration or sweating.

Primary contact dermatitis

An acute or chronic inflammation caused by contact with such primary irritants as chemical and biologic substances for example, caustic liquids, detergents, mineral oils, solvents, salts, secretions, and excretions. The type and degree of the dermatosis reaction depends upon a variety of factors, including: the nature and physical and chemical properties of the substance; the degree and the time of exposure; and the skin type and the genetic and chemical makeup of the person. Fair skinned people, and those who constantly expose their skin to water are more prone to develop contact dermatitis.

Allergic contact dermatitis

An acute or chronic inflammation caused by an allergic sensitivity; this form of dermatitis is a manifestation of a type 4 delayed hypersensitivity response. The allergen is an environmental substance, which may or may not be readily identifiable, and one to which the person has become sensitized. Chemicals found in plants, animal products, metals, rubber, and especially commercial dyes are commonly implicated in this form of dermatitis. The duration, frequency, and type of exposure to the allergen determines the degree of the allergic response.

Investigative procedures

Physical examination will indicate the characteristic skin eruption and the distribution of the lesions, in conjunction with a complete personal history, will be relative to the type of eczematous dermatitis present. In atopic dermatitis the patient will exhibit ichthyosis and xeroderma, there will be a family history of allergies, and immunofluorescence will show an elevated serum IgE. With contact dermatitis the patient interview should be structured to identify any known substances that cause a reaction on contact; in many cases the primary or sensitizing agents may not be readily identifiable and an intricate process of elimination may be required. A patch test is usually positive to the allergen in allergic contact dermatitis. However, care must be taken not to perform the procedure during an acute presentation of dermatitis as anaphylactic shock may occur.

Nursing management

Nursing management is as for any patient with a skin condition (see page 758) with emphasis on reducing exposure to the irritant. Management of pruritus will require innovative nursing care and support to reduce further skin breakdown from the patient scratching himself, for example, cotton gloves can be worn at night. Plastic-wrap film applied to areas covered with creams will prevent the early removal of the cream by clothing or bed linen. The patient will need support with maintaining a positive body image during the acute stages.

Psoriasis

Psoriasis is a chronic, recurrent disease of keratin synthesis that is marked by proliferation of the epidermis resulting in well-circumscribed, elevated, erythematous papules and plaques covered by a layer of silvery scales. Removal of the plaques reveals a deep red base covered with a thin membrane which bleeds easily.

The condition varies widely in severity and distribution; some persons find it to be no more than an isolated cosmetic nuisance, whereas others are severely afflicted and debilitated by the disease. A sudden onset of small, round lesions that may be extremely itchy, may be preceded by a streptococcal infection some 10 days previously. Alternatively, secondary infection may manifest in pustular lesions. If prolonged vasodilation is present, usually from overly aggressive therapy, the patient presents with diffusely red, hot, and massively scaling skin; this exfoliative form predisposes the patient to temperature and fluid imbalances.

It has a familial tendency, usually appears between the ages of 10 and 40 years, affects both sexes equally, and is characterized by a course of recurring remissions and exacerbations. Emotional and environmental stressors have been known to trigger attacks and spontaneous remission may occur.

Characteristically, psoriatic lesions are found on the back, buttocks, extensor surfaces of arms and legs, and the scalp; however nail beds, axillae, face and eyebrows may be involved. It is not uncommon for the patient to also have an associated arthropathy (psoriatic arthritis) which is almost identical to rheumatoid arthritis, however testing for the rheumatoid factor is negative.

Personal history and physical examination revealing characteristic lesions usually confirms the diagnosis, however, skin biopsy may be required in a minority of cases.

No cure has been found for psoriasis, however many persons achieve considerable remission with the use of occlusive dressings, topical corticosteroids, keratolytics, and coal tar preparations. Specific photochemotherapy with exposure to short-wave (UV-B) or long-wave (UV-A) ultraviolet light is currently the treatment of choice for most instances of widespread psoriasis, especially for instances of severe, refractory disease. The photosensitizer, dithranol, is used concurrently. This regime retards the rapid epidermal proliferation and enables the body's normal inflammatory response to prevail.

FOLLICULAR AND GLANDULAR SKIN DISORDERS

Acne vulgaris

Acne is an inflammatory disorder of the pilosebaceous follicles of the face and upper trunk, and is characterized by comedones (blackheads), pustules, papules, or nodular lesions which may resolve to leave ugly, pitted scars. It is a disorder

of puberty but may occur as early as 8 years or as late as 30 years of age. Acne tends to affect males more frequently than females. Most acne sufferers have a skin more greasy than normal and acne development is confined to areas where large sebaceous glands exist. The condition is worse during winter, and emotional stressors have been known to precipitate an acute flare-up. Acne improves markedly in summer due to the healing properties of sunlight. Hormonal influence is believed to be responsible for premenstrual flare-ups in young women.

The activation of sebaceous glands due to androgenic stimulation at puberty accompanied by hyperkeratinization of the hair follicle leads to follicle obstruction. The blockage causes retention of sebum, cells, detritus, and colonization of the anaerobe Corynebacterium acnes. Comedones form and are either open (blackheads) or closed (whiteheads). The comedones enlarge with retained sebum, keratinous material, and bacteria, and these either discharge onto the epidermis, forming pustules, or the base extends to the dermis and results in papule and cyst development. Rupture of the follicle may result spontaneously or be due to trauma, such as squeezing the comedone. The deeper the skin lesion the more likely that scarring will occur. Chronic, recurring lesions produce unsightly acne scars.

The success of treatment is largely dependent on gaining the person's cooperation especially in avoiding expressing the comedone. Most adolescents do not seek medical advice and self-treat with over the counter preparations that may or may not be effective. Many hope that they will grow out of acne as they get older and if the condition does not respond to treatment they may develop severe concerns with body image and social relationships.

Regular cleansing with soap and water should be encouraged and squeezing comedones or debriding pustules should be avoided. Males with acne should be advised not to use electric shavers as these harbour bacteria and tend to reinfect areas. Instead the person should be encouraged to use disposable blade razors and to alternate their use to ensure maximum drying of the blade in between use. Alternating peeling agents such as benzoyl peroxide 10%, and vitamin A cream have produced good results; however, it is important to note that the pH of any substances used in combination must be matched in order for them to be effective. Unless contraindicated, regular exposure of acne areas to sunlight should be encouraged, and the use of an ultraviolet lamp or a short course of deep X-ray therapy may be recommended. The use of long-term antibiotics in some cases of severe acne may be indicated but is still highly controversial.

Rosacea

Acne rosacea is a chronic inflammatory disease of facial skin often associated with seborrhoea and occurring commonly in middle-aged persons. Diffuse erythema occurs, inflamed papules and pustules are present, telangiectasia form, and there is a tendency to flushing of the skin. The cause is unknown but excessive exposure to ultraviolet or infra-red rays is thought to play a large role in its development.

The papules and pustules characteristically erupt on the nose and cheeks and then spread to involve the rest of the face and exposed pate. Lymphoedema causes the skin to appear shiny and the disorder is distinguishable from acne vulgaris by the lack of comedones and scars, the age of the person at onset, and in that sunlight usually aggravates the condition. The majority of sufferers are well controlled on low-dose oral tetracycline therapy combined with low-potency topical steroid ointments.

BACTERIAL SKIN INFECTIONS

Streptococcal cellulitis

This is an acute, intensely inflamed infection of the subcutaneous tissue. It is characterized by a rapidly occurring onset of a red, hot, painful, tense swelling of the affected tissue, usually involving an extremity. It most commonly follows a localized trauma, such as a puncture wound, laceration, or a friction blister on a foot or heel. The border that separates affected and normal tissue is poorly defined, lymphadenitis and lymphadenopathy are common, and dependence of the affected limb increases the severity of the oedema.

In almost all cases of streptococcal cellulitis, the patient is admitted to hospital for total rest, elevation of the affected limb, and high-dose antibiotic therapy, usually via the intravenous route. Aggressive therapy is mandatory to prevent permant lymphatic impairment as circulation to the limb is usually compromised with this condition.

Erysipelas

This is a superficial form of streptococcal cellulitis that classically affects the abdominal wall in infants and the face in children and adults. Less commonly, the lower limb is involved.

Erysipelas is characterized by a rapidly spreading erythema with a very well-defined area of demarcation between affected and normal tissue. The affected tissue is bright red, oedematous, hot to touch, and extremely painful. It is often accompanied by high fever, rigors, general malaise, headache, nausea, and back pain.

As the most common infecting organism is *Streptococcus pyogenes*, penicillin is the drug of choice and may be ordered orally in mild or early cases; IM or IV penicillin will be ordered in more severe instances of erysipelas. Cooling compresses may give local relief until antibiotic therapy is successful.

Staphylococcal furunculosis

Furunculosis (boils) is severe infection of hair follicles caused by *Staphylococcus aureus* strains that are usually resistant to penicillin and the tetracyclines. Carbuncles may develop if adjacent follicles are involved or if chronic furunculosis develops. Folliculitis is a less painful form.

Poor hygiene, stress, chronic illness or debility, and work and environmental factors may predispose to infection. When furuncles burst the purulent exudate is an important source of auto- and cross infection and any lesion that leads to scratching and picking has the potential to develop into a furuncle. Should antibiotic therapy be delayed it may be necessary to incise and drain large furuncles.

Education of the patient regarding the prevention of re-infection is often necessary to break the cycle of recurrent furunculosis. Should incision and drainage be necessary, health teaching regarding care of the wound will be the responsibility of the nurse.

Impetigo

Impetigo contagiosa is a superficial, highly contagious skin eruption occurring primarily in infants and children. Its bullous form is caused by coagulase-positive *Staphylococcus aureus*; nonbullous impetigo is caused by the Beta-haemolytic Streptococcus. Ecthyma is an ulcerative form of impetigo caused by the streptococcus.

The lesions most commonly occur in the perioral area, the nares, ears, and axillae, and begin as small vesicles which spread rapidly, forming clusters of pus-filled bullae. Once the bullae rupture, thin, sticky, brown crusts form in the area of distribution of the clusters.

Nursing care consists of removing the crusts with warmed olive oil and then applying the ordered antibacterial topically; oral antibiotics are also usually ordered. Antibiotics are used to prevent secondary infection, re-infection, and cross infection to other children, but the use of gentle washing and debridement techniques along with light dressings are as effective. Once the lesions are clean and the crusts have lifted they may be dried by using povidone iodine solution.

Staphylococcal scalded skin syndrome (SSSS) is a severe exfoliation of skin following impetigo in young infants and results in red, moist, denuded skin similar in appearance to a severe scald. This is a medical emergency and the infant requires immediate hospitalization and aggressive care with antistaphylococcal antibiotics, intravenous fluids, electrolytes and plasma globulins, and heat regulation to combat the losses due to the extensive skin exfoliation.

Leprosy

Leprosy is a bacterial skin infection caused by the *Mycobacterium leprae*. Leprosy (Hansen's disease) presentation is determined by the patient's immunity. People with high but incomplete resistance develop tuberculoid leprosy, and those with no resistance develop nodular lepromatous disease (lepromatous leprosy). Borderline (dimorphous) leprosy is said to exist when a diagnosis of either form is not definitive. Leprosy is not highly contagious and a person must live continuously and closely with a sufferer to run a risk of cross infection. Most people have a natural immunity although leprosy is endemic among Australian Aboriginals of the Northern Territory.

Although primarily a tropical disease, its incidence is rising in countries such as the United Kingdom and Australia, and is seen widely in North America, due primarily to a more mobile world population. The increase in the refugee population in each of these countries has further contributed to the rise in incidence in this and other diseases.

The mycobacterium attacks the peripheral nervous system and in particular the ulnar, radial, posterior popliteal, anterior tibial, and facial nerves. Damage to small nerves results in skin lesions. Large nerve damage results in motor nerve disease, weakness and pain, leading to anaesthesia, paralysis, or atrophy and deformities, for example, claw hand, and foot drop result. Scarring and contractures occur as injury, ulceration, and infection lead to disuse of the deformed part. Severe systemic disease if left untreated will result in mutilation of the extremeties.

The drug dapsone is specific for the treatment of all types of leprosy no matter the staging of the disease and only in a few cases is intolerance a problem. Rifampicin has been shown to be superior in effect but resistance of the mycobacterium has reduced its use as a sole means of therapy. Drug therapy must continue for at least 2, and in some cases 4 years. Leprosy can be cured but the disfiguration is irreversible.

Nursing management is aimed at preventing injury to the affected extremeties and patient education to minimise the effects of the disease. These may be achieved by, for example, adequately padding and splinting affected areas, and ensuring that skin lesions are dressed aseptically; teaching the patient the importance of maintaining his drug therapy, and inspecting at least daily anaesthetized extremities to ensure early treatment of areas of tissue erosion.

FUNGAL SKIN INFECTIONS

Dermatophytosis (ringworm)

Infection by dermatophytes (fungi) results in the clinical condition of tinea. Tinea infections may affect the scalp (tinea capitis), body (tinea corporis), nails (tinea unguium), feet (tinea pedis), groin (tinea cruris), and skin of the beard (tinea barbae). Tinea is a fairly contagious disease and transmission can occur directly from contact with infected skin lesions, or indirectly from contact with, for example, infected clothing, bath towels, or contaminated shower recesses. Tinea corporis and/or capitis is a common childhood infection and may reach epidemic proportions in individual schools. It is not uncommon for children to become infected from contact with domestic cats.

Tinea corporis produces the characteristic ringworm lesion: a reddened, pruritic, and scaly lesion with a well defined, advancing border. Tinea pedis causes scaling and blistering of the skin between the toes and is otherwise known as athlete's foot. Other sites of tinea usually result in reddened, raised, pruritic lesions that may also show vesicle and pustule formation.

Diagnosis is usually made on inspecting the lesions but can be confirmed by skin scrapings for microscopy. Griseofulvin orally is specific to the dermatophyte but tinea pedis requires complementary topical therapy to effect a cure.

Nursing management primarily involves patient education to improve hygiene and diet, to correctly apply topical medications, and to reduce the likelihood of re-infection or transmission to others.

Candidiasis

Overgrowth of the yeast *Candida albicans* is responsible for the development of candida infections ('thrush'). It more commonly occurs in diabetics, pregnant women, obese persons, patients on cytotoxic chemotherapy and those on antibiotic therapy. Candidiasis is most commonly the cause of vulvo-vaginitis and of severe nappy rash in infants; and oral 'thrush' is not an uncommon occurrence in some patients.

The lesions may be bright red and accompanied by pustules, or even denuded when they occur in skin folds, and form cream-coloured patches on mucous membrane. Intense pruritus is a feature and re-infection via the genito-oral route is common if scratching cannot be controlled.

Antibiotic therapy can so alter the normal flora of the gut that candida can overgrow as a consequence. Persons ordered a course of antibiotics should be advised to either eat natural (living) yoghurt daily or to take an associated course of oral vitamin B for the duration of the antibiotic therapy. Either measure maintains the normal flora Lactobacillus and prevents the overgrowth of the Candida. Topical nystatin orally or vaginally will usually effect a cure and the topical application of natural (living) yoghurt is also effective.

VIRAL SKIN INFECTIONS

Herpes simplex

Herpes simplex is a recurrent viral infection caused by the herpes simplex type I or type II viruses, which are extremely widespread infectious agents. Type I virus causes cold sores and these almost exclusively appear on the face and lips; type II virus is most commonly transmitted venereally as genital herpes (see page 669).

Lesions begin as localized areas of itchiness and tingling, and then eruption of the turbid vesicles occurs. After the vesicles rupture, crusts develop and left untreated the lesions will heal within 7–10 days.

Following a primary infection of herpes simplex a person becomes a carrier for life, regardless of antibody activity to the virus. There is, therefore, no cure and treatment is symptomatic with the use of analgesia and antipyretics in the acute stage. Avoidance of irritant foodstuffs during the acute attack and encouragement of cold drinks and ice to suck will provide considerable relief. Antiviral agents in the form of topical creams have had limited results, being of most use if the eye is involved as an infection site. Children with atopic eczematous dermatitis should be protected from contact with herpes simplex virus, because they are at great risk of developing a generalized herpetic infection; this has a high morbidity and mortality rate in these children. Complications of herpes simplex infection are not common but when they occur the most likely is herpetic meningitis (see page 220).

Herpes zoster ('shingles')

Herpes zoster is an acute inflammation in the distribution of a dorsal root ganglion, caused by infection with the Varicella zoster virus. The vesicular skin lesions erupt unilaterally and follow a segmental skin band (dermatome) supplied by the dorsal root ganglion. The virus is reactivated, having lain dormant in the ganglion since a childhood episode of chickenpox (varicella). The mechanism of reactivation is unknown and commonly follows periods of stress, trauma, malignancy, and local radiation, for example sunburn. It more commonly affects adults and usually occurs after the age of 40 years.

The outbreak of skin lesions is preceded by fever, general malaise, and then pruritus, paraesthesia, hyperaesthesia and severe pain over the distribution of the affected nerve root. Fluid or pus filled vesicles appear within 2 days and burst within 10 days, when they dry and form scabs. They may become infected and lymphadenopathy may develop. Occasionally the cranial nerves are involved and rarely a generalized CNS infection may develop.

Post herpetic neuralgia is a complication seen most commonly in the elderly; this leads to intractable neuralgic pain that may persist for years. Blindness may result should the facial nerve be involved.

There is no known cure and medical and nursing management is symptomatic. Antiviral agents, in the form of topical creams, must be applied within hours of the vesicles developing to be of any success. The primary goals of care are to relieve pain and pruritus and to prevent infection of the vesicles. Pain is best controlled with the use of oral aspirin and codeine, and the topical application of a local anaesthetic agent. Pruritus is best managed by the liberal application of calomine lotion and the local anaesthetic is best applied in combination with the lotion. Drying agents are of value in hastening the resolution of

the condition once vesicles rupture and cytotoxic paints may occasionally be used.

The patient must be instructed to avoid scratching the lesions and to apply cold compresses when the vesicles rupture. The patient is advised to inspect the lesions for any signs of infection and he can be reassurred that once the inflammation has run its course the herpetic pain will subside.

Warts

Warts (verrucae) are common, benign viral infections that can appear on almost any part of the skin, and they occur most commonly in children and young adults. Genital warts (see page 660) are transmitted by sexual contact and are an increasingly more common form of venereal disease among Australians.

The human papilloma virus is the causative agent and the mode of transmission is by direct contact. Most warts spontaneously disappear whilst others disappear readily with treatment and some persist regardless of treatment.

Unless the wart is unduly large, unsightly, or causes problems (for example, the wart bleeds after catching on clothing) it is usually left untreated. Warts on the soles of the feet (plantar warts) are usually removed surgically as they commonly cause problems with gait. Curettage followed by cautery is the most common medical treatment used. Many OTC preparations are available for self-treatment, the commonest being the silver nitrate stick. Many alternative therapies (for example thistle milk) have been tried but in the long run most warts disappear within 5 years.

PARASITIC SKIN INFESTATION

Scabies

Scabies is an intensely pruritic, maculopapular, pustular skin eruption resulting from a burrowing infestation of the female acarid (mite) *Sarcoptes scabiei var hominis* (Fig. 75.1). It is transmitted by skin contact or venereally, and infestation is usually predisposed by overcrowding and poor hygiene; however, it not unusually occurs in schools and can reach endemic proportions. The

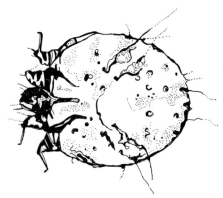

Fig. 75.1 Scabies mite.

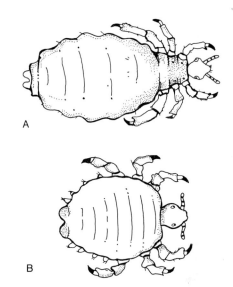

Fig. 75.2 A – Head louse. **B** – Pubic louse.

female acarid burrows under the skin and lays her eggs; the larvae then emerge, copulate, and reburrow under the skin. The presence of the acarid, eggs, and burrows cause a sensitivity reaction and red nodular skin lesions erupt. Mites that live on birds (especially starlings) also infect humans and such infestation results following the departure of birds from a nest somewhere in the house, usually the roof. The mites leave the nest during darkness, track down to and bite the sleeping person, then return to the bird's nest before light. Insecticide spraying of the mites whilst tracking, plus removal of the bird's nest is sufficient to cease the infestation.

In adults the palms of the hands, soles of the feet, and the face are usually free of lesions whereas in children these are the most common sites.

Diagnosis is suspected by the characteristic lesions, history of poor hygiene, or exposure to carriers and is confirmed by finding the mite and/or eggs in skin scrapings; the acarid can be seen with a powerful hand lens.

Treatment with pediculicide creams and/or lotions must be preceded by bathing with soap and water. Benzyl benzoate, crotamiton, dieldrin, and gamma benzene hexachloride are pediculicides in common use. The nurse must make sure that the patient, or parent, understands the need to wear clean clothing and to ensure clean bedding post treatment; failure to improve general hygiene will result in reinfestation. Clothing should be treated as for pediculosis corporis (see page 768).

Pruritus persisting following treatment is commonly due to either mite sensitization or to contact dermatitis from repeated use of pediculicides; topical steroids may therefore be necessary. Secondary bacterial infection of skin lesions is more common in warmer climates and systemic antibiotics will be prescribed in this instance.

Pediculosis

Pediculosis is a skin infestation of parasitic forms of lice: *Pediculus humanus capitis* (head lice) (Fig. 75.2A) cause pediculosis capitis; *Pediculus humanus corporis* (body lice) cause pediculosis corporis; and *Phthirus pubis* (pubic/crab lice) (Fig. 75.2B) cause pediculosis pubis ('crabs').

Head lice are the most common of the species and are caused predominantly by overcrowding and poor personal hygiene. Children are affected more commonly than adults and young girls are affected more often than boys. Transmission is via shared clothing, combs, hairbrushes, hats and scarves. Schools are likely reservoirs of the louse and outbreaks of infestation among school children are common.

Body lice live in the seams of clothing and infestation is most often associated with the prolonged wearing of the same clothes, as may happen during winter. They more commonly infest adults and are seen most often in the elderly and homeless. Spread is via shared clothing and bedding. Pubic lice infest the pubic hair and infestation may spread to involve the eyelashes, eyebrows, and body hair on areas such as the axilla and chest. Pediculosis pubis is usually spread via sexual intercourse or via contact with infected clothes, bath towels, or bedding.

Lice feed on human blood by biting the skin of the host and they lay their eggs (nits) in body hair or in the fibres of clothes. The louse injects saliva containing a toxin and anticoagulants into the bite and a purpuric spot results. Severe infestation results in an intensely pruritic, excoriated, erythematous, macular skin rash. Diagnosis is confirmed by finding the lice and/or nits in hair or clothing; lice and nits are macroscopic.

Prior to treatment using pediculicide creams or lotions the patient must bathe using soap and water to remove as many lice from the body as possible. The pediculicide is applied and a fine-toothed comb used to remove nits from the hair; the treatment should be repeated within 1 week. Where practicable, infested clothing, bedding, and personal articles should be destroyed by burning; laundering of bedding and clothes will prevent reinfestation and the use of a hot iron or drycleaning will destroy nits in cloth fibres. The nurse must make sure that the patient, or parent, understands the need to wear clean clothing and to ensure clean bedding post treatment; the failure to improve general hygiene will result in reinfestation.

IMMUNOLOGICAL SKIN REACTIONS

Urticaria ('hives')

Urticaria is an episodic, allergic skin eruption that is usually self-limiting and produces multiple, circumscribed, smooth, raised, pinkish, pruritic weals. These weals develop very suddenly, usually last only a few days, and then disappear leaving no visible trace. Urticaria is most commonly caused by allergic, infective, pharmacological, or physical reactions.

Angioneurotic oedema is a severe form of urticaria which produces much deeper and larger weals usually involving the skin of the face, eyelids, lips, hands, feet, or genitals and the mucous membrane of the mouth and throat. If the angioneurotic oedema produces glottal or laryngeal oedema then asphyxiation may result.

When the cell membranes of mast cells are destroyed the cells release histamine, resulting in vasodilation and increased vascular permeability; erythema, oedema, pruritus, and weals develop. In angioneurotic oedema the amount of histamine released is so great that capillary permeability is widespread and profound hypovolaemia and hypotension results from a massive fluid shift. The hypotensive state produces a reflex vasoconstriction and traps the fluid in the periphery resulting in extreme oedema and prostration.

Allergy to particular foodstuffs, food preservatives and colourings, insect stings, inhaled allergens such as animal dander, house dust, cosmetic powders; parasitic worm infestations; drug hypersensitivity (anaphylaxsis); and extreme sensitivity to stimulants such as cold, heat, water, or sunlight can all produce histamine release and therefore urticaria.

The treatment obviously depends on ascertaining the triggering factor, and then eradicating the cause, for example, prescribing anthelmintics. The patient should learn to avoid the cause, for example, known food allergens, and cover exposed skin surfaces with either clothing or UV cream when in direct sunlight. He should wear a drug-alert bracelet in the case of a known drug hypersensitivity. If avoidance of the trigger factor is impossible, the patient may require desensitization.

If the symptoms of urticaria are severe enough to incapacitate the patient then the nurse will need to provide symptom relief. Pruritus can be controlled with the liberal use of antipruritic creams and lotions. However, many of these agents contain corticosteroids to help reduce the wealing tendency, and these should be applied strictly as ordered to lessen cutaneous absorption of the steroid. Oral antihistamines remain the major form of therapy and can be prescribed on a regular or intermittent basis to control the symptoms of pruritus, weals, and oedema during periods of known contact with trigger factors. The nurse must ensure that the patient understands that histamines have the effect of making him drowsy and he should not operate a vehicle or drink alcohol whilst taking the medication.

Extreme angioneurotic oedema as seen in severe drug anaphylaxis is a medical emergency and the nurse must be prepared to assist in the resuscitation of the patient. Airway management is critical as laryngeal or glottal oedema will result in asphyxiation if the condition is left untreated. Resuscitation aims at reversing the process of hypovolaemia and peripheral oedema by first increasing cardiac output with parenteral adrenalin and then reducing the histamine effect with parenteral antihistamines and corticosteroids. Blood pressure then rises and fluid returns to the vascular compartment, further stabilizing the blood pressure and reversing the peripheral oedema. Only in the event that these measures fail to work within 3 minutes would it be necessary to consider tracheostomy for airway management. Oxygen via mask is administered and an intravenous line is established for further drug administration. IV fluids must be strictly monitored as cardiac failure is a danger if large volumes of fluid are administered prior to the reversal of the fluid shift. When treated quickly the process of reversal is as dramatic as the onset of the attack. Following recovery the aims of treatment are as for any patient with urticaria.

Erythema multiforme

A widespread skin eruption, erythema multiforme is usually caused by a reaction to circulating immune complexes produced by viruses (especially herpes simplex), bacteria (most commonly the streptococcus), and drugs (long acting sulphonamides, the penicillins, and barbiturates). A maculopapular rash develops and involves the hands, forearms, and lower parts of the legs. Distinct lesions then develop, which are raised areas surrounded by an erythematous ring the centre of which may be purpuric, contain vesicles or bullae, or become crusted.

The condition is known as Stevens-Johnson syndrome when the skin eruption is severe, bullae appear, and the reaction involves the mucous membrane of the mouth, eyes, and genitalia. This syndrome is a severe illness and is accompanied by pyrexia, lymphadenopathy, and polyarthritis.

In uncomplicated erythema multiforme the treatment is the simple application of a topical antipruritic cream or lotion, and an oral antihistamine. Topical antibiotic cream may be necessary for treating ulcerated lesions, and oral antibiotics should be necessary only if widespread infection of the lesions occurs. In Stevens-Johnson syndrome the nurse will be required to manage the febrile patient and bullous lesions will need dressing as they rupture. Corticosteroids may be prescribed and mouth washes will be necessary if mucosal ulceration has occurred.

Uncomplicated erythema multiforme is usually managed by the physician in the community and hospitalization is only necessary when secondary infection of the lesions occurs. Stevens-Johnson syndrome frequently proves fatal as the patient will totally desquamate unless the condition is recognized and treated virtually instantaneously.

Pemphigus

Pemphigus is an autoimmune reaction, the cause of which is unknown. In this disorder, there are circulating IgG immunoglobulins which are sensitized against epidermal intercellular substance and this can be demonstrated with immunofluorescence in over 90% of patients. It is a chronic, blistering disease and presents as superficial and deep bullae that rupture exuding a clear or purulent fluid, then become scaly and malodorous. Many forms of pemphigus occur but the most common is pemphigus vulgaris, which initially causes extremely painful oral lesions. Pemphigus vulgaris commonly affects the elderly or the debilitated.

The treatment of choice is the IV use of corticosteroids and immunosuppressive agents and the nurse will be responsible for caring for a patient who is at risk of infection due to his immune suppressed state (see page 405). Wet compresses or soothing cool baths assist in obtaining topical relief and scrupulous mouth care must be provided. A nutritional and appetizing diet consisting of very soft food must be encouraged and aids in tissue repair; fluid balance will require initial management via the IV route.

NEOPLASTIC DISORDERS OF SKIN

Tumours of the skin are quite common. The majority of skin lesions are benign and many of these occur with increasing age. Unless the lesion is cosmetically disfiguring it is usually left untreated. Common benign lesions include moles, freckles, lentigines, seborrhoeic warts, dermatofibromas, squamous papillomas, corns, and skin tags.

Malignant lesions of the skin account for nearly 2% of all malignancies and occur most commonly in Caucasians and in persons who are exposed to high levels of UV radiation. Australia rates as the country with the highest incidence of skin cancer due largely to the continued exposure of fair skinned people to sunlight. Common malignant lesions include squamous cell carcinoma, basal cell carcinoma, and malignant melanoma.

Benign skin lesions

Moles (pigmented naevi) occur as a result of a dermal accumulation of melanocytes and are thought to be an inherited characteristic. They commonly occur in young adults, disappear with advancing age, and only on very rare occasions undergo malignant transformation. Naevi of vascular origin (strawberry naevi) occur more commonly in young infants, may grow to a large size during the first year of life and then shrink, disappearing before puberty.

Birth marks (port wine stains) occur most commonly on the face, are present at birth, grow proportionately in size, and do not fade with age. The introduction of laser beam therapy has produced fairly reasonable cosmetic results in the treatment of large, disfiguring birth marks.

Freckles (ephelides) most commonly occur in fair skinned persons when exposed to UV radiation. Freckles become increasingly darker and more prominent when continually exposed to sunlight.

Lentigines are light brown pigmented areas that commonly occur on skin exposed to sunlight, for example, the dorsum of the hand; they increase in incidence with age and are known as liver spots. When they occur in children they are commonly a feature of an inherited disorder and exposure to UV radiation is not implicated in their development.

Squamous papilloma is a warty growth of keratinocytes and a seborrhoeic wart is a basal cell papilloma. Both are raised, rough, brown growths that cause concern mainly because of their unsightliness.

Dermatofibromas are firm, skin coloured nodules that are thought to occur in response to either an insect bite or minor skin trauma.

Corns are cone-shaped, overgrown, and hardened epidermis that are produced by friction or pressure. The corn's point is in the deeper layers of the dermis and this usually necessitates removal by a qualified podiatrist. They occur on the feet, on or between toes, and can cause severe discomfort if left untreated.

Skin tags (fibroepithelial polyps) develop mainly on the skin of the neck and in the axillae; affect middle-aged women more than men; and occur most commonly in brunettes. They are usually tiny but if large the pedicle can be cut using cautery.

Should a benign lesion require excision this is usually performed, whilst the person is an outpatient, using cautery, curettage, or cryosurgery. The nurse must ensure that the patient receives instruction on the care of the skin following excision of a lesion, with emphasis on preventing infection. The nurse must also participate in education of those patients with skin disorders that may undergo malignant transformation. Advice is given that if a mole changes in colour, shape, size, or texture, or if it begins to itch, ulcerate, or bleed, then medical advice should be sought. Health education in the community should also concentrate on making all citizens aware of the dangers of exposing their skin to excessive sunlight and advice should be given to wear a hat, shirt, and sunscreen during the summer months to reduce the incidence of skin cancer.

Malignant skin lesions

Squamous cell carcinoma

Squamous cell carcinoma (SCC) is an invasive carcinoma that presents as a nodule and grows rather slowly on a firm indurated base. It most commonly develops on skin exposed to sunlight and usually does not undergo metastasis; the exception is SCC of the lips and/or ears which can be highly metastatic lesions with a poor prognosis. If left untreated the nodule ulcerates and forms a characteristic eroded, cauliflower-type lesion.

The size, location, and invasiveness of the tumour will determine the treatment modality but invariably lesions are excised and treated with follow-up radiotherapy. Surgical excision is usually very wide and the patient will require plastic repair to the defect and skin grafting is common. When treated early SCC has high cure and low recurrence rates; preventative measures against constant skin exposure to sunlight can further diminish recurrence. Nursing measures are aimed at preventing recurrence through patient education and in preventing secondary infection in the wound following excision and plastic surgical repair of the defect.

Basal cell carcinoma

Basal cell carcinoma (BCC) is the most common malignancy in fair skinned people; it appears nearly always after 50 years of age; it is also known as a rodent ulcer; and it is the most likely cause of skin lesions occurring in the elderly. A BCC begins as a small, smooth papule and then enlarges to a rounded lesion with pearly nodules in a rolled edge. Telangiectasia develop across the lesion's surface and sometimes there is a central ulcer covered by a crust which, when removed, reveals the characteristic pearly edge.

BCC develop on skin areas exposed to prolonged sunlight and are most commonly found on the face and dorsum of the hand. They rarely undergo metastasis but, if left untreated, they will erode underlying tissue and may even penetrate bone as in the case of a large BCC of the forehead. A BCC is commonly diagnosed when the patient seeks medical advice for local trauma to an existing small lesion, for example, prolonged bleeding of a BCC lesion traumatized whilst shaving.

Medical and nursing intervention is the same as for SCC and if treated early BCC can be completely eradicated. Patient education to reduce exposure to sunlight can result in a radical reduction in BCC recurrence.

Malignant melanoma

Malignant melanoma is a tumour arising from melanocytes and, whilst less common than SCC or BCC, it is increasingly being seen in Australia which carries the highest incidence rate in the world for this tumour. Early diagnosis, when the melanoma is confined to either the epidermis or the papillary layer, followed by wide block dissection carries a high cure rate with a low rate of recurrence. However, as many patients with melanoma present with a deep lesion that has undergone metastasis, excision is not as successful and recurrence is high, and therefore prognosis in these instances is poor.

Only in 25% of malignant melanoma does the tumour arise from a pre-existing mole and the risk of a mole becoming malignant is thought to be in the order of 1 : 1 000 000. Several predisposing factors in its development have been identified and these include: protracted exposure of skin to sunlight; fair skinned, red or blonde haired people with blue eyes who sunburn easily; familial tendency; hormonal factors in which pregnancy increases melanoma incidence; and past history of, as recurrence rates are high. Males tend to develop malignant melanoma on head, neck, and back regions whereas women are more likely to develop lesions on their legs. Melanomas can occur in other areas and these less commonly include the conjunctiva, choroid of the eye, bladder, pharynx, mouth, anus, or vagina.

Anti-Cancer Council education programmes have concentrated on advising people to seek medical advice should they notice any change in a wart or mole or should they discover a new skin lesion that appears to be undergoing continued change. Any skin lesion that starts to grow, darken, bleed, ulcerate, form a crust, develop a patchy change in or become darker in colour, or extend pigment beyond the edge of the original lesion, should be investigated. It is usual for the entire lesion, plus a wide margin of normal skin and any clinically involved lymph nodes, to be excised during biopsy. The width of the lesion's margin is usually indicative of its depth, and the wider the excision the less likely the recurrence. Radiotherapy, chemotherapy, and immunotherapy are usually reserved for deeper lesions that have undergone metastasis and their use is usually only of value in palliation therapy.

The nurse must be prepared to care for a patient who has undergone wide surgical excision and skin grafting of the wound defect (see page 780). Depending upon the location of the lesion, extensive alteration may have occurred to body image and/or limb function and the nurse will be required to assist the patient accordingly. Psychological support for the patient, and his significant others, is crucial in helping them to cope with the diagnosis, radical surgery, and/or palliative treatment and to assist in relieving anxiety. Prior to discharge, the nurse must ensure that the patient understands the need for constant follow up as recurrences are common and metastases may occur up to 5 years post-excision.

DISORDERS OF HAIR FOLLICLES

Each hair follicle undergoes repeated growing (anagen) and resting (telogen) phases with the anagen phase occurring over 2–3 years and the telogen phase lasting a few months. The average person's scalp contains approximately 100 000 hairs and at any one stage 5–15% of these are in the telogen phase. Once the hair is shed, the anagen phase recommences spontaneously although this may be stimulated by plucking hair from its follicle. Should a person suffer a major illness then the tendency is for more hairs to enter the telogen phase; there may, therefore, be considerable hair loss (telogen effluvium) at this time but regrowth follows within a few months.

Common baldness is seen most often in men and less so in women and its onset can be any time following puberty. Baldness is androgen linked and most women with baldness have raised androgen levels. Treatments abound, and hair transplantation appears to be the most successful, however caution should be used in patient referral as this procedure is extremely expensive. The oral administration of anti-androgens has been reasonably effective in treating female baldness but is contraindicated in males due to the side-effects of feminization.

Alopecia (hair loss of the scalp) may be associated with an underlying disease state or may be primary (alopecia areata). Alopecia secondary to malabsorption, drug reactions, or cytotoxic chemotherapy is reversible and regrowth occurs once the primary condition is treated or cytotoxic drug administration ceases. Alopecia secondary to hypothyroidism or iron deficiency anaemia is less likely to be reversed on treatment of the primary condition.

Alopecia areata occurs equally in men and women and may present at any age. There is usually a familial tendency, and the relationship of either autoimmune disease or stress to its development is still being explored. Hair loss usually occurs in well demarcated patches that become totally bald, leaving a smooth white patch of scalp skin which is otherwise normal in structure. Characteristic of this condition is the finding of 'exclamation mark' hairs in an otherwise normal scalp. Regrowth normally occurs within weeks or months but the hair is initially white and develops pigmentation as regrowth progresses. Occasionally hair loss occurs in other sites, for example eyelashes and eyebrows, and areas may remain bald for many years.

In nearly all instances of hair loss, reassurance and psychological support are paramount treatment strategies for the nurse. Acceptance of the altered body image may take a long time and the patient may even require referral for wig fitting if the condition fails to rectify itself in a short period of time. Topical and intradermal corticosteroids have been used with limited effect.

DISORDERS OF THE NAILS

Nail infection (paronychia) and ingrowing toenails are common afflictions of the nail beds.

Paronychia

Paronychia affects the fingernails and can be acute or chronic. Acute paronychia is caused by a bacterial infection (commonly *S. aureus*) of the proximal nail fold and is most often seen in nail biters with a damaged cuticle; chronic paronychia usually affects persons who have their hands frequently immersed in water. It is common among nurses, and is usually due to an overgrowth of *C. albicans*. The degree of inflammation around the nail fold can be quite severe and extremely painful.

Treatment is primarily aimed at promoting cuticle regrowth and reducing inflammation. The patient must understand the need to keep the affected fingers dry at all times but that the prolonged wearing of rubber gloves will only intensify the problem due to their occlusive nature. Oral antibiotics will be prescribed for acute paronychia and antifungal creams will be topically applied for chronic paronychia. The patient must continue treatment until regrowth of the cuticle is established.

Ingrown toenails

Ingrown toenails are most frequently seen in the great toes of young adults and are primarily due to a large lateral nail fold compounded by ill-fitting shoes, hyperhidrosis, or incorrect cutting of the nail. A nail spicule may also be present, growing into the nail fold and increasing the degree of pressure and inflammation. The nail fold is extremely red and swollen and the entire toe may become inflamed preventing the wearing of shoes. The chronic inflammation produces granulation tissue which serves to increase the problem.

Treatment aims to reduce the inflammation using potassium permanganate washes and topical antibiotic creams. Granulation tissue is usually removed by cautery or cryotherapy; nail spicules are excised; and in many instances the entire nail is removed. Wedge resection of the toenail or total nail bed ablation is required if the condition persists.

76

Nursing the patient with burns

Chris Game

The skin is the largest organ in the body and has a role in a range of vital functions which include: preventing the loss of body fluids; controlling body temperature; protecting against the invasion of microorganisms and hence protecting against infection; secreting waste products; producing vitamin D; and providing the sensory input of touch. Additionally, the skin's cosmetic role contributes to the shaping of an individual's self concept.

A burn of the skin is an extremely common form of accidental injury. Fortunately, the majority of burns are minor and do not require any sophisticated medical or nursing treatment. Accurate statistics describing the mortality rate from serious burns are not available, but it is known that burns are the third major cause of accidental death in children under the age of 10 years. Furthermore, there is no reliable data on the psychological, economic, and social impact of serious burn injury on those who survive.

In the case of a serious burn, the degree to which the person's physical condition is compromised is largely dependent upon the relative size of the burn. Children, having a greater body surface area in proportion to their body mass than adults, can become profoundly dehydrated by only a very small burn; a similarly sized burn in an adult may not even necessitate admission to hospital for treatment. The larger the area burnt the greater the likelihood that scarring will result; if scarring is widespread then plastic repair to achieve both functional and cosmetic rehabilitation will be necessary.

In some patients with burns, death may be due to factors other than the burn wound itself: smoke inhalation, overwhelming septicaemia, negative nitrogen balance, and loss of the will to live are primary causes. Nearly 70% of all burns result from fire and of these the greatest number are due to the ignition of clothing or other fabrics such as bedding. It is interesting to note that of all burns, regardless of type or cause, nearly 80% occur in the home.

TYPES AND CAUSES OF BURNS

Thermal burns are by far the most common type and of these flame is the leading cause. Flame burns due to fires in the home or the bush, and following motor vehicle accidents or the improper use or storage of petroleum products are the most common. Children playing with matches, malfunctioning electrical equipment, ignition of clothing from an unguarded fire place or heater, kitchen accidents, and smoking in bed are the most likely cause of fires in the home. Other thermal burns include flash burns especially from the ignition of gas from a leaking bottle, scalds from hot liquids, the touching of hot surfaces, and the spilling of molten metal; scalds are an extremely common burn in young children.

Other types of burns include chemical, electrical, friction, and radiation. Chemical burns most commonly result from contact with, or ingestion or inhalation of, strong acids or alkalis. Electrical burns from faulty wiring, contact with high voltage lines, cutting through power lines, or more rarely lightning strikes, occur with less frequency. When an electric current passes through the body, it produces two burn sites – a small burn at the point of entry and a larger burn at the exit site of the current. Friction, or abrasion, burns are commonly seen following accidents or as a result of physical violence. Radiation burns as a result of sunburn occur more frequently in Australia than in many other countries. Damage effected by freezing tissue, for example frostbite or after prolonged exposure to cold, is similar to the damage sustained when a burn occurs and the care of the skin of such a patient is the same as for treating the patient with burns.

ASSESSMENT

When assessing a person who has suffered a burn, a variety of factors will be used to determine the severity of the burn wound and the type of treatment necessary. These factors include: the depth of the burn, the area of body surface burned, the type and cause of the burn, the location on the body of the burn, the patient's age, and his previous medical history. It is also important to gain a description of the burn incident as this may assist in determining the severity of the burn and any complications that may be anticipated. Questions that may elicit such information when the patient is brought to the hospital include:

• How long was the person in contact with the burn agent?
• What was the causative agent?
• How much protection was afforded by clothing?
• Was the wound contaminated with dirt, debris, soiled clothing, or dirty water?

Burn depth

Burns are classified according to the depth of tissue damage and the internationally accepted classifications are: superficial; partial thickness, either superficial or deep; and full-thickness burns (Fig. 76.1). Since, on initial inspection, it is extremely difficult to assess accurately the true extent of the damage, caution should be exercised when estimating and reporting the depth of any burn. The prognosis, especially in relation to the likely need for skin grafting, is often uncertain.

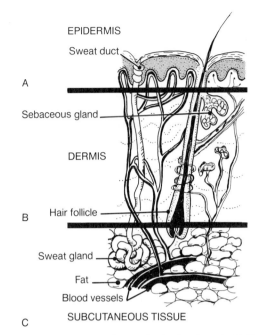

Fig. 76.1 Classification of burn depth. **A** – Superficial. **B** – Partial thickness. **C** – Full-thickness.

Superficial

A superficial burn is a burn of the epidermis only which is manifested by erythema ranging from mild to severe, and may or may not be accompanied by blistering. If blisters are present these vesicles have very thin walls and burst easily making the burn surface moist. The skin will blanche with only mild pressure and, in the absence of blistering, quickly becomes dry and taut over the burn area. Superficial burns are extremely painful and hypersensitive and are marked by tingling sensations; during the first 72 hours, only mild irritation from clothes or light breezes can cause extreme discomfort or pain. Maximum pain relief for a superficial burn is achieved by cooling the burn area, with, for example, a cryogel pack. This form of treatment is highly effective as the cryogel will not freeze at 0°C and remains pliable and can therefore be moulded over the wound. As healing commences, the burn area will desquamate within 3–7 days depending on burn size. Scarring does not occur although permanent changes to skin colour of the burn area may result.

Partial thickness

A partial thickness burn is a burn that extends to the dermis and may involve the superficial or deep dermal structures. A superficial, partial thickness burn is characterized by: erythema and blanching due to excessive vasodilation; extensive thick-walled blisters over the burn area; severe oedema of the limb or surrounding tissues; extreme pain and hypersensitivity due to exposure of nerve endings; and extreme sensitivity to cold air.

Epithelialization and healing will occur within 14 days and hair regrowth is usually normal as hair follicles and sweat glands in the deep dermis are usually not involved in the burn. However, abnormal skin texture and colouring results and scarring of the burn area is common.

A deep, partial thickness burn may extend through as much as 85% of the dermis and be clinically indistinguishable from a full-thickness burn. A deep, partial thickness burn is usually characterized by: severe oedema; a reddened, moist, shiny base or a dry base with a thin eschar (burn slough/scab); and extreme pain and hyper-sensitivity as for a superficial, partial thickness burn. If allowed to heal naturally, epithelialization will be extremely slow and healing may take as long as 28–30 days depending upon the burn depth and whether hair follicles and sweat glands remain. Spontaneous healing results in a thin-skinned, poorly pigmented and hairless defect, which may contain hypertrophic scar tissue. To reduce the likelihood of infection and/or ugly scarring, skin grafting is preferred to natural healing.

It should be noted that a partial thickness burn, regardless of depth, may become a deeper or full-thickness wound if treated inappropriately or if severe infection occurs within the burn.

Full-thickness

A full-thickness burn extends through the epidermis and dermis and involves deeper tissue layers with destruction of subcutaneous fat, muscle, nerve, and even bone. This type of burn is characterized by: white, deep red, brown, or blackened and charred skin; oedema of the limb or surrounding tissues; a dry eschar due to severe tissue dehydration; exposure of underlying struc-

tures; and a complete loss of pain sensation and temperature discrimination in the burn area due to the destruction of nerve endings. The person with a full-thickness burn has relatively little pain when compared to the person with a lesser burn.

Except at skin edges, epithelialization and hair regrowth cannot occur. Destruction of blood vessels leads to ischaemia, necrosis, and eschar formation; necrotic tissue usually suppurates and sloughs after 2–3 weeks. As spontaneous healing is impossible, debridement of the eschar and skin grafting must be used to minimize the development of excessive scar tissue and to replace the destroyed tissue. However, in the case of full-thickness burns even with skin grafting, scarring deformities will result and functional loss can also be anticipated.

Body surface area burned

It is essential to estimate the total of the body surface area (BSA) burned as this factor is basic to determining likely fluid loss and therefore fluid replacement regimens. The person can be quickly assessed using the 'Rule of Nines' (Fig. 76.2) in which each area of the body is expressed as a percentage that, when totalled, equals 100%. However, more precise formulae have been devised to assess BSA burned in children and accurate fluid replacement in adults. These formulae vary widely between burn units and the nurse should become familiar with the formula used in the individual acute care facility.

Type and cause of the burn

The degree of damage will be influenced by the circumstances of the burn. If a flame burn occurred in an enclosed space, or if the victim fled with burning clothing, associated inhalation burns should be suspected. A scald will vary according to contact time, and with the temperature and viscosity of the liquid involved; for example, boiling oil or fat will do more damage than does boiling water. A burn's location may seriously effect the severity and treatment of the injury. Burns located around the head, neck and chest invariably impair ventilatory capacity either by restriction of the thoracic musculature or by

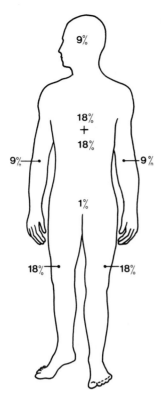

Fig. 76.2 The 'rule of nines' for calculating extent of burns. The front and back of the trunk are each assigned 18%, and the perineal area 1%.

involvement of the mucous membrane of the respiratory tract in smoke or chemical inhalation. Burns involving the chest and back have a high mortality due to the large BSA involved and burns involving the face usually require long periods of hospitalization due to the necessity for extensive plastic repair. Burns involving the perineum and buttocks commonly increase the time of hospitalization as these areas are prone to repeated infection.

Patient age and previous medical history

Children under 2 years of age and persons over 60 years of age rarely survive an extensive burn of more than 50% BSA. In these patients BSA is proportionally greater in relation to body mass since both groups have less subcutaneous fat; therefore burns are usually deeper and relatively more extensive. Greater BSA also increases the rate of fluid loss and irreversible burns shock is

a common cause of death in the very young and the old.

A fit and healthy person will withstand the effects of burns shock far better than a person who has a history of co-existing systemic disease. Additionally a severe burn may exacerbate a previously well controlled systemic disease, which further complicates management.

When assessing a patient's burn it is not unusual to obtain a photograph of the patient showing the extent of his burn injury. This pictorial record is then used as a baseline against which to assess recovery.

FIRST AID MANAGEMENT

The first aid management of a burn aims to: prevent extension of the burn; relieve pain; and reduce the likelihood of contamination. Prior to transport to hospital these aims can be simply achieved by removing the person from the burn agent and wrapping the burn in a clean cotton garment or towel, or wrapping the person in a clean sheet. It is imperative to protect the burn from air to relieve pain and prevent the loss of body heat.

Extension of the burn can be minimized by the gentle application of a constant trickle of cool running water. This first aid measure will also assist in pain relief and in the prevention of contamination of the wound.

Only in the case of chemical burns should clothing be removed to prevent further contact with the burn agent before the burn is irrigated. Removing clothing from a flame burn victim may result in profound desquamation. Ointments should not be applied as these may compromise subsequent burn treatment, and the person must not be given any fluid until assessed in hospital.

Children and the elderly, regardless of severity of burn, and all persons with burns in excess of 10% BSA should be transferred immediately to hospital. A person is normally admitted to an acute care facility for further burn management if: he is under 5 years or over 50 years; the burn involves more than 10% BSA and is at least partial thickness; the burn involves the face, hands, feet, or is circumferential; or if there are associated injuries.

BURNS SHOCK

Patients with burns in excess of 10% BSA will experience burns shock in varying degrees. When a burn occurs intense vasodilation results and fluid is lost into and below the burn area. If skin is intact, as in superficial burns, blistering will result and it is not unusual for extensive scalding to produce blisters that contain many litres of body fluid. When skin is destroyed in the burn, fluid will be lost directly from the body in the form of cell fluid, plasma, or even blood in the case of full-thickness burns.

Compensation will cause peripheral vasoconstriction in an attempt to preserve circulating blood volume and the patient will undergo the physiological changes seen in hypovolaemic shock (see Chapter 11). Even small burns in children and the elderly can produce profound fluid loss due to their disproportionately large BSA in relation to their body mass. It is imperative that fluid replacement occurs quickly in all burn patients. Many different formulae exist for estimating fluid replacement in burn patients and the nurse should become familiar with the formulae used in the acute care facility.

The amount and type of fluid required is determined by the type and extent of the burn, the rate at which fluid is being lost from the extracellular fluid compartment, the type of fluid loss, and the age and physical condition of the patient. Normally half the total fluid required for the first 24 hours is infused during the first 8 hours of treatment in an attempt to reduce burns shock and prevent renal shutdown. Most regimes aim to restore the individual's normal fluid balance within 24 hours and then to maintain that balance via the IV route until the patient can take adequate fluids orally.

MEDICAL, SURGICAL, AND NURSING MANAGEMENT

Recovery from a serious burn injury is a slow and painful process, punctuated by repeated episodes in the operating room, and often characterized by periods of profound anxiety and depression.

The patient with a burn injury therefore requires highly skilled medical and nursing care and will, in the majority of instances, be admitted to a specialist burns unit in an acute care facility. This chapter will identify only the basic principles of burn care which must be applied to assist in the recovery of the patient and to minimize the development of any complications.

If the burn area exceeds 20% of BSA the patient should be isolated and nursing procedures instituted to avoid any unnecessary contamination of the burn wound. To reduce excessive cross-infection, all staff should observe strict handwashing procedures and wear protective clothing, including gloves and masks, when providing direct care. Intact skin and mucous membrane is the body's primary defence against invading microorganisms and when this defence is lost the patient must be protected against infection at all times until healing has taken place. The type of bed on which the patient is nursed will vary between units and in nearly all instances sterile bed linen is utilized. The environment should be kept warm as the patient is usually nursed unclothed and covered only by bed linen. Loss of body heat may be minimized by the use of heat shields.

Any burn has the potential to cause severe psychological stress for the patient as his concept of body image will be altered in some way. This is especially true if the burn involves the patient's face, head, neck, or arms or legs. Isolation increases the degree of psychological stress and dependence experienced by the patient and, as the nurse is in almost constant attendance, she/he will be largely responsible for maintaining the patient's optimistic outlook.

The nurse will be responsible for the management of the fluid replacement and for observing the effects of rapid fluid replacement therapy in the patient. In the majority of patients a central venous line will be established for fluid therapy. His vital signs must be recorded regularly and observation of tissue turgor, urine output, and central venous pressure must also be recorded. Where possible the patient is weighed to establish a baseline from which to compare the effects of fluid replacement and subsequent recovery. An indwelling urinary catheter will be inserted as an accurate record of urine output is mandatory for estimating fluid replacement and for monitoring patient response to fluid therapy and recovery from burns shock. The nurse must ensure that the drainage system remains patent and free of contamination so as to avoid the development of a urinary tract infection.

Pain relief is usually obtained by covering the burn with a topical agent; however, narcotic analgesics may be required in the first few days until topical therapy is established. Sedation may be required in the severely burned patient, especially if assisted mechanical ventilation is indicated. Tetanus toxoid is usually administered to the severely burned patient on admission to minimize colonization of *Clostridium tetani* in necrotic tissue.

A nasogastric or nasoenteric tube is usually inserted as a precaution to minimize the development of a neurogenic paralytic ileus (see page 532). Until his condition stabilizes, the patient usually receives nutrients in the form of hyperalimentation via the central venous infusion (see page 470). A diet high in protein and carbohydrates is essential to promote tissue healing and prevent muscle wasting. Dietary requirements are determined by the patient's general physical condition, body weight, and BSA burned. Daily weighing of the patient is usually necessary to ensure adequate dietary control.

Prior to any topical therapy to the burn area, wound swabs are taken to establish whether any invasion of bacteria has occurred – it is normal for bacteria to colonize in burn wounds as the protective skin layer has been destroyed. Specimens of body fluids and swabs of body orifices are also obtained prior to the commencement of any antibiotic therapy. Regular wound swabs are usually taken throughout the recovery period to monitor the extent of any wound contamination or wound sepsis.

The burn wound is cleaned and any debris or material removed and then a topical agent is usually applied. The use of occlusive versus nonocclusive dressings varies widely between burns units.

In the case of the patient with a circumferential burn, initial burn oedema may be so great that the eschar constricts to the underlying tissues. This is especially dangerous in circumferential burns of the trunk as ventilatory insufficiency may develop.

Escharotomy, which involves a vertical incision through the tight, dead eschar layer, may be required to allow skin expansion whilst oedema forms. The nurse must ensure that aseptic techniques are maintained when caring for escharotomy sites as these may easily become infected.

Where possible the patient is fully immersed in a bath daily, as this allows for the easier removal of the topical agent, softening of the eschar, and permits less painful physiotherapy to ensure full range of movement is retained in all joints. However, the nurse must ensure that the bath water is kept warm so that the patient does not lose body heat. Stringent cleaning of the bath will minimize the risk of cross-infection. Some patients find bathing extremely painful, and some physicians discourage bathing for the patient with extensive burns as sodium loss may occur.

Topical agents vary but the most common agents used are silver sulphadiazine and mafenide acetate creams. The cream is applied in a layer 3–5 mm thick over the entire burn surface. It is applied using either a sterile spatula or, preferably, by a hand covered with a sterile glove. Depending upon the location of the burn it may then be covered by an occlusive dressing. Preferably the burn is not covered and the cream is reapplied as necessary throughout the day. The creams are effective against a wide range of bacteria, promote tissue regeneration, penetrate and soften eschar, promote eschar separation, protect the burn from sensitivity to air, and are painless and easy to apply. In a minority of patients sensitization to the drug occurs and prohibits its use.

Once the patient's condition has stabilized, debridement of dead tissue must occur before healing of the underlying tissue can take place. Eschar can be removed in a variety of ways including:

● Primary excision wherein the burn wound is surgically excised down to viable tissue and a skin graft applied to the defect. It is usually performed within the first week of a burn, before granulating tissue is present in large amounts.
● Surgical debridement, which involves the removal of necrotic tissue by the use of a dermatome, a surgical knife, or more commonly by a combination of scrubbing and scalpel paring.

• Mechanical debridement in which wet saline dressings are used to soften the eschar so that it can be removed. If wet-to-dry dressings are used the saline softens the eschar which then adheres to the dressing as it dries. On removal of the dressing, adherent eschar is pulled away. Wet-to-wet dressings allow painless softening of the eschar so that it can be lifted with forceps and then trimmed away from the wound. Daily bathing is an even more effective method of wet-to-wet dressing debridement.

Primary excision and surgical debridement promote more rapid healing but have disadvantages in that they require multiple surgical procedures under general anaesthesia. Proteolytic enzymes may be utilized to digest necrotic tissue but these can lead to destruction of healthy tissue.

Skin grafting

Deep partial thickness and full-thickness burns require skin grafting to ensure healing with as little scarring as possible. Xenografts or heterografts, using pig skin, may be used in the early stages of burns to provide a cover to the burn wound and promote debridement of eschar prior to final grafting. Homografts from cadavers are used in some instances but their use is restricted by the paucity of donors. Most commonly autografts, from elsewhere on the patient's body, are used to cover burn wounds. Autografts will not suffer rejection and when a free graft is placed over a raw burn wound it will adhere quickly and, as long as it is protected, it will not move or break its adherence. Grafts may be thick or thin, but the thinner the graft the more likely its survival.

The split-thickness skin graft (SSG) is the most common form of graft used and is a thin sheet of skin comprising epidermis and dermis. It is removed from the donor site using a dermatome and is then cut into small patches which are laid irregularly over the granulating wound area. Tissue fluid of the burn wound bathes the patch graft and although some contraction of the graft occurs, adherence commences within minutes.

The donor site is usually wrapped in saline gauze until haemostasis is effected. Prior to the patient leaving the OR the saline gauze is removed and the donor site is dressed with a single layer of paraffin gauze and enclosed in a firm cotton dressing held in place with a firmly wrapped crepe bandage. The donor site should not be touched until the paraffin gauze detaches – usually after 14 days – and the nurse must ensure that the donor site remains dry during this period. The progress of healing at the donor site can be inspected by carefully lifting the edges of the wound dressings. When it is obvious that the paraffin gauze has detached, the patient should be allowed to gently remove the donor site dressing whilst that body part is immersed in a bath. The donor site is normally painful for at least 48 hours after grafting and it is common for the patient to be prescribed a narcotic analgesic for pain relief. Following removal of the dressing the donor site should be kept pliant with the administration of a moisturizing cream.

The SSG patch grafts may be sutured in place or covered with a pressure dressing to prevent fluid accumulation and graft separation. More commonly the SSG is left open and the nurse should ensure that the wound area is protected from friction and pressure of clothes and bed linen. The graft should be frequently inspected and where necessary the graft should be 'rolled' to prevent accumulation of fluid between the graft and granulation tissue. This fluid will prevent the graft 'taking' and will result in separation. To roll a graft, the nurse, utilizing an aseptic technique, gently rolls a sterile applicator over the graft from the centre outwards thereby expressing any fluid that may have accumulated. A successful graft will 'take' within 72 hours and, as long as it is protected from infection or shearing movements, it will survive to cover the defect. Within 3 months the patient should be able to discriminate pain and temperature over the graft area.

The nurse should appreciate that pain is a feature of healing for a burn patient, and that this pain may produce reluctance to participate in the treatment regime. The nurse will therefore need to enlist the patient's aid in planning a daily schedule which allows for treatment procedures (such as dressing changes, bathing, or therapy) to be conducted under analgesic cover, but which also leaves the patient alert and able to respond appropriately at meal times and during visiting hours. Effective nutrition and contact with significant others are key elements in the lengthy process of physical and psychological repair for the burn patient.

Allied paramedical care

Other members of the health team are vitally important for the patient's survival and ultimate rehabilitation to a quality lifestyle. The physiotherapist must plan and supervise the patient's rehabilitation schedule to ensure that muscle wasting and joint contractures are minimized. The occupational therapist will be required to assist in retraining for activities of daily living and for modification of the home environment where necesary. The dietitian is responsible for ensuring that the patient's diet includes the nutrients and kilojoules necessary for maximum tissue repair. The social worker may be required to advise on lifestyle changes, especially if alternative employment is envisaged. The patient will be faced with an extensive period of rehabilitation and will require the maximum input of all the health team members if he is to succeed in his recovery.

COMPLICATIONS OF BURNS

The most common cause of death in patients with burns is overwhelming infection or septicaemia. The more extensive the burn the more likely the patient will be to suffer a combination of complications; however, infection of the burn area leading to septicaemia is the most difficult complication to control. Ventilatory insufficiency due either to the effects of the burn agent (for example, smoke inhalation) or to infection (for example, pneumonia) is also a leading cause of death post-burn.

The development of a Curling's (stress) ulcer is a common occurrence in the majority of patients who suffer extensive deep partial or full-thickness burns. It is known that burn sepsis increases the probability of Curling's ulcer, in that with the resolution of wound sepsis gastric mucosa also recovers. The medical and nursing management of the patient with a Curling's ulcer is as for the patient with a peptic ulcer (see page 492).

Psychological distress is common in burn patients. A severe burn can have devastating consequences. The circumstances surrounding the burn event, the sudden disruption of normal life, the pain, the slow process of repair, apprehension about likely scarring and disfigurement, and the need for reframing of body image may all have a profound effect on the patient's psychological well-being.

The nurse should expect to assist the patient to work through a variety of reactions which may include: blame, guilt, anger, grief, withdrawal, dependence on nursing staff, and possibly even reluctance to integrate into the wider world as healing progresses. Many patients with burns to over 60% BSA find their perceived future intolerable and cannot bear the thought of protracted plastic reconstructive surgery. Some patients may 'give up' their will to live and succumb to overwhelming infection. Burn patients and their significant others require extensive counselling and psychological support from all health team members, and the nurse working in a specialist burns unit is a constant source of encouragement and advice for patients.

ANTICIPATED OUTCOME

A severe burn is a life-threatening event, and the more extensive the burn the higher the potential mortality rate – especially in the young and the elderly. However, specialist burns units, with dedicated resuscitation, topical, surgical, rehabilitation and reconstructive techniques, have greatly increased the chances of successful treatment and return to the community for most patients.

The nurse should ensure that the patient and significant others fully understand the need for special care of the donor and graft sites following discharge – for many years in some cases. Protective measures include:

● The avoidance of sunburn, irritants, friction, and abrasions to the wound area
● The regular application of softening creams
● The constant wearing of specially tailored pressure garments to help avoid keloid scarring.

Some patients will require regular follow up after discharge, and all should be offered an introduction to a burns support group which can assist in the process of rehabilitation.

77

Disorders of the immune system

Chris Game

INTRODUCTION

The leucocyte and plasma protein population of cells is the body's primary response against any attack by foreign bodies or cellular mutation. Macrophages, lymphocytes, and immunoglobulins (antibodies) are responsible for first recognizing an invading organism or foreign protein as being abnormal, then mounting an attack, destroying the foreign matter, and finally programming the immune system to recognize the invader should it again gain entry (Fig. 77.1).

Macrophagacytic leucocytes (macrophages) are the front line defence against invasion by foreign organisms. Macrophages engulf and phagocytoze the invading organisms, thereby preventing an infection from occurring, or they assist in the transfer of the organism's antigen to the lymph glands where specialized lymphocytes are activated to destroy the antigen. The mechanisms by which the immune system operates is extremely complex but can be best described by following the sequence of events that occur whenever a virus invades a person for the first time.

Viruses must reach body cells (usually via the circulation) and gain entry in order to survive, replicate, and cause disease; viruses are intracellular obligate parasites. As viruses enter the circulation, macrophages engulf and consume some of the virus particles and transfer the virus antigen to their own surface. Also circulating with these macrophages are T-lymphocytes which are programmed to 'read' the antigen on the macrophage surfaces. Once 'read', the T-lymphocytes bind to the macrophages and become activated as helper T-lymphocytes. The helper T-cells then multiply and proceed to the spleen and/or lymph nodes where they are responsible for stimulating the body to produce further cellular and chemical weaponry against the invading virus particles.

In particular, helper T-cells stimulate the production of killer T-cells which are sensitized to recognize and kill only the invading virus. Also, helper T-cells stimulate the production of B-lymphocytes which are responsible for binding their antibodies to the viral antigens as well as for differentiating into antibody secreting plasma cells; antibodies being Y-shaped protein molecules. These B-cells normally reside in the spleen and/or lymph nodes until stimulated to replicate by helper T-cells.

During the period of T- and B-cell stimulation/production, many virus particles will have successfully gained entry into body cells where they are able to live and replicate; this successful entry is signified either by the clinical presentation of disease or the subclinical activation of the immune system.

Body cells invaded by viruses are in turn invaded by B-cells and killer T-cells. The latter cause the destruction of the cell membranes with the consequent exposure of the active virus to the B-cell antibodies. These antibodies are able to neutralize the viruses in one of two ways, either by binding directly to the surfaces of the viruses which then prevent them from attacking other body cells, or by tagging the body cell containing the virus in such a way that it is recognized and destroyed by killer T-cells or chemical reactions of the body. In this process infected body cells are also destroyed. Macrophages rejoin the scene to phagocytoze and remove the debris from the infection site.

Once the infection is brought under control by

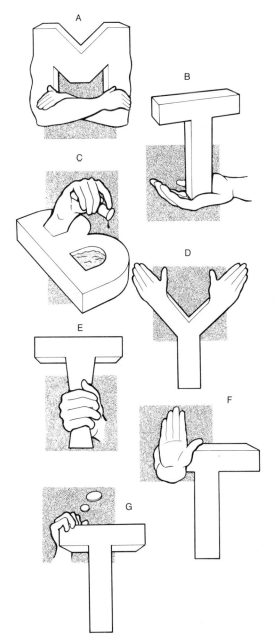

Fig. 77.1 Schematic representation of component cells of the immune system. **A** – Macrophage. **B** – Helper T cell. **C** – B cell. **D** – Antibody. **E** – Killer T-cell. **F** – Suppressor T-cell. **G** – Memory T-cell

the T- and B-cells, circulating helper T-cells stimulate the activation of suppressor T-lymphocytes which in turn quell the response of the B-cells and killer T-cells. This suppressor T-cell

biofeedback method is essential to prevent cellular destruction from becoming uncontrolled.

Once the viral attack has been fought and overcome by the immune system, specialized lymphocytes known as memory B-cells and memory T-cells are left circulating throughout the blood stream and lymphatic system. These memory cells may last for many years and are responsible for ensuring that the body generates a rapid response should the invading organism ever regain entry. Consequently, further attacks of disease specific to that organism either do not occur, or occur only in a mild form.

Optimal immune response can occur either naturally or artificially. Natural immunity can be actively gained by experiencing the actual disease as produced by the invading organism, for example a clinical attack of rubella; or be acquired passively, for example the transfer of maternal immunoglobulins to the neonate across the placental membrane. Artificial immunity is actively gained through vaccination regimens, for example Triple Antigen, tetanus toxoid, rubella vaccine; or acquired passively, for example tetanus antitoxin, hepatitis immunoglobulin. It should be noted that killer T-lymphocytes are, in the main, activated against viral invasion and mutating cancerous body cells, whereas bacterial invasion is mainly fought with antibodies.

DISORDERS OF THE IMMUNE SYSTEM

Disorders of the immune system are usually the result of an immunodeficiency, either inherited or acquired, of T- or B-lymphocytes; of an immunoproliferation, usually of B-lymphocytes; or of an autoimmune nature.

Immunodeficiency disorders include hypogammaglobulinaemias, acquired immunoglobulin deficiency, sarcoidosis (see page 373), leprosy (see page 764) and AIDS (Acquired Immune Deficiency Syndrome, see page 784). Immunoproliferative disorders include multiple myeloma (see page 413), lymphoma and Burkitt's lymphoma (see page 410), leukaemia (see page 394), and amyloidosis.

Autoimmune disease results in a lack of control of the immune system leading to an 'anti-self' response in which the system destroys body cells as if they were foreign proteins. The exact mechanism of disruption to the immune system, or the identification of the cells responsible for the self destruction, is as yet unknown and millions of dollars are spent annually in research of this area.

Autoimmune disorders are classified as being either organ specific or nonorgan specific. The former include Hashimoto's thyroiditis, pernicious anaemia (see page 383), gastritis type A (see page 491), diabetes mellitus type IB (see page 252), pemphigus (see page 769), myasthenia gravis (see page 212), sympathetic ophthalmia, and chronic active hepatitis (see page 433). Disorders thought to be caused in part by autoimmune responses include amyotrophic lateral sclerosis (Lou Gehrig's disease, see page 215), multiple sclerosis (MS, see page 199), and ulcerative colitis (see page 516). Nonorgan specific autoimmune disorders include systemic lupus erythematosus (SLE, see page 786), discoid lupus erythematosus (DLE, see page 787), systemic sclerosis (scleroderma), dermatomyositis and rheumatoid arthritis (see page 726).

As AIDS and SLE clearly demonstrate the effects of the immune system out of control both of these disorders will be covered in detail in this chapter. The immune system dysfunction as a basis in the cause of other disease states is covered with the specific disorder elsewhere in this text.

ACQUIRED IMMUNE DEFICIENCY SYNDROME (AIDS)

In the USA during the early 1980s, previously healthy homosexual males were being diagnosed with overwhelming opportunistic infections, most commonly *Pneumocystis carinii* pneumonia. The peculiarity of this particular infection is that this organism is normally nonpathogenic in humans. Additionally, some patients were also found to have an unusual form of skin cancer (Kaposi's sarcoma), or a central nervous system lymphoma and these were occurring out of all proportion to the rate in the general population. As increasing numbers of patients were diagnosed, the new syndrome Aquired Immune Deficiency Syndrome (AIDS) was identified along with the risk groups in the population. Initially only homosexual men,

particularly Americans, were identified but by the mid 1980s patients from all population groups were being diagnosed throughout the world.

Pathophysiology and statistical incidence

The causal agent that renders the patient immune deficient has been identified as one of: human T-cell lymphotropic virus Type III (HTLV-III), lymphadenopathy-associated virus (LAV), or AIDS-associated retrovirus (ARV). These viruses are now collectively described as Human Immune Virus (HIV).

AIDS virus is endemic in parts of Africa and in Haiti and cases have occurred in these countries in which homosexual practices are not relevant. It has been estimated that 10 000–12 000 people per year will die of AIDS in America alone by 1990 and that there will be 30 000 new cases diagnosed each year. In Australia, by mid-1987 there had been 562 people diagnosed with AIDS and the death rate stood at 55%, that is, 308 deaths. It is estimated that at least 15 new cases will be diagnosed and that approximately 500 people will test antibody-positive each month. AIDS attracts more government funding for research per year than does any other single disorder and this is mainly due to the alarming rate of increase in the disease's incidence since its identification.

The mode of transmission is via body fluids, especially semen and blood, and doubt still exists as to whether saliva and vaginal secretions are capable of causing transmission. The high risk groups include persons with multiple sex partners who do not use safe-sex practices; bisexual men; prostitutes; intravenous drug users, especially if they share contaminated needles; and persons receiving blood and blood products, for example, haemophiliacs. Infants are not immune from AIDS and may be exposed whilst in utero, during birth, or after birth; however, most infants with AIDS have parents from a high-risk group or have received the virus via contaminated blood. In Australia homosexual and bisexual men still constitute at least 85% of all diagnosed cases.

Once exposed to HIV, the body produces antibodies to the virus antigen and these can be identified by serological testing. Being AIDS antibody-positive indicates exposure to the virus and the potential for the development of the full blown syndrome. HIV has the capacity to remain dormant within normal body cells until such time as it is activated, and the mechanism of activation is not yet known. Once activated, HIV renders the person immune deficient by attacking and destroying helper T-lymphocytes, thus virtually stripping the immune system of its capacity to mount any response to any invasion by a microorganism. This then exposes the patient to any opportunistic infection or disorder, and most AIDS patients initially present with a history of insidious onset of an overwhelming infection. Organisms normally symbiotic, nonpathogenic, or only mildly pathogenic in humans are commonly the cause of the overwhelming infection in AIDS patients. The mortality rate for patients with the full blown active stage of AIDS is universally quite high and increases if the patient has Kaposi's sarcoma either alone or in combination with pneumocystis infection. Most AIDS patients die within 3–5 years of diagnosis, having experienced minimal remission with even the most aggressive medical therapies. The major causes of death are either overwhelming infection or cerebrovascular accident due to either haemorrhage, emboli, or extension of lymphoma.

As awareness of AIDS and immunological testing of persons in high-risk groups increases, it has become apparent that many persons exposed to HIV suffer from some of the constitutional symptoms and signs of AIDS but do not have the opportunistic infections or tumours that are present in the patient diagnosed with AIDS. These patients are said to have an AIDS-related complex (ARC) and such categorization is important for identifying high-risk persons who may later develop the full AIDS syndrome.

Clinical manifestations

The majority of patients present with an overwhelming opportunistic infection which is most likely to be pulmonary in origin, such as *Pneumocystic carinii* pneumonia. Other opportunistic pulmonary infections may be caused by cytomegalovirus (CMV), Aspergillus fungi, mycobacterium, or the Legionella bacteria. The patient usually describes a slow onset of a nonproductive cough accompanied by fever, vague chest pain, and shortness of breath.

The patient with an opportunistic infection of the gastrointestinal tract will usually describe the symptoms of low volume diarrhoea, weight loss, abdominal discomfort and pain. If initial symptoms are ignored by the patient, he may ultimately present with high-volume diarrhoea, severe malabsorption, extreme weight loss, and cachexia resembling the terminal stages of carcinomatosis. The most likely causative organism is the *Cryptosporidium protozoa*. Opportunistic infections of the central nervous system are most likely due to invasion by CMV, *Toxoplasma gondii*, *Candida albicans*, or mycobacterium. However, severe neurological involvement is usually due to a central nervous system lymphoma. The patient may present with a history of severe headaches, altering conscious states, personality changes, convulsions, or focal sensory or motor disorders. A few patients may present initially with a pyrexia of unknown origin and have no other indications of a localized infection. The causative organism in this case is usually CMV, another invading virus group, or a bacterial complex. Gastrointestinal and/or pulmonary infections may later superimpose.

Nearly a third of all patients with AIDS present with a malignancy which is most commonly in the form of Kaposi's sarcoma. This consists of bluish-brown, slowly growing plaques or nodules that involve the skin of the face, trunk, and arms. It is not unusual for there to be systemic organ involvement as well as lesions of the buccal cavity. In non-AIDS Kaposi's sarcoma, the lesions are almost always restricted to the skin of the lower extremities.

By definition, a patient with an ARC presents with at least 2 symptoms of AIDS, most commonly diarrhoea and fever, and must also have at least 2 laboratory findings consistent with an AIDS diagnosis, for example, diminished helper T-cells and a leucopenia. As well, patients with an ARC do not demonstrate an opportunistic infection or the presence of a malignancy.

Investigative procedures

The patient's clinical and social history, including sexual activity, is usually indicative of the disorder.

Confirmation of AIDS is made with immunological testing to identify opportunistic infection and/or malignancy, and the diminution of helper T-cells; plus virological studies to determine the presence of the HIV.

Medical management

Medical intervention is aimed at eradicating opportunistic infection, effecting a remission for those patients with a malignancy, resuscitation of the severely cachexic patient, and bolstering the patient's immune system.

Only a few of the opportunistic infections respond to any antimicrobial therapy and even then the degree of response is usually only minimal. The drugs prescribed need to be fairly potent, for example, co-trimoxazole, amphotericin B and acyclovir, and the rate of adverse drug reaction in these patients is also high. Consequently relapse is common and a fatal overwhelming infection results. Cytotoxic chemotherapy to control malignancy has achieved remission of the cancer in some patients, but to be successful early diagnosis is essential. In recent times some success at bolstering the patient's immune system has been achieved in a few AIDS units worldwide. Treatment has concentrated on the use of interferon, interleukin 2, AZT, thymic hormones, and bone marrow transplantation. However, these measures are still experimental and as yet no cure for AIDS has been demonstrated.

The severely cachexic patient will require intensive and aggressive medical therapy to overcome the effects of malabsorption, fluid and electrolyte losses, and body systems dysfunction.

Nursing management

The nurse will be responsible for providing care to a patient who is severely immunodeficient (see page 405), is in most cases suffering from severe malabsorption (see page 504), is in the terminal stages of the AIDS disease process, and who requires considerable support both emotionally and physically. As well, the nurse must liaise with both the patient and his significant others/care givers regarding his ongoing care and physical comfort. Many AIDS patients, fearing the stigma of the disease and rejection by health care workers, are showing an increased desire to live out their remaining time at home in the care of loved ones and friends. In response to this need, community health groups are setting up home care support services for these patients and their care givers. Increasingly, nurses are taking on the role of liaison between the patient and the health care system.

Prevention of AIDS

Health education of the community at large is the primary means of controlling the spread and incidence of AIDS. The teaching of safe-sex techniques is of paramount importance and government spending on community education programmes is increasing worldwide. It has been clearly demonstrated that people in monogamous relationships practising safe-sex, including homosexuals, have a significantly lower risk of contracting AIDS. Therefore education centres on encouraging people to use condoms and to restrict the number of their sex partners, as well as discouraging oral-genital sex practices and having intercourse with known contacts or antibody-positive persons.

It is an offence in most countries to knowingly donate contaminated blood and most blood donation collection agencies now test all donated blood for HIV or antibodies. Regular screening of prostitutes is slowly being implemented, however the control of the shared use of contaminated needles by drug addicts remains a major public health problem.

When handling the blood, semen, or other body fluids of any patient the nurse should wear gloves and/or other protective clothing to prevent the absorption of the antigen through the skin or minor lacerations.

SYSTEMIC LUPUS ERYTHEMATOSUS

Systemic lupus erythematosus (SLE) is a multisystem disease that is characterized by the deposition of fibrinoid material in blood vessel walls and in connective tissue. Widespread vasculitis produces characteristic symptoms and signs and the presentation is highly variable in that the disease may range from mild to severe and may even be fatal. Commonly, the skin, central nervous system, and kidneys are involved. Lupus affecting the skin only is called discoid lupus erythematosus (DLE). The person has high titres of antinuclear antibodies and other autoantigens. SLE is further characterized by recurring remissions and exacerbations. Post pubescent females are nearly 10 times more likely to suffer SLE than are males, who appear to have a hormone-based resistance to the onset of SLE.

The cause of SLE is unknown but the most common theory is that it is autoimmune in that the body produces autoantigens, for example antinuclear antibody (ANA), which form antigen-antibody complexes and lead to self-cell destruction. Alternatively, predisposing factors have been identified which make a person susceptible to developing SLE. These factors include infection (especially streptococcal or viral), extreme physical or mental stress, overexposure to sunlight or UV rays, pregnancy, and following vaccinations. As well, some drugs have been thought responsible for either triggering or aggravating SLE, and these include hydralazine, phenytoin, sulphonamides, procainamide, and oral contraceptives. As SLE has shown a familial pattern in some cases, genetic origins are also under investigation.

Clinical manifestations

The symptoms and signs that most commonly cause the patient to seek medical advice include joint pain and stiffness, which usually involves the hands, feet, and large joints. Although the joints show the inflammatory process of arthritis it is rarely deforming. There is usually associated muscle weakness and tenderness.

Facial rash aggravated by exposure to sunlight is probably the most characteristic feature of SLE. This 'butterfly' pattern facial erythema may range from mild erythema to discoid lesions (plaques).

Generalized constitutional upsets occur often. These include general aches and pains, and malaise; abdominal pain, nausea, vomiting, diarrhoea, anorexia, and weight loss; and fatigue, low grade fevers, and chills. Females may complain of irregular periods or amenorrhoea.

On presentation the patient may also be found to be suffering from one or more of the following:

1. Raynaud's phenomenon, vasculitis, peripheral neuropathy, venous thrombosis, necrotic ulcers or digital gangrene
2. Patchy alopecia, oral or nasopharyngeal ulcerations
3. Pleuritis, myositis, carditis, dependent oedema
4. Migraine, convulsions, psychoses
5. Haemorrhagic tendencies
6. Proteinuria (> 3.5 g/day), glomerulonephritis, excessive casts in urine.

Investigative procedures

All patients suspected of having SLE should be ordered a full blood examination which will most likely demonstrate an anaemia, leucopenia, and thrombocytopenia. The ESR is usually elevated and most patients have a hypergammaglobulinaemia. ANA and LE cells are usually present on indirect immunofluorescence on nucleated tissue, and the anti-DNA test is positive in patients with active disease. As anti-DNA correlates extremely well with SLE activity it is the definitive test used in monitoring the effect of the disease to treatment.

Microscopy and culture of urine may show haematuria, casts, protein, and infecting organisms.

Chest X-ray may demonstrate pulmonary and cardiac involvement and ECG will confirm the type of conduction defect.

Renal biopsy is usually performed to determine the extent of renal involvement and to assist in the staging of the disease.

Medical management

Patients with mild presentation of SLE rarely require little more than: aspirin to control the symptoms of arthritis; topical corticosteroid creams for skin lesions; and encouragement to cover exposed skin areas with protective clothing and/or sunscreens when in the sun.

Oral corticosteroid drugs remain the medical intervention of choice for patients who have systemic disease, acute generalized exacerbations of the disease, or who have severe involvement with vital organ systems. It is not uncommon for the patient to be initially prescribed up to 60 mg prednisone in such situations and for there to be a remarkable response within 48 hours. As soon as symptoms begin to abate the steroid dose is tapered and, wherever possible, the patient is maintained on as low a dose as is necessary to maintain symptom control. Most physicians prefer an alternate day dosage of steroids to daily doses, as this produces fewer side-effects.

Immunosuppressive agents are sometimes used either when vital organs are involved in the acute disease process or as an alternative to steroid therapy.

Nursing management

Nursing management is aimed at assessing the patient throughout all phases of treatment, providing physical care for symptom relief, emotional support, and health education. The nurse is responsible for observing the patient for any of the constitutional symptoms that may arise and for providing symptomatic relief, for example: aspirin administration for joint pain, fever, and chills; small frequent meals of foods preferred by the patient, although a low-sodium, low-protein diet may be indicated if renal involvement occurs; application of topical creams to reduce skin irritation; application of heat to reduce joint stiffness and to relieve joint pain; and ensuring an adequate rest and exercise ratio to prevent fatigue.

The nurse should observe the patient's skin, mucous membranes, and urine, and monitor vital signs and record (and where necessary report) signs of systemic involvement of the disease, for example, dyspnoea, chest pain, hypertension, dependent oedema, haematuria, weight gain, increasing size of skin lesions or alopecia patches, headaches, convulsions, or personality changes.

The patient should be advised of the expected effects of the steroid therapy and of the possible side-effects. She should be advised never to alter the dose unless under medical orders and to never abruptly cease steroids. The nurse should be prepared to provide emotional support for the patient who will have an obvious alteration to her concept of body image.

Anticipated outcome

Now that serological testing has improved, most cases of SLE are diagnosed prior to major organ damage occuring. The advent of earlier treatment has meant that most patients are able to lead a near normal life style with a near normal life expectancy. Severe renal and/or central nervous system involvement is accompanied by an extremely poor prognosis with a high mortality.

SECTION L – REFERENCES AND FURTHER READING

Texts

Ackerman A B 1984 The lives of lesions: chronology in dermatopathology. Masson, New York

Amos W M G 1981 Basic immunology. Butterworths, London

Anderson J R (ed) 1976 Muir's textbook of pathology, 10th edn. Edward Arnold, London

Anthony C P 1984 Structure and function of the body. Mosby, St Louis

Arndt K A 1983 Manual of dermatologic therapeutics, with essentials of diagnosis, 3rd edn. Little, Brown & Co, Boston

Barker D J 1979 Essentials of skin disease management. Blackwell Scientific, Oxford

Creager J G 1982 Human anatomy and physiology. Wadsworth, California

Fisher A A 1986 Contact dermatitis, 3rd edn. Lea & Febiger, Philadelphia

Fitzpatrick T B, Freeberg I M 1987 Dematology in general medicine: textbook and atlas, 3rd edn. McGraw-Hill, New York

Havard M 1986 A nursing guide to drugs, 2nd edn. Churchill Livingstone, Melbourne

Holmes H N, Johnson P, Shinehouse P M 1985 Immune disorders: nurse's clinical library. Springhouse, Pennsylvania

Luckmann J, Sorensen K C 1980 Medical-surgical nursing: a psychophysiologic approach, 2nd edn. Saunders, Philadelphia

Macleod J 1987 Davidson's principles and practice of medicine, 15th edn. Churchill Livingstone, Edinburgh

Moschella S L, Hurley H J 1985 Dermatology, 2nd edn. Saunders, Philadelphia

Read A E, Barritt D W, Langton Hewer R 1986 Modern medicine, 3rd edn. Churchill Livingstone, Edinburgh

Roitt I M 1985 Immunology. Churchill Livingstone, Edinburgh

Rook A (ed) 1970 Textbook of dermatology. Blackwell, Oxford

Rook A et al (eds) 1986 Practical management of the dermatologic patient. Lippincott, Philadelphia

Rook A et al (eds) 1986 Textbook of dermatology, 4th edn. Mosby, St Louis

Sauer G C 1985 Manual of skin diseases, 5th edn. Lippincott, Philadelphia

Sneddon I B 1983 Practical dermatology, 4th edn. Edward Arnold, London

Society of Hospital Pharmacists of Australia 1985 Pharmacology and drug information for nurses, 2nd edn. Saunders, Sydney

Solomons B 1983 Lecture notes on dermatology, 5th edn. Blackwell Scientific, Oxford

Stewart P T 1982 Microbiology and immunology for the health team. John Wiley, Brisbane

Stone J (ed) 1985 Dermatologic immunology and allergy. Mosby, St Louis

Storlie F J (ed) 1984 Diseases: nurse's reference library, 2nd edn. Springhouse, Pennsylvania

Weir D M 1983 Immunology: an outline for students of medicine and biology. Churchill Livingstone, Edinburgh

Wells J V 1986 Clinical immunology illustrated. Williams & Wilkins, Sydney

Journals

Bayley E W, Smith G A 1987 The three degrees of burn care. Nursing 87 17 : 3 : 34–41

Brosnan S 1986 Our first home care AIDS patient: Maria. Nursing 86 16 : 9 : 37–39

Burrell C J, Davis K G 1985 The blood story, Part II: AIDS. The Australian Nurses Journal 14 : 7 : 45–47

Byrne M, Feld M 1984 Preventing and treating decubitus ulcers. Nursing 84 14 : 4 : 55–57

Cohen M R 1985 Drug-induced anaphylaxis. Nursing 85 15 : 2 : 43

Conrad F L 1983 Tips for treating corrosive burns. Nursing 83 13 : 2 : 55–57

Crovella A C 1985 The person behind the disease. Nursing 85 15 : 9 : 42

Deglin J H, Walters J K 1984 Anaphylactic shock: as soon as you see it – stop it. Nursing 84 14 : 9 : 6–8

Dhundale K, Hubbard P M 1986 Home care for the AIDS patient: safety first. Nursing 86 16 : 9 : 34–36

Duggan D, Smith R C, Hastemink R J 1983 Nutritional support for the burn patient. The Australian Nurses Journal 13 : 10 : 39–40, 48

Fidler R 1983 Complement assays. Nursing 83 13 : 6 : 17–19

Fine M 1986 AIDS and the nurse. Part 3. The Australian Nurses Journal. 15 : 7 : 43–44

Goble H, Kovcoulidis T, Pollett B, Whitbourn G 1986 AIDS and the nurse Part 1. The Australian Nurses Journal 15 : 7 : 37–41, 62

Guarda N P, Peterson J Z 1986 Screening for HIV antibodies. Nursing 86 16 : 11 : 28–29

Hayman L L 1983 Varicella. Nursing 83 13 : 4 : 41

Herrmann C S 1983 Performing intradermal skin tests the right way. Nursing 83 13 : 10 : 509–53

Holderman M C 1984 Skin problems: a guide for making "rash" decisions. Nursing 84 14 : 11 : 22–23

Hurt R A 1985 More than skin deep: guidelines on caring for the burn patient. Nursing 85 15 : 6 : 52–57

Kennedy M 1987 AIDS coping with the fear. Nursing 87 17 : 4 : 45–46

Kerr P, Sudano L 1986 AIDS and the nurse. Part 2. The Australian Nurses Journal 15 : 7 : 42, 62

Marvin J A 1983 Planning home care for burn patients. Nursing 83 13 : 8 : 11–13

Nurse's Reference Library 1983 Anaphylaxis: five steps for fast treatment. Nursing 83 13 : 11 : 6

Pollett B 1987 AIDS: Australia's response. The Australian Nurses Journal 16 : 7 : 49–51

Popkin B 1983 Caring for the AIDS patient – fearlessly. Nursing 83 13 : 9 : 50–55

Prigel C L B 1987 How to spot melanoma. Nursing 87 17 : 6 : 60–62

Randall B J 1986 Reacting to anaphylaxis. Nursing 86 16 : 3 : 34–39

Reckling J B, Neuberger G B 1987 Understanding immune system dysfunction. Nursing 87 17 : 9 : 34–41

Searle L 1985 Honoring the personal side of chronic illness. Nursing 85 15 : 11 : 52–57

Shannon M L 1984 5 Famous fallacies about pressure sores. Nursing 84 14 : 10 : 34–41

Taylor D L 1984 Immune response: physiology, signs, and symptoms. Nursing 84 14 : 5 : 52–54

Taylor D L 1984 Anaphylaxis: physiology, signs, and symptoms. Nursing 84 14 : 6 : 44–45

Watts B 1987 Operation cover up. The Australian Nurses Journal. 17 : 4 : 56–57

Appendix 1: Sample nursing assessment form

NURSING ASSESSMENT FORM

Assessment must be completed by an RN, or checked by an RN if conducted by a student of Nursing.
A full assessment must be made on all patients, except those defined as 'short-term' or 'day-only'.

Date _____ Time _____ Name _____ Age _____
Prefers to be called _____ Location of assessment _____
Interviewed/assessed by _____

Mode of admission _____ Accompanied by _____
History, X-rays with patient? _____ Reason for admission _____
Major health complaint(s) _____

Duration of this problem/onset _____ Admission diagnosis _____

Previous hospitalizations/illnesses: Date _____ Where hospitalized _____

Type of illness or surgery and outcome _____
_____
_____

Family health history: Diabetes _____ Cardiac _____ Cancer _____
Renal _____ TB _____ COAD _____
Asthma _____ Epilepsy _____ Psychiatric _____
Other _____

Social history of : Alcohol _____ Smoking _____ Drug abuse _____
Allergies (what type of reaction) _____

Medications:

Name	With patient?	Dose & time	Time of last dose	Patient's understanding of effect

Nursing assessment on a systems basis:
T _____ P _____ R _____ BP _____ Height _____ Weight _____
Urinalysis _____
Diet _____
Neurological _____
Respiratory _____
Gastrointestinal _____
Genitourinary _____
Reproductive (incuding breast) _____
Musculoskeletal _____
Skin _____

Prostheses: Spectacles _____ Contact lenses _____ Dentures _____ Other _____

Activities of daily living and patterns of behaviour: Hygiene _____
Rest/sleep _____ Activity status _____
Elimination habit _____ Meals/diet _____
Health practices _____
Typical daily profile _____

Information obtained from: Patient _____ Significant other _____ Relationship to patient _____
Previous records _____

Comments _____
_____
_____

Signature _____ Checked by (if applicable) _____

Appendix 2: Sample postoperative nursing care plan

Identified problem/need: 'Nursing diagnosis'	Objective	Nursing actions	Evaluation
1. Pain from abdominal wound and position of drainage tubes (actual)	To be pain-free at all times	• Sit upright with back and leg supports • Splint wound when repositioning and during breathing and coughing exercises • Splint drain tubes at dressing change Administer ordered analgesia strictly every 3 hours	Day 1 – Has had minimal pain since return from the OR Day 2 – States that he is happy with the management of his pain Appears to be gaining relief from pain
2. Unable to state his needs as he does not speak English (actual)	To be able to communicate all his needs whenever necessary	• Use nonverbal methods of communication • Use translation lists and picture cards • Use hospital interpreter service when plan is designed, implemented and evaluated	Day 1 – States via interpreter that he feels that at most times he is understood, and can understand what the staff expect of him Day 2 – Is able to communicate his needs and understands nursing actions
3. Restricted mobility due to painful arthritic joints (actual)	To achieve independence within his limitations, before his date of discharge	• Allow all the time that is necessary to let him perform those activities of daily living of which he is capable • Intervene only when he has reached his limitations or he requests help • Administer ordered anti-inflammatory drugs	Day 1 – Needs assistance with all movement Day 2 – Needs assistance only to wash/shower, and to dress Day 2 – Appears to be gaining relief from the recommencement of his drug therapy
4. Anxiousness brought on by his fear of the unknown and how he will cope with the surgery (potential)	To understand hospital and preoperative routine and the implications of the surgery	• Involve family members in all care planning • Use interpreter services as much as possible • Arrange for visit by OR nurse preop. Arrange contact with the migrant support services • Explain all procedures simply, but in detail • Let him voice his fears	Day 1 – States, through wife, that he knows what is expected of him Day 2 – Appears to be coping and progressing well postop. Day 2 – States, via interpreter that he is happy about his progress and has no worries
5. Deep vein thrombosis due to obesity and postoperative immobility (potential)	To avoid development of venous stasis or thrombosis	• Active leg & feet exercises hourly whilst RIB • No pillows under knees or calves Offer oral fluids hourly • Explain why he should not cross his legs whilst he is RIB • Ambulate ASAP • Commence 7560 kJ reduction diet when tolerating oral foods	Day 1 – Wife states that he understands the need for his exercises Day 2 – Showing no signs of venous stasis or a deep vein thrombosis Day 2 – States, via interpreter that he is happy with diet

Index

Neurological status assessment,
   149–151
   autonomic function, 150–151
   cranial nerve function, 150, 151
   mental state evaluation, 149–150
   motor function, 150
   reflex activity, 150
   sensory function, 150
Neuromotor disease
   Parkinson's disease, 194
   myasthenia gravis, 212–215
Neurones, 147–148
Neuropathy, 202–204
   diabetic *see* Diabetes mellitus
   parenchymatous, 202–203
   Schwann cell dysfunction, 203
   vascular induced, 203
Neurotransmitters, 149
Neutropenia, 393–394
   antirheumatic drugs and, 729
   bone marrow transplantation and,
      404–405
   leukaemia and, 399
Nodule, skin, 755
Noncompliance, 16–19
Nonspecific urethritis, 563, 667
   epididymo-orchitis and, 644
Nonverbal communication, 14–15
Norepinephrine, 267
   see also Catecholamines
Nursing assessment, 5
   form, 790
   preoperative, 34
Nursing care plan, 6, 7, 791
Nursing diagnosis, 6
Nutrition
   and osteomalacia, 749
   and the elderly, 135–136
   coeliac disease, 505
   dumping syndrome and, 502
   gastrointestinal, 467–468
   in gout, 74
   in osteoporosis, 745
   intravenous, 470
   iron deficiency anaemia, 381
   oesophagitis and, 483, 484
   postoperative, 52–53
   preoperative, 33, 34
   vomiting and, 461–462
   wound healing, and 59
   see also Malabsorption, Obesity

Obesity
   hypertension and, 284
   osteoarthritis and, 717, 718
   postoperative care, 51
   surgery, 503
   Turner's syndrome and, 272
   vascular disorders and, 288
      atherosclerosis, 281, 282
Obstructive airways disorders, 362–368
Obstructive jaundice, 427
   acute pancreatitis and, 450
   cholelithiasis and, 444

hepatitis and, 434, 435
   pancreatic carcinoma and, 453
Occlusive arterial disease, 292–297
   surgery, 294–297
Occlusive venous disease, 297–301
Oedema, 82
Oesophageal cancer, 488–489
Oesophageal dilatation, 484
Oesophageal disorders, 482–490
   achalasia of the cardia, 485–486
   aphagia, 490
   dysphagia, 489–490
   hiatus hernia, 486–488
   inflammatory disorders, 488–484
   neoplasm, 488–489
   trauma, 484–485
Oesophageal reflux
   hiatus hernia and, 487
   peptic ulcer and, 494
Oesophageal trauma, 484–485
Oesophageal varices, bleeding,
      430–431
   anaemia and, 381
   hepatic encephalopathy and, 439
   liver failure and, 436, 438
   massive haemorrhage, 331
   Sengstaken-Blakemore tube, 430,
      431–432
   spleno-renal shunt, 431, 432
Oesophagitis
   acute corrosive, 482
   chronic atrophic, 482–483
   recurrent reflux, 483–484
   subacute infective, 482
Oestrogen, 262, 270, 271, 272, 638,
      639, 675, 744
Oligodendroglia, 148
Oligodendroglioma, 189
Ophthalmia neonatorum, 666
Opportunistic infection, 784, 785
Oral hypoglycaemic drugs, 254–255
Orchitis, 644
   tuberculosis of urinary tract and,
      570
Orthopaedic surgery, 702–705
Osmosis, 77
Osmotic pressure, 77
   dehydration and, 80
Osteitis fibrosa cystica, 249
Osteoarthritis, 717–719
   dislocation/subluxation and, 696
   fracture and, 714
   joint replacement surgery, 704
   Paget's disease and, 748, 749
Osteoclastoma, 739
Osteogenic sarcoma, 739
   Paget's disease and, 749
Osteogenesis imperfecta, 698
Osteoid osteoma, 739
Osteoma, 739
Osteomalacia, 749–750
   malabsorption syndromes and, 506
Osteomyelitis, 736–737
   respiratory streptococcal infection
      and, 349

Osteoporosis, 133, 744–746
   chronic renal failure and, 598, 600
   Cushing's syndrome and, 263, 264
   fracture treatment, 746
   malabsorption syndromes and, 506
   multiple myeloma and, 413, 414
   pathological fracture and, 698
   rheumatoid arthritis and, 730, 732
   spinal cord injury and, 169
   systemic corticosteroids and, 730
Osteotomy, 719
Ostomy club, 474
Otitis media
   acute coryza and, 348
   tonsillitis and, 349
Ovarian neoplasm, 655–656
   virilism/hirsutism and, 273
Ovaries, 634
Ovulation, 636
Oxygen
   arterial blood gas analysis, 88
   carriage in blood, 86–87
   therapy, 91
   toxicity, 91–92
   utilization, 87–88
Oxyhaemoglobin, 87
   dissociation curve, 87, 88
Oxytocin, 230, 232, 237, 675

Pacemaker insertion, 324
Paget's disease, 746–749
Pain, 114–122
   assessment, 117, 121
   associated autonomic phenomena,
      116
   central, 116
   chronic, spinal cord injury and, 169
   cultural aspects, 12
   deep visceral, 116
   gastrointestinal disorders, 462–463
   iatrogenic aspects, 117
   incisional, 462
   intermediate, 115–116, 119
   loss of protective responses with
      anaesthesia, 45–46
   neurovascular assessment and, 707
   peripheral, 114–116
   psychogenic, 116
   psychological modification, 116–
      117
   referred, 462, 675
   superficial, 114–115, 119
   'wind', postoperative, 462–463
Pancreas, 425–426
Pancreatic abscess
   acute pancreatitis and, 450, 451
   chronic pancreatitis and, 452
Pancreatic calculi, 449, 452
Pancreatic carcinoma, 453
   obstructive jaundice and, 427
   secondary diabetes and, 252
Pancreatic disorders, 251–261, 449–
      454
   malabsorption and, 506, 507